W9-AGE-379

SYNOPSIS OF
PSYCHIATRY
Behavioral Sciences
Clinical Psychiatry

FIFTH EDITION

SENIOR CONTRIBUTING EDITOR

ROBERT CANCRO, M.D., MED.D.Sc.

Professor and Chairman, Department of Psychiatry,
New York University School of Medicine;
Director, Department of Psychiatry, University Hospital
of the New York University Medical Center;
Director, Department of Psychiatry, Bellevue Hospital,
New York, New York; Director, Nathan S. Kline Institute for
Psychiatric Research, Orangeburg, New York

CONTRIBUTING EDITOR

JACK A. GREBB, M.D.

Assistant Professor of Psychiatry, New York University
School of Medicine; Assistant Attending Psychiatrist,
Bellevue Hospital; Guest Investigator,
Laboratory of Cellular and Molecular Neuroscience,
The Rockefeller University, New York, New York;
Research Associate, Nathan S. Kline
Institute for Psychiatric Research, Orangeburg, New York

Dedicated to our wives
Nancy Barrett Kaplan
and
Virginia Alcott Sadock
without whose help and sacrifice
this textbook would not have been possible

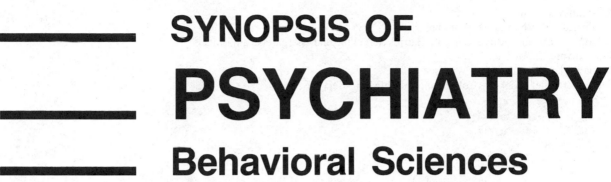

SYNOPSIS OF
PSYCHIATRY
Behavioral Sciences
Clinical Psychiatry

Fifth Edition

HAROLD I. KAPLAN, M.D.

Professor of Psychiatry, New York University School of Medicine; Attending Psychiatrist, University Hospital of the New York University Medical Center; Attending Psychiatrist, Bellevue Hospital, New York, New York

BENJAMIN J. SADOCK, M.D.

Professor and Vice Chairman, Department of Psychiatry, New York University School of Medicine; Attending Psychiatrist, University Hospital of the New York University Medical Center; Attending Psychiatrist, Bellevue Hospital, New York, New York

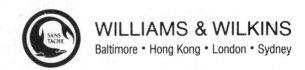

WILLIAMS & WILKINS
Baltimore • Hong Kong • London • Sydney

Editor: Nancy Collins
Associate Editor: Victoria M. Vaughn
Copy Editors: Suzanne Boyd Enright, Harriet Serenkin, and Margaret Yamashita
Design: JoAnne Janowiak
Illustration Planning: Lorraine Wrzosek
Production: Rachel Hockett, Cobb/Dunlop Publishing Services, Inc.

Copyright © 1988
Williams & Wilkins
428 East Preston Street
Baltimore, MD 21202, USA

All rights reserved. This book is protected by copyright. No part of this book may be reproduced in any form or by any means, including photocopying, or utilized by any information storage and retrieval system without written permission from the copyright owner.

Accurate indications, adverse reactions, and dosage schedules for drugs are provided in this book, but it is possible that they may change. The reader is urged to review the package information data of the manufacturers of the medications mentioned.

Printed in the United States of America

First Edition 1972
Second Edition 1976
Third Edition 1981
Fourth Edition 1985

ISBN 0-683-04518-0

87 88 89 90 91
1 2 3 4 5 6 7 8 9 10

Preface

Modern-day psychiatry emphasizes the humane and compassionate aspects of medicine. This textbook is dedicated to that humanism which is often lost in technically based modern-day medical practice. Equally, the interaction between medical school faculty and students requires a high level of empathic concern if we are to avoid producing computer-like robotic physicians.

In the United States, psychiatry is the only medical school course consistently taught throughout the four years of the curriculum. If taught properly, this course should be a dramatic reminder to all of medicine of its mission—diagnosis, treatment, and the elimination of pain, suffering, and disease through the treatment of the whole person.

This edition of the *Synopsis of Psychiatry* represents a departure from previous editions in that it is being published before rather than after the new edition of the *Comprehensive Textbook of Psychiatry*. The rapid and substantial changes in the field are such that a new and timely publication of the *Synopsis* was deemed necessary. Among those events were the publication of the revision of the third edition of the American Psychiatric Association's *Diagnostic and Statistical Manual of Mental Disorders* (DSM-III-R), the major advances in the neural sciences and, finally the curriculum changes in the medical schools of the United States where this textbook is used. When the new edition of the *Comprehensive Textbook of Psychiatry* is published, it will incorporate the above mentioned changes in much greater detail for the practicing psychiatrist and psychiatric resident.

This *Synopsis* contains many of the highlights of the forthcoming edition of the *Comprehensive Textbook of Psychiatry*. This book serves as a guide to that edition, which enables the student to read about any subject in more depth written by an expert in the area. Additionally, there is much content that is original and new, written by the authors specifically for this *Synopsis* and synthesized and adapted for student use. This *Synopsis* is therefore a complete and up-to-date revision with new emphases for the practice of psychiatry of the 1990s.

CHANGES IN THIS EDITION

New Format. This book is being published in a new format—both as a larger volume that covers the basic behavioral sciences and all of the clinical psychiatric disorders, and a smaller text that covers the clinical psychiatric disorders alone. The first format provides the student with a book that can be used throughout the entire four years of medical school. The second is of use to the student who requires a textbook covering clinical psychiatry alone. We believe such flexibility in choice will admirably meet the needs of a wide variety of readers from psychiatry, psychology, psychiatric social work, psychiatric nursing, occupational and recreational therapy, and other mental health professionals.

New and Updated Sections. The section *The Brain and Behavior* appears for the first time in this edition. It provides extensive coverage of the fields of neurochemistry, neurophysiology, psychoimmunology and psychoendocrinology, which represent the cutting edge of psychiatry.

Other new and changed areas include the role of laboratory tests in psychiatry, attachment theory; aggression; ethology; socioeconomics of health care; ethics; grief therapy; and statistics to name but a few. The chapters on child and adolescent psychiatry have been heavily rewritten and the sections on psychopharmacology have been thoroughly updated. In addition, the authors have included a series of clinical case vignettes in an appendix to this volume, which illustrate many of the various psychiatric syndromes described herein. These cases have been derived from the *DSM-III Casebook* published by the American Psychiatric Association, and have been updated by the authors to correlate with DSM-III-R.

The *Synopsis* forms one part of a tripartite system developed by the authors to facilitate the teaching of psychiatry and the behavioral sciences. Another part of that system is the *Comprehensive Textbook of Psychiatry*, soon to appear in the fifth edition, which is global in depth and scope but is hardly as portable as this book. The final part of this effort is the *Study Guide and Self-Examination Review of the Synopsis of Psychiatry*, which consists of multiple-choice questions and answers derived from and keyed to this edition of the *Synopsis of Psychiatry*. A book of multiple-choice questions gives recognition to the importance and contributions of the National Board of Medical Examiners and the American Board of Psychiatry and Neurology on whose published curricula all of our books are based. Their examinations are given in multiple-choice question format; this is the type of question and teaching technique used in the *Study Guide*, which is recommended as a companion volume to be used with this textbook.

While the authors recognize the enormous importance and positive contributions of those Boards, there is controversy about their influence and power, albeit constructive, on our educational system. Similarly, the nosology used in this textbook is based on the revised third edition of the American Psychiatric Association's *Diagnostic and Statistical Manual of Mental Disorders* (DSM-III-R), which is the "law of the land" in American psychiatry.

While the authors have reservations about the utility and validity of DSM-III-R, which is an innovative but questionable improvement over the previous manual, DSM-III, the student must know DSM-III-R until it is predictably changed when the next version, DSM-IV, is published. *Synopsis* is neither a review book nor an outline of psychiatry and it is much more than a diagnostic manual. It is a comprehensive, thoroughly eclectic, and fully integrated textbook, which is what the field of psychiatry both deserves and requires.

In the preparation of this edition we have been most fortunate to enlist the assistance of Jack Grebb, M.D., Assistant Professor of Psychiatry at New York University Medical Center, who served in the capacity of Contributing Editor. Dr. Grebb is an outstanding academic, research, and clinical psychiatrist.

We especially want to thank Virginia Alcott Sadock, M.D., Clinical Associate Professor of Psychiatry and Director of Graduate Education in Human Sexuality at New York University Medical Center. As in all our previous books, including the *Comprehensive Textbook of Psychiatry,* she has served as assistant to the editors and actively participated in every editorial decision. Her enthusiasm, sensitivity, comprehension, and depth of psychiatric knowledge were of immeasurable importance to the authors. She has ably represented not only the viewpoint of women in medicine and psychiatry but also has made many contributions to the content of this textbook. We are deeply appreciative of her outstanding help and assistance.

Wayne Green, M.D., Associate Professor of Clinical Psychiatry and Peter Kim, M.D., Professor of Psychiatry, both at New York University Medical Center provided important help in the area of child psychiatry, which was heavily rewritten in this edition.

Peter M. Kaplan, M.D., Fellow in Child Psychiatry at Columbia University College of Physicians and Surgeons, served as a key assistant to the editors in the preparation of this book. Not only did he represent the viewpoint of the modern-day medical student and psychiatric resident but he helped enormously in all aspects of the production of this textbook. He made particular contributions in the fields of psychopharmacology and child psychiatry, which are his areas of specialization.

A skilled and devoted technical staff was necessary to complete the enormous task involved in the production of this book. We want to thank Phillip Kaplan, M.D., Nancy Barrett Kaplan, James Sadock, Victoria Sadock, and Hilary Slaven for their assistance.

We would like to express our thanks to Lynda Abrams who performed a variety of tasks in an outstanding manner that contributed to the publishing of this book. Her unique organizing abilities combined with her capacity to work prodigiously and with alacrity helped to make this venture feasible. We also want to thank Amy Brown who assisted the authors. Her intelligence and cheerful disposition made working with her a great pleasure. Rebecca Jones, M.D. helped coordinate the new DSM-III-R nomenclature into the text and Brian Shaw provided important library research.

Robert Cancro, M.D., Professor and Chairman of the Department of Psychiatry at New York University Medical Center participated as Senior Contributing Editor of this edition. Dr. Cancro's commitment to psychiatric education and psychiatric research are recognized throughout the world. He has been an important source of great inspiration to the authors and has contributed immeasurably to this and previous editions. Dr. Cancro is renowned as a researcher, clinician, and educator. He is a much valued and highly esteemed mentor to the authors and it is a very special privilege to work closely with him. Dr. Cancro has developed a department that represents the very best in American psychiatry. The fruitful and stimulating exchange of ideas between Dr. Cancro and the faculty, residents, medical students, and other professionals at New York University creates a unique blend of academic and clinical psychiatry for which he is responsible. Our collaboration and association with this outstanding American educator has contributed immeasurably to the new ideas and directions shaping this textbook.

Harold I. Kaplan, M.D.
Benjamin J. Sadock, M.D.

New York University Medical Center   December 1987
New York, New York

Contents

vii

1

History of Psychiatry

INTRODUCTION

Psychiatry is the branch of medicine that deals with mental disorders—diseases, manifestations of which are primarily behavioral or psychological. Psychiatry was the last specialty to be incorporated into medicine. Although the study of human behavior is as old as recorded history, it was only within the last 200 years that mental disorders were considered within the province of medicine.

The history of psychiatry is, at the same time, the history of civilization. As man increased his knowledge of the world around him, he also increased his knowledge of the world within. The major workers in the field of psychiatry, their contributions, and major events are described in Table 1.

Table 1
Major Workers in Psychiatry and Their Contributions

Name	Date	Country	Publications	Significant Contributions
Hippocrates of Cos (ca. 450–355 B.C.)		Greece	*Hippocratic Writings* (Pelican Classics, 1978)	Diseases caused by imbalance in four humors (blood, phlegm, yellow bile, black bile); melancholia caused by excess black bile; hysteria caused by wandering uterus; look for natural causes of epilepsy, called the "sacred disease"; dietary treatment of illness
Plato (427–347 B.C.)		Greece	*The Dialogues of Plato*, trans. B. Jowett, (New York, Random House, 1937)	In *Timaeus, Phaedrus,* and *The Republic*, described two kinds of madness: that in which the appetitive soul lost the domination of the rational soul; and madness inspired by the gods, "divine madness"
Aristotle (384–322 B.C.)		Greece	W. D. Ross, *Aristotle,* 6th edition, 1955	In *De Anima* and other "psychological" works, described the affections of desire, anger, fear, courage, envy, joy, hatred, and pity
Galen of Pergamum (130–200 A.D.)		Asia Minor (Turkey) in the Roman Empire	*On the Affected Parts,* trans. and ed. Rudolph Siegel (Basel, S. Karger, 1976)	Consolidated the thoughts of Hippocrates, Plato, and Aristotle; idea that depression was caused by excess

Table 1 *continued*

Name	Date	Country	Publications	Significant Contributions
				of black bile was influential until the 19th century
St. Augustine (345–430 A.D.)		Tageste (Numidia, North Africa)	*Confessions*, trans. E. B. Pusey, (New York, The Modern Library, 1949)	His *Confessions* was the first book centering on psychological introspection
Avicenna (980–1037 A.D.)		Persia	*A Treatise on the Canon of Medicine of Avicenna*, (London, O. C. Gruner, 1930)	His *Canon of Medicine* recognized that certain physical diseases were caused by emotional upsets, and was widely read by Christian and Mohammedan physicians
Constantius Africanus (ca. 1020–1087)		Carthage, North Africa	Constantino L'Africano, *Della Melancolia*, (Rome, 1959)	His *Melancolia* made observations on delusional thinking, and from the first medical school at Salerno spread Galenic ideas on depression throughout Western Europe
Bartholomaeus Anglicus (13th century)	1250?	Paris, France	*De Proprietatibus Rerum*, (London, 1535)	One of the earliest attempts to localize mental diseases and functions to different parts of the brain
Henry Kramer and James Sprenger (15th century)	1486	Germany	*Malleus Maleficarum* (Witches' Hammer)	Influential in causing persecution of individuals for witchcraft
Paracelsus (ca. 1493–1541)	1520	Austria	*Diseases Which Lead to a Loss of Reason*	Psychiatric illnesses not caused by demons but are natural diseases, new classification of diseases, treatment of diseases with chemicals (absence of psychotherapy)
Juan Louis Vives (1492–1540)	1538	Spain	*De Anima et Vita* (Of Soul and Life)	Described the importance of psychological associations and their influence in forming emotions. A forerunner of Freud
Johann Weyer (1515–1588)	1563	Holland	*De Prestigiis Daemonum* (The Deception of Demons)	Influential in refuting *Malleus Maleficarum*
Juan Huarte de San Juan (ca. 1530–1592)	1574	Spain	*The Examination of Men's Wits*	An early account of differences in temperaments and dispositions

Table 1 *continued*

Name	Date	Country	Publications	Significant Contributions
Timothy Bright (?1551–1615)	1586	England	*A Treatise of Melancholia*	The first treatise by an English physician on mental illness. Divided melancholy into that caused by humoral imbalance, and that caused by psychological factors. Similar to present-day classification
Giambattista Porta (1535–1615)	1586	Italy	*De Humana Physiognomia*	Gave to physiognomy the role of at least a pseudoscience
Felix Plater (1536–1614)	1602, 1614	Switzerland	*Practice of Medicine, Observations of Diseases Injurious to Body and Mind*	New classification of diseases based on symptoms, causes, and treatments; careful description of all known psychiatric and organic diseases; the first physician to separate medicine from philosophy and make it a branch of natural science
Edward Jorden (1569–1632)	1603	England	*A Brief Discourse of a Disease Called the Suffocation of the Mother*	First book in English by a physician, delineating hysteria as a sex-linked disease, imitating other diseases
Robert Burton (1577–1640)	1621	England	*The Anatomy of Melancholy*	The most famous book on psychiatry in the 17th century. A comprehensive presentation of all previous medical-psychological thought on melancholy, also drawing on the nonmedical literature of Western civilization
William Harvey (1578–1657)	1628	England	*De Motu Cordis* (The Motion of the Heart)	In his discovery of the circulation of the blood, Harvey emphasized that mental emotions affect the movements of the heart
Paolo Zacchia (1584–1659)	1621–1650	Italy	*Questiones Medico-Legales*	This held that a physician, rather than a priest or lawyer, should evaluate a patient's responsibility for disturbed behavior. The beginning of forensic psychiatry
Thomas Sydenham (1624–1689)	1682	England	"Dissertatio epistolaris . . ." in *The Entire Works of Dr. Thomas*	Gave a comprehensive picture of the many symptoms of hysteria,

Table 1 *continued*

Name	Date	Country	Publications	Significant Contributions
			Sydenham newly made English, 1742	believing that in the form of "hypochondriacal complaints" it could exist in the male, and that it was caused by disturbed animal spirits
Thomas Willis (1622–1675)	1683	England	*Two Discourses Concerning the Soul of Brutes*	Summarized what was known about major psychiatric illnesses. Recognized differences in illnesses where there was gross brain disease and where brain seemed normal, attributing latter to disturbed animal spirits. Attributed hysteria to disturbed animal spirits acting on the brain, not to a wandering uterus
George Ernest Stahl (1660–1734)	1707, 1708	Germany	*Theoria Medica Vera, De Animi Morbis*	Theory of animism. The soul, anima, maintains functions of body in health and disease; psychiatric illness caused either by inhibitions of anima, or diseases of body
George Chyne (1671–1743)	1733	England	*The English Malady or, a treatise of nervous diseases*	Depression thought to be caused by gluttony and intemperance, and called "the English Malady"
Simon Andre Tissot (1728–1797)	1758	Switzerland	*Onanism*	First medical discussion of masturbation, emphasizing the pathological effects of excessive masturbation
William Battie (1703–1776)	1758	England	*A Treatise on Madness*	First physician who made insanity his full work, raised "the mad business" to a respected specialty, and first used "madness" in the title of his book
Boissier de Sauvages (1706–1767)	1763–1770	France	*Nosologia Methodica*	Nosology divided diseases into classes based on symptoms; although speculative and artificial it stimulated a rethinking of concepts of disease

Table 1 *continued*

Name	Date	Country	Publications	Significant Contributions
John Aiken (1747–1822)	1771	England	*Thoughts on Hospitals*	First book on hospitals in which "lunatic hospitals" were discussed
Franz Anton Mesmer (1734–1815)	1779	Austria, France	*Memoire sur la Découverte du Magnetism Animal*	Showed that when a mental therapist used (so called) "animal magnetism" it could cure cases of psychiatric illness. This led to the discovery of hypnosis
Vincenzo Chiarugi (1759–1820)	1789	Italy	*Regulations of the Hospitals of Santa Maria Nuova and of Bonifazio*	One of the first attempts to treat the insane inmates of asylums humanely and without restraints
William Cullen (1710–1790)	1800	Scotland	*Nosology, or a systematic arrangement of diseases*	A great eighteenth-century nosologist who first used the term "neurosis" and its adjective "neurotic," to describe mental diseases
Philippe Pinel (1745–1826)	1801	France	*A Treatise on Insanity in Which are Contained the Principles of a New and More Practical Nosology of Mental Disorders*	Classified mental illness into four main forms, and established a new humane treatment for inmates of insane asylums which he called "the moral treatment of insanity"
Johann Reil (1759–1813)	1803	Germany	*Rhapsodies about the Application of Psychotherapy to Mental Disturbances*	"The founder of rational psychotherapy," recognizing the therapeutic value of institutional surroundings, music, psychodrama, and occupational therapy; first used the word "psychiatry," and founded the first psychiatric journal
Benjamin Rush (1745–1813)	1812	USA	*Medical Inquiries and Observations upon the Diseases of the Mind*	First general book on psychiatry in America. Rush was regarded as the father of American psychiatry and the most famous American physician of his time; signer of Declaration of Independence
Thomas Sutton (?1767–1835)	1813	England	*Tracts on Delirium Tremens*	First description of alcoholic delirium tremens

Table 1 *continued*

Name	Date	Country	Publications	Significant Contributions
William Tuke (1732–1822); Samuel Tuke (1784–1857) grandson of William Tuke; Daniel Hack Tuke (1827–1895) youngest son of Samuel Tuke; John Charles Bucknill (1817–1895)	1796–1858	England	*Description of the Retreat, an Institution near York, for Insane Persons of the Society of Friends,* by Samuel Tuke, (York, 1813); *A Manual of Psychological Medicine Containing the History, Nosology, Description, Statistics, Diagnosis, Pathology, and Treatment of Insanity,* by Daniel Tuke and Bucknill, (London, 1858)	William Tuke founded the York Retreat, for "moral treatment" of mentally ill Quakers, in 1796. Samuel Tuke's *Description of the Retreat* influenced asylum treatment in England, Europe, and the USA. The *Manual* of Daniel Tuke and Bucknill was the first comprehensive textbook of psychiatry
Joseph Adams (1756–1818)	1814	England	*A Treatise on the Supposed Hereditary Properties of Diseases . . . Particularly in Madness and Scrofula*	First book on "the hereditary properties of diseases." Argued it was not a disease that was inherited but a susceptibility to disease, therefore prevention and cure were possible
Franz Joseph Gall (1758–1828), Johann Gaspar Spurzheim (1776–1832)	1815	Austria, Germany	*The Physiognomical System of Drs. Gall and Spurzheim; founded on an anatomical and physiological examination of the nervous system in general and of the brain in particular*	The beginning of "phrenology"; with its mapping parts of the brain, defining their psychological functions, and then making psychological and psychotherapeutic predictions
Johann Christian Heinroth (1773–1843)	1818	Germany	*Disturbances of the Mind*	First systematic textbook of psychiatry that attempted to formulate an actual clinical system of psychotherapy. Heinroth was the first to use the word "psychosomatic" and the first to hold a chair in psychological medicine in the University of Leipzig
Robert Gooch (1784–1830)	1829	England	*An Account of . . . Diseases Peculiar to Women*	First account of postpartum psychosis
Amariah Brigham (1789–1849)	1832	USA	*Remarks on the Influence of Mental Cultivation upon Health*	Pioneer in social psychiatry, supervised patient activity programs today called recreational or occupational therapy; Founded and edited *American Journal of Insanity* (1844), today *American Journal of Psychiatry*

Table 1 *continued*

Name	Date	Country	Publications	Significant Contributions
James Prichard (1786–1848)	1835	England	*A Treatise on Insanity and Other Disorders Affecting the Mind*	Standard textbook of psychiatry, covering all the literature on all known diseases; described "moral insanity," later called psychopathic personality
Jean Etienne Dominique Esquirol (1782–1840)	1838	France	*Des Maladies Mentales Consideres sous les rapports Medical, Hygienique et Medico-Legal*	First coined the term "hallucination," described idiocy, classified insanities into monomania (partial insanity) and general delirium, and recognized both emotional and organic causes of illness
Isaac Ray (1807–1881)	1838	USA	*Treatise on Medical Jurisprudence of Insanity*	Founded American forensic psychiatry
James Braid (1795–1860)	1843	England	*Neurypnology; or, the Rationale of Nervous Sleep . . .*	This "entirely separated hypnotism from animal magnetism," and began the study of hypnotic phenomena
Wilhelm Griesinger (1817–1868)	1845	Germany	*Mental Pathology and Therapeutics*	Proclaimed that psychiatric diseases are brain diseases and that psychiatry had become a medical specialty; founded specialty of "neuropsychiatry"
J. Moreau de Tours (1804–1884)	1845	France	*Du Haschich et de L'alienation Mentale*	Described the effects of his taking hashish and became the first psychiatrist to experience a drug-induced psychosis
Pliny Earle (1809–1892)	1848	USA	*History, Description and Statistics of the Bloomingdale Asylum for the Insane*	This book established a pattern of reporting the statistics on Asylum inmates which was followed by other asylums
Walter Cooper Dendy (1794–1871)	1853	England	"Psychotheria, or the Remedial Influence of Mind" in *Journal of Psychological Medicine and Mental Pathology*, 1853, 6:268	First introduced the term "psychotherapeia" (today "psychotherapy"), which he defined as "prevention and remedy of [disease] by psychical influence," and which he predicted would become valuable in psychiatry

Table 1 *continued*

Name	Date	Country	Publications	Significant Contributions
Jean Pierre Falret (1794–1870), Jules Baillarger (1809–1890)	1854	France	First Baillarger, "La Folie à Double Forme"; then Falret "La Folie Circulaire", two weeks later, both in *Bulletin de l'Académie Imperiale de Medecine*, 1853–1854, 19, 340–52, 382–400	The association of melancholia and mania in the same patient had been observed but not named by an American psychiatrist, Rufus Wyman, in 1830. Kraepelin, in 1896, then named this illness manic-depressive psychosis
Thomas Kirkbride (1809–1883)	1854	USA	*On the Construction, Organisation, and General Arrangements of Hospitals for the Insane*	Set a standard for mid-nineteenth century care of the chronic insane which still commands respect today
John Conolly (1794–1866)	1856	England	*The Treatment of the Insane Without Mechanical Restraints*	Conolly's work for the "non-restraint system" marked the success of a movement which began with Pinel and created a new approach to insanity throughout the civilized world
George Robinson (1821–1875)	1859	England	*On the Prevention and Treatment of Mental Disorders*	First book that introduced the idea of looking "beyond the precincts of the asylum" in order to prevent mental illness
Gustav Theodor Fechner (1801–1887)	1860	Germany	*Elements of Psychophysics*	Established the relationship between the intensity of stimuli and sensory reactions. Fechner was called the founder of experimental psychology
Benedict-Augustin Morel (1809–1873)	1860	France	*Traite des Maladies Mentales*	Cases of insanity and other mental illnesses caused by inherited mental degeneration, becoming worse from one generation to the next
Thomas Laycock (1812–1876)	1860	England	*Mind and Brain . . .*	Mentioned "unconscious functional activity of the brain," but did not further develop this
Forbes B. Winslow	1860	England	*On Obscure Diseases of the Brain and Disorders of the Mind*	First to mention "psychical diagnostic tests" (psychological tests), and the psychiatric interview

Table 1 *continued*

Name	Date	Country	Publications	Significant Contributions
Cesare Lombroso (1836–1909)	1864	Italy	"Genio e Follia" ("genius and insanity"), Prefazione al corso di clinica psichiatica Milano: Chiusi, 1864	Emphasized the relation between geniuses and abnormal mental traits
Henry Maudsley (1835–1918)	1867	England	*The Physiology and Pathology of the Mind*	Attempted to integrate psychology, reflex neurophysiology, and psychiatry into a single synthetic whole
Ewald Hecker (1843–1909)	1871	Germany	"Die Hebephrenie," *Archive für Pathologische Anatomie und Physiologie*, vol. LII, 1871	First description of hebephrenia (later a subgroup of dementia praecox)
Jean M. Charcot (1825–1893)	1871	France	*L'Hysteria; Textes Chosis et Presentes par E. Trillat*	Vivid presentation of hysterical symptoms, including their occurrence in men as well as women
Karl Kahlbaum (1828–1899)	1874	Germany	*Die Katatonie oder das Spannungsirresein* (Berlin, 1874)	First description of Catatonia (later a subgroup of dementia precox)
George Miller Beard (1839–1883)	1880	USA	*A Practical Treatise on Nervous Exhaustion (Neurasthenia)*	Neurasthenia—a disease of mental and physical exhaustion—replaced the previous diagnosis of hypochondriasis; became prevalent in the American and European middle classes
Richard von Kraft-Ebbing (1840–1902)	1886	Germany	*Psychopathia Sexualis*	Described homosexuality and sex porversions, coining terms "sadism" and "masochism," claiming some were caused by degeneration and stimulated research in sex
Herman Emminghaus (1845–1904)	1887	Germany	*Psychic Disturbances of Childhood*	First textbook of child psychiatry
S. S. Korsakov (1854–1900)	1890	Russia	"Eine Psych. Storung Combiniert Mit Multipler Neuritis," *Allg.Zeitschr.f.Psych*. vol. XLVI, 1890	"Korsakov's psychosis": commonly caused by chronic alcoholism; manifested by multiple neuritis, disorientation, and loss of memory with pseudoreminiscences
Emil Kraepelin (1855–1926)	1899	Germany	*Psychiatrie: Ein Lehrbuch für Studirende und Aerzte*, 6th edition	The major psychoses were divided into two groups: dementia precox, which deteriorated to dementia, and manic-depressive psychosis, which did not deteriorate

Table 1 _continued_

Name	Date	Country	Publications	Significant Contributions
John Hughlings Jackson (1835–1911)	1870–1900	England	_Selected Writings of John Hughlings Jackson,_ (London, 1931–1932)	For several decades he developed the thesis that psychiatric symptoms were a regression from higher functions which were the product of evolution. The symptoms resulted from activating more primitive functions
Sigmund Freud (1856–1939)	1900–1905	Austria	_The Interpretation of Dreams, Three Essays on Sexuality_	Discovered the manifestations of the unconscious and how to use these in treating psychiatric patients; and infantile sexuality, and how these accounted for adult sexual dysfunctions; founded psychoanalysis
Morton Prince (1854–1929)	1905	USA	_The Dissociation of a Personality_	Early account of a "multiple personality," emphasizing techniques of hypnosis and manifestations of the unconscious
Clifford Beers (1876–1943)	1908	USA	_A Mind that Found Itself_	Account of experiences in psychiatric hospitals which stimulated the "mental hygiene" movement in America
Pierre Janet (1859–1947)	1910	France	_Les Névroses (The Neuroses)_	Originated the concept of "psychasthenia," a weakness in the nervous system which resulted in parts of consciousness being split off and forming dissociative, hysterical, or obsessive-compulsive symptoms
Eugen Bleuler (1857–1939)	1911	Switzerland	_Dementia Praecox or the Group of Schizophrenias_	Coined name "schizophrenia" and described its symptoms
Hideyo Noguchi (1876–1928)	1913	USA	H. Noguchi and J. W. Moore, "A Demonstration of the Treponema Pallidum in the Brain in Cases of General Paralysis," _J.Exp.Med.,_ vol. XVII	The definitive demonstration—after a century of controversy—that the syphilitic organism causes general paresis, the first time that the etiology of a major psychosis became known
William Alanson White (1870–1937), Smith Ely Jelliffe (1866–1945)	1915	USA	_Diseases of the Nervous System: A Textbook of Neurology and Psychiatry_	Represented an important new view, integrating neurologic, biological, psychiatric, and psychoanalytic concepts

Table 1 *continued*

Name	Date	Country	Publications	Significant Contributions
				It went through many editions and was standard in many medical schools. Jelliffe was called "the father of psychosomatic medicine"
Alfred Adler (1870–1937)	1917	Austria	*Study of Organ Inferiority and its Psychical Compensations*	First psychoanalytic defector from Freud; founded the school of Individual Psychology and coined the terms "life style", and "inferiority complex"
Hermann Rorschach (1884–1922)	1921	Switzerland	*Psychodiagnostik*	Rorschach's inkblot test revealed unconscious motivations and ego defenses against these, and was used for psychiatric diagnosis. It stimulated the development of other "projective" diagnostic tests
Elmer Ernest Southard (1876–1920)	1922	USA	*The Kingdom of Evils Psychiatric Social Work . . . With a Classification of Social Evils,* by Southard and Mary C. Jarrett (social worker)	Emphasized that a psychiatrist should know the entire social environment, both past and present, of the patient, and that for this the aid of a social worker is needed
Ernst Kretschmer (1888–1964)	1924	Germany	*Constitution und Character*	Linked two body types to psychoses: *leptosome* (aesthenic) to schizophrenic; *pyknic* (rotund) to manic depressive
Julius Wagner von Jauregg (1857–1940)	1917–1927	Austria	*Therapeutic Malaria,* 1927, by G. de Rudolf	During the decade 1917–27 he showed that general paresis patients underwent remissions when treated with malaria. For the time it was the most successful organic treatment of a psychosis. For this he became, in 1927, the first psychiatrist to receive the Nobel Prize. In the 1940s penicillin became the treatment of choice for paresis
Ivan Petrovich Pavlov (1849–1936)	1903–1936	Russia	*Lectures on Conditioned Reflexes,* ed., H. Gantt, 1941	In the last years of his life he attempted to show how conditioned reflexes influenced normal and pathological thought. In America this

Table 1 *continued*

Name	Date	Country	Publications	Significant Contributions
				influenced the work of J. B. Watson, "the father of behaviorism."
Karen Horney (1885–1952)	1937	Germany up to 1932, then USA	*The Neurotic Personality of Our Time*	Opposed Freud's theory of the castration complex in women, and his emphasis on the oedipal complex and sexuality as influencing neurosis; argued that neurosis was influenced by the society in which one lived.
Albert Deutsch (1905–1961)	1937	USA	*The Mentally Ill in America, A History of Their Care and Treatment from Colonial Times*	In its time, the most scholarly and influential history of the subject that had appeared
Franz Kallman (1897–1965)	1938	Germany, and after the 1930s, USA	*The Genetic Theory of Schizophrenia*	Indicated that the hereditary factor is relevant in schizophrenia and established the first full-time genetic department in a psychiatric institution in America
Ugo Cerletti (1877–1963), Lucio Bini (1908–1964)	1938	Italy	"Old and New Information About Electroshock," *Amer.J.Psychiat.*, 107, 1950, (Cerletti)	Electroshock was first used in 1938 as a way of producing convulsions, which it was hoped would alleviate psychosis: first in schizophrenia, and then in manic-depressive psychosis. It was soon observed to be more effective in the latter illness, and (with modifications) is still in use today.
Gregory Zilboorg (1891–1959)	1941	Russia to 1918, then USA	*A History of Medical Psychology*, in collaboration with George W. Henry, 1941	The first comprehensive history of psychiatry in English by two American historians
Leo Kanner (1894–1981)	1943	USA	"Autistic Disturbances of Affective Content", *The Nervous Child*, 2:217, 1943	The first account of "early infantile autism," in 1935 Kanner published *Child Psychiatry*, the first textbook on the subject in English
Helene Deutsch (1884–1982)	1945	Europe up to 1935, then USA	*The Psychology of Women*	Her two-volume work was for several decades the most comprehensive Freudian view of the life cycle of womanhood. She also named and described the psychology

Table 1 *continued*

Name	Date	Country	Publications	Significant Contributions
				of the "as if" personality; an apparently normal individual who gives a good semblance of adaptation to reality, yet is actually devoid of genuine emotion
Melanie Klein (1882–1960), Anna Freud (1895–1983)	1932–46	Austria, then England since 1930s	*The Psycho-Analysis of Children*, Klein, 1932; *The Psycho-Analytical Treatment of Children*, Anna Freud, 1946	Two different ways of applying psychoanalysis to children which have stimulated present-day English and American schools of child psychiatry
John Cade (1912–1981)	1949	Australia	"Lithium salts in the treatment of psychotic excitement," *Medical Journal of Australia*, 36:349, 1949	In his article Cade was the first to observe that lithium quieted manic patients, and that their mania returned when lithium was stopped. After the development of methods of controlling lithium's toxicity through measuring its blood levels it became used in the treatment of manic-depressive disease
Erik H. Erikson (1902–)	1950	Europe, USA since 1930s	*Childhood and Society*	In this book Erikson restated in a new way Freud's concepts of infantile sexuality, and developed concepts of adult: "identity," "identity vs. role diffusion," and "identity crisis." He has also applied psychoanalytic concepts to American cultural life and American political history
Jean Delay (1907–) Pierre Deniker (1917–)	1952	Paris, France	Delay and Deniker: "Le Traitment des Psychoses par une Méthode Neurolytique Dérivée de L'hibernothérapie," *C. R. Congrès Med. Alién. Neurol. France* 50:497	In their first reports on chlorpromazine to French psychiatrists, Delay and Deniker emphasized how patients were quieted, like animals in hibernation, and called the drug "hibernotherapie." Chlorpromazine then became a factor in reducing the number of asylum patients
Maxwell Jones (1907–)	1953	England	*Therapeutic Community* (Basic Books, 1953)	In this book Jones delineates the interactions of the mental patient with the communities in and outside of the hospital and the need for support

Table 1 *continued*

Name	Date	Country	Publications	Significant Contributions
				from groups of patients and patient's families. It heralded a period of psychiatric advance that was called "social psychiatry," which was the title of the English edition of Jones's book
Harry Stack Sullivan (1892–1949)	1953	USA	*The Interpersonal Theory of Psychiatry,* ed. by Perry and Gawel	The interpersonal theory held that an individual's impulses and strivings cannot be studied in and for themselves, but only as they are made manifest in an interpersonal situation. Sullivan also coined the terms "participant observer" (the therapist needs to be aware not only of the overt and covert behavior of the patient but also of his own reactions); "consensual validation" (the awareness by both patient and therapist of the terminology they are using); "parataxic distortion" (the patient's distortion of the "real" person of the therapist out of the necessities of his personality structure)
Carl Gustav Jung (1875–1961)	1921–55	Switzerland	*Psychological Types,* 1921; *Two Essays on Analytical Psychology,* 1912–28; *The Structure and Dynamics of the Psyche,* 1916–52; *The Archetypes and the Collective Unconscious,* 1934–55	After separating from Freud, Jung founded the school of analytical psychology, developing new psychotherapeutic approaches and concepts of the unconscious (especially the "collective unconscious") and new personality types such as introvert and extrovert
Adolf Meyer (1866–1950)	1957	USA	*Psychobiology: A Science of Man* by Adolf Meyer, ed. by E. Winters and E. M. Bowers, 1957	Psychobiology viewed the patient as a biological and psychological unity who became mentally ill because of internal pathology and maladaptations to the environment. In his "Common-Sense Psychiatry" he treated patients with psychotherapy administered by psychiatrists and social work-

Table 1 *continued*

Name	Date	Country	Publications	Significant Contributions
				ers in community clinics. He used the term *ergasia* (based on the Greek root for "work") to designate mentally integrated activity, and then an ergasia terminology to describe diseases. He foreshadowed the dynamic community psychiatry of the contemporary USA.
Roland Kuhn	1958	Switzerland	"The Treatment of Depressive States with G22355 (Imipramine Hydrochloride)," *Am. J. Psych.*, 115:459, 1958	An early account of treating over 500 psychiatric patients, over a 3-year period, with imipramine (Tofranil) and finding that it had potent antidepressant action. This was then followed by the development of other effective antidepressant medications
Joint Commission on Mental Illness and Mental Health (1955–1961)	1961–63	USA	*Action for Mental Health*, 1961; *Community Mental Health Centers Act of 1963*	*Action for Mental Health*, prepared by the Joint Commission on Mental Illness and Mental Health, recommended psychiatric deinstitutionalization of the care of the mentally ill: that their care be shifted from large mental hospitals into community mental health clinics. De-Institutionalization then became a reality with the passage of the *Community Mental Health Centers Act of 1963*, in October 1963
William H. Masters (1915–) Virginia E. Johnson (1925–)	1966–71	USA	*Human Sexual Response*, 1966; *Human Sexual Inadequacy*, 1970	Some of the changes in sex information and attitudes which followed the publication of the two books of Masters and Johnson included: demonstration that female capacity for orgasm greatly exceeds that of most men and that throughout history society has inhibited women's sexuality; sexuality continues, with changes, into old age; most sexual dysfunction is amenable to some form of treatment. Since 1970 there has been a

Table 1 *continued*

Name	Date	Country	Publications	Significant Contributions
				proliferation of sex therapies
American Psychiatric Association (APA), and National Gay Task Force (NGTF)	1973–74	USA	*Homosexuality and American Psychiatry: The Politics of Diagnosis,* Ronald Bayer, 1981	In 1973, in the light of new clinical information and under political pressure from the NGTF, the APA changed its diagnosis of homosexuality from a disease into a condition which would only be considered a disease if it was subjectively disturbing to an individual. APA members protested this decision, but in a 1974 APA referendum it was sustained by 58% vote. The controversy over the nature of homosexuality continues and its causes remain largely unknown
Jacques Lacan (1901–1981) "The French Freud"	1968–78	France	*The Language of the Self: The Function of Language in Psychoanalysis,* by Lacan, trans. A. Wilden 1968; *Psychoanalytic Politics: Freud's French Revolution,* trans. Sherry Turkle, 1978.	Lacan emphasized language and the need to make contact with the prelanguage period in the unconscious, and rejected the standard 50-minute analysis for sessions that were sometimes 10, 5, or even 3 minutes. Founded his own school of psychoanalysis, described as a return to Freud. At the time of his death there were, reportedly, about 5,000 Lacanian analysts in France. He was the most influential figure in French psychiatry. His ideas were influential in literature, language, linguistics, economics, mathematics; he was an integral part of the political left
Heinz Kohut (1913–1981)	1971–79	Austria until 1940, then USA	*The Analysis of the Self* (1971), *The Restoration of the Self* (1977), "The two analyses of Mr. Z", *Int.J.Psychoanal.,* 60:3–27, 1979; "Heinz Kohut's Self Psychology: An Overview", H. Baker and M. Baker, *Am.J.Psych.,* 144:1–9, 1987	Kohut originated the psychoanalytic school of self-psychology, which delineated a new group of developmental needs, and three new views of transferences as: mirroring, idealizing, and alter ego

The aforementioned listing was prepared by Ralph Colp, Jr., M.D.

The challenge of the 1980s and beyond is to further the gains in neurochemistry and neurophysiology while, at the same time, maintaining the humanistic side of psychiatry. The future of psychiatry is brighter than ever before. The 21st century will use new knowledge from the basic behavioral sciences to better understand the causes of mental illness and to develop new and more effective treatments.

References

Ackerknecht E H: *A Short History of Psychiatry*. Hafner Publishing Co., New York, 1968.

Alexander F G, Selesnick S T: *The History of Psychiatry*. Harper & Row, New York, 1966.

Blain D, Barton D: *The History of American Psychiatry: A Teaching and Research Guide*. American Psychiatric Association, Washington, DC, 1979.

Detre T: The Future of Psychiatry. Am J Psychiatry *144*(5):621, 1987.

Deutsch A: *The Mentally Ill in America: A History of Their Care and Treatment from Colonial Times*. Columbia University Press, New York, 1949.

Ducey C, Simon B: Ancient Greece and Rome. In *World History of Psychiatry*, J G Howell, editor. Brunner and Mazel, New York, 1975.

Ellenberger H F: *The Discovery of the Unconscious: The History and Evolution of Dynamic Psychiatry*. Basic Books, New York, 1970.

Goldstein I, editor: *Historic Deviation of Modern Psychiatry*. McGraw-Hill, New York, 1966.

Menninger K: Psychiatry and medicine. Bulletin of the Menninger Clinic, 1936. Bull Menninger Clin *50*(5):419, 1986.

Mora G: The history of psychiatry: Its relevance for the psychiatrist. Am J Psychiatry, *126*:957, 1970.

Mora G, Brand J, editors: *Psychiatry and Its History*. Charles C Thomas, Springfield, Ill, 1970.

Reich J, Black D W, Jarjona D: Architecture of research in psychiatry 1953 to 1983. Arch Gen Psychiatry *44*(4): 311, 1987.

Schneck J M: *A History of Psychiatry*. Charles C Thomas, Springfield, Ill, 1960.

2

The Physician-Patient Relationship

The physician-patient relationship is the core of the practice of medicine. It concerns all physicians and needs to be evaluated in all patients. Although personality factors are most significant when emotional and mental problems are the core of the illness, they also affect the care of the patient with organic disease. A good relationship, even more than a cure, is expected by the patient; it is typical of patients to be tolerant of the therapeutic limitations of medicine. Physicians work with sick people, not only with disease syndromes. A medical aphorism holds that there are no diseases; there are only sick people. Therefore, it is incumbent on all physicians, regardless of specialty, to consider the nature of the relationship, the psychodynamic factors in themselves and in their patients that influence the relationship, and the manner in which good rapport can be achieved.

Rapport is the spontaneous, conscious feeling of harmonious responsiveness that promotes the development of a constructive therapeutic relationship. It implies that there is an understanding and trust between doctor and patient. With rapport, the patient feels accepted, even though he may think his assets are outnumbered by his liabilities. Frequently, the physician is the person to whom the patient can talk about things he cannot talk about with anyone else. Most patients feel that they can trust physicians, especially psychiatrists, to keep secrets. This confidence must not be betrayed. The patient's feeling that someone knows him, understands him, and accepts him is a source of strength for him.

THE PHYSICIAN'S ATTITUDE TOWARD THE PATIENT

Failure of the physician to establish good rapport accounts for much of the ineffectiveness in the care of patients. Alexis Carrel pointed out that the young physician all too often loses sight of the whole man and instead regards the patient as the corpse dissected by the anatomist, the cells and fluids studied by the physiologist, or the consciousness observed by the psychiatrist. However, a live patient presents a new factor that the medical student's first patient, the cadaver, did not have: transference. The young physician may, in turn, develop a countertransference, that is, an emotional reaction to the patient based on the physician's own needs and conflicts. The physician identifies with the patient to a greater or lesser degree. Physicians

consciously or unconsciously know something about the patient's needs, for everyone has been sick, at least as a child. Thus, the physician develops empathy, which means that he has the capacity to put himself in the patient's place to such a degree that he is able to experience the meaning of the patient's feelings, wishes, and thoughts.

If a physician dislikes a patient, he is prone to be ineffective in dealing with him. Emotion breeds counteremotion. For example, if the physician is hostile, the patient becomes more hostile; the physician then becomes even angrier, and there is rapid deterioration of the relationship. If the physician can rise above such emotion and handle the resentful patient with equanimity, there may be a victory in the interpersonal relationship, and the patient may become loyal and cooperative. Physicians are bound to like some patients more than others. It is not uncommon for physicians to be emotionally upset by certain personalities or illnesses. However, it is important to try to give all possible understanding to each patient's situation. If the physician feels antagonism, he should try to evaluate the basis for this feeling.

THE PATIENT'S REACTION TO THE PHYSICIAN

The reaction of the patient to the physician is apt to be a repetition of the attitude he has had toward previous physicians or to parents, teachers, or other persons in authority who have figured prominently in his life. His reaction may be positive, negative, or ambivalent. One type of patient may expect the doctor to do something (e.g., prescribe medication or perform surgery) while he remains the passive recipient. Another patient may be more active and cooperate more fully in his treatment. This doctor-patient model of mutual participation is more important in chronic diseases such as multiple sclerosis and diabetes than in acute illnesses such as pneumonia.

In some respects, the role of the psychiatrist is different from that of the traditional physician. Because the customary role of the physician is one of taking action and giving advice, patients are sometimes reluctant to tell their stories to a psychiatrist. Patients come to the psychiatrist with the expectation that all of their difficulties will be promptly resolved with no further effort on their part except for a passive compliance with the physician's directions. Although it is easy for the patient to identify the psychiatrist with another person in his life when there are realistic similarities, the transference needs are so great at times that unrealistic factors suffice. For example, a young person can easily look upon an older psychiatrist as a father figure. When unresolved conflicts with the father are strong, even a woman examiner may be identified with personality characteristics of the father.

The words and deeds of the doctor have a power far beyond the commonplace because of his unique authority and the patient's dependence on him. What the particular physician feels has a direct bearing on the emotional and physiological reactions of the patient. One patient repeatedly had high blood pressure when examined by a physician he considered cold, aloof, and stern. He had normal blood pressure when seen by a physician he regarded as warm, understanding, and sympathetic.

Not only individual experiences but broad cultural attitudes of patients affect their reactions. In one survey of 700 patients, there was substantial agreement among the patients that physicians do not have the time or inclination to listen to and consider the patient's feelings, that they do not have enough knowledge of the emotional problems and of the socioeconomic background of the family, and that they increase fear by giving explanations in technical language. As psychosocial and economic factors exert a profound influence on human reactions, it is desirable for the physician to have as much understanding as possible of the patient's subculture. Differences in social, intellectual, and educational status have been found to interfere seriously with rapport. Understanding—or lack of understanding—of the patient's beliefs, use of language, and attitudes toward illness influences the character of the physician's examination.

THE INTERRELATIONSHIP

It has been pointed out that there is a core of the howling, enraged child in most patients—even in "good patients," an expression that usually means cooperative patients. The physician is required to cope with the patient's aggressions. Counteraggressions also arise, but they are usually sublimated rather than expressed directly, as they were in the days when Dr. Willis flogged the psychotic George III, with the considered approval of a good part of the medical profession. The physician's unconscious guilt, an outgrowth of his incapacity to deal with the patient and his illness, may be alleviated by an accusatory approach or method of questioning, which carries the implication that the patient is responsible for his illness.

Gaining conscious insight into the relationship between the physician and the patient requires constant evaluation. The better understanding the doctor has of himself, the more secure he feels and the better able he is to modify destructive attitudes. The doctor needs to empathize, but not to the point of assuming the burdens of his patients. He should be able to leave behind the problems of his patients when away from the office or the hospital. Otherwise, he will be handicapped in his efforts to help the sick person, who needs sympathy and understanding but not sentimentality.

The physician is prone to some defensiveness, partly with good reason, for many innocent doctors have been sued, attacked, and even killed because they did not give some patients the satisfactions they unconsciously desired. As a protective, defensive pattern, the psychiatrist may habitually assume a defensive attitude toward all patients. Although such rigidity may create the image of thoroughness and efficiency, it is frequently inappropriate to the particular patient and situation. Greater flexibility leads to a responsiveness to the subtle interplay between two individuals.

The physician must avoid side-stepping issues that, although they are important to the patient, he finds boring or difficult to deal with because of his own sensitivities, prejudices, or peculiarities. For example, one medical student insisted on questioning a patient about her relationship with her 23-year-old son. It was evident from the playback of a tape-recorded interview that she wished to talk about her problem with her husband. When the patient was later interviewed by the supervising doctor, she said: "The medical student was a nice fellow, but I could see he was having trouble with his mother. It made me understand my own son more."

In such a complex interaction as the interview, mistakes are usually not disastrous to the relationship if they are relatively infrequent. When the patient senses interest, enthusiasm, and good will on the part of the interviewer, he is apt to be tolerant of considerable inexperience.

GENERAL CONSIDERATIONS

The attitudes of both the patient and the physician are significant in determining the type of interview or examination and its success. The patient comes to the doctor for expert assistance. He may have a relatively realistic attitude characterized by some insight, awareness of the limitations of medical knowledge and skill, trust and confidence in a properly chosen physician, and capacity to cooperate. On the other hand, he may, like a helpless child, yearn for a parental type of guidance and may expect magic from the doctor. When there is such immature involvement on the part of the patient, the doctor should try to dissipate these beliefs through a straightforward approach and analysis of the medical problem.

For instance, if the patient has questions, they should be answered frankly. Explanations in keeping with the patient's capacity to understand should be given. Such factors as intelligence, sophistication in regard to personality reactions, and degree and type of illness should influence the vocabulary and content of the physician's response. Every effort should be made to convey to the belligerent patient both understanding and tolerance for his feelings.

The status of the examiner in the professional hierarchy influences some patients. Those who have had problems with authority may talk most easily to those of lesser status, and those who need to have their security bolstered require attention from someone of recognized reputation.

A knowledge of psychodynamics is of great use in helping to comprehend what is going on and in altering one's approach to the patient. For example, if the patient is overbearing, it is likely that he is frightened. The interviewer needs to cope with this underlying fear in order to dissipate the overcompensatory anger. If the patient feels the doctor has empathy, he is likely to talk more freely. It is frequently possible to capitalize on the patient's sense of humor in getting him to talk more easily. Smiling with him helps him feel a sense of rapport. (Needless to say, laughing at him alienates him.)

Another aphorism in medicine is: Let the patient tell his story, he is giving you the diagnosis. Accordingly, the doctor should allow the patient to freely express his thoughts, feelings, and complaints. Listening is a valuable tool. It encourages the patient to expand on his thoughts and enables him to bring up relevant topics. Attention must be paid to what the patient omits as well as to what he says. Undue emphasis or exaggeration, overt signs of emotion, and changes in manner and tone of voice may give clues to a distortion. For example, when a woman volunteers to a psychiatrist that her husband is absolutely perfect, her statement should raise suspicions about the soundness of the marital adjustment. But it is not advisable to challenge such dogmatic and emotionally charged statements immediately. These areas can be fully explored later, when the patient feels more secure with the psychiatrist. Misrepresentation and misperception of the facts due to conscious denial or lack of awareness can be clarified gradually.

Evaluating the social pressures existing in the patient's earlier life helps the doctor better understand the susceptibility of the patient, for personality reactions, healthy or unhealthy, are the result of a constant interplay of biological, sociological, and psychological forces. Each stress leaves behind some trace of its influence and continues to manifest itself throughout life in proportion to the intensity of its effect and the susceptibility of the particular human being. Stresses or strains that are producing emotional reactions should be determined to the extent possible. The significant point may not be the stress itself but what that particular stress means to the person.

References

Balint M: *The Doctor, the Patient, and the Illness.* International University Press, New York, 1964.

Brett A S, et al.: When patients request specific interventions: Defining the limit of the physician's obligation. N Engl J Medicine, Nov. 1986; 315(21)p. 315.

Engel G L: The clinical application of the biopsychosocial model. Am J Psychiatry, *137*:535, 1980.

Freud S: The dynamics of transference. In *The Standard Edition of the Complete Works of Sigmund Freud. 12*:99, Hogarth Press, London, 1958.

Freud S: Recommendations to physicians practicing psychoanalysis (1912). In *The Standard Edition of the Complete Psychological Works of Sigmund Freud. 12*:109, Hogarth Press, London, 1974.

Korsch B, Negrete V: Doctor-patient communication. Sci Am, *227*:66, 1972.

Lane F E: Utilizing physician empathy with violent patients. Am J. Psychother *40*(3):448, 1986.

Leigh H, Reiser M F: *The Patient: Biological, Psychological, and Social Dimensions of Medical Practice.* Plenum Press, New York, 1980.

Quill T: Partnerships in patient care: a contractual approach. Ann Intern Med 98:228, 1983.

Reiser D E, Rosen D H: *Medicine as a Human Experience.* University Park Press, Baltimore, 1984.

Reiser D E, Schroder A K: *Patient Interviewing: The Human Dimension.* Williams & Wilkins, Baltimore, 1980.

Wilson J: Patients' wants vs. patients' interests. J Med Ethics *12*(3):127, 1986.

3

Human Development Throughout the Life Cycle

3.1

An Overview of the Life Cycle and Normality

All human beings go through a sequence of periods that have been categorized by a variety of terms—prenatal; infancy, toddler, preschool, school period; early, middle, and late adolescence; early, middle, and late adulthood (old age). There is, however, no standard language that clearly defines these phases, although each has its own character, qualities, and crises. Taken together, these stages imply that there is an order to the course of human life, in spite of the fact that each person's life is unique. The charting of the life course from birth to death is essential to complete understanding of the complexities of human behavior and is especially useful in predicting the difficulties that arise in the course of human development.

LIFE CYCLE

The fundamental assumption of all life cycle theories is that development occurs in successive, clearly defined stages. This sequence is considered to be invariant; that is, it occurs in a constant order in every life whether or not all stages are completed. A second assumption is the *epigenetic principle,* first described by Erik Erikson, which maintains that each stage of the life cycle is characterized by events or crises that must be satisfactorily resolved in order for development to proceed smoothly. If resolution is not achieved within a given life period, the epigenetic model states that all subsequent stages reflect that failure in the form of physical, cognitive, social, or emotional maladjustment. A third notion is that each stage contains a dominant feature, a complex of features, or a crisis point that distinguishes it from phases that either precede or follow.

The most significant differences between various models of the human life cycle involve the developmental criteria cited. For instance, individual schemes may emphasize such diverse elements as biological maturity, psychological capacities, adaptive techniques, defense mechanisms, symptom complexes, role demands, social behavior, and cognitive style. Another common difference between life cycle theories involves language: There is no standard vocabulary to describe the major developmental phases. A

phase of the life cycle may be described by terms such as stage, season, period, era, epoch, and life stage. In general, though, those terms are conceptually congruent and can be used interchangeably.

Contributions to Life Cycle Theory

Current thinking about the human life cycle has been shaped by a handful of highly influential sources. The dominant work on the subject remains the developmental scheme introduced by Freud in 1915. Freud's theory, which focused on the childhood period, was organized around his libido theory. According to Freud, childhood phases of development correspond to successive shifts in the investment of sexual energy to areas of the body usually associated with eroticism: the mouth, the anus, and the genitalia. Accordingly, he discerned developmental periods that were classified as follows: oral phase, birth to 1 year; anal phase, age 1 to 3 years; and phallic phase, age 3 to 5 years.

Freud also described a fourth period, latency, which extends from age 5 years until puberty. Latency is marked by a diminution of sexual interest, which is reactivated at puberty. The basic outlook expressed by Freud was that successful resolution of those childhood phases is essential to normal adult functioning. By comparison, what happens in adulthood is of comparatively little consequence.

Many followers of Freud modified or built upon his conceptualizations while adhering to his focus on sexual energy as the quality that distinguishes the stages of development. Karl Abraham, for example, subdivided the phases of psychosexual development and linked certain adult personality types to difficulties in resolving one of those specific periods.

Melanie Klein, while she adhered to Freud's basic formulations, saw developmental events as occurring more rapidly. The basic premise of Klein's work—like that of Freud's and Abraham's—is that internal processes are the fundamental determinants of personality development and, so, are the moving forces in the human life cycle.

Carl Jung, on the other hand, viewed external factors as playing an important role in personal growth and adaptation. He further held that personality development occurs throughout life—it is not firmly determined by early childhood experiences.

Harry Stack Sullivan took that view even farther. He approached the issue of the life cycle by stating that human development is largely shaped by external events, specifically by social interaction. His influential model of the cycle states that each phase of development is marked by a need for interaction with certain other people. The quality of that interaction influences the personality of the person. Sullivan distinguished the stages or eras of normal development as follows: Infancy, birth to the beginning of language (1½ to 2 years); childhood, language to the need for compeers (2 to 5 years); juvenile era, the need of compeers and the beginning of formal education to preadolescence (5 to 9 years); preadolescence, the beginning of the capacity for intimate relationships with peers of the same sex until genital maturity (9 to 12 years); adolescence, the eruption of true genital interest to the patterning of sexual behavior, and maturity, the establishment of a fully human or mature repertoire of interpersonal relationships, the development of self-respect, and the capacity for intimate and collaborative relationships and loving attitudes.

Erik Erikson accepted Freud's theory of infantile sexuality, but also saw developmental potentials at all stages of life. Indeed, Erikson constructed a model of the life cycle consisting of eight stages that extend into adulthood and old age. The succession of stages is summarized below, along with the dominant issue or maturational crisis that arises during each period according to Erikson:

1. Oral-sensory stage: trust versus mistrust
2. Muscular-anal stage: autonomy versus shame and doubt
3. Locomotor-genital stage: initiative versus guilt
4. Stage of latency: industry versus inferiority
5. Stage of puberty and adolescence: ego identity versus role confusion
6. Stage of young adulthood: intimacy versus isolation
7. Stage of adulthood: generativity versus stagnation
8. Stage of maturity: ego integrity versus despair

Margaret Mahler, who studied early childhood object relations, made a significant contribution to the understanding of personality development. She described the separation-individuation process, resulting in a person's subjective sense of separateness from the world around him. The separation-individuation phase of development begins in the fourth or fifth month of life and is completed by age 3 years. Mahler delineated four subphases of the separation-individuation process:

1. DIFFERENTIATION. The child is able to distinguish between self and other objects.
2. PRACTICING PERIOD. In the early phase, the child discovers the ability to physically separate himself from his mother by crawling and climbing but still requires the mother's presence for security. The later phase is characterized by free, upright locomotion (7 to 10 months until 15 to 16 months).
3. RAPPROCHEMENT. Increased need and desire for the mother to share the child's new skills and experiences. Also, a great need for the mother's love (16 to 25 months of age).
4. CONSOLIDATION. Achievement of a definite individuality and attainment of a certain degree of object-constancy (25 to 36 months of age).

Other approaches, emphasizing neither the psychodynamic nor the environmental aspects of development, have also influenced the study of the life cycle. Jean Piaget presented elaborate formulations about the qualitative differences in cognition during development. His work has been instrumental in elucidating the development of thought processes. He discerned four major periods of intellectual development: sensorimotor, birth to 2 years; preoperational, 2 to 7 years; concrete operations, 7 to 11 years; and formal operations, 11 years through adulthood.

One important study has been conducted by Daniel Levinson and his co-workers at Yale University. That study set out to clarify the issues and characteristics of male personality development in early and middle adulthood. A total of 40 men were studied, whose ages at the start of the investigation ranged from 35 to 45 years; the resulting observations caused Levinson to postulate a new scheme of the adult phases of the life cycle. He suggested that the life cycle is composed of four major eras, each lasting about 25 years, with some overlap, so that a new era is starting as the previous one is ending. Levinson was able to identify a typical age of onset, that is, the age at which an era most frequently begins. The evolving sequence of eras and their age spans as described by Levinson are: childhood and adolescence, birth to 22 years; early adulthood, 17 to 45 years; middle adulthood, 40 to 65 years; and late adulthood, 60 years and beyond. Levinson also identifies 4- to 5-year transitional periods between eras, which function as boundary zones during which a person terminates the outgoing era and initiates the incoming one.

A second major study of adulthood has been reported by George Vaillant, who studied a group of 95 men over a period of 35 years. Some of the results of the investigation are summarized here:

A happy childhood was found to correlate significantly with positive traits in middle life. That was manifested by few oral-dependent traits, little psychopathology, the capacity to play, and good object relations.

Vaillant noted that a hierarchy of ego mechanisms was constructed as the men advanced in age. Defenses were organized along a continuum that reflected two aspects of the personality, immaturity/maturity and psychopathology/mental health. It was found that the maturity of defenses was related to both psychopathology and objective adaptation to the external environment. Moreover, there were shifts in defensive style as a person matured.

Vaillant concluded that adaptive styles mature over the years and that the maturation depends more on development from within than on changes in the interpersonal environment. He also concluded that the model of the life cycle outlined by Erikson appeared valid.

NORMALITY IN PSYCHIATRY

Psychiatrists have always been interested in psychopathology and abnormality. Only recently, however, has there been a concerted effort to define mental health and normality. It was understood implicitly that mental health could be defined as the opposite of mental illness. Given such an assumption, the absence of gross psychopathology was often equated with normal behavior. A number of recent trends have cast doubt on the usefulness of this assumption and have made it increasingly important for psychiatrists to provide more precise concepts and definitions of mental health and normality.

As psychiatrists move out of their consulting rooms and hospital wards into the community, they come into contact with segments of the population not previously seen. Psychiatrists have become increasingly involved in agency consultation; they are called on to make decisions about who is healthy rather than who is too sick for a given position. Interest in evaluating the outcome of psychiatric therapeutic endeavors has also brought the issue of mental health into focus. Indeed, one of the weaknesses of much work on assessing therapeutic outcome has related to vagueness of concepts of normality and mental health.

Four Perspectives of Normality

The many theoretical and clinical concepts of normality seem to fall into four functional perspectives. Although each perspective is unique and has its own definition and description, the perspectives do complement each other, and together they represent the totality of the behavioral- and social-science approaches to normality. The four perspectives are: normality as health, normality as utopia, normality as average, and normality as process.

Normality as Health. The first perspective is basically the traditional medical psychiatric approach to health and illness. Most physicians equate normality with health and view health as an almost universal phenomenon. Behavior is assumed to be within normal limits when no manifest psychopathology is present. If all behavior were to be put on a scale, normality would encompass the major portion of the continuum, and abnormality would be the small remainder.

This definition of normality correlates with the traditional model of the doctor who attempts to free his patient from grossly observable signs and symptoms. To this physician, the lack of signs or symptoms indicates health. In other words, health in this context refers to a reasonable rather than an optimal state of functioning. In its simplest form, this perspective is illustrated by John Romano, who states that a healthy person is one who is reasonably free of undue pain, discomfort, and disability.

Normality as Utopia. The second perspective conceives of normality as that harmonious and optimal blending of the diverse elements of the mental apparatus that culminates in optimal functioning. Such a definition clearly emerges when psychiatrists or psychoanalysts talk about the ideal person or when they discuss their criteria for successful treatment. This approach can be traced directly back to Freud, who, when discussing normality, stated, "A normal ego is like normality in general, an ideal fiction."

Although this approach is characteristic of a significant segment of psychoanalysts, it is by no means unique to them. It can also be found among psychiatrists and among psychologists.

Normality as Average. The third perspective is commonly employed in normative studies of behavior and is based on the mathematical principle of the bell-shaped curve. This approach conceives of the middle range as normal and of both extremes as deviant. The normative approach based on this statistical principle describes each individual in terms of general assessment and total score. Variability is described only within the context of total groups, not within the context of one individual.

Although this approach is more commonly used in psychology and biology than in psychiatry, psychiatrists recently have been using pencil-and-paper tests to a much larger extent than in the past. Not only do psychiatrists use the results of I.Q. tests, the Rorschach test, and the Thematic Apperception Test (TAT), but they also construct their own tests and questionnaires. In this model, one assumes that the typologies of character can be statistically measured.

Normality as Process. The fourth perspective stresses that normal behavior is the end result of interacting systems. Based on this definition, temporal changes are essential to a complete definition of normality. In other words, the normality-as-process perspective stresses changes or processes rather than a cross-sectional definition of normality.

Investigators who subscribe to this approach can be found in all the behavioral and social sciences. Most typical of the concepts in this perspective is Erikson's conceptualization of epigenesis of personality development and the eight developmental stages essential in the attainment of mature adult functioning.

New Directions in Studies of Normality

Although there is growing awareness of the importance of clarifying the various perspectives on normality, there is also an increasing effort to develop empirical research in this area. These new developments are seen in almost all aspects of behavioral science, but the following areas are most prototypical of the new directions: psychoanalysis, human development, social and community psychiatry, and psychiatric research.

Psychoanalysis. In addition to their growing involvement in linking normality and social process, psychoanalysts have continued their long-term interest in elucidating the vicissitudes of the normal psychopathology of everyday life. Psychoanalysts have increasingly demonstrated their interest in normal adaptation to the social environment.

Hartmann has been a prime mover of this trend by conceptualizing autonomous functions of the ego and the ego's conflict-free sphere. The concept of autonomous and conflict-free functions of the ego has intensified clinical exploration of the mechanisms whereby some individuals lead a relatively normal life in the presence of extraordinary external experiential trauma. Discussing the average expectable environment, Hartmann has provided a framework wherein the molding of character structure in specific contexts is more easily understood.

Erikson's work also serves as a bridge linking developmental stages and social process. His concept of modal adaptive tasks at phase-specific stages of life provides a process analysis of normal behavior and a cross-sectional analysis of behavior throughout life. Thus, it becomes possible to establish specific modes of adaptation.

For a summary of psychoanalytic concepts of normality, see Table 1.

Human Development. In the area of human development, Anna Freud delineated aspects of normal growth and development in children. Like Erikson, she has been interested in empirical research directed toward helping to clarify how children cope with the variety of adaptive tasks. The understanding of child development has been advanced by a number of longitudinal studies. In addition, a great

Table 1
Psychoanalytic Concepts of Normality

Theorist	Characteristics
S. Freud	Normality is an ideal fiction; every ego approximates that of the psychotic to a greater or lesser extent.
K. Eissler	Absolute normality cannot be obtained because the normal person must be totally aware of his thoughts and feelings.
M. Klein	Normality is characterized by strength of character, the capacity to deal with conflicting emotions, the ability to experience pleasure without conflict, and the ability to love.
E. Erikson	Normality is the ability to master the periods of life: trust vs. mistrust; autonomy vs. doubt; initiative vs. guilt; industry vs. inferiority; identity vs. role confusion; intimacy vs. isolation; generativity vs. stagnation; and ego integrity vs. despair.
L. Kubie	Normality is the ability to learn by experience, to be flexible, and to adapt to a changing environment.
H. Hartmann	Conflict-free ego functions represent the person's potential for normality; the degree the ego can adapt to reality and be autonomous is related to mental health.
K. Menninger	Normality is the ability to adjust to the external world with contentment and to master the task of acculturation.
A. Adler	The person's capacity to develop social feeling and to be productive are related to mental health; the ability to work heightens self-esteem and makes one capable of adaptation.
R. E. Money-Kryle	Normality is the ability to achieve insight into one's self, which is never fully accomplished.
O. Rank	Normality is the capacity to live without fear, guilt, or anxiety and to take responsibility for one's own actions.

deal of data is being collected on individual growth and development throughout life. Populations not studied heretofore have been examined closely, and the findings have been reported precisely.

The studies by Offer and Sabshin on adolescents are prototypic of this trend. These investigators have studied a group of young adolescents throughout their high school years. The group was selected by means of a questionnaire, and psychiatric interviews have been conducted with a modal sample throughout the high school years. One group of normal teenagers is being studied over a period of time. Three normal types of development have been identified: continuous growth, surgent growth, and tumultuous growth. Although persons typical of these types are different, they are placed along a continuum of normality. Offer and Sabshin have formulated an operational definition of normality that is not absolute but, rather, is descriptive of one type of middle-class adolescent population. The criteria best describing the teenagers are: (1) almost complete absence of gross psychopathology, severe physical defects, and severe physical illness; (2) mastery of previous developmental tasks without serious setbacks; (3) ability to experience affects flexibly and to actively resolve their conflicts with reasonable success; (4) relatively good object relationships with parents, siblings, and peers; and (5) feeling a part of a larger cultural environment and being aware of its norms and values.

It is important to note that the developmental approach is also being used for adults by Vaillant and others. Studies of adaptation to marriage, to parenthood, to work, and to leisure activities have become increasingly prominent. Precise empirical studies are being conducted regarding developmental problems in the period of involution and decline.

A controversial view has been taken by Thomas Szasz, who believes that the concept of mental illness should be abandoned entirely. He also states that normality can be measured only in terms of what people do or do not do and that it is actually a problem of ethics.

The development of geriatrics has moved in a more normative direction. The deficit-focused orientation of earlier studies in gerontology has been replaced, to a significant extent, by a normative framework that asks, in effect, "How do older people cope with the adaptational tasks of the 60s, the 70s, and beyond?"

Social and Community Psychiatry. The evolution of social and community psychiatry has given even broader possibilities to studying normative populations. As psychiatrists and their collaborators have moved into the community, they have become involved in providing services for and conducting research with populations not heretofore seen by mental health professionals. Epidemiologic investigations have become increasingly precise and sophisticated. One of the pioneering studies in the epidemiology of illness and health was carried out by Alexander Leighton. This attempt to ascertain the degree of sickness and health in a large population serves as a paradigm for investigations of a variety of target populations. In general, community psychiatry involves investigation and service to meet the mental health needs of a functional or geographic community.

One important model for such community psychiatry activity is carried out in the Woodlawn Mental Health Center. At this center, studies have been conducted on all of the children entering first grade in the public and the parochial schools within a particular area. The investigators have been interested in the ratings of adaptation and maladaptation by the teachers, the parents, and the mental health researchers for this entire population. They are also interested in carrying out follow-up studies to determine the long-term impact of changes in experimental groups on the ultimate rating of adaptation and maladaptation.

It is impressive to note that this primary preventive approach combines the interest of child development with community psychiatry. This merging of two trends within the mental health field has great promise in helping to clarify definitions of adaptation and normality as well as maladaptation and abnormality.

Psychiatric Research. Psychiatric research has shown a resurgence of interest in the question of the use of controls for a variety of psychiatric investigations. Although a number of studies have focused on the emotional problems of volunteers for psychiatric experimentation, there is a general awareness that greater precision is necessary in selecting controls for a specific psychiatric research question.

Although many investigators have become engaged in studies of controls or normal samples in the context of elucidating an experimental question regarding psychopathology, a host of new investigations have been undertaken to study normal populations as such. Prototypic of this trend is Roy Grinker's presentation of a sample of homoclites—a word he uses in order to avoid the term "normal" or "healthy." His sample included an overwhelming number of persons who ordinarily would not have been seen in a psychiatrist's office. They represent well-adjusted individuals whose aspirations and capacities fall within a comparable range of each other.

Psychiatrists are currently studying the ways individuals adapt to a variety of situational stresses. The stresses vary from adjustment to physical illness and physical hardships (such as astronauts undergo) to adaptation to marriage, parenthood, leisure, and aging.

Psychologists are using standardized tests such as the Minnesota Multiphasic Personality Inventory (MMPI) to measure normality. Vaillant's work on the types of ego defenses used, ranging from primitive to mature, are also a measure of normality. Finally, normality as a biological, psychological, or social concept is always relative and must be viewed within the context of the society in which it is studied.

References

Colorusso C A, Nemiroff R A: *Adult Development: A New Dimension in Psychodynamic Theory and Practice.* Plenum Press, New York, 1981.
Erikson E: *Childhood and Society.* W W Norton, New York, 1959.
Fagan J R, et al.: Selective screening device for the early detection of normal or delayed cognitive development in infants at risk for later mental retardation. Pediatrics 78(6):1021, 1986.
Freud A: *The Ego and the Mechanisms of Defense.* International University Press, New York, 1966.
Freud S: Analysis terminable and interminable (1937). In *The Standard Edition of the Complete Psychological Works of Sigmund Freud,* vol 23. Hogarth Press and the Institute of Psycho-Analysis, London, 1974.
Hartmann H: *Ego Psychology and the Problem of Adaptation.* International Universities Press, New York, 1958.
Kellam S E, Branch J D. *Mental Health and Going to School: The Woodlawn Program of Assessment, Early Intervention, and Evaluation.* University of Chicago Press, Chicago, 1975.
Leighton D C, MacMillan A M, Harding J S, et al.: *The Stirling County Study of Psychiatric Disorder and Socio-Cultural Environment,* vol 3, *The Character of Danger.* Basic Books, New York, 1963.
Lidz T: *The Person: His and Her Development Throughout the Life Cycle.* Basic Books, New York, 1976.
Maziadi M, Cote R, Boutin P, et al.: *Temperament and Intellectual Development: A Longitudinal Study from Infancy to Four Years.* Am J Psychiatry 144(2):144, 1987.
Offer D, Sabshin M: *Normality and the Life Cycle.* Basic Books, New York, 1984.
Valliant G E, editor: *Empirical Studies of Ego Mechanism and Defense.* American Psychiatric Assoc. Press, Washington, DC, 1986.

3.2 ——————
Infancy and Childhood

Understanding the nature and process of infant and child development has always been a challenge. Questions involve the degree to which developmental potentials and patterns are present at conception and the effect that the prenatal and postnatal environment have in modifying them. The infant is not a tabula rasa—a blank slate—whose personality is developed through experience. Rather, the child is endowed with inborn responses that interact with the environment to produce new and different behaviors. The concept of *epigenesis* takes into account genetics, environmental experience, and the child's capacity to structure and restructure experience at each stage of development. The myriad events subsumed under child development begin at conception and are influenced by pregnancy, intrauterine development, and childbirth (the prenatal period).

PRENATAL EVENTS

Pregnancy and Childbirth

Pregnancy produces marked biological, physiological, and psychological changes in the woman. Most women are positive about pregnancy, especially if it was planned in conjunction with a loving partner; however, 10 percent of all children born are unwanted at conception, and an additional 20 percent, though desired, are not wanted at the particular time of conception. A woman's psychological conflicts concerning pregnancy most often involve assuming the mothering role. If her own mother was a poor role model, the woman's sense of maternal competence may be impaired, leading to a lack of confidence before and after the birth of her baby.

Twenty to 40 percent of women report emotional disturbance or cognitive dysfunction in the postpartum period. Many experience the so-called postpartum blues, a normal state consisting of feelings of sadness, dysphoria, frequent tearfulness, and clinging dependency. These feelings, which may last several days, have been variously ascribed to the rapid change in hormone levels, the stress of childbirth, and the awareness of the increased responsibility motherhood brings. A somewhat similar syndrome has been described in fathers who develop mood changes during their wives' pregnancy or after the baby is born. Such fathers are affected by several factors: added responsibility, diminished sexual outlets, decreased attention from the wife, and believing that the child represents a binding force in an unsatisfactory marriage. In rare cases (1 to 2 per 1,000 deliveries), a postpartum psychosis may develop in the mother characterized by severe anxiety, hallucinations, or delusions.

In the psychologically healthy woman, pregnancy is one expression of her sense of self-realization and identity as a woman. Negative attitudes about pregnancy are associated with a fear of childbirth or of the mothering role. Some women view pregnancy as a way of diminishing self-doubts concerning their femininity or as a means of reassuring themselves that they are able to conceive.

Pregnancy and Marriage

The effects of pregnancy on marriage vary. Sexually, some women experience an increased sex drive as pelvic vasocongestion produces a more sexually responsive state. Some women no longer fear pregnancy and are more responsive. Other women lose interest in sex altogether or have diminished desire owing either to physical discomfort or to a psychological mind set that associates motherhood with asexuality. That association can also occur in men who have a madonna complex, who view the pregnant woman as someone sacred, not to be defiled by the sexual act; some men find the pregnant body ugly. Intercourse may be erroneously regarded by either person as potentially harmful to the developing fetus; coitus may be avoided for that reason. Most obstetricians place no prohibitions on coitus until 4 to 5 weeks antepartum; this abstinence may also put a strain on the marriage. Studies have shown that if a man has an extramarital affair, it will most likely occur during the last trimester of the wife's pregnancy.

The prospective wife-mother and husband-father have to redefine their roles both as a couple and as individuals. Relationships with friends and relatives face readjustments. Each has to deal with new responsibilities as a care-giver to the newborn as well as to the spouse. The new parents must reevaluate how they choose to earn and spend their income. Accustomed to gratifying each other's dependency needs, the couple also must attend to the unremitting needs of the newborn infant and developing child. While most couples respond positively to meeting these demands, some do not.

Fetal Development

The fetal nervous system is highly susceptible to damage from a variety of causes: viral infections, toxoplasmosis, cytomegalic inclusion disease, alcoholism in the mother, maternal opioid abuse or malnutrition. Over 150 identified inborn errors of metabolism (e.g., galactosemia and phenyl-ketonuria) have been identified in neonates. Nutritional deficiencies in protein are associated with growth defects, mental retardation, and prematurity. Chromosomal abnormalities, such as Down's syndrome and Tay-Sachs disorder, may occur but are subject to intrauterine diagnosis and therapeutic abortion.

Other factors that influence intrauterine development include an excess or deficiency of maternal circulating hormones. Congenital hypothyroidism occurs in infants whose mothers are thyroid deficient; the condition is reversible. In an effort to prevent miscarriage, the administration of androgens affects sex differentiation in the fetus, so that female infants may have masculinized organs, such as an enlarged clitoris or a hypoplastic uterus. Diethylstilbestrol (DES), once given to pregnant women to prevent abortion, has been found to produce cervical dysplasia in female children born to those mothers. Through the production of adrenal hormones, maternal stress may also influence the newborn. Mothers with a high anxiety level are more likely to produce babies who are hyperactive, irritable, have sleep disorders, low birth weight, and feed poorly. Fetal alcohol syndrome affects infants born to alcoholic mothers and is characterized by delayed growth and developmental abnormalities. Smoking during pregnancy is associated with lower than average infant birth weight. Infants born to mothers addicted to narcotics go through a true withdrawal syndrome at birth. If the mother is exposed to severe radiation during the first 20 weeks of her pregnancy, the baby will be born with gross deformities. Maternal rubella during the first trimester has been associated with severe mental retardation, deafness, and microcephaly in 50 percent of infants born to those mothers. Acquired immune deficiency syndrome (AIDS) is transmitted from infected mothers to the fetus.

CHILDBIRTH

The latest available statistics (1987) indicate that there were 3,615,000 babies born in the United States and a birth rate of 15.4 per 1,000 population. Advances in prenatal and perinatal care have reduced the infant death rate to about 12 per 1,000 live births (down from 20 infant deaths per 1,000 live births in 1970).

The overwhelming majority of babies are born in a hospital with a physician in attendance, but free-standing birthing centers with access to a hospital are an alternative for some couples. There has been a steady increase in the number of babies born by Caesarean section—from about 5 percent in the 1960s to about 20 percent in the 1980s. Some of this increase is the result of the fear of malpractice. Through this procedural change, prolonged labor that is hazardous to the fetus is avoided. Analgesic drugs given to the mother during labor enter the fetal bloodstream and sedate the newborn infant. A drug that depresses the mother's nervous system affects the sucking reflex of the infant, sometimes for a few days.

Childbirth is a potentially hazardous time for both mother and child. A premature birth increases the risk of mental retardation, behavior problems, emotional disorders, and sensorimotor problems such as dyslexia. Prematurity occurs when the birth weight is under 2,500 grams or the gestation period is less than 34 weeks. Prematurity is correlated with lower socioeconomic groups, poor maternal nutrition, and teenage pregnancy and accounts for 7 percent of all births. Higher socioeconomic status correlates negatively with infant mortality.

Genetic Counseling

Genetic counseling provides patients and their families with direct medical knowledge in the field of genetics. This type of counseling is indicated when there is even the remotest possibility of a genetically based disorder in the family. A couple may ask about the chances of their first child being schizophrenic, or a person whose father had Huntington's disease may be concerned about developing the disease. In the first instance, schizophrenia is transmitted in a multifactorial manner so the couple can be told that the highest risk, about 40 percent, is to the offspring of two schizophrenic parents. If one parent has schizophrenia, the risk is in the 10- to 15-percent range. If only the brother or sister of one member of the couple is ill, the risk for their children is probably in the 2- to 3-percent range, not appreciably greater than the risk for the general population. In the case of Huntington's disease, which follows Mendelian rules of inheritance, a person whose parent has the disorder has a 50-percent chance of developing the disease. Since the age of onset varies, the longer one lives without becoming ill, the lower the remaining risk. Recently, a chemical test for determining gene carriers for Huntington's disease was developed, so that persons can now use this knowledge when deciding on marriage and parenthood.

Prenatal Diagnosis and Its Implications

Genetic counseling depends on prenatal diagnosis in many cases. Techniques used include amniocentesis (transabdominal aspiration of fluid from the amniotic sac), ultrasound examinations, x-rays, fetoscopy (the direct visualization of the fetus), fetal blood and skin sampling, and chorionic biopsy. With this vast array of techniques, about 2 percent of the total number of cases tested are positive for some abnormality. In addition to a family history of a disorder with genetic loading, prenatal diagnosis is commonly offered to older pregnant women. A problem in the routine use of diagnostic tests is that some carry a risk. About 5 percent of patients who undergo fetoscopy, for example, have a miscarriage. Amniocentesis, usually performed between the 14th and 15th week of pregnancy, causes fetal damage or miscarriage in less than 1 percent of cases.

Genetic counseling requires that the clinician be aware of a person's level of maturity, individual conflicts, defense mechanisms, and ego strengths and weaknesses. The counselor has to be ready to deal with depression, anger, anxiety, and other complex emotions related to the issues at hand.

CHILD DEVELOPMENT

Normal child development may be approached from a variety of perspectives. Freud's theories, discussed in detail in Section 7.1, described five psychosexual stages of development—oral, anal, phallic, latency, and genital—derived from the analysis of adults with various types of psychopathology. Based on direct observation of children, other psychoanalysts elaborated on many of Freud's theories. For Erik Erikson, one of these theorists, human development can be understood only if one takes into account the social forces that influence and interact with the developing person. Erikson's five childhood psychosocial stages of trust, initiative, autonomy, industry, and identity correlate with Freud's psychosexual stages. In addition, Erikson added three stages—intimacy, generativity, and integrity—which extend beyond young adulthood into old age. These eight stages have both positive and negative aspects, have specific emotional crises, and are affected by the interaction of the person's biology, culture, and society. Each stage has two possible outcomes, one positive or healthy and the other negative or unhealthy. Under ideal circumstances, the crisis is resolved when the person achieves a new and higher level of functioning at the positive end of the particular stage. According to Erikson, most persons do not achieve perfect positive polarity, but fall more toward the positive than the negative pole. A third major model is Jean Piaget's theory of cognitive (intellectual) development. By conducting intensive studies of the way children think and behave, Piaget formulated a theory of cognition, which he divided into four stages—sensorimotor, preoperational, concrete, and formal operational. Piaget's theories are reviewed in Section 5.1.

According to Erikson, Freud, and Piaget, the infant grows by predetermined steps through various stages. In this epigenetic view of development, each stage has its own characteristics and needs, and must be negotiated successfully before it is possible to go on to the next level. The sequence of stages is not automatic; rather it depends on both central nervous system growth and life experience. There is ample evidence that an unfavorable environment can delay some of the developmental stages; however, particularly favorable environmental stimulators can accelerate one's progress through the stages.

In view of the several different models for conceptualizing the phases of development (Table 1), it has become customary to organize the developmental stages in chronological order as follows: infancy; toddler period; preschool period; school period or middle years; early, middle, and late adolescence; and early, middle, and late adulthood (old age).

Infancy (Birth to 15 Months)

Neural Organization. The development of the human brain occurs predominantly during postnatal life, although some brain function in utero has been demonstrated through the response of a fetal encephalogram to sound stimuli. The weight of the human brain is about 350 grams in an infant and 1,450 grams at full development; this represents a fourfold increase in the neocortex and a lesser increase in the motor and association areas. During early development, there is enormous growth in the number and branching of dendrites and a multiplication of synaptic junctions.

Infants are born with a number of reflexes, many of which were once needed for survival. Other survival systems—breathing, sucking, swallowing, and circulatory and temperature homeostasis—are relatively functional at birth. Sensory organs, however, are incompletely developed. Further differentiation of neurophysiologic functions depends on an active automatic process of stimulatory reinforcement. Higher order capabilities arise from the differentiation and interrelation of the organism's initial given capacities.

Bonding and Attachment. As sensory development proceeds, there is for all social organisms a parallel task of fashioning a tie between the newborn and its species. Ethologists have demonstrated, primarily in birds, that there is a critical period shortly after birth during which the newborn becomes imprinted on a moving, sound-producing object. This bond elicits following behavior from the newborn. For all of its undoubted importance, imprinting has not been demonstrated conclusively in man or in other primates.

Harry Harlow. Harry Harlow studied social learning and the effects of social isolation in monkeys. Harlow placed newborn rhesus monkeys with two different types of surrogate mothers—one wire-mesh and the other wire-mesh covered with terry cloth. The monkeys preferred the terry cloth mothers that provided contact and comfort. When frightened, cloth-mother-raised monkeys showed intense clinging behavior and appeared to be comforted, whereas wire-mother-raised monkeys gained no comfort and appeared disorganized. Both types of surrogate-reared monkeys were subsequently unable to adjust to life in a monkey colony and had extraordinary difficulty in learning to mate. When impregnated, the females failed to mother their young. These behavioral peculiarities were attributed to the isolates' lack of mothering in infancy. For further discussion, see Section 5.5.

John Bowlby. John Bowlby studied the attachment of infants to mothers and concluded that early separation of infants from

Table 1
A Synthesis of Developmental Theorists

Age (Years)	Margaret Mahler	John Bowlby	Sigmund Freud	Erik Erikson	Jean Piaget
0–1	NORMAL AUTISTIC PHASE: (Birth to 4 weeks) - state of half-sleep, half-wake - major task of phase is to achieve homeostatic equilibrium with the environment NORMAL SYMBIOTIC PHASE: (3–4 weeks to 4–5 months) - dim awareness of caretaker, but infant still functions as if he and caretaker are in state of undifferentiation or fusion - social smile characteristic (two-four months) THE SUBPHASES OF SEPARATION-INDIVIDUATION PROPER FIRST SUBPHASE DIFFERENTIATION: (5 to 10 months) - process of hatching from autistic shell, i.e., developing more alert sensorium that reflects cognitive and neurological maturation - beginning of comparative scanning, i.e., comparing what is and what is not mother - characteristic anxiety: stranger anxiety, which involves curiosity and fear (most prevalent around 8 months)	PHASE I: (Birth to 8–12 weeks) - infant's ability to discriminate one person from another is limited to olfactory and auditory stimuli - to any person in infant's vicinity, infant will: - orient to that person - have tracking movements of the eyes - grasp and reach - smile - babble - stop crying on hearing voice or seeing face — these behaviors, by influencing the adult's behavior, are likely to increase time the baby is in proximity to mother (adult) PHASE II: (8-12 weeks to 6 months or much later, according to circumstances) - continuation of Phase 1 activities but more marked in relation to mother more specifically	ORAL PHASE: (Birth to 1 year) - Major site of tension and gratification is the mouth, lips, tongue - includes biting and sucking activities	BASIC TRUST VS BASIC MISTRUST: (ORAL SENSORY) (Birth to 1 year) - Social mistrust demonstrated via ease of feeding, depth of sleep, bowel relaxation - depends on consistency and sameness of experience provided by caretaker - second six-months teething and biting moves infant "from getting to taking" - weaning leads to "nostalgia for lost paradise" - if *basic trust* is strong, child maintains hopeful attitude	SENSORIMOTOR PHASE (Birth to 2 years) - Intelligence rests mainly on actions and movements coordinated under "*schemata*," (Schema is a pattern of behavior in response to a particular environmental stimulus.) - Environment is mastered through *assimilation* and *accommodation* (Assimilation is the incorporation of new environmental stimuli. Accommodation is the modification of behavior to adapt to new stimuli.) - *Object Permanence* is achieved by age 2 yrs. Object still exists in mind if disappears from view; search for hidden object - reversibility in action begins

SECOND SUBPHASE PRACTICING: (10 to 16 months)
- beginning of this phase marked by upright locomotion—child has new perspective and also mood of elation
- mother used as home base
- characteristic anxiety: separation anxiety

THIRD SUBPHASE: RAPPROCHEMENT: (16 to 24 months)
- infant now a toddler—more aware of physical separateness, which dampens mood of elation
- child tries to bridge gap between himself and mother—concretely seen as bringing objects to mother
- mother's efforts to help toddler often not perceived as helpful, temper tantrums typical
- characteristic event: rapprochement crisis: wanting to be soothed by mother and yet not be able to accept her help
- symbol of rapprochement: child standing on threshold of door not knowing which way to turn in helpless frustration
- resolution of crisis occurs as child's skills improve and child able to get gratification from doing things himself

PHASE III: (6–7 months and continues throughout second and into third year)
- attachment to mother-figure evident:
- following departing mother
- greeting her on her return
- using her as base from which to explore
- waning of friendly, undifferentiated responses to others
- treating of strangers with caution, alarm, withdrawal

PHASE IV: (from 24 months and beyond)
mother figure seen as independent
- object, persistent in time and space
- more complex relationship with mother develops—"partnership" between
- mother and child develops where child acquires insight into mother's feelings and motives
- child observes mother's behavior and what influences it

AUTONOMY VS. SHAME AND DOUBT: (MUSCULAR-ANAL) (1 year to 3 years)
- Biologically includes learning to walk, feed self, talk
- Muscular maturation sets stage for "holding on and letting go"
- Need for outer control, firmness of caretaker prior to development of autonomy
- Shame occurs when child is overtly self-conscious via negative exposure
- Self-doubt can evolve if parents overly shame child, e.g. about elimination

ANAL PHASE: (1 year to 3 years)
- Anus and surrounding area is major source of interest
- Acquisition of voluntary sphincter control (toilet training)

PRE-OPERATIONAL PHASE: (2 to 7 years)
- Appearance of symbolic functions, associated with language acquisition
- Egocentrism: all events center around child, magical thinking
- Thinking is pre-logical and nonreversible with absence of conservation of matter
- Animism: belief that inanimate objects are alive, i.e. have feelings and intentions
- "Imminent justice": belief that punishment for bad deeds is inevitable

INITIATIVE VS. GUILT: (LOCOMOTOR GENITAL) (3 to 5 years)
- Initiative arises in relation to tasks for the sake of activity, both motor and intellectual
- Guilt may arise over goals contemplated (especially aggressive)
- Desire to mimic adult world; involvement in oedipal struggle leads to resolution via social role identification
- Sibling rivalry frequent

Table 1 *continued*

Age (Years)	Margaret Mahler	John Bowlby	Sigmund Freud	Erik Erikson	Jean Piaget
3–4	FOURTH SUBPHASE: OBJECT CONSTANCY: (24 months to 36 months) - child better able to cope with mother's absence and engage substitutes		PHALLIC-OEDIPAL PHASE: (3 years to 5 years) - Genital focus of interest, stimulation, and excitement	INDUSTRY VS. INFERIORITY: (LATENCY) (6 to 11 years) - Child is busy building, creating, accomplishing - Receives systematic instruction as well as fundamentals of technology - Danger of sense of inadequacy and inferiority if child despairs of his tools/skills and status among peers - Socially decisive age	CONCRETE (OPERATIONAL) PHASE: (7 to 11 years) - Emergence of logical (cause-effect) thinking, including reversibility and ability to sequence and serialize - Understanding of part/whole relationships and classifications - Child able to take other's point of view - Conservation of number, length, weight and volume
4–5	- child can begin to feel comfortable with mother's absences by knowing she will return - gradual internalization of image of mother as reliable and stable - through increasing verbal skills and better sense of time, child can tolerate delay and endure separations		- Penis is organ of interest for both sexes - Genital masturbation common - Intense preoccupation with *castration anxiety* (fear of genital loss or injury) - *Penis envy* (discontent with one's own genitals and wish to possess genitals of male) seen in girls in this Phase - *Oedipus Complex* universal: child wishes to have sex and marry parent of opposite sex and simultaneously be rid of parent of same sex		
5–6			LATENCY PHASE: (from 5–6 years to 11–12 years) - State of relative quiescence of sexual drive with resolution of Oedipal complex		

FORMAL (ABSTRACT) PHASE:
(11 years through end of adolescence)
- Hypothetical-deductive reasoning, not only on basis of objects but also on basis of hypotheses or of propositions
- Capable of thinking about one's thoughts
- Combinative structures emerge, permitting flexible grouping of elements in a system
- Ability to use two systems of reference simultaneously
- Ability to grasp concept of probabilities

IDENTITY VS. ROLE DIFFUSION:
(11 years and through end of adolescence)
- Struggle to develop ego identity (sense of inner sameness and continuity)
- Preoccupation with appearance, hero worship, ideology
- Group identity (peers) develops
- Danger of role confusion, doubts about sexual and vocational identity
- Psychosocial moratorium, stage between morality learned by the child and the ethics to be developed by the adult

- Sexual drives channeled into more socially appropriate aims (i.e. school-work and sports)
- Formation of superego, one of three psychic structures in mind which is responsible for moral and ethical development, including conscience
- (Other two psychic structures are ego, which is a group of functions mediating between the drives and the external environment, and
- the id, repository of sexual and aggressive drives
- The id is there at birth and the ego develops gradually from rudimentary structure present at birth)

GENITAL PHASE
(from 11 to 12 years and beyond)
- Final stage of psychosexual development—begins with puberty and the biological capacity for orgasm but involves the capacity for true intimacy

6-11

11+

Table by Sylvia Karasu, M.D. and Richard Oberfield, M.D.

their mothers had severe negative effects on the child's emotional and intellectual development. He described attachment behavior which develops during the first year of life; it is characterized by the maintenance of physical contact between the mother and child when the child is hungry, frightened, or in distress. Bowlby's theories are further discussed in Section 5.2.

Social deprivation syndromes and maternal neglect. Investigators, especially René Spitz, have long documented the severe developmental retardation that accompanies maternal rejection and neglect. Infants in institutions, characterized by low staff-to-infant ratios and frequent turnover of personnel, tend to display marked developmental retardation even with adequate physical care and freedom from infection. The same infants, placed in adequate foster or adoptive care, undergo marked acceleration in development.

Fathers and attachment. Babies become attached to fathers as well as to mothers, but the attachment is different. Generally, mothers hold babies for caretaking, and fathers hold babies for purposes of play. Given a choice between either parent after separation, the infant usually will go to the mother, but if the mother is unavailable, he will turn to the father for comfort.

Stranger anxiety. A fear of strangers is first noted in infants at about 26 weeks of age, but does not develop fully until about 32 weeks. At the approach of a stranger, infants cry and cling to mother. Babies exposed to only one caregiver are more likely to have stranger anxiety than those exposed to a variety of care-givers.

Separation anxiety, which occurs between 10 and 16 months, is related to stranger anxiety but not identical to it. Separation from the person to whom the infant is attached precipitates separation anxiety. Stranger anxiety, however, occurs even when the infant is in the mother's arms. The infant learns to separate as it starts to crawl and move away from the mother—but the infant constantly looks back and frequently returns to the mother for reassurance.

Margaret Mahler described a developmental phase called symbiosis during which the infant feels fused with the mother or the mother's breast. It extends from the age of 3 to 4 weeks to 4 to 5 months, at which point the separation individuation phase occurs. Individuation is characterized by the child's perception of itself as a distinct person, separate from the mother.

Temperamental Differences. There are strong suggestions of inborn differences between infants. There is a wide variability among individual infants in autonomic reactivity and temperament. Stella Chess and Alexander Thomas identified the following nine behavioral dimensions from which reliable differences could be obtained:

1. Activity level—the motor component present in a given child's functioning
2. Rhythmicity—the predictability of such functions as hunger, feeding pattern, elimination, and sleep-wake cycle
3. Approach or withdrawal—the nature of the response to a new stimulus, such as a new food, toy, or person
4. Adaptability—the speed and ease with which a current behavior is able to be modified in response to altered environmental structuring

5. Intensity of reaction—the amount of energy used in mood expression
6. Threshold of responsiveness—the intensity level of stimulation required to evoke a discernible response to sensory stimuli, environmental objects, and social contacts
7. Quality of mood—pleasant, joyful, friendly behavior as contrasted with unpleasant, crying, unfriendly behavior
8. Distractibility—the effectiveness of extraneous environmental stimuli in interfering with or in altering the direction of ongoing behavior
9. Attention span and persistence—the length of time a particular activity is pursued by the child (attention span) and the continuation of an activity in the face of obstacles (persistence)

The ratings on individual children showed considerable stability over a 25-year follow-up period. Researchers were able to discern a relationship between the initial characteristics of the infant, the mode of parental management, and the subsequent appearance of symptoms.

Impact of Infant Care. Clinicians are starting to view the infant as an important actor in the family drama, one who, in part, determines its course. The behavior of the infant serves to control the behavior of the mother, just as the mother's behavior modulates the infant's. The calm, smiling, predictable, good infant is a powerful reward for tender maternal care. The jittery, irregular, irritable infant tries a mother's patience. If a mother's capacities for giving are marginal, such traits may cause her to turn away from her child and thus complicate the child's already inadequate beginnings.

Parental fit. The concept of parental fit refers to how well the mother (or father) relates to the newborn or developing infant and takes into account temperamental characteristics of both parent and child. As mentioned above, each newborn has innate psychophysiologic characteristics which are known collectively as temperament. Chess and Thomas also identified a range of normal temperamental patterns from the difficult child at one end of the spectrum to the easy child at the other end. Difficult children, who make up 10 percent of all children, have a hyperalert physiologic makeup. They react intensely to stimuli (cry easily at loud noises), sleep poorly, eat at unpredictable times, and are difficult to comfort. Easy children, comprising of 40 percent of all children, are regular in eating, eliminating, and sleeping, are flexible, are able to adapt to change and to new stimuli with a minimum of distress, and are easily comforted when they cry. The other 50 percent of children are mixtures of those two types. The difficult child is harder to raise and places greater demands on the parent. Chess and Thomas used the term "goodness of fit" to characterize the harmonious and consonant interaction between a mother and child in their motivations, capacities, and styles of behavior. Poorness of fit is characterized by dissonance between parent and child which is likely to lead to distorted development and maladaptive functioning. The difficult child must be recognized because parents of such infants often develop feelings of inadequacy and believe that something they are doing wrong accounts for the difficulty in sleeping, eating, and problems in comforting the child. In addition, a majority of such children develop emotional disturbances later in life.

Spacing of Children. For women in the United States, 10 percent of conceptions that lead to live births are considered to be unwanted, and 20 percent are wanted but considered to be ill-timed. The implications of these figures are that some couples may be poorly prepared or may feel guilty about not wanting to be parents at that particular time. It is desirable that pregnancy be a planned event and that the spacing of children be mutually agreed upon. The number of children in a typical family is two, as opposed to four around the beginning of the century. Repeated childbearing prevents adequate recuperation from the birth process and places the mother at risk for complications and injury. The new mother requires time to adapt; this period may range from a few weeks to several months. The demands of other children at home can be extremely taxing, and the family may be stressed beyond its capacity if those children are also young.

Studies of children from large families (four or five children) show that they are more likely to develop conduct disorders and have a slightly lower level of verbal intelligence than children from small families. Decreased parental interaction and discipline may account for these findings.

Birth order. The effects of birth order are variable. First-born children are more achievement oriented and perform better academically than second and third children. Parents tend to be more involved, but they are also more anxious about caregiving with firstborn children than with later children. Second and third children have the advantage of the parents' previous experience. If children are spaced too closely together, however, there may not be enough "lap time" for each. Finally, the arrival of new children in the family affects not only the parents but the siblings as well. Firstborn children may resent the birth of a new sibling who threatens their sole claim on parental attention. In some cases, regressive behavior such as enuresis or thumb sucking occurs.

In general, the oldest child achieves the most and is the most authoritarian; the middle child usually receives the least attention in the home and may develop strong peer relationships to compensate; and the youngest child may receive too much attention and be spoiled.

Developmental Landmarks. Arnold Gesell has described developmental schedules that outline the qualitative sequence of motor, adaptive, language, and personal-social behavior of the child from the age of 4 weeks to 6 years. These milestones of development allow for comparison between the development of a particular child and a normative standard. Gesell's schedules are widely used in both pediatrics and child psychiatry. Table 2 details the sequence of normal behavioral development from birth through the preschool period.

Language development. At birth, infants are able to make noises such as crying, but they do not vocalize until about 8 weeks. At that time, guttural or babbling sounds occur spontaneously, especially in response to the mother. The persistence and further evolution of the child's vocalizations depend on parental reinforcement. Language development occurs in well-delineated stages, as outlined in Table 3.

Piaget's view of cognition from birth to 2 years. Jean Piaget formulated a theory of intellectual development which views cognition as a special instance of biological adaptation. In Table 4, the sensorimotor period is discussed. Piaget divided this period from birth to 2 years into six subgroups or stages.

Emotional development. The stages of emotional development parallel those of cognitive development. Indeed, it is the caretaking person who provides the major stimulus for both aspects of mental growth. The human infant is totally dependent on adult caretakers for sheer survival. Through this regular and predictable interaction, an affectional tie between infant and caretaker develops. The infant's behavioral repertoire expands as a consequence of the caretaker's social responses to its behaviors (Figure 1).

Erikson's stage of basic trust vs. basic mistrust (birth to 1 year). Erikson wrote in *Growth and Crisis of the Healthy Personality*: "For the first component of a healthy personality I nominate a sense of basic trust which I think is an attitude toward oneself and the world derived from the experience of the first year of life. Trust is the expectation that one's needs will be taken care of and that the world or outer providers can be relied upon."

This period is also known as the oral stage because the mouth is the most sensitive zone of the body during this time. Finding the nipple, sucking, and taking in nutrients fill the child's primary needs. The trust-inducing mother attends to those needs assiduously, thus laying the groundwork for the infant's future positive expectation of the world. The loving parent also attends to the infant's other senses—sight, touch, hearing. Through this interaction, the baby either develops the feeling of trust that his wants will be satisfied, or if the mother is not attentive, the baby develops the mistrustful sense that he is not going to get what he wants.

Toward the second half of the first year, the oral crisis occurs. At this point, the infant's teeth develop and a drive to bite occurs. From simply being a passive recipient, the infant becomes active. If the infant bites too aggressively, however, the nipple is taken away. As a result, the child learns that he can influence the environment and begins to develop a sense of himself as an individual, separate from the environment. In our culture, weaning from the breast or bottle begins toward the end of this phase. Erikson believed that this separation is the basis of a sense of sorrow or nostalgia. However, if basic trust is strong, the child develops a sense of hope and optimism.

An impairment of basic trust leads to basic mistrust. An affectionate loving mother or surrogate mother who gives consistent, high quality care provides the basis for the development of trust. Prolonged separation from the mother at this time can lead to depression, hospitalism, anaclitic depression, or a depressive tone that becomes part of the person's adult character structure.

Toddler Stage (15 Months to 2½ Years)

The second year of life is marked by acceleration of motor and intellectual development. The ability to walk confers on the toddler a degree of control over his own actions; this mobility enables the child to determine when to approach and when to withdraw. The acquisition of speech profoundly extends the child's horizons. Typically, the child learns to say "no" before he learns to say "yes." The toddler's negativism plays a vital part in the development of independence. If persistent, however, this oppositional behavior connotes a problem.

Table 2
Landmarks of Normal Behavioral Development*

Age	Motor and Sensory Behavior	Adaptive Behavior	Personal and Social Behavior
Birth to 4 Weeks	Hand to mouth reflex, grasping reflex, Rooting reflex (turning cheek toward touch) Moro reflex (digital extension when startled), sucking reflex, Babinski reflex (toes spread when sole of foot is touched) Differentiates sounds (orients to human voice) and sweet and sour tastes Visual tracking Fixed focal distance of 8 inches	Anticipatory feeding approach behavior at 4 days	Responsiveness to mother's face, eyes, and voice within first few hours of life Endogenous smile Independent play (until 2 years)
Under 4 weeks	Makes alternating crawling movements Moves head laterally when placed in prone position	Responds to sound of rattle and bell Regards moving objects momentarily	Quiets when picked up Impassive face
4 weeks	Tonic neck reflex positions predominate Hands fisted Head sags but can hold head erect for a few seconds Visual fixation stereoscopic vision (12 weeks)	Follows moving objects to the midline Shows no interest and drops objects immediately	Regards face and diminishes activity Responds to speech Smiles preferentially to mother
16 weeks	Symmetrical postures predominate Holds head balanced Head lifted 90 degrees when prone on forearm Visual accommodation	Follows a slowly moving object well Arms activate on sight of dangling object	Spontaneous social smile (exogenous) Aware of strange situations
28 weeks	Sits steadily, leaning forward on hands Bounces actively when placed in standing position	One-hand approach and grasp of toy Bangs and shakes rattle Transfers toys	Takes feet to mouth Pats mirror image Starts to imitate mother's sounds and actions
40 weeks	Sits alone with good coordination Creeps Pulls self to standing position Points with index finger	Matches two objects at midline Attempts to imitate scribble	Separation anxiety manifest when taken away from mother Responds to social play, such as "pat-a-cake" and "peek-a-boo" Feeds self cracker and holds own bottle
52 weeks	Walks with one hand held Stands alone briefly	Seeks novelty	Cooperates in dressing
15 months	Toddles Creeps up stairs		Points or vocalizes wants Throws objects in play or refusal
18 months	Coordinated walking, seldom falls	Builds a tower of three or four cubes	Feeds self in part, spills Pulls toy on string

Table 2 *continued*

Age	Motor and Sensory Behavior	Adaptive Behavior	Personal and Social Behavior
18 months (*continued*)	Hurls ball Walks up stairs with one hand held	Scribbles spontaneously and imitates a writing stroke	Carries or hugs a special toy, such as a doll Imitates some behavioral patterns with slight delay
2 years	Runs well, no falling Kicks large ball Goes up and down stairs alone Fine motor skills increase	Builds a tower of six or seven cubes Aligns cubes, imitating train Imitates vertical and circular strokes Develops original behaviors	Pulls on simple garment Domestic mimicry Refers to self by name Says "no" to mother Separation anxiety begins to diminish Organized demonstrations of love and protest Parallel play (plays side by side but does not interact with other children)
3 years	Rides tricycle Jumps from bottom steps Alternates feet going up stairs	Builds tower of nine or 10 cubes Imitates a three-cube bridge Copies a circle and a cross	Puts on shoes Unbuttons buttons Feeds self well Understands taking turns
4 years	Walks down stairs one step per tread Stands on one foot for 5 to 8 seconds	Copies a cross Repeats four digits Counts three objects with correct pointing	Washes and dries own face Brushes teeth Associative or joint play (plays cooperatively with other children)
5 years	Skips, using feet alternately Usually has complete sphincter control Fine coordination improves	Copies a square Draws a recognizable man with a head, body, limbs Counts 10 objects accurately	Dresses and undresses self Prints a few letters Plays competitive exercise games
6 years	Rides two-wheel bicycle	Prints name Copies triangle	Ties shoelaces

*Table adapted from Arnold Gesell, M.D., and Stella Chess, M.D.

The second year of life is a period of increasing social demands on the child. Toilet training serves as a paradigm of the general training practices of the family—that is, the mother who is overly severe in this area is likely to be punitive and restrictive in others as well.

Parallel to the changing tasks for the child are changing tasks for the parents. In infancy, the major responsibility for parents is to meet the infant's needs in a sensitive and consistent fashion, without anticipating and fulfilling all the needs so that the child never experiences tension. Some tension is desirable. The parental task at the toddler stage requires firmness about the boundaries of acceptable behavior and encouragement of the progressive emancipation of the child. Parents must be careful not to be too authoritarian at this stage. Children must be allowed to operate for themselves and be able to learn from their mistakes. And they must be protected and assisted when the challenges are beyond their abilities.

Erikson's Stage of Autonomy vs. Shame and Doubt (1 to 3 Years). As previously noted, the child in the second and third years of life learns to walk alone, to feed himself, to control the anal sphincter, and to talk. It is this muscular maturation that sets the tone for this stage of development. Autonomy refers to the child's sense of mastery over himself and over drives and impulses. The toddler gains a sense of his separateness from others. "I," "you," "me," and "mine" are common words used by the child during this period. The child has a choice of holding on or letting go, of being cooperative, or of being stubborn. The term "terrible twos" refers to the willfulness of children in this stage of development.

This period coincides with Freud's anal stage of development. For Erikson, this is the time for the child to either retain feces—holding in—or eliminate feces—letting go—both behaviors having an effect on the mother. Too rigorous toilet training, which is commonplace in our society and requires a "clean, punctual, and deodorized body," can produce an overly compulsive personality that is stingy, meticulous, and selfish. Known as anal personalities, such persons are parsimonious, punctual, and perfectionistic.

If the parents permit the child to function with some autonomy and are supportive without being overprotective, the toddler gains self-confidence and feels he can control himself and his world. But if the child either is punished for being autonomous or is overcontrolled, he feels angry and ashamed. If the parents show approval when the child

Table 3
The Development of Language

Age and Stage of Development	Mastery of Comprehension	Mastery of Expression
0–6 months	Shows startle response to loud or sudden sounds Attempts to localize sounds, turning eyes or head Appears to listen to speakers, may respond with smile Recognizes 'warning,' 'angry,' and 'friendly' voices Responds to hearing own name	Has vocalizations other than crying Has differential cries for 'hunger,' 'pain' Makes vocalizations to show 'pleasure' Plays at making sounds Babbles (repeats a series of sounds)
7–11 months *Attending to language stage*	Shows listening selectivity (voluntary control over responses to sounds) Listens to music or singing with interest Recognizes 'no,' 'hot,' his own name Looks at pictures being named for up to 1 minute Listens to speech without being distracted by other sounds	Responds to own name with vocalizations Imitates the melody of utterances Uses jargon (his own 'language') Has gestures (shakes head for no) Has exclamation ('oh-oh') Plays language games (pat-a-cake, peek-a-boo)
12–18 months *Single word stage*	Shows gross discriminations between dissimilar sounds (bell *vs.* dog *vs.* horn *vs.* mother's or father's voice) Understands basic body parts, names of common objects Acquires understanding of some new words each week Can identify simple objects (baby, ball, etc.) from a group of objects or pictures Understands up to 150 words by age 18 months	Uses single words (mean age of first word is 11 months, by age 18 months, child is using up to 20 words) 'Talks' to toys, self, or others using long patterns of jargon and occasional words Approximately 25% of utterances are intelligible All vowels articulated correctly Initial and final consonants often omitted
12–24 months *Two-word messages stage*	Responds to simple directions (Give me the ball) Responds to action commands (Come here, sit down) Understands pronouns (me, him, her, you) Begins to understand complex sentences ('When we go to the store, I'll buy you some candy')	Uses two-word utterances ('mommy sock', 'all gone', 'ball here') Imitates environmental sounds in play ('moo', 'rrmm, rrmm', etc.) Refers to self by name, begins to use pronouns Echoes two or more last words of sentences Begins to use three-word 'telegraphic' utterances (all gone ball, me go now) Utterances 26% to 50% intelligible Uses language to ask for needs
24–36 months *Grammar formation stage*	Understands smaller body parts (elbow, chin, eyebrow) Understands family name categories (grandma, baby) Understands size (the little one, big one) Understands most adjectives Understnds functions (why do we eat, why do we sleep)	Uses 'real' sentences with grammatical function words (can, will, the, a) Usually announces intentions before acting 'Conversations' with other children, usually just monologues Jargon and echolalia gradually drop from speech Increased vocabulary (up to 270 words at 2 years, 895 at 3 years) includes slang Speech 50–80% intelligible P, b, m articulated correctly Speech may show rhythmic disturbances
36–54 months *Grammar development stage*	Understands prepositions (under, behind, between) Understands many words (up to 3500 at 3 years, 5500 at 4 years)	Correct articulation of n,w,ng,h,t,d,k,g Uses language to relate incidents from the past Uses wide range of grammatical forms:

Table 3 *continued*

Age and Stage of Development	Mastery of Comprehension	Mastery of Expression
	Understands cause/effect (What do you do when you're hungry?, cold?) Understands analogies (Food is to eat, milk is to ___)	plurals, past tense, negatives, questions 'Plays' with language: rhymes, exaggerates Speech 90% intelligible, occasional errors in the ordering of sounds within words Able to define words Egocentric use of language rare Can repeat a 12-syllable sentence correctly Some grammatical errors still occur
55 months on *True communication stage*	Understands concepts of number, speed, time, space Understands left/right Understands abstract terms Is able to categorize items into semantic classes	Uses language to tell stories, share ideas, and discuss alternatives Increasing use of varied grammar; spontaneous self correction of grammatical errors Stabilizing of articulation of f,v,s,z,l,r,th, and consonant clusters Speech 100% intelligible

Reprinted with permission from Rutter M, Hersovl (eds). *Child and Adolescent Psychiatry.* **Blackwell Publications, London, 1985.**

shows self-control, self-esteen is enhanced and a sense of pride develops. Parental overcontrol or loss of self-control, also called muscular and anal impotence by Erikson, produces a sense of doubt and shame. Shame implies that one is looked down on by the outside world. It exploits the child's sense of being small as one stands upright for the first time. Feeling small, the child is easily shamed by poor parenting experiences. Too much shaming causes the child to feel evil or dirty and may pave the way for delinquent behavior. In effect, the child is saying, "If that's what they think of me, that's the way I'll behave."

Sexual Development. The forerunners of sexual differentiation are evident from birth, when parents start dressing and treating infants differently due to the expectations evoked by sex typing. Through imitation, reward, and coercion, the child assumes the behaviors that the culture defines as appropriate for its sexual role. The child exhibits curiosity about anatomical sex. If this curiosity is recognized as healthy and is met with honest and age-appropriate replies, the child acquires a sense of the wonder of life and is comfortable with his own role in it. If the subject of sex is taboo and the child's questions are rebuffed, shame and discomfort result. By the age of 2½ years, the child develops a sense of gender identity—that is, whether he is a boy or a girl. In general, play is determined by gender; boys play with guns, and girls play with dolls and doll houses.

At this stage, children are likely to struggle for the exclusive affection and attention of their parents. This struggle includes rivalry both with siblings and with one or another parent for the star role in the family. Although children are beginning to be able to share, they do so with reluctance. If the demands for exclusive possession are not effectively resolved, the result is likely to be jealous competitiveness in relations with peers and lovers. The fantasies aroused by the struggle lead to fear of retaliation and displacement of fear onto external objects. In an equitable, loving family, the child elaborates a moral system of ethical

Table 4
Overview of Piaget's Sensorimotor Period of Cognitive Development

Age	Characteristics
1. Birth–2 months	Uses inborn motor and sensory reflexes (sucking, grasping, looking) to interact and accommodate to the external world
2. 2–5 months	Primary circular reaction—coordinates activities of own body and five senses (e.g., sucking thumb), reality remains subjective—does not seek stimuli outside of its visual field; displays curiosity
3. 5–9 months	Secondary circular reaction—seeks out new stimuli in the environment; starts both to anticipate consequences of own behavior and to act purposefully to change the environment; beginning of intentional behavior
4. 9 months–1 year	Shows preliminary signs of object permanence; has a vague concept that objects exist apart from itself; plays peek-a-boo; imitates novel behaviors
5. 1 year–18 months	Tertiary circular reaction—seeks out new experiences; produces novel behaviors
6. 18 months–2 years	Symbolic thought—uses symbolic representations of events and objects; shows signs of reasoning (e.g., uses one toy to reach for and get another); attains object permanence

Table adapted from Ginsburg H P: Jean Piaget. In *Comprehensive Textbook of Psychiatry,* **ed 4, H I Kaplan and B J Sadock, editors, p 179. Williams & Wilkins, Baltimore, 1985.**

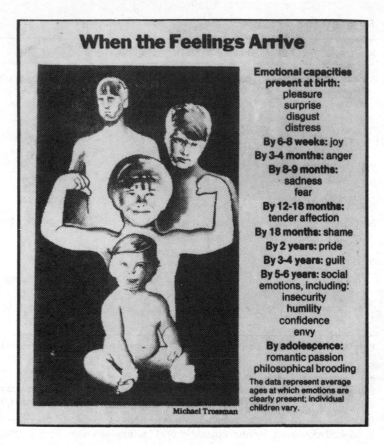

Figure 1. Emotional development from infancy through adolescence. From Joseph Campas at the University of Denver, and other researchers. Used with permission of the New York Times Company, 1984.

rights. Parents need to set realistic limits on the toddler's behavior, balancing between punishment and permissiveness. According to Piaget, the toddler period spans the sensorimotor and preoperational stages of development. At approximately age 2½, the toddler enters the preschool years and leaves babyhood for childhood.

Preschool Child (2½ to 6 Years)

This period is characterized by marked physical and emotional growth. Somewhere between 2 and 3 years of age, children reach half of their adult height. The 20 baby teeth are in place at the beginning of this stage, and by the end, they begin to fall out.

The child relates to others in new ways. The birth of a sibling (a common occurrence during this period) tests the preschool child's capacity for further cooperation and sharing. It also may evoke sibling rivalry, which is most likely to occur at this time. Sibling rivalry is dependent on child-rearing practices. Favoritism, for any reason, is a common outcome of such rivalry. Children who get special treatment because they are either gifted, defective in some way, or of a preferred gender are likely to be the recipient of angry feelings from siblings. The experience with siblings may influence the growing child's relationships with peers and authority. If, for example, the needs of the new baby prevent the mother from attending to the firstborn child's needs, a problem may result. If not handled properly, the displacement of the firstborn can be a traumatic event.

Play and Social Behavior. In the preschool years, the child begins to distinguish reality from fantasy, and play reflects this growing awareness. Games of "let's pretend" are popular and help test real life situations in a playful manner. Dramatic play in which the child acts out a role such as that of a housewife or truck driver is common. One-to-one play relationships advance to more complicated patterns with rivalries, secrets, and two-against-one intrigues. A child's play behavior reflects his level of social development.

Between 3 and 6 years of age, growth can be traced through drawings. The first drawing of a person is a circular line with marks for mouth, nose, and eyes; ears and hair are added later; next, arms and sticklike fingers appear; then legs. The last to appear is a torso in proportion to the rest of the body. The intelligent child is able to deal with greater detail. Drawings express creativity throughout the child's development. They are representational and formal in early childhood, make use of perspective in middle childhood, and become abstract and affect-laden in adolescence. Drawings also reflect a person's body image concepts as well as sexual and aggressive impulses.

Imaginary companions. Imaginary companions most often appear during the preschool years, usually in the form of persons. Imaginary companions may also be things such as toys that are anthropomorphized. Some studies indicate that up to 50 percent of children between the ages of 3 and 10 years have imaginary companions at one time or another. Their significance is not clear but they are usually friendly, relieve loneliness, and reduce anxiety in the child. In most instances, imaginary companions disappear by age 12, but they may occasionally persist into adulthood.

School

The term "preschool" for the age group of 2½ to 6 years may be a misnomer because many of these children are in preschool nurseries. Many working mothers must place their children in such nurseries or in day care centers. Preschool education can be of value; however, too great a stress on academic advancement beyond the capabilities of the child can be counterproductive.

For Piaget, this is the preoperational phase (more specifically 2 to 7 years), during which time children begin to think symbolically. In general, however, their thinking is egocentric, as in the sensorimotor period; they cannot place themselves in the position of another child and are incapable of empathy. Preoperational thought also is intuitive and prelogical; children in this stage do not understand cause-effect relationships.

Children between ages 3 and 6 years are very aware of the genitalia and of the differences between the sexes. In their play, doctor-nurse games allow children to act out their sexual fantasies. Their awareness of their bodies extends beyond the genitalia. There is a preoccupation with illness or injury, so much so that this period has been called the "Band-Aid" phase; every injury needs to be examined and taken care of by a parent.

Freud described children during this phase as being in the phallic stage of development; infancy represented the oral phase and toddlerhood, the anal stage. During this phase, pleasure is connected with the genital area. It is the time of the Oedipus complex, when children have sexual impulses toward the opposite-sex parent and want to eliminate the same-sex parent, wishes for which punishment is expected. The punishment feared by boys is castration. Castration anxiety leads the boy to give up his mother as a love object, to repress his impulses toward her, to identify with his father, and in the process to form a superego. The Electra complex holds that the girl wishes to have exclusive love of her father and to replace her mother; the daughter resolves this conflict by identifying with her mother. Lack of a penis is considered evidence of castration. Freud believed that girls develop penis envy as a result and want to possess their father in order to obtain his penis. The little girl's urge to marry the father and have a baby therefore represented the desire for a penis.

Erikson's Stage of Initiative vs. Guilt (3 to 5 Years). As children approach the end of the third year, they are able to initiate both motor and intellectual activity. Whether this initiative is reinforced depends on how much physical freedom children are given and how well their intellectual curiosity is satisfied. If toddlers are made to feel inadequate about their behavior or interests, they may emerge from this period with a sense of guilt about self-initiated activity. Conflicts over initiative can prevent developing children from experiencing their full potential and can interfere with their sense of ambition which develops during this stage.

During this period, the child's growing sense of sexual curiosity is manifested by engaging in group sex play or touching one's own genitalia or those of a peer. If not made an issue by the parents (Erikson gives the example, "If you touch it, the doctor will cut it off."), these childhood impulses are eventually repressed and reappear during adolescence as part of puberty. If too much is made of these impulses by the parent, the child may become sexually inhibited.

The child is able to move independently and vigorously by the end of this stage. By playing with peers, the child learns how to interact with others. If aggressive fantasies have been managed properly (neither punished nor encouraged) the child develops a sense of initiative and ambition.

At the end of this stage of initiative versus guilt, the child's conscience (Freud's superego) becomes established. The child learns not only that there are limits to one's behavioral repertoire (for example, that a boy cannot sleep with his mother or murder his father), but that aggressive impulses can be expressed in constructive ways such as healthy competition, playing games, and using toys—even toy weapons. The development of conscience sets the tone for the moral sense of right and wrong. Excessive punishment, however, can restrict the child's imagination and initiative. The child who develops too strong a superego, with an all-or-nothing quality, may insist as an adult that other persons adhere to his moral code and therefore may become a "great potential danger to himself and to his fellow men." If the crisis of initiative is successfully resolved, a sense of responsibility, dependability, and self discipline develops in the personality.

The Middle Years (6 to 12 Years)

During this period, the child enters kindergarten and elementary school. The formal demands for academic learning and accomplishment become major determinants of further personality development. This is the stage that Freud called the latency period. The Oedipus complex should be resolved, the child having relatively good control over instinctual drives. Successful resolution of the Oedipus complex accounts for superego development. When the superego is formed, the child is able to make moral judgments and to understand society's expectations. Moreover, the child is able to deal with the emotional and intellectual demands that are being placed on him by the environment, particularly in the school.

The girl has identified with her mother. Instead of wanting the father as a love object, the daughter now directs her energy toward wanting somebody like him. It is still culturally acceptable, however, for the girl to remain attached to the father during latency, although not with the same degree of emotional intensity.

In latency, girls as well as boys make new identifications with other adults such as teachers and counselors. These identifications may so influence the girl that her goals of wanting to marry and have babies as her mother did may be combined with a desire for a career, postponed, or abandoned entirely.

Some girls in latency act as if they are still in the oedipal stage. A girl who is unable to identify with the mother or whose father is overly attached, may become fixated at a 6-year-old level and as a result, may fear men, women, or both, or become seductively close to them. In either case, she will not be seen as normal during these school-age years. A similar situation may occur in the boy who enters latency without having resolved his Oedipus complex. The child may have been unable to identify successfully with his father because the father was aloof, brutal, or absent. Perhaps, the mother prevented the boy from identifying with his father by being over-protective or by binding the son too closely to herself. As a result, the child may enter latency with a variety of problems. The male child may be fearful of men, unsure of his sense of masculinity, unwilling to leave the mother (which may be manifested by a school phobia), or he may lack initiative and be unable to master school tasks, which then present as academic problems.

School Refusal. In some children, the refusal to go to school usually occurs at this time, generally as a result of separation anxiety. A fearful mother may transmit her own fear of separation to the child, or a child who has not resolved his dependency needs panics at the idea of separation. School refusal usually is not an isolated problem; such children typically avoid many other social situations.

The school-age period is a time in which peer interaction assumes major importance. Interest in relationships outside the family take precedence over those within the family. A special relationship exists, however, with the same-sex parent, with whom the child identifies and who is now a role model. At this time, the child idealizes the same-sex parent and wants to be like that parent.

Empathy and a concern for others begin to emerge early in this stage, so by the time the child is 9 or 10, he has well developed capacities for love, compassion, and sharing. Although sexual feelings are repressed, emotions regarding sexual differences begin to emerge as either excitement or shyness with the opposite sex. The school-age child prefers to interact with children of the same sex. This period has been referred to as a psychosexual and psychosocial moratorium, or latency period—a lull between the preschool child's oedipal strivings and the adolescent's pubescent sexual impulses. The moratorium is characterized by an absence of overt sexual behavior which, according to Freud, is sublimated and expressed in other abilities such as sports, studies, and nonsexual peer activities.

Physical and Cognitive Development. Improved gross motor coordination and greater muscle strength enable the child to write with fluency and draw more artistically. The child is also capable of complex motor tasks and activities such as tennis, gymnastics, golf, baseball, and skateboarding. Language is used to express complex ideas with relationships among a number of elements. There is a tendency for logical exploration to dominate fantasy and an increased capacity for self-regulation.

From Piaget's perspective, this phase is the stage of concrete operations, during which a child's conceptual skills develop, and thinking becomes more organized and logical. Toward the end of this period, the child begins to think in more abstract terms.

Erikson's Stage of Industry vs. Inferiority (6 to 11 Years). Erikson's fourth stage is the school-age period, during which the child begins to participate in an organized program of learning. In all cultures, children receive formal instruction at about the age of 6; in Western culture, the child learns to be literate and technical. In other societies, learning may involve becoming familiar with tools and weapons.

Industry, the ability to work and to acquire adult skills, is the keynote of the stage. The child learns that he is able to make things and, most important, able to master and complete a task. If too great an emphasis is placed on rules, regulations, "shoulds or oughts," the child will develop a sense of duty at the expense of a natural desire to work. The productive child learns the pleasure of work completion and the pride of doing something well.

A sense of inadequacy and inferiority, the potential negative outcome of this stage, results from several sources: The child may be discriminated against at school; the child may be told he is inferior; the child may be overprotected at home or excessively dependent on the emotional support of the family; or the male child may compare himself unfavorably to his father. Good teachers and good parents who encourage their children to value diligence, productivity, and to persevere in a difficult enterprise are bulwarks against a sense of inferiority.

To Erikson, this stage is socially decisive because the child learns how to work with others and develops a sense of division of labor and equality of opportunity. It is equivalent to Freud's latency period because biological drives are dormant and peer interaction prevails.

OTHER ISSUES IN CHILDHOOD

Dreams and Sleep

Dreams in children can have a profound effect on behavior. During the child's first year of life, when the differentiation between reality and fantasy has not yet been fully achieved, the dream may be experienced as if it were or could be true. The child has strong reactions to dreams; they are either viewed with pleasure or, as is most often reported, with fear. The dream content is to be seen in connection with the life experience of the child, the developmental stage, the mechanisms used during dreaming, and the child's sex.

Disturbing dreams peak when the child is 3, 6, and 10 years old. The 2-year-old child may dream about being bitten or chased; at the age of 4, there are many animal dreams, and people are introduced who either protect or destroy. At age 5 or 6, dreams of being killed or injured, of flying and being in cars, and of ghosts become more prominent, exposing the role of conscience, of moral values, and of increasing conflicts around these themes. In early childhood, aggressive dreams rarely seem to occur; instead, it is the dreamer who is in danger, which may reflect the child's dependent position. By about the age of 5, children realize that their dreams are not real, and by age 7, they know that dreams are created by themselves.

At certain periods, a child wakes from sleep disturbed by the content of the dream and extremely frightened; the child is unwilling to return to sleep unless comforted by a parent. *Pavor nocturnus* (night-terrors) is a severe form of fright in which the content of the dream overwhelms reality so that the child remains frightened by the dream for an extended period of time. During night-terrors, the child remains in an in-between state from which he cannot be fully aroused. The child does not appear to recognize the people in his room, and even though the child's eyes are open, the dream seems to continue.

Between the ages of 3 and 6 years, it is normal for a child to want to keep the bedroom door open or a light burning, so that he can either maintain contact with his parents or view the room in a more realistic and less fearful way. At times, the child resists going to sleep in order to avoid dreaming. Disorders associated with falling asleep, therefore, are often connected with the dream experience. Rituals are set up as protective devices designed to make safer the withdrawal from the world of reality into the world of sleep.

Somnambulism, or sleep walking, may occur. Very often, the content of the dream seems to release motor discharge, and the child goes to those persons and places that can offer him protection.

Periods of rapid eye movements (REM) take place about 60 percent of the time during the first few weeks of life, during which the infant sleeps two thirds of the time. Premature babies spend even more time asleep. The sleep-wake cycle of newborns is about three hours long. The dream-to-sleep ratio is quite stable among adults: 20 percent of sleeping time is spent dreaming. Even in newborns, there is brain activity similar to that of the dreaming state. It is doubtful, however, that dreaming is possible before speech—that is, before the existence of mental representations of the outside world.

Effects of Divorce on Children

Children living in homes in which divorce has occurred is commonplace. Over 20 percent of all children in America live in homes in which one parent (usually the mother) is the sole head of household. Forty-five percent of all children born in any given year can expect to live with only one parent before they reach the age of 18 years. The age of the child at the time of divorce affects the reaction to divorce. Immediately after the divorce, there is an increase in behavioral and emotional disorders in all age groups. Three- to 6-year-old children do not understand what is actually happening, and those that do often assume that they are responsible for the divorce in some way. If divorce occurs when the child is between 7 and 12 years, school performance generally declines. Older children, especially adolescents, comprehend the situation and believe that they could have prevented the divorce had they intervened in some way—in effect, serving as a surrogate marriage therapist—but they are still hurt, angry, and critical of the parents' behavior. Some children harbor the fantasy that the parents will be reunited at some future date. Such children show animosity toward a parent's real or potential new mate because they are forced to recognize that a reconciliation will not take place. Recovery and adaptation from the effects of divorce usually takes 3 to 5 years, but about a third of children from divorced homes have lasting psychological trauma. Among boys, physical aggression is a common sign of distress. Adolescents tend to spend more time away from the parental home after divorce. Suicide attempts may occur as a direct result of the divorce; one of the predictors of suicide in adolescence is the recent divorce or separation of the parents. Children who adapt well to divorce do so if each parent makes an effort to continue to relate to the child in spite of the child's anger. To facilitate this recovery, the divorced couple also must avoid arguing with one another and demonstrate consistent behavior toward the child.

Stepparents. When remarriage occurs, the child must learn to adapt to the stepparent. That adaptation is usually difficult, especially if the stepparent is nonsupportive or resentful of the stepchild or favors his or her own natural children. A natural child born to the new mother or father—a stepsibling—sometimes receives more attention than a stepchild and, as a result, is the object of sibling rivalry.

Adoption. Adoption is defined as the process by which a child is taken into a family by one or more adults who are not the biological parents but are recognized by law as the child's parents. In 1981, it was estimated that approximately 2.5 million persons under the age of 18 years were adopted. Fifty-two percent of the children were adopted by persons not related to them by birth or marriage, and the remainder were adopted by relatives or stepparents. The majority of adopted children were born out of wedlock, and 40 percent of all such children were born to mothers aged 15 to 19 years.

Most children are told they are adopted between the ages of 2 to 4 years, to avoid the possibility of the child learning about his adoptive status from extrafamilial sources, which might leave him feeling betrayed by the adoptive parents and abandoned by the biological parents.

Emotional and behavior disorders have been reported to be higher among adopted children than nonadopted children; aggressive behavior, stealing, and learning disturbances are higher among adopted children as well. The later the age of adoption, the higher the incidence and more severe the degree of behavior problems.

Throughout childhood and adolescence, children may be preoccupied with fantasies of two sets of parents. The adopted child may split the two sets of parents into "good" parents and "bad" parents. There is usually a strong desire to know the biological parents, and some children pattern themselves after their fantasies of their absent biological parents, creating a conflict with their adoptive parents.

References

Brodzinsky D M, Schechter D, editors: *The Psychology of Adoption*. Oxford University Press, New York, 1988

Brodzinsky D M, Schechter D, Brodzinsky A M: Children's knowledge of adoption. Developmental change and implications for adjustment. In *Thinking About the Family: View of Parents and Children*, R Ashmore, D. Brodzinsky, editors. Erlbaum, Hillsdale, NJ, 1986.

Call J D, editor: Normal development. In *Basic Handbook of Child Psychiatry*, J D Noshpitz, editor, vol. 1. Basic Books, New York, 1979.

Call J D, Galenson, E, Tyson, R L, editors: *Frontiers of Infant Psychiatry*, vol I, II. Basic Books, New York, 1983, 1984.

Erikson E H: *Childhood And Society*, ed 2, W W Norton, New York, 1963.

Fraiberg S H: *The Magic Years—Understanding and Handling the Problems of Early Childhood*. Scribners, New York, 1959.

Greenspan S I, Greenspan, N T: *First Feelings—The Emotional Care of Infants and Young Children*. Viking Press, New York, 1985.

Gruber H E, Voneche J J: *The Essential Piaget*. Basic Books, New York, 1977.

Lewis M: *Clinical Aspects of Child Development*, ed 2, p. 3. Lea & Febiger, Philadelphia, 1982.

Lidz T: *The Person—His and Her Development Throughout the Life Cycle*, p 79. Basic Books, New York, 1976.

Mahler, M S, Pine, F, Bergman, A: *The Psychological Birth of the Human Infant*. Basic Books, New York, 1975.

Needle R: Interpersonal influences in adolescent drug use . . . the role of older siblings, parents, and peers. Internat J Addict 21(7):739, 1986.

3.3

Adolescence

INTRODUCTION

Adolescence is a period of variable onset and duration that marks the end of childhood and lays the foundation for maturity. Development occurs on three levels—biological, psychological, and social, all of which are significantly interrelated. Biologically, onset is signaled by the final acceleration of skeletal growth and the beginnings of sexual development; psychologically, onset is characterized by an acceleration of cognitive growth and personality formation; socially, it is a period of intensified preparation for the forthcoming role of young adulthood. Indeed, the end of this period occurs when the adolescent is accorded full adult prerogatives, the timing and amount of which vary among societies. In the United States, the long period of study required for specialized occupational roles delays for many the age of self-support, the opportunity for marriage, and the age of creative contribution to society—all attributes of the adult role.

In many cultures, the onset of adolescence is clearly signaled by puberty rites, usually by having the adolescent perform feats of strength and courage. In technologically advanced societies, however, the end of childhood and the requirements for adulthood are not clearly defined. In such circumstances the adolescent undergoes a more prolonged and, at times, confused struggle to attain independent adult status.

It is useful to distinguish between puberty, which is a physical process of change characterized by the development of secondary sex characteristics, and adolescence, which is a psychological process of change. Under ideal circumstances, the processes are synchronized. When puberty and adolescence do not occur simultaneously, the adolescent has to cope with added stresses.

Adolescence can be divided into three stages—early, middle, and late. The age divisions of each phase are somewhat arbitrary, and the stages often overlap.

EARLY ADOLESCENCE (11 TO 14 YEARS)

The biological changes of puberty are initiated and controlled by complex interactions between the gonadal and adrenal systems and the hypothalamic-pituitary axis. The activity of hormones produces the clinical manifestations of puberty, which are traditionally categorized as primary and secondary sex characteristics. The primary characteristics are those directly involved in coitus and reproduction, the reproductive organs and the external genitalia. The secondary characteristics include breast development and hip enlargement in females and facial hair growth and change of voice pitch in males. In both sexes, most adult levels of hormones are achieved by the age of 16; but, girls begin puberty at an average age of 11 and boys, at age 13. The characteristic increase in height and weight also occurs earlier in girls than in boys, so that by age 12, girls are both taller and heavier than boys.

Precocious or delayed growth, acne, obesity, enlarged mammary glands in boys, and inadequate or overabundant breast development in girls are some examples of deviations from the expected patterns of maturation. Although they may be without medical significance, they often lead to psychological damage. At this period, adolescents are extremely sensitive to the opinions of peers and are constantly comparing themselves to others. Any deviation, real or imagined, can lead to feelings of inferiority, low self-esteem, and loss of confidence.

Because girls enter puberty 2 years earlier than boys, they may begin dating and having sexual intercourse at an earlier time. Each year, teenagers obtain 300,000 legal abortions and give birth to about 600,000 babies. In certain subcultures, teenagers view pregnancy as a rite of passage into adulthood. The girl who is depressed, insecure about her attractiveness, or the product of a divorced or otherwise conflicted home is more likely to become pregnant than the adolescent from a more stable background.

Freud referred to adolescence as the period of genitality in which the libido or sexual energy, which has remained latent during the preadolescent years, is revived. The sex drive is triggered by certain androgens such as testosterone, that are at higher levels during adolescence than at any other time of life. According to Masters and Johnson, the peak of the male sex drive occurs between 17 and 18 years of age. The early adolescent vents his libidinal urges most often through masturbation, a safe way to satisfy sexual impulses.

The early adolescent is still attached to the family, and there is sometimes a resurgence of oedipal feelings and even sexual fantasies toward the opposite-sex parent. In general, these thoughts and feelings are repressed and the adolescent's sexuality is directed outward; crushes, hero-worship, and idealization of movie and music stars are characteristic of this stage.

The school experience also accelerates and intensifies the degree of separation from the family. More and more, the adolescent exists in a world that the parents are unfamiliar with and do not share. Home is only a base. The real world is the school, and the most important relationships are with those persons of similar ages and interests.

Adolescent Culture

The peer group—its membership constantly shifting, its roles never formally defined—is a vital agency for social growth and change. Here, for the first time, the adolescent forms significant relationships that lack the familiarity and security of those with parents and siblings. The peer group represents challenge and opportunity to a powerful degree. Where do the adolescents fit in? What roles can they play? To what degree will they be accepted or rejected? What changes need to take place? What changes can take place? These are all critical questions, and their importance is played out in the shifting relationships of peer group society.

The peer group is an informal institution, different for each adolescent. For most adolescents, there is a core made up of a small number of sustained and emotionally significant friendships; radiating out from that core are numbers of less well-defined contacts with persons who may come and go and who are of greater or lesser importance in the adolescent's life. Sometimes, the peer group has a more defined nature—the gang, the athletic team, the social club—but more often, it is only a loose confederation held together by shared interests and the strength of friendship pairings. With distinctive jokes and phrases and unique ways of dressing and thinking, the peer group is an anticipation of the experience of individual identity that lies ahead. For the time being, however, there is the safety in numbers and the protection that the group affords its members.

Inherent in the nature of the peer group is the capacity for great social pressure carried out in a context of basic acceptance and support. This social pressure is a powerful force that does much to shape adolescent character and values. The demand for conformity to the group ideal is extreme.

According to Piaget, the child's thinking at the beginning of adolescence becomes more abstract, conceptual, logical, and future oriented. The child is entering the age of formal operations, which comes to fruition during adolescence. With the ability for formal thought and abstract reasoning, the adolescent discovers new facts, experiences, and feelings. Many adolescents are stimulated by this awakening and show remarkable creativity.

Some may write poetry, possibly for the only time in their lives. Others may find expression in writing, music, art, or other forms of creativity. Often brilliant and talented young people lose this excitement and creativity by adulthood. Creativity may also manifest itself in such areas as gymnastic or athletic ability, abstract mathematics, philosophy, debating, or journalism. As with other expressions, these avenues of creativity may disappear with the end of adolescence. In some instances, the unusual ability may be more precocity than talent; that is, such adolescents perform in an amazingly competent fashion at a much earlier age than their peers. This creativity may no longer appear outstanding, however, when their peers finally catch up.

MIDDLE ADOLESCENCE (14 TO 17 YEARS)

Two major biological events occur during this period. Boys finally catch up to and surpass girls in height and weight, and menarche (the onset of menstruation) has taken place in the majority of girls. Consequently, issues of sexuality, body image, pregnancy, male and female stereotypic roles, popularity, and identity are among the myriad and often overwhelming preoccupations and concerns of the adolescent during this stage.

In middle adolescence, sexual behavior and experimentation with a variety of sexual roles are common. Heterosexual crushes, often with an unattainable person of the same or older age, are common. Homosexual experiences may also occur at this time but are usually transient. Many adolescents need reassurance about the normality of an isolated homosexual experience and confirmation that it is not an indication of a permanent homosexual orientation.

While many adolescents experiment with sex at an early age, recent surveys indicate that the average age for first sexual intercourse in both sexes is 16 years. There is a trend in this society toward greater and more frequent sexual activity at earlier ages. A decade ago, for example, the average age for first sexual intercourse was eighteen, and only 55 percent of females had had sexual intercourse by that time. Currently, 80 percent of males and 70 percent of females have engaged in coitus by age 19.

LATE ADOLESCENCE (17 TO 20 YEARS)

The major cognitive event of adolescence is the development of the capacity for abstract logical thought, which Piaget called formal operations. It begins in early adolescence at age 11 or 12 and reaches its peak by late adolescence, when one is able to make deductions—to take separate facts and bits of data and derive general concepts from them. Thinking is no longer limited to the immediate, concrete environment, but is concerned with the larger world.

Piaget understood intelligence to result from the interaction between the growing organism and the changing environment. By late adolescence, the neural structure of the adolescent is complete, and a person constantly accommodates to the changing environment, not only of things, but of ideas. Consequently, the adolescent is concerned with humanitarian issues, morals, ethics, religion, judgment, and world issues. The potential for formal operational thought is limitless in terms of a person's ability to understand the world and one's place in it, but only a few reach their full potential. Most adolescents and adults function somewhere between the concrete and the formal operational stage. In general, those adolescents who go on to college are stimulated to function on a formal operational level; whereas, those who enter the work force after high school are less likely to have a need for the abstract conceptualization of that type of thinking.

For most people, developing a well defined sense of morality is a major accomplishment of late adolescence and adulthood. Morality is defined as conformity to shared standards, rights, and duties. There is, however, the possibility of conflict between two socially accepted standards, and the person learns to make judgments based on an individualized sense of conscience. There is a moral obligation to abide by established norms, but only to the degree that they serve human ends. This stage of development internalizes ethical principles and the control of conduct.

Resolution of Dependency and Identity

The psychosocial process of adolescence is often conceptualized in terms of the need to address two major tasks: (1) moving from a dependent to an independent person and (2) establishing an identity. Both tasks are dealt with during adolescence but extend into adulthood and must be reworked throughout the life cycle.

Dependency to Independence. A major task of adolescence is to move from being a dependent to an independent person. The initial struggles often revolve around the established concepts of sex roles and identification. Old techniques that the child used earlier to master separation may return.

Negativism reappears. "No, I can do it myself. Don't tell me how long my hair can be. Don't tell me how short my skirt can be." This negativism is a renewed attempt to tell first parents and then the world that these growing persons have minds of their own. Again, negativism becomes an active verbal way of expressing anger. Adolescents may seize almost any issue to show that they have a mind separate from that of their parents. Parents and adolescents may argue about the choice of friends, peer groups, school plans and courses, or points of philosophy and etiquette. Members of each generation recall how clothes, hairstyles, and other external badges—the more shocking the better—were used to show parents that their children now had minds of their own.

Slowly, adolescents begin to blend many different values from all kinds of sources into their own existing values. By young adulthood, a new conscience or superego is established. The compatibility and flexibility of this new superego strengthen one's ability to handle and express feelings and emotions in relationships. All through life, one's superego has to be able to change and grow in order to accommodate new life situations.

As adolescents begin to feel independent of their families and as the families support and encourage this emerging maturity, the question of the 3- to 6-year-old is heard once again: "Who am I?"

Erikson's Stage of Identity vs. Role Diffusion (11 to 20 Years). Developing a sense of identity is the main task of this period, which coincides with puberty and adolescence. Identity is defined as the person knowing who he is and where he is going. Healthy identity is built on the individual's success in passing through the first three psychosocial stages and identifying with either healthy parents or parent surrogates.

Identity implies a sense of inner solidarity with the ideas and values of a social group. The adolescent is in a psychosocial moratorium between childhood and adulthood during which various roles are tested. The individual may make several false starts before deciding on an occupation or may drop out of school to return at a later date to complete a course of study. Moral values may change, but eventually an ethical system is consoliated into a coherent organizational framework.

An identity crisis occurs at the end of adolescence. Erikson calls this a normative crisis because it is a normal event. But failure to negotiate this stage is abnormal and leaves the adolescent without a solid identity. The person suffers from identity diffusion or role confusion, characterized by not having a sense of self and of being confused about one's place in the world. Role confusion may manifest itself by behavioral abnormalities such as running away, criminality, or overt psychosis. The adolescent may defend against role diffusion by joining cliques, cults, or identifying with folk heroes.

Occupational Choice. Occupational choice stems from the question, "Where am I going?" Both men and women need to feel independent, autonomous, and content with their vocational choice. The adolescent is beleaguered by peers, parents, teachers, counselors, as well as subconscious forces in attempting to decide on a vocation. Whether or not opportunities exist for further schooling certainly plays a role in the decision. Extended schooling delays entrance into the adult world. In a recent survey of college graduates, 30 percent went on to some type of postcollege graduate education. Those adolescents who are unable to continue schooling are severely hampered in establishing a satisfactory vocational identity. Many are fated for lives of economic and emotional depression.

The psychological basis for a sense of individual worth as an adult rests on the acquisition of competence during adolescence. A sense of competence is acquired by experiencing success in a task that our society views as important. The sustained motivation necessary for mastering a difficult work role is possible only when there is a real likelihood of fulfilling that role in adult life and of having it respected by others.

References

Adelson J B: The mystique of adolescence. In *Childhood Psychopathology,* S I Harrison, J F McDermott, editors, p. 214. International Universities Press, New York, 1972.

Blos P: *On Adolescence—A Psychoanalytic Interpretation.* Free Press, New York, 1962.

Coles, R: *Erik Erikson—The Growth of His Work.* Little, Brown & Co, Boston, 1970.

Freud, A: *Adolescence.* Psychoanalytic Study Child, *13*:255, 1958.

GAP: *Normal Adolescence,* no. 68. Group for the Advancement of Psychiatry, New York, 1968.

Lidz, T: *The Person—His and Her Development Throughout the Life Cycle,* p 306. Basic Books, New York, 1976.

Mussen, P H, Conger J J, Kagan, J, et al.: Adolescence. In *Essentials of Child Development and Personality.* Harper & Row, New York, 1984.

Newcomb, M D: *Life Change Events Among Adolescents.* J. Nervous Mental Dis 175:280, 1986.

Offer D, Ostrov E, Howard K I: *The Mental Health Professional Concept of Normal Adolescents.* Arch Gen Psychiatry *38*:149, 1981.

Sarnoff C A: *Latency.* Aronson, New York, 1976.

3.4 _____
Adulthood

INTRODUCTION

Adulthood may be divided into three major periods: young or early adulthood, middle adulthood, and late adulthood or old age. Much of psychiatry is concerned with phenomena that occur during adulthood—marriage, child rearing, work, divorce, illness, and other stresses. Adulthood is a time of great change, sometimes dramatic, at other times subtle, but continuous. The individual must be capable of adapting to the ever-changing demands that this longest part of the life cycle requires.

Various workers concentrated on studying the phases of adulthood in addition to earlier developmental periods. Carl Jung referred to age 40 as the noon of life and believed that adulthood needed to be understood with the same precision as the early stages of life. Erik Erikson described three tasks to be mastered during adulthood—intimacy, generativity, and integrity.

EARLY ADULTHOOD (END OF ADOLESCENCE TO 40 YEARS)

Early adulthood is characterized by the peaking of biological development, the assumption of major social roles, and the evolution of an adult self and life structure. During late adolescence, the young person leaves home and functions more independently. Relationships with the opposite sex become more serious, and the quest for intimacy begins. This transitional period into early adulthood involves a variety of important events: high school graduation, entry into college, and leaving home. The twenties are spent, for the most part, exploring options for occupation, marriage, or alternative relationships, and making commitments in various areas. The choices made in the late teens and early twenties, however, are tentative at best; the young adult may make several false starts before a lasting commitment is reached.

Occupation

Social class, gender, and race affect the pursuit and development of a particular occupational choice. Blue-collar workers generally enter the work force directly from high school; white-collar workers and professionals usually enter the work force after college or professional school.

Women often exhibit one of two patterns in their twenties: Work for pay is the central component of their life structure, family being absent or secondary, or marriage and family is primary and career absent or secondary. Housewives and mothers face particular problems if they decide to work. These women are expected to continue to take care of child rearing and housework, maintain the marital relationship, and at the same time deal with the demands of a career. In general, men are still not expected to "juggle" the roles of husband, father, and worker. Some changes are occurring in these gender expectations, but they are not sufficient to upset the stereotype of the working woman having to be Supermom and Superwife at the same time.

Ninety percent of all females have to work to support themselves. Economic necessity as well as personal desire now prompt the homemaker to enter the labor force, which may not have been a consideration in the past. Dual-career families, in which both the husband and wife have jobs, constitute more than 50 percent of all families. When employers do not recognize family-oriented needs such as flexible working hours, negotiable leaves, and shared or part-time jobs, they contribute to family stress.

Members of racial minorities are frequently burdened with lower class status that limits their opportunities for rewarding and satisfying work. They frequently begin their twenties with hopes of becoming successful, but are often disappointed in this endeavor later in life.

A healthy adaptation to work provides an outlet for creativity, satisfactory relationships with colleagues, pride in accomplishment, and increased self-esteem. Job satisfaction is not wholly dependent on money. In contrast, maladaptation can lead to dissatisfaction with oneself and with the job, insecurity, decreased self-esteem, anger, and resentment at having to work. Symptoms of job dissatisfaction are a high rate of job changes, absenteeism, mistakes at work, accident proneness, and even sabotage.

Unemployment. The effects of unemployment transcend those of loss of income; the psychological and physical tolls are enormous. The incidence of alcoholism, homicide, violence, suicide, and mental illness rises with unemployment. The person's core identity, which is so often tied to occupation and work, is seriously damaged when a job is lost, be it through firing, attrition, or early or regular retirement.

Erikson's Stage of Intimacy vs. Self-Absorption or Isolation (20 to 40 Years)

Classical psychoanalysis, with its emphasis on the early years of human development, was not overly concerned with this period, which extends from late adolescence through early middle age. Erikson pointed out that an important psychosocial conflict can arise during this stage and that, as in previous stages, success or failure depends on how well the groundwork has been laid in earlier periods and on how the young adult interacts with the environment. The intimacy of sexual relations, friendships, and all deep associations are not frightening to the individual with a resolved identity crisis. In contrast, the person who reaches the adult years in a state of continued role confusion is unable to become involved in intense and long-term relationships. Without a friend or a partner in marriage, this person may become self-absorbed and self-indulgent; if so, a sense of isolation may grow to dangerous proportions.

In true intimacy, there is mutuality. This word is reminiscent of the first stage of life. If a child achieves initiative in genitality, the sensual pleasure of childhood merges with the idea of genital orgasm, and the young adult is able to make and share love with another person. Through the crisis of intimacy versus isolation, a person transcends the exclusivity of earlier dependencies and establishes a mutuality with an extended and more diverse social group.

Marriage and Commitment

Most Americans marry in their mid-twenties; however, the marriage rate is going down, and an increasing number of marriages in the United States end in divorce. Most of these divorced persons marry again, which indicates that the marital unit still provides the means for sustained intimacy, perpetuating the culture, and gratifying interpersonal needs.

At about age 30 young adults are likely to feel a need to take life more seriously. Many young adults ask themselves at this time whether the life they have is the one they really want. This period of reappraisal is called the "age 30 transition" by Levinson. Some young people who feel their lives are going well, reaffirm their commitments and experience a smooth transition at this time. Others, however, may experience a major crisis, manifested by marital problems, job changes, and psychiatric symptoms, such as anxiety and depression.

Parenthood

By age thirty, most persons have established families and have to deal with a variety of parent-child problems. In addition to the economic burden of raising a child (estimated to be over $100,000 for a middle-class family whose child goes to college), there are emotional costs as well. The child may reawaken conflicts in the parent that they themselves had as children, or the child may have a chronic illness which challenges the emotional resources of the family. In general, men are more concerned with their work and advancement in their occupation than with child rearing. Women are more concerned about their role as mothers; however, this emphasis is changing dramatically for both sexes as more women enter the job market. At about the age of 35, many women dramatically change the course of their lives. As their children get older, they reenter the work force to resume their career or start a career for the first time.

MIDDLE ADULTHOOD (40 TO 65 YEARS)

The ages used to define this period vary among different theorists. Typically, this period is known as "middle age." The task of terminating early adulthood involves a process of reviewing the past, considering how one's life has gone, as well as what the future will be like. With regard to occupation, many persons may begin to experience the gap between early aspirations and current achievements. They may wonder if the life style and commitments they chose in early adulthood are worth continuing. They may feel that they would like to live the remaining years in a different, more satisfying way without knowing exactly how. As children grow up and leave home, the parental roles change; at this time, people redefine their roles as husbands and wives as well.

There are important gender changes at this time. Many women, no longer needing to nurture young children, develop attitudes that have been considered masculine (e.g., becoming independent, competitive, and aggressive). Men, on the other hand, may develop qualities that have traditionally been considered feminine (e.g., expressive, dependent, and emotional). The new balance of the masculine and feminine in the self may be valuable in that it enables a person to relate more effectively to someone of the opposite sex.

Erikson's Stage of Generativity vs. Stagnation (40 to 65 Years)

During the decades that span the middle years of life, the adult chooses between generativity and stagnation. Generativity does not only refer to a person's having or raising children, but also includes a vital interest outside the home in establishing and guiding the oncoming generation or in improving society. The childless can be generative if they develop a sense of altruism and creativity. But most individuals, if able, will want to continue their personalities and energies "in the production and care of common offspring." Wanting or having children, however, does not ensure generativity. The parents need to have achieved successful identities themselves to be truly generative.

The adult who has no interest in guiding or establishing the oncoming generation is likely to look obsessively for intimacy that is not truly intimate. Such people may marry and even produce children, but all within a cocoon of self-concern and isolation. Those persons pamper themselves as if they were the children and become preoccupied with themselves. They may lack belief in the species. Indeed, parents who do not truly believe life in a given society to be worthwhile may find that their children absorb that message only too well, the result being a lack of grandchildren.

The Mid-Life Crisis

As men and women enter their middle 40s or early 30s, there is controversy as to whether or not a mid-life

crisis is inevitable. Seventy to 80 percent of men have a moderate to severe crisis at this time, which consists of a sudden drastic change in work or marital relationship, severe depression, increased use of alcohol or drugs, or a shift to an alternate life style. Persons in this state feel that their resources are inadequate to manage the stresses of their life. They feel they are growing old and have to deal with death. The association of this awareness with the feeling of panic or depression constitutes the syndrome of a mid-life crisis. There are normal turning points during middle age which are mastered without distress. It is only when life events are so severe or so unexpected—such as the death of a spouse, the loss of a job, or a serious illness—that the person experiences an emotional disorder of such proportion to warrant the term "mid-life crisis." Men and women who are most prone to mid-life crisis tend to come from families characterized by one or more of the following during their adolescence: parental discord, withdrawal by the same sex parent, anxious parents, impulsive parents with a low level of sense of responsibility.

The Male and Female Climacterium

The decrease in physiologic function in men and women has been called a climacterium. For women the menopausal period is considered to be the climacterium and may start anywhere from the 40s to the early 50s. Bernice Neugarten studied this period and found that over 50 percent of the women described the menopause as an unpleasant experience; however, a significant portion of women felt that their lives had not changed in any significant way. Since they no longer had to worry about becoming pregnant, several women reported feeling freer after the menopause than they had felt before its onset. Generally, the female climacterium has been stereotyped as a sudden or radical psychophysiologic experience. However, it is more often a gradual experience as estrogen secretion decreases with changes in the flow, timing, and eventual cessation of the menses. Vasomotor instability (hot flashes) may occur and the menopause may extend over a period of several years. Some women experience anxiety and depression, but usually one's premenopausal personality structure predisposes the person to the menopausal syndrome.

Another phenomenon described at this time has been called the empty nest syndrome, a depression that occurs in men and women when their youngest child is about to leave home. Most parents, however, perceive the departure of the youngest child as a relief rather than a stress. If no compensating activities have been developed, particularly by the mother, some of these parents become depressed.

As persons approach the age of 50, they more clearly define what they want from work, family, and leisure. Some persons may enter a period of decline at this time. Those men who may have reached their highest level of advancement in work may experience disillusionment or frustration when they realize they can no longer anticipate new work challenges. For the woman who has invested herself completely in the mothering role, this period of life leaves one with no suitable identity after the children leave home. Sometimes social rules become rigidly established; less freedom in life style and a sense of entrapment may lead to depression and a loss of confidence at this time. There may also be unique financial burdens in middle age resulting from pressure to care for aged parents, at one end of the spectrum, and one's own young children at the other.

Levinson describes a transitional period between the ages of 50 and 55, during which a developmental crisis may occur if the person feels incapable of changing an intolerable life structure. While there is no single event that characterizes this transition, the physiologic changes that begin to appear may have a dramatic impact on the person's sense of self. There is, for example, a decrease in cardiovascular efficiency that accompanies aging; but chronological age and physical infirmity are not linear. Those who exercise regularly, do not smoke, and eat and drink in moderation are able to maintain their physical health and emotional well-being. George Vaillant followed a group of Harvard freshmen into middle age and found a strong correlation between physical health and emotional health. In addition, those persons who had the poorest psychological adjustment during college years had a high incidence of physical illness in middle age.

An inability to deal with changes in body image prompt many men and women to undergo cosmetic surgery in an effort to maintain a youthful appearance. Although Masters and Johnson clearly demonstrated that enjoyable sexual activity (including coitus) may continue well into old age, a decline in sexual functioning may occur. For some persons, however, the erroneous belief that vigorous sexual activity is the prerogative of youth is sufficient to interfere with their normal physiological sexual response.

Middle age is the period when one frequently feels overwhelmed by stimuli and by too many obligations and duties, but it is also a time of great satisfaction for most persons. People have lived long enough to have developed a wide array of acquaintances, friendships, and relationships. The satisfaction a person expresses about his network of friends is predictive of positive mental health. Some social ties, however, may be a source of stress if demands are made upon the person that cannot be met or that assault the person's self-esteem. Power and leadership are most generally possessed by the middle-aged, and if one's health and vitality remain intact, it is truly the prime of life.

DIVORCE: A MAJOR PROBLEM OF ADULTHOOD

Divorce is a major crisis of adult life which is on the rise. During 1986, an estimated 1.1 million couples divorced, an increase of 3 percent over 1985.

Types of Separation That Accompany Divorce

Paul Bohannan has described types of separation that take place at the time of divorce.

Psychic Divorce. In psychic divorce, the love object is given up, and a grief reaction about the death of the relationship occurs. Sometimes a period of anticipatory mourning sets in before the divorce actually occurs. Separating from a spouse forces the person to become autonomous, to change from a position of dependency. This separation may be difficult to achieve, especially if both persons are used to being dependent on one another (as normally happens in marriage) or if one was so dependent as to be

afraid or incapable of becoming more independent. Most persons report feelings such as depression, ambivalence, and mood swings at the time of the divorce. Studies indicate that the process of recovery from divorce takes about two years. At this time the ex-spouse may be viewed neutrally, and each spouse accepts his or her new identity as a single person.

Legal Divorce. This process involves going through the courts so that each of the parties is remarriageable. Seventy-five percent of divorced women and 80 percent of divorced men remarry within three years of divorce. No-fault divorce, in which neither person is judged to be the guilty party in the divorce, has become the most widely used legal mechanism for divorce.

Economic Divorce. The division of the couple's property between them and economic support for the wife are major concerns. Many men who are ordered by the courts to pay alimony or child support flout the law, which has become a major social problem.

Community Divorce. The social network of the divorced couple changes markedly. A few relatives and friends are retained from the old communities and new ones are added. The task of meeting new friends is often difficult for divorced persons, who may realize how dependent they were on the spouse for social exchange.

Coparental Divorce. This refers to separation of a parent from the child's other parent. Being a single parent is very different from being a married parent.

Single-Parent Homes

There are over 30 million families with one or more children under the age of 18, and of these, 20 percent are single-parent homes in which the female is the sole head of the household. Although the majority of these children are left in the care of their mothers, who are awarded custody by the courts in the divorce proceedings, others are abandoned by their fathers. Among black families with one or more children under 18, almost 48 percent are headed by women with no spouse present.

Children in one-parent families are characterized by a higher incidence of academic underachievement and emotional problems. When mothers are forced to work following divorce or abandonment, their children are at further risk from emotional problems because the working mother cannot devote sufficient time to the care of the child. A small number of children in single-parent homes are precocious, their maturity fostered by having to take on increased responsibilities at a young age.

Custody

The parental right doctrine is a concept in law that awards custody to the most fit natural parent and attempts to ensure that the best interest of the child is served. Most often, custody is awarded to the mother, but in about 5 percent of cases, custody is awarded to the father.

Types of custody include (1) joint custody, in which the child spends equal time with both parents, which is becoming increasingly common; (2) split custody, in which siblings are separated and each parent has custody of one of the children; and (3) single custody, in which the child lives solely with one parent, the other parent having rights of visitation which may be limited in some ways by the court.

Problems may surface in the parent-child relationship with the custodial parent or the noncustodial parent. The presence of the custodial parent in the home represents the reality of the divorce, and this parent may become the target of the child's anger. The parent under such stress may not be able to deal with the child's increased needs and anger at this time.

The noncustodial parent must cope with limits placed upon time spent with the child. This parent loses the day-to-day gratification, as well as the responsibilities involved with parenting. Emotional distress is common to both the parent and child. Joint custody offers a solution with some advantages; however, it requires a high degree of maturity on the part of the parents and can present some problems. Parents must separate their child-rearing practices from their postdivorce resentments, and they must develop a spirit of cooperation regarding the rearing of the child. They must also have the ability to tolerate frequent communication with an ex-spouse.

Reasons for Divorce. Divorce tends to run in families and is higher in couples who marry as teenagers or come from different socioeconomic backgrounds. Marriage is psychologically unique, and so is each divorce. If a person's parents were divorced, he may choose to resolve a marital problem in the same way—through divorce. Expectations of the spouse may be unrealistic. One partner may expect the other to act as an all-giving mother or as a magically protective father. The parenting experience places the greatest strain on a marriage. In surveys of couples with and without children, those without children report getting more pleasure from their spouse than those couples with children. Illness in the child creates the greatest strain of all, and in marriages where a child has died through illness or accident, over 50 percent end in divorce.

Other causes of marital distress are problems concerning sex and money. Both areas may be used as a means of control, and withholding sex or money is a means of expressing aggression. There is also less social pressure to remain married. The easing of divorce laws and the declining influence of religion make divorce a more acceptable course of action today.

Extramarital Intercourse. Adultery is defined as voluntary sexual intercourse between a married person and someone other than his or her spouse. Studies report that by middle age, 60 percent of men and 40 percent of women have had at least one extramarital affair. For men, their first extramarital affair is often associated with their wife's pregnancy, during which time coitus may be interdicted. Most of these incidents are kept secret from the spouse and, if known, rarely account for divorce. This event, however, may serve as the catalyst for basic dissatisfactions in the marriage to surface, which then may lead to its dissolution. Adultery may decline as concern about potentially fatal sexually transmitted diseases such as AIDS begins to serve as a sobering deterrent.

References

Arthur M B, Bailyn L, Levinson D J: *Working with Cancers*. Center for Research in Career Development, Columbia University, New York, 1984.

Colorusso C A, Nemiroff R A: *Adult Development—A New Dimension in Psychodynamic Theory and Practice*. Plenum Press, New York, 1981.

Hornstein G A: The structuring of identity among midlife women as a function of their degree of involvement in employment. J Personality *54*(3):551, 1986.

Kimmel D C: *Adulthood and Aging—An Interdisciplinary Developmental View*. John Wiley & Sons, New York, 1974.

Krause N: Stress and sex differences in depressive symptoms among older adults. J Gerontol *41*(6):727, 1986.

Levinson, D J: *A Conception of Adult Development*. Amer Psychologist *41*:3, 1986.

Levinson, D J, Damow, C N, Klein E B, Levinson M H, McKeeb A: *The Seasons of a Man's Life*. Alfred A. Knopf, New York, 1978.

Lidz, T: *The Person—His and Her Development Throughout the Life Cycle*, p 392. Basic Books, New York, 1976.

Lusski W, et al.: Effective elderly adjustment. J Am Geriatr Soc *34*(10):764, 1986.

Neugarten B L: *Personality in Middle and Late Life*. Atherton, New York, 1964.

Ortega Y, Gassel J: *Man and Crisis*. W W Norton, New York, 1958.

Vaillant G E: *Adaptation to Life*. Little, Brown & Co., Boston, 1977.

Van Gennep, A: *The Rites of Passage*. The University of Chicago Press, Chicago, 1960.

3.5 _____
Late Adulthood and Old Age

Late adulthood, the so-called geriatric period, is usually considered to begin at age 65. In spite of the sober reminders of one's mortality as illness and death affect friends and loved ones, more people are living longer now, a phenomenon which has been called a triumph of survivorship rather than a cause for despair. Gerontology—the study of aging—has become a new field of specialization.

DEMOGRAPHICS

In 1900, the average life expectancy was 47 years, and only 4 percent of the population was over age 65. By the year 2020, the average life expectancy will be 77 years, and 20 percent of the population will be over age 65. In addition, by the year 2000, there will be 17 million persons over age 75—the so-called "old old" whose number is increasing faster than that of persons between age 65 and 75—the "young old." In the last 50 years, the number of senior citizens has doubled.

There are more women than men in the geriatric group because of the higher death rate among men. In 1950, men had a greater life expectancy than women, but that is now reversed; women live 10 years longer than men. Currently, there are approximately ten women for every seven men over the age of 65. The life expectancy of blacks is shorter than that of whites. Among white men, there will be 41 expected deaths per 1000 persons; whereas among black men, there will be 51 expected deaths per 1000.

More older people, both black and white, live in central parts of cities and in rural locations. Florida has the highest proportion of elderly residents, 20 percent of its population comprised of the aged. California, New York, Pennsylvania, and Illinois are other states with large numbers of the elders.

BIOLOGY OF AGING

The process of aging is known as senescence and results from a complex interaction of genetic, metabolic, hormonal, immunologic, and structural factors acting on molecular, cellular, histologic, and organ levels. In general, however, the aging of a person is the aging of cells. The most commonly held theory is that each cell has a genetically determined life span during which it can replicate itself a limited number of times after which it dies. Structural changes in cells occur with age. In the central nervous system, for example, age-related cell changes occur in neurons, which show signs of degeneration. In senility (characterized by severe memory loss and a loss of intellectual functioning), signs of degeneration are much more severe and are known as neurofibrillary degeneration, seen most commonly in Alzheimer's disease.

Changes in the structure of DNA and RNA are also found in aging cells; the cause has been attributed to genotypic programming, x-rays, chemicals, and food products, among others. There is probably no single cause of aging. All areas of the body are affected to a lesser or greater degree, and changes vary from person to person.

A progressive decline in many bodily functions includes decreases in cardiac output and stroke volume, glomerular filtration rate, oxygen consumption, cerebral blood flow, and vital capacity. There is a thickening of the optic lens associated with an inability to accommodate (presbyopia), and progressive hearing loss, particularly in the higher frequencies.

Many immune mechanisms are altered with impaired T-cell response to antigens and an increase in the formation of autoimmune antibodies. These altered immune responses probably play a role in aged persons' susceptibility to infection and possibly even to neoplastic disease. Some neoplasms show a steadily increasing incidence with age, most notably cancer of the colon, prostate, stomach, and skin.

The anatomic changes of aging include a decrease in height, reduction in overall muscle mass, deepening of the thoracic cage, and other changes such as graying of hair and lengthening of the nose and ears. Osteoporosis and osteoarthritis are common. Changes in body weight occur which represent an increase in body fat. Men tend to gain weight until about age 50 and then gradually lose it; women usually gain weight until age 70 before this loss occurs. The heart may increase in size and weight and contain lipofuscin pigment derived from lipids. Blood vessels in the heart and throughout the body show an increased amount of collagen and altered elastin. Atrophic gastritis, hiatal hernia, and diverticulosis occur, as does general wrinkling of the skin, loss of subcutaneous fat, decrease in melanin, and loss of sweat glands.

There are variable changes in endocrine function. For example, post-menopausal estrogen levels decrease, producing breast tissue involution and vaginal epithelial atrophy. Testosterone levels begin to decline in the sixth decade; however, there is an increase in follicle stimulating hormone and luteinizing hormone.

In the central nervous system, there is a decrease in brain weight, ventricular enlargement, and neuronal loss of approximately 50,000 per day, with some reduction in cerebral blood flow and oxygenation. If severe enough, significant mental deterioration (e.g., senile dementia) occurs. However, this is not the inevitable outcome of old age; it is present in only about 10 percent of persons over age 65. More commonly found is a slight decline in cognitive function in the elderly. In longitudinal studies of men between ages 60 and 70, no significant decrease in intelligence was detected. The learning of new material, however, takes longer for the elderly, and they are susceptible to memory impairment. In the elderly, memory impairments affect immediate, recent, and remote memory, in descending order. The aged who maintain normal cognitive func-

tion are most often from the middle or upper socioeconomic groups, are better educated, have higher intelligence, and are in good general physical and emotional health.

Longevity is influenced by a variety of factors. Heredity has the highest correlation: Persons whose parents were long-lived live longer. Obesity contributes to increased mortality, and a prudent diet low in saturated fats is desirable. Life-style qualities such as regular sleep patterns (between 6 and 8 hours is optimal), moderate and regular exercise, and abstinence from smoking, coffee, and alcohol are associated with longevity. Some studies have demonstrated that persons who have the equivalent of one ounce of alcohol per day live longer; but such studies have not been sufficiently replicated. Regular medical check-ups, particularly breast examinations in women over 40 and proctoscopy for men over 50, are useful for early diagnosis of potentially curable cancers that might otherwise shorten life. Those persons who are married, who are from higher rather than lower socioeconomic groups, who are working or, if in retirement, are contributing productively to society also live longer.

DEVELOPMENTAL TASKS OF OLD AGE

Erikson's Stage of Integrity vs. Despair and Isolation (Over 65 Years)

In Erikson's eighth stage of the life cycle, the conflict exists between integrity, the sense of satisfaction one feels in reflecting on a life productively lived, and despair, the sense that life has had little purpose or meaning. Late adulthood can be a contented period, a time to enjoy grandchildren, to contemplate one's major efforts, and perhaps to see the fruits of one's labor being put to good use by younger generations. Integrity allows for an acceptance of one's place in the life cycle and of the knowledge that one's life is one's own responsibility.

In regard to one's parents, there is an acceptance of who they are or were and an understanding of how they lived their lives.

However, there is no peace or contentment in old age unless one has achieved intimacy and generativity. Without generativity, there is no sense of purpose and no conviction that one's life has been purposeful. Without that conviction, there is fear of death and a sense of despair or disgust. Misanthropes and others who are contemptuous of people are in the state of despair.

Adaptation to Stress

The essence of aging is an increased vulnerability to stress of all kinds—biological, psychological, and social. Older people are less likely to attempt new occupational challenges, whether by choice or for lack of opportunity. They must, however, deal with loss through death of friends, loved ones, and especially spouses, the most stressful loss of all.

Recent studies have found that concern about physical health is related not only to age. Most persons have a characteristic level of anxiety about their health. If excessive, it is diagnosed as hypochondriasis, but there is no higher incidence of hypochondriasis in the aged than in early or middle adulthood. Age-related concerns in the elderly are realistic, as they relate to actual disease and physical changes that are likely to be affected by old age, such as vision, hearing, and genitourinary function. Urinary incontinence, for example, is a common complaint. Some studies have shown that up to 50 percent of the institutionalized elderly have some degree of incontinence.

Socioeconomics. Poverty is typically associated with old age. Thirty percent of older persons live in substandard housing, and 20 percent are living below the poverty level. Insufficient money also limits the quantity and quality of food purchases; it is estimated that 10 percent of the elderly have nutritional deficiencies. There are, of course, the remaining majority who are adequately housed and economically secure. The number of elderly who actually work, however, is dropping. One myth about older persons is that they are unproductive and unable to contribute in the workplace. However, elders have demonstrated that their reliability, productivity, and rates of absenteeism and accidents are no higher than those of younger workers. Slightly more than 20 percent of men and less than 10 percent of women over age 65 are working. Retirement programs, social security, and pension plans are the financial incentives that have contributed to that decline. With the passage of the Age Discrimination in Employment Act and its amendments, mandatory retirement at age 70 is no longer legal in many fields. That may slow the decline in the number of employed older workers.

Retirement. Retirement allows the older person to have more time for leisure pursuits, and many benefit from this newly found freedom. For others, however, retirement is a negative experience. They may feel increasingly dependent on others—especially if retirement results in economic problems—or they may be unable to find new activities and interests that contribute to their self-esteem as did a productive work experience. A second myth about the aged is that most live in institutions: only 5 percent of those below age 85 live in nursing homes, and 20 percent of persons over age 85 live in such institutions.

Social and Sexual Activity. Healthy older persons usually maintain a level of social activity that is only slightly changed from that of earlier years. For many old age is a period of continued intellectual, emotional, and psychological growth. In some cases, however, physical illness or the death of friends may preclude continued social interaction. Moreover, as the person experiences an increased sense of isolation, there is the possibility of depression. There is growing evidence that maintaining social activities is of value for physical and emotional well-being. Having contact with younger persons is also important because the older person can pass on cultural values and provide care services to the younger generation and, so, maintain a sense of usefulness that contributes to self-esteem.

It is estimated that approximately 70 percent of males and 20 percent of females over 60 are sexually active. Sexual activity is limited by the absence of an available partner. Longitudinal studies have demonstrated that sex drive does not decrease as men and women get older; in fact, some report an increase in sex drive. Masters and Johnson reported sexual functioning of individuals in their 80s. Expected physiologic changes in men include a longer time period for erection to occur, decreased penile turgidity, ejaculatory seepage; in women decreased vaginal lubrication and vaginal atrophy are associated with lower estrogen levels. A significant finding was that the more active one's sex life was in early adulthood, the more likely it was to be active in old age.

EMOTIONAL PROBLEMS OF THE AGED

Loss is the predominant theme that characterizes the emotional experiences of older people. An elderly person must deal with the grief of multiple losses (death of spouse, friends, family, and colleagues), change of work status and prestige, and decline of physical abilities and health. Losses in every aspect of late life cause older persons to expend enormous amounts of emotional and physical energy in grieving, resolving grief, and adapting to the changes that result from loss. Depression is a maladaptive response to loss, which, in the elderly, may mimic senile dementia. In addition to the classic signs of depression such as appetite and sleep disturbances, loss of interest in outside events, self-deprecatory remarks, and thoughts that life is no longer worth living, the person may show memory impairment, difficulty in concentrating, poor judgment, and irritability.

There is a higher incidence of suicide in the aged (80 per 100,000 population). The suicide of aged persons is perceived differently by surviving friends and family members, depending on gender: men are thought to have been physically ill and women are thought to have been mentally ill.

References

Anderson J E, editor: *Psychological Aspect of Aging*. American Psychological Association, Washington, DC, 1956.

Busse E W, Pfeiffer E, editors: *Behavior and Adaptation in Late Life*. Little, Brown & Co., Boston, 1969.

Butler R N: *Why Survive? Being Old in America*. Harper & Row, New York, 1975.

Butler R N, Lewis M I: *Aging and Mental Health—Positive Psychosocial and Biomedical Approaches*, ed 3. C V Mosby Co, St. Louis, 1982.

Eisdorfer C, Lawbon, M P: *The Psychology of Adult Development and Aging*. American Psychological Association, Washington, DC, 1973.

Gutmann D: Psychoanalysis and aging—a development view. In G H Pollock, S I Greenspan, editors: *The Course of Life—Psychoanalytic Contributions Toward Understanding Personality Development*, vol. 3. US Department of Health and Human Services, Mental Health Study Center, Adelphi, Maryland, 1981.

Jacobs S C, et al.: Bereavement and catecholamines. J Psychosom Res *30* (4):489, 1986.

Lidz T: *The Person—His and Her Development Throughout the Life Cycle*, p 517. Basic Books, New York, 1976.

Nemiroff R A, Calorusso C A: *The Race Against Time—Psychotherapy and Psychoanalysis in the Second Half of Life*. Plenum Press, New York, 1985.

Pollock G M: Aging or aged—development or pathology? S N S I Greenspan, G, M, Pollock, editors: *The Course of Life—Psychoanalytic Contributions Toward Understanding Personality Development*, vol 3. U.S. Department of Health and Human Services, Mental Health Study Center, Adelphi, Maryland, 1981.

Statistical Abstracts of the United States, ed 106. US Department of Commerce, US Bureau of Census, Washington, DC, 1986.

3.6 _____
Thanatology: Death and Bereavement

INTRODUCTION

Mankind is mystified by death and fears and feels wholly vulnerable to the forces that represent and bring about this state. In some respects, medicine attempts to explain the facts about death as much as it provides relief from suffering and sickness. A medical aphorism is that a physician never saves a life but only postpones a death.

Thanatology may be defined as that discipline that investigates death, dying, grief, mourning, bereavement, and fatal illness.

MEANING OF DEATH

Through the ages, many meanings have been associated with the mystery of death. It is the inevitable end of the life cycle, and as Erikson has noted, death is the fruit of a life fully lived. It should be accepted as a natural part of the life cycle, not as a source of despair or fear. This equanimity about death is not achieved unless intimacy, generativity, and integrity are experienced first.

From a psychosocial view, death may be timely or untimely. From a statistical viewpoint, *timely death* implies that one's expected survival and actual life span are approximately equal. Timeliness means that the choice of when to die coincides with its occurrence. Most people want to live as long and as well as possible. But when it is no longer possible to live without extraordinary distress, many become willing to die. *Untimely death* refers to (1) premature death of a very young person, (2) sudden, unexpected death, or (3) catastrophic death associated with violence or accident and utter meaninglessness. Death has also been described as intended (wherein the person plays a role in his suicide), unintended (due to trauma or disease), and subintended (hastened by substance abuse, alcoholism, or cigarette smoking in which the patient may be expressing an unconscious wish to die).

LEGAL ASPECTS OF DEATH

According to law, the physician must sign a death certificate that attests to the cause of death (e.g., congestive heart failure, pneumonia). The physician must also classify death as being from natural, accidental, suicidal, homicidal, or unknown causes. Anyone who dies unattended by a physician must be examined by the appointed medical examiner, coroner, or pathologist to determine the cause of death. In some cases, a psychological autopsy is performed; for example, a determination is made whether a patient died because he was pushed or jumped from a high building. Each situation has obvious medicolegal implications.

ATTITUDES TOWARD IMPENDING DEATH

Various thanatologists have identified stages of death or of dying. Seldom does any dying patient follow a regular series of responses that can be clearly identified; no established sequence is applicable to all patients. The following five stages proposed by Elizabeth Kübler-Ross are widely used.

Stage 1—Shock and Denial

Upon being told that one is dying, there is an initial reaction of shock. The patient may appear dazed at first and may then refuse to believe the diagnosis or deny that anything is wrong. Some patients never pass beyond this stage and may go from doctor to doctor until they find one who supports their position.

Stage 2—Anger

Patients become frustrated, irritable, and angry that they are ill. A common response is, "Why me?" They may become angry at god, their fate, a friend, or a family member. The anger may be displaced onto the hospital staff or doctor, who are blamed for the illness. Patients in this stage are difficult to manage. The doctor who has difficulty dealing with dying patients may withdraw from the patient or transfer the patient to another doctor's care.

Stage 3—Bargaining

The patient may attempt to negotiate with physicians, friends, or even god, that in return for a cure, the person will fulfill one or many promises, such as giving to charity or attending church regularly.

Stage 4—Depression

The patient shows clinical signs of depression—withdrawal, psychomotor retardation, sleep disturbances, hopelessness, and, possibly, suicidal ideation. The depression may be a reaction to the effects of the illness on his life (e.g., loss of job, economic hardship, isolation from friends and family) or it may be in anticipation of the actual loss of life that will occur shortly.

Stage 5—Acceptance

The patient realizes that death is inevitable and accepts the universality of the experience. Under ideal circumstances, the patient is courageous and is able to talk about his death as he faces the unknown. Those persons who have strong religious beliefs and are convinced of a life after death can find comfort in these beliefs and in the ecclesiasticism: Fear not death, remember those who have gone before you and those who will come after.

CARING FOR THE DYING PATIENT

The major task of the physician caring for the dying patient is to provide compassionate concern and continuing support for that patient. To visit with the patient regularly, to maintain eye contact, and to listen to what the patient has to say are the hallmarks of appropriate care. It is necessary that the doctor be aware of his own attitudes toward death and dying. Some physicians enter medicine because of an unconscious fear of death, which they attempt to deal with by intellectualization; they provide the patient with the minute and often unnecessary details as well as the day to day vicissitudes of the illness. What is most important is to be tactfully honest. Most patients want their doctors to be truthful with them; for example, they prefer to know that they have cancer. Honesty, however, does not preclude hope. If 85 percent of patients with a particular disease die within 5 years, then 15 percent are still alive after that time. Still, some patients do not want to know the facts of their illness. The doctor may ask how much a patient wants to know about the illness and should respond to the patient's wishes.

The patient, his family, and the hospital staff vary in the extent of their knowledge of the patient's illness. In one classification, four patterns of awareness may exist: *open awareness*, in which staff, family, and patient are completely aware of the diagnosis, treatment, and prognosis of the illness; *mutual pretense awareness*, in which those same persons know, but pretend not to know; *suspected awareness*, in which everyone knows except the patient, who suspects that such is the case; and *closed awareness*, in which everyone except the patient knows. There is a trend in hospitals toward open awareness when it can be tolerated by all concerned; but some terminally ill patients may choose not to know their condition, and that wish should be respected.

Other measures that need to be considered are pain management (which should be vigorous in the terminally ill); not taking personally complaints of a patient who may be in the anger phase of dying; and helping the members of the dying patient's family to deal with their feelings about the patient's illness. Finally, it is necessary to anticipate the wishes of the patient and his family regarding the use of life-sustaining procedures. A patient may ask that his life not be prolonged by artificial means (e.g., Do Not Resuscitate (DNR) if he is in extremis). Living wills are legal documents in which patients give instructions to their physicians about withholding such life support measures.

In 1986, the American Medical Association said that doctors could withhold all means of life-prolonging medical treatment, including food and water, from patients in irreversible comas, provided there are adequate safeguards to confirm the accuracy of the diagnosis. The decision is made in conjunction with the patient's family or legal guardians. In these cases, the physician lets a terminally ill patient die; the physician does not intentionally cause death. A person is brain dead when he suffers irreversible cessation of the functions of the entire brain, including the brain stem.

DEATH AND CHILDREN

The preschool child under age 5 is aware of death, not in the abstract sense but as a separation similar to sleep. Between the ages of 5 and 10 years, there is a developing sense of inevitable human mortality; the child first fears that his parents may die and that he will be abandoned. After age 10, death is conceptualized as something that may happen to the child as well as to the parent. As opposed to those in some other parts of the world, middle-class adults in the United States tend to shield children from a knowledge of death. The air of mystery with which death is surrounded in such instances may create irrational fears in children, just the opposite of what is intended.

Children with fatal illness create major emotional stresses on the care-givers, be they parents, relatives, hospi-

tal staff, or physicians. A consistent, trusted person is essential in providing optimal care for the dying child. The separation of the child from its mother is as traumatic an event for the hospitalized child as the illness itself; perhaps, even more so. As Bowlby pointed out, the mother (or an equally valued and familiar care-giver) rooming in with the hospitalized child can help alleviate the child's anxiety and facilitate necessary medical care.

GRIEF, MOURNING, AND BEREAVEMENT

These terms apply to the psychological reactions of those who survive a significant loss. *Grief* refers to the subjective feelings that are precipitated by the death of a loved one. The term is used synonymously with *mourning*, although in the strictest sense, mourning refers to the processes by which grief is resolved. *Bereavement* literally means to be deprived of someone by death and refers to being in the state of mourning. Regardless of the fine points that may differentiate these terms there are sufficient similarities in the experience of grief or bereavement to warrant its characterization as a syndrome that has signs, symptoms, a demonstrable course, and an expected resolution.

Characteristics of Normal Grief

Initial grief is often manifested as a state of shock that may be expressed as a feeling of numbness and a sense of bewilderment. This apparent inability to comprehend what has happened may be short lived. It is followed by such expressions of suffering and distress as sighing and crying, although in Western culture, this expected feature of grief is less common among men than among women. Other physical expressions of grief may include the following: feelings of weakness, decreased appetite, weight loss, and difficulty concentrating, breathing, and talking. Sleep disturbances may include difficulty going to sleep, waking up during the night, or awakening early. Dreams of the deceased often occur, the dreamer awakening with a sense of disappointment in finding that the experience was only a dream.

Self-reproach is not unusual, although it is less common and less intense in normal grief than in pathological grief. These thoughts usually center on some relatively minor act of omission or commission toward the deceased. A phenomenon known as survivor guilt occurs in persons who are relieved that the death is someone else's and not their own. The survivor sometimes believes that he should have been the person who died. Forms of denial occur throughout the entire period of bereavement; often the bereaved person inadvertently thinks or acts as if the loss had not occurred. Efforts to perpetuate the lost relationship are evidenced by an investment in objects that were treasured by the deceased or that remind the grief-stricken person of the deceased (linkage objects).

A sense of the deceased's presence may be so intense as to constitute an illusion or a hallucination; in normal grief, however, the person recognizes the inaccuracy of this perception. As part of what has been labeled *identification phenomena*, the person may take on the qualities, mannerisms, or characteristics of the deceased person, as if to perpetuate that person in some concrete way. This maneuver can reach potentially pathological expression with the development of physical symptoms similar to those experienced by the deceased or to ones suggestive of the illness from which the deceased died.

John Bowlby hypothesized four stages of bereavement. An early phase of numbness or protest (stage 1) that may be interrupted by outbursts of distress, fear, or anger is soon followed by a phase of yearning and searching for the lost figure (stage 2). This stage, which may last several months or even years, is characterized by preoccupation with the lost person and a physical restlessness. Weeping and anger are characteristic expressions of this search. Gradual recognition and integration of the reality lead to a subsequent phase of disorganization and despair (stage 3). Restlessness and aimlessness may now characterize inefficient and ineffective efforts to initiate and perpetuate productive patterns of behavior, interpersonal or otherwise. Finally, with the establishment of new patterns, objects, and goals, the bereaved person reaches a phase of reorganization (stage 4), during which grief recedes and is replaced by cherished memories.

Bowlby theorized that many effects of the mourning process can be understood as signs of separation anxiety, elicited by the death of a loved one and the disruption of the attachment and affectional bond. Although attachment behavior is especially characteristic of children, it remains active throughout life. Attachment behavior leads to separation anxiety when the person loses the object of the attachment, be it parent, spouse, friend, or other person with whom affectional bonds are made.

C. M. Parkes described five stages of bereavement. (1) *Alarm*, a stressful state manifested by physiologic changes such as a rise in blood pressure and heart rate, is somewhat similar to Bowlby's first stage of protest, fear, and anger. (2) *Numbness* is a state in which the person appears to be superficially unaffected by the loss but is in reality protecting himself from feeling the acute distress produced by the loss. (3) *Pining* or searching, the person looks for or is constantly reminded of the lost person. The illusions or hallucinations of the deceased mentioned above may occur during this phase (sometimes called pseudoillusions or pseudohallucinations because the person immediately recognizes them as such). This phase resembles Bowlby's second stage of yearning and searching for the lost figure. (4) In *depression*, the bereaved feels hopeless about the future, cannot go on living, and tends to withdraw from family and friends; and (5) the final stage of *recovery* and *reorganization* in which the person recognizes that his life will continue with new adjustments and different goals.

Length of Grief

Because there are great variations between individuals, the various signs, symptoms, and phases of mourning and bereavement described above are not as discrete as their characterizations might imply. Nevertheless, the diverse manifestations of grief usually tend to subside over time. Traditionally, grief expends itself within 1 or 2 years, as the person has the opportunity to experience the entire calendar year at least once without the lost person. It has become increasingly apparent that the signs and symptoms of grief may persist much longer than 1 or 2 years and that the person sometimes continues to have various grief-related feelings, symptoms, and behavior through life. Eventually, however, most persons return to a state of productivity and relative well-being.

Bereavement in Children

Bowlby studied the bereavement process in children. It is similar to that of adults, especially once the child is able to understand the irrevocability of death. The mourning process resembles that of separation in that there are three phases, protest, despair, and detachment. In the *protest* phase, which may last a week, the child has a strong desire for the mother or other caregiver who died and cries for her return; in the *despair* phase, the child begins to feel hopeless about her return, crying is intermittent, and withdrawal and apathy set in. In the *detachment phase,* the child begins to show a reawakening of interest in his surroundings and starts looking for substitute adult figures with whom to become involved. In dealing with the bereaved child, the physician should recognize the child's need to find a person who will substitute for his mother. The child may transfer his need for a mother to several adults rather than to one. If no consistent person is available severe psychological damage to the child may result, so that he no longer looks for or expects intimacy in any relationship. The importance of managing grief reactions in children is highlighted by the increased evidence that depressive disorders and suicide attempts occur more frequently in adults who in early childhood experienced the death of a parent.

Delayed, Inhibited, or Denied Grief. Delayed, inhibited, or denied grief refers to the absence of the expression of grief at the time of the loss, when it ordinarily would be expected. In some instances, grieving simply is delayed until it no longer can be avoided. Often, the first reaction to an unexpected loss is temporary shock or denial.

Individuals vary greatly in their need to hide their grief. Familial and cultural influences affect how the mourner behaves in public. The "stiff upper lip" admired by one group contrasts dramatically with the weeping, wailing, and fainting that another group accepts as the norm. Hence, it may be difficult to gauge the extent of another's grief from outward appearances unless one has some understanding of the person's background.

Grief that is inhibited or denied expression is potentially pathogenic because the person avoids dealing with the reality of the loss. A false euphoria may prevail, suggesting that bereavement is on a pathological course. Inhibited or denied grief reactions contain the seeds of such unfortunate consequences as experiencing persisting physical symptoms similar to those of the deceased or unaccountable reactions on the anniversary of the loss or on occasions of significance to the deceased. Denied or inhibited grief also may reach expression by being displaced to some other loss that, although seemingly insignificant in its own right, may symbolize the original loss. Overreaction to another person's trouble may be one manifestation of displacement.

Finally, it must be recognized that some relationships, regardless of their public appearance, are sufficiently negative to render reduced or absent grief a totally normal and appropriate response. In these cases, the consequences of the death of a spouse or parent may be decidedly positive for the survivor.

Anticipatory Grief. The concept of anticipatory grief applies to grief expressed in advance of a loss that is perceived as inevitable, as distinguished from grief that occurs at or after the loss. By definition, anticipatory grief ends with the occurrence of the anticipated loss, regardless of what reactions follow. Unlike conventional grief, which diminishes in intensity with the passage of time, anticipatory grief may increase in intensity as the expected loss becomes more imminent. In some instances, particularly when the occurrence of the loss is delayed, anticipatory grief may be expended, and the inidividual shows fewer manifestations of acute grief when the actual loss occurs. Once anticipatory grief has been expended, it may be difficult for the bereaved to reestablish the prior relationship; this phenomenon is experienced with the return of persons long gone, from combat or concentration camps, and of persons thought to have been dead.

Grief vs Depression.   Both grief and depression may be manifested by sadness, crying, and tension expressed as either psychomotor retardation or psychomotor agitation. Decreased appetite, weight loss, diminished sexual interest, and withdrawal from outside activities are also common to both conditions. As the loss becomes more remote, however, the grief-stricken person shows shifts of mood from sadness to a more normal state and finds increasing enjoyment in life's experiences. Self-blame generally centers on what was done or not done in relation to the lost person, whereas the self-accusation of depressed persons is more likely to involve being bad, worthless, even evil. The general demeanor of a grief-stricken person intuitively elicits sympathy, support, and consolation from others, to which the person shows some responsiveness and appreciation. In contrast, the complaints and laments of the depressed person may irritate and annoy the listener. In normal grief, the response is accepted as appropriate and normal by both the grieving person and others; in depression, the response readily conveys the notion that something is not right about what is going on. People who have experienced previous depressions are more likely to experience depression, rather than normal grief, at the time of a major loss; the person's clinical history, therefore, may be helpful in judging a current reaction. Depressed persons threaten suicide more often than grieving persons who, except in unusual instances—for example, physically dependent and aged persons—do not seriously wish to die even if they claim that life is unbearable. Marked feelings of worthlessness, extended functional impairment, and psychomotor retardation argue more for a major depression than for uncomplicated bereavement.

Psychodynamics

In 1917 Freud wrote, in *Mourning and Melancholia,* that normal grief (mourning) resulted from the withdrawal of the libido from its attachment to the lost object. In mourning, the loss is clearly perceived, but in abnormal grief (melancholia), the lost object is not really given up but is incorporated within the psyche and is the object of ambivalent feelings of love and hate. The negative feelings are now expressed against the self, and the person becomes depressed, develops low self-esteem, feels worthless, and becomes self-accusatory with possible delusional expectations of punishment. Freud's distinction between mourning and melancholia is still considered valid; that is, an exaggerated loss of self-esteem is not part of normal grieving. Other psychoanalytic theorists have stressed the role of unconscious dynamics in grief reactions. The greater the role of unconscious factors (e.g., anger toward the deceased), the more likely is an abnormal grief reaction. Karl Abraham described the introjection of an ambivalently loved lost object and the subsequent direction of anger toward the in-

trojected object. Anger, now expressed against the self because the object and self are indistinguishable, eventually becomes psychologically "metabolized." The end of mourning occurs with the symbolic defecation of the metabolized object.

Uncomplicated grief is viewed as a normal response in light of the predictability of its symptoms and its course. Compelling evidence suggests that during bereavement, the person is in a vulnerable physical state of biological disequilibrium. Clinical evidence and research findings support the hypothesis that bereavement may be a factor in the development of a wide range of physical and emotional disorders, including fatal illness.

Comparisons of close relatives of deceased persons with relatives of living persons (matched for age, sex, and marital status) indicate that bereaved relatives have a much higher mortality rate during the first year of bereavement, the greatest risk being for widowed people. A relationship also has been shown between the place where a person dies and the subsequent mortality of bereaved relatives, e.g. the risk of a close relative dying during the first year of bereavement is significantly greater when the death occurred at some place other than home. Widows during bereavement have a much higher consultation rate for all causes than before the loss of a spouse. Aged persons, in particular, tend to express their reactions in terms of somatic symptoms.

The Physician's Role

The physician has an important role to play in dealing with bereaved spouses, relatives, and friends. First, the physician may have to prepare the family for the possibility that a loved one may die. In the event of the person's death, the physician should encourage the ventilation of feelings. If this emotional expression is inhibited, in all likelihood these feelings will be expressed in a more intense manner at a later date. Outcomes of bereavement are most favorable if the grief-stricken person can interact with others who share or empathize with their feelings of loss. Persons in normal grief seldom seek psychiatric help because they accept their reactions and behavior as appropriate. Accordingly, the attending physician should not routinely recommend that the bereaved see a psychiatrist unless a markedly divergent reaction to the loss is noted. For example, under usual circumstances the bereaved will not make a suicide attempt. Should that occur, psychiatric intervention is indicated. When professional assistance is sought, it usually involves a request for sleeping medication from the family physician. A mild sedative to induce sleep may be useful in these situations; but there is rarely an indication for antidepressant medication or antianxiety agents in normal grief. It can be argued that the bereaved must go through the mourning process, however painful it may be, for successful resolution to occur. To "narcotize" the patient with drugs interferes with a normal process that ultimately can lead to a favorable outcome.

GRIEF MANAGEMENT AND THERAPY

Because grief reactions may develop into depressive reactions or pathological mourning, specific counseling sessions for the bereaved are often of value. Grief therapy is becoming an increasingly important field. In regularly scheduled sessions, the person is encouraged to talk about feelings of loss and about the deceased. Many bereaved persons have difficulty recognizing angry or ambivalent feelings toward the deceased, and it is important that these feelings be expressed.

During grief therapy, an attachment to the therapist usually occurs, which provides the bereaved with temporary support until a new sense of confidence about the future develops. The therapist gradually encourages the patient to take on new responsibilities and develop a sense of autonomy. In order to do grief therapy, the therapist must be comfortable dealing with the issues of death and dying and be able to handle such intense emotional reactions as sadness, anger, guilt and self-denigration. In addition, grief therapy requires that the therapist be active; one must participate in the decision-making process with the patient, especially in those decisions that direct the patient toward greater independence.

Grief therapy need not be conducted only on a one-to-one basis; group counseling can also be effective. Self-help groups have value in certain cases. About 30 percent of widows and widowers report that they become isolated from friends, withdraw from a social life, and thus, experience feelings of isolation and loneliness. The self-help group offers companionship, social contacts, and emotional support, eventually enabling its members to reenter society in a meaningful way.

Bereavement care and grief therapy have been most effective with widows and widowers. The necessity for this type of therapy stems, in part, from the contraction of the family unit. Previously, extended family members were able to provide the needed emotional support and guidance during the mourning period.

Grief in Parents of Deceased or Malformed Infants

Parents react to a child's death or the birth of a malformed infant in stages similar to those described in terminal illness by Kübler-Ross: shock, denial, anger, bargaining, depression, and acceptance. Sudden death is more traumatic than a prolonged death, because anticipatory grief can occur in the latter case. In these instances, a parent may become overprotective toward the child or shower the child with gifts that were previously denied. The physician should have regular contact with the parents and, as in grief therapy described above, allow them to talk about their feelings and about their child. The stress of dealing with the child's death may cause a marriage which has had conflicts to disintegrate. One parent may blame the other for the child's fatal illness, especially if there is some hereditary basis for the disease. The physician should be alert to these patterns of dissention. Some studies indicate that up to 50 percent of marriages in which a child dies or is malformed end in divorce.

THE HOSPICE MOVEMENT

A hospice is a domicile in which care is provided for dying patients; its primary emphasis is on the physical and psychological comfort of the terminally ill. Such care may also be provided in a institution or at home.

The hospice movement began in the early 1960s when Dame Cicely Saunders established a small residential unit to care for the terminally ill. At present, there are about 1,700 such units in the United States. Most hospices are sponsored by hospitals or are affiliated with home health-care agencies; some are approved by Medicare, which reimburses patients for hospice care. A multidisciplinary team approach is used with a staff composed of physicians, psychiatrists, social workers, and trained volunteers.

There are many positive features to the hospice program. A supervised organized routine provides intensive care for both the patient and the family; control of pain is a primary goal, and narcotics are given without the fear of addiction; and finally, group support is provided for the patients, who are not as isolated as they are in general hospitals.

Because attention is given to the bereavement process, hospice care also helps prevent pathological grief reaction from occurring in surviving family members. The *burn-out syndrome*, in which care providers become uninterested and irritable with the terminally ill patient who requires almost constant attention, is rarely seen. If the patient is in home hospice care, visiting nurses provide important relief for overburdened family members.

Medicare pays for hospice care if the patient's doctor states that the patient has a life expectancy of 6 months or less. In one study by C. M. Parkes, however, it was shown that predictions concerning the length of survival for patients referred to a hospice did not correlate with actual length of survival. Doctors were able to state only that patients with incurable cancer would die within a relatively short period of time and could not be more precise.

The hospice movement is in its ascendency, especially since it costs more to keep a terminally ill patient in a general hospital than it does to provide hospice benefits. It is also a more compassionate and humane method for managing preterminal and terminal patients.

References

Bowlby J: *Process of mourning.* Internat J Psychoanalysis *42*:317, 1961.
Freud S: Mourning and melancholia (1917). In *The Standard Edition of the Complete Psychological Works of Sigmund Freud,* vol. 14. Hogarth Press London, 1957.
Gonda T A, Ruark, J E: *Dying Dignified—The Health Professional's Guide to Care.* Addison-Wesley, Menlo Park, CA, 1984.
Kübler-Ross E: *On Death and Dying.* Macmillan, New York, 1969.
Kutscher A, Carr A, Kutscher L, editors: *Principles of Thanatology.* Columbia University Press, New York, 1987.
Leming M R, Dickinson, G E: *Understanding Dying, Death and Bereavement.* Holt, Rinehart and Winston, New York, 1985.
Lindemann E: *Symptomatology and management of acute grief.* Amer J Psychiatry *101*:141, 1945.
Osterweis M, Solomon F, Green M, editors: *Bereavement—Reaction Consequences and Care.* National Academy Press, Washington, DC, 1984.
Parkes C M, Weiss R S: *Recovery from Bereavement.* Basic Books, New York, 1983.
Zisook S, DeVaul, R: *Unresolved grief.* Amer J Psychoanal *45*:370, 1985.

4

The Brain and Behavior

4.1

Neuroanatomy and Neuropsychiatry

GROSS ANATOMY

The central nervous system (CNS) of an adult human consists of the brain and spinal cord. The adult human brain weighs approximately 1350 grams. The peripheral nervous system (PNS) consists of the cranial nerves, spinal nerves, and peripheral ganglia. The PNS brings sensory information to the CNS and conducts motor information from the CNS. Even this simple division of the nervous system into the CNS and PNS is not so straightforward because, for example, the cranial nerves, considered part of the PNS, have their originating nuclei in the CNS. The autonomic nervous system (ANS) innervates the internal organs. Sensory receptors in these peripheral organs also relay information back to the CNS, either directly, via afferent nerves, or indirectly via released hormones (e.g., atriopeptin from the heart). These anatomic connections are central to an understanding of psychosomatic disorders.

In the CNS, gray matter contains the cell bodies while white matter consists mainly of myelinated axons. There are, however, a few neuronal cell bodies in white matter. The three areas of gray matter are cerebral cortex, cerebellar cortex, and the subcortical cerebral and cerebellar nuclei. The right and left cerebral hemispheres are connected by the corpus callosum as well as other smaller commissural tracts. The cerebral cortex itself is heavily folded with gyri (convolutions) and fissures (sulci or grooves). The medulla oblongata, pons, and mesencephalon together make up the brain stem.

Within each cerebral hemisphere, there is a lateral ventricle which is divided into the anterior horn, central part, posterior horn, and temporal horn. Both lateral ventricles are continuous with the third ventricle through the interventricular foramina of Monro. The third ventricle (in the diencephalon) is connected to the fourth ventricle (in the rhombencephalon) through the cerebral aqueduct that courses through the mesencephalon.

The ventricular system is filled with cerebrospinal fluid (CSF). CSF is produced by the choroid plexuses in the lateral ventricles and within the brain parenchyma itself. The CSF leaves the ventricular system via the median aperture of Magendie and the two

lateral apertures of Luschka; it then is absorbed into the venous system through the arachnoid villi. *Hydrocephalus* results from a disorder of CSF drainage, which causes CSF pressure to increase. On computed tomographic (CT) scans, dilated ventricles can indicate its presence. *Normal-pressure hydrocephalus* can present with urinary incontinence, gait disturbances, and dementia. The CSF has a volume of approximately 125 ml in the normal adult; approximately 500 ml is made each day. The total volume of CSF, therefore, is replaced approximately four times each day. Because it reflects neurochemical activity in the brain, the CSF is a source of research information in psychiatry. It should be remembered, however, that metabolites from the spinal cord may significantly contribute to the CSF, and that neurotransmitter metabolites from deep brain structures may not reach the CSF efficiently. When evaluating research data based on CSF measurements, another consideration is the possibility of a rhythmic variation with time (e.g., diurnal) of the chemical being measured.

The brain and spinal cord are covered by the meninges. The dura mater, attached to the inside of the skull, is the strongest of the coverings. Beneath dura mater are arachnoid and pia mater, the latter attached to the brain's surface. Between arachnoid and pia mater is the subarachnoid space that is filled with CSF. A *subdural hematoma* usually results from trauma that tears a vein and causes relatively slow accumulation of blood beneath the dura mater. An *epidural hematoma* usually results from trauma tearing an artery, resulting in a rapid and life-threatening accumulation of blood between the dura mater and the skull. *Meningitis* is an infection and inflammation of one or more of the meningeal layers.

NEURONS AND GLIA

Neurons

The neuron, or nerve cell, is the basic functional unit of the nervous system. There is a large diversity of neuronal types, varying in size, shape, number of incoming and outgoing synapses, and chemistry.

The neuronal cell body is also called the soma or perikaryon. Classically, the two projections from the cell body are the axon and the dendrite. The axon arises from the cell body or from the base of one of the main dendrites. The initial axon segment, the axon hillock, is the actual site of initiation for the action potential in many neurons. The axon hillock is unmyelinated, even if the remainder of the axon is myelinated. The myelin sheath is interrupted over the course of the axon at the nodes of Ranvier. The myelination stops at the distal end of the axon, where the axon may branch and enlarge at its tips. These terminal enlargements are called the axon terminals or boutons and are the sites of presynaptic neurotransmitter release. Within the axon terminals are the synaptic vesicles that contain neurotransmitter substances. There are different types of synaptic vesicles, varying in size, shape, and other characteristics. These different types of vesicles often contain different neurotransmitters and, conceivably, differentially respond to stimulation of the axon terminal.

There may be none, one, or many unmyelinated dendrites emerging from the cell body. Most dendrites receive neurotransmitter messages from an axon. The dendrites usually are profusely branched and studded with small spikes, called dendritic spines, that are the sites of synaptic connection.

Glia

Glia, glial cells, or neuroglia are synonymous terms for a class of nonneuronal cells in the nervous system. There are four types of glial cells in the CNS (astrocytes, oligodendrocytes, ependyma, and microglia) and two types in the PNS (Schwann and satellite cells). The astrocytes provide structural support to neurons and are the major cell type in glial scar tissue in the CNS. The astrocytes also may serve an important role in isolating the receptive surfaces of neurons. The oligodendrocytes, the myelin-forming cells of the CNS, may perform a nurturing role for neurons. Both astrocytes and oligodendrocytes are involved in phagocytosis. The ependyma line the brain ventricles and the central canal of the spinal cord. Their surface is covered with cilia whose beating facilitates the movement of CSF. In addition to their functional support of neurons, glial cells may have a direct and critical role in neuronal activity. Glia contribute to the blood-brain permeability barrier, which is the semipermeable barrier between the blood vessels and brain, so constructed that many chemical compounds are unable to pass from the blood into the brain. The ability of a chemical to pass into the brain is based on its molecular size, electrical charge, solubility, and the presence in the blood-brain barrier of specific transport systems for the compound. The blood-brain permeability barrier also affects the ability of compounds to leave the CNS. The biogenic amine neurotransmitters (e.g., dopamine) are metabolized into acidic metabolites and are removed from the CNS by a transport system in the choroid plexus. The drug probenecid often is used in psychiatric research because it blocks this transport system, causing the buildup of CSF amine metabolites that then can be measured.

CEREBRAL CORTEX

The cerebral cortex contains approximately 70 percent of the neurons in the CNS. The cerebral cortex also is the area of brain that is more developed in humans than in any other animal. Because of these factors, the cerebral cortex has been the main focus of much psychiatric research and theory. Although the cerebral cortex is critically important, many other brain areas also are involved in "higher cognitive functions."

The cerebral cortex receives direct or indirect afferent input from almost every other area of brain. The cortex is reciprocally connected to the thalamus, so it has the potential to modify incoming sensory information. The output of the cerebral cortex is motor activity; it is also involved in the production of thoughts and feelings.

The cerebral cortex can be divided according to a variety of characteristics, including anatomy, cytoarchitecture, and modality. It is divided anatomically into four lobes—frontal, temporal, parietal, and occipital (see Figs. 1, 2). The longitudinal cerebral fissure separates the right and left cerebral hemispheres at the midline. The central sulcus (fissure of Rolando) separates the frontal lobe from parietal lobe. The lateral cerebral sulcus (fissure of Sylvius) marks the superior border of the temporal lobe, demarcating temporal and frontal lobes. The occipital lobe, located at the posterior end of the brain, is separated from the parietal lobe by an imaginary line running down from the parietal-occipital sulcus.

Another way to divide the cerebral cortex is on the basis of cytoarchitecture, the differential arrangement of neuron layers within the cortex. There are six classically defined layers in the cerebral cortex. The presence or absence and relative thickness of each of these layers distinguish different cytoarchitectural areas of the cerebral cortex. Brodmann, in 1909, described 47 different areas of cortex based on cerebral cytoarchitecture (Fig. 3).

Dividing the cerebral cortex by modality produces motor, sensory, and association areas. The primary motor cortex is anterior to the central sulcus in the precentral gyrus (Brodmann's area 4). Anterior to the primary motor cortex are the supplementary motor cortex and premotor cortex (Brodmann's area 6). The primary sensory cortex is modality specific, so the visual primary cortex is along the calcarine fissure in the occipital lobe (Brodmann's area 17), the auditory primary cortex is in Heschl's gyrus in the temporal lobe (Brodmann's areas 41 and 42), and the somatosensory primary cortex is in the postcentral gyrus in the parietal lobe (Brodmann's areas 1, 2, and 3). Sensory association cortex can be unimodal, polymodal, or supramodal. There are three major areas of supramodal association cortex: parietal-temporal-occipital (probably involved in sensory evaluation and language); prefrontal (probably involved in cognitive planning and motor activity), and limbic (probably involved in memory and emotion).

Interhemispheric Connectivity and Laterality

The most obvious gross features of the brain are the two cerebral hemispheres. They are connected via the corpus callosum, anterior commissure, hippocampal commissure, posterior commissure, and habenular commissure. It is believed that only the associational cortex projects information through the commissures.

The "dominant" hemisphere is the one organized to express language. The left hemisphere is dominant in 97 percent of the population, including 99 percent of right-handed persons and approximately 60 percent of left-handed persons. Language dominance is not completely synonymous with hand dominance, and there are a few persons who have mixed dominance for language. Psychological studies of persons with unilateral brain trauma or epileptic lesions have led to many theories about hemispheric functions. In addition to language ability, the left hemisphere has been described as being the rational half of the

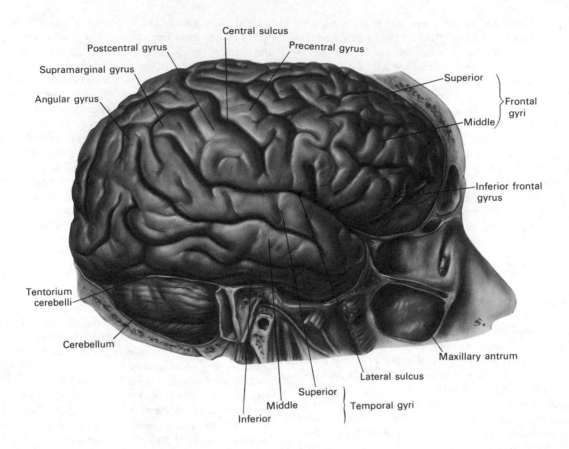

Figure 1. Lateral view of the brain exposed in the skull to show topographical relationships. (From Carpenter M B, Sutin J: *Core Text of Neuroanatomy,* ed 3, p 21. Williams & Wilkins, Baltimore, 1985.)

brain, concerned with analytic, sequencing, abstracting, and logistical abilities. Damage to the left hemisphere, which occurs in strokes, is thought to result in clinical depression more often than is damage to the right hemisphere. The right hemisphere is thought to be more involved with perceptual, visual-spatial, artistic, musical, and synthetic cortical activity. It is involved with both the perception and expression of affective content, including the perception of social cues.

Corpus Callosum Syndromes. Sectioning (i.e., cutting) the posterior portion of the corpus callosum prevents written language, seen by the right hemisphere, from getting to the left-hemisphere language centers and results in *alexia.* Sectioning of the anterior portion of the corpus callosum prevents the right motor and sensory cortices from communicating with the language and praxis areas of the left hemisphere. This results in an inability to write with the left hand, an inability to name unseen objects placed in the left hand, and a generalized *apraxia* of the left hand. Complete sectioning of the corpus callosum has been performed surgically in some patients in an attempt to prevent the spread of seizure activity. Essentially the procedure produces two independent hemispheres. Such patients have been tested by presenting information to only one hemisphere at a time. The test results support the

concepts of differential hemispheric functioning that were derived from clinical studies of patients with trauma and epilepsy.

Frontal Cortex

The frontal lobes can be divided anatomically into superior, middle, and inferior frontal gyri (Figure 1). Functionally, frontal lobes can be divided into motor cortex, premotor cortex, and prefrontal associational cortex. On the medial aspect of frontal cortex (Figure 2), the cingulate gyrus wraps around the corpus callosum and is connected to the amygdala, anterior thalamus, and septum. It receives afferents from the sensory association cortex and projects to the midbrain and to supplementary motor and basal ganglia. The cingulate gyrus is sometimes considered an area of the frontal-limbic cortex.

The functions of cortical areas are deduced from the results of lesions. Table 1 describes major behavioral and psychological symptoms of cortical injury. In general, frontal cortex is involved in motor behavior, expressive language, ability to concentrate and attend, reasoning and thinking, and orientation to time, place, and person. The prefrontal cortex also has a complex involvement in the evaluation of sensory information. It is possible to localize functions to a somewhat specific area of cortex; however, this

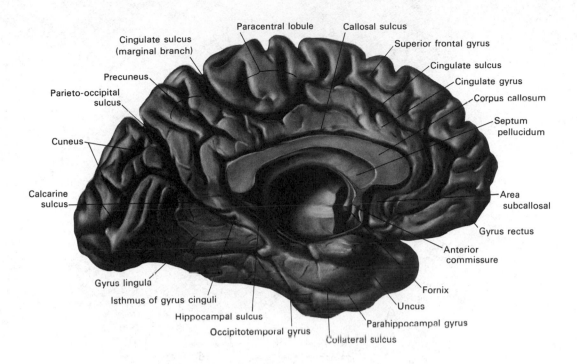

Figure 2. Medial surface of the cerebral hemisphere with diencephalic structures removed. (From Carpenter M B, Sutin J: *Core Text of Neuroanatomy,* ed 3, p 26. Williams & Wilkins, Baltimore, 1985.)

localization does not mean that a specified area of cortex is the only one associated with the function or that it is not involved in other processes within the cerebral cortex. Localization of functions within the cerebral cortex means only that a specific area has a particularly important role in that process.

Two general patterns of symptoms have been related to two different frontal lesions—a *dorsolateral convexity syndrome* and an *orbitomedial syndrome*. The dorsolateral cortex has diverse connections to other cortical and subcortical areas. Afferents are received from sensory association areas of the inferior parietal and temporal cortex as well as from the dorsomedial nucleus of the thalamus. Efferents are reciprocal to afferents and also are sent to hypothalamus, hippocampus, and basal ganglia. Lesions of the dorsolateral prefrontal cortex have produced apathy, decreased drive, poor grooming, psychomotor retardation, decreased attention, and if the dominant hemisphere is affected, aphasia. This syndrome is somewhat similar to so-called negative-symptom schizophrenia, and, indeed, evidence from brain imaging techniques has suggested this area of cortex as a potential lesion site in a subgroup of patients with schizophrenia.

The orbitomedial frontal cortex is closely linked to the limbic system and is reciprocally innervated by the dorsomedial nucleus of the thalamus and amygdala as well as by the frontal lobes. Efferents also project to the rostral brain stem. Lesions of this area of cortex result in withdrawal, fearfulness, lability of mood, explosiveness, loss of inhibitions, and occasional violent outbursts. Some of these patients seem similar to patients with severe bipolar illness.

Temporal Cortex

The lateral aspect of the temporal lobe has three gyri—superior, middle, and inferior (Figure 1). The primary functions of temporal cortex include language, memory, and emotion. Because lesions of the temporal cortex can lead to symptoms resembling those of psychiatric conditions (e.g., hallucinations, delusions, mood disturbances) this area has received particular attention in psychiatric research. The most common causes of temporal lobe lesions are stroke, trauma, and tumor. CNS infections with herpes virus show a particular predilection toward temporal lobes. Bilateral lesions of temporal lobes lead to dementia. Lesions of the dominant temporal lobe lead to euphoria, auditory hallucinations, delusions, thought disorders, decreased ability to learn new material, and poor verbal comprehension. Lesions of the nondominant temporal lobe lead to dysphoria, irritability, and cognitive deficits including decreased visual and musical ability.

Epilepsy. Epilepsy is a disorder characterized by paroxysmal dysfunction of brain tissue, as indicated by synchronous, high-voltage electrical discharges during seizure activity. Some initial positron emission tomography (PET) studies have shown that epileptic foci are hypometabolic interictally. An epileptic focus may be in any cortical area or even subcortical nuclei. Epilepsy is included under the Temporal Cortex heading because complex partial epilepsy (also known as temporal lobe epilepsy or psychomotor epilepsy) is perhaps the most relevant of the epilepsies to psychiatry. It is important, however, for the psychiatrist to consider other types of epilepsy in the differential diagnoses of psychiatric presentations (e.g., focal

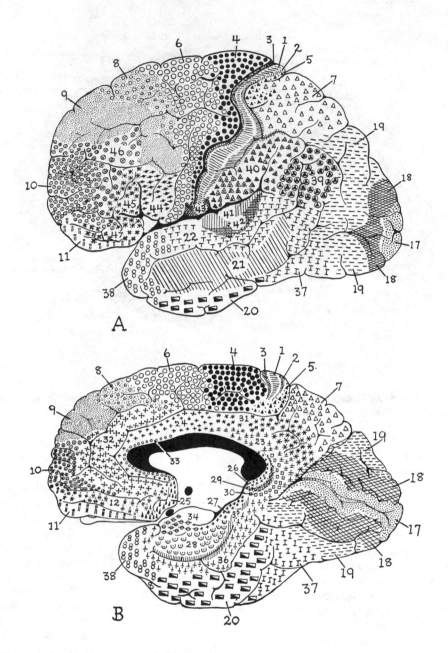

Figure 3. Cytoarchitectural map of the human cerebral cortex. (*A*) Convex surface; (*B*) medial surface (after Brodmann, '09). (From Carpenter M B, Sutin J: *Core Text of Neuroanatomy,* ed 3, p 355. Williams & Wilkins, Baltimore, 1985.)

frontal epilepsy when a patient presents with a thought disorder).

Complex partial epilepsy. There are some notable parallels between complex partial epilepsy (as well as other epilepsies) and psychiatric conditions. Primary complex partial epilepsy is an idiopathic condition, often without demonstrable anatomical or biochemical pathophysiology. Onset is during childhood and early adolescence, and there is a genetic predisposition to its development. Approximately 1 percent of the population have epilepsy, and the disorder has significant psychosocial consequences. Seizure activity is usually not constant, and anticonvulsant medication helps control seizure activity; however, anticonvulsant medications may have adverse side effects that affect behavior and cognition.

Complex partial epilepsy is the most common form of epilepsy in adults, affecting about three in 1,000 persons. A discussion of the phenomenology of complex partial epilepsy can be divided into preictal, ictal, postictal, and interictal events. Preictal events (auras) include autonomic sensations (e.g., fullness in stomach, blushing, changes in respiration), cognitive sensations (e.g., déjà vu, jamais vu, forced thinking, dreamy states), affective states (e.g., fear, panic, depression, elation), and, classically, automatisms (e.g., lip smacking, rubbing, chewing). The ictal event is characterized by brief, disorganized, and inhibited behavior. Violence is very rare during a complex partial epileptic attack. Patients are amnestic for behavior during the seizure. Following the ictus, there is a postictal period of confusion. In patients with complex partial epilepsy, a

Table 1
Major Behavioral and Psychological Symptoms of Cortical Injury

Lobe	Functions	Dysfunctions*
Frontal	-Reciprocally connected with motor, sensory, and emotional brain areas -Controls contralateral movement -Produces speech (dominant hemisphere) -Critical to personality, abstract thinking, memory, concentration, judgment, and other higher mental functions	-Frontal lobe syndrome that may include: inappropriate or uninhibited behavior, irritability and labile affect, depression and flat affect, lack of motivation, difficulty with attention, memory and other cognitive deficits -Peculiar facetious sense of humor (Witzelsucht) -Aphasia (dominant hemisphere) -Ipsilateral motor abnormalities
Temporal	-Memory (especially hippocampus) -Sexual and aggressive behavior -Comprehension of language -Interpretation of gustatory and olfactory sensations -Major component of limbic system	-Memory impairment (bilateral) -Language comprehension -Control of sexual and aggressive drives -Fluent aphasia (dominant hemisphere) -Klüver-Bucy syndrome
Parietal	-Receives and identifies sensory information from tactile receptors -Processes visual and auditory sensations Praxis	-Dominant: Alexia, agraphia, anomia, idiokinetic and kinesthetic apraxias, dyscalculia, anomia, right-left disorientation, astereognosis -Nondominant: Impaired spatial abilities, denial of illness (anosognosia), inability to recognize body parts (autopagnosia), dressing, constructional, and kinesthetic apraxias, astereognosis, left spatial neglect
Occipital	-Interpretation of visual images -Visual memory	-Disturbed spatial orientation (metamorphopsia) -Visual illusions -Visual hallucinations -Blindness -Symptoms may simulate hysteria

*The actual dysfunction is related to the specific area of the lobe that is lesioned.

seizure focus can be found on an electroencephalogram (EEG) in approximately 50 percent of patients. Performing the EEG with both sleep deprivation and sphenoidal or nasopharyngeal leads may increase the percentage slightly.

The major focus of research and clinical concern in complex partial epilepsy has been on interictal neuropsychological changes, which can be mistaken for a psychiatric disorder. Personality changes are evidenced by increased scores on the paranoia and schizophrenia scales of the Minnesota Multiphasic Personality Inventory (MMPI). There is also an increased incidence of dissociative experiences, fugue states, and multiple personality disorders. Other characteristics include hyposexuality, increased religiosity and philosophic interests, and hypergraphia. There may be an increased incidence of interictal violence among patients with complex partial epilepsy. These episodes of violence, however, are often planned and remembered by the patient. Affective changes, particularly depression, have been reported in patients with complex partial epilepsy, and there is an increased incidence of suicide in these patients. Finally, the incidence of schizophrenia-like psychoses is 10 percent to 30 percent. The symptoms often include paranoid delusions and hallucinations, and the risk factors include female sex, left-handedness, the onset of seizures during puberty, and a left-sided lesion. These psychoses do not respond well to anticonvulsants, and neuroleptics often must be used.

Kindling. Kindling is the electrophysiologic process in which repeated subthreshold stimulation of a neuron eventually generates an action potential. At the organ level, repeated subthreshold stimulation of an area of the brain results in the generation of a seizure. The clinical observation that anticonvulsants (e.g., carbamazepine, valproic acid) sometimes are useful in the treatment of mood disorders, particularly bipolar disorder, has given rise to the theory that the pathophysiology of mood disorders may involve kindling in the temporal lobes.

Side Effects of Anticonvulsant Medications. Many psychiatric patients also have epileptic disorders and are treated with both psychotropic drugs and anticonvulsants. The epileptogenesis of psychotropic drugs has been overstated in the past, although reasonable caution is still advised. The neuropsychiatric effects of anticonvulsants, however, have been underemphasized, and most of these drugs are associated with measurable cognitive deficits and lethargy at therapeutic doses.

Parietal Cortex

The gross anatomy of the parietal cortex includes the postcentral gyrus, superior parietal lobule, and inferior parietal lobule (Figures 1 and 2). The inferior parietal lobule includes the supramarginal gyrus and angular gyrus. The parietal lobes contain the associational cortices for visual, tactile, and auditory input, and, therefore, are involved in the intellectual processing of sensory information. The left parietal lobe has a preferential role in verbal processing; the right parietal lobe has a greater role in visual-spatial processing. Gerstmann's syndrome has been attributed to lesions of the dominant parietal lobe; it includes agraphia, calculation difficulties, right-left disorientation, and finger agnosia. Two symptoms of nondominant parietal lesions are denial of illness (known as anosognosia) and neglect of the left side. Classically, a person with a right-sided parietal stroke may deny that he has a paralyzed left arm and also may completely ignore the left side of his body (e.g., not washing it).

Occipital Cortex

The occipital cortex consists of the superior and inferior occipital gyri, as well as the cuneus and lingual gyri (Figure 2). The occipital lobes are the primary sensory cortex for visual input, and the major sign of a lesion in one lobe is impairment on visual field testing. Total destruction of the occipital cortex results in cortical blindness. More subtle dysfunction, however, can result in distortion of images, persistent after-images, and loss of depth perception. Some of these symptoms may be similar to those seen in psychiatric conditions and may cause the clinician to miss the diagnosis of a neurologic disorder of the occipital lobes. *Anton's syndrome* is associated with bilateral occlusion of the posterior cerebral arteries, resulting in cortical blindness and denial of blindness. The occurence of visual hallucinations in patients with occipital epileptic foci has also been reported.

Aphasias. Frontal, parietal, and temporal lobes are involved in the reception and production of language. Aphasias are not only of classic neurologic interest, vis-à-vis localization of cortical function, they also provide some insight into thought disorders of psychiatric patients, which most often present as disorganized speech. Broca's area (anterior or motor speech center) is located in the frontal lobe and controls the production of speech. Lesions of Broca's area leave comprehension unimpaired, but produce a productive aphasia in which the speech is telegraphic and agrammatical. Wernicke's area (posterior or sensory speech center) is located in the temporal lobe and is involved with the comprehension of speech. Lesions of Wernicke's area result in fluent or receptive aphasia, in which the patient cannot understand the spoken word although he has fluent but incoherent speech. Broca's area and Wernicke's area are connected by the arcuate fasciculus. Lesions of the arcuate fasciculus ("conduction" aphasias) result in symptoms resembling Wernicke's aphasia with the addition of an anomia (the inability to name objects) probably due to lesions in the angular or supramarginal gyrus. It is of clinical interest that lithium is sometimes associated with anomic difficulties, even in doses within therapeutic ranges.

Although most attention has been focused on the dominant hemisphere in speech production, regional cerebral blood flow studies have shown increased blood flow to the nondominant hemisphere during speech. The nondominant hemisphere has a parallel role in the prosody of language, the emotional inflections in speech, as it is received and produced. Patients with frontal nondominant lesions are not able to inflect their speech with affect, and patients with posterior nondominant lesions are not able to comprehend the prosody of another person's speech. Other aphasias described in standard neurology texts include transcortical motor, transcortical sensory, mixed transcortical, global, and thalamic aphasia. The language areas serve as a model system of how regions of the brain interact to serve a single function.

AMYGDALA, HIPPOCAMPUS, AND LIMBIC SYSTEM

The amygdala and hippocampus are groups of neurons within the temporal lobe. They are major components of the "limbic system" and have been implicated in the production of memory, emotions, and violent behavior.

Anatomy

Amygdala. The amygdaloid complex is in the dorsomedial portion of the temporal lobe, just anterior to the inferior horn of the lateral ventricle (Figure 4). The amygdala is a heterogeneous structure with a large basolateral group of nuclei and a smaller corticomedial nuclear group. The basolateral group is connected to the cerebral cortex and striatum. Parts of the corticomedial nuclear group are continuous with the olfactory cortex, whereas other parts are connected to the hypothalamus and brain stem. Reciprocal cortical input to the amygdala comes from frontal and temporal sensory association areas as well as from the olfactory bulb and cortex. The principal connections between the amygdala and hypothalamus are the stria terminalis and the ventral amygdaloid fugal projection. The amygdala also connects with the corpus striatum, thereby allowing the limbic system direct access to the motor system. There are connections from the amygdala to the thalamus and also afferent projections from the dopaminergic, noradrenergic, and serotonergic nuclei located in the brain stem.

Hippocampal Formation. The hippocampus lies along the floor and medial wall of the temporal horn of the lateral ventricle. The hippocampal formation consists of the hippocampus, dentate gyrus, and subiculum, a region of temporal cortex. The hippocampus is reciprocally connected to cortical sensory areas via the entorhinal cortex of the parahippocampal gyrus. The hippocampus also sends efferent projections to the septum, anterior thalamus, and hypothalamus.

Limbic System. In 1939, James Papez proposed that a reverberating circuit, consisting of hippocampus, hypothalamus, anterior thalamus, and cingulate gyrus, was the CNS localization for emotions; he referred to this area as the limbic system (also known as Papez circuit). Most current models of the limbic system include the amygdala and septal area. Other neuronatomic areas (Fig. 5) have since been shown to be part of the limbic system. Many parts of the basal ganglia are connected to the limbic system, a fact which helps to explain the simultaneous presence of a movement disorder and an emotional disorder in some patients

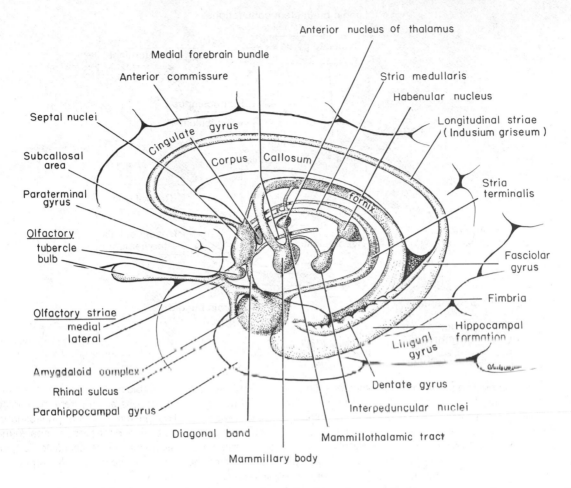

Figure 4. Semischematic drawing showing the anatomic relationships of amygdala, hippocampus, other components of the limbic system, and part of the olfactory pathway. (From Carpenter M B, Sutin J: *Core Text of Neuroanatomy*, ed 3, p 329. Williams & Wilkins, Baltimore, 1985.)

(e.g., Huntington's chorea, psychomotor retardation in depression).

Clinical Considerations

Various parts of the limbic system have been associated with emotions, sex drive, eating behavior, rage, violence, memory, and motivation. The *Klüver-Bucy* syndrome is caused by bilateral destruction of the amygdala and the temporal lobes, and presents with hypersexuality, pica, and great docility. Because there are reciprocal connections between the amygdala and sensory cortex, it is possible that the destruction of the amygdala would disconnect sensory information from affect. The hippocampus is thought to be involved in memory and motivation, although the data supporting this have been questioned. In patients with *Wernicke-Korsakoff's* syndrome (thiamine deficiency often involved with alcoholism), the poor short-term memory may be related to the observed neuropathology in the hippocampal area, including the dentate gyrus.

A connection between violence and the limbic system is suggested by the docility of animals with lesion of the amygdala as well as by animal experiments that have shown rage reactions to amygdalar stimulation. Lesions of the amygdala and anterior temporal lobes have been clinically correlated with a variety of behaviors in humans including symptoms similar to schizophrenia, depression, and mania. In summarizing the vast literature on animal studies, it is reasonable to conclude that the cerebral cortex, limbic system, and brain stem are involved in the production of rage and violence in humans. It is of clinical interest that a history of brain trauma and the presence of abnormal EEGs are very common in populations of violent children and prisoners. As previously discussed, violence is rarely thought to be an ictal event. Violence, rather, may result from a more chronic dysregulation of the pertinent neuroanatomic substrates.

BASAL GANGLIA

It was formerly thought that the basal ganglia were involved simply in the initiation and control of movement. It now seems clear that the basal ganglia are involved in a number of cerebral disorders, including psychosis, depression, and dementia.

Limbic brain stem connections

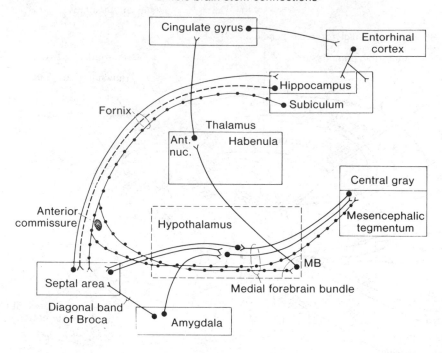

Figure 5. Schematic block diagram of major interconnections of the "limbic system." The limbic system contains structures in thalamus, hypothalamus, brain stem, cerebral cortex, as well as deep brain nuclei. Projections arising from the subiculum (dotted lines) pass via the fornix to the septal area, hypothalamus, and mesencephalic tegmentum. Fibers projecting in the fornix from the hippocampal formation are shown in dashed lines; projections from the septal area to the hippocampal formation are shown in solid lines. Entorhinal cortex (Brodmann's area 28) is the olfactory association area; the septal nuclei lie beneath the septum pellucidum and anterior to the anterior commissure. MB indicates the mamillary bodies. (From Carpenter MB, Sutin J: *Core Text of Neuroanatomy*, ed. 3, p 341. Williams & Wilkins, Baltimore, 1985.)

Anatomy

For most neuroanatomists, the basal ganglia includes the corpus striatum, substantia nigra, subthalamic nucleus, and substantia innominata. The corpus striatum is divisible into striatum and globus pallidum. The striatum consists of caudate nucleus and putamen, which are sometimes grouped together as the lentiform nucleus. The striatum is reciprocally connected to sensory association areas as well as to the limbic system; the globus pallidus is continuous with the pars compacta of the substantia nigra. The pars reticularis of the substantia nigra contains the dopaminergic cells that project to the striatum. Although not considered part of the basal ganglia, the ventral tegmental area is medial to the substantia nigra and contains the dopaminergic neurons that project to the cortex and limbic system. The substantia innominata is a poorly defined group of cells that is related to the amygdala, lateral hypothalamus, and globus pallidus. The basal nucleus of Meynert sometimes is considered part of the substantia innominata. This nucleus contains a group of cholinergic neurons that project to the cortex. It has been suggested that these neurons degenerate into some forms of dementia (e.g., Alzheimer's, Parkinson's, Down's). The subthalamic nucleus is caudal to the substantia nigra, and lesions to this nucleus result in hemiballismus.

Clinical Considerations

The major clinical observation regarding disorders of the basal ganglia is that, in addition to disorders of movement, disorders of thought processes, affect, and cognition are very common. The psychiatric symptoms are as much a result of the organic lesion as are the neurologic symptoms. Basal ganglia disorders are the neurologic disorders most associated with symptoms of psychosis. Untreated schizophrenic patients show many subtle movement disorders (extreme openings and closings of the eyes, flaring of the nares, grimacing and pouting with the mouth, protrusion of the tongue, and shaking of the head) that imply an involvement of the basal ganglia.

Parkinson's Disease. Parkinson's disease is pathologically characterized by destruction of the dopaminergic cells in the substantia nigra. There is also a degeneration of cells in the ventral tegmental area and the locus ceruleus. This degeneration leads to tremor, muscle rigidity, bradykinesia, stooped posture, and a festinating gait. The onset is most often between the ages of 40 and 60 years, and the etiology is usually idiopathic. Parkinson's syndrome can be caused by encephalitis, carbon monoxide poisoning, or head injury. The recent description of Parkinson's disease caused by the ingestion of MPTP (a contaminant of an illicitly made synthetic heroin) has raised the possibility that some forms of idiopathic Parkinson's disease actually may be environmentally induced. The more general implication of this research is that a variety of environmental agents could be toxic to limited neuronal populations. Clinical psychiatrists often are presented with parkinsonian symptoms resulting from the adverse effects of neuroleptics that block the dopaminergic transmission from the substantia nigra to the striatum.

Depression and dementia are more common in Parkinson's patients than would be expected by chance or is explainable by the psychosocial factors of the disorder. The incidence of depression in Parkinson's disease has been reported to be between 50 percent and 90 percent and is more common in males. Consistent with this clinical observation is the hypothesis that there is decreased dopaminergic activity in unipolar depression, and that levodopa, the major treatment for Parkinson's disease, has been reported to elevate mood in normal volunteers. Up to 60 percent of patients on chronic, long-term treatment with levodopa develop serious psychiatric symptoms, including confusion and psychoses. This observation is consistent with a theory of hyperdopaminergic activity in schizophrenia. Dementia is present in 30 percent to 80 percent of Parkinson's disease patients. This dementia may be similar to that seen in Alzheimer's disease, a correlation that is supported by the common presence of basal ganglia–related movement disorders in many patients with Alzheimer's disease.

Huntington's Disease. Huntington's disease is an autosomal-dominant movement disorder with complete penetrance. A recent development in neuropsychiatry is the application of molecular genetic techniques to Huntington's disease. The neuropathology consists of atrophy of the caudate nuclei, which can be visualized by CT in some patients. The peak age of onset is around 40 years, and the disorder is characterized by a deteriorating course of chorea, dementia, depression, and psychosis. Many neurotransmitters have been investigated in this disorder, but the results are still inconclusive. There is, perhaps, an increase in the peptide somatostatin in the caudate and globus pallidus.

Dementia is the presenting symptom in about 10 percent of cases, and at least 90 percent of patients develop dementia during their illness. Depression is the major psychiatric symptom in Huntington's disease (approximately 40 percent of patients), and suicide is a major complication of this disorder. Psychosis is reported in approximately 20 percent of cases, but many other psychiatric disorders have been described.

Wilson's Disease. Wilson's disease, or hepatolenticular degeneration, is an autosomal-recessive disorder resulting in diminished levels of ceruloplasmin, a copper-binding enzyme, and the subsequent deposition of copper in both the liver and the lenticular nuclei. Clinically, this disease results in liver dysfunction and CNS signs, including irritability, depression, psychosis, and dementia. Clinical signs include jaundice, Kayser-Fleischer rings in the cornea, blue "moons" on the fingernails, and a wide flapping tremor of the arms. In addition, such patients often experience rigidity, dysarthria, and dysphagia.

Fahr's Syndrome. Fahr's syndrome, also called idiopathic calcification of the basal ganglia, is a rare hereditary disorder, presenting with a parkinsonian movement disorder, neuropsychiatric symptoms, and calcification of the basal ganglia on CT. There is a bimodal curve for age of onset, patients about age 30 presenting with psychosis that progresses to dementia and patients about age 50 presenting with dementia. This syndrome has a close clinical resemblance to negative-symptom schizophrenia and is

important both in differential diagnosis and theoretical formulations.

Subcortial Dementia. This concept relates to the presence of dementia in the above movement disorders. Previously, dementia had been thought to be pathognomonic for cerebral cortical injury. It is now appreciated that lesions of the basal ganglia often present with dementia that is accompanied by abnormal movements, psychomotor retardation, apathy, and an absence of other cortical signs (e.g., aphasias). In addition to the diseases discussed above, progressive supranuclear palsy and spinocerebellar degeneration may present with subcortical dementia.

HYPOTHALAMUS AND PITUITARY

The hypothalamus and pituitary comprise the "master endocrine gland," thereby functioning as a major integrating and output system for the entire CNS. In addition to its role in endocrine regulation, the hypothalamus often is considered part of the limbic system and is involved in appetite and sexual regulation. Because clinical observations indicate that many endocrine disorders have psychiatric symptoms and that many psychiatric disorders have endocrine dysregulations, psychiatrists have been examining the anatomy of this region carefully. The hypothalamus appears also to have a major role in the control of biological rhythms and immune system regulation.

Anatomy

The hypothalamus is located in the diencephalon, beneath the thalamus and on either side of the third ventricle. Although the hypothalamus contains many nuclear groups, four of these nuclei are of particular relevance to mental functioning—the mamillary bodies of the middle hypothalamic nuclei and the suprachiasmatic, supraoptic, and paraventricular nuclei of the anterior hypothalamic nuclei. For psychiatry, the most important pathways are the fornix, connecting the hippocampal formation with the mamillary bodies, and the stria terminalis and ventral amygdalofugal pathway, connecting the amygdala with the hypothalamus. The mamillothalamic tract connects the mamillary bodies to anterior thalamus. The mesolimbic dopamine pathway, as well as ascending noradrenergic, serotonergic, and cholinergic pathways from the brain stem (the medial forebrain bundle) have terminations in the hypothalamus.

The pituitary (hypophysis) consists of the anterior pituitary (adenohypophysis) and posterior pituitary (neurohypophysis). The supraopticohypophyseal tract contains the axons from the supraoptic and paraventricular nuclei that project to the posterior pituitary, where they release vasopressin and oxytocin into the venous drainage of the posterior pituitary. The ventromedial and infundibular nuclei of the medial hypothalamic nuclei, as well as other basomedial hypothalamic nuclei, project their axons into the pituitary stalk, where they terminate on the capillaries of the hypophyseal portal veins. These nuclei release inhibiting and releasing hormones that control the emission of trophic hormones from the anterior pituitary.

Clinical Considerations

The hypothalamus and pituitary are involved in the regulation of the endocrine and autonomic nervous system and the control of eating behavior, sexual activity, body temperature, and the sleep-wake cycle. Various nuclei of the hypothalamus project sympathetic and parasympathetic nuclei to the brain stem and regulate and coordinate the autonomic nervous system. This hypothalamic involvement in the autonomic nervous system implicates it in psychosomatic disorders. There is extensive synaptic input into the hypothalamus from the amygdala, hippocampus, and brain stem. The hypothalamic regulation of temperature may be the anatomic focus of pathology in neuroleptic malignant syndrome, a life-threatening complication of neuroleptics involving autonomic dysregulation and hyperthermia.

Control of Eating Behavior. Many studies of animals have shown that destruction of the ventromedial hypothalamus results in hyperphagia and obesity, and that destruction of lateral hypothalamus results in anorexia and starvation. These areas of hypothalamus have been called the satiety center and the appetitive center, respectively, and represent relatively high concentrations of pathways relevant to the particular behavior. The limbic system and prefrontal cortex are also involved in eating behavior.

THE THALAMUS

The thalamus develops with and is intimately and reciprocally connected to the cerebral cortex and limbic system. Although once described as merely a "relay station" for sensory information, the thalamus clearly integrates and processes information at a very sophisticated level.

Anatomy

The thalamus is located above the hypothalamus and consists of many nuclei that project to diverse areas. The anterior nucleus receives input through the mamillothalamic tract and projects to the cingulate cortex, thereby being an integral part of the limbic system. The dorsomedial group is reciprocally innervated by the prefrontal cortex and receives input from other thalamic nuclei and the amygdala. The lateral and medial geniculate bodies receive input from visual and auditory pathways, respectively. The ventral nuclei receive input from the basal ganglia and cerebellum and project to the motor cortex. The output of these ventral areas is also affected by converging input from limbic and cerebral cortical structures.

Clinical Considerations

The thalamus is critical in the perception of pain. Pain receptors (nociceptors) in the periphery project to the spinal cord, where they synapse in the dorsal horn and ascend in spinothalamic and spinoreticulothalamic tracts. The ventroposterolateral and ventroposteromedial nuclei serve as focal points for the transmission of this information onto somatosensory cortex (Brodmann's areas 1, 2, and 3) in the parietal cortex. Tumors or vascular lesions of the thalamus can produce severe pain syndromes. Other areas are involved in the control of pain sensation. The periaqueductal region of the midbrain and nucleus raphe magnus of the medulla project onto dorsal horn ascending neurons and can inhibit the transmission of pain sensation to the thalamus. These regions have high concentrations of opiate receptors, and it is likely that the endogenous opioids (e.g., enkephalins, endorphins) are involved as neurotransmitters in this region for the control of pain. Some studies have suggested that release of endorphins in this area is the molecular basis for the therapeutic effects of placebos and acupuncture.

CEREBELLUM

The cerebellum consists of the cerebellar cortex, midline cerebellar vermis, and deep cerebellar nuclei (dentate, emboliform, globose, and fastigial). The cerebellum is involved in the control of movements and postural adjustment. The cerebellum projects reciprocally to the cerebral cortex, limbic system, brain stem, and spinal cord. It is therefore possible that the cerebellum is involved in "higher" mental functions as well. Some recent animal studies have shown that parts of the cerebellum are necessary for the acquisition of conditioned responses. Atrophy of the vermis has been a controversial abnormality on CT in patients with schizophrenia, bipolar disorder, and epilepsy. There are case reports of cerebellar tumors and vascular events presenting as psychiatric disorders.

BRAIN STEM

The brain stem is comprised of the mesencephalon, pons, and medulla oblongata. The most basic functions of this area concern respiration, cardiovascular activity, sleep, and consciousness. This area, however, also is the site of the ascending biogenic amine (dopamine, noradrenalin, serotonin) pathways to higher brain areas. These ascending biogenic amine pathways have been called the medial forebrain bundle.

RETICULAR ACTIVATING SYSTEM

The reticular system is a loosely organized network of neurons coursing up the midline of the brain stem. These neurons receive input from ascending sensory neurons, cerebellum, basal ganglia, hypothalamus, and cerebral cortex, and send projections to the hypothalamus, thalamus, and spinal cord. Stimulation of this area activates the cortex into a state of alert wakefulness. Psychiatric disorders in which motivation and level of arousal are impaired may involve pathology in this region.

BRAIN IMAGING

Brain imaging techniques allow assessment in vivo of structural and functional neuroanatomy. The practice of clinical neurology has been revolutionized by CT and magnetic resonance (MR) imaging of the brain. The pneumoencephalogram now is of historical interest only, and the usefulness of the skull x-ray is largely confined to the assessment of trauma. Computer-analyzed quantitative electroencephalography (QEEG), regional cerebral blood flow (CBF), and positron emission tomography (PET) allow assessment in vivo of CNS function. These techniques, therefore, serve as a technological bridge between neuroanatomy and neurochemistry. Psychiatric research has benefited from these investigational tools, and it is likely that brain imaging techniques will improve the practice of clinical psychiatry.

Computed Tomography

Computed tomography (CT) is based on x-ray technology. X-ray photons are emitted from their source, pass through the tissue being studied, and are detected by a radiographic film. The more a tissue absorbs the x-radiation, the lighter it will appear on the film; the less it absorbs, the darker it will appear. Gray and white matter are indistinguishable on CT scans. In psychiatric research, studies have focused on enlargement of ventricles, cortical atrophy, cerebellar atrophy, reversal of normal brain asymmetries, and brain density measurements. Although the major focus of CT research in psychiatry has been on schizophrenia, brain abnormalities observed with CT have been reported for other psychiatric disorders, including some cases of mood disorders and anorexia nervosa. The specificity of CT abnormalities is not as important, perhaps, as the observation that there is objective CT evidence in some psychiatric patients of a neuropathological process involving loss of brain mass.

Magnetic Resonance Imaging

Magnetic resonance imaging (MRI), previously called nuclear magnetic resonance (NMR) imaging, utilizes magnets and radio waves instead of x-radiation to produce an image. Although still not commonly available in hospitals, MRI has better spatial resolution and more potential applications than CT and is an excellent method for differentiating gray and white matter, visualizing CSF, and estimating the size of ventricles.

Quantitative Electrophysiology

Electroencephalograms (EEGs) and evoked potentials (EPs) are measured by electrodes attached to the scalp. They record the electrical activity in the topmost layers of the cerebral cortex. The frequency, amplitude, and distribution of waveforms on the tracings are the major parameters of EEG interpretation. Visual inspection of an EEG also can reveal paroxysmal events such as epileptic spikes. The major frequency bands of the EEG are delta (<4 Hz), theta ($4-8$ Hz), alpha ($8-13$ Hz), and beta (>13 Hz). Alpha is the rhythm seen in an eyes-closed resting state.

Evoked potentials, also called evoked responses, measure brain activity following discrete stimulation. These include somatosensory evoked potentials (SEPs), visual evoked potentials (VEPs), and auditory evoked potentials (AEPs). These recordings are made by repeatedly presenting the patient with the same stimulation (a flashing light for VEPs, for instance) and measuring the EEG activity for the following second. The resulting EEG records are "averaged" and a relatively smooth tracing of peaks and troughs is obtained.

Computer analysis of EEG and EP data provides a summation of the amount and amplitude of an EEG frequency and gives a graphic representation of wave forms; it produces a topographic map that displays the varying power of an EEG frequency over the surface of the brain. This technique allows researchers to identify particular regions of the brain and specify frequencies of EEG activity that differentiate between groups of patients and groups of control subjects.

Evaluation of Cerebral Blood Flow

The amount of blood flowing to a region of the cortex is positively correlated to the metabolic activity of that region. Xenon[131] is an inert, γ-emitting gas, that, when inhaled by a subject, distributes itself to the blood. When γ-ray detectors are placed in an ordered array over the scalp of the subject, it is possible to measure how much blood is flowing to different parts of the brain. CBF has the advantages of exposing the patient to less radiation than PET and of being less expensive. The technical procedures of CBF testing can be combined with psychological testing during the measurement of blood flow.

Positron Emission Tomography

PET allows assessment of structural and functional CNS information in vivo. Unstable isotopes of drugs and chemicals are made in a cyclotron and are administered to individuals to be tested by PET. The first application of this technology was with radiolabeled 2-deoxyglucose, an analogue of glucose that is taken up by neurons according to their metabolic activity. PET scans of subjects injected with 2-deoxyglucose reflect which areas of the brain are more active. A more recent application of this technology has been to label receptor-binding ligands with positron-emitting isotopes.

References

Chozick B S: The behavioral effects of lesions of the hippocampus: A Review. Internat J Neuroscience 22:63, 1983.

Chozick B S: The behavioral effects of lesions of the amygdala: A review. Internat J Neuroscience 29:205, 1986.

Cummings J L: *Clinical Neuropsychiatry.* Grune & Stratton, Orlando, 1985.

Haber S N: Neurotransmitters in the human and nonhuman primate basal ganglia. Hum Neurobiol 5(3):159, 1986.

Heimer L: *The Human Brain and Spinal Cord.* Springer-Verlag, New York, 1983.

Irwin M, Daniels M, Bloom E T, Smith T L, Weiman H: Life events, depressive symptoms, and immune function. Am J Psych 144(4):437, 1987.

Kuhar M J, Scuza E B, Unnerstall A B, Neurotransmitter receptor mapping by autoradiography and other methods. *Ann Rev Neuroscience* 9:27, 1986.

Morihisa J M, editor: *Brain Imaging in Psychiatry.* American Psychiatric Press, Washington, DC, 1984.

Pincus J M, Tucker G J: *Behavioral Neurology,* 3rd ed. Oxford, New York, 1975.

Riklan M, Levita, E: Psychological studies of thalamic lesions in humans. J Nervous Mental Dis 250:251, 1970.

Schneider J S: Basal ganglia role in behavior: Importance of sensory gating and its relevance to psychiatry. Biol Psychiatry 19:1643, 1984.

Stuss J T, Benson D F: Neuropsychological studies of the frontal lobes. Psycholog Bull 95:3, 1984.

4.2 ————

Neurochemistry and Neurophysiology

INTRODUCTION TO NEUROTRANSMISSION

It is thought that the behavioral effects of most known psychotropic drugs (as well as those of electroconvulsive therapy, [ECT]) are mediated through neurotransmitter receptors that affect neurotransmission. The simplest model of neurotransmission involves a presynaptic neuron that releases a neurotransmitter. The neurotransmitter diffuses across a synaptic cleft and binds to a specific receptor that initiates a series of molecular events in the postsynaptic neuron (Figure 1).

The first step in neurotransmission involves transport of the necessary molecules down the axon to the axon terminal. The axon terminals for biogenic amine neurotransmitters contain mitochondria (energy-supplying organelles) and enzymes involved in the synthesis and the degradation of the neurotransmitter. Some neurons, in contrast, secrete peptide neurotransmitters, which are synthesized in the cell body and transported down the axon. Waste products of neurotransmission are transported back to the cell body, where they are further processed and secreted into the bloodstream.

Once "primed," the axon terminal "waits" until it is signalled by an action potential carried down the axonal membrane. The resulting depolarization of the axon terminal causes calcium ions to enter the nerve terminal through calcium channels. The rise in intraneuronal calcium initiates a series of molecular events causing synaptic vesicles that contain neurotransmitters to migrate toward the neuronal membrane, fuse with the membrane, and release their contents into the synaptic cleft. Once released, the neurotransmitter molecules can diffuse across the synaptic cleft and bind to a postsynaptic receptor. The released neurotransmitter substance is inactivated by diffusing away from the synapse into the extracellular fluid or by active reuptake into the neuron (or a glial cell), followed by degradation by enzymes.

Each neuron receives many synaptic inputs. Some of these synaptic connections may be excitatory, that is, they contribute to the depolarization of the receiving neuron; others may be inhibitory, that is, they hyperpolarize the neuron, thereby increasing the electrical potential difference. The task of the postsynaptic neuron is to integrate multiple incoming signals.

The neuronal cell membrane is a complex regulatory mechanism for the functions of the cell. The membrane is a sea of phospholipids, organized as a bilayer with the hydrophobic ends of the molecules pointing toward each other. Within this lipid bilayer are cholesterol and protein molecules. Some proteins are embedded in the external or internal surface of the membrane. For example, neurotransmitter receptors, proteins that are located on the outside surface of the membrane, transmit their message to another protein (e.g., an enzyme) located on the inside surface of the membrane. Other proteins, such as ion channels, extend the entire width of the membrane. Cholesterol molecules within the membrane tend to keep the lipid molecules relatively fixed and orderly.

SYNAPSES

There is not just one type of synapse. A synapse can be chemical (also called humoral) or electrical. Chemical synapses use a neurotransmitter as the message, whereas electrical synapses (more commonly called gap junctions) use electric current (i.e., a flow of charged ions). Some synapses, called conjoint synapses, use both messages.

The most conventional types of synapses are the axodendritic and axosomatic synapses, in which the axon of the presynaptic neuron synapses with a dendrite or the cell body of the postsynaptic neuron. In axoaxonic synapses, the presynaptic axon synapses with

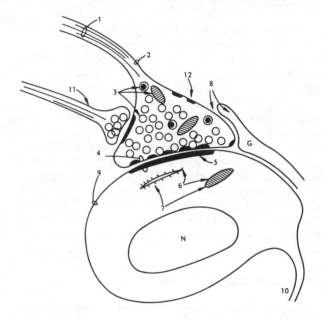

Figure 1. Twelve steps in the synaptic transmission process are indicated in this idealized synaptic connection. Step 1 is transport down the axon along microtubules. Step 2 involves the electrically excitable membrane of the axon. Step 3 involves the synthesis and storing of the neurotransmitter. Step 4 includes the actual release and reuptake of the neurotransmitter. Step 5 is the postsynaptic receptor that triggers the response of the postsynaptic cell to the transmitter. Step 6 shows the organelles within the postsynaptic cells which respond to the receptor trigger. Step 7 is the interaction between genetic expression of the postsynaptic nerve cell and the cytoplasmic organelles that respond to neurotransmitter action. Step 8 includes the enzymes present in the extracellular space and within glia for catabolizing excess neurotransmitter released from the nerve terminals. Step 9 includes the electrical portion of the nerve cell membrane which, in response to various neurotransmitters, is able to integrate the postsynaptic potentials. Step 10 is the continuation of the information transmission by which the postsynaptic cell sends information to its cell body. Step 11 indicates that the release of neurotransmitter is subjected to modification by a presynaptic (axo-axonic) synapse. Step 12 indicates presynaptic autoreceptors that respond to the neurotransmitter released by the neuron itself. (Modified from Cooper J R, Bloom F E, Roth R H: *The Biochemical Basis of Neuropharmacology*, ed 5, p 42. Oxford University Press, New York, 1986.)

the axon hillock or axon terminal of the postsynaptic neuron. Two recently identified synapses are dendrodendritic and dendroaxonic. Both types probably are involved in local modulation of synaptic function and do not elicit postsynaptic action potentials. (To complicate matters, "nonsynaptic" neurons probably exist, as well. These neurons have axon terminals that release neurotransmitters into the extracellular fluid or the cerebrospinal fluid and, therefore, do not have synapses with specific neurons.)

NEUROMESSENGERS

"Neuromessenger" is a generic term for neurotransmitters, neuromodulators, and neurohormones. *Neurotransmitters* are the classic neuromessengers that are released rapidly by the presynaptic neuron, diffuse across the synaptic cleft, and have either an excitatory or inhibitory effect on a postsynaptic neuron. *Neuromodulators* also bind to specific receptors but are conceptualized as "tuning" or "grading" the response of the postsynaptic cell to the neurotransmitter. *Neurohormones* are chemical messengers released by neurons into the bloodstream.

There are three classes of neurotransmitters—biogenic amines, amino acids, and peptides (Figure 2). The biogenic amines (monoamines) consist of three catecholamines (dopamine, norepinephrine, and epinephrine), an indoleamine (serotonin), a quaternary amine (acetylcholine), and an ethylamine (histamine). The biogenic amines account only for 5 percent to 10 percent of the synapses of the human brain, whereas the amino acid neurotransmitters may account for up to 60 percent of the synapses.

Dale's law states that the same neurotransmitter is released by all processes of a single neuron. This law now includes the fact that a single neuron can contain more than one neurotransmitter. This observation is referred to as the *coexistence of neurotransmitters*. For example, a neuron may contain a biogenic amine neurotransmitter as well as a peptide neurotransmitter.

Receptors

Receptors are proteins in the neuronal membrane that are in part exposed to the extracellular fluid and specifically recognize neuromessengers. Receptors may be postsynaptic or presynaptic. In an axodendritic synapse, for example, the receptors on the receiving dendrite are postsynaptic. The receptors on the axon itself are presynaptic. They are called presynaptic autoreceptors if they bind a neurotransmitter that their parent neuron releases, or they are called presynaptic heteroreceptors if they bind a neurotransmitter released by some other neuron.

The concepts of supersensitivity and subsensitivity are applied to receptors. These properties signify that a specific neuron is more or less sensitive, respectively, to a constant amount of neurotransmitter. Such regulation of a synaptic response could involve three receptor-related changes. First, the number of receptors available for neurotransmitter binding could increase or decrease. Second, the affinity of

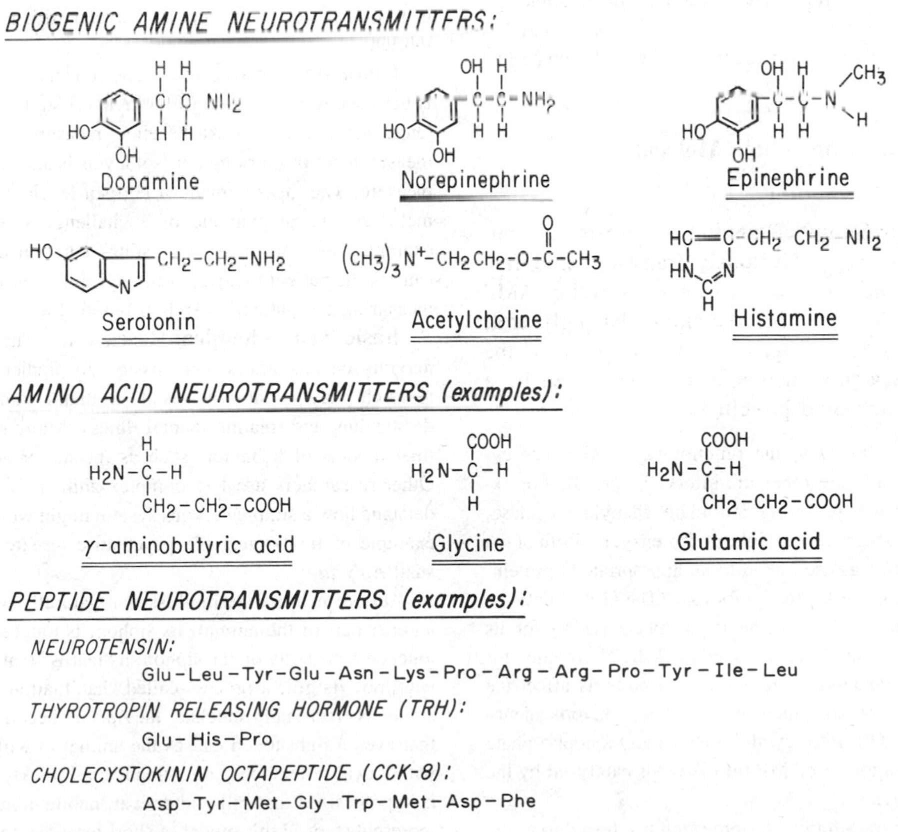

Figure 2. The three classes of neurotransmitters.

the receptor could increase or decrease. Third, the mechanism by which the receptor translates its message into the neuron could be more or less efficient. All three of these changes are examples of neuronal plasticity.

The evolution of the receptor message into an intraneuronal biological response involves translating the first message (e.g., the neuromessenger, hormone, or nerve impulse) into a second message (e.g., cAMP, cGMP, calcium ion). As part of the receptor protein or, more frequently, as a second protein in the membrane, there is an "effector" component to the receptor complex. This effector is either an enzyme or an ion channel. When a receptor is stimulated, it can then, for example, activate adenylate cyclase to produce cAMP or open chloride channels to change the neuronal electric potential. In many receptor complexes there is a modulator component (e.g., G-protein) intercalated between the receptor and effector components. The modulator component may bind a neuromodulator or other molecule that affects its functioning. The interactions of these three components involve changes in the shapes of the proteins and movement of the proteins within the neuronal membrane.

Receptor research has contributed significantly to the explosion of knowledge about neurotransmitters, particularly peptide neurotransmitters. Starting with a known ligand (e.g., heroin), it is possible to demonstrate the presence of specific and saturable receptors in human tissue. Once a receptor has been identified, one can hypothesize that endogenous substances exist to activate that receptor. Furthermore, these endogenous compounds may be *agonists* (excitatory to the receptor) or *antagonists* (inhibitory to the receptor). This type of research has demonstrated, for example, the presence of benzodiazepine binding sites in the brain and has motivated the exploration for endogeneous benzodiazepine-like compounds.

Interneuronal Neurotransmitter Molecular Biochemistry

Researchers' current understanding is that first messengers (e.g., dopamine) are variously translated into five different intracellular *second messengers*—cyclic AMP (cAMP), cyclic GMP (cGMP), calcium, diacylglycerol, and inositol triphosphate (Figure 3). In many cases, the third messenger is a protein that is phosphorylated by a second messenger-activated protein kinase.

Two receptors are linked to the functioning of adenylate cyclase, one excitatory and the other inhibitory (Figure 3). For example, dopamine type-1 receptors stimulate adenylate cyclase, whereas dopamine type-2 receptors inhibit this enzyme. Both of the dopamine receptor proteins are linked to an appropriate G protein, either G_s for stimulation or G_i for inhibition. (The G protein is so named because it requires guanosine triphosphate [GTP] for its actions. G proteins are sometimes referred to as the N proteins, for nucleotide-binding regulatory protein.) The G proteins affect the activity of adenylate cyclase, which, when active, converts adenosine triphosphate (ATP) into cyclic adenosine monophosphate (cAMP). The deactivation of cAMP into AMP is catalyzed by the enzyme phosphodiesterase.

The second major transducing system often is referred to as the phosphatidyl inositol system (Figure 3). This system is currently known to have only a stimulatory receptor. The receptor acts through a G protein to stimulate an enzyme (a phosphodiesterase) that converts phosphatidylinositol 4, 5-biphosphate (PIP_2) into diacylglycerol (DG) and inositol triphosphate (IP_3). IP_3 causes an increase in the concentration of calcium ions within the neuron, probably by inducing the release of Ca^{2+} from smooth endoplasmic reticulum. Both DG and IP_3 are metabolized quickly within the neuron. IP_3 is converted back into PIP_2 through a series of enzymatic steps, the last of which involves the enzyme inositol-1-phosphatase; this enzyme is inhibited by lithium, thereby limiting the amount of PIP_2 available for signal transduction.

Many proteins in the neuron exist in two states—active and inactive. Research suggests that a major mechanism for switching proteins "on and off" is protein phosphorylation. Two classes of enzymes, protein kinases and phosphatases, respectively, put on and remove a phosphate group from a protein molecule. The protein kinases themselves are activated by second messengers.

Research Approaches to Neurotransmission in Neuropsychiatry

Assessing Neurotransmission in Disease States. The most common approach to assessing neurotransmission status in disease states is to measure one of the following variables: neurotransmitter synthesizing enzymes, neurotransmitters, or neurotransmitter metabolites. These substances can be measured in patients by collecting blood, urine, or CSF. A variation of this same research methodology is to measure neurotransmitter receptor number and affinity in patients' nonneuronal tissue such as platelets or white blood cells. These measures provide a first approximation of neurotransmitter status in the CNS. It also is possible to measure neurotransmitter and receptor characteristics in brain tissue post-mortem.

Challenge Strategies. The concept of challenge strategies is germane to many areas of biologic research in psychiatry. Challenge strategies contrast baseline measures. For instance, the measurement of morning cortisol levels is an example of a baseline measure. The measurement of cortisol levels in response to dexamethasone is an example of a challenge strategy. For another example, one can measure "resting" cerebral blood flow, or one can ask the patient to do a psychological test as a "challenge" while measuring the patient's cerebral blood flow.

Basic Neurochemical Research. The complexity of the nervous system makes it impossible to predict which avenues of research may eventually result in major clinical gains in understanding and treating mental illness. Many researchers use animal models of behavior, such as the motor activity of rodents. Other researchers use less complex animals in an attempt to understand how a simple nervous system might work. The best known example of this strategy in psychiatric research involves the sea snail *Aplysia*.

Aplysia is a marine mollusk that naturally withdraws its gill if another part of the animal, its siphon, is touched. If the animal is touched repeatedly on the siphon, it "learns" that it does not have to withdraw its gill, a process called "habituation." If, however, the siphon is electrically shocked, the *Aplysia* becomes "sensitized," so that even a light touch causes the animal to withdraw its gill; this withdrawal reflex does not extinguish as quickly as it did before. It is hypothesized that gill withdrawal, habituation, and sensitization represent steps in this model of short-term memory. Both sensitization and habituation are correlated with changes (i.e., plasticity) in the amount of neurotransmitter released from specific neurons.

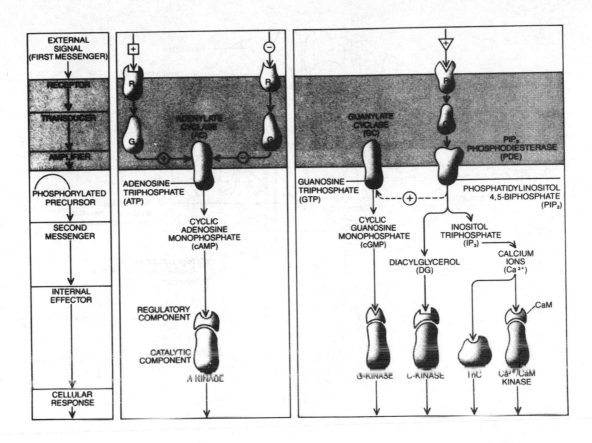

Figure 3. Known signal pathways in cells are few in number. In functional terms they share a sequence of events *(left)*. External messengers arriving at receptor molecules in the plasma membrane *(gray)* activate a closely related family of transducer molecules, which carry signals through the membrane, and amplifier enzymes, which activate internal signals carried by "second messengers." The pathway employing the second messenger cAMP (middle) has stimulatory (R_S) and inhibitory receptors (R_i), which both communicate with the amplifier adenylate cyclase (AC) by way of stimulatory or inhibitory transducers called G proteins because they require guanosine triphosphate (GTP) to function. Adenylate cyclase converts ATP into cAMP. The other major pathway (right) is not known to recognize inhibitory external signals. It employs a stimulatory G protein to activate its amplifier, a phosphodiesterase (PDE) enzyme. The enzyme converts phosphatidylinositol 4,5-biphosphate (PIP_2) into a pair of second messengers, diacylglycerol (DG) and inositol triphosphate (IP_3). In turn, IP_3 induces the cell to mobilize still another messenger, calcium ions (Ca^{2+}). Moreover, the pathway somehow induces the amplifier guanylate cyclase (GC) to convert GTP into the second messenger cyclic guanosine monophosphate (cGMP). In general, the second messengers bind to the regulatory component of a protein kinase, a class of enzymes that activate a cellular response by adding phosphate (PO_4) groups to particular proteins. Calcium binds to a family of proteins including calmodulin (CaM) and troponin C (TnC). In turn, CaM activates a protein kinase; TnC stimulates muscle contraction directly. (From Berridge M J: The molecular basis of communication within cells. Sci Am *253*:142, 1985.)

Dopamine

CNS Dopaminergic Tracts. There are three dopaminergic tracts of relevance to neuropsychiatry (see Fig. 4). The neurons of the nigrostriatal tract have their cell bodies in the pars compacta of the substantia nigra and project their axons to the corpus striatum. This tract is involved in the initiation and coordination of movement; in Parkinson's disease it degenerates. Parkinsonian side effects of antipsychotics are caused by blockade of postsynaptic dopamine receptors receiving input from this tract.

The tuberoinfundibular tract has its cell bodies in the arcuate nucleus and periventricular area of the hypothalamus and projects to the infundibulum and anterior pituitary. Dopamine acts as a release inhibiting factor in this tract by inhibiting the release of prolactin from the anterior pituitary. Patients who take antipsychotic drugs have elevated prolactin levels because the block-

ade of dopamine receptors eliminates these inhibitory effects of dopamine.

The mesolimbic-mesocortical tract has its cell bodies in the ventral tegmental area and projects its axons widely to the neocortex and limbic system. It is tempting to assign a role in emotional expression to this tract because of its projection to the neocortex and limbic system, brain areas thought to be involved in complex behavior.

The Dopaminergic Synapse. The dopaminergic terminal requires tyrosine for the production of dopamine. Tyrosine is converted to 3,4-dihydroxyphenylalanine (DOPA) by tyrosine hydroxylase. Tyrosine hydroxylase is the rate-limiting enzyme for the synthesis of dopamine and is under regulatory control by protein kinases. DOPA is converted into dopamine by an aromatic amino acid de-

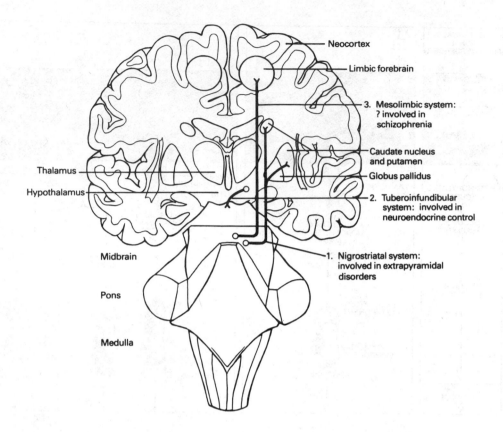

Figure 4. CNS dopaminergic tracts. (From Sachar E J: Disorders of thought: The schizophrenic syndromes. In *Principles of Neural Science*, ed 2, E R Kandel, J H Schwartz, editors, p 713. Elsevier, New York, 1985, by permission.)

carboxylase. Dopamine is then taken up and stored in vesicles. Reserpine interferes with the uptake and storage of dopamine in synaptic vesicles. Upon stimulation, the dopaminergic neuron releases dopamine into the synaptic cleft. Although it was thought that amphetamine primarily induced the release of dopamine, it is now known that the major effect of amphetamine is to block the reuptake of dopamine and norepinephrine.

Once in the synaptic cleft, dopamine interacts with presynaptic and postsynaptic dopamine receptors. Dopamine dissociates from the receptor and is actively taken back up into the presynaptic neuron. Free dopamine in the presynaptic neuron is metabolized by monoamine oxidase (MAO), which is located in mitochondria. (There are two types of MAO in the CNS—MAO_A, which selectively metabolizes norepinephrine and serotonin and MAO_B, which more selectively metabolizes dopamine.) MAO metabolism of dopamine produces DOPAC, which is further metabolized by catechol-o-methyltransferase (COMT) to produce homovanillic acid (HVA). Dopamine also may be metabolized, in reverse order, by COMT and MAO in the synaptic cleft. HVA is the dopamine metabolite that is most often measured in psychiatric research.

Dopamine Receptors. D_1 receptors stimulate adenylate cyclase, and D_2 receptors inhibit adenylate cyclase. Both D_1 and D_2 receptors are located on postsynaptic neurons. The clinical potency of neuroleptics is most closely correlated with their binding affinity to D_2 receptors. D_2 receptors are the only type of dopamine receptor found in the pituitary. D_2 receptors are also located presynaptically where they function to down-regulate the amount of dopamine synthesized within the axon terminal. Presynaptic D_2 receptors do not exist in the tuberoinfundibular pathway or the

mesocortical pathway. It has been suggested that the absence of these D_2 autoreceptors in the mesocortical pathway is the neurochemical basis for the clinical observation that tolerance does not develop to the antipsychotic effects of these drugs.

Dopamine and Antipsychotics. Both the clinical effects and the adverse effects of antipsychotics result from the blockade of dopaminergic receptors. There is a time delay between the blockade of dopamine receptors and the development of maximal clinical antipsychotic activity, although the biochemical explanation for this delay is currently unknown. The parkinsonian and other adverse motor system effects of antipsychotics relate to their blockade of dopaminergic neurotransmission, presumably in the nigrostriatal tract. Tardive dyskinesia has been hypothesized to result from a compensatory development of supersensitive postsynaptic dopamine receptors following chronic blockade.

Dopamine and Psychopathology

The dopamine hypothesis of schizophrenia. The dopamine hypothesis of schizophrenia states that the symptoms of schizophrenia are caused by hyperactivity of the dopaminergic system. The major evidence for this hypothesis is the clinical efficacy of dopamine blocking agents, such as the phenothiazines, in the treatment of schizophrenia. The two main problems with this hypothesis are (1) antipsychotics are clinically effective in treating almost all agitated and psychotic states, regardless of whether they are related to schizophrenia, and (2) other biochemical evidence supporting a dopaminergic overactivity in schizophrenia (e.g., measurement of dopamine metabolites or receptors) has not been consistently supportive of the hypothesis.

Dopamine and mood disorders. It has been hypothesized that some patients with mania may have dopaminergic overactivity, and that some patients with depression may have dopaminergic hypoactivity. This hypothesis is supported by some clinical observations. Parkinson's patients receiving L-dopa, a precursor of dopamine, have been reported to become hypomanic, and, in fact, L-dopa has been reported to be useful in treating retarded depressions. There also have been reports of state-related tardive dyskinesia that worsens when a patient is depressed (presumably with low dopamine) and improves during mania (presumably with high dopamine). Biochemical evidence has demonstrated that dopamine metabolites are elevated in some manics and decreased in some depressed patients.

Norepinephrine and Epinephrine

CNS Noradrenergic Tracts. The largest population of noradrenergic neurons in a single identified location is the locus ceruleus in the pons (Figure 5). The axons of these neurons, along with the axons of more loosely scattered noradrenergic neurons in the brain stem, ascend in the medial forebrain bundle to the cerebral cortex, limbic system, thalamus, and hypothalamus. Some evidence exists that the more ventral pathways ascend into the lateral hypothalamus and may regulate affect, whereas the more dorsal pathways ascend to the cerebral cortex and are involved with attention and alertness. Noradrenergic pathways also descend in the

spinal cord from these neurons. Adrenergic (epinephrine-containing) neurons are much rarer and less well studied than noradrenergic neurons.

The Noradrenergic (Adrenergic) Synapse. The noradrenergic terminal uses the same enzymes to make dopamine as the dopaminergic neuron. The noradrenergic neuron, however, has dopamine-β-carboxylase that converts dopamine into norepinephrine. Norepinephrine is converted to epinephrine by phenylethanolamine-N-methyltransferase (PNMT) in adrenergic neurons. Noradrenaline is taken up and stored in synaptic vesicles, a process that is blocked by reserpine. Norepinephrine is released when the synaptic vesicle fuses with the presynaptic membrane. Once in the synaptic cleft, norepinephrine interacts with noradrenergic receptors. The metabolic steps for norepinephrine are similar to those for dopamine; the most significant metabolic product from CNS norepinephrine is 3-methoxy-4-hydroxyphenylglycol (MHPG).

Noradrenergic Receptors. The two classes of noradrenergic receptors are α and β, each of which has two subtypes. Alpha$_1$ receptors are postsynaptic, and α_2 receptors are thought to be mainly presynaptic. It is useful clinically to know that presynaptic α_2 receptors are more sensitive to α-adrenergic agonists than are postsynaptic α_1 receptors. β_1 and β_2 receptors are located postsynaptically and also may be located presynaptically. It is currently believed that postsynaptic β receptors are the primary receptors for locus ceruleus input.

Norepinephrine and Psychotropics. Both the tricyclic antidepressants (TCAs) and the monoamine oxidase inhibitors (MAOIs) affect the noradrenergic system. The

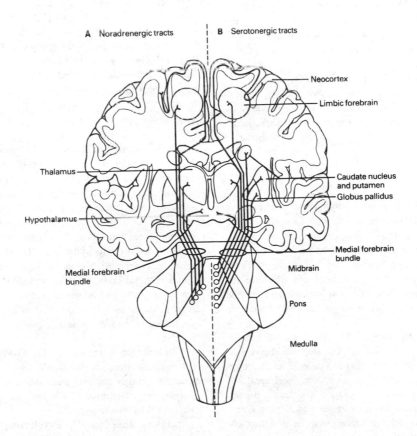

A Noradrenergic tracts   **B** Serotonergic tracts

Neocortex
Limbic forebrain
Thalamus
Caudate nucleus and putamen
Globus pallidus
Hypothalamus
Medial forebrain bundle
Medial forebrain bundle
Midbrain
Pons
Medulla

Figure 5. CNS ascending noradrenergic (*A*) and serotonergic (*B*) tracts. (From Sachar E J: Disorders of feeling: affective diseases. In *Principles of Neural Science*, ed 2, E R Kandel, J H Schwartz, editors, p 721. Elsevier, New York, 1985, by permission.)

acute effect of TCAs is to block reuptake of norepinephrine and serotonin; the acute effect of MAOIs is to block the metabolism of norepinephrine and serotonin. Thus, both antidepressants acutely increase the concentration of these biogenic amines in the synaptic cleft. The acute effects of both antidepressants (but especially the tertiary TCAs—doxepin, amitriptyline, and imipramine) include the blockade of α_1 receptors, causing sedation and postural hypotension. Blockade of α_1 receptors by antipsychotics also produces these side effects. A unique side effect of MAOIs occurs when a patient being treated with this drug eats tyramine-rich food, thereby promoting an adrenergic surge that can result in a life-threatening hypertensive crisis.

Two other drugs of interest are clonidine and propranolol. Clonidine is an alpha-agonist, which selectively stimulates presynaptic α_2 receptors. Clonidine has been used with partial success in a variety of neuropsychiatric disorders, including opiate withdrawal. Propranolol is one of a class of β-blocking drugs; in addition to being antihypertensive, these drugs have been reported to be clinically useful in treating lithium-induced tremor and social phobias.

Norepinephrine and Mood Disorders. The major hypothesis regarding norepinephrine is the monoamine hypothesis of mood disorders, which states that depression is the result of too little noradrenergic and/or serotonergic activity and that this activity is increased by TCAs and MAOIs. There are three major problems with this original hypothesis: (1) there is a three- to four-week delay between the acute biochemical effects of increasing synaptic norepinephrine and serotonin and the clinical effect of reduced depression; (2) there are drugs that are potent reuptake blockers (e.g., cocaine) that are not effective antidepressants; and (3) newly developed antidepressants that have no reuptake blockade activity or MAOI–like activity are clinically effective as antidepressants. The most recent theory is that the therapeutic effect of all antidepressant treatments (TCAs, MAOIs, ECT, sleep deprivation) is produced by a decrease in the number of postsynaptic β receptors and decreased responsiveness of serotonin receptors. These receptor changes are seen approximately 3 weeks after initiation of treatment, thereby correlating with the time course of clinical improvement.

Serotonin

CNS Serotonergic Tracts. Serotonergic neurons have their cell bodies in the upper pons and midbrain, specifically, the median and dorsal raphe nuclei, caudal locus ceruleus, area postrema, and interpeduncular area. These neurons project to the basal ganglia, limbic system, and cerebral cortex (Figure 5). These neurons also project down the spinal cord and modulate the transmission of sensory pain input. These spinal cord tracts may be the site of action for serotonergic antidepressants that have been used to control pain.

The Serotonergic Synapse. The serotonergic terminal is similar to those of the catecholamines. The amino acid precursor tryptophan is converted into serotonin (also called 5-hydroxytryptamine) by tryptophan hydroxylase and an amino acid decarboxylase. The serotonin is stored in synaptic vesicles, a process that is blocked by reserpine. Serotonin is released into the synaptic cleft upon synaptic stimulation. Once inside the synaptic cleft, serotonin binds to serotonergic receptors. The major mechanism of deactivation of serotonin is reuptake into the presynaptic

terminals. Serotonin is metabolized by MAO (preferentially type A) to 5-hydroxyindoleacetic acid (5-HIAA).

Serotonergic Receptors. S_1 and S_2 receptors are differentiated primarily by the relative selectivity of S_1 receptors for serotonin and S_2 receptors for spiperone (an antipsychotic). Both receptor types respond to serotonin in vivo. It appears that S_1 receptors mediate the inhibitory actions of serotonin, while S_2 receptors are excitatory. S_1 receptors have been further subtyped into S_{1A}, which may function as serotonergic autoreceptors, and S_{1B}. Some serotonergic receptors stimulate adenylate cyclase, and others appear to act through the phosphatidyl inositol system.

Serotonin and Psychotropics. Catecholamines and serotonin are interrelated. Antidepressants, for example, affect both noradrenergic and serotonergic synapses. Most tricyclic antidepressants (except desipramine) acutely block serotonin reuptake and chronically (after about three weeks) down-regulate postsynaptic serotonin receptors. L-tryptophan affects the serotonergic system by supplying more of the amino acid precursor, thereby pushing the pathway to synthesize more serotonin. L-tryptophan has been used both as a hypnotic and as an antidepressant.

Serotonin and Psychopathology. Serotonin has been implicated in mood disorders, anxiety, violence, and schizophrenia. The acute effects of TCAs and MAOIs to increase the availability of serotonin (and norepinephrine) in the synaptic cleft led to the inclusion of serotonin in the monoamine hypothesis of mood disorders. Imipramine binding sites (a neurochemical label of serotonin reuptake sites) in platelets have been reported to be decreased in depressed patients and in the postmortem brains of patients who committed suicide. The involvement of serotonin in violence is supported by findings of decreased concentrations of CSF 5-HIAA in patients with anxiety disorders and suicide attempts. The major reason to suspect dysregulation of serotonin in schizophrenia was data that suggested the serotonergic synapse was the primary site of action for lysergic acid diethylamide (LSD). Both the complexity of the biochemical actions of LSD and the dissimilarity between LSD-induced and schizophrenic symptoms argue against this hypothesis.

Acetylcholine

CNS Cholinergic Tracts. In humans, there is a group of cholinergic neurons in the nucleus basalis of Meynert that projects to the cerebral cortex and limbic system. These neurons degenerate in dementing conditions, including Alzheimer's disease, Down's syndrome, and Parkinson's disease. There also is a group of cholinergic neurons in the reticular system that project to the cerebral cortex, limbic system, hypothalamus, and thalamus.

The Cholinergic Synapse. The cholinergic terminal synthesizes acetylcholine from acetyl-CoA and choline with the enzyme acetyltransferase. Once acetylcholine is released, it interacts with its receptors and is then degraded to choline and acetate by acetylcholinesterase. The choline is taken back up into the presynaptic nerve terminal where it can be resynthesized into acetylcholine.

Cholinergic Receptors. The two types of cholinergic receptors are nicotinic and muscarinic, based on their selective preference for nicotinic and muscarinic drugs, respectively. Muscarinic receptors are antagonized by atropine, and nicotinic receptors are antagonized by d-tubocurarine.

Acetylcholine and Psychotropics. Anticholinergic drugs are used to treat the parkinsonian side effects of antipsychotics. Many psychotropics (especially low-potency antipsychotics and tricyclic antidepressants) block muscarinic receptors, thereby causing the side effects of blurred vision, dry mouth, constipation, and difficulty initiating urination. Excessive blockade of CNS cholinergic receptors causes confusion and delirium. This condition is seen when patients take illicit drugs laced with scopolamine or when a patient is treated simultaneously with too many drugs with anticholinergic effects (e.g., thioridazine, amitriptyline, and benztropine).

Acetylcholine and Psychopathology. Cholinergic pathophysiology has been implicated in movement disorders (e.g., Parkinson's disease, Huntington's disease, and tardive dyskinesia) because of the effectiveness of cholinergic agents in treating some of these conditions. The degeneration of cholinergic neurons in the nucleus basalis of Meynert has prompted the hypothesis that such degeneration is a specific pathology for dementia. Acetylcholine has been implicated in the pathophysiology of mood and sleep disorders, with an overactivity of cholinergic pathways suggested in depression. Myasthenia gravis is an autoimmune disorder in which the body selectively destroys peripheral muscarinic receptors. The autoimmune destruction of a specific subclass of receptors should be considered as a possible pathophysiologic mechanism for some psychiatric disorders.

Histamine

Histaminergic cells are found in the hypothalamus and project to the cerebral cortex, limbic system, and thalamus. Histamine receptors are divided into two classes. H_1 receptors act through adenylate cyclase, guanylate cyclase, and phosphatidyl inositol H_1 receptor blockade is the mechanism of action for allergy medications and also contributes to the psychotropic-induced side effects of sedation, weight gain, and hypotension. H_2 receptors activate adenylate cyclase. Doxepin, a tricyclic antidepressant, is a powerful blocker of histamine receptors and has been used, like cimetidine, to treat peptic ulcer disease.

Amino Acids

In addition to being the structural building blocks of proteins, amino acids have many other roles in intraneuronal metabolism. There is evidence that amino acids function as neurotransmitters similar to the biogenic amines. The amino acids are probably the neurotransmitters in 60 percent to 70 percent of the synapses in the brain. The best studied amino acid neurotransmitter is γ-aminobutyric acid (GABA), an inhibitory amino acid neurotransmitter. Other inhibitory amino acids are glycine and probably taurine and β-alanine. Excitatory amino acids include glutamic acid, aspartic acid, and probably cysteine and homocysteic acid.

γ-Aminobutyric Acid (GABA). The two identified long GABA–ergic tracts are the neurons that project from the corpus striatum to the substantia nigra and the cerebellar Purkinje cells that project out of the cerebellum. Local GABA–ergic interneurons exist in the cerebral and cerebellar cortices, as well as in the hypothalamus, where they may play a regulatory role in the neuroendocrine system.

In the GABA–ergic synapse, GABA is synthesized by the actions of glutamic acid decarboxylase (GAD) and degraded by GABA–transaminase (GABA–T). There are two types of GABA receptors—GABA$_A$ and GABA$_B$. GABA$_A$ receptors seem to be limited to a postsynaptic distribution on dendrites and cell bodies. The GABA$_A$ receptor complex consists of a GABA recognition site, a benzodiazepine binding site, and a chloride ion channel. The binding of a benzodiazepine to a benzodiazepine binding site increases the affinity of the GABA binding site for GABA. Endogenous ligands may exist for the benzodiazepine binding site. Theoretically, there could be endogenous benzodiazepine agonists (e.g., diazepam binding inhibitor (DBI)) that reduce anxiety and endogenous benzodiazepine antagonists (e.g., GABA-modulin) that create anxiety. Barbiturates also seem to act through the GABA$_A$ receptor by prolonging the length of time the chloride channel is open. A third drug that is used to treat epilepsy, valproic acid, increases GABA–ergic activity by inhibiting the actions of GABA–T.

GABA and Psychopathology. The clinical efficacy of benzodiazepines in treating anxiety has led to the hypothesis that too little GABA activity may be the molecular pathophysiologic basis for anxiety. In addition, decreased GABA activity may be involved in the pathophysiology of epilepsy, since a number of anticonvulsants increase GABA activity. GABA–ergic neuronal loss has been reported in Huntington's disease and Parkinson's disease; and tardive dyskinesia may involve the GABA–ergic system. Finally, it has been hypothesized that schizophrenia could result from an underactivity of GABA–ergic inhibition on dopaminergic and noradrenergic neurons.

Other Amino Acids. Other amino acid neurotransmitters include glycine and glutamic acid. Glycine functions as an inhibitory neurotransmitter within the spinal cord. Glutamic acid is an excitatory neurotransmitter; it may be the neurotransmitter for both the primary afferent nerve endings in the spinal cord and the cerebellar granule cells. Excitatory amino acid neurotransmitters may be involved in the pathophysiology of epileptic and neurodegenerative disorders.

Peptide Neurotransmitters

Neuroscience research is producing an explosion of information about peptide neurotransmitters, also called neuroactive peptides. Approximately 50 neuroactive peptides already have been identified (Table 1), and some investigators have suggested that as many as 300 different neuroactive peptides may exist. Peptides act as neurotransmitters or neuromodulators and coexist in axon terminals with other neurotransmitters, such as the biogenic amines or amino acids.

A peptide is a short protein consisting of less than 100 amino acids. The peptide neurotransmitters are stored in vesicles in the axon terminals, released by a calcium-dependent mechanism, and bind to peptide-specific receptors. Research evidence now suggests that peptide action is terminated by degradative peptidases in the synaptic cleft.

The major known difference between peptide neurotransmitters and other neurotransmitters is in their synthesis. Biogenic amines and amino acids are made in the nerve terminals by the actions of enzymes on available substrates. Peptides, on the other hand, are made in the neuronal cell body through the transcription and translation of a genetic message coded on DNA.

Selected Peptide Neurotransmitters

Endogenous opioids. Animal and human studies suggest that the endogenous opioids, which include the endorphins (α, β, and γ), are involved in mediating the effects of stress and pain. There is controversial evidence implicating these peptides in mood and schizophrenic disorders. Clinical studies using synthetic opioid agonists and antagonists (e.g., naloxone) have suggested potential clinical applications.

Table 1
CNS Neuroactive Peptides

Adrenocorticotropic hormone (ACTH)
Androgens
Angiotensin I, II, and III
Bombesin
Bradykinin
Calcitonin
Cardioexcitatory peptide
Carnosine
Cholecystokinin
Corticotropin-releasing hormone (CRH)
Cortisol
Endogenous opioids
Estrogens
Follicle-stimulating hormone (FSH)
Gastrin
Gastrin-inhibiting peptide
Glucagon
Gonadotropin-releasing hormone (GRH)
Growth hormone
Growth hormone–releasing factor
Insulin
Luteinizing hormone (LH)
Melanocyte-inhibiting factor
Melanocyte-stimulating hormone
Melatonin
Motilin
Neural growth factor
Neuronal polypeptide
Neuropeptide Y
Neurotensin
Oxytocin
Prolactin
Prolactin-inhibiting hormone (possibly dopamine)
Prolactin-releasing hormone
Progesterone
Secretin
Sleep-inducing peptide
Somatostatin
Substance K
Substance P
Thyroid hormones
Thyrotropin-releasing hormone (TRH)
Thyroid-stimulating hormone (TSH)
Vasoactive intestinal peptide
Vasopressin

ACTH and Corticotropic Releasing Hormone (CRH). Although these peptides are part of the limbic-hypothalamic-pituitary-adrenal axis, they also serve as neurotransmitters outside the hypothalamus. Specifically, they may be involved in the regulation of stress, mood, and memory.

Cholecystokinin (CCK). CCK has been reported to coexist with GABA and dopamine, thereby implying a potential pathophysiologic role in schizophrenia. CCK also has been implicated in eating and movement disorders.

Neurotensin. This peptide coexists with dopamine and norepinephrine and may be a modulator of dopaminergic neurotransmission. It has been postulated, therefore, that neurotensin may be involved in the pathophysiology of schizophrenia.

Somatostatin. Somatostatin has been strongly implicated by postmortem studies to be involved in the pathophysiology of Huntington's disease and Alzheimer's disease. Clinical studies have suggested a role for somatostatin in mood disorders.

Substance P. Substance P coexists with acetylcholine and serotonin; it appears to be the primary neurotransmitter in many primary afferent sensory neurons and in the striatonigral pathway. Substance P neurotransmission, therefore, has been suggested as a possible pathologic mechanism underlying pain syndromes, movement disorders (particularly Huntington's disease), and mood disorders.

Vasopressin. Vasopressin may modulate the effects of norepinephrine and potentially may be involved in mood disorders. Parallel to ACTH and CRH, vasopressin has an independent role as a neurotransmitter in addition to its role in the hypothalmic-posterior pituitary axis.

Vasoactive Intestinal Peptide (VIP). This peptide neurotransmitter coexists with acetylcholine and has been implicated in the pathophysiology of dementia and mood disorders.

PSYCHOENDOCRINOLOGY, PSYCHOIMMUNOLOGY, AND CHRONOBIOLOGY

There are three systems in the body that are "designed" so that different parts of each system can mutually communicate with other parts—the nervous, endocrine, and immune systems. All three systems change in both predictable and unpredictable fashions with the passage of time and are responsive to changes in the environment. The study of the periodic variation of biological functions of the body is known as chronobiology.

The action of the endocrine and immune systems are relevant to psychiatry. Both endocrine disorders (e.g., Cushing's disease) and immune disorders (e.g., systemic lupus erythematosus) can have neuropsychiatric symptoms—even as the presenting symptoms. Conversely, endocrine and immunologic abnormalities are seen in psychiatric disorders.

Psychoneuroendocrinology

Psychoneuroendocrinology studies the interactions between the nervous system and the endocrine system. The major endocrine systems and their target tissues are diagrammed in Figure 6. The neuroendocrine axes can be conceptualized as starting in the hypothalamus where they receive input from the cerebral cortex and limbic system. Each component in the neuroendocrine axes can feed back onto any of the other components, including the cerebral cortex and limbic system.

Endocrine Axes

Anterior pituitary. The cortex and limbic system affect the hypothalamus so that the hypothalamus transmits releasing and inhibiting factors to the anterior pituitary which in turn releases trophic hormones into the peripheral circulation. Most of these trophic hormones then cause a peripheral organ to release a hormone. The adrenal axis is the best understood and is now appreciated to be more complex than was previously thought. Specifically, both vasopressin and corticotropin-releasing hormone (CRH) control the release of hormones from the anterior pituitary. Moreover, both β-endorphin and adrenocorticotropin (ACTH) are released together from the same pituitary cells. Recent investigations have begun to subtype depressed patients according to whether cortisol, β-endorphin, or both hormones escape suppression by dexamethasone in the dexamethasone suppression test (DST).

Posterior pituitary. Vasopressin (also called antidiuretic hormone) and oxytocin are synthesized in both the supraoptic and paraventricular nuclei. Vasopressin is involved with the control of blood pressure and fluid and electrolyte balance. Its release is stimulated by pain, stress, morphine, and barbiturates and is inhibited by alcohol. Oxytocin, released in the female by suckling, stimulates glandular contraction in the breast. Oxytocin also stimulates uterine contractions during delivery.

Pineal. The pineal contains many peptides (e.g., vasopressin, LHRH) in addition to its principal hormone, melatonin, which is secreted in the dark and suppressed in the light. Melatonin is synthesized from serotonin by the actions of two enzymes: serotonin-N-acetylase and 5-hydroxyindole-O-methyltransferase.

Regulation and Testing of Neuroendocrine Interactions. The release of hypothalamic and pituitary peptides and hormones is affected by biogenic amine neurotransmitters; one example is the interaction between estrogens and dopamine receptors. Estrogens have mixed dopaminergic and antidopaminergic effects in the CNS. Although estrogens do not bind to dopamine receptors, they increase the number of dopamine receptors and decrease the amount of dopamine in the nigrostriatal, mesolimbic, and tuberoinfundibular pathways. The co-administration of neuroleptics and estrogens has an additive effect on the increase in dopamine receptor number. These interactions are reflected clinically. Tardive dyskinesia is more frequent in women than in men, with a higher prevalence in postmenopausal women. The concomitant use of estrogen-containing birth control pills and neuroleptics increases the incidence of neuroleptic-induced motor system symptoms. In female parkinsonian patients, L-dopa–induced dyskinesias improve with estrogens, and chorea has been reported as a complication of both pregnancy and birth control pills.

Endocrine assessment. There are two basic approaches to assessing neuroendocrine function: to measure baseline or "resting" values of various peptides and hormones and to challenge the axis with some stimulus. Each level of the axis can be challenged, and when the assays are available, the response of different levels of the axis can be measured. Psychological stress (e.g., taking an examination) can challenge the suprahypothalamic areas. Insulin-induced hypoglycemia is believed to represent a fairly pure hypothalamic challenge. The pituitary can be challenged by the administration of exogenous releasing and inhibiting peptides, and the peripheral glands can be challenged by the administration of exogenous trophic hormones. Many factors can affect the results of these tests; these factors include alcohol withdrawal, administration of other drugs (including some psychotropics), and malnutrition (as is seen in anorexia nervosa). An abnormal neuroendocrine chal-

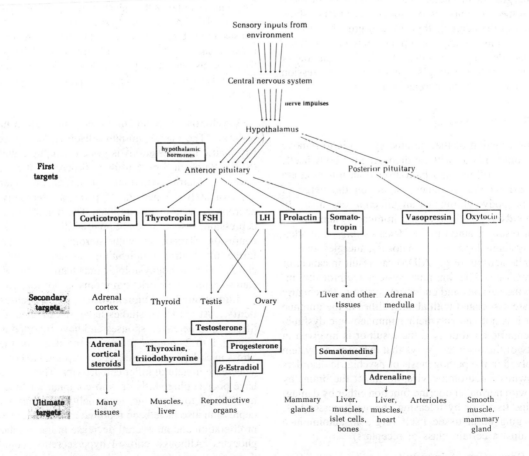

Figure 6. The major endocrine systems and their target tissues. (From Lehninger A L: *Principles of Biochemistry,* p 722. Worth, New York, 1982, by permission.)

lenge test conducted under appropriately controlled conditions indicates a dysregulation of the axis, thus demonstrating an objective dysfunction of the CNS.

Psychiatric Abnormalities in Endocrine Disorders. Classic psychiatric symptoms are observed in many endocrine syndromes. Cushing's syndrome involves psychiatric symptoms in 40 percent to 90 percent of patients. The most commonly seen symptom is depression, and suicide attempts occur in approximately 10 percent of patients. The administration of endogenous steroids (e.g., ACTH for multiple sclerosis) also causes depression and is associated with hypomania, emotional lability, and even psychosis. Addison's disease involves depression in approximately 40 percent of patients; apathy, fatigue, and occasionally psychosis characterize its symptoms. Although anxiety is the hallmark of hyperthyroidism, apathetic hyperthyroidism, characterized by depression, can be seen in elderly patients. Hypothyroidism is most commonly associated with depression and some anxiety. Some female patients with autoimmune thyroiditis may present only with symptoms of depression. Both hyperparathyroidism and hypoglycemia are associated with anxiety and depression.

Endocrine Dysregulation in Psychiatric Syndromes. Third ventricle enlargement has been noted in some schizophrenic patients and suggests lesions in the surrounding hypothalamus. Such lesions cause endocrine dysregulation, and research data indicate a dysregulation of the gonadal, growth hormone, and adrenal axes in these patients. Some patients with mood disorders show dysregulation in the adrenal, thyroid, and growth hormone axes. There is an interesting conceptual continuum between endocrine disorders and mood disorders. As an example of this continuum, both Cushing's syndrome and depression have dysregulations of the adrenal axis.

Psychoneuroimmunology

The basic function of the immune system is to remove pathogens from the body without damaging the body itself. The erythema, swelling, and pain around an infection are examples of how the immune system, on the verge of damaging the body, eliminates an infecting organism. In more serious dysregulations of the immune system, overactivity can result in autoimmune diseases (e.g., myasthenia gravis, systemic lupus erythematosus), allergies, or anaphylaxis; underactivity (e.g., AIDS) can result in cancer or serious infections. The immune system reciprocally interacts with the nervous and endocrine systems. Psychiatric conditions are associated with abnormalities in the immune system, but it is not known whether immunologic dysfunction in psychiatric conditions is the result or is involved in the causality of the disorder. Ways that the immune system can be involved in the pathogenesis of psychiatric disorders are by allowing a neurotoxic virus to infect the brain, by interfering with normal endocrine function either by damaging endocrine tissue or by releasing chemical messengers, or by damaging brain tissue itself (e.g., an autoimmune reaction against a certain class of receptors).

Neural Regulation of Immunity. Animal studies have shown that lesions of the hypothalamus, hippocampus, and pituitary all result in fairly specific dysfunctions of the immune system.

The principal neurochemical messengers for this regulation are thought to be norepinephrine, β-endorphin, met-enkephalin, and cortisol. Increased immune function has been correlated with a decrease in norepinephrine in the hypothalamus (presumably functioning as an inhibitory neurotransmitter) and an increase in cell firing (measured by implanted electrodes). The lymphocytes may communicate back to the brain through the release of chemical messengers, including ACTH, β-endorphin, or unique lymphocyte-secreted chemicals.

Studies of animals in experimentally designed stressful situations demonstrate a decrease in lymphocyte number, a decreased proliferation in response to stimulation, and a reduction in the production of antibodies. Although true for animals in experimental paradigms of inescapable stress (e.g., foot shock without anywhere to go), these immune responses are not found in animals that have a way to stop the stressful stimulus. It also has been found that infant monkeys taken away from their mothers exhibit similar immune system dysfunction.

A series of experiments with different animal models has demonstrated that immunosuppression can be conditioned, so that upon receiving a nonbiologically relevant stimulus (e.g., bell ringing) the animal's immune response is suppressed. One of these experiments paired a conditioned stimulus (a sweet drinking solution) with an unconditioned stimulus (an immunosuppressive drug). Once conditioned, the animal, when exposed to a previously stimulating antigen in the presence of the conditioned stimulus, exhibited a blunted immune response. Therefore, the possibility exists that patients with autoimmune disorders can learn to suppress their immune response through conditioning or behavior modification. Another series of animal experiments has suggested that the left side of the brain is involved in the stimulation of the immune response and that the role of the right hemisphere is to inhibit the left hemisphere. This data may be consistent with observations that left-handed persons are more prone to autoimmune disorders.

Psychiatric Abnormalities in Immune Disorders. The classic immune disorder that presents with psychiatric manifestations is systemic lupus erythematosus (SLE). Between 5 percent and 50 percent of SLE patients have psychiatric symptoms at initial presentation, but approximately 50 percent of patients eventually develop neuropsychiatric manifestations. The major complaints are depression, insomnia, emotional lability, nervousness, and confusion. Treatment with steroids commonly induces further psychiatric complications, including mania and psychosis. The pathophysiologic mechanism by which SLE causes neuropsychiatric symptoms is not known.

Immunologic Abnormalities in Psychiatric Patients. At least two studies have investigated T-cell proliferation in bereaved spouses and have reported a decrease around 1 to 2 months following the death of the spouse. Stress in college students has been reported to correspond to a decrease in natural killer cell activity. Those students who have poor coping skills or who complain of loneliness are most likely to show the abnormality. Patients with major depression also have been reported to have decreased T-cell proliferation and an overall decrease in the number of lymphocytes. Although cortisol hypersecretion could explain these findings, there is evidence that the endocrine, immune, and nervous systems are mutually interactive and that it is not possible to draw a one-way, cause-and-effect arrow between hypercortisolemia and decreased immune function.

Schizophrenia may also be associated with immunologic abnormalities, supporting a viral hypothesis of schizophrenia. Various reports have found abnormal looking lymphocytes, decreased numbers of natural killer cells, variations in T- and B-cell function and number, and high and low levels of immunoglobulins. It is possible that either an infection results in an abnormal immune response or that an abnormal immune system allows an infection to develop. Other schizophrenia researchers have investigated the hypothesis that the disorder represents an autoimmune phenomenon caused by antibrain antibodies. This research is supported by increased skin reactivity to intradermal test antigens as well as reports of antibodies to brain proteins in the CSF from some patients with schizophrenia.

Chronobiology

Chronobiology objectively explores and quantifies mechanisms of time structure in biological systems; it is the study of biological rhythms. There are rhythms in endocrine secretion, neurotransmitter synthesis, receptor number, enzyme levels and affinities, brain electrical activity, weights of body organs, duration of cell cycle times, and ultrastructural components of cellular organelles. These rhythms can have different cycle lengths—less than a day (ultradian), approximately 24 hours (circadian), more than 1 day (infradian), approximately 1 week (circaseptan), around 1 month, and around 1 year (circannual).

There are multiple biological rhythms in a living organism. In a human, for example, these rhythms include the sleep-wake cycle, hormone levels, body temperature, and the menstrual cycle. When all of these are in correct or normal relationship to each other, the rhythms of the organism are said to be in phase. In disease states, on the other hand, one or more rhythms may become out of phase. A biological rhythm may have an abnormal phase advance, in which it begins earlier than usual, or a phase delay, in which it begins later than usual. Under experimental conditions, a phase-response curve for a biological rhythm may show whether a particular stimulation (e.g., light) causes either a phase advance or a phase delay when it is delivered at different times in the cycle (e.g., sleep-wake cycle).

Zeitgebers (time givers, time clues, synchronizers) entrain or set the biological rhythms. The principal endogenous *zeitgeber* is believed to be the suprachiasmatic nuclei of the hypothalamus. Examples of exogenous *zeitgebers* include the light-dark cycle, patterned mealtimes, and the nine-to-five work day. In the absence of exogenous clues, the period of human circadian rhythms is a bit longer than a day—24.5 hours. The implications of these rhythms include the likelihood that the response to drugs varies with time of day, the response to environmental stress varies with time, and biological measures themselves vary with time. Information about chronobiology could guide such decisions as when surgery is best performed and when best to give psychotropic or pain medications.

Chronobiological Considerations in Psychiatry. The most common and normal perturbation of chronobiology is the phenomenon of jet lag, usually presenting with fatigue and dysphoric mood. When an individual travels from east to west, he experiences a phase delay, not a large problem because the body actually "wants" a slightly longer (24.5 hours) day. Travelling west to east, however, pre-

sents a phase advance that opposes the natural tendency and particularly disrupts biological rhythms. The subjective discomfort of a phase advance may be further influenced by variations in the time that different biological rhythms take to adjust to the new schedule of exogenous clues. Shift work, including the difficult hours of interns and residents, also disrupt biological rhythms.

One theory of depression is that it represents a phase-advance disorder, as evidenced by early morning awakening, decreased latency of REM sleep, and neuroendocrine perturbations. One hypothesis is that depression occurs in some individuals when the sleep-sensitive phase of the circadian system advances from the first hours of awakening to the last hours of sleep. There is also a group of patients who appear to have a seasonal affective disorder (SAD) with the occurrence of fatigue, oversleeping, overeating, and depression during winter. These patients are more often females and relatively young (in their 20's), but this disorder may also appear in some children presenting with school problems. There is research evidence that alterations in the light-dark cycle for these patients, either by prolonged exposure to artificial light or by changing the patients' sleep-wake cycles, can relieve the symptoms. The observation that lithium and many of the TCAs and MAOIs delay rhythms in experimental animal models supports the hypothesis that depression is a phase-advance disorder.

GENETICS

Two aims of investigations in population genetics are to demonstrate the existence and relative contribution of gene-borne influences on a disorder and to determine the mode of inheritance of these influences.

Family Risk Studies

Family risk studies compare the prevalence of a psychiatric condition among relatives of the affected persons with its prevalence in the general population. Affected persons in the original group of patients are called index cases or probands. For a genetic illness, first-degree relatives (mother, father, siblings) are more likely to have the disorder of the proband than are more distant relatives.

Twin Studies

Monozygotic (MZ) twins develop from a single ovum, whereas dizygotic (DZ) twins develop from two different ova and share, on the average, no more genetic information than nontwin sibs. Twin studies are useful in separating genetic and environmental influences and in looking for protective and precipitating factors. A genetic disorder should occur (e.g., be concordant) in MZ twins more often than in DZ twins. The DZ concordance rate, moreover, should be quite similar to that for nontwin sibs. Furthermore, for a genetic illness, first-degree relatives should be more likely to have the disorder of the proband than more distant relatives.

Adoption Studies

Adoption studies attempt to assess what effect the environment has on the expression of genes. The most powerful adoption studies involve MZ twins reared apart in adoptive households. Theoretically, differences in the expression of diseases then can be attributed to the environment. One problem with this interpretation, however, is that the MZ twins may have been subjected to significantly different environments before the adoption. These differences could even have begun in utero, where the twins may have received different levels of hormones or other nutrients.

Molecular Genetics

From DNA to Proteins. The organism's complete set of genes is referred to as its genome. The human genome consists of 23 pairs of chromosomes, one member of each pair being inherited from each parent. There are 22 pairs of somatic chromosomes and one pair of sex chromosomes (XX for females, XY for males). The chromosomes consist of deoxyribonucleic acid (DNA) tightly packed in a organized fashion. In addition, chromosomes contain proteins (histones and nonhistone proteins) that are believed to be involved in the folding and organization of the DNA within the chromosome. The complete set of chromosomes define the genotype, not only of an individual cell, but also of every cell in that organism. Each cell, however, expresses only a portion of that genotype to produce its unique characteristics, called its phenotype. A cerebellar Purkinje neuron and a thalamic neuron from a given person, for example, have the same genotype but differ in their phenotypic expressions.

The gene is the unit of functional information on the chromosome. It is easiest to conceptualize a gene as containing the information necessary to produce a functional protein or proteins. The only exception to this concept is that some genes produce either rRNA (ribosomal RNA) or tRNA (transfer RNA), both involved in the synthesis of proteins.

Application to Psychiatric Research. The development of recombinant DNA technology, which is synonymous with the concept of "genetic engineering," has generated a great deal of excitement in the field of genetics.

Both phrases refer to the ability to manipulate DNA and RNA so that both the messages and the expression of the messages can be manipulated experimentally.

Specific abnormal proteins in idiopathic psychiatric disorders have not been identified. Psychiatric research approaches the isolation of these proteins by employing the molecular genetic technique of identifying restriction fragment length polymorphisms (RFLPs). RFLPs are an inherited variation in the lengths of restriction fragments produced by exposure of the DNA to restriction endonucleases. It is possible to measure these restriction patterns for each individual and to look for specific patterns of RFLPs found in patients with a particular disease. The identification of an RFLP localized at the terminal region of the chromosome 4 short arm served as a genetic marker in patients with Huntington's disease. Having isolated a fragment of DNA that is associated with a disease it is possible to use this DNA in the diagnosis of the disease (including prenatal and presymptomatic diagnosis). Through the use of genetic markers, it may be possible to identify and localize the genes involved in a disease process, thereby allowing the molecular and cellular pathophysiology of the disease to be understood, potentially treated, and perhaps prevented.

References

Browning M D, Huganir R, Greengard P: Protein phosphorylation and neural function. J Neurochem 45:11, 1985.

Jaeckle R S, Kathol R G, Lopez J F, Meller W H, Krummel S J: Enhanced adrenal sensitivity to exogenous cosyntropin (ACTH α^{1-24}) stimulation in major depression. Arch Gen Psych 44(3):233, 1987.

Krieger D T: Brain peptides: What, where and why? Science 222:975, 1983.

Pauly J E: Chronobiology: Anatomy of time. Am J Anat 168:365, 1983.

Press G D, Green J P: Histamine as a neuroregulator. Ann Rev Neurosci 9:209, 1986.

Rosenberg R N: Molecular genetics, recombinant DNA techniques, and genetic neurological disease. Ann Neurol 15:511, 1984.

Sanger D J: Minireview: GABA and the behavioral effects of anxiolytic drugs. Life Sci 36:1503, 1985.

Smith C K, Barish, J, Correa, J, Williams R M: Psychiatric disturbance in endocrinological disease. Psychosomat Med 34:69, 1972.

Tecoma E S, Huey, L Y: Psychic distress and the immune response. Life Sci 26:1799, 1985.

Tricklebank M D: The behavioral response to 5-HT receptor agonists and subtypes of the central 5-HT receptor. Trends Pharmacol Sci 10:403, 1985.

5

Contributions of the Psychosocial Sciences to Human Behavior

5.1

Jean Piaget

The noted Swiss psychologist Jean Piaget (1896–1980) formulated a comprehensive theory of cognitive or intellectual development in which he described how children think and acquire knowledge. He derived his theories from direct observations of children's behavior and by questioning children about their thinking. Piaget learned as much about how children think from their wrong answers as from their right answers. He referred to his theory of development as *genetic epistemology* because it studied the acquisition and modification and growth of abstract ideas and abilities based on an inherited or biological substrate. There is a replacing of physical acts and experiences by mental ones, suggesting a continuum between physical and mental functioning.

Central to Piaget's theory is the concept of *epigenesis*, which holds that growth and development occur in a series of stages, each of which is built upon the successful mastery of the one that comes before. Every stage occurs at a certain age, and the child demonstrates a higher level of thinking during each successive stage of development.

THE PROCESS OF ADAPTATION

Adaptation is the ability of the person to adjust to the environment through two complementary processes: *assimilation* and *accommodation*. Assimilation is a subjective process that involves the filtering of the world through one's own system of knowledge—a taking in of new experience through the person's established mental structure. Accommodation involves the adjustment of one's knowledge to the reality demands of the environment by reorganizing or modifying the existing cognitive structure. Taken together, they enable the infant or child to adapt to the outside world and react with increasingly complex patterns of awareness and behavior called *organization*.

Organization is both biological and psychological, and all species inherit the ability to organize, which is different for different species: Birds organize flying and babies organize crawling.

Organization varies for each individual, but its function is constant. For instance, every baby crawls in his own way, but crawling is constant.

STAGES IN THE DEVELOPMENT OF INTELLIGENCE

Piaget described four major stages leading to the capacity for adult thought. Each stage is a necessary prerequisite for the one that follows. The rate at which different children move through different stages, however, varies with their native endowment and environmental circumstances. The four stages are: (1) sensorimotor stage, (2) stage of preoperational thought, (3) stage of concrete operations, and (4) stage of formal operations.

Sensorimotor Stage (Birth to 2 Years)

Piaget used the term "sensorimotor" to describe this stage because the infant first begins to learn through sensory observation and gains control of his motor functions through activity, exploration, and manipulation of the environment. Piaget divided this stage into six substages, which are discussed in Section 3.2. From the outset, biology and experience blend to produce learned behavior. For example, infants are born with a sucking reflex. A type of learning occurs when an infant alters the shape of the mouth and discovers the location of the nipple. A stimulus is received and a response results, accompanied by a sense of awareness called a *schema* or elementary concept. As the infant becomes more mobile, one schema is built upon another, and new and more complex *schemas* are developed. The spatial, visual, and tactile world of the infant expands during this period, and the child actively interacts with the environment using previously learned behavior patterns. For example, having learned to use a rattle, the infant shakes a new toy like the rattle he has already learned to use. The infant also will use the rattle in new ways.

The critical achievement of this period is the development of *object permanence*. This term defines the child's ability to understand that objects have an existence independent of his involvement with the object. The child learns to differentiate himself from the world and is able to maintain a mental image of an object even though it is not present and visible.

Also, at about this time (approximately 18 months), infants begin to develop mental symbols and use words, a process known as *symbolization*. Infants are able to create a visual image of a ball or a mental symbol or the word "ball" to stand for or signify the real object. Such mental representations allow children to operate on new conceptual levels. The attainment of object permanence marks the transition from the sensorimotor stage to the preoperational stage of development.

Stage of Preoperational Thought (Intuitional Stage; 2 to 7 Years)

During this stage, the child uses symbols and language more extensively than in the sensorimotor stage. Thinking and reasoning is on an intuitive level in that the child learns without the use of reasoning. The child is unable to think logically or deductively and concepts are primitive; he can name objects, but not classes. Preoperational thought is midway between socialized adult thought and the completely autistic Freudian unconscious. Events are linked not by logic but by juxtaposition. Early in this stage, if the child drops a glass and it breaks, there is no sense of cause and effect. The child believes the glass was ready to break, not that he broke it. Also, the child is unable to grasp the sameness of an object in different circumstances; the same doll in a carriage, a crib, or a chair is perceived to be three different objects. During this time, things are represented in terms of their function. For example, a child would define a bike as "to ride" and a hole as "to dig."

In this phase, children begin to use language and drawings in more elaborate ways. From one-word utterances, two-word phrases made up of either noun plus verb or noun plus objective develop. A child may say "Bobby up" or "Bobby eat."

Children in the preoperational phase are unable to deal with moral dilemmas, although they have a sense of what is good and what is bad. For example, when asked, "Who is more guilty: the person who breaks one dish on purpose or the person who breaks ten dishes by accident?" the young child usually answers that the latter is more guilty because he broke more dishes.

During this period children are described as being *egocentric*. They see themselves as the center of the universe, have a limited point of view, and are unable to take the role of the other person. The child is unable to modify behavior for someone else. For example, the child is not being negativistic when he does not listen to commands to be quiet because his brother has to study. Instead, egocentric thinking prevents an understanding of his brother's point of view.

During this stage, children also employ a type of magical thinking, called *phenomenalistic causality,* in which events that occur together are thought to cause one another (e.g., thunder causes lightning, bad thoughts cause accidents). In addition, the child demonstrates *animistic thinking,* which is the tendency to endow physical events and objects with psychological attributes, such as feelings or intentions.

Stage of Concrete Operations (Operational Stage; 7 to 11 Years)

This stage is so named because in this period the child operates and acts upon the concrete, real, and perceivable world of objects and events. Egocentric thought is replaced by *operational thought,* which involves attending to and dealing with a wide array of information outside the child. Therefore, a child can now see things from someone else's perspective. Children in this stage begin to use limited *logical thought processes* and are able to serialize, order, and group things in classes based on common characteristics. Syllogistic reasoning, in which a logical conclusion is formed from two premises, occurs during this period; for example, all horses are mammals (premise), all mammals are warm blooded (premise), therefore, all horses are warm blooded (conclusion). Children are able to reason and follow rules and regulations. They are able to regulate themselves and begin to develop a moral sense and a code of values.

Children who become overly invested in rules may show obsessive-compulsive behavior; children who resist a code of values often seem willful and inactive. The most desirable developmental outcome for this period is for the child to attain a healthy respect for rules and to understand that there are legitimate exceptions to rules.

Conservation is the ability to recognize that even though the shape and form of objects may change, the objects still maintain or conserve other characteristics that enable them to be recognized as the same. For example, if a ball of clay is rolled into a long and thin sausage shape, the child will recognize that there is the same amount of clay in the two forms. An inability to conserve (which is characteristic of the preoperational stage) is observed when the child declares that there is more clay in the sausage-shaped form because it is longer. The child in this stage realizes that the act of reshaping the clay into a ball reverses the act of stretching it—a concept known as reversibility.

The task of the 7- to 11-year-old is to organize and order what is occurring in the real world. Dealing with the future and its possibilities occur in the formal operational stage.

Stage of Formal Operations (11 Through End of Adolescence)

This period of cognitive development is characterized by the young person's ability to think abstractly, to reason deductively, and to define concepts (hypotheticodeductive thinking). This stage is so named because the person's thinking operates in a formal, highly logical, systematic, and symbolic manner. Formal operations is also characterized by skills in dealing with permutations and combinations. The young person can grasp the concept of probabilities. The adolescent attempts to deal with all possible relations and hypotheses in order to explain data and events. During this stage, language use is complex, follows formal rules of logic, and is grammatically correct. *Abstract thinking* is demonstrated by the adolescent's interest in a variety of issues: philosophy, religion, ethics, and politics.

Because young people can reflect on their own and other people's thinking, they are prone to self-conscious behavior. As the adolescent attempts to master new cognitive tasks, there may be a return of egocentric thought, but on a higher level. For example, adolescents may think that they can accomplish everything or change events by thought alone.

Not all adolescents enter the stage of formal operations at the same time or to the same degree. Depending on the capacity of the individual, some may not reach the stage of formal operational thought at all and remain in the concrete operational mode throughout life.

APPLICATIONS TO PSYCHIATRY

Piaget's theories have psychiatric implications. The hospitalized child who is in the sensorimotor stage has achieved object permanency and, so, suffers from separation anxiety. Such a child is best off if the mother is allowed to stay in the room overnight. The preoperational child, unable to deal with concepts or abstractions, benefits more from role-playing proposed medical procedures or situations than by having them described verbally in detail. For example, if the child is to receive intravenous therapy, it might be useful to act out the procedure using a toy intravenous set and dolls. Also, since the child in the preoperational stage does not understand cause and effect, physical illness may be interpreted as punishment for bad thoughts or deeds. Because the child has not yet mastered the capacity to conserve and does not understand the concept of reversibility (which normally occurs during the concrete operational stage), he cannot understand that a broken bone can mend or that blood lost in an accident can be replaced.

The clinician must also be aware that the thinking of the adolescent during formal operations may appear to be overly abstract when it is, in fact, a normal developmental stage. A picture of adolescent turmoil may not herald a psychotic process but it may well be the result of the normal adolescent coming to grips with his newly acquired abilities to deal with the unlimited possibilities of the surrounding world.

Finally, it is important to remember that adults under stress can regress cognitively as well as emotionally. Their thinking can become preoperational, egocentric, and sometimes animistic.

References

Lane R O, Schwartz G E: Levels of emotional awareness: A cognitive developmental theory and its application to psychopathology. Am J Psych *144*(2):p133, 1987.

Piaget J: *Judgement and Reasoning in the Child.* Harcourt, New York, 1926.

Piaget J: *The Language and Thought of the Child.* Routledge and Kegan Paul, London, 1926.

Piaget J: *The Moral Judgement of the Child.* Harcourt, New York, 1932.

Piaget J: *Play, Dreams, and Imitation in Childhood.* W W Norton, New York, 1951.

Piaget J: *The Origins of Intelligence in Children.* International University Press, New York, 1952.

Piaget J: *Logic and Psychology.* Basic Books, New York, 1957.

Piaget J, Inhelder B: *The Psychology of the Child.* Basic Books, New York, 1969.

Piaget J: *Genetic Epistemology.* Columbia University Press, New York, 1973.

Piaget J, Inhelder B: *Memory and Intelligence.* Basic Books, New York, 1973.

Piaget J: *The Grasp of Consciousness.* Harvard University Press, Cambridge, MA, 1976.

5.2 _____
John Bowlby

The British psychoanalyst John Bowlby born in 1907 (now living in England), formulated a theory of attachment. *Attachment* refers to the emotional tone between the developing child and the *outer-provider* or *care-giver,* the person primarily responsible for the infant's care and toward whom the infant directs his emotional energies. Attachment to a specific stable figure—the mother in most societies—is crucial to healthy development. According to Bowlby, attachment occurs when there is a "warm, intimate and continuous relationship with the mother in which both find satisfaction and enjoyment." Infants tend to attach to one person—they are *monotropic*—but multiple attachments may also occur, and attachment may be directed toward the father or a surrogate. Attachment is a gradually developing phenomenon; it results in one person wanting to be with a preferred person, who is perceived as stronger, wiser, and able to reduce anxiety or distress.

Attachment occurs during the first year of life and has a reciprocal quality in that infant and mother attach to one another. The term *bonding* is sometimes used synonymously with attachment, but they are actually different phenomena. Bonding refers to the mother's feelings for her infant and differs from attachment because a mother does not normally rely on her infant as a source of security—a requirement of attachment behavior. There has been a great deal of research on the bonding of mother to infant, which occurs when there is skin-to-skin contact between the two or when other types of contact are made, such as voice or eye contact. Some workers have concluded that a mother who has skin-to-skin contact with her baby immediately after birth shows a stronger bonding pattern and may provide more attentive care than the mother who does not have this experience. Some researchers have even proposed a critical period immediately after birth, during which such skin-to-skin contact must occur if bonding is to take place. This is a much disputed concept because many mothers are clearly bonded to their infants and display excellent maternal care even though they did not have this contact immediately postpartum. Humans are also able to develop so-called representational models of their babies in utero or even before conception. This type of representational thinking may be equally as important to the bonding process as skin, voice, or eye contact.

Attachment behavior is reinforced by signs of distress, or signal indicators, which elicit a behavioral response in the mother. Crying is the primary signal, and although the infant cries most often from hunger, the mother generalizes the crying stimulus to represent distress from pain, frustration, or anger. Other signs that reinforce attachment are smiling, cooing, and looking.

As the developing child becomes attached to the care-giver or mother, he will cry when the mother goes away. The meaning of the separation depends on the child's developmental level and the stage of attachment that exists.

In the first stage, sometimes called the *preattachment stage* (birth to 8 weeks), the baby orients to the mother, follows her with its eyes over a 180° range, and turns toward and moves rhythmically with her voice. In the second phase, sometimes called *attachment-in-the-making* (8 to 10 weeks to 6 months), the infant becomes attached to one or more persons in the environment. Separation from a particular person is not a problem for the infant in either of these stages, providing his needs are satisfied. In the next stage, sometimes called *clear-cut attachment* (6 months through adulthood), the infant cries and shows other signs of distress when separated from the care-giver or mother (this may occur as early as 3 months in some infants). Upon being returned to the mother, the infant stops crying and clings, as if to gain further assurance of the mother's return. Sometimes, seeing the mother after separation is sufficient for crying to stop. As children grow, there is a critical distance from the mother beyond which point they experience distress.

Bowlby's theory of *anxiety* holds that the child's sense of distress during separation is perceived and experienced as anxiety. Any stimuli that alarm the child and cause fear (such as loud noises, falling, or cold blasts of air), mobilize signal indicators (such as crying), which cause the mother to respond in a caring way by cuddling and reassuring the baby. The ability of the mother to relieve the infant's anxiety or fear is fundamental to the increasing attachment in the infant or child. *Security*—the opposite of anxiety—occurs when the mother is close to the child and the child experiences no fear.

A syndrome known as maternal deprivation, also called hospitalism by René Spitz or anaclitic depression, occurs in some children under 2 years old who are placed in institutions and separated from their mothers for long periods of time (over three months). A predictable set and sequence of behavior patterns can be observed in these children: (1) *protest*, in which the child protests against the separation by crying, calling out, and searching for the lost person; (2) *despair*, in which the child appears hopeless about the mother ever returning; and (3) *detachment*, in which the child emotionally separates himself from the mother. Bowlby believes this sequence involves ambivalent feelings toward the mother; the child both wants her and is angry at her for her desertion.

The child in the detachment stage responds in an indifferent manner when the mother returns; the mother has not been forgotten, but the child is angry at her having gone away in the first place and fears that it may happen again. Some of these children develop affectionless personalities, characterized by emotional withdrawal, little or no feeling, and a limited ability to form affectionate relationships. Bowlby suggested a Darwinian evolutionary basis for attachment behavior; it ensures that adults protect their young. Ethological studies show that subhuman primates and other animals show attachment behavior patterns that are presumed to be instinctual and governed by inborn tendencies. An instinctual attachment system is seen in *imprinting*, in which certain stimuli are capable of eliciting innate behavior patterns during a critical period of the animal's behavioral development; thus, the infant offspring becomes attached to its mother at a critical period early in its development. The presence of imprinting behavior in humans is highly controversial. However, bonding and attachment behavior during the first year of life closely approximate it.

Bowlby's theories have had an immense impact on understanding normal and abnormal child development. Failure-to-thrive syndromes, psychosocial dwarfism, depression, delinquency, academic problems, and borderline intelligence have been traced to negative attachment experiences. When maternal care was deficient because the mother was mentally ill, the child was institutionalized for a long period, or the primary object of attachment died, emotional damage to the child occurred. Bowlby originally thought that the damage was permanent and invariable; but he revised his theories to take into account the time at which separation took place, the type and degree of the separation, and the level of security the child had experienced prior to the separation.

RECENT ADVANCES IN ATTACHMENT THEORY

A great deal of research has been done by followers of Bowlby that supports and expands on his observations, particularly the theory that there is an evolutionary, genetic basis for human infants becoming attached to their principal care-givers. Mary Ainsworth has shown that the interaction between the mother and her baby during the attachment period significantly influences the baby's current and future behavior. Patterns of attachment also vary among babies; for example, some babies signal or cry less than others. Sensitive responsiveness to infant signals, such as cuddling the baby when he cries, causes infants to cry less in later months rather than reinforcing crying behavior. Close bodily contact by the mother when the baby signals for her also is associated with the growth of self-reliance, rather than a clinging dependence, as the baby grows older. Less responsive mothers produce more anxious babies, and these mothers are characterized as having lower I.Q.s and being emotionally immature and younger than more responsive mothers.

Attachment behavior persists throughout life—from the cradle to the grave—as Bowlby hypothesized. Clinical studies demonstrated attachment behavior in school-age children, adolescents, and adults. College students, away from home for the first time, made good social adjustments if their early attachments to care-givers were secure. Low self-esteem, poor social relatedness, and emotional vulnerability to stress were associated with less secure attachments during the first year of life. Ainsworth concluded that humans continue to be attached to their parents, regardless of whether or not their early attachments were optimal. She also found that attachments occur to various other persons such as teachers, relatives, coaches, or older siblings—especially when attachments to the parent was poor or inadequate. Such attachment figures are cast in the parental role and may be mentors or even therapists. By inspiring trust, these individuals provide a secure base from which the person gains confidence in himself and in his ability to deal with the outside world. Thus, the new attachment figure promotes a corrective emotional experience.

Affectional bonds that later develop between people have attachment components to them. The sharing of experience is important in a variety of attachment bonds between persons other than parent-child, such as siblings, friends, relatives, and marital pairs. What makes the adult attachment bond unique is that it provides a sense of security, a sense of being needed, and a sense of being able to give. The absence of the attachment figure makes the person feel lonely or anxious. Bowlby reported that reactions to the death of a parent or spouse can be traced to the nature of the person's past and present attachment to the lost figure. When a lack of demonstrable grief occurs, it may be due to real experiences of rejection and lack of closeness in the relationship; the person may even consciously offer an idealized picture of the deceased. This individual usually tries to present himself as an independent type, for whom closeness and attachment mean little.

References

Ainsworth M D S: Attachments across the life span. Bull NY Acad Med 61:792, 1985.
Bowlby J: *Maternal Care and Mental Health. World Health Organization,* Geneva, 1951.
Bowlby J: The nature of the child's tie to his mother. Internat J Psychoanal 39:350, 1958.
Bowlby J: *Attachment and Loss,* vols I, II, III. Basic Books, New York 1969, 1973, 1980.
Klaus M H, Kennell J H: *Parent-Infant Bonding,* ed 2. C V Mosby, St. Louis, 1982.
Klaus M H, Kennell J H: *Bonding: The Beginnings of Parent-Infant Attachment.* C. V. Mosby, St. Louis, 1983.
Osofsky J D, editor: *Handbook of Infant Development.* John Wiley & Sons, New York, 1979.
Papovsek K H, Papovsek M: The Evolution of parent-infant attachment: New psychobiological perspectives. In *Frontiers of Infant Psychiatry,* J D Can, editor, vol. II, p 276. W B Saunders, Philadelphia, 1984.

5.3 ————
Learning Theory

Learning can be defined as a change in behavior that results either from practice or from previous experience. It is assumed that learning represents a permanent change. Learning is inferred from observed performance that manifests itself as behavior. Therefore, learning and performance are related.

Most theorists believe that practice alone is not sufficient to produce learning. Instead, there must be some type of association between a stimulus and a response that causes learning to occur. The association may vary to include the satisfaction of a basic need, such as food, or a more complex need, such as approval.

There are three major theories of learning: (1) conditioning, based upon the link between stimulus and response; (2) cognition, based upon insight and experience; and (3) social learning, based upon interpersonal interaction, role modeling, and identification.

CONDITIONING LEARNING THEORY

Two types of conditioning have been described: classical and operant.

Classical Conditioning

Ivan Pavlov (1849–1936), the Russian physiologist and Nobel prize winner, observed in his work on gastric secretion that a dog salivated not just when food was placed in its mouth, but also at the sound of the footsteps of the person coming to feed the dog, even though the dog could not see

or smell the food. He analyzed these events and called the flow of saliva that occurred with the sound of footsteps a *conditioned response* (CR); that is, a response that could be elicited under certain conditions by a particular stimulus. In a typical Pavlovian experiment, a *stimulus* (S) that had no capacity to evoke a particular type of response before training, does so after consistent association with another stimulus. For example, under normal circumstances, a dog will not salivate when a bell is sounded. If bell sounds are always followed by the presentation of food, however, the dog ultimately pairs the bell and food. Eventually, the bell sound alone elicits salivation (CR). Because the food naturally produces salivation, it is referred to as an *unconditioned stimulus* (UCS). Salivation, a response that is reliably elicited by food (UCS), is referred to as an unconditioned response (UCR). The bell, which was originally unable to evoke salivation but came to do so when paired with food, is referred to as a *conditioned stimulus* (CS). Classical conditioning is most often applied to responses mediated by the autonomic nervous system.

Classical conditioning is diagrammed as follows:

Before conditioning
Food (UCS)——————→ Salivation (UCR)
Bell (CS) paired with food (UCS) ——→ Salivation (UCR)
After conditioning
Bell (CS)————————————→ Salivation (CR)

Extinction. Extinction is the eventual disappearance of a conditioned response. It occurs when the conditioned stimulus is constantly repeated without the unconditioned stimulus. In the above example, extinction occurs if the bell (CS) is presented repeatedly without being paired with food (UCS). Eventually, salivation (CR) would not occur when the bell sounded, and extinction would have taken place. However, extinction is not a complete destruction of the conditioned response. If an animal is rested after extinction, the conditioned response returns but is less strong than before, a phenomenon known as *partial recovery.*

The American psychologist John B. Watson (1878–1958) used Pavlov's theory of classical conditioning to explain certain aspects of human behavior. In 1920, Watson described how he produced a phobia in an 11-month-old boy called Little Albert. At the same time that the boy was shown a white rat that he initially did not fear, a loud frightening noise was sounded. After several such pairings, Albert became fearful of the white rat, even though no loud noise was present. Watson and his colleagues obtained the same results using a white rabbit, and eventually, the response was generalized to any furry object. Many theorists believe that this process accounts for the development of childhood phobias in general; that is, they are learned responses based on classical conditioning.

Generalization. Generalization refers to the process whereby a conditioned response is transferred from one stimulus to another. Animals respond to stimuli that are similar to the original conditioned stimulus. A dog conditioned to respond to a bell will also respond to the sound of a tuning fork. Generalization is one theory used to explain higher learning because it enables one to learn similarities. For example, a street sign will be recognized whether or not it is on a pole, building, or curb. There is sufficient stimulus similarity for generalization to occur.

Discrimination. Discrimination is the process of recognizing and responding to the differences between similar stimuli. If the two stimuli are sufficiently different, the animal can be taught to respond to one and not the other; for example, an animal can learn to respond to different bells. In higher learning, a child learns to discriminate four-legged animals (the common stimulus) into dogs, cats, cows, and other quadrupeds.

Learning can be viewed as a balance of generalization and discrimination. Some disorders of thinking may stem from difficulties with these two processes. For example, a person may have had a traumatic experience as a child involving a person with a moustache. The transfer of those negative feelings to all men with moustaches is an example of both faulty discrimination and generalization.

Operant Conditioning

B. F. Skinner, born in 1904, proposed a theory of learning and behavior known as operant or instrumental conditioning. In classical conditioning, the animal is passive or restrained. In operant conditioning, however, the animal is active and behaves in a way that produces a reward. For example, a monkey that randomly presses various levers will be conditioned to that lever that, when pressed, releases a reward of food. Pressing the lever then becomes the conditioned response (CR). The reinforcement is controlled by the behaving organism in that it must produce a response in order to receive a reward. For example, a rat receives the reinforcing stimulus (food) only if it gives the response of pressing a lever. In addition to food, approval, praise, good grades, or any other response that satisfies a need in the animal or person can serve as a reward. In operant conditioning, behavior is reinforced by the experimenter. Operant conditioning is related to trial-and-error learning, described by the American psychologist, Edward L. Thorndike (1874–1949). In trial-and-error learning one attempts to solve a problem by trying out a variety of actions until one proves successful—a freely moving organism behaves in a way that is *instrumental* in producing a reward. For instance, a cat in a Thorndike puzzle box must learn to lift a latch in order to escape from the box. Operant conditioning is sometimes called instrumental conditioning for that reason. Thorndike's law of effect states that certain responses are reinforced by reward, and the organism learns from these experiences. There are four kinds of instrumental or operant conditioning: primary reward conditioning, escape conditioning, avoidance conditioning, and secondary reward conditioning. They are described in Table 1.

Respondent and Operative Behavior. Skinner described two types of behavior: (1) *respondent behavior,* behavior that results from known stimuli (e.g., the knee jerk reflex to patellar stimulation or the pupillary constriction to light); and (2) *operant behavior,* which is independent of a stimulus (e.g., the random movements of an infant or the aimless movements of a laboratory rat in a cage). Skinner took advantage of operant behavior by placing one of those rats in a Skinner box (named after him, its developer). The rat was deprived of food and randomly pressed a bar. At some point in the experiment, food was released by the experimenter when the bar was pressed. The food *reinforced* the bar pressing, which increased or decreased in rate depending on the level of reinforcement given by the experimenter. A reinforcer is anything that maintains a response or increases its strength. It is

Table 1
Four Kinds of Operant or Instrumental Conditioning

1. Primary reward conditioning	Simplest kind of conditioning. The learned response is instrumental in obtaining a biologically significant reward, such as a pellet of food or a drink of water
2. Escape conditioning	The organism learns a response that is instrumental in getting him out of some place he prefers not to be
3. Avoidance conditioning	The kind of learning in which a response to a cue is instrumental in avoiding a painful experience. A rat on a grid, for example, may avoid a shock if he quickly pushes a lever when a light signal goes on
4. Secondary reward conditioning	The kind of learning in which there is instrumental behavior to get at a stimulus which has no biological utility itself but which has in the past been associated with a biologically significant stimulus. For example, chimpanzees will learn to press a lever to obtain poker chips, which they insert in a slot to secure grapes. Later they will work to accumulate poker chips even when they are not interested in grapes

used synonymously with the term reward; however, some workers make this distinction: Responses are reinforced; individuals are rewarded.

Reinforcement Schedule (Programming). Reinforcers are described as *primary* when they are independent of previous learning (e.g., the need for food or water) or *secondary* when based on previous learning that has led to rewards (e.g., money, grades). In operant conditioning, it is possible to vary the schedule of reward or reinforcement given to a behavioral pattern—a process known as programming. The intervals between reinforcements may be *fixed* (e.g., every third response rewarded) or *variable* (e.g., sometimes the third response is rewarded; other times, the sixth). A continuous reinforcement schedule, in which every response is reinforced, leads to the most rapid acquisition of a behavior. When the response is reinforced only a fraction of the time the behavior occurs, it is called *partial reinforcement*. Partial or intermittant reinforcement is very effective in maintaining behavior and is resistant to extinction. For example, a person's use of a gambling slot machine is more continuous when the reward is partially reinforced, that is, when money is won at variable times. That procedure keeps the gambler guessing or trying to anticipate when a payoff will occur. The strength of operant learning is reflected in how frequently an animal responds. A high response frequency indicates strong operant learning. A decrease in frequency indicates that extinction is occurring. Table 2 illustrates various reinforcement schedules used in operant conditioning and the effects of these schedules on behavior.

In operant conditioning *positive reinforcement* refers to the process by which certain consequences of a response increase the probability that the response will occur again. Food, water, praise, and money are positive reinforcers. *Negative reinforcement* de-

Table 2
Reinforcement Schedules in Operant Conditioning

Reinforcement Schedule	Example	Behavioral Effect
Fixed ratio (FR)	Reinforcement occurs after every 10 responses 10:1 ratio; 10 bar presses release a food pellet	Rapid rate of response to obtain greatest number of rewards. Animal knows that next reinforcement depends on certain number of responses being made.
Fixed interval (FI)	Reinforcement occurs at regular intervals (e.g., every third hour)	Animal keeps track of time. Rate of responding drops to near 0 after reinforcement and then increases at about expected time of reward.
Variable ratio (VR)	Variable reinforcement occurs (e.g., after the third, sixth, then second response, and so on)	Generates fairly constant rate of response because probability of reinforcement at any given time remains relatively stable (e.g., slot machines)
Variable interval (VI)	Reinforcement occurs after variable intervals (e.g., every 3, 6, and then 2 hours) similar to VR	Response rate does not change between reinforcement. Animal responds at steady rate in order to get reward when it is available; common in trout fisherman

scribes the process by which a response that leads to the removal of an aversive event increases that response. For example, a teenager mows the lawn in order to avoid his parents' complaints, or an animal jumps off a grid in order to escape a painful shock. Any behavior that enables one to avoid or escape a punishing consequence will be strengthened.

Negative reinforcement is not punishment. *Punishment* is an aversive stimuli (e.g., a slap) that is presented specifically to weaken or supress an undesired response. Punishment reduces the probability that a response will recur.

Aversive Control. Aversive control or conditioning is a form of operant conditioning in which the organism changes its behavior to avoid a painful, noxious, or aversive stimulus. Electric shocks are common aversive stimuli used in laboratory experiments. Any behavior that avoids an aversive stimulus is reinforced as a result.

Escape Learning and Avoidance Learning. Negative reinforcement is related to two types of learning, *escape learning* and *avoidance learning*. In escape learning, the animal learns a response to get out of some place where he does not want to be (e.g., an animal jumps off an electric grid whenever it is charged). Avoidance learning requires an additional response. The same rat on the grid will learn to avoid a shock if it quickly pushes a lever when a light signal goes on. To move from escape learning to avoidance learning, an *anticipatory response* is necessary to prevent the punishment from occurring. Escape learning and avoidance learning are two forms of aversive control. Behavior that terminates the source of aversive stimuli is strengthened and maintained.

Shaping Behavior. Shaping involves changing behavior in a deliberate and predetermined way. By reinforcing those responses that are in the desired direction, shaping occurs. If the experimenter wants to train a seal to ring a bell with its nose, he can give a food reinforcement as the animal's random behavior brings

its nose nearer to the bell. The closer the time of the reinforcement to the operant behavior, the better the learning.

Adventitious Reinforcement. Responses that are reinforced accidentally by coincidental pairing of response and reinforcement are adventitious. Such events may have clinical implications in the development of phobias or other neurotic behavior.

Application of Conditioning Theory to Psychiatry

In 1950, Joseph Wolpe defined anxious behavior as persistent habits of learned or conditioned responses acquired in anxiety-generating situations. In using the term, "habit," Wolpe drew upon Clark I. Hull's concept of learning as being mediated by central nervous system activity. If a response inhibitory to anxiety can occur in the presence of anxiety-evoking stimuli, then it will weaken the connection between these stimuli and the anxiety response. Wolpe referred to this process as *reciprocal inhibition*. Relaxation, for example, is considered to be incompatible with anxiety and, therefore, is inhibitory to it.

Anxiety Hierarchy. Wolpe developed a method of therapy known as *systematic desensitization,* the goal of which is to eliminate maladaptive anxiety and behavior. To accomplish this goal, Wolpe asked his patient to imagine the least disturbing item on a list of potentially anxiety-evoking stimuli and then to proceed up the list to the most disturbing stimuli. For example, a patient with a fear of heights would rank the sight of a tall building lower in the anxiety hierarchy than standing on a high ledge; *being* on the tenth floor of a building would fall somewhere in between. In the relaxed state (usually induced by hypnosis, but sometimes induced by drugs), the patient is instructed to visualize the least anxiety-producing situation; if that visualization does not produce anxiety, the person moves up the hierarchy. Eventually, the patient is desensitized to the source of anxiety.

Tension Reduction Theory. John Dollard and Neal Miller attempted to reconcile behavioral theory and Freudian psychodynamics by stressing the commonalities between the two. Subscribing to the *tension-reduction* theory of behavior, they see behavior as motivated by the organism's attempt to reduce tension produced by unsatisfied or unconscious drives. Freud's pleasure principle is a tension-reducing force and consequently, is a strong motivator. If repressed, fear is learned and is transformed into anxiety. In either case, it acts as an acquired drive; thus, a person's behavior may be motivated by an attempt to reduce fear. Early childhood events may be traumatic (that is, may cause anxiety). If such events are repressed, the adult may avoid situations that are likely to stimulate anxiety, but may be completely unaware of those avoidance patterns. Therapy, in part, is an unlearning process. The organism learns that certain behaviors can reduce anxiety, and avoidance patterns are replaced by approach patterns.

Learned Helplessness Model of Depression. A laboratory animal may be classically conditioned to accept a painful stimulus when restrained. Such restraint eventually teaches the animal that there is no way to avoid the aversive stimulus. A condition known as *learned helplessness* develops when an organism learns that there is no behavioral pattern that can influence the environment. The learned helplessness paradigm has been used to explain depression in humans who feel helpless, without options, and unable to control events.

Brain Stimulation and Reinforcement. When certain areas of the hypothalamus are electrically stimulated, intense pleasure is experienced by both animals and man. Nonhuman primates were provided with a method by which they could stimulate pleasure centers in their brains. The animals preferred stimulating themselves to eating or drinking. In human beings, similar phenomena occur, and in one case, a patient stimulated his brain 1,000 times in a six-hour period until he was forced to stop.

COGNITIVE LEARNING THEORIES

Cognition is defined as the process of obtaining, organizing, and utilizing intellectual knowledge. Cognitive learning theories focus on the role of understanding. Mental operations are performed by the person, and bits of information are stored in memory to be retrieved at some later time. Cognition implies an understanding of the connection between cause and effect, between action and the consequences of that action. *Cognitive strategies* are mental plans used by a person to understand self and environment.

Depressed patients have a cognitive strategy that focuses on what is wrong, rather than what is right. A form of cognitive therapy developed by Aaron Beck for the treatment of depression teaches patients to recognize and value their assets and alerts them to the cognitive pattern that causes their depression. Beck described the cognitive triad that exists in depression as consisting of a person's (1) negative view of self, (2) negative interpretation of experience, and (3) negative expectation of the future.

Many theorists, such as Piaget, define a series of stages in cognitive growth. Another approach toward cognition is termed *information processing,* which refers to a sequence of mental operations involving input, storing, and output of information. Cognition involves calling up and processing relevant information from stored memory.

SOCIAL LEARNING THEORIES

Social learning theory relies on role modeling, identification, and human interactions. A person can learn by imitating the behavior of another person; but personal factors are involved. If the role model is not someone the person likes, imitative behavior is not likely to occur. Social learning theorists combine operant and classical conditioning theories. For example, although observation of models may be a major factor in the learning process, imitation of the model must be reinforced or rewarded if the behaviors are to become part of the person's repertoire.

Albert Bandura is a major proponent of the social learning school. Behavior occurs as a result of the interplay between cognitive and environmental factors, a concept known as *reciprocal determinism*. Persons learn by observing others, intentionally or accidentally, a process known as *modeling* or learning through imitation. The person's choice of a model is influenced by a variety of factors, such as age, sex, status, and similarity to oneself. If the chosen model reflects healthy norms and values, the person develops *self-efficacy,* the capacity to adapt to normal everyday life and to threatening situations. It is possible to eliminate negative behavior patterns through behavior modification by having a person learn alternate techniques from other role models.

NEUROPHYSIOLOGY OF LEARNING

One of the first theorists to approach the neurophysiologic aspects of learning was Clark I. Hull (1884–1952), who developed a drive-reduction theory of learning. Hull postulated that neurophysiological connections are established in the central nervous system that reduce the level of a drive (e.g., obtaining food reduces hunger). An external stimulus stimulates an efferent system and elicits a motor impulse. The critical connection is between the stimulus and the motor response, which is a neurophysiologic reaction that leads to what Hull called a habit. Habits are strengthened when a response leads to a further reduction in the drive associated with the aroused need.

By exploring the human brain, researchers such as Broca and Wernicke identified specific areas of the brain involved in the development and retention of speech and language. Electrical stimulation of certain brain sites evoked vivid mental imagery in patients. Also, lesions of the amygadaloid nucleus in animals have been demonstrated to interfere with learning.

Learning produces changes in the structure and function of nerve cells. In one study, monkeys that were trained to use a particular finger to obtain food, showed hypertrophy of the area of the brain responsible for finger control. In the study of the snail aplysia by Eric Kandel, synaptic connections were altered as a result of learning.

The neurobiological basis of learning is located in the structures of the brain involved in forming and storing information. These structures include the hippocampus, the cortex, and the cerebellum. One hundred billion neurons in the brain are involved in forming memories, including a layer of 4.6 million cells in the hippocampus.

Learning begins with the senses taking in an environmental stimulus that is eventually transformed into a memory trace or memory link. An electrical or chemical impulse passes through the neuron when the brain receives information, which triggers the formation of connections between synapses. Animal experiments have demonstrated an increase in synaptic connections when learning occurs.

Long-term memories are retained longer than short-term memories owing to the increased time such memories have had to link up with a number of locations in the cortex. The more connections, the better the chance of contacting a neural pathway leading to the memory. Repeated reliving of a memory enhances its permanence.

Storage is the key to a good memory. Relating material to something that is already known creates more pathways and increases the storage power. Processing information at a semantic level involves more of the mind than rote memorization. This information decays at a slower rate than information memorized on a superficial level, without meaning and comprehension.

Memory is divided into short term and long-term memory. Short-term memory, also called "working memory" or "buffer memory," is very adversely affected by chronic emotional stress and lack of "effort" due to psychological exhaustion or too much input. Short-term memory and long-term memory differ in the amount of information that can be stored. The capacity of short-term memory is limited (five to nine bits of information), however, the process of retrieving specific memories may be forgotten.

Smell and emotion may underlie long-term memories. Scent conveys information through the olfactory nerve to the hippocampus, which plays a role in the control of emotions. Learning and memory are affected by stress. The increase in adrenaline resulting from stress can enhance learning, but if stress is too great, learning is inhibited. A person's mood affects the learning and recall of material; that is, learning material while in a happy mood enhances memory, and the person recalls material better while in a happy mood. Some childhood memories survive. They are usually those associated with the period when the child learned to speak, between the ages of 3 and 5 years. Before that time, memories associated with traumatic events or with smell are most likely to be remembered.

Perception

According to a generally accepted definition, perception is the process of organizing and interpreting sensory data by combining them with the results of previous experience. This definition indicates that perception is a complex process involving the past as well as the present and an external stimulus as well as an internal response. Much of perception is learned behavior.

Organization. A great deal of the work on the influence of the stimulus field in perception has been done in the area of vision. This is probably because what is perceived visually is strongly determined by the ordering of the

stimulus components in space, and this ordering is rather easy to manipulate. For example:

****

is a row of 16 asterisks. By manipulating the spatial relationships, one can enhance the probability that they will be seen as eight pairs of asterisks:

** ** ** ** ** ** ** **

Such situations led to the enunciation of the principle that the whole is different from the sum of its parts. One explanation of this principle defines stimulus organization, or *Gestalt,* as an additional property of the stimulus. A basic way of perceiving is to place a figure against a background. The figure then has shape, distance, and perspective.

Selectivity. Far more stimuli than a person can be aware of or respond to are available for perception at any given instant. These stimuli impinge simultaneously and through many different channels. But, the perceptual process is a central one, and only a limited amount of the available information can be processed at one time. Therefore, a process of selectivity becomes operative. Some stimuli are perceived, some are not; some that are perceived are responded to, and some are not.

Some objective and many subjective factors govern the operation of this selectivity; both the stimulus field and the attributes of the perceiver determine what is perceived. One important objective factor is the strength of the stimulus. A strong stimulus is more likely to be perceived than a weak one. Another objective factor that governs what is perceived is timing. A stimulus that begins an instant before a second stimulus may be perceived to the exclusion of the second.

Individual Development and Experience. A person tends to perceive more important stimuli rather than less important ones. Since the attribute of importance is based on individual experience and interests, two people in the same situation may perceive very different things. What each perceives is a function of personal learning and experience. For example, the letter A is simply a pattern of lines to someone who does not know the alphabet.

An experience that predisposes an individual to certain types of perceptions is called a *set*. The more ambiguous the stimulus, the more its perception is determined by the set of proclivities of the subject. And the stronger the set of the individual, the more it determines one's perception. The meaning attributed to a particular stimulus by a given person is a function of the ambiguity of the stimulus and the strength of that person's set.

The major application of these principles in psychiatry has been in projective testing, in which ambiguous stimuli are presented and subjects' responses are analyzed in terms of their emphasis and patterning. A description of the subject's personality in terms of perceptual proclivities is extrapolated from this analysis. Perhaps the best known projective test is the Rorschach test, a collection of ten inkblots.

Many experiments have indicated that people can be influenced in their own perceptual judgments of others. The degree of influence depends on the consistency of others' judgments, the status of the other judges, and the expertise attributed to them.

Motivation

Motivation is a state of being that produces a tendency toward some type of action. That state may be a state of deprivation (e.g., hunger), a value system, or a strongly held belief (e.g., religion). In the mediation of learning and perception, biological mechanisms play an important role in motivating behavior. The organism tries to maintain homeostasis or internal balance against any disturbance of equilibrium (e.g., the thirsty animal is motivated to find water and drink). Social motives, such as the need for recognition and achievement, also account for behavioral patterns (e.g., studying hard to get good grades). However, the intensity of motivation to achieve at any task in any particular situation is determined by at least two factors: the achievement motive (desire to achieve), and the likelihood of success.

There are marked individual differences in the values placed on objects and goals. Some students strive for As; others depreciate the importance of grades, placing higher value on intellectual satisfactions or on extracurricular activities. The expectancy factor refers to the subjective probability that, with the expenditure of sufficient effort, the object may be acquired or the goal reached.

Cognitive dissonance means incongruity or disharmony with respect to such matters as expectation and actuality. An example of cognitive dissonance is the unwillingness of a person to believe that a car for which he or she paid a great deal of money, or which is considered to be a status symbol, could have anything wrong with it or be defective in any way. In general, dissonance occurs when there is a palpable disparity between two experimental or behavioral elements. It is postulated that cognitive dissonance produces an uncomfortable tension state (like hunger) that is motivating. The chief distinguishing feature of a cognitive approach to motivation is that cognitive motivation theorists focus on perceptual and informational aspects of the total stimulating situation. They tend to deal with physiologic arousal in terms of stimuli generated by the physiologic processes.

Attribution theory is also a cognitive approach; in essence, it is concerned with how people perceive the motivations of others. The basic assumption is that an individual is motivated to attain a cognitive mastery over the environment.

Freud's writings were probably the most powerful single influence initiating scientific investigations of human motivation. From Freud's observations, it was plain that a full understanding of the causes of human behavior could not be gained from conscious introspections alone. Clearly, much of behavior is determined by unconscious mental activities, activities that the person is unaware of and, consequently, cannot report on.

References

Bandura A, Walters R H: *Social Learning and Personality Development.* Holt, Rinehart & Winston, New York, 1963.
Dollard J, Miller N E: *Personality and Psychotherapy.* McGraw Hill, New York, 1950.
Dunn A J: Neurochemistry of learning and memory: An evaluation of recent data. Ann Rev Psychol *33*:343, 1980.
Hilgard E R, Bower G H: *Theories of Learning,* ed 3. Appleton-Century-Crofts, New York, 1966.
Hull C L: *Principles of Behavior. An Introduction to Behavior Therapy.* Appleton-Century-Crofts, New York, 1943.
Mowrer O H: *Learning Theory and Behavior.* Wiley, New York, 1960.
Pavlov I P: *Conditioned Reflexes.* Oxford, London, 1927.
Rescorla R A, Holland P C: Behavioral studies of associative learning in animals. Ann Rev Psychol *33*:265, 1982.
Skinner B F: *Science and Human Behavior.* Macmillan, New York, 1953.
Wolpe J: The genesis of neurosis. S Afr Med J *24*:613, 1950.

5.4 _____
Aggression

Aggression is any form of behavior directed toward the goal of harming or injuring another creature that is motivated to avoid such treatment. Aggression also implies intent to do harm, which must be inferred from events that precede or follow acts of aggression. In some cases, establishing the presence of an intention to harm others is relatively simple. Aggressors often admit their desire to harm their victims and express disappointment if the attempt fails.

THEORETICAL PERSPECTIVES

Aggression as Instinctive Behavior

Freud's View. In his early writings, Freud held that all human behavior stems either directly or indirectly from *eros*—the life instinct—whose energy, or libido, is directed toward the enhancement or reproduction of life. In this framework, aggression was viewed simply as a reaction to the blocking or thwarting of libidinal impulses. As such, it was neither an automatic nor an inevitable part of life.

After the tragic events of World War I, Freud gradually came to adopt a somewhat gloomier position regarding the nature of human aggression. He proposed the existence of a second major instinct—*thanatos,* the death force—whose energy is directed toward the destruction or termination of life. According to Freud, all human behavior stems from the complex interplay of this instinct with eros and the constant tension between them.

Because the death instinct, if unrestrained, would soon result in self-destruction, it was hypothesized that through other mechanisms, such as displacement, the energy of thanatos is redirected outward, so that it serves as the basis for aggression against others. In Freud's view, aggression stems primarily from the redirection of the self-destructive death instinct away from the person and toward others.

Lorenz's View. According to Konrad Lorenz, aggression that causes physical harm to others springs from a fighting instinct that humans share with other organisms. The energy associated with this instinct is spontaneously produced in organisms at a more or less constant rate. The probability of aggression increases as a function of the amount of stored energy and the presence and strength of aggression-releasing stimuli. Aggression is inevitable, and at times, spontaneous eruptions occur.

Aggression as an Elicited Drive

The drive theory of aggression proposes that (1) the drive is elicited by external, situational conditions (e.g., frustration, loss of face, physical pain) and (2) its arousal ultimately leads to overt forms of aggression against others. The best-known statement of this perspective is the frustration-aggression hypothesis, first proposed by John Dollard in 1939. According to this view, frustration—the blocking of ongoing goal-directed behavior—leads to the arousal of a drive whose primary goal is that of harming some person or object. This drive, in turn, leads to attacks against various targets, especially against the source of the frustration.

Aggression as Learned Social Behavior

This perspective regards aggression primarily as a learned form of social behavior—one that is acquired and maintained in much the same manner as other forms of activity. According to Bandura, neither innate urges toward violence nor aggressive drives aroused by frustration and other conditions is the root of human aggression. Rather, they engage in assaults against others because (1) they acquired aggressive responses through past experience, (2) they receive or anticipate various forms of reward for performing such actions, or (3) they are directly instigated to aggression by specific social or environmental conditions. In contrast to both instinct and drive theories, the social learning perspective does not attribute aggression to one or a few potential causes. It suggests that the roots of such behavior are quite varied in scope, involving aggressors' past experience and learning as well as a wide range of external, situational factors. For example, soldiers receive medals for killing enemy troops during times of war, and professional athletes attain widespread admiration and large financial rewards by competing in an aggressive manner (Table 1).

Evolutionary Biology of Aggression

In the evolutionary framework, aggressive behavior is not viewed as the result of a specific kind of process, such as a drive, an innate tendency, an eliciting stimulus, or something learned. Rather, it is an evolved capacity that can be developed. Its functions include: securing preferential or exclusive access to such vital resources as space, shelter, food, reproduction, and, defense of oneself, those in whom one has direct genetic investment (e.g., offspring, parents), and selected nonkin.

The implications of this framework for understanding human aggression is as follows: First, in many situations, aggression may be adaptive. People, as well as animals, often display aggression in situations wherein valuable resources and essential functions are perceived to be threatened (e.g., competition for food or a mate, property encroachment, favors not repaid). Second, the form of aggression differs in the situations described above (e.g., throwing a rock, hand-to-hand combat, waiting for a predator to behave in a certain way). Third, for any given instance of aggression, the contributions of physiologic, psychological, and contextual factors vary.

DETERMINANTS OF AGGRESSION

Social Determinants

Frustration. If 100 persons were stopped at random on the street and asked to name the most important single cause of aggression, most would reply with one word: frustration. Many would indicate that the single most potent means of inciting human beings to aggression is the thwarting of their goals. Widespread acceptance of this view stems mainly from John Dollard's frustration-aggression hypothesis. In its original form, this hypothesis suggested that (1) frustration always leads to some form of aggression and (2) aggression always stems from frustration.

It is now clear, however, that frustrated persons do not always respond with aggressive thoughts, words, or deeds. They may actually show a wide variety of reactions, ranging from resignation, depression, and despair, to attempts to overcome the source of their frustration. It is also apparent that not all aggression results from frustration. People (e.g., boxers, football players) act aggressively for many reasons and in response to many different stimuli.

A careful examination of existing evidence suggests that whether frustration increases or fails to enhance overt aggression depends largely on two factors. First, it appears that frustration increases aggression only when the frustration is quite intense. When it is mild or moderate, aggression may fail to be enhanced. Second, growing evidence suggests that frustration is more likely to facilitate aggression when it is perceived as arbitrary or illegitimate rather than when it is viewed as deserved or legitimate.

Direct Provocation from Others. Existing evidence suggests that physical abuse or verbal taunts from others often serve as powerful elicitors of aggressive actions. Once aggression begins, it often shows an unsettling pattern of escalation; as a result, even mild verbal slurs or glancing blows may initiate a process in which stronger and stronger provocations are exchanged.

Exposure to Aggressive Models. A link between aggression and exposure to televised violence has been noted. The more televised violence children watch, the greater their level of aggression against others. The strength of this relationship appears to increase over time, pointing to the cumulative impact of media violence. The processes that account for the effects of filmed or televised violence on the behavior of children are outlined in Table 2.

Environmental Determinants

Effects of Air Pollution. It has been reported that exposure to noxious odors, similar to the ones produced by chemical plants and other industries, may increase personal irritability and, therefore, aggression. This effect appears to be true only up to a point. If the odors in question are truly foul, aggression appears to decrease—perhaps because escape from the unpleasant environment becomes a dominant tendency among the persons involved.

Effects of Noise. Several studies have reported that individuals who are exposed to loud and irritating noise direct stronger assaults against others than do persons who are not exposed to such environmental conditions.

Effects of Crowding. Some studies suggest that overcrowding may produce elevated levels of aggression; other investigations have failed to obtain evidence for such a link. In situations where typical reactions are negative (e.g., annoyance,

Table 1
Three Contrasting Theoretical Perspectives on Human Aggression

Theory/Perspective	Assumed Source of Human Aggression	Possibility of Preventing or Controlling Such Behavior
Instinct theory	Innate tendencies or instincts	Low: aggressive impulses constantly generated; impossible to avoid
Drive theory	Externally elicited aggressive drive	Low: external sources of aggressive drive very common (e.g., frustration) and impossible to eliminate
Social learning theory	Present social or environmental conditions plus past social learning	Moderate to high: appropriate changes in current social and environmental conditions, or in reinforcement contingencies, can reduce or prevent overt aggressive actions

Baron R A: Aggression. In *Comprehensive Textbook of Psychiatry,* ed 4, H I Kaplan, B J Sadock, editors, p 216. Williams & Wilkins, Baltimore, 1985.

irritation, frustration), crowding may enhance the likelihood of aggressive outbursts.

Situational Determinants

Heightened Physiological Arousal. Some research indicates that heightened arousal stemming from such diverse sources as participation in competitive activities, vigorous exercise, and exposure to provocative films enhance overt aggression.

Sexual Arousal and Aggression. Recent investigations suggest that the impact of sexual arousal on aggression strongly depends on the type of erotic materials employed to induce such reactions and on the precise nature of the reactions themselves. When the erotica viewed by subjects is mild in nature, such as photos of attractive nudes, aggression is reduced. When they are more explicit, such as films of couples engaged in various acts of love making, aggression is enhanced.

Erotic materials inducing mild levels of arousal and largely positive feelings among participants have been found to reduce their subsequent levels of aggression. In contrast, erotica inducing strong arousal plus negative feelings has been observed to enhance overt aggression. Thus, it appears that the impact of sexual arousal upon overt aggression can indeed be understood by reference to two basic psychological mechanisms: the level of such arousal itself, and the positive or negative feelings accompanying such excitement.

Pain as an Elicitor. Physical pain may serve to arouse an aggressive drive—the motive to harm or injure others. Such drive, in turn, may find expression against any available target, including ones not in any way responsible for the aggressor's discomfort. This hypothesis may explain why persons exposed to aggression may act aggressively toward others.

Hormones, Drugs, and Aggressive Behavior

Aggression has been linked in animals with testosterone, progesterone, luteinizing hormone, renin, β-endorphin, prolactin, melatonin, norepinephrine, dopamine, epinephrine, acetylcholine, serotonin, 5-hydroxyindoleacetic acid, and phenylacetic acid, among others.

Some studies have related the level of aggression to the androgen insensitivity syndrome (in which there is defective binding of androgens to proteins resulting in male offspring who have a feminine appearance) and to the adrenogenital syndrome (in which the mother's adrenal cortex exposes the fetus to elevated adrenal androgens resulting in masculinization), as evidenced by an increase in rough-and-tumble play in masculinized girls.

Considering drugs and chemicals, the following generalizations appear to hold: Small doses of alcohol inhibit aggression and large doses facilitate it; barbituate effects are similar to those of alcohol; aerosols and commercial solvent effects (acute) also resemble alcohol's effects; anxiolytics generally inhibit aggression, although paradoxical aggression is sometimes observed; opiate dependence (but not opiate intoxication) is associated with increased aggression, as is the use of stimulants, cocaine, hallucinogens, and nearly toxic doses of marijuana.

Neuroanatomy and Aggressive Behavior

Anger, rage, and increased irritability are frequent during certain stages of Korsakoff's syndrome and Huntington's chorea, diseases that directly affect the brain. Encephalitis lethargica and rabies also are associated with increases in aggression. There is evidence suggesting that the following kinds of lesions are associated with increased aggression: irritable focal lesions; certain forms of epilepsy, particularly temporal lobe and psychomotor; temporal lobe tumors; anterior hypothalamic lesions; frontal lobe lesions; abnormal discharges in the medial amygdala and mesencephalic tegmentum; and, dominant-hemisphere lesions. While lesions establish that particular anatomical structures are important in mediating aggression, some structures may be more essential than others.

Animal studies indicate that stimulation of the lateral and medial hypothalamus result in different types of aggression and that the amygdala has a critical role in aggression. Very small experimental surgical extirpations of the amygdala have caused members of normally aggressive species such as wild cats to become quite tame. Amygdolotomy has been tried experimentally on humans for the treatment of unpredictable violence, sexual delinquency and anhedonia.

Table 2
Mechanisms Underlying the Impact of Televised or Filmed Violence on the Behavior of Viewers

Mechanism	Description of Effects
Observational learning	Viewers acquire new means of harming others not previously present in their behavior repertoires
Disinhibition	Viewers' restraints or inhibitions against performing aggressive actions are weakened as a result of observing others engaging in such behavior
Densensitization	Viewers' emotional responsivity to aggressive actions and their consequences—signs of suffering on the part of victims—is reduced. As a result, they demonstrate little, if any, emotional arousal in response to such stimuli

From Baron R A: Aggression. In *Comprehensive Textbook of Psychiatry*, ed 4, H I Kaplan, D J Sadock, editors, p 219. Williams & Wilkins, Baltimore, 1985.

PREVENTION AND CONTROL OF AGGRESSION

Punishment as a Deterrent

Punishment is sometimes effective as a deterrent to overt aggression. Research findings suggest that the frequency or intensity of such behavior can often be sharply reduced by even mild forms of punishment such as social disapproval; but there appear to be strong grounds for doubting that punishment always, or even usually, produces such effects.

The recipients of punishment often interpret it as an attack against them. To the extent that this is so, individuals may respond even more aggressively. Strong punishment is more likely to provoke desires for revenge or retribution than to instill lasting restraints against violence in the subject. Persons who administer punishment may serve as aggressive models for those on the receiving end of such discipline, and as noted earlier, exposure to such models may potentiate violent acts. There is some indication that punishment, because of the conditions under which it is usually administered (a long while after the aggression is committed) only temporarily reduces the strength or frequency of aggressive behavior. Once punishment is discontinued, aggressive acts quickly reappear. For these reasons, it seems likely that direct punishment often backfires and actually enhances, rather than inhibits, the dangerous actions it is designed to prevent.

Catharsis

For many years it has been widely believed that providing angry persons with an opportunity to engage in expressive but noninjurious behaviors reduces their tension or arousal and weakens their tendency to engage in overt and potentially dangerous acts of aggression. These effects embody the catharsis hypothesis. Although Freud accepted the existence of such catharsis, he was relatively pessimistic about its usefulness in preventing overt aggression. At present, the benefits of catharsis are mixed. It may help some people discharge aggression while others may become more aggressive as a result.

Training in Social Skills

A major reason why many persons become involved in repeated aggressive encounters is that they lacking basic social skills. They do not know how to communicate effectively and, so, adopt an abrasive style of self-expression. Their ineptness in performing such basic tasks as making requests, engaging in negotiations, and lodging complaints often irritate friends, acquaintances, and strangers. These severe social deficits seem to ensure that they will experience repeated frustration, and that they will frequently anger those with whom they have direct contact. One technique for reducing the frequency of such behavior may involve providing such persons with the social skills that they so sorely lack. Social skills training has been applied to diverse groups of persons, including highly aggressive teenagers, police, and even child-abusing parents. In many cases, dramatic changes in the targeted behaviors have been produced (e.g., enhanced interpersonal communication, improved ability to handle rejection and stress), and reductions in aggressive behavior related to these shifts have frequently been observed. These results are encouraging and suggest that training in appropriate social skills can offer a promising approach to the reduction of human violence.

The Induction of Incompatible Responses

Empathy. When aggressors attack other persons in face-to-face confrontations they are often exposed to signs of pain and suffering on the part of their victims. One reaction to such feedback may be the arousal of empathy and a subsequent reduction in further aggression. In several experiments, exposure to signs of pain or discomfort on the part of the victim has been found to inhibit further aggression by male participants.

Humor. Informal observation suggests that anger can often be reduced through exposure to humorous material, and some laboratory studies support this proposal. It appears that several types of humor, presented in several different formats, may induce reactions or emotions incompatible with aggression among the persons who observe them.

Other Incompatible Responses. Many other reactions may also prove to be incompatible with anger or overt aggression. As noted above, mild sexual arousal sometimes operates in this fashion. Similarly, feelings of guilt concerning the performance of aggressive actions may often reduce such behavior. There is also some indication that participation in absorbing cognitive tasks such as solving mathematics problems may induce reactions incompatible with anger or aggressive actions.

Drug Treatment

Current reports suggest that different types of drugs as well as different types of clinical monitoring (e.g., blood pressure, EEG) are essential for optimal treatment of aggressive persons suffering from psychiatric disorders. The current findings may be summarized as follows: lithium carbonate appears to be a drug of major promise for some populations of violent patients, especially delinquent adolescent boys; anticonvulsants occasionally reduce seizure-induced forms of aggression and they may have the same effect on nonepileptics; antipsychotic medications appear to reduce aggression in both psychotic and nonpsychotic violent patients; antidepressants may be effective in reducing violence in some depressed patients; minor tranquilizers appear to have a limited role in reducing aggression; and, antiandrogen agents may be effective in the treatment of the aggressive sex offenders. β-blockers and stimulants may be effective in aggressive children. And, electroconvulsive therapy may be effective in selected patients.

References

Bandura A: *Aggression: A Social Learning Analysis.* Prentice-Hall, Englewood Cliffs, NJ, 1973.

Baron R A: *Human Aggression.* Plenum, New York, 1977.

Berkowitz L, Cochran S T, Embree M C: Physical pain and the goal of aversity stimulated aggression. J Pers Soc Psychol *40:*587, 1981.

Berkowitz L, Donnerstein E: External validity is more than skin deep: Some answers to criticisms of laboratory experiments. Am Psychol *37:*245, 1982.

Dollard J, Doob L, Miller N, Mowrer O H, Sears R R: *Frustration and Aggression.* Yale University Press, New Haven, CT, 1939.

Goldstein A P, Carr E G, Davidson W S, Wehr P: *In Response to Aggression.* Pergamon Press, New York, 1981.

Liebert R M, Sprafkin J N, Davidson E S: *The Early Window: Effects of Television on Children and Youth,* ed 2. Pergamon Press, New York, 1982.

Lorenz K: *On Aggression.* Bantam Books, New York, 1966.

Toch H: *Violent Men.* Schenkman Publishing, Cambridge, MA, 1980.

Zillmann D: *Connections Between Sex and Aggression.* Erlbaum Associates, Hillsdale, NJ, 1984.

5.5 ———————
Ethology and Experimental Disorders

Ethology is the systematic study of animal behavior. Originally, ethologists were interested primarily in the detailed analysis of the behavior of intact animals in their natural environment or in closely related environments. Direct observation was the basic technique for behavioral measurement. With the passage of time, ethologists added experimental modifications to the natural environment and initiated experimental laboratory investigations. Ethology is particularly relevant for psychiatry because findings of animal studies can shed light on human behavior.

IMPRINTING

Imprinting refers to the early, rapid, specific, and persisting learning, seen particularly in birds, by which the newborn animal becomes attached to the mother and, by generalization, to members of its own species. The phenomenon was described in 1935 by Konrad Lorenz, who observed that goslings responded to him as to the parental object if he presented himself before them when they were newly hatched. Lorenz concluded that species recognition is imprinted on the nervous system of young animals during the first period of exposure after hatching (Figure 1).

The imprinting phenomenon implies that there is a specific time in the animal's development when it is most

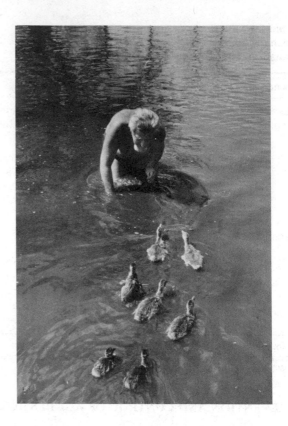

Figure 1. In a famous experiment, Lorenz demonstrated that goslings would respond to him as if he were the natural mother. (Reprinted by permission from Hess E H Imprinting: An effect of early experience. Science *130:* 133, 1959.)

susceptible to the formation of social bonds with fellow species members. This period usually occurs quite early in the life of the animal. Eckhard Hess suggested that imprinting research added a certain degree of substance to Freud's theory of developmental periods in the life of the human child. Imprinting has also reinforced the concept that early institutionalization has adverse effects on later behavior; the human infant's environment must satisfy certain minimal requirements of social interaction during the first year of life for normal development to occur.

Another pioneer in ethology was Niko Tinbergen, who emphasized the relationship between hormonal states and environmental factors in producing so-called instinctive responses. Tinbergen applied some of his concepts to the treatment of autistic children.

ANIMAL MODELS OF PSYCHOPATHOLOGY

Pharmacologic Experimentation

With the emergence of biological psychiatry, many researchers have utilized pharmacological means to produce syndrome analogues in animal subjects. Two classic examples are the reserpine model of unipolar depression and the amphetamine psychosis model of paranoid schizophrenia. In the depression studies, animals given the norepinephrine-depleting drug reserpine exhibited behavioral abnormalities analogous to those of major depression in humans. The behavioral abnormalities produced were generally reversed by antidepressant drugs. These studies tended to corroborate the theory that unipolar depression in humans is, in part, the result of diminished levels of norepinephrine. Similarly, animals given amphetamines acted in a stereotyped, inappropriately aggressive, and apparently frightened manner that was similar to paranoid psychotic symptoms in humans. Both of these models are currently thought to be too simplistic in their concepts of etiology, but they remain as early paradigms for this type of research.

Studies were done on the effects of catecholamine-depleting drugs on monkeys during separation and reunion periods. These studies showed that catecholamine-depletion and social separation can interact in a highly synergistic fashion, yielding depressive symptoms in subjects for whom mere separation or low-dose treatment by itself is not sufficient to produce depression.

Environmental Experimentation

A number of researchers, including Ivan Pavlov in Russia and W. Horsley Gantt and H. S. Lidell in America, studied the effects of stressful environments on animals such as dogs and sheep. Pavlov produced a phenomenon in dogs which he labeled *experimental neurosis,* by use of a conditioning technique that led to symptoms of extreme and persistent agitation. The technique involved teaching dogs to discriminate between a circle and an ellipse and then progressively diminishing the difference between the two. Gantt used the term *behavior disorders* to describe the reactions he elicited from dogs forced into similar conflictual learning situations. Lidell described the stress response he obtained in sheep, goats, and dogs as *experimental neurasthenia,* which was obtained in some cases by merely doubling the number of daily test trials in an unscheduled manner.

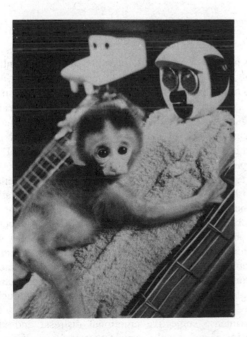

Figure 2. An infant rhesus monkey clinging to a cloth-covered surrogate mother.

The *learned helplessness model* of depression, developed by Martin Seligman, is a good example of an experimental disorder. Dogs were exposed to electric shocks from which they could not escape. The dogs eventually "gave up," making no attempt to escape new shocks. This apparent giving up generalized to other situations, and eventually the dogs always appeared to be helpless and apathetic. Because the cognitive, motivational, and affective deficits displayed by these dogs resembled symptoms common to human depressive disorders, learned helplessness, although controversial, was proposed as an animal model of human depression. Research on subjects with learned helplessness and the expectation of inescapable punishment has discovered brain release of endogenous opiates, destructive effects on the immune system, and elevation of the pain threshold.

A social application of this concept involves school children who have learned that they fail in school no matter what they do—they view themselves as helpless losers and this self-concept causes them to stop trying. Teaching them to persist may reverse this process with excellent results in self-respect and school performance.

STUDIES OF DEVELOPMENTAL PROCESSES IN NONHUMAN PRIMATES

An area of animal research that has important relevance to human behavior and psychopathology is longitudinal study of nonhuman primates. Monkeys have been followed from birth to maturity, not only in their natural habitats and laboratory facsimiles, but also in laboratory settings that involve differing degrees of social deprivation early in life. Social deprivation has been produced through two predominant conditions: *social isolation* and *separation. Socially isolated* monkeys are raised in varying degrees of isolation and are not permitted to develop normal attachment bonds. Monkeys that are *separated* are taken from their primary caretaker and thereby experience a disruption in an already developed bond. Social isolation techniques illustrate the impact of an infant's early social environment on subsequent development, while separation techniques illustrate the effects of loss of a significant attachment figure. The name most associated with the isolation and separation studies is Harry Harlow. A summary of Harlow's work is presented in Table 1.

In a series of experiments, Harry Harlow separated rhesus monkeys from their mothers during their first weeks of life. During this time, the monkey infant is dependent on its mother for nourishment and protection, as well as for physical warmth and emotional security, "contact comfort," as Harlow first termed it in 1958. Harlow substituted a surrogate mother made from wire or cloth for the real mother. The infants preferred the cloth-covered surrogate mother that provided contact comfort to the wire-covered surrogate that provided food but no contact comfort (Figure 2).

Rehabilitation of Abnormal Behavior in Primates

In 1972, Stephen Suomi demonstrated that isolates could be rehabilitated if they were exposed to monkeys that would promote physical contact without threatening the isolates with aggression or overly complex play interactions. These monkeys were called "therapist" monkeys. To fill such a

Table 1
Social Deprivation in Nonhuman Primates

Type of Social Deprivation	Effect
Total isolation (not allowed to develop caretaker or peer bond)	Self orality, self-clasping, very fearful when placed with peers, unable to copulate. If impregnated, females are unable to nurture young (motherless mothers). If isolation goes beyond 6 months no recovery is possible
Mother-only reared	Fail to leave mother and explore. Terrified when finally exposed to peers. Unable to play or to copulate
Peer-only reared	Engage in self-orality, grasp one another in clinging manner, easily frightened, reluctant to explore, timid as adults, play is minimal (see Figure 3)
Partial isolation (can see, hear, and smell other monkeys)	Stare vacantly into space, engage in self-mutilation, stereotyped behavior patterns
Separation (taken from caretaker after bond has developed)	Initial protest stage changing to despair 48 hours after separation; refuse to play. Rapid reattachment when returned to mother

therapeutic role, young normal monkeys were chosen that would play gently with the isolates and approach and cling to them. Within 2 weeks, the isolates were reciprocating the social contact, and their incidence of abnormal self-directed behaviors began to decline significantly. By the end of the 6-month therapy period, the isolates were actively initiating play bouts with both the therapists and each other, and most of their self-directed behaviors had disappeared. These isolates were observed closely for the following 2 years, and it was found that their improved behavioral repertoires did not regress over time. The results of this and subsequent monkey therapist studies have underscored the potential reversibility of early cognitive and social deficits at the human level. These studies also have served as a model for developing therapeutic treatments for socially retarded or withdrawn children.

Several investigators have argued that social separation manipulations with nonhuman primates provide a compelling basis for developing animal models of depression and anxiety. Some monkeys react to separations with behavioral and physiologic symptoms very similar to those seen in depressed human patients; both electroconvulsive therapy (ECT) and tricyclic antidepressant drugs are effective in reversing the symptoms in monkeys. It is also true that not all separations produce depressive reactions in monkeys, just as separation does not always precipitate depression in humans, young or old.

Individual Differences in Reactions to Social Situations

Recent research has revealed that some rhesus monkey infants consistently display fearfulness and anxiety in situations when similarly reared peers demonstrate normal exploratory behavior and play. These situations generally involve exposure to some kind of novel object or situation. Once the object or situation has become familiar, any behavioral differences between these anxiety-prone or timid infants and their more outgoing peers disappear. These individual differences, however, appear to be quite stable during development. Infant monkeys at 3 to 6 months of age that are at

high risk for fearful or anxious reactions tend to remain at high risk for such reactions, at least until adolescence.

Long-term follow-up study of the above monkey subjects has revealed some interesting behavioral differences between fearful and nonfearful females when they become adults and have their first infants. Fearful female monkeys that grow up in socially benign and stable environments typically become fine mothers; however, fearful females who have reacted to frequent social separations during childhood with depression are at high risk for maternal dysfunction; more than 80 percent of these mothers either neglect or abuse their first offspring. Yet, nonfearful females who encounter the same number of social separations but do not react to any of these separations with depression subsequently turn out to be good mothers.

SENSORY DEPRIVATION

The history of sensory deprivation and its potentially deleterious effects evolved from instances of aberrant mental behavior in explorers, shipwrecked sailors, and prisoners in solitary confinement. Toward the end of World War II, startling confessions, induced by brainwashing prisoners of war, caused a rise of interest in this psychological phenomena brought about by the deliberate diminution of sensory input.

To test the hypothesis that an important element in brainwashing is prolonged exposure to sensory isolation, Hebb and his co-workers brought solitary confinement into the laboratory and demonstrated that volunteer subjects—under conditions of visual, auditory, and tactile deprivation for periods of up to seven days—reacted with increased suggestibility. Some of the subjects also showed characteristic symptoms of the sensory deprivation state: anxiety, tension, inability to concentrate or organize one's thoughts, increased suggestibility, body illusions, somatic complaints, intense subjective emotional distress, and vivid sensory imagery—usually visual, sometimes reaching the proportions of hallucinations with delusionary quality.

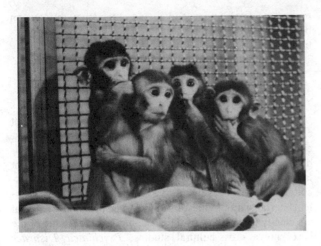

Figure 3. Mutual clinging among peer-reared rhesus monkey infants.

Theories of Sensory Deprivation

Psychological Theories. Anticipating psychological explanations, Freud wrote, "It is interesting to speculate what could happen to ego function if the excitations or stimuli from the external world were either drastically diminished or repetitive. Would there be an alteration in the unconscious mental processes and an effect upon the conceptualization of time?"

Indeed, under conditions of sensory deprivation, the abrogation of such ego functions as perceptual contact with reality and logical thinking brings about confusion, irrationality, fantasy formation, hallucinatory activity, and wish-dominated mental reactions. In the sensory deprivation situation, the subject becomes even more dependent on the experimenter and must trust him for the satisfaction of such basic needs as feeding, toileting, and physical safety. It has been suggested that a patient undergoing psychoanalysis is in a kind of sensory deprivation room (e.g., soundproofed, dim lights, couch) in which primary-process mental activity is encouraged through free association.

Physiological Theories. The maintenance of optimal conscious awareness and accurate reality testing depends on a necessary state of alertness. This alert state, in turn, depends on a constant stream of changing stimuli from the external world, mediated through the ascending reticular activating system in the brain stem. In the absence or impairment of such a stream, as occurs in sensory deprivation, alertness falls away, direct contact with the outside world diminishes, and impulses from the inner body and the central nervous system may gain prominence. For example, idioretinal phenomena, inner ear noise, and somatic illusions may take on a hallucinatory character.

Other Theories.

Personality. Personality theories do not attempt to explain the phenomena of sensory deprivation, but rather the variation in these phenomena from subject to subject. For example, why do some volunteers in experiments quit sooner than others? Different approaches are offered by different investigators—introversion-extroversion, body-field orientation, and optimal stimulation level.

Expectation. These hypotheses involve social influences, including the important role played by the experimenter. Modern researchers place great emphasis on anticipation, instructional set, and the demand characteristics of the experimental situation (tacit and overt suggestion).

Cognitive. These theories stress that the organism is an information-processing machine whose purpose is optimal adaptation to the perceived environment. Due to insufficient information, the machine is unable to form a cognitive map, against which current experience is matched. Disorganization and maladaptation are the result. In order to monitor one's own behavior and attain optimal responsiveness, the organism must receive continuous feedback. Without this feedback, the person is forced to project outward idiosyncratic themes that have little relationship to reality. This situation is similar to that of many psychotics.

References

Barabasz A F: Restricted environmental stimulation and the enhancement hypnotizability: Pain, EEG alpha, skin conductance and temperature responses. Int Clin Exp Hypn *30*:147, 1982.

Barash D P: *Sociobiology and Behavior,* ed 2. Elsevier, New York, 1982.

Borrie R A, Suedfeld P: Restricted environmental stimulation therapy in a weight reduction program. J Behav Med *3*:147, 1980.

Fine T H, Turner J W, Jr: The effect of brief restricted environmental stimulation therapy in the treatment of essential hypertension. Behav Res Ther *20*:567, 1982.

Harlow H F: The nature of love. Am Psychol *13*:673, 1958.

Lorenz K Z: *The Foundations of Ethology.* Springer-Verlag, New York, 1981.

Pavlov I P: Conditioned Reflexes (GV Arrep, trans.). Oxford University Press, London, 1927.

Pitman R K, Kolb B, Orr S P, Singh M: Ethological study of facial behavior in non-paranoid and paranoid schizophrenic patients. Am J Psych *144*(1):99, 1987.

Suedfeld P, Ballard E J, Murphy M: Water immersion and flotation: From stress experiment to stress treatment. J Environ Psychol *3*:147–155, 1983.

Suomi S J: Social development in rhesus monkeys: Consideration of individual difference. In *The Behaviour of Human Infants,* A Oilverio, M Zappella, editors. Plenum Press, New York, 1983.

Suomi, S J, Harlow H F: Social rehabilitation of isolate-reared monkeys. Dev Psychol *6*:487, 1972.

5.6 _____

Anthropology and Psychiatry

Anthropology is the study of culture, which can be defined as the sum of what individual members of a community learn from generations of accumulated social experience. Culture includes manners, customs, tastes, skills, language, beliefs, and all the other patterns of behavior that are part of organized social life. It is *traditional* in that social practices are passed from generation to generation. Culture also encompasses the notion of a group of persons sharing a system of action and beliefs capable of persisting longer than the life span of any one individual, a group whose adherents come from the sexual reproduction of the group members. In that sense, every culture is *historical* and *genetic*. A culture also possesses a value system of good, bad, desirable, and undesirable behavioral patterns and can be examined from both a *psychological* and *normative* view, in terms of how the majority adapt to stresses unique to a particular culture.

PSYCHOANALYTICAL ANTHROPOLOGY

Beginning with *Freud*, psychoanalysts have applied their insight to cultural data. In 1913, in *Totem and Taboo*, Freud described earliest man as a group of brothers who killed and devoured their violent primal father. That criminal act and the so-called totem meal made the brothers feel guilty. Consequently, they set up rules formulated so that similar acts would never occur again; these rules were the beginning of social organization. *Carl Jung's* writings include many anthropological references, especially to archeology and mythology. In *Symbols and Transformations,* written in 1912, Jung traced patients' fantasies back to man's earliest artifacts. Neither Freud nor Jung had field experience, but *Erik Erikson,* for example, did. Erikson is best known for his psychocultural biographies of Gandhi and Martin Luther and for the 1950 book *Childhood and Society,* in which he attempted to integrate individual psychosexual development with cultural influences. Many of his conclusions were based on his experiences with the Pine Ridge Indians in the Dakotas and the Yurok Indians in Oregon.

George Devereux studied American Plains Indians and provided insights into the problems that arise in dealing with patients from diverse ethnic backgrounds. In the 1930s and 1940s, *Abram Kardiner* worked with the concept of *national character,* suggesting that each culture is associated with a common (or at least widely shared) personality structure. Kardiner believed that the adult Russian personality, for example, was characterized by depressive and manic traits. Other such generalities about national character were set forth by various workers, but those descriptions were often used to foster political, ideological, or discriminatory attitudes and, so, have fallen out of favor. The current consensus is that a clinically meaningful prediction about one's personality cannot be made on the basis of nationality alone. But as *Ruth Benedict* wrote in *Patterns of Culture,* personality types may reflect a culture's configuration because people are malleable and they assume a society's expected behavior pattern.

Bronislaw Malinowski and *Margaret Mead* were among the group of anthropologists who examined the psychoanalytic concept that adult personality and mental functioning are largely determined during childhood. Malinowski examined childhood and adult sexuality in the Trobriand Islanders and claimed that he found no evidence of the Oedipus complex, which at the time was believed to be universal. Margaret Mead examined gender and sex-role behavior. She observed three tribes in New Guinea and found different patterns of sex-role behavior for men and women in each tribe. According to Mead, behavior is relative, and a society can create deviancy by either condoning or condemning certain behavior patterns. Mead believed the Oedipus complex to be a useful concept in its widest meaning, which is that in all societies adults are involved in the growing child's sexual attitudes, especially toward the parent of the opposite sex.

Child-Rearing Practices

Studies of child-rearing practices among different cultures have concluded the following: (1) indulgence in early infancy is an extremely important determinant of adult mental health; (2) the nurture of the child by various care-givers, in addition to the mother, is not harmful; (3) a wide variety of child-rearing practices are found in different cultures; and (4) the major influences on personality development revolve around love-hate and dependence-independence issues rather than the control of sexual behavior. The basic relationship, however, between child-rearing patterns and subsequent adult personality in complex societies, such as the United States, has not yet been elucidated. In this country, there are cycles of permissiveness and constraint, reward and punishment, and a general tendency to focus on bowel and bladder training as important child-rearing practices.

CROSS-CULTURAL STUDIES

Cross-cultural studies examine and compare different cultures along a number of parameters: attitudes, beliefs, expectations, memories, opinions, roles, stereotypes, prejudices, and values. Usually, the cultures studied use different languages and have different political organizations. Cross-cultural studies are subject to extreme bias owing to problems in translation. Questions have to be asked in ways that are clearly understood by the group under study. One of the best known cross-cultural studies, *Psychiatric Disorder Among the Yoruba* by Alexander Leighton, was his attempt to replicate in Nigeria the Stirling County study he had conducted in Canada. The study was criticized because not only did it fail to distinguish psychophysiological symptoms from those associated with infections, parasites, and nutritional diseases, but it assumed that the same indicators for sociocultural disintegration in Stirling County could be used among the Yoruba. Other studies have confirmed that psycholinguistics—the study of language and its communicative functions—must be taken into account if cross-cultural approaches are to have validity. All cultures are relative; that is, each must be examined within the context of its own language, customs, and beliefs. Various cultures assign different roles depending on status. Research has shown that there is a high incidence of depression among adult women in Kikuyu society, who are subject to heavy role demands. There is also a high prevalence of schizophrenia among last-born sons in rural Ireland because of the stresses linked to that role.

Diagnoses of mental disorders have been conducted among various cultures by the World Health Organization. The International Pilot Study of Schizophrenia confirmed that schizophrenia exists among all groups studied (e.g., Nigerians, Danes, Laotians, Celts, Croatians, Hutterites, South Pacific Tongans, and Taiwanese) and are constant across cultures. Outcome studies of patients with schizophrenia, however, are not reliable because some societies (unlike the United States) do not stigmatize persons with mental illness who are quickly reintegrated into the society. A major difficulty in cross-cultural diagnosis is the bias due to the researcher's cultural background, which can be reduced if careful attention is given to translation and to the attitude of the examiner.

ETHNOGRAPHY

In the anthropological tradition, ethnography (derived from the Greek word *ethnos,* meaning race or people) refers to an inductive method of describing cultural forms through the examination of a series of cases. Ethnographers document phenomena by various methods, such as the examination of written records, folk tales, and myths; linguistic analysis; interviews with key informants; collections of life histories; questionnaire surveys; psychological tests; and, most important, participant observation.

United States Culture

The United States is a multiethnic country, but the values of the white middle class predominate. The numerous subgroups that represent waves of immigration over the years have influenced our culture, but not to such an extent that those groups have lost their identity. They have been partially *acculturated;* that is, they have assumed characteristics of the larger or more advanced society. But, they have not been *assimilated;* that is, their unique cultural traits have not disappeared totally. Recognized minority subcultures in this country include Hispanics (Mexican Americans, Puerto Ricans, Cuban Americans), Asian Americans (Chinese, Japanese, Korean, Pacific Islanders), Afro-Americans, and native Americans (American Indians, Eskimos).

As of the 1980 census, the resident population in the United States by race and national origin was as follows: white, 188 million; black, 26 million; American Indian (including Eskimo), 1.4 million; Chinese, 806,000; Filipino, 775,000; Japanese, 701,000; Asian Indian, 361,000; Korean, 354,000; Vietnamese, 262,000; Americans of Spanish origin, 14.5 million.

It is extremely hazardous to attempt to describe ethnic characteristics of a culture. The risk of stereotyping is great, and, as mentioned above, the concept of national character is controversial among contemporary anthropologists. Nevertheless, U.S. society has been described as having certain characteristics against which the ethnic groups in this country are compared. Table 1 lists the characteristics attributed to the national character of the United States.

Some subcultures approximate the U.S. national character more than others, and some characteristics are more highly valued and prevalent within a particular ethnic group than in the culture as a whole. Hispanics, for example, value the nuclear family and place greater emphasis on having more, rather than fewer, children. Asian-Americans place an extremely high value on education; although they make up about 1 percent of the general population, they represent about 15 to 20 percent of college students. Another example is that of filial piety, a strong value among Chinese-Americans, in which parents expect their children to care for them in their old age.

The nuclear family of mother, father, and children is a universal unit in all cultures. The extended family, in which grandparents, parents, children, and relatives all live under the same roof, is no longer common in the United States, but it is still prevalent in less industrialized cultures. Functions of the extended family such as caring for the sick and elderly have been taken over by institutions.

In the United States over 85 percent of men and women between the ages of 35 and 45 are husband or wife in a nuclear family. Even though close to one out of two marriages ends in divorce, a majority of persons remarry and create a new nuclear unit. In fact, serial monogamy, in which persons remarry after divorce while remaining faithful to the spouse during the course of the marriage, is a noticeable trend. Other family figurations are outlined in Table 2.

Table 1
American Cultural Characteristics

1. Nuclear family unit valued highly with few children; financially independent by age 18
2. Bowel and bladder training important in child-rearing
3. Personal hygiene emphasized, neatness valued
4. Self-reliance and rugged individualism valued
5. Avoidance of dependency role, especially after age 65; unwillingness to be cared for by children
6. Ambivalence about overt expressions of sexuality
7. Ownership of own home desirable
8. Hard work will be rewarded
9. Collective approach to solving common problems
10. Upward social mobility desirable

Table 2

Type of Family Systems	Characteristics
Monandry	Woman with one husband
Polyandry	Woman has multiple husbands at once; biological father generally unknown, all males in family take paternal responsibility
Polygamy	Husband has multiple wives at once; woman's status inferior to man's; pecking order among wives exists in some forms, one claiming more rights than others
Patrimony	Property is inherited from the father
Patronymic	Bride takes the groom's name; son takes the name of the father
Patrilocal	Fathers arrange marriages of sons and daughters by making contracts with other fathers; wife resides with the family of tribe of her husband
Patrilineal	Kinship or descent through the father
Matrilineal	Kinship or descent through the mother
Polygamy	The practice of having many or several spouses (especially wives) at once
Bigamy	The crime of marrying while one has a wife or husband still living from whom one is not divorced
Monogamy	Marriage with only one person at a time
Matrilocal	Married couple lives in home of bride
Neolocal	Married couple sets up new home independent of mother and father
Bilineal	Both male and female parents are considered equal in regard to descent

A modern ethnographic approach in Western subcultures is demonstrated by the 1971 study of a predominantly black ghetto in a large northern U.S. city. The researchers studied the community by living in it and by experiencing ghetto life directly. They progressed from being observer-participants to active participants in community life, becoming partisans who openly identified with the population under study. The scientific motivation for their study was to examine the patterns usually ascribed to persons living in a culture of poverty. They found that 83 percent of black families were conventional male-headed households and that the social structure beyond the family level consisted of a multiplicity of local institutions, such as churches, social clubs, and political organizations. Since then, a radical change has occurred: In 1983, only 42 percent of black families were made up of two parents with a male head of household.

Culture Change

Persons deal with culture change either by moving into a different culture or by staying put while the culture changes around them. When change is acute and sweeping the adaptive mechanisms of individuals and of their social support may be overwhelmed. *Culture shock* is characterized by anxiety or depression, a sense of isolation, derealization, and depersonalization. Culture shock is minimized if persons are part of an intact family unit and if they are prepared for the new culture in advance. It is preferable if refugees, for example, are clustered in a few central locations rather than dispersed throughout the nation.

Studies have demonstrated a higher rate of psychiatric hospitalization in the United States, for immigrants, especially young men, than for the native-born. There also appears to be a higher incidence of paranoid symptoms among immigrant groups, which may be related to their differences (color, language, habit) from the larger society. Acute psychotic episodes that occur among Third World immigrants in this country usually have clear-cut precipitating factors, are recurrent, and have a good prognosis.

MEDICAL ANTHROPOLOGY

Medical anthropology focuses on the practice of medicine and the cultural aspects of providing and receiving health care. The study of culture, attitudes, and beliefs has a special importance for psychiatry and medicine. For example, an effective prevention program for alcoholism involves changing attitudes and values about drinking. Similarly, the success of antismoking campaigns depends on altering attitudes about tobacco. Cultural aspects of health care are best understood within the context of the particular culture under study.

Culture of the Mental Hospital

The physical and sociocultural environment of mental hospitals was studied in terms of its effects on patients. When disagreements concerning a patient's management occurred among staff members, patients did not do as well as when staff consensus existed. The environment of the hospital is as much a therapeutic agent as the medication a patient receives. A psychiatric hospital as described by Alfred Staunton is a small society with established hierarchical categories. Dissension or confusion about staff roles or expectations may be transmitted to patients, whose symptoms may be exacerbated as a result. The English psychiatrist, Maxwell Jones, attempted to organize the psychiatric hospital as a *therapeutic community*. Jones's primary goal was the elimination of the divisions between various mental health professions, which he believed to be artificial and harmful to the patient.

Psychosocial Model of Disease

George Engel described the biopsychosocial model for understanding disease. The biologic system deals with the anatomic, structural, and molecular influence on disease; the psychological system deals with the influence of personality, motivation, and psychodynamic factors on illness; and the social system encompasses environmental, cultural, and life stressor influence on disease. *Illness behavior* is a term used to describe the reactions of patients to developing an illness. It is affected by a patient's previous experience with disease and by the patient's cultural beliefs about the specific problem. The relationship of the illness to family processes is of major importance. Patients seek and need more family support at this time; however, their premorbid attitudes about dependency and helplessness influence their ability to ask for or to receive help. Other factors that influence the experience of illness are class status and ethnic identity. It is important, however, to avoid generalizations. The patient must be understood in terms of the specific culture or ethnic group to which one belongs. Mexican Americans and Puerto Rican Americans, for example, share as many group cultural differences as they do commonalities. Different cultures—Haitians, West Indians, Puerto Ricans, and Christian faith healers—incorporate shamans, persons who follow a divine call to healing. The clinician must find out how acculturated the patient is to the cultural mainstream of life. The influence of culture on the reporting and presentation of symptoms must be considered. A reluctance to discuss certain topics may stem from the patient's individual psychology or from adherence to the customs and etiquette of the social group.

Hispanic Americans. Mexican Americans make up the largest group (10 million) of Americans of Spanish origin and are referred to as Chicanos, particularly in the Southwestern United States, where most Mexican Americans live. They frequently receive health care from folk healers *(curanderos)* who prescribe herbs or dietary change or use magic.

Puerto Rican Americans are the second largest Hispanic group (2 million). Most live in the Northeastern states. In a study of Puerto Rican households in New York City, a significant number of adults visited folk healers or spiritists *(espiritismos)* during times of emotional crisis. Spiritism is practiced in small neighborhood centers (centros) where a medium performs magical procedures such as drawing off evil spirits that may have entered into the patient, a therapeutic process known as *trabajando la causa* (working the cause).

Asian Americans. The two largest groups of Asian Americans, Chinese and Japanese, have shown different degrees of acculturation in the United States. During World War II, internment of second-generation West Coast Japanese (Nisei) in concentration camps was imposed by the United States government. Over 100,000 people were forcibly detained, and when they regained their freedom in 1945 they were filled with fear and resentment. Chinese immigration preceded that of the Japanese, and they too were subject to discriminatory legislation. Prejudice tends to rein-force ethnic identity and retard assimilation. Since the 1960s' Civil Rights Movement, greater assimilation of Asian Americans has occurred. Nevertheless, the clinician must be aware of unique cultural behavioral patterns. For example, a Japanese patient may say yes *(hai)* as a sign of polite participation in a conversation rather than as a sign of agreement; Hawaiian patients may avoid eye contact if they were taught that eye contact is a sign of aggression; Chinese patients may smile or laugh when they are embarrassed or sad; and Pacific Islanders may miss medical sessions because it is socially acceptable to be casual about fixed dates and appoint-ments.

American Indians. Native Americans are among the most widely studied groups with the best known ethnographies. They are

Table 3
Cross-Cultural Syndromes

Diagnosis	Country Culture	Characteristics
Amok	Southeast Asia	Sudden rampage, usually including homicide and suicide; occurs in males
Bulimia	North America	Food binges, self-induced vomiting; may occur with depression, anorexia or substance abuse
Koro	Asia	Fear that the penis will withdraw into the abdomen causing death
Windigo	Native American Indians	Fear of being turned into a cannibal through possession by supernatural monster, the windigo
Piblokto (Arctic hysteria)	Eskimo	Mixed anxiety and depression, confusion, depersonalization, derealization; occurs mainly in females
Susto	Latin America	Severe anxiety, restlessness, fear of black magic and of evil eye
Empacho	Mexican and Cuban American	Inability to digest and excrete recently ingested food
Hi-Wa itck	Mohave American Indian	Anorexia, insomnia, depression, suicide associated with unwanted separation from loved one
Boufée delirantes	France	Transient psychosis with elements of trance or dream states
Reactive psychosis	Scandinavia	Psychosis precipitated by psychosocial stress; acute onset with good prognosis, premorbid personality fairly intact; in DSM-III-R known as schizophreniform psychosis
Shinkeishitsu	Japan	Syndrome marked by obsessions, perfectionism, ambivalence, social withdrawal, neurasthenia and hypochondriasis
Involutional paraphrenia	Spain, Germany	Paranoid disorder occurring in mid-life; distinct from schizophrenia but may have elements of both
Latah	Southeast Asia, Malaysia, Bantu of Africa, Ainu of Japan	Automatic obedience reaction with echopraxia and echolalia precipitated by a sudden minimal stimulus; occurs in females
Taijin-kyofusho	Japan	Anxiety, fear of rejection, easy blushing, fear of eye contact, concern about body odor
Grisi siknis	Miskito of Nicaragua	Headache, anxiety, anger, aimless running

the only ethnic group in America to have a separate medical care program administered by the federal government, the Indian Health Service. There is a long tradition of healing rituals among native Americans, who make no distinction between mental and physical illness. Illness is thought to result from a disharmony among a person's natural, supernatural, and human environments caused by culturally unacceptable behavior or by witchcraft. High rates of alcoholism and suicide are found in native Americans and Eskimos.

Black Americans. The 26 million black Americans comprise an extremely heterogeneous group, however, most belong to the lower and lower-middle socioeconomic classes. Only 20 percent hold white-collar jobs, compared to 40 percent of white workers, and the median income of black families is only about 55 percent that of white families.

Unique to certain black subgroups, such as those from Haiti, is root work or voodoo. Rites, hexes, prayers, curses, and other practices are used by shamans and witch doctors to influence health or illness. Persons undergoing a healing experience often enter a trance state, during which they are vulnerable to shamanistic suggestions. Shamans give objective reality to popular and emotionally accepted beliefs of the cultural group.

Certain generalizations about the health of black Americans can be made. They have a shorter life expectancy than whites, a higher incidence of hypertensive disease, a higher suicide rate (among young black men compared to young white men; other age cohorts have the same rates); and a higher homicide rate. Some of these differences are related to the low socioeconomic level of most blacks; in general, the poor do not utilize health care facilities as readily as the more affluent.

Christian Beliefs. The past two decades have seen a growing interest in Christian faith healing directed toward what is called sickness of the spirit, the emotions, and the body. According to certain fundamentalist groups, any form of sickness may have a demonic origin, and some cases call for prayer and exorcism in order for recovery to occur. The role of the physician is to heal through divine intervention. Some faith healers are willing to work with physicians. Others, however, believe that participation in a close-knit Christian community, participation in a bible-study group, and prayer are sufficient.

Culture-Bound Syndromes

There is a group of disorders that are found only in certain cultures or among certain groups. They often occur with little warning, their course is usually short, and their prognosis is generally favorable.

The notion of culture-bound syndromes is conceptually simple but operationally complex. Because culture is the matrix in which all biological, psychological, and social functioning operates, it follows that all psychiatric syndromes are, to some extent, culture bound. Western psychiatrists, for example, tend to view mental syndromes in Western societies as culture free; but, bulimia is as shaped by Western culture as koro is by Oriental culture. If African healers with limited Western contact were transplanted briefly to this country, they would be equally surprised by the odd symptoms of the patients here. Table 3 briefly outlines some of the culture-bound syndromes that have been described by observers with a Western frame of reference.

References

Benedict R: *Patterns of Culture.* Houghton Mifflin, Boston, 1934.
Erikson E: *Childhood and Society.* W W Norton, New York, 1963.
Favazza A, Faheem A: *Themes in Cultural Psychiatry.* University of Missouri Press, Columbia, 1982.
Freud S: *Totem and Taboo.* W W Norton, New York, 1950.
Jung C: *Symbols and Transformations,* ed 2. Princeton University Press, Princeton, 1967.
Kardiner A, Linton R, DuBois C: *The Psychological Frontiers of Society.* Columbia University Press, New York, 1945.
Kleinman A, Eisenberg L, Good B: Culture, illness, and care. Ann Intern Med, *88:*251, 1978.
Leff J: *Psychiatry Around the Globe: A Transcultural View.* Marcel Dekker, New York, 1981.
Malinowski B: *Sex and Repression in Savage Society.* Harcourt, New York, 1927.
Mollica R, Wyshak G, de Marneffe D, Khwon F, Lavelle J: Indochinese versions of the Hopkins symptom checheirt-25: A screening instrument for the psychiatric care of refugees. Am J Psych *144*(4): 497, 1987.
Westermeyer J: *Psychiatric diagnosis across cultural boundaries.* Am J Psychiatry *142:*7, 1985.

5.7 ▬▬▬▬
Epidemiology and Social Psychiatry

Psychiatric epidemiology is concerned with the pattern of occurrence of mental disorders. It deals with the distribution, incidence, prevalence, and duration of psychiatric illness with respect to the physical, biological, and social environment in which people live. Epidemiology helps to define and evaluate strategies to prevent and control disease and disability. It relies on the use of certain statistical methods that are necessary to a full understanding of the field.

DEFINITIONS

Measurements of Disease Frequency

Frequency (commonly abbreviated as f) refers to the number of cases having a certain score or characteristic. For example, if 15 persons out of 100 have a score of 50 on a 50-item psychological test of anxiety (high scores indicating extreme anxiety), and 30 persons receive a score of 25 (moderate anxiety), frequency (f) is 15 for extreme anxiety and 30 (f=30) for moderate anxiety. A table in which all score values are listed in one column with the number of individuals who received each score in the second column is called a *frequency distribution*.

Relative Frequency. Relative frequency measures the number of persons in a specific group, (e.g., sex or age) who have a disorder. Measures of disease frequency involve two major concepts, prevalence and incidence.

Prevalence. Prevalence refers to the number of cases of a disorder that exist. There are several types of prevalence.

Point prevalence. This basic measure of prevalence refers to the number of persons who have a disorder at a specified point in time. The point can be a certain day on the calendar (e.g., April 1, 1986) or any day during a particular study (e.g., the fourth day of the study), regardless of the calendar day. It is calculated as follows:

$$\text{Point prevalence} = \frac{\text{Number of persons with a disorder at a specified point in time}}{\text{Total population at a specified point in time}}$$

Period prevalence. This refers to the number of people who have a disorder at any time during a specified time period (longer than a calendar day or point in time). It is calculated as follows:

$$\text{Period prevalence} = \frac{\text{Number of persons with a disorder during a time period}}{\text{Total population during a time period}}$$

The numerator includes any existing cases at the start of the time period plus any new cases that develop during the period. Period prevalence may be used to determine the number of persons with a disorder, the number of persons in treatment, and the duration of an illness.

Lifetime prevalence. This is a measure at a point in time of the number of persons who had the disorder at some time during their lives. A potential problem with lifetime prevalence is that it is almost always based on subject recall, which can be inaccurate.

Treated prevalence. This term refers to the number of persons being treated for a disorder by counting all persons in a defined geographic area who are receiving treatment. One may measure treated point prevalence (e.g., the number of patients being treated for a disorder in a clinic on a certain day) or treated period prevalence (e.g., the number of patients being treated for a disorder at a clinic over the past year).

Cross-sectional prevalence. This refers to conducting a single assessment of prevalence at a particular point in time. It differs from a longitudinal study in which a population is studied over a long period of time.

Incidence. Incidence refers to the number of new cases occurring over a specified period of time. The most common time period used is 1 year, producing an annual incidence rate calculated as follows:

$$\text{Incidence rate} = \frac{\text{Number of new persons developing a disease (over a 1-year period of time)}}{\text{Total number of persons at risk (over a 1-year period)}}$$

A study of incidence is more difficult to perform than a study of prevalence cases because one has to exclude from the incidence numerator those persons who already have the disease; they cannot be considered as new cases. Since persons who have had the disease are no longer at risk for developing it, they also must be excluded from the denominator. A broader concept of total incidence includes those persons with a new episode of illness, regardless of whether or not there were previous episodes.

Lifetime expectancy is the total probability of a person developing a disorder during a lifetime. Prevalence and incidence vary for sex and age; thus, *sex-specific* rates and *age-specific* rates are used to express the relative frequency of cases in each category.

Risk Factors. There is an association between risk factors and a disorder that may support a causal connection. Risks may be *factor-specific* (e.g., it occurs only in one sex) or *factor-related* (e.g., it is more likely to occur in a certain environment). Factors that demonstrate a causal connection between a risk factor and a disorder are: (1) temporality—a factor precedes the disorder being studied; (2) the repeated demonstration of the same risk factor appearing in multiple studies; (3) specificity—a risk factor is associated with one disorder only; and (4) finding that the experimental intervention that eliminates the risk factor also eliminates the disorder. Determining what factor or factors account for increased risk of a disorder is one of the challenges of psychiatric epidemiology.

Relative risk. Relative risk is the ratio of the incidence of the disease among persons exposed to the risk factor to the incidence among those not exposed. For example, the relative risk of lung cancer is much greater for heavy smokers than for nonsmokers.

Attributable risk. Attributable risk is the absolute incidence of the disease in exposed individuals that can be attributed to the exposure. This measure is derived by subtracting the incidence of the disease in question among unexposed persons from its total incidence among exposed persons. For example, the lung cancer death rate for nonsmokers may be subtracted from the total community lung cancer death rate. The results would be the attributable community risk of lung cancer. Attributable risk is a useful concept because it tells what might be expected if the risk were removed. For example, on the basis of available data, the attributable risk of deaths for lung cancer could be avoided if the factor of smoking was eliminated.

ASSESSMENT INSTRUMENTS

The major obstacle to identification of cases has been the lack of an explicit set of criteria for diagnostic classification. Over the years, a variety of diagnostic procedures and assessment instruments have been developed. Table 1 lists various scales used as diagnostic criteria for schizophrenia.

Information about a subject can be collected in several ways. Medical records often are used for patients in clinical settings. Records in central data banks called *case registers* can be used. In Scandinavian countries, particularly Sweden, control data banks are extensive. An important source of information about a subject is the *direct interview,* which is a person to person interaction. *Indirect surveys* using a structured self-report form may be used, but they lack the clinical judgment of an experienced practitioner that may be necessary in some instances.

The most common assessment approach is an interview format, which may be *structured* (the same questions asked of all subjects) or *unstructured,* (the interviewer chooses his questions based upon his own clinical judgment). Several structured instruments with acceptable interrater reliability are outlined in Table 2.

An effective assessment instrument must be reliable, valid, and free of bias. *Reliability* refers to whether or not the findings of the assessment instrument or diagnostic procedure are reproducible and can be replicated when the instrument is used by different examiners *(interrater reliability)* or on different occasions *(test-retest reliability).* For example, are various clinicians referring to the same thing when they diagnose schizophrenia? *Validity* refers to

Table 1
Diagnostic Criteria Used in Schizophrenia

Scale	Key Signs & Symptoms	Course
Emil Kraepelin	Phenomenological approach with emphasis on auditory hallucinations, loosening of associations, flat affect, catatonia, negativism and autism	Impaired cognition and judgment lead to deterioration
Eugen Bleuler	Disturbance of affect, ambivalence, autism and association (the four As), hallucinations, delusions, loosening of associations	Does not necessarily lead to deterioration
Kurt Schneider	Described first-rank symptoms of audible thoughts, arguing voices, thought withdrawal and insertion, delusions, flat affect and second-rank symptoms of delusions and changes in perception (e.g., illusions)	Fluctuating course
International Classification of Disease, World Health Organization 9th edition, 1978, (ICD-9)	Distorted thinking, outer control of personality, bizarre delusions, abnormal affect, autism	Clear consciousness and intellectual capacity maintained
St. Louis Criteria (I P Feighner, et al., 1972)	Delusions, hallucinations, impaired communication, blunted affect, loose associations	No disorientation, and disease must be present for at least 6 months; chronic course
Research Diagnostic Criteria (RDC) (Spitzer, et al., 1978)	Thought broadcasting, delusions, auditory hallucinations, blunted affect. A structured interview Schedule for Affective Disorders and Schizophrenia (SADS) developed for increase in reliability; also a lifetime version (SADS-L) to include past episodes of illness; and a version for measuring change (SADS-C)	Signs must be present for at least 2 weeks. SADS-L reflects concept that disorder may have occurred in past and disease is not always active
Diagnostic and Statistical Manual, 3rd edition-Revised (DSM–III-R)	Delusions, hallucinations, loose associations, affect disturbance, incoherence, disorganized behavior	Deterioration from prior level of function but disorder may become residual; onset usually before age 45

Table 2
Commonly Used Assessment Instruments

Instrument	Condition	Interviewer	Comments
Present State Examination (PSE)	Psychotic conditions, schizophrenia	Psychiatrists	Limited to 1 month period prior to interview; can be used with computer program, CATEGO
Schedule for Affective Disorders and Schizophrenia (SADS)	Schizophrenia and affective disorders	Psychiatrists or specially trained interviewer	Variations: SADS-C measures current disorder, and SADS-L measures lifetime disorders
General Health Questionnaire (GHQ)	Medical patients with psychiatric symptoms of anxiety or depression	Self-report	Does not identify specific mental disorders
Diagnostic Interview Schedule (DIS)	Covers over 30 mental disorders including schizophrenia, affective disorders, anxiety, substance abuse, organic mental disorders, etc.	Self-report combined with specially trained interviewers	Correlates with range of DSM–III diagnostic classification; assesses symptoms over lifetime

whether or not the test measures what it is supposed to measure. Does the assessment instrument identify cases that it is designed to identity?

Validity can be broken down further into the following categories: *Criterion validity,* in which results from one test instrument are compared to the results of another test whose validity has already been established; *face validity,* which refers to the test making sense to the investigator using it; *content validity,* which refers to the test covering specific types of information that can be interpreted or scored at a later date; and *construct validity,* which refers to the test instrument being constructed so that it measures the thing that it is designed to measure. The two properties of validity and reliability are extremely important in psychiatric epidemiology, especially if one is attempting to identify a specific disorder or syndrome.

Analytic studies can also be flawed by *bias,* an error in construction that favors one outcome over another. Bias can occur if an examiner knows something about the status of the case that influences his judgment (e.g., he may know that one group is receiving medication). These potential flaws can affect the validity of a study's findings. To eliminate this kind of bias, the *double-blind method* (described below) was developed. Bias is also diminished by randomization of the sample, in which each member of the total group studied has an equal chance of being selected; for example, each person may be assigned a number from a table of random numbers.

Assessment instruments must be *sensitive,* that is, they must be able to detect the thing being evaluated (e.g., to diagnose a disorder when it is present). If an instrument detects a disorder in a person who does not have the disorder, the result is called a *false-positive,* rather than a *true-positive.* Tests must also be *specific;* that is, they must not detect things not being evaluated. For example, tests must be able to diagnose the absence of a disorder in a person who does

not have the disorder, which is called *true-negative.* If a disorder is diagnosed as absent in a person when it is present, it is called a *false-negative result.* Assessment instruments should also have good *predictive value,* which is the proportion of true-positive or true-negative tests. Predictive values indicate what percentage of test outcomes are expected to coincide with assigned diagnoses. Table 3 summarizes the interpretation of the concepts of sensitivity, specificity, and predictive value.

TYPES OF STUDIES

Studies that are carried out over a long period of time are known as *longitudinal or cohort studies.* For example, Stella Chess and Alexander Thomas studied temperamental characteristics of the same group of infants at ages 3 months, 2 years, 5 years, and 20 years. They were able to discern a relationship between the initial characteristics of the infant and a subgroup of children who eventually developed clinical psychiatric problems. A *cohort* is a group chosen from a well defined population. In this study, the cohort is the group born and studied in the year the study began.

A simpler study design is the *cross-sectional study,* which examines a group at one point in time. It looks at a "slice of the pie" and studies a cohort in terms of specific qualities that exist at the time of the study but which may or may not be present at any other time.

Cohort studies provide direct estimates of risk associated with a suspected causal factor; however, they are more time consuming and expensive to perform than case history studies, which are relatively quick and inexpensive. Cohort studies are usually started when there is ample evidence

Table 3
Definitions and Calculations for Interpreting Performance of Diagnostic Tests

Term	Definition	Calculation
True positive (TP)	Diseased person with abnormal test	
True negative (TN)	Nondiseased person with normal test	
False positive (FP)	Nondiseased person with abnormal test	
False negative (FN)	Diseased person with normal test	
Referent value	A value to which laboratory results can be referred and from which the probability of disease or predictive value can be calculated	
Sensitivity	True positive rate	$\dfrac{TP}{TP + FN} \times 100$
Specificity	True negative rate	$\dfrac{TN}{TN + FP} \times 100$
Predictive value of abnormal test (PV +)	Proportion of abnormal tests that are true positive	$\dfrac{TP}{TP + FP} \times 100$
Predictive value of normal test (PV −)	Proportion of normal tests that are true negative	$\dfrac{TN}{TN + FN} \times 100$
Efficiency	Percent of all results that are true results, whether positive or negative	$\dfrac{TP + TN}{\text{Grand Total}} \times 100$

From Greden J F: Laboratory tests in psychiatry. In *Comprehensive Textbook of Psychiatry,* ed 4, H I Kaplan and B J Sadock, editors, p 2030. Williams & Wilkins, Baltimore, 1985.

from case history studies that a relationship exists between a risk factor and a disorder. In the relationship between smoking and lung cancer, for example, many case history studies had been published prior to the first cohort study.

Studies may be *retrospective,* based on past data or past events or *prospective,* based on observing events as they occur. Retrospective studies that sample persons with or without the disorder are known as *case history* or *case control studies,* respectively. *Clinical treatment trials* are studies that compare groups of patients who are exposed to a treatment with those in a control group who are not exposed to a given treatment.

Double-Blind Study

This type of study helps eliminate bias because neither the patient nor the persons involved in the study know which, if any, treatment is being given to the patient. In drug studies, a control group of patients may receive a placebo, an inert substance prepared to resemble the active drug being tested in the experiment. A response to the placebo may represent the psychological effect of taking a pill, a response not due to any psychopharmacological property (so-called *placebo effect*). In addition, the doctor does not know the treatment given because drugs are identified by special codes unknown to him. Assessment of outcome may also be made by persons other than those administering the treatment—the so-called blind evaluators. Control subjects may also receive an alternative comparison treatment, rather than just a placebo.

Crossover Studies

This type of study is a variation of the double-blind study. The treatment group and the control or placebo group change at some point so that the placebo group gets the treatment and the initial treatment group gets the placebo. This procedure eliminates bias because if the treatment group improves in each instance and the placebo group does not, one can conclude the make-up of both groups is truly random. Each group serves as the control for the other in both trials.

Psychiatric Case Register

A case register maintains a longitudinal record of psychiatric contacts for each person receiving care in a geographically defined community. Not all areas lend themselves to a register because persons may leave the area for treatment or the population may be highly mobile. A well-maintained register is of great value in reporting accurate treated incidence rates, lifetime or period treated prevalence rates, comparative rates for different time periods for the same population, information regarding utilization of services over time, and identification of high-risk groups for further study.

DATA ANALYSIS

Descriptive and inferential statistics are used to analyze data derived from the studies described above. A brief glossary of commonly used statistical terms follows.

Analysis of Variance

A statistical technique by which sets of measurements are investigated to find out if the differences between groups are due to experimental influence or due to chance alone.

Measure of Central Tendency

A central value in a distribution around which other values are distributed. Three measures of central tendency are the mode, the median, and the mean.

Mode. The value that appears most frequently in a set of measurements.

Median. The middle value in a set of measurements. For example, in the series 2, 3, 5, 11, 21, the number 5 is the median value.

Mean. A statistical measurement derived from adding a set of scores and then dividing by the number of scores; the mean is the average score.

Chi-Square

A statistical technique whereby variables are categorized in order to determine if the difference between the distribution of scores is due to chance or to experimental factors.

Coefficient of Correlation

A term referring to the relation between two sets of paired measurements. Correlation coefficients, which may be positive, negative or curvilinear depending on whether the variations are in the same direction, the opposite direction, or both directions, can be computed in a variety of ways. The most common is the product-moment method referred to as r. Another method is rank correction (p). Correlation coefficients are intended to show degree of relation and not that one variable causes the other. The maximum value of a correlation coefficient is 1; the minimum value of 0 indicates that no relationship exists between two variables.

Critical Ratio

In a statistical study involving 30 or more subjects, the critical ratio is used to determine whether differences found between two items are larger than could be expected from chance. The term T-ratio is used in studies involving fewer than 30 subjects to determine whether differences are related to chance.

Deviation

A statistical measure representing the difference between an individual value in a set of values and the mean value in that set.

Mean Deviation

A measure of variation determined by dividing the sum of deviations in a set of variables by the number of cases involved.

Standard Deviation (SD)

A measure of variation derived by squaring each deviation in a set of scores, taking the average of these squares, and then taking the square root of the result. The standard deviation is represented by the Greek letter sigma (Σ). In a normal distribution, $\pm$ 1 SD includes 68 percent of the population; $\pm$ 2 SD includes 95 percent of the population; and $\pm$ 3 SD includes 99 percent of the population.

Standard Error

A measure of how much variation in test results is due to chance and error and how much is due to experimental influences.

Variable

A characteristic that can assume different values in different experimental situations is called a variable. In research methodology, independent variables are those qualities that the experimenter systematically varies (e.g., time, age, sex, type of drug) in the experiment. Dependent variables are those qualities that measure the influence of the independent variable or outcome of the experiment (e.g., measurement of a person's specific physiologic reactions to a drug).

Variance

A measure arrived at by squaring all the deviations in a set of measures, summing them, and then dividing them by the number of measures. Variance is helpful in analyzing how much variation is due to experimental influence and how much to chance or error influence.

Variation

A term referring to different results obtained in measuring the same phenomenon. Variation may be associated with known variables within the data or with variables that result from error or chance.

Null Hypothesis

The assumption that there is no significant difference between two random samples of a population.

EPIDEMIOLOGIC STUDIES

Major psychiatric epidemiologic research studies have been conducted over the years. The goal of each study was to determine the prevalence of psychopathology in a defined community. Persons in a particular community were interviewed directly (usually using a structured interview protocol) to determine the presence or absence of psychological symptoms. The major studies are described below.

Chicago Area

A team under the direction of R. Faris and H. Dunham examined about 35,000 admissions to mental hospitals in Chicago between 1922 and 1934. The survey reported that first hospital admissions for schizophrenia was highest among persons from the central sections of Chicago, members of the city's lowest socioeconomic class. It was also reported that rates of admission decreased as one moved away from the central areas and into more affluent communities. Faris and Dunham postulated a *drift hypothesis,* which holds that impaired persons slide down the social scale because of their illness. By contrast, a *segregation hypothesis* holds that instead of helplessly drifting downward, the schizophrenic person actively seeks city areas where anonymity and isolation protect him against the demands that more organized societies make upon him. This study helped conceptualize two additional hypotheses about mental illness: (1) the *social causation* theory, which holds that being a member of a low socioeconomic group is

etiologically significant in causing illness; and (2) the *social selection* theory, which holds that having a mental illness leads one to become a member of the lower socioeconomic group as a secondary phenomenon. In other words, the illness is caused by genetic or psychological factors and the drift downward occurs as a result.

Monroe County, New York

The Monroe County, New York psychiatric case register is an epidemiologic data file maintained by the University of Rochester School of Medicine since 1960. The case register contains information on all county residents who utilize psychiatric services. The data found that 3 percent of the county received care in mental health care facilities in the region, including the offices of private practitioners. The "newly-treated" incidence rate was less than 1 percent.

Midtown Manhattan Study

In 1954, a team directed by Thomas Rennie and Leo Srole designed and conducted a survey involving 1,660 adults sampled from a specific section of New York City. The objectives of the study were to determine the effects of demographic, social, and personal factors on mental health and illness using a structured interview conducted by nonpsychiatrists. Mental illness was rated as not present, mild, moderate, or marked. The main objective was to test the association between life stress and psychological symptoms. Some of the findings follow. There was a rise in mental disorders as age increased; 81 percent of persons from 20 to 59 years of age had symptoms that were mild to severely incapacitating, and 23.4 percent of persons in this age group were substantially impaired. Socioeconomic status was the single most significant variable affecting mental illness, persons in the lower socioeconomic group having six times as many symptoms as those from the higher groups.

New Haven Study

In 1950, A. B. Hollingshead and F. C. Redlich studied the relation of social class to the prevalence of treated mental illness in New Haven, Connecticut. Their studies included a census of psychiatric patients, a survey of the population at large, the community, a study of psychiatrists, and a controlled case study. Analysis of the data revealed a definite relationship between social class and mental illness. Neurosis was more prevalent among persons in the higher socioeconomic groups; psychosis was more prevalent among persons in the lower socioeconomic groups. The poor were more often seen in mental health clinics than by private psychiatrists. In addition, low socioeconomic status, occupational instability, and downward mobility were associated with the highest frequency of psychiatric disability. Hollingshead and Redlich devised a subgrouping of class structure in this county based on a particular level of education, occupation, and income. Their class distinctions, described in Table 4, are used widely by sociologists and epidemiologists. A more recent New Haven study used a structured diagnostic interview in order to make specific diagnoses. A major finding of that study was that

15.1 percent of the adult population over age 26 showed evidence of a mental disorder, and a probable mental disorder was present in an additional 2.7 percent.

Stirling County Study

In 1952, Alexander H. Leighton conducted a psychiatric epidemiologic study of Stirling County, a Nova Scotian county of 20,000 persons. Information was recorded using structured interviews by nonclinician interviewers that was later rated by a psychiatrist. Unlike the New Haven and Midtown Manhattan surveys, subjects of the Stirling County study lived in rural areas, with persons from small villages, one small town, and many isolated farms. Male and female household heads were interviewed. The major findings were that 57 percent of persons could be identified as having a lifetime prevalence of some mental disorder, 24 percent having notable impairment, and 20 percent being in need of psychiatric attention. Women showed considerably more psychiatric disorders than did men, and psychiatric disorders were found to increase with age and degree of poverty.

Additional Epidemiologic Studies

A 1974 study by B. P. Dohrenwend described the influence of social factors in psychopathology and concluded that the highest rate of mental disorders was found in the lowest social class, confirming the findings of earlier studies of Faris and Dunham and Rennie. One interesting finding was that schizophrenia and personality disorders had a higher correlation with lower social class than did neurosis or bipolar mood disorder, the latter two being more common among the upper and upper middle social classes.

Other studies attempted to assess the influence of the early physical environment on mental illness. Benjamin Pasamanick demonstrated the relationship between prenatal factors and functional disorders in children. He also correlated season of birth and incidence of mental deficiency. Significantly more children born in the winter months were admitted to the Columbus State School in Ohio. This finding was particularly true for those children born in years when the average temperature in the third month after their conception had been the highest of the summer. This finding suggests that pregnant women may then have decreased their protein intakes to levels low enough to impair the developing brains of their unborn children. Malnourished populations have been shown to have various defects of central nervous system development.

THE NIMH EPIDEMIOLOGIC CATCHMENT AREA PROGRAM (NIMH ECA)

The NIMH–ECA project evolved from the report of the 1977 *President's Commission on Mental Health,* which highlighted the need to identify who are the mentally ill, how they are treated, and by whom. Darrel Regier and his associates at the Division of Biometry and Epidemiology of the NIMH sought to identify the percent of the population with a mental disorder. The objective was to determine what percent of the population with a mental disorder was receiving treatment in mental health settings (such as psy-

Table 4
Class Status and Cultural Characteristics of Subjects in the New Haven Study

Class	Class Status and Cultural Characteristics
I	Class I, containing the community's business and professional leaders, has two segments: a long established core group of interrelated families and a smaller upward-mobile group of new people. Members of the core group usually inherit money along with group values that stress tradition, stability, and social responsibility. Those in the newer group are highly educated, self-made, able, and aggressive. Their family relations often are not cohesive or stable. Socially, they are rejected by the core group, to whom they are, however, a threat by the vigor of their leadership in community affairs.
II	Class II is marked by at least some education beyond high school and occupations as managers or in the lesser-ranking professions. Four of five are upward mobile. They are joiners at all ages and tend to have stable families, but they have usually gone apart from parental families and often from their home communities. Tensions arise generally from striving for educational, economic, and social success.
III	Class III males for the most part are in salaried administrative and clerical jobs (51 percent) or own small businesses (24 percent); many of the women also have jobs. Typically, they are high-school graduates. They usually have economic security but little opportunity for advancement. Families tend to be somewhat less stable than in class II. Family members of all ages tend to join organizations and to be active in them. There is less satisfaction with present living conditions and less optimism than in class II.
IV	In Class IV, 53 percent say they belong to the working class. Seven of ten show no generational mobility. Most are content and make no sacrifices to get ahead. Most of the men are semiskilled (53 percent) or skilled (35 percent) manual employees. Practically all the women who are able to hold jobs do so. Education usually stops shortly after graduation from grammar school for both parents and children. Families are much different from those in Class III. Families are larger, and they are more likely to include three generations. Households are more likely to include boarders and roomers. Homes are more likely to be broken.
V	Class V adults usually have not completed elementary school. Most are semiskilled factory workers or unskilled laborers. They are concentrated in tenement and cold-water-flat areas of New Haven or in suburban slums. There are generally brittle family ties. Very few participate in organized community institutions. Leisure activities in the household and on the street are informal and spontaneous. Adolescent boys frequently have contact with the law in their search for adventure. There is a struggle for existence. There is much resentment, expressed freely in primary groups, about how they are treated by those in authority. There is much acting out of hostility.

chiatric clinics), private psychiatrists' offices, and in such nonpsychiatric settings as general medical treatment centers and internists' offices. In 1978, provisional estimates indicated that at least 15 percent of the population of the United States was affected by mental disorders in one year, and only one fifth of these persons received care from mental health specialists. Three fifths of persons with identified mental disorders were treated by primary care physicians.

A major goal of the NIMH–ECA study is to determine more specifically the prevalence of mental disorder as defined by DSM–III and DSM–III-R and to establish longitudinal data on the course of various mental disorders.

Various sites around the country are being studied to assess mental disorder prevalence, incidence, and service use from geographically defined community populations of at least 200,000 residents. Random samples are drawn to obtain completed interviews on at least 20,000 community and institutional residents. The Diagnostic Interview Schedule (DIS), which assesses the presence, duration, and severity of symptoms, is the major instrument that the trained lay interviewer used to interview each subject.

Compared with all previous studies, the NIMH–ECA study utilizes better diagnostic tools and more specific criteria to make a reliable diagnosis. These include careful clinical description, laboratory studies, family and genetic studies, and follow-up studies. Much larger samples are used than in the previously described studies.

In general, early findings of the ECA program show the following: Rates of depression are twice as high for females as for males; males are more likely than females to have alcoholism; and drug abuse is more common in persons under age 30. The most current epidemiologic and treatment findings for a specific mental disorder will be found in the chapter that discusses that disorder.

SOCIAL PROCESSES AND MENTAL DISORDER

Sociologists study social class and society, particularly the interactions of persons who constitute a group that has delimited boundaries, called a social system. Social position correlates with mental and physical illness, attitudes toward health care, and personality traits. For example, the preponderance of evidence suggests that both treated mental disorders and the symptoms of psychological discomfort are found more frequently in (1) the lower socioeconomic class, (2) among persons without meaningful social ties, (3) among those who do not have useful social roles, and (4) among those who have suffered traumatic loss of significant social ties.

SOCIAL STRUCTURE AND PERSONALITY

At every stage of life, a person is enmeshed in a structure of relationships and expectations that influences how goals and self-image are defined. The infant is born into a matrix of social relationships as well as an ongoing cultural order. They provide the infant with his initial orientations and train him for expected performances. Within this ma-

trix, the child develops characteristic ways of interpreting and responding to others. Position in society also carries an implicit social stereotype of attributed characteristics. Other people define the child in terms of his family's reputation, his social class, his ethnic group, and his religion.

The concept of social class has been variously formulated in terms of economic power, social prestige, political identification, and patterns of association. In American society, class position is most frequently characterized by occupation and education. White-collar occupations, which are usually coupled with a college education, tend to place one in the middle class; blue-collar occupations, which are coupled with a high-school education at best, tend to place one in the working class. Studies by social psychologists have shown that life styles, aspirations, and to a degree, cognition and modes of personality, coping, and defense tend to differ by class. However, a major problem with social class studies is the tendency toward broad generalization that may promote stereotypical thinking. For example, statements that characterize working class persons as impulsive and unable to delay gratification have little validity. Many studies that compare traits among class groups are related, upon careful examination, more to income than to other factors. Similarly, feelings of personal efficacy — of being in control of one's destiny and not subject to external controls — are more characteristic of the middle class than in the working class. But, a sense of autonomy and one's level of income are not unrelated. Nevertheless, behavioral science research has established that chronic life stresses occur more often in the working class than in the middle class. Moreover, working class members are more vulnerable to stressors than are members of the middle class.

LIFE CRISES

Although the most general formulations of life stress have not greatly illuminated the understanding of mental disorders, a number of studies of life crises suggest a correlation with mental illness. Studies of schizophrenic patients, for example, suggest that specific life changes in the weeks immediately preceding breakdown frequently serve as precipitants of the onset of schizophrenia. In one study, it was found that in the 3 weeks before onset of a schizophrenic episode, 60 percent of schizophrenic patients experienced objectively confirmable events that impinged directly on themselves or on close relatives. The comparable figure for a control group was only 19 percent. Other investigators have shown that life changes are associated with symptoms and with a number of physical ailments.

In the Midtown Manhattan study mentioned above, life stress was taken into account in the following categories: economic deprivation, single-parent homes, medical illness, social isolation, concern about work. A correlation between psychiatric symptoms and life stresses was found. In a well-known study by T. H. Holmes and B. Rahe, point values were assigned to various life changes that required the person to change or adapt (see Table 5). If a critical number of events happened to a person during a one year period, he was at risk for some type of medical or psychiatric illness. Of those people who accumulated 300 points

Table 5
The Social Readjustment Rating Scale*

Life Event	Mean Value
1. Death of spouse	100
2. Divorce	73
3. Marital separation from mate	65
4. Detention in jail or other institution	63
5. Death of a close family member	63
6. Major personal injury or illness	53
7. Marriage	50
8. Being fired at work	47
9. Marital reconciliation with mate	45
10. Retirement from work	45
11. Major change in the health or behavior of a family member	44
12. Pregnancy	40
13. Sexual difficulties	39
14. Gaining a new family member (through birth, adoption, oldster moving in, etc.)	39
15. Major business readjustment (merger, reorganization, bankruptcy, etc.)	39
16. Major change in financial state (a lot worse off or a lot better off than usual)	38
17. Death of a close friend	37
18. Changing to a different line of work	36
19. Major change in the number of arguments with spouse (either a lot more or a lot less than usual regarding child rearing, personal habits, etc.)	35
20. Taking on a mortgage greater than $10,000 (purchasing a home, business, etc.)[†]	31
21. Foreclosure on a mortgage or loan	30
22. Major change in responsibilities at work (promotion, demotion, lateral transfer)	29
23. Son or daughter leaving home (marriage, attending college, etc.)	29
24. In-law troubles	29
25. Outstanding personal achievement	28
26. Wife beginning or ceasing work outside the home	26
27. Beginning or ceasing formal schooling	26
28. Major change in living conditions (building a new home, remodeling, deterioration of home or neighborhood)	25
29. Revision of personal habits (dress, manners, associations, etc.)	24
30. Troubles with the boss	23
31. Major change in working hours or conditions	20
32. Change in residence	20
33. Changing to a new school	20
34. Major change in usual type or amount of recreation	19
35. Major change in church activities (a lot more or a lot less than usual)	19
36. Major change in social activities (clubs, dancing, movies, visiting, etc.)	18
37. Taking on a mortgage or loan less than $10,000 (purchasing a car, TV, freezer, etc.)	17
38. Major change in sleeping habits (a lot more or a lot less sleep or change in part of day when asleep)	16
39. Major change in number of family get-togethers (a lot more or a lot less than usual)	15
40. Major change in eating habits (a lot more or a lot less food intake or very different meal hours or surroundings)	15
41. Vacation	15
42. Christmas	12
43. Minor violations of the law (traffic tickets, jaywalking, disturbing the peace, etc.)	11

*From Holmes T: Life situations, emotions, and disease. J Acad Psychosom Med *19:* 747, 1978.
[†] This figure no longer has any relevance in light of inflation; what is significant is the total amount of debt from all sources-Ed.

in 1 year, about 80 percent were at risk of illness in the near future.

Recent work, however, indicates that external events may not, in and of themselves, be sufficient to cause mental illness. Rather, a combination of genetic and experiential factors have to exist in order for illness to occur. This *vulnerability theory* presumes that the occurrence of illness depends on such factors as child-rearing practices, physical disorders, psychological stressors, genetics, and adverse social stressors. Each person has a personal threshold of vulnerability and innate ability to tolerate stress. It had been thought that any response could be conditioned to any

stimulus. It is now known that conditioning associations occur on the basis of the "principle of preparedness" (that is, organisms are biologically prepared to make some associations more easily than others). This factor is important in conditioned states of sickness, such as reactions to radiation therapy (i.e., some patients are more likely than others to get ill from this treatment).

Hans Selye, who developed the major theories of stress and illness, did not view stress as always being a negative factor in a person's life. Only when stress overwhelms the person and produces distress did he consider it to be damaging. Similarly, Holmes and Rahe's work has been reviewed in terms of whether the life change was viewed as pleasant or unpleasant, wanted or unwanted, and expected or unexpected. The quality of the stress and the effect of change on the person's life is as important as the nature of the life event itself.

References

Breslau M, Davis G C: Chronic stress and major depression. Arch Gen Psychiatry *43*:309, 1986.

Dohrenwend B P, Dohrenwend B S: Perspectives on the past and future of psychiatric epidemiology (The 1981 Rema Lapouse Lecture). Am J Public Health *72*:127, 1982.

Eisenberg L: Psychiatry and society. New Engl J Med *296*:903, 1977.

Fenton W S, Robinowitz C B, Leaf P J: Male and female psychiatrists and their patients. Am J Psychiatry *144*(3):358, 1987.

Hollingshead A B, Redlich F C: *Social Class and Mental Illness.* John Wiley & Sons, New York, 1958.

Regier D A, Goldberg I D, Taube C A: The de facto U.S. mental health services system: A public health perspective. Arch Gen Psychiatry *35*:685, 1978.

Robins L N: Epidemiology: Reflection on testing the validity of psychiatric interviews. Arch Gen Psychiatry *42*:918, 1985.

Robins L N, Helzer J E, Croughan J, Ratcliff K S: National Institute of Mental Health diagnostic interview schedule: Its history, characteristics, and validity. Arch Gen Psychiatry *38*:381, 1981.

Srole L, Langner T S, Michael S T, Opler M K, Rennie T A C: *Mental Health in the Metropolis: The Midtown Manhattan Study.* McGraw-Hill, New York, 1962.

Weissman M M, Klerman G L: Epidemiology of mental disorders: Emerging trends in the United States. Arch Gen Psychiatry *35*:705, 1978.

5.8 —————
Community Psychiatry and Mental Health

DEFINITION OF COMMUNITY PSYCHIATRY

Community psychiatry is the branch of psychiatry that develops and maintains organized programs for the promotion of mental health, the prevention and treatment of mental disorders, and the rehabilitation of former psychiatric patients. It requires that the psychiatrist relate to the community at large instead of, or in addition to, the individual. Other terms used for community psychiatry are community mental health, preventive psychiatry, outreach psychiatry, and public health psychiatry. It has been called the "third psychiatry revolution" (the first being the age of enlightenment following the middle ages and the second being the development of psychoanalysis).

DEVELOPMENT OF COMMUNITY PSYCHIATRY

In 1963, Congress passed the Community Mental Health Centers Act, which provided funds for the construction of community mental health centers (CMHC) with specified catchment areas (geographic regions with a population of 75,000 to 200,000). Each CMHC must provide five basic psychiatric services: inpatient care, emergency services (on a 24-hour basis), community consultation, day care (including partial hospitalization programs, halfway houses, after-care services, and a broad range of outpatient services), and research and education. By the early 1980s, the CMHC movement had made a major impact on mental health services and on the practice of psychiatry and the other mental health professions. At that time there were about 800 such centers in operation with over half in urban areas. Currently, because of severe financial constraints, the CMHC function is severely limited.

In 1981, a block grant program was created to provide federal funds to states for drug abuse, alcohol abuse, and other mental health programs. Several states established community support systems to help furnish needed mental health services; these programs are currently available nationwide. In spite of these efforts, state mental hospitals still utilize the majority of state-allocated mental health dollars. Financial limitations have interfered with the block grant programs and state programs.

CHARACTERISTICS OF A CMHC

Commitment

Commitment to a population implies a responsibility for planning. Commitment suggests (1) that the plan should identify all the mental health needs of the population, inventory the resources available to meet these needs, and organize a system of care; (2) a responsibility for involving the citizens and political figures in the planning process; (3) that prevention is at least as important as direct treatment; and (4) that the responsibility is to all persons in the population, including children, the aged, minorities, the chronically ill, the acutely ill, and those who live in geographically remote areas.

The requirement that mental health services be located close to the patient's residence or place of work makes it easier for people to get to a treatment site. Furthermore, this proximity enables illness to be identified earlier, making it more likely that hospitalization, when required, is brief.

Services

The community mental health movement views community mental health as a total system, rather than a single service. It has proposed a number of services suited to the needs of those served. The original legislation called for five required services—emergency services, outpatient services, partial hospitalization, inpatient services, and consultation-education services. Public Law 94-63 required the addition of services for children, services for the aged, screening before hospitalization, follow-up services for those who had been hospitalized, transitional housing services, alcoholism services, and drug abuse services.

The community mental health team includes psychiatrists (including child psychiatrists), clinical psychologists, psychiatric social workers, psychiatric nurses, necessary administrative help and clerical staff, and occupational and recreational therapists for inpatient and partial hospitalization programs. Links to welfare workers, clergy, family agencies, schools, and other human services groups also are maintained.

Long-Term Care

Stemming from concerns about fragmentation of care and the tendency to keep patients hospitalized or unnecessarily restricted to one type of service, community mental health programs encourage continuity of care. This continuity of care enables a single clinician to follow a given patient through emergency services, hospitalization, partial hospitalization as a transition to the community, and outpatient treatment as follow-up. It also provides an exchange of information and team responsibility for the patient when different therapists, for reasons of convenience or economy, treat the patient in several different settings. A free exchange of clinical information between centers and a liaison between different agencies are also part of the total system of care.

Community Participation

The community should participate in decisions about its mental health care needs and programs, instead of having them solely defined by professionals. Mental health services are sensitive to the needs of those served if the public is actively involved. The expectation is that mental health services are more apt to be used when knowledgeable persons interpret and educate the community about their availability.

Consultation

Consultee-centered work focuses on the person receiving the consultation, and ranges from attention to or even treatment of the emotional problems of the consultee to using knowledge about human behavior to help the consultee achieve his or her professional goals with the program and its patients. Program-centered consultation focuses on the total system or program, offering whatever assistance the mental health professional can give in regard to programs, systems, and agencies.

Evaluation and Research

Evaluation refers to the process of obtaining information about the total community mental health program and its effect on persons, institutions, and communities. Program evaluation should also provide feedback to the planners and decision makers, so that the operating programs can be modified and new ones planned. It is now a required activity on which federally funded centers have to spend at least 2 percent of their budgets. Research may focus more specifically on key issues, rather than on the total program. The problem addressed may be a particular disorder or treatment method.

PREVENTION IN PSYCHIATRY

The prevention of mental disorders is based on public health principles and has been divided into primary, secondary, and tertiary prevention. The goal of preventive efforts is to decrease the onset (incidence), duration (prevalence), and residual disability of mental disorders.

Primary Prevention

The goal of primary prevention is to prevent the onset of a disease or disorder thereby reducing its incidence (number of new cases occurring in a specific period of time). This goal is accomplished by eliminating etiological agents, reducing risk factors, enhancing host resistance, or interfering with the mode of disease transmission. For some physical disorders the identification and modification of one or more of these factors has revolutionized the health care of the population. These successes are best exemplified by the virtual elimination of many infectious diseases and vitamin deficiency states as well as the reduction of certain forms of cancer, heart, and lung disease.

Examples of primary prevention to help the individual cope include mental health education programs (e.g., parent training in child development and alcohol and drug education programs); efforts at competence building (e.g., Head Start and other enriched day care programs for disadvantaged children, Outward Bound); development and utilization of social support systems to reduce the effects of stress on persons at high risk (e.g., widow-to-widow programs); anticipatory guidance programs to assist people in preparing for expected stressful situations (e.g., counseling of Peace Corp volunteers); and crisis intervention following the occurrence of stressful life events such as bereavement, marital separation and divorce, individual traumas, or group disasters.

Primary prevention also aims at eradicating stressful agents and reducing stress. Such programs include prenatal and perinatal care to decrease the incidence of mental retardation and organic brain disorders in children (e.g., improved nutrition and abstinence from alcohol and drugs during pregnancy, improved obstetrical practices, specific dietary modification for neonates vulnerable to phenylketonuria); stricter lead elimination laws to reduce the incidence of lead encephalopathy; modification of divorce, adoption, and child abuse laws to provide a healthy environment for child development; enrichment or replacement of institutional settings for infants, children, and the elderly; modification of certain risk factors for mental disorders that appear to be associated with low socioeconomic status; and genetic counseling to parents with a high risk for chromosomal abnormalities to prevent unwitting conception of compromised infants; and efforts to reduce the spread of certain sexually transmitted diseases (e.g., AIDS, syphilis) among the sequelae of which are mental disorders.

Several studies have found that some of the negative psychological effects on children from socially and economically disadvantaged environments can be reduced through special educational programs designed to build their overall competence level. Research on hospitalism among infants reared in emotionally sterile institutions indicates that enrichment of these institutions or placement of infants with caring adoptive families immediately after birth can eliminate this syndrome. Another study demonstrated that interventions with the children of psychotic parents made them less withdrawn, anxious, and inhibited than a control group of children who did not receive services.

Secondary Prevention

Secondary prevention is defined as early identification and prompt treatment of an illness or disorder with the goal of reducing the prevalence (total number of existing cases) of the condition by shortening its duration.

The experiences in military psychiatry in World War II and the Korean War renewed interest in secondary prevention. Military personnel observed that treatment duration could be considerably reduced and its effectiveness increased by treating soldiers with combat-induced mental disorders promptly, near the front. This procedure enabled soldiers to maintain ties to the social support of their military units, with the expectation that they would recover quickly. It became clear that these three principles—immediacy, proximity, and expectancy—could be applied in a civilian context. Thus, by providing rapid treatment of emerging mental disorders in the social milieu of the patient's home community with the expectation than he can improve, a clinician can facilitate a patient's recovery.

A large number of secondary prevention services have been established in this country's CMHCs, including emergency services, outpatient clinics, day treatment programs, and community-based inpatient units. To what extent these services have actually fulfilled the secondary preventive goal of reducing the community's prevalence of mental disorders is unknown. The research in this area is sparse, inconclusive, and often utilizes a number of case episodes—persons in treatment and length of treatment rather than illness duration as measures of outcome. However, the evidence that rapid treatment of certain mental disorders (e.g., affective disorders, anxiety disorders, acute psychoses) can reduce the duration of illness episodes suggests that the increased availability of treatment services through the CMHC system, in conjunction with the development of more effective psychological and pharmacological treatments, may well have reduced the community prevalence of some of these conditions. There is also growing evidence that when economic barriers are removed, through insurance and prepaid health plans, more people with mental disorders seek earlier treatment, which should lead to a reduction in the duration of some disorders and fulfill the goal of secondary prevention.

Tertiary Prevention

The goal of tertiary prevention is to reduce the prevalence of residual defect or disability due to illness or disorder. In the case of psychiatric conditions, tertiary prevention involves rehabilitative efforts to enable those who have a chronic mental illness to reach the highest level of functioning feasible.

The disabilities associated with chronic mental illness represent major social, economic, and public health problems. In the United States, they afflict more than 3 million people, are extremely costly, and create immense suffering for the affected persons, their families, and society. Although the term "chronic mental illness" has traditionally been associated with older patients who have a long history of mental hospitalization, it recently has been broadened to include younger adults with a variety of mental disorders who have grown up in the era of deinstitutionalization, many of whom have never been hospitalized but whose ability to lead productive controlled lives in the community is severely impaired.

The broad range of services necessary for community-based tertiary prevention include comprehensive emergency services; acute inpatient facilities; partial hospitalization; outpatient programs that provide medication monitoring; psychosocial, individual, group, and family therapies; a continuum of supervised living arrangements that afford increasing self-reliance; psychosocial peer and family support organizations; case management

services to link patients to income support agencies (e.g. SSDI, welfare, Medicaid) and provide aggressive outreach services to patients reluctant to keep in contact with the treatment system; and a variety of social and vocational rehabilitation programs. Such programs enable the chronically mentally ill person to be managed on an outpatient basis instead of being confined to an institution.

Over the past 30 years, most patients have been discharged from state institutions (or deinstitutionalized). Since 1955, the public hospital census has declined by 80 percent, and most chronic mental patients now live outside of hospitals. Although anecdotal evidence from CHMC site visits suggests that many chronic patients are living more satisfying lives with less residual impairment in the community than when they resided in state hospitals, there are very few methodologically sound follow-up studies.

While the goals of tertiary prevention have been partially reached for many chronic patients, for others deinstitutionalization has meant an absence of adequate services, transinstitutionalization to custodial nursing homes or within the penal system, repetition in the community of the barrenness and isolation that characterized life in custodial state hospitals, deprivation of the most basic human necessities (e.g. shelter, adequate nutrition, medical care), and repeated, brief trips through the revolving door of short-term inpatient management. Several studies have clearly demonstrated that without an active, multifaceted treatment system that is willing to assume ongoing responsibility for all facets of the patient's care, chronic mental patients will regress in the community as they did in the state hospital. One of the major problems faced by chronic patients is that their illness interferes with their coping skills, rendering them particularly likely to drift downward into even more stressful, impoverished environments. The end result is an increase in homeless persons in urban areas.

References

Angermeyer M C, Glink B, Majcher-Angermeyer A: Stigma perceived by patients attending modern treatment settings. Some unanticipated effects of community psychiatry. J Nervous Mental Dis *175*(1):4, 1987.

Avison W R, Nixon Speechley K: The discharged psychiatric patient: A review of social, social-psychological and psychiatric correlates of outcome. Am J Psychiatry *144*(1):10, 1987.

Barrett J, Rose R M: *Mental Disorders in the Community*. Guilford Press, New York, 1986.

Beiser M, Shore J H, Peters R: Does community care for the mentally ill make a difference? Am J Psychiatry *142*:1047, 1985.

Berlin R M, Kales J D, Humphrey F J, Kales A: The patient care crisis in community mental health centers: A need for more psychiatric involvement. Am J Psychiatry *138*:450, 1981.

Borus J F: Strangers bearing gifts: A retrospective look at the early years of community mental health center consultation. Am J Psychiatry *141*:868, 1984.

Caplan G: *Principles of Preventive Psychiatry*. Basic Books, New York, 1964.

Chacko R C, editor: *The Chronic Mental Patient in a Community Context*. American Psychiatric Press, Washington, DC, 1985.

Friedman M J, West A N: Current need versus treatment history—Predictors of use of outpatient psychiatric care. Am J Psych *144*(3):355, 1987.

Jones M: *The Therapeutic Community*. Basic Books, New York, 1953.

Klein D C, Goldston S E: *Primary Prevention: An Idea Whose Time Has Come*. US Government Printing Office, Washington, DC, 1977.

Langley D G, Berlin I N, Yarvis R M: *Handbook of Community Mental Health*. Medical Examination Publishing Co, Garden City, NY, 1981.

Okin R L, Dolnick J A, Pearsall D T: Patients' perspectives on community alternatives to hospitalization: A follow-up study. Am J Psychiatry *140*:1460, 1983.

Schrader J L. The Alaska mental health lands. Am J Psych *144*(1):107, 1987.

Strayhorn J M, Jr.,: Control groups for psychosocial intervention outcome studies. Am J Psych *144*(3):275, 1987.

5.9 ————
Socioeconomic Aspects of Health Care

The World Health Organization (WHO) defines health as: the state of complete physical, mental, and social well being and not merely the absence of disease. In its effort to promote health, the American health care delivery system attempts to provide and maintain high quality medical care for all of its citizens while advancing medical research and technology. The current emphasis on health care is on prevention and health promotion as well as treatment and diagnosis of medical disorders. Increasing health care costs have become significant obstacles in fulfilling these objectives. The focus on efforts to control these costs affects the distribution of health care funds, delivery of health care services, and reimbursement mechanisms for these services.

Both social and economic factors significantly affect the health status and delivery of health services to our nation. Studying the qualities of a population that influence its health, illness, and death is invaluable when assessing current health care requirements, designing future facilities and programs, and allocating dollars to optimize the provision of adequate services.

SOCIAL FACTORS

Life-Style

Life-style and personal habits are major factors in the cause of illness and death in the United States, accounting for about 70 percent of all illness, both mental and physical. Obesity, for example, is related to heart disease and diabetes, and a person's weight bears a direct relation to habit patterns.

Many cancer deaths have been related to both poor dietary habits and the chewing and smoking of tobacco. Over the last 20 years, the smoking rate for women has been rapidly approaching that for men; 35 percent of men and 30 percent of women smoked cigarettes in 1983. The increase in lung cancer among women has parallelled this rise in smoking behavior. For women 55 to 70 years of age, lung cancer is the primary cause of death due to cancer.

Regular physical activity has a positive effect on stress reduction. It is also useful in treating and preventing such mental problems as anxiety and depression and such physical problems as obesity, heart disease, diabetes, and high blood pressure. A trend in this country over the last two decades indicates that while the number of adults involved in a daily exercise regimen is rising, less than half of school-age children are exercising on a daily basis.

Age

The incidence of illness is affected by age. Eighty-six percent of persons over 65 years of age have one or more chronic conditions. The three leading chronic conditions of old age are arthritis, hypertension, and heart disease. Hearing impairments, diabetes, cataracts, and varicose veins also are common chronic problems. Mental health problems increase with age, as well. While chronicity is a factor among the elderly, young persons are more predisposed to acute illnesses. The three most common acute medical problems, across age groups, are upper respiratory conditions, influenza, and injuries.

Age influences the utilization of all health care services. Both younger persons (age 20 to 30) and persons over 65 tend to have more illnesses and health care needs than persons in middle adulthood. Young children's health care habits are often modeled after those of their parents. Prior experiences with health care influence future attitudes and behavior.

Socioeconomic Status (SES)

A person's SES is not based solely on income but includes such factors as education, occupation, and living expenses. The incidence of physical illness is affected by SES. Persons in low SES groups are more likely to be afflicted with hypertension, arthritis, upper respiratory illness, speech difficulties, and eye diseases. There is a reduced life expectancy for lower SES persons, as longevity is positively correlated to SES level.

There is a positive correlation between SES and mental health; consequently, high SES persons have better mental health than persons of low SES. With regard to the incidence of psychopathology, some studies have found a slightly higher percentage of bipolar disease among higher SES persons and a greater number of schizophrenic persons in lower SES groups.

Sex

Regardless of age, women seek health care and are hospitalized more often than men. Women are most frequently hospitalized for childbirth, heart disease, and cancer, whereas men are hospitalized for heart disease, cancer, and fractures. The three leading chronic conditions that can limit activity for men are heart conditions, followed by arthritis, and impairment of the back or spine; for females, they are arthritis, heart conditions, and hypertension.

Race

Race affects the utilization of health care facilities. In 1984, approximately ten times as many visits were made to physicians' offices by white persons as by blacks. The rates of such chronic conditions as obesity, diabetes, heart disease, hypertension, and arthritis are higher among blacks than whites.

Environment

The environment contributes to approximately one quarter of today's health problems. The exposure to such environmental risks as toxic waste, natural disasters, lead, asbestos, dioxins, is a major source of disease and death in man. Approximately 75 percent of all carcinogens come from the environment.

With regard to mental health, there is a general rise in mental disorders among people as their environment changes from the suburban community to the inner city.

MORTALITY TRENDS

The health status and health needs of a population can be assessed by examining general health trends, including death rates, causes of death, and longevity. The existence of certain medical disorders influences the need for particular health care delivery systems, programs, and personnel. A population's general health status determines the overall need for services and dollars.

In 1984, the death rate accross all age groups in the United States was 547.7 per 100,000. This is the lowest level ever recorded. It compares to the rate of 585.8 in 1980 (a 7 percent reduction) and 1,779 in 1900 (a 69 percent reduction). The causes of death have varied through the years. Pneumonia, tuberculosis, and gastrointestinal disease were the three leading causes of death at the beginning of the 20th century. In 1983, the three leading causes of death were heart disease, cancer, and stroke, in decreasing order. While psychiatric illness does not play a major role in the mortality rate, it is probably the major factor in the morbidity rate and is also a major cause of days lost from work.

Mortality rates differ considerably by race and sex. Females have lower mortality rates than males in all age groups, but the difference has been decreasing in recent years. Racial minorities within a given population have higher death rates than the majority population.

The primary cause of death for each of the different sex and race groups is heart disease. The mortality rate for heart disease, cancer, and stroke is greatest among black males and is higher for males than females.

The most common cause of death among adolescents and young adults (age 15 to 24) is accidents; approximately three fourths of these fatalities occur in automobiles. Homicide and suicide are the second and third leading causes of death, respectively, in this age group. For children under age 14, the leading causes are accidents, cancer, and congenital anomalies, in that order. The three leading causes of infant death are congenital anomalies, respiratory distress syndrome, and sudden infant death syndrome, in decreasing order. The mortality rate for white infants is about half as high as that for black infants (9.7 versus 19.2 deaths per 1,000).

In the United States, life expectancy of all age, sex and race groups has been steadily increasing since the turn of the century. In 1984, the average life expectancy from birth was 74.7 years. Black males have the shortest life expectancy from birth (65.5 years). White males (71.8 years), black females (73.7 years), and white females (78.8 years) all live longer than black males. Although life expectancy of females is greater than that of males (78.3 years versus 71.1 years), this difference has been diminishing in recent years. The differential attributable to race has lessened as well. The reduction is more significant for black females than for black males.

UTILIZATION OF HEALTH CARE RESOURCES

In the last decade, 75 percent of adults have been in a hospital at least once, women being hospitalized more often than men. Rates of hospitalization for all illness increase with age. The average general hospital stay across specialties is 7.8 days, which represents a reduction over the last decade. A slight increase in hospital use, however, has been reported for children and elderly persons during the last 5 years. At present, there is a 10 percent oversupply of hospital beds in this country, particularly in urban areas; the expense of maintaining the beds continues even if they are empty. The health care staff is the largest component of hospital costs.

Physician services tend to be underutilized. Twenty-five percent of the population does not see a physician at all in a given year. Of the 75 percent who do, most are very young or old, or are women, and they average about five visits a year. Physician visits may take place in the doctor's office (56 percent), hospital outpatient departments, including the Emergency Room (15 percent), and over the telephone (16 percent). As family income rises, the rates of office and phone consultations increase and the rate of hospital outpatient visits decreases. The five leading reasons for office visits are general examination, prenatal examination, throat problems, hypertension, and postoperative visits, in descending order of frequency.

HEALTH CARE DELIVERY SYSTEMS AND PROVIDERS

Hospitals

The hospital is the institutional provider of general medical and surgical services in the United States health care system. According to the WHO, hospitals must have a physician staff, offer continuous medical and nursing care to patients, and maintain inpatient facilities. The classification of hospitals may be based on ownership, length of stay, or nature of service. See Table 1 for an overview of important aspects of hospital organization. Since hospitals consume the biggest percentage of health dollars, their utilization is the focus of current cost-containment strategies.

Nursing Homes

In 1982, there were approximately 14,500 nursing homes in the United States with approximately 1,500,000 beds. Classified by the intensity of care they offer, nursing homes range from nursing care homes, which employ one or more nurses and provide nursing care to most of the residents, to domiciliary care homes, which provide personal and domiciliary care services. Nursing home care will be of increasing importance in this country because people are living longer. In the year 2000, about 50 percent of our population will be at least 50 years old; in 1982, this number was only 26 percent. Approximately 8 percent ($32 billion) of national health care dollars are spent on nursing home care each year.

Table 1
Aspects of Hospital Organization*

Criteria	Voluntary Hospital	Investor-Owned Hospitals	State Mental Hospital System	Municipal Hospital System	Federal Hospital System	Special Hospital
Patient population	All illnesses	All illnesses, although hospital may specialize	Mental illness	All illnesses	All illnesses	70 percent of facility must be for single diagnosis
Number of hospitals	5,843	757	277 (140,000 beds nationally)	Variable per city	342	150
Profit orientation	Nonprofit	For profit	Nonprofit	Nonprofit	Nonprofit	For profit or nonprofit
Ownership	Private management board	Private corporation; may be owned by MDs	State	City government	Federal government	Private or public
Affiliation	1200 church-affiliated; remainder are privately owned or university sponsored	May be owned by large chains such as Hospital Corporation of America or Humana Corporation	Free-standing or affiliated with various medical schools	Voluntary teaching hospitals and medical schools	Department of Defense (190); Public Health Service, Coast Guard, Prison, Merchant Marine, Indian Health Service; Veterans Administration (129)	Optional affiliation with medical schools
Other	Provide bulk of care in U.S.	Increasing in importance nationally	Deinstitutionalization—number of patients has been reduced	Most physicians at municipal hospitals are employed by their affiliated medical school	V.A. Hospitals usually have affiliations with medical schools	Less regulated than other types of hospitals (see note 5)

*Notes (1) To be designated a teaching hospital, at least four types of approved residencies must be maintained, and an affiliation with a medical school must be maintained. (2) As of 1982, there were 364 state-operated facilities and approximately 14,600 private facilities for the mentally retarded. (3) In 1983 there were 154 investor-owned for profit hospitals for psychiatric patients in the United States. That number is growing. The total number of psychiatric hospitals (public and private) is about 564. (4) Short-term hospitals have an average patient stay of less than 30 days; long-term, an average of longer duration. (5) Special hospitals include obstetrics and gynecology; eye, ear, nose, and throat; etc. They do not include psychiatric hospitals or substance abuse hospitals.

Private Practice

Most physicians in America are in traditional autonomous office-based practices, and the majority of patients receive health care in the physician's private office. Physicians utilize their own facilities and equipment to provide a variety of health care services.

Private practices are organized in one of three ways: independent, partnership, and group. Independent or solo practitioners comprise a significant part of the health care delivery system today. A physician in an independent private practice works for himself and provides personalized service to patients.

In a partnership, the overhead (office, personnel, equipment expenses) is shared by the two or more physicians. The patients, in contrast, may or may not be "shared" by the doctors; the practice may remain independent in this respect.

Group practice is gaining popularity in the United States. The American Medical Association defines group practice as the delivery of medical services by three or more physicians who are formally organized to provide care, consultation, diagnosis, and treatment. The group shares the use of equipment and personnel, and income from the medical practice is distributed among the members of the group.

Group practices may consist of a single specialty or be multidisciplinary in nature and thereby deliver a greater variety of services to the patient. As with the partnership, the group practice offers the physician economic benefits and fewer working hours. The group practice also enables the physician to maintain a more regular work schedule. The ability to form ongoing doctor-patient relationships diminishes, however, as the number of patients increase. Recently, private practitioners have been more inclined to move away from independent practice to participate in group practices and, to a lesser extent, partnerships.

In private practice, patients pay for services directly or through third-party payers, that is, insurance companies. As economic conditions change, however, office-based physicians are joining, at an increasing rate, prospective (prepayment) reimbursement systems, as described in the next sections.

Health Maintenance Organization (HMO)

An HMO is an organized system of providing comprehensive (both inpatient and outpatient) health care in all specialties, including psychiatry. Members enroll in the plan and pay a prepayment, or capitation fee, to cover all health care services for a fixed period of time (a month or a year). There are currently about 300 HMOs in the United States (up from 175 in 1976), with an enrollment of approximately 15 million people.

By employing a capitation or prospective payment method, the HMO is assuming a more dominant role in U.S. health care. The primary reason for the popularity of the HMO is that it decreases health care costs by limiting the number of new hospitalizations and discharging patients from the hospital earlier. The emphasis on prevention and health promotion, and on performing as much diagnosis and therapy as possible on an outpatient basis also help to control expenses.

There are three types of HMOs. (1) In the Staff Model, physicians receive a salary to provide services in the HMO's own facility. (2) In the Group Model, health care is furnished by one or more groups of doctors; payment is received on a contractual basis at a predetermined rate. Physicians in Staff and Group Models often own stock in their HMO. (3) The Individual Practice Association (IPA) is also referred to as the Network Model. The HMO negotiates with individual physicians to receive a capitation fee for providing services to each IPA member seen in their private offices. Physicians retain their office-based private practices when they join an IPA.

Preferred Provider Organization (PPO)

Similar to the HMO, this type of alternative delivery organization employs a prospective payment system. In the PPO, however, a corporation or insurance company forms an agreement with a particular group of community hospitals and doctors to supply health services to PPO members at a previously determined lower rate. Patients who enroll in a PPO select their physician from among the list of participating doctors, which includes both specialists and primary care physicians. Inpatient care is received at one of the designated hospitals, and this too is done at the patient's chosen facility. There are about 200 PPOs in the United States at this time.

HEALTH MANPOWER

There are approximately 30,000 psychiatrists among the 500,000 physicians in the United States, and while the number is adequate, the problem is in their distribution. High physician-patient ratios exist in the Northeast and in California; but low concentrations are the norm in the Southern and Mountain States. Psychiatrists tend to be concentrated in major urban areas.

Primary care physicians number about 35 percent of all doctors and are usually defined as general practitioners, family practitioners, internists, and pediatricians. Primary care has been defined as a type of medical care delivery which emphasizes first-contact care and assumes ongoing responsibility for the patient in both health maintenence and therapy of illness. Many believe that psychiatry also should be classified as a primary care specialty. This is not currently the case.

When projections are made through the 1990s, there are shortages, balances, and surpluses in the overall numbers of physicians and physicians in various specialties. In the United States, for example, it is believed that there will be an oversupply of 70,000 physicians by 1990 and that this number will be as high as 145,000 at the turn of the century. However, in 1990, 48,000 psychiatrists will be needed in this country, but only 38,000 will be trained. The only other fields in which there will be a shortage are emergency medicine and preventive medicine. Other specialties will be in surplus; for example, 24,000 surgeons will be needed in 1990, and 35,000 will be available. Other fields in which there will be a similar surplus are neurology, ophthalmology, obstetrics and gynecology, internal medicine, and neurosurgery. Fields in which supply will equal demand in 1990 include dermatology, family practice, otolaryngology, and pediatrics.

HEALTH CARE COSTS

The provision of adequate services to the American public in a cost-effective manner is a critical concern. Spending for all types of health care, including the care of the mentally ill, continues to escalate. The growth rate of health care expenditures continues to outdistance the pace of growth of the economy. Health care has become increasingly expensive owing to inflation, population growth, and advanced technology.

In 1984, approximately $387 billion or 10.6 percent of the gross national product, was spent for health care. Mental illness accounts for a large proportion of this expenditure. Although the 9.1 percent rise in 1984 in national health care expenditures was its smallest increase in about 25 years, health care spending constituted a growing share of the GNP over the same time period.

Government spending is on the rise. Owing in part to Medicare and Medicaid's implementation in 1967, the federal government's monetary contribution to health care has grown from about 10 percent in 1965 to about 30 percent in 1984. Overall, the government pays approximately 40 percent (30 percent federal, 10 percent state) of personal health care expenditures. Private funds account for the other 60 percent through direct payments (28 percent), private health insurance (31 percent), and industry and philanthropy (1 percent).

Representing approximately 41 percent of expenditures, hospitals utilize the largest proportion of health care dollars. Physicians' fees are about 20 percent of costs, followed by nursing homes, drugs, and dental services. In general, hospital costs and general medical care services have risen at a far greater rate than physicians' fees.

As many as 85 percent of Americans have some form of health insurance, which covers approximately 80 percent of hospital costs and 60 percent of physicians' services, except in the case of psychiatry. Twenty-five percent of hospital costs to the patient represent laboratory tests and imaging, and the remaining costs are for administration, nursing, drugs, and other support services.

BASIC CONCEPTS OF PSYCHIATRIC HEALTH CARE DELIVERY

Because psychiatry is a branch of medicine, the psychiatrist must be familiar with the problems of the medical establishment such as regulation organization, reimbursement, and cost containment.

Regulation and Organization of Hospital Standards and Programs

There is a group of agencies such as the Joint Commission on Accreditation of Hospitals (JCAH) and the Liaison Committee on Medical Education (LCME) that influence the standards of hospital care and performance. In addition to governmental regulations (city and state health rules) with which hospitals must comply, the JCAH inspects hospitals every 2 years. The JCAH also is responsible for determining the requirements for hospital accreditation. Hospital reimbursements from Medicare and Medicaid are contingent on meeting these standards. This accreditation, however, is done on a

voluntary basis. The LCME and the Liaison Committee on Graduate Education are charged with accrediting medical schools and residency training programs, respectively. The two accrediting committees review their respective education and training programs every 4 years; this procedure is voluntary.

Currently, there is a trend toward monitoring all the hospitals in a community as a single health entity and community resource. That means that each unit does not have the prerogative to develop new facilities without concern for the services offered by the other hospitals in the area.

Utilization Review. This in-house evaluation process was created to ensure that institutions provide efficient, quality health care that meets patients' needs. The members of the utilization review committee consist of hospital administrators, doctors, and nurses. The committee reviews each patient's chart within a specified number of days of admission. The appropriateness of admission, treatment strategies, and length of hospital stay are reviewed to facilitate the patient's discharge. Through this process, the utilization review committee determines whether a particular admission was really indicated and whether the hospital stay was longer than necessary. A hospital must conduct utilization reviews to be eligible for JCAH accreditation.

Professional Standards Review Organization (PSRO). The PSRO was set up by the federal government to review and to monitor care received by patients that is paid for with government funds. PSROs have been established by local medical associations and serve several functions. They attempt to ensure high quality care, control costs, determine maximum lengths of stay by patients in hospitals, conduct utilization reviews, and censure physicians who do not adhere to established guidelines. The PSRO may conduct a medical audit to retrospectively evaluate the quality of care by carefully examining charts. The PSRO is made up of doctors elected by local medical societies.

Peer Review Organization (PRO). In the early 1980s, the PRO replaced the PSRO as the federal review organization for hospitals receiving Medicare funds. In order to promote compliance with federal guidelines for health and hospital care, the PRO conducts independent utilization reviews and quality-of-care studies, validates Diagnosis Related Group (DRG) assignments, and reviews hospital admissions and readmissions.

Federally mandated and funded, the PROs have greater authority than the PSROs. PROs can impose sanctions on hospitals for inadequate care. They can even recommend the termination of federal funding to hospitals that consistently violate federal standards. In addition, PROs can adjust or refuse payment for health services that they consider unnecessary.

The PRO operates on a statewide level and can be either for profit or nonprofit in nature. In order to reduce costs, a PRO is chosen through a competitive bidding process from among qualified, physician-sponsored organizations.

Health Systems Agency (HSA). These nonprofit organizations are mandated by the federal government and set up on a statewide basis. HSAs promote or limit the development of health services and facilities depending on the needs of a particular locality or state. They are made up of consumers and have considerable power in medicine. For example, before one can build a new hospital or conduct extensive renovations on an existing one, the HSA must approve a Certificate of Need (CON). In order to receive a CON, the necessity for a new facility in a specified locale must be established. HSAs control capital expenditures, and, therefore, the availability of health resources. In each state, HSAs develop both long- and short-term goals and plans, approve health care proposals requesting federal funding, review existing facilities and services, and suggest future construction and renovation projects based on their findings.

Reimbursement Programs

Medicare (Title 18). Under the Federal Social Security Act, Medicare is a federally funded health insurance program. It provides both hospital and medical insurance for persons 65 years or older and to persons with certain disabilities (e.g., blindness, renal disease). Medicare is comprised of two parts. Part A covers inpatient hospital care, home health services, dialysis, and nursing home care after hospitalization. Funding is derived from a federal trust fund, which, in turn, receives its funds from social security taxes. Part B is optional medical insurance that can be purchased by the patient to cover such services as physicians' fees, medical supplies, home health care, outpatient hospital care, and therapy services. Benefits and eligibility standards of Medicare are uniform throughout the United States.

Medicaid (Title 19). Mandated by the federal government, Medicaid is an assistance program for certain needy and low-income persons. It is financed by both federal and state governments, but each state defines its requirements for eligibility and is responsible for their administration. Although benefits vary from state to state, federal provisions require that Medicaid cover inpatient and outpatient hospital care (including psychiatric care), physician's services, laboratory tests, diagnostic imaging, home health care services, and nursing home care. Additional services may be provided at the state's option.

Blue Cross Association (BCA). This association of over 80 independent insurance plans around the country pays primarily for inpatient hospital service. Blue Shield pays for physician services during the patient's hospital stay. In contrast to commercial insurance carriers, BCA is a nonprofit organization whose premiums cover administrative expenses and benefits and provide a reserve to cover financial losses. It is regulated by state insurance departments. Benefits for psychiatric services are limited compared to those for other medical illnesses, though inpatient psychiatric care is less limited than outpatient care.

Self-Pay. Persons contract with commercial insurance companies to cover both inpatient and outpatient costs, including physicians' fees, diagnostic procedures, and laboratory tests. For this type of insurance, self-pay patients pay a premium that may be based on (1) an experience rating determined by one's risk or prior record for reimbursement on insurance claims or (2) a community rating system in which each participant pays the same premium because the plan's cost is divided equally among group members.

Owing to increased claim costs of private insurance companies, cost control strategies are being employed to reduce financial risk and increase profits. By utilizing such procedures as benefit maximums for a given year, deductibles, and copayments, health insurance companies can limit increases in premium rates while still covering most of the costs incurred by the patient.

Cost Containment

As protection against soaring health care expenditures, government and commercial insurance programs have enacted measures to limit spending. Two such mechanisms are described below.

Diagnosis Related Group (DRG). A DRG is a classification system consisting of 470 disease categories. In the 1970s, DRGs were developed at Yale University as a way to help health care personnel determine the appropriate length of hospitalization for any given patient. The assignment of a patient to a DRG category is based on principal diagnosis, treatment procedures, personal attributes (e.g., age, sex), complications, and discharge status.

In 1983, the federal Health Care Financing Administration adopted DRGs as the method for repaying hospitals for Medicare services. Most states now use this prospective payment system, whereby a hospital is reimbursed for patient care based on a predetermined rate for each diagnostic category. An advantage of a prospective price system is that hospitals and physicians must deliver health services with greater efficiency in order to conserve resources and funds. The hospital knows in advance the dollar amount it will be reimbursed for each DRG, and it will make money if the actual cost of treatment is less than this designated price. The institution assumes a monetary loss, however, if the costs of hospitalization exceed this amount.

Criticisms of the DRG system include the concern that necessary but cost-ineffective medical services and programs will be eliminated. It is also feared that if the service provider anticipates that adequate treatment will cost more than the assigned rate, patients either will be prematurely released or refused care.

Claims Review. This method of peer review consists of the examination of claims for the reimbursement of treatment after it has been rendered. It has the disadvantage of being a decision to pay or not pay after the treatment has been given. Insurance companies and governments have been doing claims reviews for many years. Traditionally, it has consisted of the examination of a claim by a clerk, with determination of eligibility by nonprofessionals. When a claim for psychiatric treatment payment is turned down and appealed or when a claim is for a large amount, in the past the claim was reviewed by a single psychiatric consultant, who was an employee of the insurance company concerned. That system resulted in idiosyncratic decisions that may or may not have reflected local practice quality. In many instances, guidelines for insurance companies were developed without any input from practicing psychiatrists. As a result, psychiatric societies are now willing to help develop criteria for claims review and have been willing to nominate committees to serve as claims reviewers (peer reviewers) for insurance plans and government systems.

The first level of claims review generally consists of a clerical examination to determine whether the bill shows the necessary administrative information and whether the claimant is, indeed, insured. There is no determination of appropriateness of care. The second level of claims review is generally done by trained personnel, often nurses. Here the claims reviewer compares the treatment rendered with previously established criteria of treatment that have been agreed on as appropriate for the condition. The second-level reviewer may approve payment for the claim. If the second-level reviewer has questions or if the treatment is considered inappropriate according to the criteria, the claim is reviewed by a third-level group or a true peer review committee. Here there is a professional determination of the appropriateness of care. The peer review committee—one or more psychiatrists review each claim—may approve or disapprove. There are levels of appeal for the practitioner who is dissatisfied with the committee determination. The appeals process often goes to a special committee of the county or state medical society.

The most extensive system of claims review has been developed by the American Psychiatric Association under a contract with CHAMPUS (Civilian Health and Medical Plans for United States Armed Forces) of the Department of Defense. A national advisory group developed criteria and procedures for the review of both inpatient and office treatment. The criteria and procedures provide for all three levels of review. Peer review committees have been established throughout the United States to function through the central office of the American Psychiatric Association. Claims are reviewed initially by clerks and then by second-level trained reviewers. They go to a committee of peers when professional determinations about the appropriateness of treatment are needed. Only a peer review committee can deny a claim on the basis of professional necessity for that care, but clerks and second-level reviewers can deny a claim for administrative reasons.

This poor and inequitable claims review system leads to clerical bureaucracy and interference in the doctor-patient relationship, which may result in poor medical care.

References

Culliton B J: Health care economics: The high cost of getting well. Science *200*:883, 1978.

Freiman M P, Mithcell J B, Rosenbach M L. An analysis of DRG-based reimbursement for psychiatric admissions to general hospitals. Am J Psych *144*(5):p. 603, 1987.

Grant I, Yager J, Sweetwood H L: Life events and symptoms. Arch Gen Psychiat *39*:599, 1982.

Health: United States. US Department of Health and Human Services, Washington, DC, 1985.

Iglehart J K: The new era of prospective payment for hospitals. N Engl J Med *307*:1288, 1982.

McGuire T G, Dickey B, Shively G E, Strumwasser I: Differences in resource use and cost among facilities treating alcohol, drug abuse, and mental disorders: Implications for design of a prospective payment system. Am J Psych *144*(5):616, 1987.

Manning W G, Jr, Wells K B, Benjamin B: Use of out-patient mental health services over time in a health maintenance organization and fee-for-service plans. Am J Psych *144*(3):283, 1987.

Mitchell J B, Dickey B, Liptzin B, Sederer L I: Bringing psychiatric patients into the medicare prospective payment system: Alternatives to DRG's. Am J Psychiatry *144*(5):610, 1987.

National Data Book and Guide to Sources: Statistical Abstracts of the United States, ed 106. U S Department of Commerce, U S Bureau of the Census, Washington, DC, 1986.

Relman A S: The new medical-industrial complex. N Engl J Med *303*:963, 1980.

Rogers D E, Blendon R J, Moloney T W: Who needs Medicaid? N Engl J Med *307*:13, 1982.

Steven R S, Epstein A M: Institutional responses to prospective payment based on diagnostic-related groups. N Engl J Med *312*:621, 1985.

Syme S L, Berkman L F: Social class, susceptibility and sickness. Am J Epidemiol *104*:1, 1976.

Wennberg J E, McPherson K, Caper P: Will payment based on diagnostic-related groups control hospital costs? N Engl J Med *311*:295, 1984.

5.10 ▬▬▬▬
Ethics in Psychiatry

Ethics involves a set of moral principles that determine what is right or wrong and good or bad. For physicians and psychiatrists, these issues affect almost every aspect of their work, especially how their professional responsibilities and opinions relate to the values of their patients, their patients' families, and the society at large. Common ethical issues in psychiatry include such areas as competence, confidentiality, informed consent, involuntary hospitalization, right to treatment, right to refuse treatment, duties to third parties, and regulation of treatment.

COMPETENCE

A frequent source of ethical concern for the psychiatrist is the extent to which mental disorders impair the competence of patients to make decisions. Although law and ethics demand respect for patients' rights and preferences, psychiatric patients may have limited capacity to make choices for themselves. The problems of competence are glaring in the case of severely mentally ill patients. More subtle is the question of competence in neurotic, or "healthier," psychiatric patients. Given the complex nature of unconscious mental life and the defense mechanisms, can the psychiatrist simply rely on the patient's manifest declarations? For example, a patient may authorize or even request the psychiatrist to disclose confidential information to family members, employers, lawyers, or others for motives that are unclear or even obviously pathological, symptomatic of the intrapsychic and interpersonal disturbances for which the patient seeks treatment. The psychiatrist is then faced with an ethical as well as a clinical dilemma: Should the patient's request be respected, or should the best interests of the patient as perceived by the psychiatrist be protected? Each case must be evaluated individually and thoroughly.

TREATMENT

Several ethical principles may serve as the basis for psychiatric intervention. Perhaps the most familiar is the principle of *beneficence* (do good and avoid harm). Many psychiatric treatments, however, are not without risks and side effects. As a result, it is often necessary to turn to the weaker *utilitarian* principle (benefits must outweigh costs). Another principle frequently introduced is *respect for persons*. Although the principles of beneficence, utility, and respect for persons sometimes mutually reinforce each other, at other times, they conflict. Thus, to treat a person's depression may be beneficial, but to treat against a competent person's will fails to respect the person's right to make a decision. However, treatment of an incompetent person may be beneficial and, at the same time, show respect by restoring the person's capacity for self-determination. It is clear that the criteria for and the assessment of *competence* play a central role in determining whether an intervention is ethically justified.

Another ethical principle that is especially relevant to the ethics of mental health policy is *justice,* understood in this context as a fair distribution and application of psychiatric services. Justice in the sense of fair procedures enters into the justification for involuntary hospitalization and treatment of persons who, as a result of mental illness, are dangerous to themselves or others.

PROFESSIONAL CODES

In recent years, there has been increased interest in the use of professional codes of ethics as a standard of criticism and as a means to regulate professional misconduct. Local chapters of psychiatric societies and psychoanalytic institutes have strengthened their enforcement mechanism for dealing with complaints against their members. For example, much attention has been given to complaints against psychiatrists who have allegedly exploited their patients, especially through sexual contact. This behavior is both unethical and illegal. The action of professional ethics committees does not prevent patients from pursuing legal actions against their psychiatrists, and some have done so successfully.

Many critics of professional ethics note, however, that professional ethics codes, in psychiatry and in other professions, have little impact on education, on advanced training, or on routine professional practice. And others question the efficacy of the enforcement mechanism for the codes because of the lack of sanctions against or public disclosures about psychiatrists who have acted unethically. At the same time, psychiatrists who are brought before the ethics committee sometimes feel badly treated by their colleagues, especially if they have already been legally penalized for misconduct.

INVOLUNTARY TREATMENT

The principle of beneficence is invoked to justify treatment of some persons against their will. If a person has a mental disorder that constitutes a danger to self or others, the law permits involuntary treatment. The legal ground for treatment of persons dangerous to others is to protect public safety; the legal basis for treatment of suicidal or gravely disabled persons is to protect lives or safety. In both cases, the ethical basis is to benefit the patient by treating the mental disorder.

But there are legal and ethical limits. Involuntary patients have a right to a judicial review of the grounds for their confinement and treatment. Because involuntary treatment restricts a person's liberty and personal choice, the law requires that it be done for good reasons. Moreover, the hospitalization may not be indefinite, as it was prior to the late 1960's. From an ethical perspective, involuntary treatment is permitted on a time-limited trial basis to determine whether the treatment is beneficial. The law usually permits longer periods of involuntary treatment for persons who are more dangerous to others than to themselves. But in both cases, the benefits of treatment must accrue within a finite time. Otherwise, even a dangerous patient may not be held and treated against his will. A voluntary and consenting patient can be treated as long as it is deemed medically necessary.

Some mentally disordered, disruptive, and dangerous patients cannot benefit from treatment unless their behavior and the underlying psychoses can be brought under control. Sedation or restraint may be unavoidable. At the same time, it is important to emphasize that behavior control alone is not a sufficient goal of ethical psychiatric care. It may, in some instances, be all that can be achieved; sometimes mental illness defies psychiatry's best efforts to control it. But treating the mental illness, restoring competence and ability to function, and helping the mentally ill person cope with or even conquer mental illness are the ultimate goals of psychiatric intervention.

INFORMED CONSENT

For more than 25 years, the legal doctrine of *informed consent* has increasingly dominated discussions about the doctor-patient relationship. American law reflects strong popular beliefs about deep cultural commitments to self-determination. To permit competent adults to make important personal choices about life style, career, relationships, and other values is one way to demonstrate respect for persons. It is understandable, then, why psychiatrists must guard against the tendency to dominate the patient's decision making.

The legal doctrine of informed consent is a crude reminder that psychiatrists must respect the rights of patients, including their right to be informed and to make treatment choices. The law does not, however, provide guidance about the more complex and subtle ethical responsibility to show respect for one's patients, especially when their competence is compromised, to some degree, by their illness. The ethical task of the psychiatrist must be carried out first by the manner in which the patient (or prospective patient) is treated. To show respect is to listen, to try to understand, and to avoid stereotyping and premature diagnosis. Respect is further conveyed by the way the psychiatrist talks, tries to explain, and seeks to provide realistic options to patients, even questionably competent ones. Physicians must take precautions against assuming that patients are incompetent to decide for themselves until proven otherwise or protected by courts. Respect for patients is achieved by reciprocity, communication, and concern, not by domination.

At the very least, all patients should be told the nature of their illness as well as treatment options and side effects. The extent of choice about and among treatments will vary in accordance with patients' competence. Those who are competent may choose for themselves; those who are incompetent may require an authorized substitute to choose in concert with or on behalf of them. Respect for persons incorporates and goes beyond informed consent. It is unfortunate that so much emphasis has been placed on informed consent—its rituals, documentation, and difficulties—at the expense of the higher ethical standard of respect for persons.

RIGHT TO HEALTH CARE

After years of debate about the right to health care, it is clear that public and professional opinions remain divided. Some believe that health care is a right to which all persons are equally entitled. Others think that health care is a privilege that must be privately purchased. Still others believe that some amount of health care should be provided for those with significant health care needs who are unable to obtain them with their own resources, if not as a matter of right as an act of benevolence. Various proposals for national health insurance, catastropic health insurance, health insurance of the indigent, among others, have been considered, and some coverage for certain categories of needy persons in the United States is made available through Medicare, Medicaid, and other special programs. It is clear, however, that many persons' psychiatric needs are covered inadequately or not at all. Moreover, current trends do not appear to be moving toward better provision of psychiatric services for underserved populations or even the middle class. Instead, psychiatric services, both inpatient and outpatient, are restricted by federal and state programs. Private insurance seems to be moving toward reductions of psychiatric coverage as well. The trends are toward less outpatient coverage, fewer visits, and reduced long-term care. All this points toward serious ethical problems in the allocation of psychiatric services.

PRIVACY, CONFIDENTIALITY, AND PRIVILEGE: RECURRENT ETHICAL CONCERNS

The idea of *privacy* refers to limiting the access of others to one's body or mind, including dreams, fantasies, thoughts, or beliefs. Privacy in the law is sometimes linked to freedom from intrusion by the state or third persons and also designates a domain of personal decision, usually about such matters as personal associations, abortion, or bodily integrity. Thus, the notion of privacy has multiple, complex meanings. *Confidentiality* concerns the communication of private information from one person to another in a setting where it is expected that the recipient of the information, such as a psychiatrist, will not ordinarily disclose the information to a third person. Patients normally want and expect confidentiality because the private information revealed to psychiatrists is often sensitive, troubling, or shameful. *Privilege* refers to the right of patients, or psychiatrists on their behalf, to assert that certain confidential information may not be disclosed in a judicial or quasijudicial setting.

Unauthorized disclosure by a psychiatrist of confidential patient information is a serious violation of professional ethics. Discussion of a particular patient for purposes of supervision is permissible if safeguards protect confidentiality. But gossiping about patients, even if names are withheld, is unethical. It is potentially harmful, disrespectful, and unfair to patients.

Another area in which patient confidentiality is compromised is in the use of patient information in case reports, both published and unpublished. Case reports in teaching institutions, professional meetings, books, and journals sometimes violate patient confidentiality. Psychiatrists have an obligation not to disclose identifiable patient information (and, perhaps, any descriptive patient information) without appropriate informed consent.

As a final point, one of the most controversial legal and ethical issues in the past decade concerns limitations on confidentiality to protect public safety. Two areas of concern in which law and ethics intersect with confidentiality are child abuse reporting laws and duties to protect potential victims of dangerous patients. It is now legally required in all states that psychiatrists, among others, who have reason to believe that a child has been the victim of physical or sexual abuse must make an immediate report to an appropriate agency. In this situation, confidentiality is decisively limited by legal statute on the grounds that potential or actual harm to vulnerable children outweighs the value of confidentiality in a psychiatric setting. Although there are many complex psychodynamic nuances that accompany the required reporting of suspected child abuse, it is generally agreed that such reports are ethically justified.

A more controversial area concerns the duties of psychiatrists who have dangerous patients to protect threatened third parties. The Tarasoff case (described in Chapter 47 on Forensic Psychiatry) in California ruled that psychotherapists have a duty to take reasonable steps to protect threatened third parties from dangerous patients. Patient confidentiality is limited to the extent that a psychiatrist must disclose otherwise confidential communications. Despite protests from the psychiatric community that such a legal duty to third parties undermines the integrity of the psychiatrist-patient relationship and violates the patient's right to confidentiality, several states have adopted some version of the Tarasoff rule. Consequently, psychiatrists must cope with the practical ethical difficulties of trying to protect third parties while minimizing damage to the therapeutic relationship. Many psychiatrists have reported that potentially violent situations can be defused by careful clinical responses aided by legal, ethical, and psychiatric consultation, adequate communication with patients, and cooperation with law enforcement agencies.

References

American Psychiatric Association: *The Principles of Medical Ethics.* American Psychiatric Press, Washington, DC, 1981.

American Psychoanalytic Association: *Principles of Ethics for Psychoanalysts.* American Psychoanalytic Association, New York, 1983.

Bloch S, Chodoff P, editors: *Psychiatric Ethics.* Oxford University Press, Oxford, 1984.

Culver C, Gert B: *Philosophy and Medicine.* Oxford University Press, New York, 1982.

Jonsen A R, Siegler M, Winslade W J: *Clinical Ethics,* ed 2. Macmillan, New York, 1986.

Karasu T B: The ethics of psychotherapy. Am J Psychiatry *137*:1502, 1980.

Katz J: *The Silent World of Doctor and Patient.* Free Press, New York, 1985.

Kentsmith D K, Sallady S A, Miga P A: *Ethics in Mental Health Practice.* Grune & Stratton, Orlando, 1986.

Ross J W, Bayley, Sister C, Michel V, Pugh D: *The Handbook for Hospitals Ethics Committees.* American Hospital Association, Chicago, 1986.

Tancredi L, Weisstub D: Law, psychiatry, and morality: Unpacking and muddled prolegomenon. Internat J Law Psychiatry, *9*:1, 1986.

6

Psychology and Psychiatry: Psychometric Testing

6.1

Psychological Testing of Intelligence and Personality

Psychological tests provide a fairly objective picture of a person's intelligence and personality and include a psychodynamic formulation of the ways in which the mind functions. The tests can also be used to help in the diagnosis of mental disorders and to provide guidelines for treatment.

Most of the commonly used assessment instruments are standardized against normal controls, who are required to respond to the same stimuli or set of questions. The responses are tabulated into a normal distribution pattern against which new subjects are compared. When responses are limited, that is, when the subject is required to answer in some fixed response pattern (e.g., yes or no, true or false), standardization is used to insure that any variability that occurs is in the subject and not in the test.

Related to the standardization of any test are the available data that presumably demonstrate whether the test is valid and reliable. Reliability refers to the reproducibility of results; validity refers to the concept of whether or not the test measures what it purports to measure.

CLASSIFICATION OF TESTS

Tests are classified in various ways as follows:

Objective tests. Objective tests are typically pencil-and-paper tests based on specific items and questions. They yield numerical scores and profiles easily subjected to mathematical or statistical analysis. An example is the Minnesota Multiphasic Personality Inventory (MMPI).

Projective tests. These tests present stimuli whose meaning is not immediately obvious; that is, some degree of ambiguity forces the subject to project his own needs into the test situation. The projective tests presumably have no right or wrong answers. The person being tested must give meaning to the stimulus in accordance with his own inner needs, drives, abilities, and defenses. Examples include the Thematic Apperception Test (TAT), Draw-a-Person test, Rorschach test, and Sentence Completion test.

Individual or group tests. Tests may be administered individually or given simultaneously to a group. Individual testing has the advantage of providing an opportunity for the examiner to evaluate rapport and motivational factors as well as to observe and record the patient's behavior during testing. Careful timing of responses is also possible. Group tests, on the other hand, are usually more easily administered and scored.

Battery tests. A number of individual tests used together make up a psychological battery. The test battery can give more information about different areas of function than an individual test and can increase the level of confidence if there is a positive correlation between them. The Halstead-Reitan is an example of a test battery.

INTELLIGENCE TESTING

Intelligence can be defined as a person's ability to assimilate factual knowledge, to recall either recent or remote events, to reason logically, to manipulate concepts (either numbers or words), to translate the abstract to the literal or the literal to the abstract, to analyze and synthesize forms, as well as to deal meaningfully and accurately with problems and priorities deemed important in a particular setting. There are tremendous individual differences in intelligence.

Alfred Binet introduced the concept of the mental age (M.A.), which is the average intellectual level of a particular age. The intelligence quotient (I.Q.) is the ratio of M.A. over C.A. (chronological age) multiplied by 100 to do away with the decimal point; it is represented by the following equation:

$$I.Q. = \frac{M.A.}{C.A.} \times 100$$

When chronological and mental ages are equal, the I.Q. is 100, that is, average. Since it is impossible to measure increments of intellectual power past the age of 15 by available intelligence tests, the highest divisor in the I.Q. formula is 15. One way of expressing the relative standing of an individual within his group is by percentile. The higher the percentile, the higher one's rank within a group. For example, if a person is at the 80th percentile level, he exceeds 80 percent of the group in the trait measured and is exceeded by the remaining 20 percent. An I.Q. of 100 corresponds to the 50th percentile in intellectual ability for the general population.

As measured by most intelligence tests, I.Q. is an interpretation or classification of a total test score in relation to norms established by some group. The I.Q. is a measure of present functioning ability, not necessarily of future potential. Although under ordinary circumstances the I.Q. is stable throughout life, there is no absolute certainty about its predictive properties. A person's I.Q. must be examined in light of past experiences as well as future opportunities.

The I.Q. itself is no indicator of the origins of its reflected capacities, genetic (innate) or environmental. The most useful intelligence test must measure a variety of skills and abilities, including verbal and performance, early learned and recently learned, timed and untimed, culture-free and culture-bound. No intelligence test is totally culture-free, although tests do differ significantly in degree.

Wechsler Adult Intelligence Scale (WAIS)

The WAIS is the best standardized and most widely used intelligence test in clinical practice today. It was constructed by David Wechsler at New York University Medical Center and Bellevue Psychiatric Hospital. The test comprises 11 subtests made up of six verbal subtests and five performance subtests, yielding a verbal I.Q., a performance I.Q., and a combined or full-scale I.Q. Intelligence levels are based on the assumption that intellectual abilities are normally distributed (in a bell-shaped curve) throughout the population (see Table 1 for a classification of intelligence scores). Verbal and performance I.Q.s, as well as the full-scale I.Q., are determined by the use of separate tables for each of the seven age groups (from 16 to 64 years) on which the test was standardized. Variability in functioning is revealed through both discrepancies between verbal and performance I.Q.s and by the scatter pattern between the subtests.

The following subtests are described in the order in which they are presented to the subject:

Information. This subtest covers general information and general knowledge and is subject to cultural variables. Persons from lower socioeconomic groups with little schooling do not perform as well as those from higher socioeconomic groups with more schooling.

Comprehension. This subtest measures the subject's ability to adhere to social conventions and to understand social judgment by asking about proverbs and how one ought to behave under certain circumstances.

Arithmetic. Ability to do arithmetic and other simple calculations is reflected on this subtest, which is adversely influenced by anxiety and poor attention and concentration.

Similarities. This subtest covers the ability to abstract by asking subjects to explain the similarity between two things. It is a sensitive indicator of intelligence.

Digit span. Immediate retention is measured in this subtest. The subject is asked to learn a series of two to nine digits, which are immediately recalled both forward and backward. Anxiety, poor attention span, and brain dysfunction interfere with recall.

Vocabulary. The subject is asked to define 35 vocabulary words of increasing difficulty. Intelligence has a high correlation with vocabulary, which is related to level of education. Idiosyncratic definitions of words may give clues to personality structure.

Picture completion. This subtest initiates the performance part of the WAIS and consists of completing a picture that is missing a part. Visuoperceptive defects become evident when mistakes are made.

Table 1
Classification of Intelligence by I.Q. Range

Classification	I.Q. Range
Profound Mental Retardation (MR)*	Below 20 or 25
Severe MR*	20–25 to 35–40
Moderate MR*	35–40 to 50–55
Mild MR*	50–55 to approx 70
Borderline	70–79
Dull Normal	80 to 90
Normal	90 to 110
Bright Normal	110 to 120
Superior	120 to 130
Very Superior	130 and above

*According to DSM-III-R

Block design. This subtest requires the subject to match colored blocks and visual designs. Brain dysfunction involving impairment of left-right dominance interferes with performance.

Picture arrangement. The subject is required to arrange a series of pictures in a sequence that tells a story (e.g., a person committing a crime). In addition to testing performance, this subtest provides data about the subject's cognitive style.

Object assembly. The subject has to assemble objects, such as the figure of a woman or an animal, in their proper order and organization. Visuoperception, somatoperception, and manual dexterity are tested.

Digit symbol. In this final subtest of the WAIS, the subject is given a code that pairs symbols with digits. The test consists of matching a series of digits to their corresponding symbols in as little time as possible.

Each subtest is influenced by a variety of factors that have to be taken into account for accurate interpretation. Educational background affects the information and vocabulary subtests. Arithmetic and memory for digits is adversely affected by anxiety. A disparity between the verbal and performance test (usually greater than 15 points) may be indicative of psychopathology and requires further testing.

Designed in 1939, the original WAIS has gone through several revisions. A scale for children ages 5 through 15 years has been devised (the WISC—Wechsler Intelligence Scale for Children) as well as a scale for children ages 4 to 6½ years (WPPSI—Wechsler Preschool and Primary Scale of Intelligence). In practice, the WAIS, WISC, or WPPSI is used as part of a battery of psychological tests.

PERSONALITY TESTING

In most psychiatric settings, the tests in the psychological test battery are individually chosen in terms of how well they contribute to a psychodynamic formulation of personality functioning. Behavior is often motivated by forces that vary as to their accessibility to awareness and behavioral expression. The need for a battery of tests arises not because of the possible invalidity of any single test, but because different tests detect different levels of functioning and because the relationships between tests reflect the person's multilevel system of functioning.

Rorschach Test

With the possible exception of the WAIS, the Rorschach test is the most frequently used individual test in clinical settings throughout the United States. The Rorschach was devised by Hermann Rorschach, a Swiss psychiatrist, who began around 1910 to experiment with ambiguous inkblots. A standard set of ten inkblots serve as stimuli for associations. In the standard series, the blots, are reproduced on cards 7 by 9 ½ inches and are numbered from I to X. Five of the blots are in black and white; the remainder include colors. The cards are shown to the patient in a particular order. A record is kept of the patient's verbatim responses, along with initial reaction times and total time spent on each card. After completion of what is called the free-association phase, an inquiry phase is conducted by the examiner to determine important aspects of each response that will be crucial to its scoring.

Scoring of responses converts the important aspects of each response into a symbol system related to location areas, determinants, content areas, and popularity.

Location. Location is scored in terms of what portion of the blot was used as the basis for a response (e.g., the whole blot, a common detail of the blot, an unusual detail of the blot, or an area of white space). Attention to the whole blot with accurate form perception reflects good organizational ability and high intelligence. Overattention to detail is common in obsessive and paranoid subjects.

Determinants. The determinants of each response reflect what there was about the blot that made it look the way the patient thought it looked (e.g., form, shading, color, movement either of humans or animals, inanimate movements, or combinations of these determinants with varying emphasis). Overemphasis on form suggests rigidity and constriction of the personality. Color responses relate to the emotional reactions of the person to the environment and to the control of affect.

Content. Responses are scored in terms of the content they reflect—human, animal, anatomy, sex, food, nature, and so forth. In general, content areas reflect breadth and range of interests.

Popularity. Certain responses to the different cards are more popular than others.

Interpretation. The Rorschach is particularly useful as an aid in diagnosis. The thinking and association patterns of the subject are brought more clearly into focus because the ambiguity of the stimulus provides relatively few cues about what are conventional, standard, or normal responses. Proper interpretation, however, requires a great deal of experience. There is a high reliability among experienced clinicians who administer the test. In proper hands, it is extremely useful, especially in eliciting psychodynamic formulations, defense mechanisms, and subtle disorders of thinking.

The Rorschach elicits data that can aid in differential diagnosis, particularly in evaluating whether or not a thought disorder exists. For example, patients with schizotypal or borderline personalities are characterized by idiosyncratic thought, peculiarities of language, and unconventional thinking.

Thematic Apperception Test (TAT)

The TAT was designed by Henry Murray and Christiana Morgan as part of the normal personality study conducted at the Harvard Psychological Clinic in 1943. It consists of a series of 30 pictures and one blank card. Not all of the pictures are used. The choice depends on what conflict area one wishes to clarify with a peculiar patient. Examples of TAT pictures are a young woman seated on a couch looking up at an older man, a man standing beside a nude woman in a bed, and a gray haired man looking at a younger man.

Although most of the pictures depict people and all are representational (making the test stimuli more structured than the inkblots of the Rorschach test) there is ambiguity in each pictures. Unlike the Rorschach blots, to which the patient is asked to associate, the TAT requires that the patient construct or create a story.

As the test was originally conceived, an important aspect of each story was the figure (the hero) with whom the subject seemed to identify and to whom he was presumably attributing his own wishes, strivings, and conflicts. The characteristics of people other than the hero were considered to represent the subject's views of other people in his environment. It is assumed that all the figures in a TAT story are equally representative of the subject, with the more accepted and conscious traits and motives attributed to figures closest to the subject in age, sex, and appearance and the more unacceptable and unconscious traits and motives attributed to figures most unlike the subject.

The stories must be considered from the standpoint of unusualness of theme or plot. Whether the patient is dealing with a common or an uncommon theme, however, his story reflects his own idiosyncratic approach to organization, sequence, vocabulary, style, preconceptions, assumptions, and outcome. TAT cards have different stimulus values and can be assumed to elicit data pertaining to different areas of functioning. Generally, the TAT is more useful as a technique for inferring motivational aspects of behavior than as a basis for making a diagnosis.

Sentence Completion Test (SCT)

The SCT is designed to tap the patient's conscious associations to areas of functioning in which the psychologist may be interested. It is composed of a series (usually 75 to 100) of sentence stems, such as "I like . . .," "Sometimes I wish . . .," that the patient is asked to complete in his own words.

Most frequently, some time pressure is applied, and the patient is instructed to write down the first thing that comes to mind. In other instances the text is administered verbally by the examiner, similar to the word-association technique. Sentence stems vary in their ambiguity, hence some items serve more as a projective test stimulus ("Sometimes I . . ."). Others more closely resemble direct-response questionnaires ("My greatest fear is . . .").

With the individual protocol, most psychologists use an inspection technique, noting particularly those responses that are expressive of strong affects, that tend to be given repetitively, or that are unusual or particularly informative in any way. Areas where denial operates are often revealed through omissions, bland expressions, or factual reports ("My mother is a woman"). Humor may also reflect an attempt to deny anxiety about a particular issue, person, or event. Important historical material is sometimes revealed directly ("I feel guilty about the way my sister was drowned").

Word-Association Technique

The word-association technique was devised by Carl Jung, who presented stimulus words to patients and had them respond with the first word that came to mind. After the initial administration of the list, some clinicians repeat the list, asking the patient to respond with the same words that he used previously; discrepancies between the two administrations may reveal associational difficulties. Complex indicators include long reaction times, blocking difficulties in making responses, unusual responses, repetition of the stimulus word, apparent misunderstanding of the word, clang associations, perseveration of earlier responses, and ideas or unusual mannerisms or movements accompanying the response. Because it is easily quantified, the test has continued to be used as a research instrument, although its popularity has diminished greatly over the years.

Minnesota Multiphasic Personality Inventory (MMPI)

The MMPI is a self-report inventory that is the most widely used and most thoroughly researched of the objective personality assessment instruments. It was developed in 1937 by Starke Hathaway, a psychologist, and J. Charnley McKinley, a psychiatrist. The tests consists of 550 statements—such as "I worry about sex matters," "I sometimes tease animals," "I believe I am being plotted against"—to which the subject must respond with "true," "false," or "cannot say." The test may be used in card or booklet form, and several programs exist to process the responses by computer.

The MMPI gives scores on ten standard clinical scales, each of which was derived empirically (that is, homogeneous criterion groups of psychiatric patients were used in developing the scales). The items for each scale were selected for their ability to separate medical or psychiatric patients from normal controls.

Clinical Scales. The clinical scales are numbered and are often referred to by number, rather than by name, particularly in coding deviantly high scores. It should be noted that a high score on a particular scale does not mean that the person has that illness. For example, a high Sc score does not indicate that the patient is necessarily schizophrenic. An accurate interpretation requires great experience with the test and some understanding of the social, educational and class background from which the patient comes. Recent evidence suggests that religion and race are both potential variables in MMPI responses. The scales are as follows:

1. Hypochondriasis (Hs) scale. Thirty-three items having to do with bodily function and malfunction reflect abnormal concern over bodily health. Although the scale rises slightly in the presence of actual physical disease, it is also a character scale for pessimism and irritability. Physically ill patients generally score higher on the depression scale.

2. Depression (D) scale. The 60 items relate to such things as worry, discouragement, hopelessness, and low self-esteem. Depression is frequently the highest scale in the profiles of

psychiatric patients. As a mood scale, it may fluctuate widely over time and often reflects changes in outlook that occur with improvement in psychotherapy.

3. Hysteria (Hy) scale. Sixty items refer either to specific somatic complaints or to a happy acceptance of things in general (denial). High scorers on this scale use repression as a defense mechanism and are emotionally immature, demanding, and concerned about bodily functions.

4. Psychopathic deviate (Pd) scale. The 50 items in this scale reflect asocial behavior characterized by interpersonal withdrawal. High scorers are angry at normal social conventions and are impulsive. Low scorers tend toward conformity.

5. Masculinity-femininity (Mf) scale. The 60 items have to do with culturally accepted attitudes about male and female roles. In both sexes, scores are correlated with aggressiveness, passivity, aesthetic interests, personal awareness, and emotional sensitivity. High scores on this scale should not be taken as an indication of homosexuality, although they may reflect a lack of identification with culturally prescribed masculine and feminine roles.

6. Paranoia (Pa). These 40 items have to do with being easily hurt or complaints of persecution and suspiciousness. Combined with a high score on the schizophrenic scale, an elevation on this scale is often found in paranoid schizophrenia. True paranoiacs, however, may sometimes score low rather than high, thus avoiding detection.

7. Psychasthenia (Pt) scale. Forty items relating to narcissism, magical thinking, and sadomasochistic tendencies, this scale is a general measure of anxiety, self-concern, and self-doubt. Marked elevations on this scale correlate highly with an obsessive-compulsive defense system. This scale is sensitive to almost all psychiatric problems, although in a nonspecific way.

8. Schizophrenic (Sc) scale. The 78 items cover social and family alienation, bizarre emotions, delusions, somatic symptoms, influence of external agents, peculiar bodily dysfunction, dissatisfaction, and depression. High scorers have fundamental questions about their own identity and may be confused about their lives. Difficulties in thinking and communication are also found with high scores on this scale.

9. Hypomania (Ma) scale. The 46 items are generally related to expansiveness, egotism, and irritability. Moderate-range scorers may be enthusiastic, outgoing, and pleasant; increasingly higher scores reflect a likelihood of maladaptive hyperactivity and flightiness.

10. Social distance (Si). Seventy items relate to social participation, including lack of confidence, worry, and interpersonal anxiety.

The MMPI also has several scales that increase the validity of the test:

1. Lie scale (L). Fifteen items identify persons who attempt to present an overly perfectionistic view of themselves by giving false answers.

2. Frequency scale (F). Sixty-four items have to do with unconventional beliefs or eccentric attitudes. A high score indicates persons who are characterized by unusual or bizarre thinking or who wish to put themselves in a bad light. In some cases, a high score means that they fail to understand the instructions of the test.

3. Correction scale (K). Thirty items were selected to be a measure of guardedness or defensiveness in test-taking attitude. High scorers are people who cannot tolerate suggestions that they are insecure, have difficulty in social relations, or do not have well-ordered lives.

An F–K index or ratio is sometimes used to indicate whether or not a person is faking (i.e., trying to look extremely well-adjusted by denying problems or trying to look more emotionally ill by exaggerating problems).

Interpretation. Although the MMPI was designed as an objective personality test, the individual scales cannot be taken at face value. It is necessary to relate each scale to the other scales to obtain an accurate profile, which is best done by a person with extensive testing experience. The MMPI is most effectively used in conjunction with other information about the patient, especially clinical interviews. Currently, work is being done to restandardize the MMPI based upon a contemporary sample of normal people. Questions and language are being updated to reflect current cultural views.

Bender (Visual Motor) Gestalt Test

The Bender-Gestalt test is a test of visual motor coordination, useful for both children and adults. It was designed by Lauretta Bender, New York University Medical Center and Bellevue Psychiatric Hospital in 1938, who used it to evaluate maturational levels in children. Developmentally, a child below the age of 3 years is generally unable to reproduce any of the test's designs meaningfully. Around 4 years of age, the child may be able to copy several designs, but poorly. At about age 6, the child should produce some recognizable, though still uneven, representations of all the designs. By age 10 and certainly by age 12, his copies should be reasonably accurate and well orga-

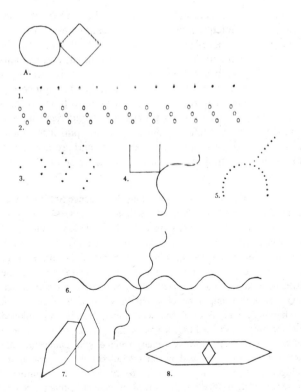

Figure 1. Test figures from the Bender Visual Motor Gestalt Test, adopted from Wertheimer. (From Bender, L. *A Visual Motor Gestalt Test and Its Clinical Use.* Research Monograph, no. 3, American Orthopsychiatric Association, New York, 1938.)

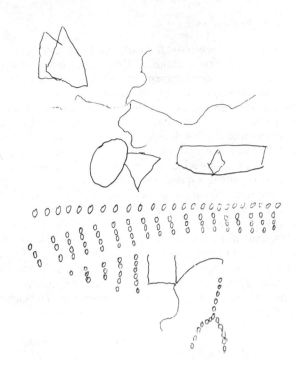

Figure 2. Bender-Gestalt drawings of a 57-year-old brain-damaged female patient.

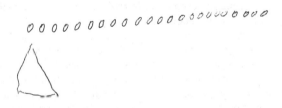

Figure 3. Bender-Gestalt "recall" of the 57-year-old brain-damaged female patient in the above figure.

nized. Bender also presented studies of adults with organic brain defects, mental retardation, aphasias, psychoses, neuroses, and malingering.

The test material consists of nine separate designs, adapted from those used by Wertheimer in his studies in Gestalt psychology. Each design is printed against a white background on a separate card (Figure 1). Presented with unlined paper, the patient is asked to copy each design with the card in front of him. There is no time limit. This phase of the test is highly structured and does not investigate memory function, because the cards remain in front of the patient while he copies them. Many clinicians include a subsequent recall phase, in which (after an interval of 45 to 60 seconds) the patient is asked to reproduce as many of the designs as he can from memory. This phase not only investigates visual memory but also presents a less structured situation, since the patient must now rely essentially on his own resources. It is often particularly helpful to compare the patient's functioning under the two conditions.

Probably, the Bender-Gestalt test is used most frequently with adults as a screening device for signs of organic dysfunction. Evaluation of the protocol depends on the form of the reproduced figures and on their relationship to each other and to the whole spatial background (Figures 2 and 3).

Draw-a-Person Test

The Draw-A-Person test (DAP) was first used as a measure of intelligence in children. Detail was correlated with intelligence and developmental level. It has since become more useful as an adult test. The test is easily administered, usually with the instructions, "I'd like you to draw a picture of a person; draw the best person you can." After the completion of the first drawing, the patient is asked to draw a picture of a person of the sex opposite to that of his first drawing. Some clinicians use an interrogation procedure in which the patient is questioned about his drawings. ("What is he doing?" "What are his best qualities?") Modifications include asking for a drawing of a house and a tree (House-Tree-Person Test), of one's family, and of an animal.

A general assumption is that the drawing of a person represents the expression of the self or of the body in the environment. Interpretive principles rest largely on the assumed functional significance of each body part. Most clinicians use drawings primarily as a screening technique, particularly for the detection of brain damage.

INTEGRATION OF TEST FINDINGS

The integration of test findings into a comprehensive, meaningful report is probably the most difficult aspect of psychological evaluation. Inferences from different tests must be related to each other in terms of the confidence the psychologist holds about them and of the presumed level of the patient's awareness or consciousness being tapped.

Most psychologists follow some general outline in preparing a psychological report, such as: test behavior, intellectual functioning, personality functioning (reality-testing ability, impulse control, manifest depression and guilt, manifestations of major dysfunction, major defenses, overt symptoms, interpersonal conflicts, self-concept, affects), inferred diagnosis, degree of present overt disturbance, prognosis for social recovery, motivation for personality change, primary assets and weaknesses, recommendations, and summary.

References

Anastasi A: *Psychological Testing,* ed 5. Macmillan, New York, 1968.
American Psychological Association: *Standards for Educational and Psychological Tests and Manuals.* American Psychological Association, Washington, DC, 1974.
Caligan R C, Offord K P: Revitalizing the MMPI: The development of contemporary norms. Psychiatric Ann *15*:558, 1985.
Cronbach L: *Essentials of Psychological Testing.* Harper & Row, New York, 1960.
Exner J E: *The Rorschach: A Comprehensive System,* vols 1, 2, and 3. John Wiley & Sons, New York, 1982.
Halstead W: *Brain and Intelligence: A Quantitative Study of the Frontal Lobes.* University of Chicago Press, Chicago, 1947.
Lezak M D: *Neuropsychological Assessment,* ed 2. Oxford, New York, 1983.
Matarazzo J D: *Wechsler's Measurement and Appraisal of Adult Intelligence.* ed 5. Oxford, New York, 1972.
Rorschach H: *Psychodiagnostik.* Bircher, Bern, 1921.
Wechsler D: *WAIS-R Manual.* Psychological Corporation, New York, 1981.
Zimmerman I, Woo-Sam J: *Clinical Interpretation of the Wechsler Adult Scale.* Grune & Stratton, New York, 1973.

6.2 _____
Neuropsychiatric Tests of Brain Function

INTRODUCTION

Disease or injury at the higher levels of the central nervous system is likely to be manifested in disturbances in mentation, feelings, and conduct. Thus, neuropsychological assessment is an integral part of clinical neurologic evaluation, particularly when the question of disease involving the cerebral hemispheres is raised.

To a considerable degree, the aspects of behavior sampled by clinical observation and by neuropsychological tests are the same—for example, speed of response, level of comprehension, and use of language—but the test procedures assess these aspects of behavior with greater reliability and precision. The tests sample other aspects of behavior, such as visual memory and psychomotor skill, that are not readily elicited in the general examination. Thus, neuropsychological tests both validate the impressionistic findings of the general clinical examination and provide additional information about other aspects of intellect and personality.

GENERAL INTELLIGENCE AND DEMENTIA

Patients with cerebral disease may show an overall behavioral inefficiency and may be unable to meet the diverse intellectual demands associated with the responsibilities of daily life. Dementia implies an overall impairment in mental capacity with a consequent decline in social and economic competence. There are clinically distinguishable types of dementia—for example, an aphasic type, an amnesic type, a type showing prominent visuoperceptual and somatoperceptual defects, and a relatively pure type manifesting impairment in abstract reasoning and problem solving within a setting of fairly intact linguistic and perceptual capacity.

In this country, the Wechsler Adult Intelligence Scale (WAIS) is by far the most widely used test battery to assess general intelligence in adult subjects. In its clinical application, a number of procedures have been used to evaluate the possibility of a decline in general intelligence that may be attributable to the presence of cerebral disease. The most direct approach is to compare the patient's obtained age-corrected I.Q. score with the age-corrected I.Q. score that might be expected in view of his educational background, cultural level, and occupational history. An obtained I.Q. below the expected I.Q. may raise the question of the presence of cerebral disease. However, many patients with unquestionable cerebral disease do not show an overall decline in general intelligence of sufficient severity to be reflected in a significant lowering of their WAIS I.Q. score. Consequently, this procedure may be expected to yield a fair proportion of false-negative results.

A variant of this procedure is to compare obtained and expected I.Q. scores on the WAIS performance scale, which consists, for the most part, of nonverbal and relatively novel tasks. This comparison has proved to be practically as useful as the comparison of full-scale I.Q. scores.

Since it has been found, at least in nonaphasic patients, that certain types of performance tend to be more seriously affected by cerebral damage than are others, a second approach has been to compare performance level of presumably less sensitive tasks with that on more sensitive tasks. Thus, verbal scale I.Q. is compared to performance scale I.Q.; performance on a set of insensitive tests, such as information or picture completion, is compared with performance on a set of sensitive tests, such as arithmetic or block designs.

REASONING AND PROBLEM SOLVING

Impairment of the capacity for abstract reasoning and reduction in behavioral flexibility when confronted with an unfamiliar situation are well known behavioral characteristics of the brain-damaged patient. Special tests have been devised to measure reasoning and problem solving, but one must first rule out language and perceptual handicaps as causes of defective performance.

MEMORY

Impairment of various types of memory, most notably short-term and recent memory, is a prominent behavioral deficit in brain-damaged patients, and it is often the first sign of cerebral disease and of aging. Memory is a comprehensive term that covers the retention of all types of material over different periods of time and involves diverse forms of response. Consequently, the neuropsychological examiner is more inclined to give specific memory tests and evaluate them separately than to use an omnibus battery that provides a brief assessment of a large variety of performances and yields a single score.

Immediate memory may be defined as the reproduction, recognition, or recall of perceived material within a period of not more than 5 seconds after presentation. It is most often assessed by digit repetition and reversal (auditory) and memory-for-designs (visual) tests. Both an auditory-verbal task, such as digit span or memory for words or sentences, and a nonverbal visual task, such as memory for designs or for objects or faces, should be given to assess the patient's immediate memory. Patients can also be asked to listen to a standardized story and to repeat the story as closely as possible to what they heard. Patients with lesions of the right hemisphere are likely to show more severe defects on visual nonverbal tasks than on auditory verbal tasks. Conversely, patients with left hemisphere disease, including those who are not aphasic, are likely to show more severe deficits on the auditory verbal tests with variable performance on the visual nonverbal tasks.

Recent memory refers to events over the past few days and can be tested by asking the patient what he had for breakfast and who visited with him in the hospital. *Recent past memory* refers to the retention of information over the past few months. The patient can be asked questions about current events.

Remote memory is the ability to remember events in the distant past. It is commonly believed that remote memory is well preserved in patients who show pronounced defects in recent memory. However, the remote memory of senile and amnesic patients is usually significantly inferior to that of normal persons of comparable age and education. Even patients who appear to be able to recount their past fairly accurately, on close examination, will show gaps and inconsistency in their recital.

Clinical investigators have developed and used standardized objective tests for the assessment of remote memory. These tests require the patient to identify past presidents or the photographs of public figures who were prominent in past decades and to recall public events that occurred many years before the onset of the patient's illness. The results have been that patients with brain disease do show impairment in remote memory, and their deficiency in recall and recognition is as severe for the oldest and most remote events as it is for less remote material.

ORIENTATION

Orientation for person or place is rarely disturbed in the brain-damaged patient who is not psychotic or severely demented; but, defects in temporal orientation, which can be considered to reflect the integrity of recent memory, are common. These defects are often missed by the clinical examiner because of the tendency to regard as inconsequential slight inaccuracy in giving the day of the week or the date of the month. However, about 25 percent of nonpsychotic patients with hemispheric cerebral disease are likely to show significant inferiority with respect to precision of temporal orientation. A simple test for orientation is outlined in Table 1.

PERCEPTUAL AND PERCEPTUOMOTOR PERFORMANCE

Many patients with brain disease show impaired ability to analyze complex stimulus constellations or inability to translate their perceptions into appropriate motor action. Unless the impairment is of a gross nature, as in visual object agnosia or dressing apraxia, or interferes with a specific occupation skill, these deficits are not likely to be the subject of spontaneous complaint. However, appropriate testing discloses a remarkably high incidence of impaired performance on visuoanalytic, visuospatial, and visuoconstructive tasks in brain-damaged patients, particularly in those persons with disease involving the right hemisphere. This type of impairment also extends to tactile and auditory perceptual task performances.

Visuoperceptive and visuoconstructive capacity, as well as somatoperceptual defects, can be assessed by tests. Double simultaneous stimulation (DSS) is tested by lightly touching one of the patient's cheeks with one hand and simultaneously touching the back of the patient's hands with the other. A patient with brain dysfunction is unable to recognize one or both of the stimuli. The DSS is a general test of defective capacity for perceptual integration.

Perceptuomotor tests often help localize the cerebral lesion. A significant portion of patients with lesions of the right hemisphere who do not show obvious impairment in language functions perform poorly on perceptual tests.

Table 1
Temporal Orientation Schedule

Administration

What is today's date? (The patient is required to give month, day, and year.)

What day of the week is it?

What time is it now? (Examiner makes sure that the patient cannot look at a watch or clock.)

Scoring

Day of week: one error point for each day removed from the correct day to a maximum of three points

Day of month: one error point for each day removed from the correct day to a maximum of fifteen points

Month: five error points for each month removed from the correct month with the qualification that, if the stated date is within 15 days of the correct date, no points are scored for the incorrect month (for example, May 29 for June 2 = four points off)

Year: ten error points for each year removed from the correct year to a maximum of 60 points with the qualification that, if the stated date is within 15 days of the correct date, no points are scored for the incorrect year (for example, December 26, 1982 for January 2, 1983 = seven points off)

Time of day: one error point for each 30 minutes removed from the correct time to a maximum of five points

From Benton A L: Psychological testing for brain damage. In *Comprehensive Textbook of Psychiatry,* ed 4, H I Kaplan, B J Sadock, editors, p 539. Williams & Wilkins, Baltimore, 1985.

LANGUAGE FUNCTIONS

Relatively minor defects in the use of language may be valid indicators of the presence of brain disease. The dominant hemisphere controls language function. The affective part of speech that conveys mood is called prosody and is controlled by the nondominant hemisphere. Fluency is tested by asking the patient to give all the words he can think of beginning with a given letter of the alphabet. Aphasic patients with left hemisphere disease fail this task. Variables influencing language tests are educational background, sex, and age. Reading and writing are also associated with the dominant hemisphere and are tested by asking the patient to read aloud from prepared material and to write his name or a brief passage. Dyslexia and dysgraphia are suspected if difficulties in performing those tasks are found.

ATTENTION AND CONCENTRATION

The capacity to sustain a maximal level of attention over a period of time is sometimes impaired in brain-damaged patients, and this impairment is reflected in oscillation in performance level on a continuous or repeated activity. There is some evidence that this instability in performance is related to electroencephalographic abnormality and that inexplicable decline in performance is related temporally to the occurrence of certain types of abnormal electrical activ-

ity. Simple reaction time provides a convenient measure of the variability and speed of simple responses.

The reaction time needed to respond to a stimulus is impaired in 40 to 45 percent of brain-damaged patients and is a sensitive indicator of overall cerebral integrity. Comparison of the reaction times of the right and left hands often provides an indication of the site of the lesion in a patient and of unilateral cerebral disease.

Behavioral flexibility is also reduced in brain-damaged patients who are unable to modify their approach to a problem in accordance with changing requirements. This was described by Kurt Goldstein as part of the catastrophic reaction first noted in brain-injured soldiers.

BEHAVIORAL INDICES OF BRAIN DAMAGE IN CHILDREN

If present, the behavioral consequences of early brain damage may take many forms, of which the hyperkinetic (or attention-deficit hyperactivity disorder) is only one. Early brain damage may result in little or no behavioral deficit, and when such deficit does appear, it is usually less severe than that caused by a comparable lesion in adults. Thus, there is reason to believe that many brain-damaged children are not identified by current methods of behavioral assessment.

General Intelligence

The most frequently used batteries are the Wechsler Intelligence Scale for Children (WISC), the Stanford-Binet, and the Wechsler Preschool and Primary Scale of Intelligence (WPPSI). A relatively low level of general intelligence is probably the most constant behavioral result of brain damage in children.

Perceptual and Perceptuomotor Performances

Many brain-damaged children with adequate verbal skills show strikingly defective visuoperceptive and visuomotor performance. The test most frequently used is copying of designs, either from a model or from memory. About 25 percent of brain-damaged school children of adequate verbal intelligence perform defectively. The task helps discriminate between brain-damaged children and those suffering from presumably psychogenic emotional disturbance.

Language Functions

There is considerable evidence that children who show gross maldevelopment of oral language abilities as compared with general mental level suffer from brain damage. Perinatal brain injury may be a causative factor in at least some cases of developmental dyslexia or more generalized learning disability. The finding of a relatively high incidence of electroencephalographic abnormality in children with learning disabilities points to the same conclusion.

Motor Performances

Motor awkwardness and inability to carry out movement sequences on command or by imitation are commonly seen in brain-damaged children. A variety of tests are available for the assessment of manual dexterity (e.g., manipulations with tweezers, paper cutting, and peg placing).

Motor impersistence—an inability to sustain an action initiated on command, such as keeping the eyes closed—is seen in a relatively small proportion of adult patients with cerebral disease. However, it is shown with remarkably high frequency by nondefective brain-damaged children. Many children with mental defects also show excessive motor impersistence, particularly those with brain damage.

COMPREHENSIVE TESTING

A number of test batteries have been developed to help in the neuropsychological and neuropsychiatric evaluation. Among these are the Luria-Nebraska and Halstead-Reitan neuropsychological test batteries.

Luria-Nebraska Neuropsychological Battery

Based upon the work of the Russian neuropsychologist, A. R. Luria, the Luria-Nebraska Neuropsychological Battery (LNNB) was developed at the University of Nebraska. The test assesses a wide range of cognitive functions: memory, motor functions, rhythm, tactile, auditory, and visual functions, receptive and expressive speech, writing, spelling, reading, and arithmetic. The test is designed for persons at least 15 years of age and a children's version for use with 8 to 12-year-olds is being developed. The LNNB is extremely sensitive for identifying specific types of problems (e.g., dyslexia, dyscalculia) rather than being limited to more global impressions of brain dysfunction. It also helps localize the various cortical zones that are involved in a particular function and is useful in establishing left or right cerebral dominance.

Halstead-Reitan Battery of Neuropsychological Tests

In the early 1940s, Ward Halstead at Chicago and his student, Ralph Reitan, developed a battery of tests that were used to determine the location and effects of specific brain lesions. The battery is composed of the following ten tests:

1. Category Test. The patient must discover the common element in a set of pictures; it measures concept function, abstraction, and visual acuity.

2. Tactual Performance Test. The patient places shapes in a form board while blindfolded and then must recall the arrangement of the board; it tests dexterity, spatial memory, and tactual discrimination.

3. Rhythm Test. The patient identifies 30 pairs of rhythmic beats as either the same or different; tests auditory perception, attention, and concentration.

4. Finger-Oscillation Test. The patient taps the index finger of each hand in a measured 10-second period; test measures dexterity and motor speed.

5. Speech-Sounds Perception Test. The patient matches 60 nonsense syllables that he hears with several printed alternatives; measures auditory discrimination and phonetic skills.

6. Trail Making Test. The patient first connects 25 numbered circles in order and then connects 25 lettered and numbered circles in order, alternating between numbered and alphabetical circles; tests visuomotor perception and motor speed.

7. Critical Flicker Frequency. The patient notes when a flickering light becomes steady; tests visual perception.

8. Time Sense Test. The patient judges, without looking, the time it takes for the second hand of a watch to make several revolutions; tests memory and spatial perception.

9. Aphasia Screening Test. The patient must name objects, read, write, calculate, draw shapes, identify body parts, perform acts, differentiate between left and right; tests a wide range of verbal and nonverbal brain functions.

10. Sensory-Perceptual Tests. The patient performs a number of tasks with his eyes closed—such as identifying where he is touched when touched on the hand and face simultaneously (simultaneous sensory stimulation test), identifies which finger is touched (finger localization), what coins are placed in the hand (stereognosis), what numbers are written on the skin (tactile perception).

In addition to the tests outlined above, objective tests, such as the Minnesota Multiphasic Personality Test (MMPI) and the Wechsler Adult Intelligence Scale, may be used. Taken together, the battery tests a variety of brain functions—perception, sensation, visuomotor integration, concept formation, abstract thought, attention, and concentration.

INTERPRETATION

In any neuropsychiatric examination, the clinician must be careful that a deviation from normal is not due to factors unrelated to neuropathology. Anxiety and depression are two major causes of cognitive dysfunction, and a careful assessment of the patient's mental state should be carried out to rule out these conditions as sources of poor performance. Other sources of error result from the patient not understanding the directions given by the examiner, problems with language, or general uncooperativeness. A summary of the many mental status cognitive tasks discussed in this section as well as others that can be used to test and localize various dysfunctions is presented in Table 2.

References

Benton A L, Hamsher K deS, Varney N R: *Contributions to Neuropsychological Assessment.* Oxford, New York, 1983.

Filskov S B, Boll T J: *Handbook of Clinical Neuropsychology.* Wiley, New York, 1981.

Gilandas A, Touyz S, Bermont P J V, Greenberg H P: *Handbook of Neuropsychological Assessment.* Grune & Stratton, Orlando, FL, 1984.

Grant I, Adams, K M: *Neuropsychological Assessment of Neuropsychiatric Disorders.* Oxford, New York, 1986.

Incagnoli T, Goldstein G, Golden C J: *Clinical Application of Neuropsychological Test Batteries.* Plenum Press, New York, 1986.

Lezak, M D: *Neuropsychological Assessment,* ed 2. Oxford, New York, 1983.

Matarazzo J D: Computerized clinical psychological test interpretations. Am Psychologist 41:14, 1986.

Moses J A: Relationship of the profile evaluation and impairment scales of the Luria-Nebraska Neuropsychological Battery to neuropsychological examination outcome. Internat J Clin Neuropsychol 7:4, 1985.

Reitan R M, Davison L A: *Clinical Neuropsychology: Current Status and Applications.* Wiley, New York, 1974.

Wishaw I Q, Kolb B: *Fundamentals of Human Neuropsychology.* W H Freeman, New York, 1985.

Table 2
Mental Status Cognitive Tasks

Task	Dysfunction	Abnormal Response	Suggested Localization
Spell "earth" backward	Concentration	Any improper letter sequence	Frontal lobes
Serial sevens	Concentration	One or more errors or longer than 90 seconds	Frontal lobes
Name the day of the week, month, year, location	Global disorientation	Any error	Frontal lobes (if memory intact)
Repeat: "No ifs, ands, or buts," "The President lives in Washington," "Methodist Episcopal," "Massachussetts"	Expressive language	Missed words or syllables; repetition of internal syllables; dropping of word endings	Dominant frontal lobe
Name common objects (e.g., key, watch, button, etc.)	Anomia	Cannot name; word approximations; describes functions rather than word	Dominant temporal lobe, angular gyrus
Conversation during examination	Receptive language	Word approximations, neologisms, word salad, stock words, tangential speech	Dominant temporal lobe
(a) Repeat four words or items (e.g., blue, chair, swim, glove)	Immediate recall	One or more errors	Temporal lobes/frontal lobes (hippocampus)
(b) Remember them after 10 minutes with interposed tasks	Recent memory	One or more errors	Temporal lobes (hippocampus, thalamus, fornix, mamillothalamic tract)
(c) Provide accurate detail and sequence of past events	Long-term memory	Significant loss of detail; confused sequence	Temporal lobes (hippocampus)
Copy examiner's hand and arm movements (each hand/arm)	Dyspraxia	Any error, mirror movements	Contralateral parietal lobe
Demonstrate use of key, hammer, flipping a coin	Ideomotorapraxia	Use of hand as object; failure to use fine hand and wrist movements; verbal overflow	Dominant parietal lobe, disconnected dominant from nondominant frontal lobe
(a) Left hand only plus some expressive language difficulty			Dominant frontal lobe or anterior corpus callosum
(b) Both hands			Dominant parietal lobe, arcuate fasciculus
Name fingers	Finger agnosia	Two or more errors; cannot identify after examiner numbers each	Dominant parietal lobe
Calculations	Dyscalculia	Errors in borrowing or carrying over when concentration is intact	Dominant parietal lobe
Write a sentence	Dysgraphia	No longer able to write cursive; loss of word structure; abnormally formed letters	Dominant parietal lobe
In individual steps, copy sentence, read it, and do what it says ("Put the paper in your pocket")	Dysgraphia, dyslexia, comprehension	No longer able to write cursively; loss of sentence structure; loss of word structure; abnormally formed letters	Dominant temporoparietal lobe
Place left hand to right ear, right elbow, right knee; same for right hand	Right/left disorientation	Two or more errors or two or more 7-second delays in carrying out tasks	Dominant parietal lobe
Copy the outline of simple objects (e.g., Greek cross, key)	Construction apraxia	Loss of gestalt, loss of symmetry, distortion of figures	Nondominant parietal lobe
Camouflaged object(s)	Visual-perception deficit	Cannot name when camouflaged, can name when clear	Occipital lobes

From Taylor M A et al: Cognitive tasks in the mental status examination. *J Nerv Ment Dis 168*:168, 1980. © 1980, The Williams & Wilkins Co., Baltimore. Used with permission.

7

Theories of Personality and Psychopathology

7.1

Sigmund Freud: Founder of Classical Psychoanalysis

INTRODUCTION

Concepts derived from psychoanalysis are applied so widely in psychiatric training and practice that they have become a fundamental part of the approach to mental and emotional disorders. Therefore, it is imperative that the student develop a clear understanding of classic psychoanalytic theory and the work of its founder, Sigmund Freud. Freud established the basis for psychodynamic thinking.

Traditionally, classical or orthodox psychoanalysis has referred primarily to Freud's libido and instinct theories; it has come to include the concepts of ego psychology as well. Essentially, psychoanalysis is based on the free association method of investigation, which yielded the data used by Freud to formulate the key concepts of unconscious motivation, psychic determinism, conflict, symbolism, and repression. One of Freud's most important contributions was the concept of the unconscious—first used to define mental material not in the field of awareness and, later, to designate a topographic device of the mind where psychic material is not readily accessible to conscious awareness.

Psychoanalytic theory, like all personality theory, is concerned primarily with the elucidation of those factors that motivate behavior. Psychoanalysis is unique, however, in that it considers these motivating forces to derive from unconscious mental processes.

LIFE OF FREUD

Sigmund Freud was born of Jewish parents on May 6, 1856, in Freiburg, a small town in Moravia, which has since become part of Czechoslovakia. When he was 4 years old, his father, a wool merchant, brought the family to Vienna where Freud lived most of his life. He was forced to flee to England in 1938, when the Nazis annexed Austria. Freud died in 1939. See Figures 1 through 3 for highlights in the life of Freud.

BEGINNINGS OF PSYCHOANALYSIS

From 1887 to 1897, the period in which Freud seriously began to study the disturbances of his hysterical patients, psychoanalysis can be said to have taken root. The emergence of psychoanalysis had a three fold aspect: as a method of investigation, as a therapeutic technique, and as a body of scientific knowledge based on an increasing fund of information and basic theoretical propositions. The early research stemmed first from Freud's initial collaboration with Josef Breuer, then increasingly out of his own independent investigations and theoretical developments.

The Case of Anna O.

Josef Breuer was a prominent Viennese physician who formed a close friendship with Freud. Breuer's treatment of "Anna O."—specifically his communication to Freud of the details of the case—was one of the factors that led to the development of psychoanalysis.

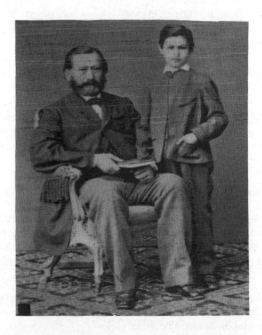

Figure 1. Sigmund Freud and his father. (Austrian Information Service, New York, N.Y.)

133

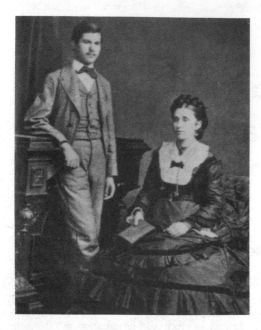

Figure 2 Sigmund Freud and his mother in 1872. (Austrian Information Service, New York, N.Y.)

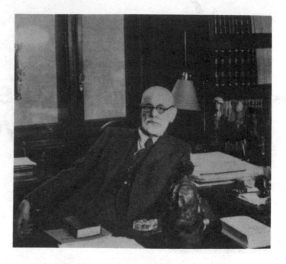

Figure 3. Sigmund Freud at his desk in his Vienna office. (Austrian Information Service, New York, N. Y.)

Breuer treated Anna O. (Bertha Pappenheim) from December 1880 to June 1882. The patient was an intelligent girl of 21 who had developed a number of hysterical symptoms in association with the illness of her father, of whom she was passionately fond. These symptoms included paralysis of the limbs, contractures, anesthesias, disturbances of sight and speech, anorexia, and a distressing nervous cough. Her illness was further characterized by two distinct phases of consciousness. During one, she was normal; during the second, she took on another, more pathological, personality. The transition between these states of consciousness was influenced by autohypnosis, which Breuer subsequently supplemented with artificial hypnosis. Anna had shared with her mother the duties of nursing her father until his death. During her altered states of consciousness, called hypnoid states, Anna was able to relate the vivid fantasies and intense emotions that she had experienced while tending to her father. To the great amazement of the patient—and Breuer—Anna's symptoms could disappear if she could recall, with an accompanying expression of affect, the circumstances under which her emotions had arisen. Once she had become aware of the value of this "talking cure," or "chimney sweeping," Anna proceeded to eliminate each of her manifold symptoms, one after another.

Studies on Hysteria

In 1895 in *Studies on Hysteria,* Breuer and Freud reported their clinical experience in the treatment of hysteria and proposed a theory of hysterical phenomena. Out of these cases, Freud constructed the following sequence of steps in the development of hysteria:

1. The patient has undergone a traumatic experience, one that has stirred up intense emotion and excitation that was intensely painful or disagreeable to the patient.
2. The traumatic experience represented to the patient some idea or ideas that were incompatible with the dominant mass of ideas constituting the ego.

3. This incompatible idea was intentionally dissociated or repressed from consciousness with a counterforce.
4. The excitation associated with the incompatible idea was converted into somatic pathways and resulted in the hysterical manifestations and symptoms.
5. What is left in consciousness is merely a mnemonic symbol; it is connected with the traumatic event only by associative links, which are frequently disguised.
6. If the memory of the traumatic experience can be brought into consciousness and the patient is able to release the strangulated affect associated with it, the affect is discharged, and the symptoms disappear in a process Freud called *abreaction.*

Freud introduced the concept of *psychic determinism,* in which mental phenomena often have antecedent causes operating on an unconscious level. All psychological events can be explained on some level by a well-defined cause and effect relationship. Most symptoms are overdetermined; a concept in which phenomena such as dreams and neurotic symptoms reflect the operation of multiple factors, particularly with regard to symbolic meaning or significance.

Free Association Method

The use of *free association* evolved very gradually from 1892 to 1895. The first step in its development came about when a patient, Elisabeth von R., remarked that she had not expressed her thoughts because she was unsure what Freud wanted to hear. From this point on, Freud no longer tried to direct the patient's thinking, but encouraged her to ignore all censorship and to express every idea that occurred to her freely and truthfully, no matter how insignificant, irrelevant, or shameful it might seem. This method of free association is enhanced by the patient lying on a couch. Free association is known as the *fundamental rule of psychoanalysis.*

Freud discovered that the patient's memory extended well beyond the traumatic event that had precipitated the onset of illness. He found that patients were able to produce memories of their childhood experiences and of long forgotten scenes and events. This discovery led to the conclusion that these memories were inhibited because they involved sexual experiences or painful incidents in the patient's life. Moreover, the recollection of such experiences could evoke intense excitement, moral conflict, feelings of self-reproach, or fear of punishment. Since these childhood experiences remained so vivid, they exerted a predisposing influence on the development of psychoneurosis. Freud continued to acknowledge the role of heredity in determining a person's future susceptibility to neurosis, but he assigned much of the responsibility for the cause of the psychoneuroses to unfavorable childhood experiences.

Freud discovered early in his practice that his patients were often unwilling or unable to recount memories that later proved to be significant. He defined this reluctance as *resistance*. Later, Freud found that in the majority of his patients, resistance was due to active forces in the mind (of which the patients themselves were often unaware) that excluded painful or distressing material from consciousness. Freud described this active force as *repression*. In a broad sense, Freud considered repression to be at the core of all symptom formation.

THEORY OF THE INSTINCTS

Freud used the term *libido* to refer to that force by which the sexual instinct is represented in the mind. He recognized that the psychosexual instinct does not originate in finished form. Rather, it undergoes a complex process or pathway of development that has many manifestations apart from the simple aim of genital union. The *libido theory* referred to the investigation of all of these manifestations and the complicated paths they might follow in the course of development. Later, Freud accorded aggression a separate status as an instinct with a distinct source. Table 1 provides a summary of psychosexual libido development.

Freud's Case History

Applying the libido theory and his theory of instincts, Freud publicized a series of psychoanalytic case histories that are both historically and psychodynamically significant. They are summarized in Table 2.

Narcissism

Before its use by psychoanalysts to indicate excessive self-love, the term *narcissism* referred to an autoerotic perversion displayed by Narcissus, the mythological Greek youth who fell in love with his own reflection. In 1908, Freud observed that in cases of dementia precox (schizophrenia), libido appeared to have been withdrawn from other persons or objects, and he concluded that excessive narcissism might account for the loss of contact with reality that typified such patients. Freud then speculated as to where this libido could have been invested. The megalomanic delusions of these patients appeared to indicate that the libido they had withdrawn from external objects was reinvested in themselves—in their own egos.

Life and Death Instincts

Freud introduced his theory of the dual life and death instincts, *Eros* and *Thanatos,* in 1920 in *Beyond the Pleasure Principle*. The life and death instincts were thought to represent the forces that underlie the sexual and aggressive instincts, respectively.

Freud defined the death instinct, or Thanatos, as the tendency of organisms and their cells to return to the inanimate state. In contrast, the life instinct, or Eros, referred to the tendency of particles to reunite or parts to bind to one another to form greater unities, as in sexual reproduction. Inasmuch as the ultimate destiny of all biological organisms, with the exception of the germ cells, was death, Thanatos was considered to be the dominant force.

Pleasure and Reality Principles

The pleasure principle, which Freud viewed as an inborn tendency of the organism to avoid pain and to seek pleasure through tension discharge, dominates infancy and childhood. In essence, the pleasure principle persists throughout life, but it must be modified by the reality principle. The demands of external reality, called the *reality principle,* necessitate the postponement of immediate pleasure, with the aim of achieving perhaps even greater pleasure in the long run. The reality principle is largely a learned function. Therefore, it is closely related to the maturation of ego functions and may be impaired in a variety of mental disorders resulting from impeded ego development.

TOPOGRAPHIC THEORY

The topographic theory, as set forth in the *Interpretation of Dreams* in 1900, represented an attempt to divide the mind into three regions: the unconscious, the preconscious, and the conscious, which were differentiated by their relationship to consciousness.

The Unconscious

The *unconscious* contains repressed ideas and affects and is characterized as follows:

1. Ordinarily, the elements of the unconscious are inaccessible to consciousness; they become conscious only through the preconscious, which excludes them by means of censorship or repression. Repressed ideas may reach consciousness when the censor is overpowered (as in psychoneurotic symptom formation), relaxed (as in dream state), or fooled (as in jokes).
2. The unconscious is associated with a particular form of mental activity that Freud called the *primary process* or primary process thinking. The primary process has as its principle aim the facilitation of wish fulfillment and instinctual discharge; thus, it is intimately associated with the pleasure principle. Primary process thinking disregards logical connections, permits contradictions to coexist, knows no negatives, has no conception of time, and represents wishes as already fulfilled. This type of thinking is characteristic of very young children, who are dedicated to the immediate gratification of their desires.
3. Memories in the unconscious lose their connection with verbal expression. However, they can reach consciousness once words are reapplied to the forgotten memory trace.

Table 1
Stages of Psychosexual Development

Oral Stage			
Definition	The earliest stage of development in which the infant's needs, perceptions, and modes of expression are primarily centered in the mouth, lips, tongue, and other organs related to the oral zone.	Objectives	To establish a trusting dependence on nursing and sustaining objects, to establish comfortable expression and gratification of oral libidinal needs without excessive conflict or ambivalence from oral sadistic wishes.
Description	The oral zone maintains its dominant role in the organization of the psyche through approximately the first 18 months of life. Oral sensations include thirst, hunger, pleasurable tactile stimulations evoked by the nipple or its substitute, sensations related to swallowing and satiation. Oral drives consist of two separate components: libidinal and aggressive. States of oral tension lead to a seeking for oral gratification, typified by quiescence at the end of nursing. The oral triad consists of the wish to eat, to sleep, and to reach that relaxation that occurs at the end of sucking just before the onset of sleep. Libidinal needs (oral erotism) are thought to predominate in the early parts of the oral phase, whereas they are mixed with more aggressive components later (oral sadism). Oral aggression may express itself in biting, chewing, spitting, or crying. Oral aggression is connected with primitive wishes and fantasies of biting, devouring, and destroying.	Pathological traits	Excessive oral gratifications or deprivation can result in libidinal fixations that contribute to pathological traits. Such traits can include excessive optimism, narcissism, pessimism (often seen in depressive states), or demandingness. Oral characters are often excessively dependent and require others to give to them and to look after them. Such individuals want to be fed, but may be exceptionally giving to elicit a return of being given to. Oral characters are often extremely dependent on objects for the maintenance of their self-esteem. Envy and jealousy are often associated with oral traits.
		Character traits	Successful resolution of the oral phase provides a basis in character structure for capacities to give to and receive from others without excessive dependence or envy. A capacity to rely on others with a sense of trust as well as with a sense of self-reliance and self-trust.
Anal Stage			
Definition	The stage of psychosexual development that is prompted by maturation of neuromuscular control over sphincters, particularly the anal sphincters, thus permitting more voluntary control over retention or expulsion of feces.	Objectives	The anal period is essentially a period of striving for independence and separation from the dependence on and control of the parent. The objectives of sphincter control without overcontrol (fecal retention) or loss of control (messing) are matched by the child's attempts to achieve autonomy and independence without excessive shame or self-doubt from loss of control.
Description	This period, which extends roughly from 1 to 3 years of age, is marked by a recognizable intensification of aggressive drives mixed with libidinal components, in sadistic impulses. Acquisition of voluntary sphincter control is associated with an increasing shift from passivity to activity. The conflicts over anal control and the struggle with the parent over retaining or expelling feces in toilet training give rise to increased ambivalence, together with a struggle over separation, individuation, and independence. Anal erotism refers to the sexual pleasure in anal functioning, both in retaining the precious feces and in presenting them as a precious gift to the parent. Anal sadism refers to the expression of aggressive wishes connected with discharging feces as powerful and destructive weapons. These wishes are often displayed in such children's fantasies as bombing or explosions.	Pathological traits	Maladaptive character traits, often apparently inconsistent, are derived from anal erotism and the defenses against it. Orderliness, obstinacy, stubbornness, willfulness, frugality, and parsimony are features of the anal character derived from a fixation on anal functions. When defenses against anal traits are less effective, the anal character reveals traits of heightened ambivalence, lack of tidiness, messiness, defiance, rage, and sadomasochistic tendencies. Anal characteristics and defenses are most typically seen in obsessive-compulsive neuroses.

Anal Stage *continued*

Character traits	Successful resolution of the anal phase provides the basis for the development of personal autonomy, a capacity for independence and personal initiative without guilt, a capacity for self-determining be-	havior without a sense of shame or self-doubt, a lack of ambivalence and a capacity for willing cooperation without either excessive willfulness or sense of self-diminution or defeat.

Urethral Stage

Definition	This stage was not explicitly treated by Freud but is envisioned as a transitional stage between the anal and phallic stages of development. It shares some of the characteristics of the preceding anal phase and some from the subsequent phallic phase.	to what extent the objectives of urethral functioning differ from those of the anal period.
Description	The characteristics of the urethral phase are often subsumed under those of the phallic phase. Urethral erotism, however, is used to refer to the pleasure in urination as well as the pleasure in urethral retention analogous to anal retention. Similar issues of performance and control are related to urethral functioning. Urethral functioning may also be invested with a sadistic quality, often reflecting the persistence of anal sadistic urges. Loss of urethral control, as in enuresis, may frequently have regressive significance that reactivates anal conflicts.	The predominant urethral trait is that of competitiveness and ambition, probably related to the compensation for shame due to loss of urethral control. In control this may be the start for development of penis envy, related to the feminine sense of shame and inadequacy in being unable to match the male urethral performance. This is also related to issues of control and shaming.
		Besides the healthy effects analogous to those from the anal period, urethral competence provides a sense of pride and self-competence derived from performance. Urethral performance is an area in which the small boy can imitate and match his father's more adult performance. The resolution of urethral conflicts sets the stage for budding gender identity and subsequent identifications.
Pathological traits		
Character traits		
Objectives	Issues of control and urethral performance and loss of control. It is not clear whether or	

Phallic Stage

Definition	The phallic stage of sexual development begins sometime during the third year of life and continues until approximately the end of the fifth year.	establishing of the oedipal situation is essential for the furtherance of subsequent identifications that will serve as the basis for important and enduring dimensions of character organization.
Description	The phallic phase is characterized by a primary focus of sexual interests, stimulation, and excitement in the genital area. The penis becomes the organ of principal interest to children of both sexes, with the lack of penis in the female being considered as evidence of castration. The phallic phase is associated with an increase in genital masturbation accompanied by predominantly unconscious fantasies of sexual involvement with the opposite-sex parent. The threat of castration and its related castration anxiety arise in connection with guilt over masturbation and oedipal wishes. During this phase the oedipal involvement and conflict are established and consolidated.	The derivation of pathological traits from the phallic-oedipal involvement are sufficiently complex and subject to such a variety of modifications that it encompasses nearly the whole of neurotic development. The issues, however, focus on castration in males and on penis envy in females. The other important focus of developmental distortions in this period derives from the patterns of identification which are developed out of the resolution of the oedipal complex. The influence of castration anxiety and penis envy, the defenses against both of these, and the patterns of identification that emerge from the phallic phase are the primary determinants of the development of human character. They also subsume and integrate the residues of previous psychosexual stages, so that fixations or conflicts that derive from any of the preceding stages can contaminate and modify the oedipal resolution.
Pathological traits		
Objectives	The objective of this phase is to focus erotic interest in the genital area and genital functions. This focusing lays the foundation for gender identity and serves to integrate the residues of previous stages of psychosexual development into a predominantly genital-sexual orientation. The	

Table 1 *continued*

Phallic Stage *continued*		
Character traits	The phallic stage provides the foundations for an emerging sense of sexual identity, of a sense of curiosity without embarrassment, of initiative without guilt, as well as a sense of mastery not only over objects and persons in the environment but also over internal processes and impulses. The resolu-	tion of the oedipal conflict at the end of the phallic period gives rise to powerful internal resources for regulation of drive impulses and their direction to constructive ends. This internal source of regulation is the superego, and it is based on identifications derived primarily from parental figures.

Latency Stage			
Definition	The stage of relative quiescence or inactivity of the sexual drive during the period from the resolution of the Oedipus complex until pubescence (from about 5–6 years until about 11–13 years).	Pathological traits	The danger in the latency period can arise either from a lack of development of inner controls or an excess of them. The lack of control can lead to a failure of the child to sufficiently sublimate energies in the interests of learning and development of skills; an excess of inner control, however, can lead to premature closure of personality development and the precocious elaboration of obsessive character traits.
Description	The institution of the superego at the close of the oedipal period and the further maturation of ego functions allow for a considerably greater degree of control of instinctual impulses. Sexual interests during this period are generally thought to be quiescent. This is a period of primarily homosexual affiliations for both boys and girls, as well as a sublimation of libidinal and aggressive energies into energetic learning and play activities, exploring the environment, and becoming more proficient in dealing with the world of things and persons around them. It is a period for development of important skills. The relative strength of regulatory elements often gives rise to patterns of behavior that are somewhat obsessive and hypercontrolling.	Character traits	The latency period has frequently been regarded as a period of relatively unimportant inactivity in the developmental schema. More recently, greater respect has been gained for the developmental processes that take place in this period. Important consolidations and additions are made to the basic postoedipal identifications. It is a period of integrating and consolidating previous attainments in psychosexual development and an establishment of decisive patterns of adaptive functioning. The child can develop a sense of industry and a capacity for mastery of objects and concepts that allows autonomous function and with a sense of initiative without running the risk of failure or defeat or a sense of inferiority. These are all important attainments that need to be further integrated, ultimately as the essential basis for a mature adult life of satisfaction in work and love.
Objectives	The primary objective in this period is the further integration of oedipal identifications and a consolidation of sex-role identity and sex roles. The relative quiescence and control of instinctual impulses allow for development of ego apparatuses and mastery skills. Further identificatory components may be added to the oedipal ones on the basis of broadening contacts with other significant figures outside the family, e.g., teachers, coaches, and other adult figures.		

Genital Stage			
Definition	The genital or adolescent phase of psychosexual development extends from the onset of puberty from ages 11–12 until the individual reaches young adulthood. There is a tendency to subdivide this stage in current thinking, into preadolescent, early adolescent, middle adolescent, late adolescent, and even postadolescent periods.		provides the opportunity for a reresolution of these conflicts in the context of achieving a mature sexual and adult identity.
Description	The physiological maturation of systems of genital (sexual) functioning and attendant hormonal systems leads to an intensification of drives, particularly libidinal drives. This produces a regression in personality organization, which reopens conflicts of previous stages of psychosexual development and	Objectives	The primary objectives of this period are the ultimate separation from dependence on and attachment to the parents and the establishment of mature, nonincestuous, heterosexual object relations. Related to this are the achievement of a mature sense of personal identity and acceptance and integration of a set of adult roles and functions that permit new adaptive integrations with social expectations and cultural values.

Genital Stage *continued*

Pathological traits	The pathological deviations due to a failure to achieve successful resolution of this stage of development are multiple and complex. Defects can arise from the whole spectrum of psychosexual residues, since the developmental task of the adolescent period is in a sense a partial reopening and reworking and reintegrating of all of these aspects of development. Previous unsuccessful resolutions and fixations in various phases or aspects of psychosexual development will produce pathological defects in the emerging adult personality. A more specific defect from a failure to resolve adolescent issues has been described by Erikson as "identity diffusion."	Character traits	The successful resolution and reintegration of previous psychosexual stages in the adolescent, fully genital phase, sets the stage normally for a fully mature personality with a capacity for full and satisfying genital potency and a self-integrated and consistent sense of identity. Such an individual has reached a satisfying capacity for self-realization and meaningful participation in areas of work, love, and in the creative and productive application to satisfying and meaningful goals and values. Only in the last few years has the presumed relationship between psychosexual genitality and maturity of personality functioning been put in question.

Table by Meissner W W: Theories of personality and psychopathology: classical psychoanalysis. In *Comprehensive Textbook of Psychiatry*, ed 4, p 360, H I Kaplan and B J Sadock, editors, Williams & Wilkins, Baltimore, 1985.

4. The content of the unconscious is limited to wishes seeking fulfillment. These wishes provide the motivating force for dream and neurotic symptom formation.

5. The unconscious is closely related to the instincts. It contains the mental representatives and derivatives of the instinctual drives, especially the derivatives of the sexual instinct.

The Preconscious

The preconscious region of the mind is not present at birth but develops in childhood. The *preconscious* is accessible to both the unconscious and the conscious. Elements of the unconscious gain access to consciousness by first becoming linked with words through the preconscious. However, one of the functions of the preconscious is to repress or censor a person's wishes and desires. The type of mental activity associated with the preconscious is called *secondary process* or secondary process thinking. In accordance with the demands of external reality and the person's moral precepts or values, such thinking is aimed at avoiding unpleasantness, delaying instinctual discharge, and binding mental energy. Secondary process thinking respects logical connections and consistency more than the primary process thinking does. Thus, the secondary process is closely allied with the reality principle that, for the most part, governs its activities.

The Conscious

Freud regarded the *conscious* as a sense organ of attention, operating in close association with the preconscious. Through attention, the person becomes conscious of perceptual stimuli from the outside world. Within the organism, however, only elements in the preconscious enter consciousness; the rest of the mind lies outside of awareness.

THE INTERPRETATION OF DREAMS

Freud first became aware of the significance of dreams in therapy; in the process of free association, patients frequently described their dreams of the previous night or of years past. He discovered that these dreams had a definite meaning, although it often was disguised. Freud found that by encouraging his patients to free associate to dream fragments, rather than to real life events, he facilitated the disclosure of unconscious memories and fantasies.

In *The Interpretation of Dreams*, published in 1900, Freud concluded that a dream, like a neurotic symptom, was the conscious expression of an unconscious fantasy or wish that was not readily accessible in waking life. He called dreams "the royal road of the unconscious." The dream images represent unconscious wishes or thoughts disguised through symbolization and other distorting mechanisms. Although dreams were considered one of the normal manifestations of unconscious activity, they bore some resemblance to the pathological thoughts of psychotic patients in the waking state.

The analysis of dreams elicits material that has been repressed or otherwise excluded from consciousness. The *manifest dream*, which embodies the experienced content of the dream that the sleeper may or may not be able to recall after waking, is the product of the dream activity. The unconscious thoughts and wishes that, in Freud's view, threaten to awaken the sleeper are described as the *latent dream* content. Freud referred to the unconscious mental operations by which the latent dream content is transformed into the manifest dream as the *dream work*. In the process of dream interpretation, Freud was able to move from the manifest content of the dream by way of associative exploration to arrive at the latent dream content, which provided it with its core meaning.

In Freud's view, a variety of stimuli initiated dreaming activity—nocturnal sensory stimuli, day residues, and repressed infantile drives. Contemporary understanding of the dream process, however, suggests that dreaming activity takes place in conjunction with the psychic patterns of central nervous system activation that characterize certain phases of the sleep cycle. What Freud thought to be initiating stimuli may, in fact, be incorporated into the dream content.

Significance of Dreams

Freud gained access to the understanding and operation of unconscious processes primarily through the study of dreams and the

Table 2
Classical Psychoneurotic Reactions of Childhood[a]

	Conversion Reaction (Dora)	Phobic Reaction (Hans)	Obsessive-Compulsive Reaction (Rat Man)	Mixed Psychoneurotic Reaction (Wolf Man)
Family history	Striking family history of psychiatric and physical illness.	Both parents treated for "neurotic conflict" but not severe.	No family history of mental illness.	Striking family history of psychiatric and physical illness.
Symptoms	Enuresis and masturbation 6–8 yrs. Onset of neurosis at 8. Migraine, nervous cough, and hoarseness at 12. Aphonia at 16. Appendicitis at 16. Convulsions at 16. Facial neuralgia at 19. Change of personality at 8 from "wild creature" to quiet child.	Compulsive questions at 3–3½ yrs., regard to sex difference. Jealous reaction to sibling birth at 3½. Overt castration threat. Overt masturbation at 3½. Overeating and constipation at 4–5. Phobic reaction at 4–5. Attack of flu at 5 worsens phobia. Tonsillectomy at 5 worsens phobia.	Naughty period at 3–4 yrs. Marked timidity following beating by father at 4. Recognizing people by their smells as a child ("Renifleur"). Precocious ego development. Onset of obsessive ideas at 6–7.	Tractable and quiet up to 3¼ yrs. "Naughty" period at 3¼–4 yrs. Phobias at 4–5 with nightmares. Obsessional reaction at 6–7 (pious ceremonials). Disappearance of neuroses at 8.
Causes	Seduction by older man. Father's illness. Father's affair.	Seductive care by mother. Sibling birth at 3½.	Seduction by governess at 4. Death of sibling at 4. Beating by father at 4.	Seduction by older sister at 3¼. Mother's illness. Conflict between maid and governess.

[a]Adapted from Freud by Anthony E J: Psychiatric disorders of childhood. II: Psychoneurotic, psychophysiological, and personality disorders. In *Comprehensive Textbook of Psychiatry,* A M Freedman and H I Kaplan, editors, p 1388. Williams & Wilkins, Baltimore, 1967.

process of their formation. He maintained that every dream somehow represents a wish fulfillment, a form of gratification of an unconscious instinctual impulse in fantasy form. In the state of suspended mobility and regressive relaxation induced by the sleep state, the dream permits a partial and less dangerous gratification of the instinctual impulse.

STRUCTURAL THEORY OF THE MIND

Freud shifted the emphasis from the topographic model to the structural model of the psychic apparatus. In 1923, the structural model was formulated and presented in *The Ego and the Id.*

From a structural viewpoint, the psychic apparatus is divided into three provinces: id, ego, and superego, which are distinguished by their different functions. The main distinction lies between the ego and the id. The *id* is the locus of the instinctual drives. It is under the domination of the primary process; therefore, the id operates in accordance with the pleasure principle, without regard for reality. The *ego,* on the other hand, represents a more coherent organization whose task it is to avoid displeasure and pain. In order to conform with the demands of the external world, the ego opposes or regulates the discharge of instinctual drives. The discharge of id impulses is further opposed or regulated by the *superego,* the third structural component of the psychic apparatus. The superego contains the internalized moral values and influence of the parental images—the conscience.

Id

Freud conceived of the id as a completely unorganized, primordial reservoir of energy, derived from the instincts and under the domination of the primary process. Freud postulated that the infant is endowed at birth with an id, that is, with instinctual drives that seek gratification. The infant does not, however, have the capacity to delay, control, or modify these drives. In coping with the external world, the infant is completely dependent on the egos of other persons in the surrounding environment.

Ego

Toward the end of his career in 1938, Freud gave his most comprehensive definition of the ego in *Outline of Psychoanalysis:*

Here are the principal characteristics of the ego. In consequence of the preestablished connection between sense and perception and muscular action, the ego has voluntary movement at its command. It has the task of self-preservation. As regards external events, it performs that task by becoming aware of stimuli by storing up experiences about them (in the memory), by avoiding excessively strong stimuli (through adaptation), and finally by learning to bring about expedient changes in the external world to its own advantage (through activity). As regards internal events in relation to the id, it performs that task by gaining control over the demands of the instinct, by deciding whether they are to be allowed satisfaction, by postponing that satisfaction to times and circumstances favorable in the external world, or by suppressing their excitations entirely. It is guided in its activity by consideration of the tension produced by stimuli, whether these tensions are present in it or introduced into it.

Freud believed that the modification of the id occurs as a result of the impact of the external world upon the drives. The pressures of external reality enable the ego to appropriate the energies of the id to do its work. In its formation process, the ego seeks to bring the influences of the external world to bear upon the id. By substituting the reality principle for the pleasure principle, the ego thereby contributes to its own development. Freud emphasized the role of the instincts in ego development, particularly the role of conflict. In the beginning, the conflict is between the id and the outside world; later, it is between the id and the ego itself.

At first, infants are unable to differentiate their own bodies from the rest of the world; the ego begins with children's ability to perceive their body as distinct from the external world.

Superego

The superego is that part of the personality that represents the internalized values, ideals, and moral attitudes of society. Its psychic functions are expressed as guilt, self-criticism, and conscience. It has a rewarding function, referred to as the ego ideal, as well as a critical and punishing function that evokes the sense of guilt. The superego comes into being with the resolution of the Oedipus complex.

Functions of the Ego

Several functions are thought to be fundamental to the ego's operation. Many advances have been made in studying the ego, and this study makes up the field of *ego psychology*.

Control and Regulations of Instinctual Drives. If the ego is to assure the integrity of the individual and to fulfill its role as mediator between the id and the outside world, the ability to delay immediate discharge of urgent wishes and impulses is essential. The development of the capacity to postpone both instinctual discharge and test reality is closely related to the progression in early childhood from the pleasure principle to the reality principle.

This progression also parallels the development of the *secondary process* or logical thinking, which aids in the control of drive discharge. The evolution of thought from the initially prelogical primary process thinking to the more logical and deliberate secondary process thinking is one of the means by which the ego learns to postpone the discharge of instinctual drives. For example, the representation in fantasy of instinctual wishes as having been fulfilled may obviate the need for urgent action that might not serve the realistic needs of the individual. The capacity to figure things out or to anticipate consequences represents thought processes that are essential for the realistic functioning of the individual.

The Relation to Reality. Freud always regarded the ego's capacity for maintaining a relationship to the external world as one of its principal functions. The character of its relationship to the external world may be divided into three components: (1) the sense of reality, (2) reality testing, and (3) the adaptation to reality.

1. *The Sense of Reality.* The sense of reality originates simultaneously with the development of the ego. Infants first become aware of the reality of their own body dimensions; over time, infants come to discern a reality outside of their bodies.

2. *Reality Testing.* The ego's capacity for objective evaluation and judgment of the external world depends on the primary autonomous functions of the ego, such as memory and perception. Because of the fundamental importance of reality testing in negotiating with the outside world, its impairment may be associated with a severe mental disorder. The development of the ability to test reality (which is closely related to the progression from the pleasure to the reality principle) and to distinguish fantasy from actuality occurs gradually. Once gained, this capacity is subject to regression and temporary deterioration in children in the face of anxiety, conflict, or intense instinctual wishes. This deterioration, however, should not be confused with the breakdown of reality testing that occurs in adult psychopathology.

3. *Adaptation to Reality.* The capacity of the ego to use the individual's resources to form adequate solutions is based upon previously tested judgments of reality. Thus, it is possible for the ego to develop good reality testing in terms of perception and grasp and, at the same time, develop an adequate capacity to accommodate one's resources to the situation. Adaptation is closely allied to the concept of mastery, in respect to both external tasks and instincts. It should be distinguished from adjustment, which may entail accommodation to reality at the expense of certain resources or potentialities of the individual. The function of adaptation to reality is closely related to the defensive functions of the ego.

Object Relations. The development of a capacity for mutually satisfying object relationships is one of the fundamental functions of the ego. The relationship with a need-satisfying adult object begins at birth and undergoes progressive development. This process may be disturbed by retarded development, regression, limitations in the capacity to develop object relationships, or, conceivably, genetic defects. The development of object relationships is closely related to the evolution of drive components and the phase-appropriate defenses that accompany them. Object constancy refers to one's capacity to maintain positive emotional attachments to a particular object while tolerating one's ambivalent feelings and acknowledging its qualities and attributes. This achievement provides the basic components for the later emergence of significant object relationships in adult life.

Internalizing experience results in internal self-images, called a key human experience in *object relations theory*. One views objects the way one views oneself. Heinz Kohut has further emphasized self experience and *synthetic functions of ego*. The synthetic function—the ego's integrative tendency to bind, unite, tolerate anxiety, coordinate, create, and simplify or generalize—is concerned with the overall organization and operation of other ego functions in the course of its operation. It reconciles conflict by delaying conflict.

Primary Autonomous Functions. Primary inborn autonomous ego functions are based on rudimentary apparatuses that are present at birth; they develop independent of the conflict with the id. Heinz Hartmann has included perception, intuition, comprehension, thinking, speaking, language, certain phases of control of motor development, learning, intelligence, and memory among the functions in this conflict-free sphere. However, each of these functions may become involved in conflict during the course of development. For example, if aggressive, competitive impulses intrude on the impetus to learn, they may evoke inhibitory reactions on the part of the ego.

DEFENSE MECHANISMS

Sigmund Freud coined the idea of defense functions in 1894. According to Freud, defense mechanisms serve to keep conflictual ideation out of consciousness.

The first systematic and comprehensive study of the defenses used by the ego was presented in Anna Freud's 1936 book, *The Ego and the Mechanisms of Defense,* which marked the beginning of ego psychology, as opposed to Sigmund Freud's older id psychology. Anna Freud (Sigmund Freud's daughter) maintained that everyone, normal as well as neurotic, used a characteristic group of defense mechanisms to varying degrees. She listed ten defense mechanisms associated with adult neuroses that were normal in children: regression, repression, reaction formation, isolation, undoing, projection, introjection, turning against the self, and reversal. The tenth defense mechanism of sublimation was normal in both children and adults.

In the early stages of psychosexual development, defense mechanisms emerge as a result of the ego's struggle to mediate between the pressures of the sexual and aggressive impulses of the id and the requirements and strictures of outside reality. At each phase of libidinal development, associated drive components evoke characteristic ego defenses. For example, introjection, denial, and projection are defense mechanisms associated with oral sadistic impulses, whereas reaction formation, such as shame and disgust, develop in relation to anal impulses and pleasures. Defense mechanisms from earlier phases of development persist side by side with those of later periods. When defenses associated with pregenital phases of development tend to become predominant in adult life over more mature mechanisms such as sublimation and repression, the personality retains an infantile cast.

Defenses are not in and of themselves pathological. To the contrary, they may serve an essential function in maintaining normal psychological well-being. Nonetheless, psychopathology may arise as a result of alterations in normal defensive functioning. Table 3 presents a brief classification and description of the most important basic defense mechanisms.

Classification of Defense Mechanisms

It will be noted from Table 3 that a considerable number of defense mechanisms has been defined by various authors. As noted above, Anna Freud classified defense mechanisms according to whether they were meant to control sexual or aggressive impulses. She also correlated them with specific psychosexual stages. For example, during the oral phase of development, denial, projection, introjection, regression, and turning against the self are important. During the anal phase, reaction formation, isolation, and undoing are crucial, and during the phallic period, repression is most significant. Sublimation is used during the latency and adult phases.

George Vaillant has further classified defenses according to the level of adaptation and use. Narcissistic defenses are used by children and psychotics. Immature defenses are used by adolescents and are seen in depression, obsessions and compulsions. Neurotic defenses are seen in adults under stress and are encountered in obsessive-compulsive and hysteric persons. Mature defenses are normal adult adaptive mechanisms. These defenses are encountered in psychologically and physically healthy adults with good marriages, successful and satisfying careers, and gratifying recreational outlets. Some overlapping of defenses may exist among these groups, for example, mature sublimation may be used by a psychotic or narcissistic defenses may be used by a mature adult.

Theory of Anxiety

For many years, Freud approached anxiety from a drive perspective, and he regarded neurotic anxiety as transformed libido. In 1926, he attacked the problem of anxiety from the standpoint of the ego. Both real anxiety and neurotic anxiety were viewed as a signal—the response of the organism to danger. In real anxiety, the threat emanated from a known danger outside the person; neurotic anxiety was precipitated by an unknown or repressed danger.

Freud distinguished two kinds of anxiety-provoking situations. In the first, for which the phenomenon of birth is the prototype, anxiety occurs as a result of excessive instinctual stimulation that the organism is unable to bind or handle. In the second, more common situation, which occurs after the defensive system has matured, anxiety arises in anticipation of danger rather than as the result of it, although the affect may be experienced as if the danger had already occurred. In these situations, the anxiety may arise because the person has learned to recognize, at a preconscious or unconscious level, aspects of a situation that were once traumatic. Anxiety serves as a signal to mobilize protective measures that avert the danger and prevent a traumatic situation from taking place. The person may use avoidance mechanisms to escape from a real or imagined danger from without, or the ego may use psychological defenses from within to guard against or reduce the quantity of instinctual excitation.

Character

In 1913, Freud made an important distinction between neurotic symptoms and character or personality traits. Neurotic symptoms come into being as a result of the failure of repression; character traits owe their existence to the success of repression or, more accurately, to the defense system that achieves its aim through a persistent pattern of reaction formation and sublimation. In 1923, Freud observed that the replacement of object attachments by identification (introjection), in which the ego internalized the lost object, also made a significant contribution to character formation. In 1932, Freud emphasized the particular importance of identification with the parents for the construction of character, particularly with reference to superego formation.

Psychoanalysis has come to regard character as the pattern of adaptation to instinctual and environmental forces that is typical or habitual for a given person. Character is distinguished from the ego in that it largely refers to styles

Table 3
Classification of Defense Mechanisms*

Narcissistic Defenses

Projection. Perceiving and reacting to unacceptable inner impulses and their derivatives as though they were outside the self. On a psychotic level, this takes the form of frank delusions about external reality, usually persecutory, includes both perception of one's own feelings in another, with subsequent acting on the perception (psychotic paranoid delusions). The impulses may derive from the id or superego (hallucinated recriminations) but may undergo transformation in the process. Thus, according to Freud's analysis of paranoid projections, homosexual libidinal impulses are transformed into hatred and then projected onto the object of the unacceptable homosexual impulse.

Denial. Psychotic denial of external reality, unlike repression, affects the perception of external reality more than the perception of internal reality. Seeing, but refusing to acknowledge what one sees, or hearing, and negating what is actually heard, are examples of denial and exemplify the close relationship of denial to sensory experience. Not all denial, however, is necessarily psychotic. Like projection, denial may function in the service of more neurotic or even adaptive objectives. Denial avoids becoming aware of some painful aspect of reality. At the psychotic level, the denied reality may be replaced by a fantasy or delusion.

Distortion. Grossly reshaping external reality to suit inner needs, including unrealistic megalomanic beliefs, hallucinations, wish-fulfilling delusions; and employing sustained feelings of delusional superiority or entitlement.

Immature Defenses

Acting Out. The direct expression of an unconscious wish or impulse in action to avoid being conscious of the accompanying affect. The unconscious fantasy, involving objects, is lived out impulsively in behavior, thus gratifying the impulse more than the prohibition against it. On a chronic level, acting out involves giving in to impulses to avoid the tension that would result from postponement of expression.

Blocking. An inhibition, usually temporary in nature, of affects especially, but possibly also thinking and impulses. It is close to repression in its effects, but has a component of tension arising from the inhibition of the impulse, affect, or thought.

Hypochondriasis. The transformation of reproach toward others arising from bereavement, loneliness, or unacceptable aggressive impulses, into self-reproach and complaints of pain, somatic illness, and neurasthenia. Existent illness may also be overemphasized or exaggerated for its evasive and regressive possibilities. Thus, responsibility may be avoided, guilt may be circumvented, instinctual impulses may be warded off.

Introjection. In addition to the developmental functions of the process of introjection, it also serves specific defensive functions. The introjection of a loved object involves the internalization of characteristics of the object with the goal of establishing closeness to and constant presence of the object. Anxiety consequent to separation or tension arising out of ambivalence toward the object is thus diminished. If the object is a lost object, introjection nullifies or negates the loss by taking on characteristics of the object, thus in a sense internally preserving the object. Even if the object is not lost, the internalization usually involves a shift of cathexis reflecting a significant alteration in the object relationships.

Introjection of a feared object serves to avoid anxiety through internalizing the aggressive characteristic of the object, and thereby putting the aggression under one's own control. The aggression is no longer felt as coming from outside, but is taken within and utilized defensively, thus turning the subject's weak, passive position into an active, strong one. The classic example is identification with the aggressor. Introjection can also be out of a sense of guilt in which the self-punishing introject is attributable to the hostile-destructive component of an ambivalent tie to an object.

Thus, the self-punitive qualities of the object are taken over and established within one's self as a symptom or character trait, which effectively represents both the destruction and the preservation of the object. This is also called identification with the victim.

Passive-Aggressive Behavior. Aggression toward an object expressed indirectly and ineffectively through passivity, masochism, and turning against the self.

Projection. Attributing one's own unacknowledged feelings to others; it includes severe prejudice, rejection of intimacy through suspiciousness, hypervigilance to external danger, and injustice collecting. Projection operates correlatively to introjection, such that the material of the projection is derived from the internalized configuration of the introjects. At higher levels of function, projection may take the form of misattributing or misinterpreting motives, attitudes, feelings, or intentions of others.

Regression. A return to a previous stage of development or functioning, to avoid the anxieties or hostilities involved in later stages. A return to earlier points of fixation embodying modes of behavior previously given up. This is often the result of a disruption of equilibrium at a later phase of development. This reflects a basic tendency to achieve instinctual gratification or to escape instinctual tension by returning to earlier modes and levels of gratification when later and more differentiated modes fail.

Schizoid Fantasy. The tendency to use fantasy and to indulge in autistic retreat for the purpose of conflict resolution and gratification.

Somatization. The defensive conversion of psychic derivatives into bodily symptoms: tendency to react with somatic rather than psychic manifestations. Infantile somatic responses are replaced by thought and affect during development (desomatization): regression to earlier somatic forms of response (resomatization) may result from unresolved conflicts and may play an important role in psychological reactions.

Turning Against the Self. Changing an unacceptable impulse that is aimed at others by redirecting it against oneself.

Table 3 *continued*

Neurotic Defenses

Controlling. The excessive attempt to manage or regulate events or objects in the environment in the interest of minimizing anxiety and solving internal conflicts.

Displacement. Involves a purposeful, unconscious shifting from one object to another in the interest of solving a conflict. Although the object is changed, the instinctual nature of the impulse and its aim remain unchanged.

Dissociation. A temporary but drastic modification of character or sense of personal identity to avoid emotional distress; it includes fugue states and hysterical conversion reactions.

Externalization. A general term, correlative to internalization, referring to the tendency to perceive in the external world and in external objects components of one's own personality, including instinctual impulses, conflicts, moods, attitudes, and styles of thinking. It is a more general term than projection, which is defined by its derivation from and correlation with specific introjects.

Inhibition. The unconsciously determined limitation or renunciation of specific ego functions, singly or in combination, to avoid anxiety arising out of conflict with instinctual impulses, superego, or environmental forces or figures.

Intellectualization. The control of affects and impulses by way of thinking about them instead of experiencing them. It is a systematic excess of thinking, deprived of its affect, to defend against anxiety caused by unacceptable impulses.

Isolation. The intrapsychic splitting or separation of affect from content resulting in repression of either idea or affect or the displacement of affect to a different or substitute content.

Rationalization. A justification of attitudes, beliefs, or behavior that might otherwise be unacceptable by an incorrect application of justifying reasons or the invention of a convincing fallacy.

Reaction Formation. The management of unacceptable impulses by permitting expression of the impulse in antithetical form. This is equivalently an expression of the impulse in the negative. Where instinctual conflict is persistent, reaction formation can become a character trait on a permanent basis, usually as an aspect of obsessional character.

Repression. Consists of the expelling and withholding from conscious awareness of an idea or feeling. It may operate either by excluding from awareness what was once experienced on a conscious level (secondary repression), or it may curb ideas and feelings before they have reached consciousness (primary repression). The "forgetting" of repression is unique in that it is often accompanied by highly symbolic behavior, which suggests that the repressed is not really forgotten. The central role of repression in the development of psychoanalytic theory and particularly the important discrimination between repression and the more general concept of defense has been discussed.

Sexualization. The endowing of an object or function with sexual significance that it did not previously have, or possesses to a lesser degree, to ward off anxieties connected with prohibitive impulses.

Undoing. A person symbolically acts out in reverse something unacceptable that has already been done; a form of magical expiatory action.

The Mature Defenses

Altruism. The vicarious but constructive and instinctually gratifying service to others. This must be distinguished from altruistic surrender, which involves a surrender of direct gratification or of instinctual needs in favor of fulfilling the needs of others to the detriment of the self, with vicarious satisfaction only being gained through introjection.

Anticipation. The realistic anticipation of or planning for future inner discomfort: implies overly concerned planning, worrying, and anticipation of dire and dreadful possible outcomes.

Asceticism. The elimination of directly pleasurable affects attributable to an experience. The moral element is implicit in setting values on specific pleasures. Asceticism is directed against all "base" pleasures perceived consciously, and gratification is derived from the renunciation.

Humor. The overt expression of feelings without personal discomfort or immobilization and without unpleasant effect on others. Humor allows one to bear, and yet focus on, what is

too terrible to be borne, in contrast to wit, which always involves distraction or displacement away from the affective issue.

Sublimation. The gratification of an impulse whose goal is retained, but whose aim or object is changed from a socially objectionable one to a socially valued one. Libidinal sublimation involves a desexualization of drive impulses and the placing of a value judgment that substitutes what is valued by the superego or society. Sublimation of aggressive impulses takes place through pleasurable games and sports. Unlike neurotic defenses, sublimation allows instincts to be channeled rather than to be dammed-up or diverted. Thus, in sublimation, feelings are acknowledged, modified, and directed toward a relatively significant person or goal so that modest instinctual satisfaction results.

Suppression. The conscious or semiconscious decision to postpone attention to a conscious impulse or conflict.

---

*Compiled and adapted from Semrad (1967), Bibring and associates (1961), and Vaillant (1971) by Meissner W W: Theories of personality and psychopathology: Classical psychoanalysis. In *Comprehensive Textbook of Psychiatry,* **ed 4, p 389. H I Kaplan and B J Sadock, editors. Williams & Wilkins, Baltimore, 1985.**

of defense and directly observable behavior rather than to thinking and feeling.

Innate biological predisposition, the interaction of id forces with early ego defenses and environmental influences, and various early identifications and imitations of other human beings leave their lasting stamp upon character. The degree to which the ego has developed a capacity to tolerate delay in drive discharge and to neutralize instinctual energy determines the degree to which such character traits will emerge in later life.

The exaggerated development of certain character traits at the expense of others may lead to character disorders or produce a vulnerability or predisposition to the psychoses.

THEORY OF NEUROSIS

Neuroses develop under the following conditions: (1) There is an inner conflict between drives and fears that prevents drive discharge. (2) Sexual drives are involved in this conflict. (3) The conflict has not been "worked though" to a realistic solution. Instead, the drives that seek discharge have been expelled from consciousness through repression or another defense mechanism. (4) The repression has merely rendered the drives unconscious; it has not deprived them of their power and made them innocuous. Consequently, the repressed tendencies—disguised neurotic symptoms—have fought their way back into consciousness. (5) A rudimentary neurosis, based on the same type of conflict, existed in early childhood.

Secondary Gains of Neurosis

The reduction of tension and conflict through neurotic illness is the primary purpose or gain of the disorder. The ego, however, may try to gain advantages from the external world by provoking pity in order to get attention and sympathy or even monetary compensation. These advantages are the secondary gains of the illness.

Each form of neurosis has its characteristic form of secondary gain. In phobias, there is a regression to childhood, when one was still protected. Gaining attention through dramatic acting out and, at times, deriving material advantages, are characteristic of conversion hysteria. In compulsive neurosis, there is frequently a narcissistic gain through pride in illness. In psychosomatic states, psychic conflicts are denied by projecting them onto the physical sphere.

TREATMENT

Freud realized that the success of treatment depended on the patient's ability to understand the emotional significance of an experience and to retain that insight. Psychoanalysis tries to bring repressed material back to consciousness. On the basis of a greater understanding of one's needs and motives, a patient may find a realistic solution to the conflict. Freud elaborated a treatment method that attaches minimal importance to the immediate relief of symptoms, moral support from therapist, and guidance counseling.

Analytical Process

The analytical process refers to the regressive emergence, working through, interpretation, and resolution of the transference neurosis. The analytical situation, on the other hand, refers to the setting in which the analytical process takes place—specifically, the positive real relationship between patient and analyst based on the therapeutic alliance. The analyst, however, assumes a passive role in this relationship.

The regression induced by the analytical situation allows for a reemergence of infantile conflicts and thus induces the formation of a transference neurosis. In the transference neurosis, the original infantile conflicts and wishes become focused on the analyst and are reexperienced. In analytical regression, earlier infantile conflicts are revived. The tendency to repeat previous conflicts is known as the *repetition compulsion*.

Techniques

The cornerstone of the psychoanalytic technique is *free association*, i.e., the patient relates freely everything that passes through his or her mind. The primary function of free association, besides the obvious one of providing content for the analysis, is to induce the necessary regression and passive dependence that are connected with establishing and working through the transference neurosis. Although it remains the basic technique and the fundamental rule that guides the patient's participation in the analysis, the use of free association in the analytical process is a relative matter. There are frequent occasions when the process of free association is interrupted or modified; defensive needs or the developmental progression taking place within the analysis affect its use.

The analysis becomes a recurring conflict between *transference, transference neurosis,* and *resistance*. Manifested by involuntary inhibitions of the patient's effort to free associate, this conflict is a repetition of the sexuality-guilt conflict that produced the neurosis itself. The analysis of resistance is the analyst's prime function and interpretation is the chief tool. The patient displaces the feelings that were originally directed toward the participants in these early events onto the analyst. The analyst alternately becomes a friend or an enemy and is, correspondingly, loved or hated. To an increasing extent, the patient's feelings toward the analyst replicate his or her feelings toward the specific people talked about. This object displacement, which is an inevitable concomitant of psychoanalytic treatment, is called *transference*. As unresolved childhood attitudes emerge during transference, patients begin to see themselves as they really are, with all their unfulfilled and contradictory needs exposed.

Modifications in Classical Analysis

Although some orthodox analysts are reluctant to prescribe psychopharmacologic agents, others do, and a number work with psychopharmacologists as consultants. A few psychoanalysts have modified time and frequency of psychoanalytic sessions.

References

Compton A: *Freud:* Objects and structure. Journal of the American Psychoanalytic Association *34:*561, 1986.

Fenichel O: *The Psychoanalytic Theory of Neurosis.* W W Norton, New York, 1945.

Freud A: *The Ego and the Mechanisms of Defense.* International University Press, New York, 1946.

Freud S: *Beyond the Pleasure Principle.* W W Norton, New York, 1961.

Freud S: *The Ego and the Id.* W W Norton, New York, 1960.

Freud S: *An Outline of Psycho-Analysis.* W W Norton, New York, 1969.

Freud S: *The Standard Edition of the Complete Psychological Works of Sigmund Freud.* vols 1–24, Hogarth Press, London, 1953–1966.

Jones E: *The Life and Work of Sigmund Freud,* 3 vols. Basic Books, New York, 1953–1957.

Zetzel E R: *The Capacity for Emotional Growth.* International University Press, New York, 1970.

Zetzel E R, Meissner W W: *Basic Concepts of Psychoanalytic Psychiatry.* Basic Books, New York, 1973.

7.2 _____

Schools Derived from Psychoanalysis and Psychology

KARL ABRAHAM (1877–1925)

Karl Abraham was one of Freud's earliest followers and the first psychoanalyst in Germany. He elaborated on Freud's stages of psychosexual development and separated the oral period into a sucking and biting phase; divided the anal period into a destructive-expulsive (anal-sadistic) and a mastering-retentive (anal-erotic) phase; and divided the phallic period into an early phase of partial genital love (true phallic phase) and a later mature genital phase. He focused on adult character development and concluded that depression is a result of fixation at the oral stage of development and that obsessional neurosis is the result of fixation at the anal-sadistic phase.

ALFRED ADLER (1870–1937)

Alfred Adler was among those who expanded upon Freud's theories to such an extent that the two men eventually were estranged. Adler turned away from the sexual theory of neurosis and focused on the instinct of aggression. His theories are collectively known as *individual psychology.*

Aggression expresses itself as a striving for power, which Adler believed to be a masculine trait. He introduced the term *masculine protest* to depict the tendency to move from a passive and feminine role to a masculine and active role.

The child's development of self-esteem is hindered by any defect in his or her bodily structure, which Adler called *organ inferiority.* He expanded upon that concept and introduced the term *inferiority complex* to refer to a sense of weakness and inadequacy that everyone is born with and must overcome. That sense of inferiority is tied to the child's oedipal strivings that can never be gratified.

According to Adler, children's *birth order* in the family affects their life-styles. The firstborn reacts against the birth of siblings and

is angry about having to give up the powerful position of being the only child. The second born wants to equal and wrest power from the first; the third born can never be displaced and will always be the youngest.

Encouragement was Adler's main therapeutic approach to help patients overcome their feelings of inferiority. As a result of consistent human relatedness, patients become more hopeful, feel less isolated, and feel more a part of society. Adler placed even greater emphasis on the patients' needs to realize their strengths and abilities and to develop a belief in their own dignity and worth.

FRANZ ALEXANDER (1891–1964)

Franz Alexander moved from his native Germany to the United States, where he founded the Chicago Institute for Psychoanalysis. He developed the concept of the *corrective emotional experience* in which patients modify the results of traumatic events of their past life in the analytic situation. Because of the positive emotional involvement with a therapist, who is supportive and trustworthy, the patients are able to master past traumas and grow from the experience. Alexander also influenced the field of psychosomatic medicine with his *specificity hypothesis* that certain organic diseases are associated with specific personality constellations.

GORDON ALLPORT (1897–1967)

Gordon Allport taught the first course in psychology of personality to be offered in an American college—Harvard. He represents the *humanistic school* of psychology, which holds that there is an inherent potential for growth and autonomous function in every person.

A sense of self is a person's only real guarantee of personal existence. Selfhood develops in stages—the early self of the infant proceeds through the awareness of the body to self-identity. For the self that is known, Allport used the term *propriem;* propriate strivings are related to the maintenance of self-esteem and self-identity. In Allport's system, *traits* are the chief units of personality structure. A trait has actual existence, and some are common to people in the same culture. Individual traits, known as *personal dispositions,* represent the essence of the personality that is unique to the individual. *Maturity* is characterized by a greatly extended sense of self and a capacity to relate warmly and intimately to others. Such persons have zest, enthusiasm, humor, insight, and security. Psychotherapy directs the person to realize those characteristics.

ERIC BERNE (1910–1970)

Eric Berne received training in classical psychoanalysis, but set aside the analytic technique to develop *transactional analysis.* A *transaction* is a stimulus from one person that produces a corresponding response in another person. If the transaction is stereotyped and predictable, it is referred to as a psychological *game,* which people learn in childhood and play throughout their lives. *Strokes* are the basic motivating factor of human behavior and consist of rewards, such as love, approval, and other positive reinforcements. Berne defined three ego states that exist within each person: (1) the *child,* which represents archaic elements that become fixed in early childhood; (2) the *adult,* which is the part of the personality capable of objectively appraising reality; and (3) the *parent*, which is an introject of the person's actual parents' values. The therapeutic process involves helping patients understand whether or not they are functioning in the adult, child, or parent mode as they interact with others. They learn to recognize the games they play. The ultimate goal is for individuals to function in the adult mode as much as possible as they relate to others.

RAYMOND CATTELL (b. 1905)

Raymond Cattell obtained his Ph.D. in England before moving to the United States. He introduced the use of *multivariate analysis* and *factor analysis*—statistical procedures that simultaneously examine the relationship among multiple variables and factors—to the study of personality. By objectively examining the person's life record using personal interviewing and questionnaire data, Cattell described a variety of traits that represent the building blocks of personality.

Traits are both biologically based and environmentally determined or learned. Biological traits include sex, gregariousness, aggression, and parental protectiveness. Environmentally learned traits include cultural ideas such as work, religion, intimacy, romance, and identity. An important concept is the *law of coercion to the biosocial mean*, which holds that society exerts pressure on genetically different individuals to conform to social norms. Thus, for example, a person with a strong genetic tendency toward dominance is likely to receive social encouragement for restraint, whereas the naturally submissive person will be encouraged toward self-assertion.

RONALD FAIRBAIRN (1889–1964)

Ronald Fairbairn was an English psychiatrist representative of the object relations school of psychiatry. The significance of object relationships for normal psychological development was fully appreciated relatively late in the development of psychoanalysis. The evolution in the child's capacity for relationships with others, which progresses from narcissism to social relationships within the family and then within the group, has been described by Anna Freud and Dorothy Burlingham. Fairbairn, along with other workers such as Michael Balint (1986–1970), discussed the early stages in the relationship of the infant with need-satisfying objects and the gradual development of a sense of separateness from the mother. Donald Winnicott (1897–1971) described the *transitional object* (e.g., blanket, teddy bear) as the link between developing children and their mothers. The child develops feelings of security from the object, which symbolizes the good breast and reduces anxiety.

The capacity for mutually satisfying object relationships is one of the fundamental functions of the ego—the part of the psychic apparatus that deals with instinctual drives via the various defense mechanisms. The ego comprises a group of functions that share the task of mediating between the instincts and the outside world. The list of basic ego functions (such as the defense mechanisms listed in Section 7.1) differ among various authors. Two workers, Herman Nunberg and Heinz Hartmann, expanded on Freud's initial concepts and described *primary autonomous ego functions* that develop independently of instincts, conflicts, and drives. These functions, considered to be *conflict-free*, include perception, intuition, comprehension, thinking, language, certain phases of motor development, learning, and intelligence. Hartmann pointed out that in spite

of being conflict-free, each of those functions may become involved in conflict during the course of development. For example, if aggressive, competitive impulses intrude on the impetus to learn, the ego may evoke inhibitory reactions. This area of study has come to be known as *ego-psychology*, which is now represented by many contemporary psychoanalysts.

SANDOR FERENCZI (1873–1935)

Sandor Ferenczi, a close associate of Freud, was a Hungarian psychiatrist who studied early childhood thinking. Infants start out with a sense of magic hallucinatory omnipotence. They then move toward the use of words and finally to acceptance of reality in which all needs cannot be gratified. The therapeutic process, known as *active therapy*, helps the patient develop an awareness of reality through active confrontations by the therapist. Ferenczi tried to shorten analysis, and he was once cautioned by Freud about the need to keep aloof from patients, especially in the sexual area.

ERICH FROMM (1900–1980)

Erich Fromm came to the United States in 1933 from Germany, where he received his Ph.D. He helped found the William Alanson White Institute for Psychiatry in the United States. Fromm identified five character types that are common to and determined by Western culture; each person may possess qualities from one or more types. They are (1) the *receptive personality*, who is passive; (2) the *exploitative personality*, who is manipulative; (3) the *marketing personality*, who is opportunistic and changeable; (4) the *hoarding personality*, who saves and stores; and (5) the *productive personality*, who is mature and enjoys love and work. The therapeutic process involves strengthening the person's sense of ethical behavior toward others and developing *productive love*, characterized by care, responsibility, and respect for another person.

KURT GOLDSTEIN (1878–1965)

Kurt Goldstein was born in Germany and received his M.D. from the University of Breslau; he was influenced by Gestalt psychology and existentialism. Every organism has dynamic properties, which are energy supplies that are relatively constant and evenly distributed. When states of tension-disequilibrium occur, the organism automatically attempts to return to its normal state. What happens in one part of the organism affects every other part, a phenomenon known as *holocoenosis*.

A major concept used by Goldstein is *self-actualization*—the genuinely creative powers inherent in each person that lead one to fulfill one's potentialities. Each person has different innate potentialities; therefore, people strive for self-actualization along different paths.

To function reasonably well, the organism must come to terms with the environment, which can produce imbalances in the system but also act as one's source of supply. As individuals' coping methods improve, their chances of self-actualization increase. When sickness occurs, self-actualization is severely disrupted. An organism's whole integrity is threatened, and responses may be rigid and compulsive. A regression to primitive levels of behavior may occur. Under major stress (e.g., damage to the brain), a *catastrophic reaction* may occur in which the person becomes agitated and fearful and refuses to perform even the simplest task due to fear of possible failure. As health returns and the person masters illness, self-actualization resumes.

KAREN HORNEY (1885–1952)

Karen Horney was an American psychiatrist who believed that a person's current personality attributes were the result of the interaction between the person and the environment and were not based on infantile libidinal strivings carried over from childhood. Her theory, known as *holistic psychology,* maintains that a person needs to be seen as a unitary whole who influences and is being influenced by the environment. She challenged the concept of the Oedipus complex and attributed excessive concern with the genitals to parental attitudes, such as maternal overconcern or rigidity regarding sexuality.

There are three concepts of the self: (1) The *actual self* consists of the sum total of experience; (2) the *real self* is the harmonious healthy person; and (3) the *idealized self* is a neurotic expectation or glorified image of what the person feels he or she should be. The *pride system* alienates the person from the real self because it overemphasizes prestige, intellect, power, strength, appearance, and sexual prowess. It can lead to self-hatred, self-contempt, and self-effacement. Horney also introduced the concept of *basic anxiety* and *basic trust*. The therapeutic process emphasizes *self-realization*, which removes distorting influences on the personality that prevent growth from recurring.

CARL JUNG (1875–1961)

Carl Jung's psychoanalytic school, known as *analytical psychology,* includes basic ideas related to, but going beyond, Freud's theories. He expands on Freud's concept of the unconscious by describing the *collective unconscious* as consisting of all mankind's common and shared mythologic and symbolic past.

The collective unconscious includes *archetypes*—representational images and configurations that have universal symbolic meaning. Archetypal figures exist for the mother, father, child, and hero, among others. Archetypes contribute to *complexes,* which are feeling-toned ideas that develop as a result of personal experience interacting with archetypal imagery. Thus, a mother complex is determined not only by the mother-child interaction, but also by the conflict between archetypal expectation and actual experience with the real woman who functions in a motherly role.

Jung noted that there are two types of personality organization: introversion and extroversion. *Introverts* focus on their inner world of thoughts, intuitions, emotions, and sensations; *extroverts* are more oriented toward the outer world, other people, and material goods. Each person has a mixture of both components. The *persona* is the mask covering the personality that the person presents to the outside world. The persona may become fixed so that the real person is hidden from himself or herself. *Anima* and *animus* are unconscious traits possessed by men and women, respectively, and are contrasted to the persona. Anima refers to a man's undeveloped femininity, whereas animus refers to a woman's undeveloped masculinity.

The aim of Jungian treatment is to bring about an adequate adaptation to reality, which involves fulfilling one's creative potentialities. The ultimate goal is to achieve *individuation,* a process that continues throughout life in which individuals develop a unique sense of their own identity. This developmental process may lead persons down new paths, which may be different from their previous positions in life.

SOREN KIERKEGAARD (1813–1855)

Soren Kierkegaard was one of the major developers of existentialism, a philosophic theory upon which the teachings of such men as Martin Heidegger (1889–1976), Jean Paul Sartre (1905–1980), and Martin Buber (1878–1965) are based. Existentialism questions methodologies that view persons as objects or theories that explain behavior on the basis of responses to stimuli. It goes beyond observable behavior and questions the purpose and nature of existence itself. Existentialism deals with what it means to be human and, in doing so, denies entirely the question of heredity versus environment as behavioral determinants. Instead, it deals with the issue of *existential anxiety,* which is our awareness of being and nonbeing, the latter suggesting an awareness of our own death. To compensate for that knowledge, we must strive for *authenticity,* the ability to live our life with dignity and self-respect. Buber made a distinction between *I-thou* and *I-it* relationships, the former being authentic in that it is subjective, whereas the latter being inauthentic because it is detached.

Existentialism has not evolved into a clear-cut therapeutic approach; however, it has influenced therapists to explore what is experienced by patients and in what manner mental phenomena present themselves to consciousness—a school known as *phenomenology.*

MELANIE KLEIN (1882–1960)

Although still close to traditional psychoanalysis, Melanie Klein modified psychoanalytic theory and techniques in various ways, particularly in its application to infants and very young children. The libido is experienced at birth as pleasurable contacts with gratifying objects, primarily the good breast. Gratifying experiences reinforce basic trust, but if experience is frustrating—especially in the first year of life—the person develops a paranoid-schizoid position characterized by isolation and persecutory fears. Oedipal strivings are experienced during the first year of life, and a longing for the good breast is displaced onto a longing for the father's penis by both sexes. Klein stressed that envy of the opposite sex occurs in both sexes; she assumed that the infant possesses an inborn knowledge of the genitals. *Splitting,* a major defense mechanism used in development, occurs when good and bad objects exist with a splitting of love and aggression between them. In the first year of life, a primitive superego exists, and if too severe, it may lead to a depressive position later in life. Klein developed an analytical play technique with children in which play was treated in a symbolic fashion, much as dreams are used in adult therapy.

HEINZ KOHUT (1913–1982)

Heinz Kohut, an important innovator in psychoanalysis, expanded Freud's concept of narcissism. Originally, the infant's energies are devoted entirely to the satisfaction of his own needs and well-being, a state known as *primary,* or *primitive, narcissism.*

Primary narcissism can be divided into two basic archaic configurations—the grandiose self and the idealized parent image. Eventually, narcissism must be modified to accommodate frustration and disappointment; otherwise, people remain unable to relate to others unless those relationships serve to gratify narcissistic needs. Kohut's theories are known as *self-psychology,* and the therapeutic process requires that patients become aware of their excessive needs for approval and self-gratification.

KURT LEWIN (1890–1947)

Kurt Lewin received his Ph.D. in Berlin. In the 1930s, Lewin came to the United States and taught at Cornell, Harvard, and the Massachussetts Institute of Technology (MIT). He adapted the field approach from physics into a concept called *field theory.* A field is the totality of coexisting parts that are mutually interdependent. Behavior becomes a function of the person and his or her environment, which together make up the *life space.* The life space represents a field in constant flux that has *valences* or needs that require satisfaction. A hungry person is more aware of restaurants than someone who has just eaten, and a person who wants to mail a letter is aware of mailboxes.

Lewin applied field theory to groups. *Group dynamics* refers to the interaction of members of a group with one another, each of whom is dependent on the other. The group is capable of exerting pressure on a person to change behavior; but the person also influences the group when change occurs.

ABRAHAM MASLOW (1908–1970)

Abraham Maslow was born in Brooklyn, New York, and completed both his undergraduate and graduate work at the University of Wisconsin. Maslow, along with Kurt Goldstein, believed in the self-actualization theory—the need to understand the totality of a person. He was also a major worker in the field of humanism.

A hierarchical organization of needs is present in each person. Among the most powerful of these needs are survival-oriented needs, such as hunger and thirst. As they are fulfilled, other less powerful needs (e.g., needs for shelter, affection, and self-esteem) become effective motivators in their turn. Self-actualization is the highest need.

A *peak experience,* frequently occurring to self-actualizers, is an episodic, brief occurrence in which a person suddenly experiences a powerful transcendental state of consciousness. During this state, a person experiences a sense of heightened understanding, an intense euphoria, an integrated nature and unity with the universe, and an altered perception of time and space. This powerful experience tends to occur most often in the psychologically healthy and may produce long-lasting beneficial effects.

ADOLPH MEYER (1866–1950)

Adolph Meyer came to the United States from Switzerland in 1892 and eventually become director of the psychiatric Henry Phipps Clinic of Johns Hopkins Medical School. Although he did not entirely reject Freud's theoretical emphasis of mental functioning, Meyer preferred to examine the verifiable and objective aspects of a person's life. His theory of *psychobiology* explained disordered behavior as reactions to genetic, physical, psycholog-

ical, environmental, and social stresses. Meyer introduced the concept of *common sense psychiatry,* focusing on ways in which the patient's current life situation could be realistically improved. He coined the concept of *ergasia* which stands for the action of the total organism. The goal of therapy is to aid patients' adjustment by helping them modify unhealthy adaptations. One of Meyer's tools was an autobiographical life chart constructed by the patient during therapy.

GARDNER MURPHY (1895–1979)

Gardner Murphy was born in Ohio and received his Ph.D. at Columbia University. He was among the first to publish a comprehensive history of psychology and made major contributions to social, general, and educational psychology.

According to Murphy, three essential stages of personality development are: (1) the stage of undifferentiated wholeness, (2) the stage of differentiation, and (3) the stage of integration. This development is frequently uneven with the occurrence of regression as well as progression along the way.

There are four inborn human needs: visceral, motor, sensory, and emergency related. These needs become increasingly specific in time as they are molded by a person's experiences in various social and environmental contexts. *Canalization* brings about those changes by establishing a connection between a need and a specific way of satisfying that need.

Murphy was interested in parapsychology. Certain phenomena, such as clairvoyance and mental telepathy, may be more normal than paranormal. States—such as sleep, drowsiness, certain drug and toxic conditions, hypnosis, and delirium—tend to be favorable to paranormal experiences. Impediments to paranormal awareness include various intrapsychic barriers, conditions in the general social environment, and a heavy investment in the ordinary types of sensory experience.

HENRY MURRAY (b. 1893)

Henry Murray was born in New York City, attended medical school there, and was a founder of the Boston Psychoanalytic Institute. He proposed the term *personology* to describe the study of human behavior. He focused on motivation, which is a need that is aroused by internal or external stimulation; once aroused, it produces continued activity until it is reduced or satisfied. He developed the *Thematic Apperception Test* (TAT), a projective technique used to reveal both unconscious and conscious mental processes and problem areas.

FREDERICK S. PERLS (1893–1970)

Gestalt theory developed in Germany under the influence of several men: Max Westheimer (1880–1943), Wolfgang Kohler (1887–1967), and Kurt Lewin (1890–1947).

Frederick "Fritz" Perls applied Gestalt theory to a type of therapy that emphasizes the current experiences of the patient in the here and now, as contrasted to the "there and then" of the psychoanalytic schools. In terms of motivation, the patients learn to recognize what their needs are at any given time and how the drive to satisfy those needs may influence their current behavior. According to the Gestalt point of view, behavior represents more than the sum of its parts. A *gestalt,* or a whole, both includes and goes beyond the sum of smaller, independent events. It deals with essential characteristics of actual experience, such as value, meaning, and form.

SANDOR RADO (1890–1972)

Sandor Rado came to the United States from Hungary in 1945 and founded the Columbia Psychoanalytic Institute in New York. His theories of *adaptational dynamics* hold that the organism is a biological system operating under hedonic control, which is somewhat similar to Freud's pleasure principle. Cultural factors often cause excessive hedonic control and disordered behavior by interfering with the organism's ability for *self-regulation.* In therapy, the patient needs to relearn how to experience pleasurable feelings.

OTTO RANK (1884–1939)

In his 1924 publication, *The Trauma of the Birth,* Otto Rank broke with Freud and developed a new theory, which he called *birth trauma.* Anxiety is correlated with separation from the mother; specifically, with separation from the womb, the source of effortless gratification. This painful experience results in *primal anxiety.* Sleep and dreams symbolize the return to the womb.

The personality is divided into impulses, emotions, and will. The child's impulses seek immediate discharge and gratification. As impulses are mastered, as in toilet training, the child begins the process of will development. If will is carried too far, pathological traits—such as stubbornness, disobedience, and inhibitions—may develop.

WILHELM REICH (1897–1957)

Wilhelm Reich's major contributions to psychoanalysis were in the area of character formation and character types. *Character armor* is a term that refers to the defenses built up by the personality that serve as a resistence to self-understanding and change. There are four major character types: (1) The *hysterical character* is sexually seductive, anxious, and fixated at the phallic phase of libido development. (2) The *compulsive character* is controlled, distrustful, indecisive, and fixated at the anal phase. (3) The *narcissistic character* is confident, arrogant, aggressive, and fixated at the phallic stage of development; if male, there is a contempt for women. (4) The *masochistic character* is long-suffering, complaining, and self-deprecatory, with an excessive demand for love.

The therapeutic process—called *will therapy*—emphasizes the relationship between patient and therapist; the goal of treatment is to help persons accept their separateness. A definite date is used for termination of therapy to protect against excessive dependence on the therapist.

HARRY STACK SULLIVAN (1892–1949)

Harry Stack Sullivan received his training in psychiatry in the 1930s during the early years of Freud's profound influence on American psychiatry; but like Adolf Meyer, under whom he studied, Sullivan insisted on formulating his concepts on observable data.

There are three modes of experiencing and thinking about the world: (1) The *prototaxic mode* is undifferentiated thought that is unable to separate the whole into parts or to use symbols. It occurs normally in infancy and is also seen in patients with schizophrenia. (2) The *parataxic mode* sees events as causally related because of temporal or serial connections. Logical relationships, however, are not perceived. (3) The *syntaxic mode* is the logical, rational, and most mature type of cognitive functioning of which an individual is capable. These three types of thinking and experiencing occur side by side in all individuals; it is the rare person who functions in the syntaxic mode exclusively.

The total configuration of personality traits is known as the *self-system,* which develops in various stages and is the outgrowth of interpersonal experiences rather than the unfolding of intrapsychic forces. During *infancy,* anxiety occurs for the first time as a result of the infant's failure to achieve satisfaction of his or her primary needs. During *childhood,* from age 2 to 5 years, the child's main tasks are to become educated as to the requirements of the culture and to learn how to deal with powerful adults. As a *juvenile,* ranging from 5 to 8 years, the child has a need for and must learn how to deal with peers. In *preadolescence,* ranging from 8 to 12 years, the development of the capacity for love and collaboration with another person of the same sex develops. This so-called "chum" period is the prototype for a sense of intimacy; in the history of schizophrenic patients, this period is often missing. During *adolescence,* major tasks include the separation from one's family, the development of standards and values, and the transition to heterosexuality.

The process of therapy requires the active participation of the therapist, who is known as a *participant observer.* Modes of experience, particularly the parataxic, need to be clarified, and new patterns of behavior need to be implemented. Ultimately, persons need to see themselves as they really are, instead of what they think they are or what they want others to think they are.

References

Adler A: In *The Individual Psychology of Alfred Adler: A Systematic Presentation in Selections from His Writings,* H L Ansbacher, R R Ansbacher, editors: Basic Books, New York, 1956.

Baker H S, Baker M N: Heinz Kohot's self psychology: an overview. Am J Psych *144:* 1, 1987.

Blum G S: *Psychodynamics: The Science of Unconscious Mental Forces,* Brooks/Cole Publishing Company, Belmont, CA, 1966.

Bromberg W: *The Mind of Man.* Harper and Brothers, New York, 1959.

Horney K: *The Neurotic Personality of Our Time.* W W Norton, New York, 1937.

Jung C G: *Memories, Dreams, Reflections.* Random House, New York, 1961.

Millon T: *Theories of Psychopathology* (part 2). Saunders, Philadelphia, 1967.

Perry H S: *Psychiatrist of America: The Life of Harry Stack Sullivan.* The Belknap Press of Harvard University Press, Cambridge, MA, 1982.

Segal H: *Melanie Klein.* Viking Press, New York, 1980.

Smith S: *Ideas of the Great Psychologists.* Harper & Row, Philadelphia, 1983.

Wyss D: *Psychoanalytic Schools, From the Beginning to the Present.* Jason Aronson, New York, 1973.

8

Clinical Examination of the Psychiatric Patient

8.1

Psychiatric Interview

INTRODUCTION

The modern psychiatric interview is based on a clear understanding of psychopathology and psychodynamics. It is not a random or arbitrary meeting between doctor and patient. The psychiatric interview is characterized by the fact that the psychiatrist is an expert in the field of mental phenomena and interpersonal relations and, accordingly, offers the patient more than a sympathetic ear. Psychiatrists demonstrate their expertise by both the questions they do and do not ask and by certain other activities discussed later in this section.

The interview may be complicated by the fact that not all psychiatric patients have voluntarily sought the physician's help, and their willingness or ability to cooperate may be impaired. Psychiatric patients may be motivated to reveal themselves in order to gain relief from their suffering; but they may also be motivated to conceal their innermost feelings and the fundamental causes of their psychological disturbance.

If patients suspect that some of the less admirable aspects of their personality are involved in their illness, they may be unwilling to disclose such material until they are certain that they will not lose the doctor's respect as they expose themselves. For this reason, the psychiatrist's relationship with the patient strongly influences what the patient tells or does not tell him or her.

FACTORS INFLUENCING THE INTERVIEW

Many factors influence both the content and the process of the interview:

The nature of the patient's symptoms and character style significantly influence the transference and the way in which the interview unfolds.

Special clinical situations—such as the patient seen on a general hospital ward, the patient with psychosomatic symptoms, the psychologically unsophisticated patient, and the emergency patient—introduce specific dimensions that shape the interview.

Technical factors, such as telephone interruptions, the use of an interpreter, note taking, and the physical space and comfort of the room, affect the interview.

The timing of the interview in the patient's illness influences the content and the process of the interview.

The interviewer's style, orientation, and experience have a significant influence on the interview. Even the timing of interjections such as "uh-huh" influence patients' production as they unconsciously seek to follow the subtle leads provided by the interviewer.

ROLE OF THE INTERVIEWER

The most important role of the interviewer is to listen and to understand the patient. This understanding is then used to establish *rapport* and develop a treatment plan based on sound clinical judgment and the individual needs of the patient. Interviewers use their own empathic responses to facilitate the development of rapport. In general, interviewers are nonjudgmental, interested, concerned, and kind. They frequently ask questions to obtain information or clarify their own or the patient's understanding. Questions can be a subtle form of suggestion; or, by the tone of voice in which they are asked, they may give the patient permission to do something. For example, the interviewer may ask, "Did you ever tell your husband how you feel about that?"

Interviewers make either implicit or explicit suggestions to the patient. They may suggest that the patient discuss major decisions before acting on them, or that it would or would not be a good idea to discuss certain feelings with important persons in his or her life. They may, at times, give patients some advice or practical suggestions about their life. Many of the interviewer's activities serve to gratify the patient's emotional need to feel protected or loved. However, on many occasions, interviewers frustrate patients' emotional needs, since they cannot realistically make the patients' problems disappear by magic or find them a better job or a better spouse.

The interviewer may offer the patient suggestions concerning specific fears or offer general reassurance, such as, "Please continue, you're doing fine."

Interviewers may, in some situations, have to set limits with patients who have trouble controlling their impulses, or they may attempt to strengthen drives with other patients who are severely repressed.

Interviewers also help to build patients' self-esteem when they focus on patients' successful achievements and talents and can reduce patients' guilt through interventions designed to mollify a harsh superego.

Interviewers offer interpretations that aim at undoing the process of repression. This process allows unconscious thoughts and feelings to become conscious, thereby enabling patients to develop new methods of coping with their conflicts without the formation of symptoms. The two preliminary steps of an interpretation are confrontation, or pointing out that the patient is avoiding something, and clarification, or formulating the area to be explored.

PRACTICAL ISSUES

Time Factors

Psychiatric interviews last for varying lengths of time. The average consultation or therapeutic interview is 30 to 50 minutes long. Interviews with psychotic or medically ill patients are often brief, since the patient may find the interview stressful after 20 minutes. However, in the emergency room, longer interviews may be required. In most situations, the patient should know in advance approximately how long the interview will last.

Patients' management of time reveals an important facet of their personality. In most cases, patients arrive a few minutes early for their appointment. An anxious patient may arrive as much as a half-hour early. If the patient arrives very early and does not seem anxious, it probably deserves some exploration during the early part of the interview. The patient who arrives significantly late creates a problem for the interviewer. The first time it occurs, the interviewer might listen to the explanation if one is offered and even respond sympathetically if the lateness was clearly due to circumstances beyond patient's control. The psychiatrist, however, should avoid making such comments such as, "That's quite all right." If the patient indicates a blatant resistance—such as, "I forgot all about the appointment"—the psychiatrist might ask, "Did you feel some reluctance about coming?" If the answer is "Yes," the psychiatrist can explore the matter further. But if the reply is "No," it is better to drop the matter for the time being. It is sometimes appropriate to comment, "Well, we'll cover as much as we can in the time remaining."

The psychiatrist's handling of time is also an important factor in the interview. Chronic carelessness regarding time indicates a lack of concern for the patient. If the psychiatrist is unavoidably detained for an interview, it is quite appropriate to express regret that the patient was kept waiting.

Space Considerations

Most patients do not speak freely unless they have privacy and are sure that their conversations cannot be overheard. Quiet surroundings offer fewer distractions for both parties than a noisy atmosphere; interruptions are undesirable except for an occasional brief telephone call, preferably not more than one during an interview.

Proper seating arrangements also facilitate the interview. Both chairs should be of approximately equal heights so that neither person looks down on the other, and it is desirable to place the chairs so that no furniture is between the doctor and the patient. If the room contains several chairs, the doctor indicates his or her own chair and then allows the patient to choose the chair in which he or she will feel most comfortable. Overly dependent patients, for example, may prefer the chair that is closest to the doctor; oppositional or competitive patients choose a chair that is farther away, often the one that is directly across from the doctor.

Note Taking

Since there is a legal and moral responsibility to maintain an adequate record of each patient's diagnosis and treatment, the need for keeping written records about patients is clear. The patient's record also aids the psychiatrist's memory. Each interviewer must decide what type of information to record and must develop a system of record keeping.

The most common practice is to make fairly complete notes during the first few sessions while eliciting historical data. After this time, most psychiatrists record only new historical information, important events in the patient's life, medications prescribed and their effects, transference or countertransference trends, dreams, and general comments about the patient's progress.

Some patients express resentment if the psychiatrist wrote no notes during the interview; they feel that what they said must not have been sufficiently important to record or that the psychiatrist was uninterested. Other patients cannot tolerate note taking; in such cases, it should be discontinued.

INTERVIEW DATA

The Patient

The interview reveals data about the patient's psychopathology, psychodynamics, personality strengths, motivation, transference, and resistance.

Frequently, a patient comes to a psychiatrist expecting the doctor to be interested only in symptoms and possible deficiencies of character. It can be reassuring for such a patient when the psychiatrist shows some interest in his or her assets, talents, and other personality strengths. Although some patients volunteer such information, others must be asked, "Can you tell me some of the things you like about yourself?" Sensitivity and proper timing are required in the asking of such questions. There is little likelihood that the patient will demonstrate a capacity for joy and pride if, just after revealing painful material, he or she is asked, "Tell me, what do you do for fun?" It is preferable to lead the patient gently away from upsetting topics, allowing the opportunity of a transition period, before exploring capacities for warmth and tenderness.

Transference. Transference is a process in which patients unconsciously and inappropriately displace onto persons in their current life those patterns of behavior and emotional reactions that originated with significant figures from their childhood. The relative anonymity of psychiatrists and their role as a parent surrogate facilitates this displacement to them. (Patients' realistic and appropriate reactions to their doctors are not transference.)

Positive transference is limited to those idealized responses that are displaced from childhood figures and are now inappropriate. The omnipotent power that the patient delegates to the physician is an example. The same principles apply in defining negative transference, which stems from children's fear, anger, or mistrust of their parents.

Realistic factors concerning the doctor can be starting points for the initial transference. Age, sex, personal manner, and social and ethnic background all influence the rapidity and the direction of the patient's responses. The patient's desire for affection, respect, and gratification of dependent needs is the most widespread form of transference.

Resistance. Resistance is defined as any behavior on the part of the patient that blocks or delays the progress of treatment. Resistance may be expressed by the patterns of communication during the interview. Silence, garrulousness, censoring or editing thoughts, intellectualization, and preoccupation with one phase of life are some examples of a patient's resistance. Arriving late, forgetting the appointment, using a minor physical illness to avoid the session, seductive behavior, and competitive behavior are other common examples of resistance.

The Interviewer

The principal tool of the psychiatric interview is the psychiatrist. Each psychiatrist brings a different personal and professional background to the interview. Their character structure, values, and sensitivity to the feelings of others influence their attitude toward other human beings, patients and nonpatients alike. Differences in the social, educational and intellectual backgrounds of the patient and the interviewer may interfere with the development of rapport. It is an advantage for the psychiatrist to acquire as much understanding and familiarity as possible with the patient's subculture.

Therapeutic Alliance. The relationship between doctor and patient is geared toward alleviating the patient's symptoms. It is made up of the doctor's analyzing ego and the healthy, observing, rational component of the patient's ego. Sometimes called the working alliance, the therapeutic alliance is based on trust, empathy, and mutual respect.

Countertransference. Countertransference may be defined as the doctor's responding to the patient as if he or she was an important figure from the doctor's past. The more the patient actually resembles figures from the doctor's past, the greater the likelihood of such reactions. Examples include becoming dependent on the patient's praise or approval, being intolerant and frustrated when the patient is angry, being exhibitionistic to court the patient's favor, being unable to see inconsistencies in certain interpretations, insisting on one's own infallibility, being critical of prior psychiatrists the patient has seen, overidentifying with the patient, experiencing vicarious pleasure from the patient's sexual or aggressive behavior, power struggles, arguing with the patient, and wishing to be the patient's child or parent. Boredom or inability to concentrate on what the patient is saying often reflects unconscious anger or anxiety on the part of the interviewer.

INITIAL INTERVIEW

Doctors obtain much information when they first meet a patient. They can observe who, if anyone, has accompanied the patient and how the patient was passing the time while waiting for the interview to begin. The physician can greet the patient by name and then introduce himself or herself. Social pleasantries such as, "It's nice to meet you" are inappropriate. If the patient is unduly anxious, the doctor may introduce a brief social comment, perhaps inquiring if he or she had any difficulty in finding the office. A natural and pleasant manner on the part of the psychiatrist is useful to make the patient feel more at ease.

Development of Rapport

Initial Greeting. A suitable beginning is to ask the patient to be seated and then inquire, "What problem brings you here?" or "Could you tell me about your difficulty?" A less directive approach is to ask the patient, "Where shall we start?" or "Where would you prefer to begin?"

It is comforting for the patient who is not self-referred to feel that the physician already knows something about the problem. For example, the psychiatrist may say, "Dr. Jones has told me that you and your wife have had some difficulties" or "I understand that you've been quite depressed." Usually, the patient continues the story; but occasionally the patient asks, "Didn't he give you all the details?" The psychiatrist can reply, "He did go into more detail than that, but I'd like to hear more about it from you."

Understanding the Patient. To establish rapport, psychiatrists must communicate a feeling of understanding to the patient. They do not wish to create the impression that they can read the patient's mind, but they do want the patient to realize that they have treated other people with similar problems and that they understand these problems— not only as neurotic and psychotic symptoms but as ordinary problems in living.

Uncovering Feelings. A helpful technique to get patients better in touch with their emotions is to ask for specific examples when patients make general statements about their lives, such as, "My husband doesn't understand me" or "My mother was too overprotective." When the psychiatrist replies, "Can you give me an example?" or "What do you remember about that?" the patient is obliged to focus on those events and, in part, to relive them.

Frequently, patients struggle to maintain control over their emotions as the reliving of upsetting experiences reawakens their accompanying affects. If the interviewer observes that the patient stops speaking and has tears in his or her eye, the doctor may comment, "It makes you sad to speak of that" or "You're trying not to cry," or "It's all right to cry." Anger is another emotion that may be difficult to acknowledge. When the patient manifests no response, the doctor may indicate that a certain experience would make most people angry.

Abrupt Transition. An abrupt transition is sometimes required after the patient has discussed a present illness.

This transition can be done with a comment such as, "We have a lot of things that we haven't discussed yet, and, if we don't move on, we may not get to them" or "Our time is limited today, and we haven't talked about your marriage."

Exploring the Past.   Depending on the amount of time available and whether there will be more than one interview, the psychiatrist plans the inquiry into the patient's past. The question of which past issues are most significant varies with the patient's problems and the nature of the consultation.

Using the Patient's Words.   Using the patient's own words not only facilitates the development of rapport but actually helps avoid the resistance of the patient who argues over terms and different shades of meaning. This technique is particularly important when the psychiatrist wishes to return to a statement that the patient made earlier in the interview. Such occasions occur when the interviewer wants to allow the patient to continue with a point he or she was developing rather than to deflect the patient by pursuing another issue that the patient raised while telling the story. It is sometimes possible to conduct an entire and thorough interview without the doctor's having to introduce a new topic, merely by developing the patient's own references.

Open- and Closed-Ended Questions.   In most situations, closed-ended questions that can be answered "Yes" or "No" tend to place an undue burden on the interviewer and allow the patient to assume little responsibility for keeping the interview moving. However, it may be necessary to ask an evasive patient for a yes or no answer on certain occasions. Even when the interviewer wants to explore a particular topic, he or she can use an open-ended question in such a way as to give the patient the greatest possible leeway in answering. For example, a patient may indicate that her husband seems distant and overly involved with his work. The interviewer can ask, "What things do you do together for fun?" or "Has he always been that way?" These questions may uncover important information, but the interviewer might have learned even more by telling the patient, "Please go on" or "Tell me more about your marriage."

Stressing the Patient.   The psychiatrist occasionally finds it necessary to conduct a stress interview to help clarify the patient's diagnosis. For example, a patient with a suspected memory deficit may be skillful at covering up a problem. The interviewer must confront the patient in the memory area in order to establish the shared awareness of the patient's incapacity. The psychiatrist may also have to confront the patient's idiosyncratic ideas in order to elicit a delusion or to reveal the extent of the patient's thought disorder.

Patient's Questions.   About five or ten minutes should be set aside near the end of the initial interview to deal with certain issues. The patient who has been crying needs some time to regain composure before leaving the office. And, a patient who has come with a written or mental list of questions for the psychiatrist needs time to ask them.

As the end of the session nears, the psychiatrist may say, "We have about ten minutes remaining. Perhaps there are some questions you would like to ask." The patient may then reveal material that has been of concern throughout the interview; obsessive patients are noted for this behavior. Most often, the patient raises questions pertaining to an illness or need for treatment.

SUBSEQUENT INTERVIEWS

A single meeting with a patient permits only a cross-sectional study. If a second interview is planned, it is a good idea to allow a few days to intervene between the first and the second interviews. The added perspective provides supplementary information concerning how the patient may react to further treatment. The subsequent interview also allows the patient to correct any misinformation provided in the first meeting. It is often helpful to start the second interview by asking the patient if he or she has thoughts about the first interview and for any reactions to the experience. Another variation of this technique is for the doctor to say, "Frequently, people think of additional things they had wanted to discuss after they have left. What thoughts did you have?"

Psychiatrists often learn something of value when they ask patients if they discussed the interview with anyone else. If the patient has done so, it is enlightening to learn the details of that conversation and with whom the patient spoke.

There is no set of rules concerning which topics are best put off until the second interview. In general, as patients' comfort and familiarity with the physician increases, they are more able to reveal the most intimate details of their lives.

The patient's relatives may provide valuable information concerning the patient that helps the physician arrive at a treatment plan more quickly. There are three important guidelines in speaking with the relatives of adult patients: one is always to see the patient first. Another is to obtain the patient's permission before speaking with a family member; comatose or severely confused patients are the only exceptions to this rule. The third rule is not to violate the patient's confidence directly or indirectly. If any information provided by the patient needs to be discussed with a family member, the psychiatrist should obtain the patient's permission first.

The only exception to the third rule arises when the life of the patient or someone else is in danger. If the psychiatrist cannot obtain the patient's permission to reveal a plan for suicide or homicide and the patient refuses hospitalization, the doctor has an obligation to advise the family and to recommend hospitalization. If the doctor cannot obtain the patient's permission to disclose such data, he or she can at least give the patient the courtesy of saying that he or she plans to disclose that information and why. Some part of the patient may be relieved, even though he or she consciously objects.

References

Enelow A J, Swisher S N: *Interviewing and Patient Care*, ed 3. Oxford University Press, New York, 1986.

Freud S: The dynamics of transference. In *The Standard Edition of the Complete Works of Sigmund Freud*, Vol 12, pg 99. Hogarth Press, London, 1958.

Garrett A M: *Interviewing: Its Principles and Methods*. Family Welfare Association of America, New York, 1942.

Gill M, Newman R, Redlich F C: *The Initial Interview in Psychiatric Practice*. International University Press, New York, 1954.

Hersen M, Turner S M: *Diagnostic Interviewing*. Plenum Press, New York, 1985.

MacKinnon R A, Michaels R: *The Psychiatric Interview in Clinical Practice*. W B Saunders, Philadelphia, 1971.

MacKinnon R A, Yudofsky S C: *The Psychiatric Evaluation in Clinical Practice*. L B Lippincott, Philadelphia, 1986.

Powdermaker F: The techniques of the initial interview and methods of teaching them. Am. J. Psychiatry *104*: 642, 1948.

Reiser D E, Schroder A K: *Patient Interviewing: The Human Dimension*. Williams & Wilkins, Baltimore, 1980.

Sullivan H S: *The Psychiatric Interview*. W W Norton, New York, 1954.

8.2 ————

Psychiatric History and Mental Status Examination

PSYCHIATRIC HISTORY

Introduction

Psychiatrists, as well as other specialists in medicine, rely on a careful history as the foundation for the diagnosis and treatment of every illness. The psychiatric history strives to convey the more elusive picture of patients' individual personality characteristics, including both their strengths and weaknesses. It provides insight into the nature of their relationships with those closest to them and includes all the important people in their past and present life. A complete story of the patient's life is impossible to obtain; however, a reasonably comprehensive picture of the patient's development, from the earliest formative years until the present, can usually be elicited.

The most important technique in obtaining the psychiatric history is to allow patients to tell their own story in their own words in the order that they feel is most important. Skillful interviewers recognize those points, as patients relate their story, at which they can introduce relevant questions concerning the areas described in the outline of the psychiatric history and the mental status examination.

The organization of this section is only for the purpose of preparing the written record.

Preliminary Identification

The psychiatrist should begin the written history by stating the patient's name, age, marital status, sex, occupation, language if other than English, race, nationality, religion, and a brief statement about the patient's place of residence and circumstances of living. Comments such as, "The patient lives alone in a furnished room" or "The patient lives with her husband and three children in a three bedroom apartment" provide adequate detail for this part. If the patient is hospitalized, a statement can be included as to the number of previous admissions for similar conditions.

Chief Complaint

The chief complaint is the presenting problem for which the patient seeks professional help. The chief complaint should be stated in the patient's own words; if the information is not supplied by the patient, the record should contain a description of the person who supplied it and his or her relationship to the patient. In many cases, the patient does not begin the story with the chief complaint. One or more sessions may be required for the physician to learn what it is that the patient finds most disturbing or why the patient seeks treatment at this particular time. In other situations, the chief complaint is provided by someone other than the patient. For example, an acutely confused and disoriented patient may be brought in by someone else who provides the chief complaint concerning the patient's confusion. Ideally, the chief complaint should give the explanation for why the patient seeks treatment now.

Personal Identification

Although a detailed description of the patient appears at the beginning of the mental status part of the record, it is useful to have a brief, nontechnical description of the patient's appearance and behavior. What is needed here is a description that would enable someone who had never met the patient identify him or her sitting in a waiting room with many other people.

History of Present Illness

During the interview, the psychiatrist must allow an adequate amount of time to explore the details of the patient's presenting symptoms. These symptoms are usually the prime reason the patient decided to consult a psychiatrist. An account of each symptom—its nature, cause, and associated features—is required. Particular attention must be paid to the first symptom and the most disabling symptoms. Most often, a relatively unstructured question such as, "How did it all begin?" leads to an adequate unfolding of the present illness. A well-organized patient is able to present a reasonably chronological account of the difficulties. However, major modifications may be necessary when interviewing a disorganized patient.

In addition, the psychiatrist should learn the details of the patient's life circumstances at the onset of the symptoms and behavioral changes that culminated in seeking assistance. The doctor should also ascertain the ways in which the patient's illness affected his or her life activities—for example, did the patient lose a job or did the spouse leave?

Previous Illness

The previous illness section is a transition between the story of the present illness and the past personal history. Here, prior episodes of emotional and mental disturbances are described. The patient's symptoms, extent of incapacity, type of treatment received, names of hospitals, length of each illness, and effects of prior treatments should all be explored and recorded chronologically. Particular attention should be paid to the first and most recent episodes, as well as to suicidal episodes. It is frequently helpful to assess the patient's past compliance with prescribed treatment at this point.

Past Medical History

The psychiatrist should note any major medical illness the patient has experienced, particularly those requiring hospitalization (e.g., surgical disorders, accidents, and complications of obstetric procedures). The cause, complications, and treatment of the illnesses, as well as the effects on the patient, should be noted. The physician must also inquire about prescribed medications. All patients should be asked about alcohol and drug use. If the patient uses or has used abusable substances, the quantity and frequency of use should be questioned. Extensive drug and alcohol use or problems associated with their use in the patient's life must be explored in great depth. For patients in certain subcultures, it is important to ask about use of specific substances (e.g., cocaine, marijuana, or heroin).

In certain settings and with certain patients, it is useful to screen for the likelihood of an organic mental syndrome. Such inquiries involve specific questions about the presence of a seizure disorder, episodes of loss of consciousness, a change in usual headache patterns, and a change in vision.

In addition to studying the patient's present illness and current life situation, the psychiatrist needs a thorough understanding of the patient's past life and its relationship to the present emotional problem.

The past history is usually divided into the major developmental periods of prenatal, infancy, early childhood, middle childhood or latency, late childhood, and adulthood.

Prenatal History. The psychiatrist considers the nature of the home situation into which the patient was born and whether the patient was planned and wanted. Were there any problems with the mother's pregnancy and delivery? Was there any evidence of defect or injury at birth?

Early Childhood. The early childhood period consists of the first three years of the patient's life. The quality of the mother-child interaction during feeding and toilet training is important. It is frequently possible to learn whether the child presented problems in these areas. Early disturbances in sleep patterns and signs of unmet needs, such as head banging and body rocking, provide clues about possible maternal deprivation. In addition, it is important to obtain a history of human constancy during the first three years. Did persons other than the mother care for the patient? Did the patient exhibit problems at an early period with stranger anxiety or separation anxiety? The patient's siblings and the details of his or her relationship to them are other areas to be explored.

The emerging personality of the child is also a topic of crucial importance. Was the child shy, restless, overactive, withdrawn, studious, outgoing, timid, athletic, friendly? The clinician should seek data concerning the child's increasing ability to concentrate, to tolerate frustration, to postpone gratification, and, as he or she became older, to cooperate with peers, to be fair, to understand and comply with rules, and to develop mature conscience mechanisms. The child's preference for active or passive roles in physical play should also be noted.

The psychiatrist should also ask the patient for his or her earliest memory and for any recurrent dreams or fantasies that occurred during the first three years.

Middle Childhood (Ages 3 to 11 Years). In this section, the psychiatrist can address such important subjects as gender identification, punishments used in the home, and who provided the discipline and influenced early conscience formation. The psychiatrist must inquire about the patient's early school experiences, especially how the patient first tolerated being separated from his or her mother. Data about the patient's earliest friendships and peer relations are valuable. The psychiatrist should identify and define the number and closeness of the patient's friends, describe whether the patient took the role of a leader or follower, and describe the patient's social popularity and participation in group or gang activities. Early patterns of assertion, impulsiveness, aggression, passivity, anxiety, or antisocial behavior emerge in the context of school relationships. A history of the patient's learning to read, as well as the development of other intellectual and motor skills, is important. A history of minimal cerebral dysfunction or of learning disabilities, their management, and their impact on the child is of particular significance. The presence of nightmares, phobias, bed wetting, fire setting, cruelty to animals, and masturbation should also be explored.

Late Childhood (Prepuberty Through Adolescence). During late childhood, people begin to develop independence from their parents through relationships with peers and in group activities. The psychiatrist should attempt to define the values of the patient's social groups and determine who were the patient's idealized figures. This information provides useful clues concerning the patient's emerging idealized self-image.

Further exploration is indicated of the patient's school history, relationships with teachers, and favorite studies and interests, both in school and in the extracurricular area. The psychiatrist should ask about the patient's participation in sports and hobbies and inquire about any emotional or physical problems that may have first appeared during this phase. Common examples include feelings of inferiority, weight problems, smoking, running away form home, and drug or alcohol use or abuse.

Psychosexual History. Much of the history of infantile sexuality is not recoverable, although many patients are able to recall curiosities and sexual games played during the ages of 3 to 6 years. The interviewer should ask how patients learned about sex and what attitudes they felt their parents had about their sexual development. The interviewer can also inquire if the patient was sexually abused during childhood.

The onset of puberty and the patient's feelings about that milestone is important. Female patients should be questioned about preparation for the onset of their menses and about the circumstances and their feelings concerning the development of secondary sexual characteristics. The adolescent masturbatory history, including the nature of the patient's fantasies and feelings about them, is of significance. The interviewer should routinely inquire about dating, petting, crushes, parties, and sex games. Attitudes toward the opposite sex should be described in detail. Was the patient shy, timid, aggressive? Or did the patient need to impress others and boast of sexual conquests? Did the patient experience anxiety in the sexual setting? Was there promiscuity? Did the patient participate in homosexual, group masturbatory, incestuous, aggressive, or perverse sexual behavior?

Religious Background. The psychiatrist should describe the religious background of both parents and the details of the patient's religious instruction. Was the family attitude toward religion strict or permissive, and were there any conflicts between the two parents over the religious education of the child? The psychiatrist should trace the evolution of the patient's adolescent religious practices to present beliefs and activities.

Adulthood.

Occupational and advanced educational history. The psychiatrist should describe the patient's choice of occupation, the requisite training and preparation, and the long-term ambitions and goals. The interviewer should also explore the patient's feeling about his or her current job and relationships at work (with authorities, peers, and, if applicable, subordinates) and describe the job history (e.g., number and duration of jobs, reasons for job changes, and changes in job status).

Social activity. The psychiatrist should describe the patient's social life and the nature of friendships, with emphasis on the depth, duration, and quality of human relations. What type of social, intellectual, and physical interests does the patient share with friends?

Adult sexuality. The premarital sexual history should include any sexual symptoms—such as anorgasmia, vaginismus, impotence, premature or retarded ejaculation, and paraphilias.

Marital history. In this section, the interviewer describes each marriage, legal or common law, that the patient has had. Significant relationships with persons with whom the patient has lived for a protracted period of time are also included. The story of the marriage should include a description of the courtship. The evolution of the relationship should be explored and should describe the areas of agreement and disagreement, including the management of money, the roles of the in-laws, attitudes toward raising children, and sexual adjustment. The topic of their sexual adjustment should include a description of how their sexual activity is usually initiated, the frequency of their sexual relations, and their sexual preferences, variations, and techniques. It is usually appropriate to inquire if either party has engaged in extramarital relationships and, if so, under what circumstances and whether the spouse knew of the affair. If the spouse did learn of the affair, it is important to describe what happened. The reasons underlying an extramarital affair are just as important as an understanding of its effect on the marriage. Attitudes toward contraception and family planning are important, and the names, ages, descriptions, and relationships of the patient to all the children should be obtained. It is important to obtain some assessment of the patient's capacity to function adequately in the parental role.

Military history. The psychiatrist should inquire about the patient's general adjustment to the military, whether he saw combat or sustained an injury, and the nature of his discharge. Was he ever referred for psychiatric consultation, and did he suffer any disciplinary action during his period of service?

Family History

A brief statement about any psychiatric illnesses, hospitalizations and treatments of the patient's immediate family members should be placed in this part of the report. In addition, the family history should provide a description of the personalities of the various people living in the patient's home from childhood to the present. The psychiatrist should also define the role each person has played in the patient's upbringing and the current relationships with the patient. Informants other than the patient may be available to contribute to the family history, and the source should be cited in the written record. Finally, the psychiatrist should determine the family's attitude toward and insight into the

patient's illness. Does the patient feel that they are supportive, indifferent, or destructive?

Current Social Situation

The psychiatrist should inquire about where the patient lives in sufficient detail to describe the neighborhood, as well as the patient's residence. He or she should include the number of rooms, the number of family members living in the home, and the sleeping arrangements. The psychiatrist should inquire as to how issues of privacy are handled, with particular emphasis on parental and sibling nudity and bathroom arrangements. He or she should ask about the sources of family income and any financial hardships. If applicable, the psychiatrist might inquire about public assistance and the patient's feelings about it. If the patient has been hospitalized, have provisions been made so that he or she will not lose a job or apartment? The psychiatrist should ask who is caring for the children at home, who visits the patient in the hospital, and how frequently.

Dreams, Fantasies, and Value Systems

Freud stated that the dream is the royal road to the unconscious. Repetitive dreams are of particular value. If the patient has nightmares, what are their repetitive themes? Some of the most common themes of dreams are food, examinations, sex, helplessness, and impotence. Fantasies or daydreams are another valuable source of unconscious material. As with dreams, the psychiatrist can explore and record all manifest details and attendant feelings.

Finally, the psychiatrist may inquire about the patient's system of values—both social and moral—including values that concern work, play, children, parents, friends, community concerns, and cultural interests.

MENTAL STATUS EXAMINATION

General Description

Appearance. This is a description of the patient's appearance and the overall physical and emotional impression conveyed to the interviewer, as reflected by posture, bearing, clothing, grooming, and dominant attitude toward the interviewer. Other aspects include the patient's degree of poise, the amount of anxiety manifested, and the manner in which it is expressed. A narrative paragraph describing these aspects should allow someone who does not know the patient to easily recognize him or her in a room full of people.

Behavior and Psychomotor Activity. This category refers to both the quantitative and qualitative aspects of the patient's motor behavior. The psychiatrist should describe any mannerisms, tics, gestures, twitches, stereotyped behavior, echopraxia, hyperactivity, agitation, combativeness, flexibility, and rigidity, as well as the patient's gait and agility.

Attitude Toward Examiner. The patient's attitude toward the examiner can be described as cooperative, friendly, attentive, interested, frank, seductive, defensive, hostile, playful, ingratiating, evasive, or guarded; any number of other adjectives can be used.

Speech Activity. This part of the report is used to describe the physical characteristics of speech. Speech can be described in terms of its quantity, its rate of production, and its quality. The patient may be described as talkative, garrulous, voluble, taciturn, unspontaneous, or normally responsive to cues from the interviewer. Speech may be rapid or slow, pressured, hesitant, emotional, monotonous, loud, whispered, slurred, or mumbled. Impairments of speech, such as stuttering and echolalia, are included in this section.

Mood, Feelings, and Affect

Mood. The psychiatrist is interested in whether the patient remarks voluntarily about feelings or whether it is necessary to ask the patient how he or she feels. Statements about the patient's mood should include depth, intensity, duration, and fluctuations.

Affective Expression. In the normal expression of affect, there is a variation in facial expression, tone of voice, use of hands, and body movements. When affect is restricted, there is a clear reduction in the range and intensity of expression. In blunted affect, there is severe reduction in the intensity of affective expression. To diagnose flat affect, one should find virtually no signs of affective expressions, the patient's voice should be monotonous, and the face should be immobile. Blunted, flat, and shallow refer to the depth of emotion; depressed, proud, angry, fearful, anxious, guilty, euphoric, and expansive refer to particular affects.

Appropriateness. The appropriateness of the patient's emotional responses can be considered only in the context of the subject matter the patient is discussing. Paranoid patients who are describing a delusion of persecution should be angry about the experiences they believe are happening to them. Anger in this context is not an inappropriate affect. Some psychiatrists have reserved the term "inappropriateness of affect" for a quality of response found in the schizophrenic patient.

Perception

Perceptual disturbances, such as hallucinations and illusions, may be experienced in reference to the self or the environment. The sensory system involved, as well as the content of the hallucinatory experience, should be described. The circumstances of the occurrence of any hallucinatory experience are important, since hypnagogic and hypnopompic hallucinations are of much less serious significance than other types of hallucinations. Feelings of depersonalization and derealization are also examples of perceptual disturbance.

Thought Process (Form of Thinking)

Stream of Thought. The patient may either have an overabundance or a paucity of ideas. There may be rapid thinking, which if carried to the extreme is called a flight of ideas. Another patient may exhibit slow or hesitant thinking.

Do the patient's replies really answer the questions asked, and does the patient have the capacity for goal-directed thinking? Is there a clear cause-and-effect relationship in the patient's explantions? Does the patient have loose associations? Disturbances of the continuity of thought involve statements that are tangential, circumstantial, rambling, evasive, or perseverative. Blocking is an interruption of the train of speech before a thought or idea has been completed; the patient indicates that he or she cannot recall what was being said or intended to be said. Circumstantiality indicates the loss of capacity for goal-directed thinking; in the process of explaining an idea, the patient brings in many irrelevant details and parenthetical comments. Distractibility is a disturbance of thought process; the patient loses the thread of the conversation and pursues tangential thoughts stimulated by various external or internal irrelevant stimuli.

Language impairments may be reflected by incoherent or incomprehensible speech (word salad), clang associations, and neologisms.

Content of Thought. Disturbances in content of thought include preoccupations, which may involve the patient's illness, environmental problems, obsessions, compulsions, and phobias. A major category of disturbances of thought content involves delusions. The content of any delusional system should be described, and the psychiatrist should attempt to evaluate its organization and the patient's conviction as to its validity. The manner in which it affects the patient's life is appropriately described in the history of the present illness. Ideas of reference and ideas of influence should also be described.

Abstract thinking is the ability of the patient to deal with concepts. Asking the patient to give the meaning of a simple proverb, "People who live in glass houses shouldn't throw stones," may reveal concrete thinking—"The glass will break."

Sensorium and Cognition

This portion of the mental status examination seeks to assess the brain function and intelligence of the patient. Although there are no pathognomonic signs, impairments in these functions increase the probability that brain disorder is present. Sensorium refers to the state of functioning of the special senses.

Consciousness. Disturbances of consciousness usually indicate organic brain impairment. The term "clouding of consciousness" describes an overall reduced awareness to the environment. A patient may be unable to sustain attention of environmental stimuli or to sustain goal-directed thinking or behavior. Clouding or obtunding of consciousness is frequently not a fixed mental state. The typical patient manifests fluctuations in his or her level of awareness of the surrounding environment. The patient who has an altered state of consciousness often shows some impairment of orientation as well, although the reverse is not true.

Orientation. Disorders of orientations are traditionally separated according to time, place, and person. Any impairment usually appears in this order; similarly, as the patient improves, the impairment clears in the reverse order. It is necessary to determine whether patients can give the approximate date. In addition, if patients are in a hospital, do they know how long they have been there? And do the patients behave as though they are oriented to the present? In questions about the patients' orientation for place, it is not sufficient that they be able to state the name and the location of the hospital correctly; they should also behave as though they know where they are. In assessing orientation for person, the interviewer asks patients whether they know the names of the people who are around them, and whether they understand their roles in relationships to them. It is only in the most severe instances that patients do not know who they are.

Concentration and Cognition. Subtracting serial 7's from 100 is a simple task that requires both concentration and cognitive capacities to be intact. It may not always be clear to the examiner whether the patient's difficulty in performing the task is due to anxiety, a disturbance of mood, some alteration of consciousness, or, at times, a combination of all three.

Memory. Memory functions have been traditionally divided into four areas: remote memory, recent past memory, recent memory, and immediate retention and recall. Recent memory may be checked by asking the patient about his or her appetite and then inquiring what was had for breakfast or for dinner the previous evening. The patient may be asked at this point if he or she recalls the interviewer's name. Asking the patient to repeat six digits forward and then backward is a test for immediate retention. Remote memory can be tested by asking the patient for information about his or her childhood that can be later verified. Asking the patient to recall important news events from the past few months checks recent remote memory.

Information and Intelligence. If the physician has detected a possible organic mental impairment, he or she can inquire whether the patient has trouble with mental tasks, such as counting the change from $10.00 after a purchase of $6.37. If this task is too difficult, easier problems may be substituted. The patient's intelligence is related to vocabulary and general fund of knowledge (e.g., the distance from New York to Paris, Presidents of the United States). Similarities between nouns (e.g., an apple and pear) or concepts (e.g., truth and beauty) is a sensitive test of intellectual capacity. The patient's education level and socioeconomic status must be taken into account.

Judgment

During the course of the history taking, the examiner should be able to assess many aspects of the patient's capacity for social judgment. Does the patient understand the likely outcome of his or her behavior and is he or she influenced by that understanding? For instance, a patient may be asked, "What would you do if you found a stamped, addressed letter in the street?"

Insight

Insight refers to patients' degree of awareness and understanding that they are ill. Patients may exhibit a complete denial of their illness, or may show some awareness that they are ill but place the blame on others, on external factors, or even on organic factors. They may acknowledge that they have an illness but ascribe it to something unknown or mysterious in themselves.

Intellectual insight is present when patients can admit that they are ill and acknowledge that their failures in adaptation are, in part, due to their own irrational feelings. However, the major limitation to intellectual insight is that the patient is unable to apply knowledge in order to alter future experiences. True emotional insight is present when patients' awareness of their own motives and deep feelings leads to a change in their personality or behavior patterns.

Reliability

The mental status part of the report concludes with the examiner's impression of the patient's reliability and capacity to report his or her situation accurately.

Recommendations

In formulating the treatment plan, the clinician should note whether the patient requires psychiatric treatment at this time and, if so, what problems and target symptoms the treatment is aimed at; what kind of treatment or combination of treatments the patient should receive; and what treatment setting seems most appropriate. If hospitalization is recommended, the clinician should specify the reasons for hospitalization, the type of hospitalization indicated, the urgency with which the patient has to be hospitalized, and the anticipated duration of inpatient care. The clinician should estimate the immediate and long-term prognosis of the patient's illness and the estimated length of treatment.

If either the patient or family is unwilling to accept the recommendations for treatment and the clinician feels that the refusal of the recommendations may have serious consequences, the patient or a parent or guardian should be invited to sign a statement that the recommended treatment was refused.

References

American Psychiatric Association: *Diagnostic and Statistical Manual of Mental Disorders,* ed III-R. American Psychiatric Association, Washington, D C, 1986.

Baker N J, Berry S L, Adler I. E: Family diagnoses missed on a clinical inpatient service. Am J Psych *144*; 630, 1987

Hayman M: Two minute clinical test for measurement of intellectual impairment in psychiatric disorders. Arch Neurol Psychiatry 47: 454, 1942.

Keller M B, Manschreck T C: The bedside mental status examination— Reliability and validity. Comp Psychiatry *22*: 500, 1981.

Lewis N D C: *Outlines for Psychiatric Examinations,* ed 3, New York State Department of Mental Hygiene, Albany, 1943.

MacKinnon R A, Michels R: *The Psychiatric Interview in Clinical Practice.* W B Saunders, New York, 1971.

Menninger K A, Mayman M, Pruyser P W, editors: *A Manual for Psychiatric Case Study,* ed 2, Grune & Stratton, New York, 1962.

Ryback R: *The Problem-Oriented Record in Psychiatry and Mental Health Care.* Grune & Stratton, New York, 1974.

Spitzer R L: Immediately available record of mental status exam: The mental status schedule inventory. Arch Gen Psychiatry *13*: 76, 1965.

Stevenson I: *The Psychiatric Examination.* Little, Brown & Co, Boston, 1969.

Strub R L, Black F W: *The Mental Status Examination in Neurology,* ed 2, F A Davis Co., Philadelphia, 1985.

Swift M. The family history in clinical psychiatric practice. Am J Psych *144*: 628, 1987.

8.3

Psychiatric Report

The following summary represents an outline the student may use to write a psychiatric report.

I. Psychiatric history

A. Preliminary identification: name, age, marital status, sex, occupation, language if other than English, race, nationality, and religion insofar as they are pertinent; previous admissions to a hospital for the same or different conditions; person or people with whom the patient lives.

B. Chief complaint: exactly why the patient came to the psychiatrist, preferably in the patient's own words; if this information does not come from the patient, note who supplied it.

C. Personal identification: brief, nontechnical description of the patient's appearance and behavior as a novelist might write it.

D. History of present illness: chronological background and development of the symptoms or behavioral changes culminating in the patient's seeking assistance; patient's life precipitating stress circumstances at the time of onset; personality when well; how illness has affected patient's life activities and personal relations—changes in personality, memory, speech; psychophysiological symptoms—nature and details of dysfunction; location, intensity, fluctuation; relationship between physical and psychic symptoms; extent to which illness serves some additional purpose for the patient when dealing with stress—secondary gain; whether anxieties are generalized and nonspecific (free floating) or are specifically related to particular situations, activities, or objects; how anxieties are handled—avoidance of feared situations, use of drugs or other activities for distraction.

E. Previous illnesses

1. Emotional or mental disturbances: extent of symptoms and incapacity, type of treatment, names of hospitals, length of illness, effect of treatment, compliance

2. Psychosomatic disorders: hay fever, rheumatoid arthritis, ulcerative colitis, asthma, hyperthyroidism, gastrointestinal upsets, recurrent colds, skin conditions

3. Medical conditions, following the customary medical review of systems, if necessary; syphilis, use of alcohol or drugs; at risk for AIDS

4. Neurological disorders: history of craniocerebral trauma, convulsions, or tumors

F. Past personal history: history (anamnesis) of the patient's life from infancy to the present to the extent that it can be recalled; gaps in history as spontaneously related by the patient; emotions associated with these life periods—painful, stressful, conflictual.

1. Prenatal history: nature of mother's pregnancy and delivery: length of pregnancy, spontaneity and normality of delivery, birth trauma, whether patient was planned and wanted, birth defects

2. Early childhood (through age 3)

a. Feeding habits: breast-fed or bottle-fed, eating problems

b. Early development—walking, talking, and teething—language development, motor development, signs of unmet needs, sleep pattern, object constancy, stranger anxiety, maternal deprivation, separation anxiety, other caretakers in home

c. Toilet training: age, attitude of parents, feelings about it

d. Symptoms of behavior problems: thumb sucking, temper tantrums, tics, head bumping, rocking, night-terrors, fears, bed-wetting or bed-soiling, nail-biting, masturbation

e. Personality as a child: shy, restless, overactive, withdrawn, persistent, outgoing, timid, athletic, friendly, patterns of play

f. Early or recurrent dreams or fantasies

3. Middle childhood (3 to 11): early school history—feelings about going to school, early adjustment, gender identification, conscience development, punishment, peer relations, nightmares, phobias, bed-wetting, fire-setting, cruelty to animals

4. Later childhood (puberty through adolescence)

a. Social relationships: attitudes toward sibling(s) and playmates, number and closeness of friends, leader or follower, social popularity, participation in group or gang activities, idealized figures; patterns of aggression, passivity, anxiety, antisocial behavior

b. School history: how far the patient progressed, adjustment to school, relationships with teachers—teacher's pet vs. rebellious, favorite studies or interests, particular abilities or assets, extracurricular activities, sports, hobbies, relationships of problems or symptoms to any school period

c. Cognitive and motor development: learning to read and other intellectual and motor skills, minimal cerebral dysfunctions, learning disabilities—their management and effects on the child

d. Adolescent emotional or physical problems: nightmares, phobias, masturbation, bed-wetting, running away, delinquency, smoking, drug or alcohol use, anorexia, bulimia, weight problems, feelings of inferiority

5. Psychosexual history (childhood through adolescence)

a. Early curiosity, infantile masturbation, sex play

b. Acquisition of sexual knowledge, attitude of parents toward sex, sexual abuse

c. Onset of puberty, feelings about it, kind of preparation, feelings about menstruation, development of secondary sexual characteristics

d. Adolescent sexual activity: crushes, parties, dating, petting, masturbation, nocturnal emissions and attitudes toward them

e. Attitudes toward opposite sex: timid, shy, aggressive, need to impress, seductive, sexual conquests, anxiety

f. Sexual practices: sexual problems, homosexual experiences, paraphilias, promiscuity

6. Religious background: strict, liberal, mixed (possible conflicts), relationship of background to current religious practices

7. Adulthood

a. Occupational history: choice of occupation, training, ambitions, conflicts; relations with authority, peers, and subordinates; number of jobs and duration; changes in job status; current job and feelings about it

b. Social activity: does patient have friends, is patient withdrawn or socializing well; kind of social, intellectual, and physical interests; relationships with same sex and opposite sex; depth, duration, and quality of human relationships

c. Adult sexuality

i. Premarital and extramarital sexual relationships

ii. Marital history: common-law marriages, legal marriages, description of courtship and role played by each partner, age at marriage, family planning and contraception, names and ages of children, attitudes toward raising children, problems of any family members, housing difficulties if important to the marriage, sexual adjustment, areas of agreement and disagreement, management of money, role of in-laws

iii. Sexual symptoms: anorgasmia, impotence, premature ejaculation, lack of desire

iv. Attitudes toward pregnancy and having children; contraceptive practices and feelings about them

v. Sexual practices: paraphilias such as sadism, fetishes, voyeurism; attitudes about fellatio, cunnilingus, and coital techniques; frequency

d. Military history: general adjustment, combat, injuries, referral to psychiatrists, veteran status, disciplinary action

G. Family history: elicited from patient and from someone else because quite different descriptions may be given of the same people and events; ethnic, national, and religious traditions; other people in the home, descriptions of them—personality and intelligence—and what has become of them since the patient's childhood; descriptions of different households lived in; present relationships between patient and other people who were in the family; role of illness in the family; history of mental illness and treatment.

H. Current social situation: where does patient live—neighborhood and particular residence of the patient; is home crowded; privacy of family members from each other and from other families; sources of family income and difficulties in obtaining it; public assistance, if any, and attitudes about it; will patient lose job or apartment by remaining in the hospital; who is caring for children.

I. Dreams, fantasies, and value systems

1. Dreams: prominent ones, if patient will tell them; nightmares

2. Fantasies: recurrent, favorite, or unshakable daydreams; hypnagogic phenomena

3. Value systems: whether children are seen as a burden or a joy; whether work is seen as a necessary evil, an avoidable chore, or an opportunity; concept of right and wrong

II. Mental Status: sum total of the examiner's observations and impressions derived from the initial interviews

A. General description

1. Appearance: body type, posture, bearing, clothes, grooming, hair, nails; healthy, sickly, angry, frightened, apathetic, perplexed, contemptuous, ill at ease, poised, old looking, young looking, effeminate, masculine; signs of anxiety—moist hands, perspiring forehead, restlessness, tense posture, strained voice, wide eyes; shift in level of anxiety during interview or abrupt changes of topic

2. Behavior and psychomotor activity: gait, mannerisms, tics, gestures, twitches, stereotypes, picking, touching examiner, echopraxia, clumsy, agile, limp, rigid, retarded, hyperactive, agitated, combative, waxy

3. Speech: rapid, slow, pressured, hesitant, emotional, monotonous, loud, whispered, slurred, mumbled, stuttering, echolalia, intensity, pitch, ease, spontaneity, productivity, manner, reaction time, vocabulary

4. Attitude toward examiner: cooperative, attentive, interested, frank, seductive, defensive, hostile, playful, ingratiating, evasive, guarded, level of rapport

B. Mood, feelings, and affect

1. Mood (a pervasive and sustained emotion that colors the person's perception of the world): how does patient say he or she feels; depth, intensity, duration, and fluctuations of mood—depressed, despairing, irritable, anxious, terrified, angry, expansive, euphoric, empty, guilty, awed, futile, self-contemptuous

2. Affective expression: how examiner evaluates patient's affects—broad, restricted, depressed, blunted or flat, shallow, anhedonic, labile, constricted, fearful, anxious, guilty; amount and range of expression; difficulty in initiating, sustaining, or terminating an emotional response

3. Appropriateness: is the emotional expression appropriate to the thought content, the culture, and the setting of the examination; note examples if emotional expression is not appropriate

C. Perceptual disturbances

1. Hallucinations and illusions: does patient hear voices or see visions; content, sensory system involved, circumstances of the occurrence; hypnagogic or hypnopompic hallucinations

2. Depersonalization and derealization: extreme feelings of detachment from one's self or the environment

D. Thought process

1. Stream of thought: quotations from patient

a. Productivity: overabundance of ideas, paucity of ideas, flight of ideas, rapid thinking, slow thinking, hesitant thinking; does patient speak spontaneously or only when questions are asked

b. Continuity of thought: do patient's replies really answer questions; are they goal directed and relevant or irrelevant; is there a lack of cause-and-effect relationships in patient's explanations; are statements illogical, tangential, rambling, evasive, perserverative; is there blocking or distractibility

c. Language impairments: impairments that reflect disordered mentation, such as incoherent or incomprehensible speech (word salad), clang associations, neologisms

2. Content of thought

a. Preoccupations: about the illness; environmental problems; obsessions, compulsions, phobias; plans, intentions, recurrent ideas about suicide, homicide, hypochondriacal symptoms, specific antisocial urges; specific questions should always be asked about suicidal ideation

b. Thought disturbances

i. Delusions: content of any delusional system, its organization, the patient's convictions as to its validity, how it affects patient's life; somatic delusions—isolated or associated with pervasive suspiciousness; mood-congruent delusions—in keeping with a depressed or elated mood; mood-incongruent delusions—not keeping with the patient's mood; bizarre delusions, such as thoughts of being controlled by external forces or thoughts being broadcast out loud

ii. Ideas of reference and ideas of influence: how ideas began, their content and the meaning the patient attributes to them

iii. Abstract thinking: disturbances in concept formation; manner in which the patient conceptualizes or handles ideas; similarities, differences, absurdities, meanings of simple proverbs, such as "A rolling stone gathers no moss"; answers may be concrete (giving specific examples to illustrate the meaning) or overly abstract (giving generalized explanation); appropriateness of answers should be noted

E. Sensorium and Cognition

1. Consciousness: clouding, somnolence, stupor, coma, lethargy, alertness, fugue state

2. Orientation

a. Time: does patient identify the day correctly; can patient approximate date, time of day; if patient is in a hospital, does the patient know how long he or she has been there; does patient behave as though he or she is oriented to the present

b. Place: does patient know where he or she is

c. Person: does patient know who the examiner is: does patient know the roles or names of the persons with whom he or she is in contact

3. Concentration: subtract 7 from 100 and keep subtracting 7's; if patient cannot subtract 7's, can easier tasks be accomplished—4 times 9; 5 times 4; whether anxiety or some disturbance of mood or consciousness seems to be responsible for difficulty

4. Memory: impairment, efforts made to cope with impairment—denial, confabulation, catastrophic reaction, circumstantiality used to conceal deficit; whether the process of registration, retention, or recollection of material is involved

a. Remote memory: childhood data, important events known to have occurred when the patient was younger or free of illness, personal matters, neutral material

b. Recent past memory: the past few months

c. Recent memory: the past few days, what did patient do yesterday, the day before; what did patient have for breakfast, lunch, dinner

d. Immediate retention and recall: ability to repeat six figures after examiner dictates them—first forward, then backward, then after a few minutes interruption; other test questions; did same questions, if repeated, call forth different answers at different times; digit-span measures; other mental functions, such as anxiety level and concentration

e. Effect of defect on patient: mechanisms patient has developed to cope with defect

5. Information and intelligence: patient's level of formal education and self-education: estimate of the patient's intellectual capability and whether patient is capable of functioning at the level of basic endowment; counting, calculation; general knowledge; questions that have some relevance to the patient's educational and cultural background

F. Judgment

1. Social judgment: subtle manifestations of behavior that is harmful to the patient and contrary to acceptable behavior in the culture; does the patient understand the likely outcome of his or her behavior and is patient influenced by this understanding; examples of impairment

2. Test judgment: patient's prediction of what he or she would do in imaginary situations; for instance, what patient would do if he or she found a stamped, addressed letter in the street

G. Insight: degree of awareness and understanding the patient has that he or she is ill

1. Complete denial of illness

2. Slight awareness of being sick and needing help but denying it at the same time

3. Awareness of being sick but blaming it on others, on external factors, or on organic factors

4. Awareness that illness is due to something unknown in patient

5. Intellectual insight: admission that patient is ill and that symptoms or failures in social adjustment are due to patient's own particular irrational feelings or disturbances without applying that knowledge to future experiences

6. True emotional insight: emotional awareness of the motives and feelings within patient and the important people in his or her life

H. Reliability: estimate of examiner's impression of patient's veracity or ability to report the situation accurately

III. Further diagnostic studies

A. Physical examination

B. Additional psychiatric diagnostic interviews

C. Interviews with family members, friends, or neighbors by social worker

D. Psychological tests as indicated: electroencephalogram, computed tomography scan, positron emission tomography, laboratory tests, tests of other medical conditions, reading comprehension and handwriting tests, tests for aphasia

IV. Summary of positive findings: mental symptoms, laboratory findings, psychological test results, if available; drugs patient has been taking, including dosage and duration of intake

V. Diagnosis: diagnostic classification according to the revised third edition of the American Psychiatric Association's *Diagnostic and Statistical Manual of Mental Disorders,* (DSM-III-R)—nomenclature, classification number, diagnoses to be ruled out; DSM-III-R uses a multiaxial classification scheme consisting of five axes, each of which should be covered in the diagnosis

A. Axis I: consists of all clinical syndromes (e.g., mood disorders, schizophrenia, generalized anxiety disorder)

B. Axis II: consists of personality disorders and specific developmental disorders

C. Axis III: consists of any existing medical or physical illness (e.g., epilepsy, cardiovascular disease, gastrointestinal disease)

D. Axis IV: refers to psychosocial stressors (e.g., divorce, injury, death of a loved one) relevant to the illness; a rating scale with a continuum of 1 (no stressors) to 6 (catastrophic stressors) is used

E. Axis V: relates to the highest level of functioning exhibited by the patient during the previous year (e.g., social, occupational, and psychological functioning); a rating scale with a continumm of 90 (superior functioning) to 1 (grossly impaired functioning) is used

VI. Prognosis: opinion as to the probable future course, extent, and outcome of the illness; specific goals of therapy

VII. Psychodynamic formulation: causes of the patient's psychodynamic breakdown—influences in the patient's life that contributed to the present illness; environmental, genetic, and personality factors relevant in determining patient's symptoms; primary and secondary gains; outline of major defense mechanisms used by the patient

VIII. Treatment plan: modalities of treatment recommended, role of medication, inpatient or outpatient treatment, frequency of sessions, probable duration of therapy; type of psychotherapy: individual, group, or family therapy; symptoms or problems to be treated

8.4 _____

Laboratory Tests in Psychiatry

Laboratory tests have come to play a more important role in psychiatry than ever before. They are of help in a variety of ways, such as screening for medical illness, improving diagnostic reliability, monitoring treatment (especially through measurement of the blood levels of psychoactive drugs), and continuing research into psychiatric illness. In this section, an overview and outline of laboratory tests used in psychiatry are presented. It should be emphasized, however, that psychiatric diagnoses cannot be made on the basis of any of these tests alone given the present state of knowledge.

BASIC SCREENING TESTS

A routine medical evaluation is indicated before initiating psychiatric treatment for the purpose of screening for concurrent disease, ruling out organicity, and establishing baseline values of functions to be monitored. Such an evaluation includes a medical history and routine medical lab tests.

NEUROENDOCRINE TESTS

Thyroid Function Tests

Several tests are available, which include testing for thyroxine (T_4) by competitive protein binding (T_4 [D]) and by radioimmunoassay (T_4 [RIA]) involving a specific antigen-antibody reaction. Over 90 percent of T_4 is bound to serum protein and is responsible for thyroid stimulating

hormone (TSH) secretion and cellular metabolism. Other thyroid measures include the free T_4 Index (FT_4I), triiodothyronine uptake, and total serum triiodothyronine measured by radioimmunoassay (T_3 [RIA]). These tests are used to rule out hypothyroidism, which can present with symptoms of depression. In some studies, up to 10 percent of patients complaining of depression and associated fatigue had incipient hypothyroid disease. Lithium can cause hypothyroidism and more rarely hyperthyroidism. Neonatal hypothyroidism results in mental retardation and is preventable if the diagnosis is made at birth.

Thyrotropin-Releasing Hormone (TRH) Stimulation Test. The thyrotropin-releasing hormone (TRH) stimulation test is indicated in patients who have marginally abnormal thyroid test results with suspected subclinical hypothyroidism, which may account for clinical depression. It is also used in patients with possible lithium-induced hypothyroidism. The procedure entails an IV injection of 500 mg of TRH, which produces a sharp rise in plasma TSH when measured at 15, 30, 60, and 90 minutes. An increase in plasma TSH of from 10 to 20 μU/mL above the baseline is normal. An increase of less than 7 μU/mL is considered a blunted response, which may correlate with a diagnosis of depression.

Dexamethasone Suppression Test

Dexamethasone is a long-acting synthetic glucocorticoid with a long half-life. Approximately 1 mg of dexamethasone is equivalent to 25 mg of cortisol. The dexamethasone suppression test is used to confirm a diagnostic impression of major depression with melancholia (DSM-III-R classification) or endogenous depression (Research Diagnostic Criteria [RDC] classification).

Procedure. The patient is given 1 mg of dexamethasone by mouth at 11 P.M. and plasma cortisol is measured at 8 A.M., 4 P.M., and 11 P.M. Plasma cortisol above 5 μg/dl (known as nonsuppression) is considered abnormal, i.e., positive. Suppression of cortisol indicates that the hypothalamic-adrenal-pituitary axis is functioning properly. Since the 1930s, dysfunction of that axis has been known to be associated with stress.

The DST can be used to follow the response of a depressed person to treatment. Normalization of the DST, however, is not an indication to stop antidepressant treatment because the DST may normalize before the depression resolves.

There is some evidence that patients with a positive DST (especially 10 μg/dL) will have a good response to somatic treatment, such as electroconvulsive therapy (ECT) or cyclic antidepressant therapy. The problems associated with the DST include varying reports of sensitivity and specificity. False positives and false negative results are common and are listed in Table 1.

Catecholamines

The serotonin metabolite 5-hydroxyindoleacetic acid (5-HIAA) is elevated in the urine of patients with carcinoid tumors and at times in patients who take phenothiazine medication or in persons who eat foods high in serotonin, e.g., walnuts, bananas, avocados. Norepinephrine, and their metabolic products—metanephrine, normetanephrine, and vanillylmandelic acid (VMA)—are found in the urine where they can be measured. Some depressed patients have a lower urinary norepinephrine to epinephrine ratio (NE:E).

Table 1
Medical Conditions and Pharmacological Agents That May Interfere with Results of the Dexamethasone Suppression Test*

False-positive results are associated with
  Phenytoin
  Barbiturates
  Meprobamate
  Glutethimide
  Methyprylon
  Methaqualone
  Carbamazepine
  Cardiac failure
  Hypertension
  Renal failure
  Disseminated cancer and serious infections
  Recent major trauma or surgery
  Fever
  Nausea
  Dehydration
  Temporal lobe disease
  High-dosage estrogen treatment
  Pregnancy
  Cushing's disease
  Unstable diabetes mellitus
  Extreme weight loss (malnutrition, anorexia nervosa)
  Alcohol abuse
False-negative results are associated with
  Hypopituitarism
  Addison's disease
  Long-term synthetic steroid therapy
  Indomethacin
  High-dosage cyproheptadine treatment
  High-dosage benzodiazepine treatment

---

*From Young M, Stanford J: The dexamethasone suppression test for the detection, diagnosis, and management of depression. Arch Int Med *100:* 309, 1984. Used with permission.

High levels of urinary norepinephrine and epinephrine have been found in some patients with posttraumatic stress disorder. The norepinephrine metabolite, 3-methoxy-4-hydroxyphenylglycol (MHPG) levels is decreased in patients with severe depressive disorders, especially in those patients who attempt suicide. The amount of 5-HIAA in cerebrospinal fluid is low in persons who are in a suicidal depression and who show antisocial, aggressive, or impulsive personality traits.

Renal Function Tests

Creatinine clearance detects early kidney damage and can be serially monitored to follow the course of renal disease. Blood urea nitrogen (BUN) is also elevated in renal disease. Lithium may cause renal damage, and serum creatinine is followed in patients taking lithium.

Liver Function Tests

Total and direct bilirubin are elevated in hepatocellular injury and intrahepatic bile stasis that can occur from phenothiazine or tricyclic medication. Certain drugs, (e.g., phenobarbital) may decrease serum bilirubin.

TESTS FOR SEXUALLY TRANSMITTED DISEASE

The Venereal Disease Research Laboratory (VDRL) test is used as a screening test for syphilis. If positive, the result is confirmed using the more specific Fluorescent Treponemal Antibody Absorption Test (FTA-ABS test), which uses the spirochete *Treponema pallidum* as the antigen. Central nervous system VDRL is measured in patients with suspected neurosyphilis. A positive HIV test indicates that the person has been exposed to infection with the virus that causes AIDS. See Chapter 12 for the psychiatric impact of HIV (Human Immunodeficiency Virus) Seropositivity and of AIDS.

PLASMA LEVELS OF PSYCHOTROPIC DRUGS

There is a trend in caring for patients on psychotropic medication to have regular measurements taken of their plasma level of the prescribed drug. For some types of drugs, such as lithium, it is essential; but for other types of drugs, such as neuroleptics, it is mainly of academic or research interest. The clinician need not practice defensive medicine by insisting that all patients receiving psychotropic drugs have blood levels taken for medicolegal purposes. In the discussion that follows, the major classes of drugs and the suggested guidelines are outlined. The current status of psychopharmacological treatment is such that the psychiatrist's clinical judgment and experience, except in very rare instances, is a better indication of a drug's therapeutic efficacy than is a plasma level determination. Moreover, the reliance on plasma levels cannot replace clinical skills and the need to maintain humanitarian aspects of patient care.

Benzodiazepines

No special tests are needed for patients taking benzodiazepines. Among those metabolized in the liver by oxidation, impaired hepatic function will increase the half-life. Baseline liver function tests (LFT) are indicated in patients with suspected liver damage. Urine testing for benzodiazepines is used routinely in cases of substance abuse.

Antipsychotics

Antipsychotics can cause leukocytosis, leukopenia, mild anemia, and, in rare cases, agranulocytosis. A baseline may be desirable; but because bone marrow side effects can occur abruptly even when the dosage of a drug has remained constant, a CBC will not be preventive. Antipsychotics are metabolized in the liver, so an LFT may be useful. Antipsychotic plasma levels do not correlate with clinical response; however, there is a possible correlation between high plasma levels and toxic side effects. Plasma levels are currently of clinical use only to detect noncompliance or nonabsorption.

Cyclic Antidepressants

An electrocardiogram (EKG) should be given before starting cyclic antidepressants to assess for conduction delays, which may lead to heart block at therapeutic levels. Some clinicians believe that all patients on prolonged cyclic antidepressant therapy should have an annual EKG. At therapeutic levels, these drugs suppress arrhythmias via a quinidine-like effect. Trazodone (Desyrel), an antidepressant unrelated to cyclic antidepressants, has been reported to cause ventricular arrhythmias.

Blood levels of cyclic antidepressants may be of use in patients in whom there is a poor response at normal dose ranges: in high-risk patients, e.g., patients with heart disease, for whom one wants to maintain the lowest possible dose and for patients for whom there is an urgent need to know whether a therapeutic or toxic plasma level of drug has been reached. Some characteristics of tricyclic drug plasma levels are as follows:

1. *Imipramine*. The percentage of favorable response correlates with plasma levels in a linear manner between 200 and 250 ng/mL but some patients may respond at a lower level. At levels over 250 ng/mL there is no improved favorable response and side effects increase.
2. *Nortriptyline*. The therapeutic window (that range within which a drug is most effective) is between 50 and 150 ng/mL.
3. *Desmethylimipramine*. Levels greater than 125 ng/mL correlate with a higher percentage of favorable response.

Procedure. The procedure for taking blood levels is as follows: Draw the blood specimen 10 to 14 hours after the last dose, usually in the morning following a bedtime dose. Patients must be on a stable daily dose for at least 5 days for the test to be valid. Some patients are unusually poor metabolizers of cyclic antidepressants and may have levels as high as 2,000 ng/mL while taking normal doses and before showing a favorable clinical response. Such patients must be monitored very closely for cardiac side effects. Patients with levels greater than 1000 ng/mL are generally at risk for cardiotoxicity.

Lithium

Patients on lithium should have baseline thyroid function tests, electrolytes, renal function tests (BUN and creatinine), and a baseline EKG. The maintenance level is 0.6 to 1.2 meq/L, although acutely manic patients can tolerate up to 1.5 to 1.8 meq/L. Some patients may respond at lower levels, whereas others may require higher levels. Toxic reactions usually occur with levels over 2.0 meq/L. Regular lithium monitoring is essential since there is a narrow therapeutic range beyond which cardiac problems and central nervous system (CNS) effects can occur.

Lithium levels are drawn 8 to 12 hours after the last dose, usually in the morning following the bedtime dose. The level should be measured at least twice per week while stabilizing the patient and then may be drawn monthly.

Carbamazepine (Tegretol)

A pretreatment CBC including platelet count should be done. Reticulocyte count and serum iron are also desirable. These tests should be repeated weekly during the first 3 months of treatment and then monthly thereafter. Carbamazepine can cause aplastic anemia, agranulocytosis, thrombocytopenia, and leukopenia. The medication should be discontinued if there are any signs of bone marrow suppression as measured with periodic CBCs.

POLYSOMNOGRAPHY

Polysomnography is a battery of tests that include an electroencephalogram (EEG), EKG, and electromyogram (EMG). It is often given with tests for penile tumescence, blood oxygen saturation, body movement, body temperature, galvanic skin response, and gastric acid. The tests are of assistance in a variety of conditions, such as insomnia, nocturnal myoclonus, sleep apnea, enuresis, somnambulism, seizure disorders, impotence, vascular headaches, gastroesophogeal reflux, and depression.

Polysomnographic findings in major depression include (1) hyposomnia, (2) shortened time between onset of sleep and onset of the first REM period (REM-latency), (3) decreased EEG slow wave (delta wave) and shorter sleep stages 3 and 4, (4) more rapid eye movements (REM density), and (5) a greater proportion of REM sleep early in the night.

ELECTROENCEPHALOGRAPHY

The electroencephalograph (EEG) measures voltages between electrodes placed on the scalp and provides a description of the electrical activity of the brain and its neurons. The EEG is used in the assessment of organic mental disorders and in the diagnosis of specific seizure disorders, space-occupying lesions, vascular lesions, and encephalopathies, among others. Characteristic changes are caused by specific drugs. EEG waves are classified as follows: beta—14 to 30 Hz (cycles per second); alpha—8 to 13 Hz; theta—4 to 7 Hz; and delta—0.5 to 3 Hz.

In grand mal seizures, there are rhythmic synchronous high-amplitude spikes between 8 and 12 Hz, which correlate with the tonic phase. After 15 to 30 seconds, spikes may become grouped and may be separated by slow waves that correlate with the clonic phase. Finally, a quiescent phase of low-amplitude delta (slow) waves occurs.

In petit mal seizures, there is the sudden onset of bilaterally synchronous generalized spike and wave patterns with very high amplitude and characteristic 3 Hz frequency.

EVOKED POTENTIALS

Evoked potential refers to the evoked response of brain electrical activity to repetitive sensory stimuli. These responses can be separated from the spontaneous EEG activity by computer-averaging techniques known as Brain Electrical Activity Mapping (BEAM), which produces a topographic color map of brain activity. Potentials can be evoked from a variety of sources: somatosensory evoked potentials (SSEP), visual evoked potentials (VEP), and auditory evoked responses (AER). Evoked potentials are clinically useful in evaluating the functional integrity of the somatosensory or special sensory pathways. Different latencies and wave patterns help to localize lesions ranging from the end organ through the nervous system to the cerebral cortex. Often, defects in these pathways are not otherwise evident.

AERs are remarkably constant and are unaffected by sleep or coma. By means of VEPs or AERs, vision and hearing can be evaluated in infants, and psychogenic defects of these special senses can be differentiated from organic diseases. Lesions of sensory pathways from the peripheral nerve, nerve root, and spinal cord show different patterns of SSEPs. Evoked potentials are being used to monitor neural pathways when patients are anesthetized during surgery and to document brain death. Some preliminary results show differences between schizophrenic patients and controls: In schizophrenic patients, there is increased asymmetric beta wave activity in certain regions, and increased delta wave activity is present and is most prominent in the frontal lobes.

RADIOISOTOPE BRAIN SCANNING

In contrast to normal brain tissue, abnormal brain tissue may retain radioisotope compounds. This retention is due to the breakdown of the blood-brain barrier (BBB) associated with organic disease. By means of scanning equipment, the gamma energies emitted by the radioisotope retained in a lesion can be recorded on X-ray film (photoscan). The radioisotope labeled with technetium (Tc^{99}) is intravenously injected from 30 minutes to 2 or 3 hours before the scanning. Scanning equipment projects signals to an image read-out oscilloscope, and the image, in turn, may be photographed. The isotope gallium (Ga^{67}) tends to be picked up in inflammatory and lymphomatous lesions.

A cerebral infarct picks up the radioactive isotope only 1 to 4 days after the onset; the zone of infarction often has a wedge-shaped appearance. Brain scans are frequently negative when the lesion is small (less than 2 cm in diameter), avascular (such as a cyst), or obscured by muscle mass or confluence of blood vessels.

Dynamic brain scanning is an additional technique. From 9 to 12 seconds after the intravenous injection of the radioactive isotope, serial pictures are taken in rapid sequence. Asymmetry in the flow of blood containing the radioisotope may be indicative of stenosis or occlusion of a carotid artery or ischemia within the cerebral zone of the artery. There is usually delayed perfusion in the area of ischemia and increased perfusion of a neoplasm. The rapid filling and emptying of an arteriovenous malformation can be seen by this method.

Radioisotope Cisternography

The radioisotope cisternography test helps to determine the rate of absorption of CSF in normal pressure hydrocephalus and is used to trace leakage of CSF. When indium (In^{111}) is injected through a lumbar puncture, the isotope diffuses through the spinal canal and into the basal cisterns in 2 to 4 hours. It is seen over the convexity of the brain in 24 hours, is predominantly parasagittal in 48 hours, and is minimally detectable at 72 hours. In patients with normal pressure hydrocephalus, due to a chronic defect impairing absorption of CSF, the radioactive isotope diffuses into the ventricles of the brain and is still seen in the ventricles after 24 hours.

Nuclear Magnetic Resonance Imaging (NMR or MRI)

Some atomic nuclei (protons) within a strong magnetic field will align and rotate within the direction of the field. When these nuclei are then exposed to radio frequency, they absorb energy from the radio frequency, after which they undergo computer analysis in order to portray a spatial image. In this way, not only detailed anatomy but also the biochemical state of the tissue can be evaluated. The MRI reveals lesions not seen by other means and is useful in evaluating demyelinating diseases, particularly multiple sclerosis.

Positron Emission Tomography (PET)

Short-lived positron-emitting elements of oxygen, carbon, and nitrogen are used to label organic compounds (e.g., glucose, amino acids, and neurotransmitters), which are then introduced into the body by injection or inhalation. The energy emitted is picked up by scintillation detectors and is computer analyzed. Using tomographic techniques, transverse sections of the brain are constructed and displayed. Quantitative data can be assessed in specific areas for functions such as blood flow, oxygen or glucose metabolism, and other complex physiological phenomena. Alterations in metabolism associated with disease and the actions of medications can be monitored in this way. An on-site cyclotron is required to prepare the short-lived radioisotopes.

Computed Tomography (CT)

Minute variations in the radiographic density of brain tissue are measured from an X-ray source and opposing sensitive detectors arrayed around the head. Tens of thousands of readings are computer processed, and the relative tissue densities of thousands of areas within one plane are then displayed on a cathode ray tube. The picture of one plane of the brain thus presented is photographically recorded. A major advance of CT scanning is that it is accurate, noninvasive, and with minimal risk of morbidity.

Most lesions larger than 0.5 cm on cross-section can be visualized by CT. In addition, ventricular size and displacement, as well as the subarachnoid space, can be seen. The cerebral cortex and basal nuclei can be visualized. In some instances, lesions may not be demonstrated by CT, either because the defect is too small or because the density of the lesion is not distinguishable from the density of the brain. Figures 1 through 7 are examples of CT's picturing cerebral neoplasm, abscess, subdural hematoma, infarct, hemorrhage, acute multiple sclerosis, and cerebral atrophy. CT scans are also useful in dementia, delirium, and in the work-up of organic mental syndrome. Enlargement of the lateral cerebral ventricles determined by CT is frequently reported in schizophrenics.

REGIONAL CEREBRAL BLOOD FLOW (rCBF)

The regional cerebral blood flow (rCBF) technique uses xenon-133 (a low energy gamma ray emitting radioisotope), which is inhaled and crosses the BB barrier freely but is inert. Detectors measure the rate at which xenon-133 is cleared from specific brain areas (gray matter clears quickly, and white matter clears slowly). The rCBF has great potential in studying diseases that have a decrease in the amount of brain tissue, e.g., dementia, ischemia,

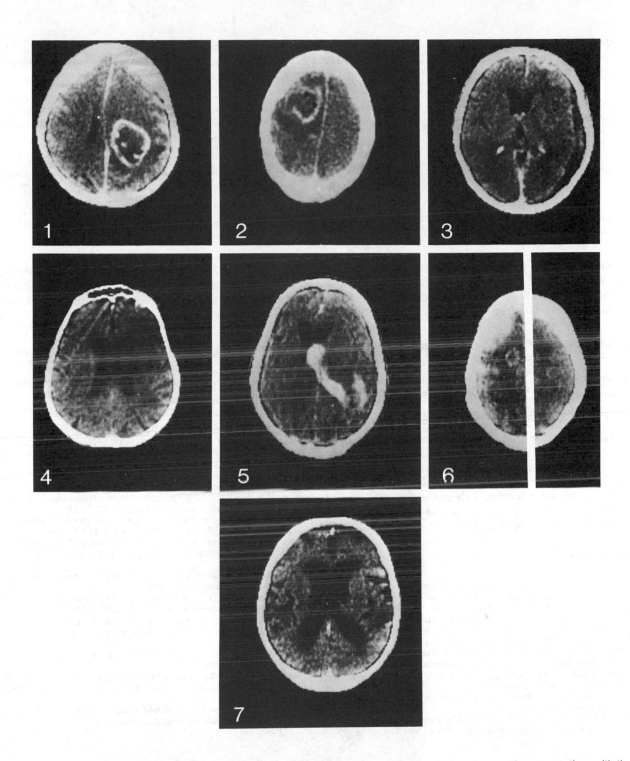

Figures 1 through 7 Computed tomograms of the head are presented as if looking down on a coronal cross-section, with the frontal area at the top and the occipital area at the bottom of the picture; the left and right sides are the same as the viewer's right and left. In the pictures, the least dense substances, such as air and cerebrospinal fluid, are the darkest; the densest areas, such as the skull and blood clots, are the lightest. Although air and clear fluid may appear equally dark and bone and blood clot may appear equally light, the great differences in the densities of these materials can be determined with the aid of the computer. (Courtesy of Norman Leeds, MD, Montefiore Medical Center, New York, NY.)

Figure 1 Cerebral neoplasm. A large mass, glioblastoma multiforme, is present within the right hemisphere. Circumferential density is enhanced by intravenous contrast, and there is adjacent edema, as manifested by rarefaction.

Figure 2 Cerebral abscess. A large left frontal abscess is enclosed by a hypervascular capsule (density enhanced by intravenous contrast) and surrounded by a zone of edema (decreased density). The tiny markedly lucent zones within the lesion represent gas produced by bacteria and indicate that this mass is an abscess, rather than a neoplasm.

Figure 3 Subdural hematoma. A chronic subdural hematoma over the right convexity has caused a ventricular shift from right to left. A small rim of increased density between the surface of the brain and the hematoma represents the membrane enclosing the hematoma. The hematoma has, for the most part, changed from dense blood clot to a less dense fluid.

Figure 4 Cerebral infarct. An old right frontal infarct is manifested by a zone of decreased density. The adjacent right lateral ventricle is, if anything, larger than the left lateral ventricle.

Figure 5 Cerebral hemorrhage. A right parietal hemorrhage has broken into the posterior horn of the right lateral ventricle. There is swelling of the right hemisphere and a shift of the ventricles from right to left.

Figure 6 *A* and *B*, acute multiple sclerosis. With intravenous contrast, multiple circular densities are seen on both the right and the left sides at slightly different levels in a patient with acute multiple sclerosis. These lesions might be mistaken for metastases were it not for the absence of mass effect. This picture is not an invariable finding in multiple sclerosis, but the lesions are even more prominent here than are those seen on sectioning of the brain at autopsy.

Figure 7 Cerebral atrophy. Cerebral atrophy is manifested in this case by both ventricular dilation and widened cortical sulci.

From Solomon S: Neurological evaluation. In *Comprehensive Textbook of Psychiatry*, H I Kaplan and B J Sadock, editors, ed 4, vol 1, p 102. Williams & Wilkins, Baltimore, 1985.

and atrophy. The test is quick, equipment is relatively inexpensive, and there is low radiation. Preliminary data show that schizophrenics may have decreased dorsolateral frontal lobe, blood flow (hypofrontality), and increased left hemisphere blood flow. No differences are found in resting schizophrenic patients. Decreased right hemisphere flow has been found in some depressed patients. The test is still under development.

References

Amsterdam J D, Schweizer E, Winokur A: Multiple hormonal responses to insulin-induced hypoglycemia in depressed patients and normal volunteers. Am J Psych *144:*170, 1987.

APA Task Force on the Use of Laboratory Tests in Psychiatry: Tricyclic Antidepressants—Blood level measurement and clinical outcome: An APA Task force Report: A J Psych 142:155, 1985.

Baldessarini R K, Arama G W: Does the dexamethasone suppression test have clinical utility in psychiatry? J Clin Psych 46:25, 1985.

Carroll B J: Dexamethasone Suppression test: A review of contemporary confusion: J Clin Psych 46:13, 1985.

Extein I, Gold M S: Psychiatric applications of thyroid Tests. J of Clin Psych 47:13 supplement, 1986.

Hall R C W, Beresford T P: *Handbook of Psychiatric Diagnostic Procedures.* vols 1, 2. S P Medical & Science Books, New York, 1984, 1985.

Holsboer F, Genken A, Stalla G K, Miller O A: Blunted aldosterone and ACTH release after human CRH administration in depressed patients. Am J Psych *144:*229, 1987.

Kiloh G L, McComas A J, Osselton J W, Upton A R M: *Clinical Electroencephalography,* Butterworths & Co, 1981.

Krans R P, Hux M, Grof P: Psychotropic drug withdrawal and the dexamethasone suppression test. Am J Psych *144:*82, 1987.

Liebowitz M R, Gorman J M, Fyer A J, Levit M: Lactate provocation of panic attacks. Archives of General Psychiatry, 42:709, 1985.

Loosen P T, Marciniak R, Thadani K: TRH-induced TSH response in healthy volunteers. Relationship to psychiatric history. Am J Psych *144:* 455, 1987.

Morihisa J, editor: *Brain Imaging in Psychiatry.* American Psychiatric Association, Washington, DC, 1984.

Perry J C, Jacobs, D: Overview: Clinical applications of the amytal interview in psychiatric emergency settings: Am J Psych *139:*552, 1982.

Reselow E D, Baxter N, Rieve R R, Barouche F: The dexamethasone suppression test as a monitor of clinical recovery. Am J Psych *144:*30, 1987.

Sternberg E: Testing for physical illness in psychiatric patients, J Clin Psychiatry *47:*3, 1986.

Thase M E, Reynolds III F, Glanz L M, Jenmnings J R, Sewitch D E, Kupfer D J, Frank E: Nocturnal penile tumescence in depressed men. Am J Psych *144:*89, 1987.

Zimmerman M, Coryell W, Pfohl B: Prognostic validity of the dexamethasone suppression test: Results of a six-month follow-up. Am J Psych *144:*212, 1987.

9

Typical Signs and Symptoms of Psychiatric Illness Defined

I. Consciousness: state of awareness

Apperception: perception modified by one's own emotions and thoughts. Sensorium: state of functioning of the special senses (sometimes used as a synonym for consciousness)

A. Disturbances of consciousness

1. Disorientation: disturbance of orientation in time, place, or person

2. Clouding of consciousness: incomplete clearmindedness with disturbance in perception and attitudes

3. Stupor: lack of reaction to and unawareness of surroundings

4. Delirium: bewildered, restless, confused, disoriented reaction associated with fear and hallucinations

5. Coma: profound degree of unconsciousness

6. Coma vigil: coma in which the patient appears to be asleep but ready to be aroused (also known as akinetic mutism)

7. Twilight state: disturbed consciousness with hallucinations

8. Dreamlike state: often used as synonym for complex-partial or psychomotor epilepsy

9. Somnolence: abnormal drowsiness seen most often in organic processes

B. Disturbances of attention: attention is the amount of effort exerted in focusing on certain portions of an experience; ability to sustain a focus on one activity

1. Distractibility: inability to concentrate attention; attention drawn to unimportant or irrelevant external stimuli

2. Selective inattention: blocking out only those things that generate anxiety

C. Disturbances in suggestibility: compliant and uncritical response to an idea or influence

1. *Folie à deux* (or *folie à trois*): communicated emotional illness between two (or three) persons

2. Hypnosis: artificially induced modification of consciousness characterized by a heightened suggestibility

II. Emotion: a complex feeling state with psychic, somatic, and behavioral components that is related to affect and mood

A. Affect: the experience of emotion expressed by the patient and observed by others. Affect has outward manifestations that can be observed. Affect varies over time, in response to changing emotional states.

1. Appropriate affect: the normal condition in which emotional tone is in harmony with the accompanying idea, thought, or speech; also further described as broad or full affect, in which a full range of emotions is appropriately expressed

2. Inappropriate affect: disharmony between the emotional feeling tone and the idea, thought, or speech accompanying it

3. Blunted affect: a disturbance in affect manifested by a severe reduction in the intensity of externalized feeling tone

4. Restricted or constricted affect: reduction in intensity of feeling tone less severe than blunted affect, but clearly reduced

5. Flat affect: absence or near absence of any signs of affective expression; voice monotonous, face immobile

6. Labile affect: rapid and abrupt changes in emotional feeling tone, unrelated to external stimuli

B. Mood: a pervasive and sustained emotion, subjectively experienced and reported by the patient; examples include depression, elation, anger

1. Dysphoric mood: an unpleasant mood

2. Euthymic mood: normal range of mood, implying absence of depressed or elevated mood

3. Expansive mood: expression of one's feelings without restraint, frequently with an overestimation of one's significance or importance

4. Irritable mood: easily annoyed and provoked to anger

5. Mood swings: oscillations between periods of euphoria and depression or anxiety

6. Elevated mood: air of confidence and enjoyment; a mood more cheerful than normal but not necessarily pathologic

7. Euphoria: intense elation with feelings of grandeur

8. Ecstasy: feeling of intense rapture

9. Depression: psychopathological feeling of sadness

10. Anhedonia: loss of interest in and withdrawal from all regular and pleasurable activities, often associated with depression

11. Grief or mourning: sadness appropriate to a real loss

12. Alexithymia: inability or difficulty in describing or being aware of one's emotions or moods

C. Other emotions

1. Anxiety: feeling of apprehension due to the anticipation of danger, which may be internal or external

2. Free-floating anxiety: pervasive, unfocused fear not attached to any idea

3. Fear: anxiety due to consciously recognized and realistic danger

4. Agitation: anxiety associated with severe motor restlessness

5. Tension: increased motor and psychological activity that is unpleasant

6. Panic: acute, episodic, intense attack of anxiety associated with overwhelming feelings of dread and autonomic discharge

7. Apathy: dulled emotional tone associated with detachment or indifference

8. Ambivalence: coexistence of two opposing impulses toward the same thing in the same person at the same time

D. Physiologic disturbances associated with mood: signs that refer to somatic (usually autonomic) dysfunction of the individual, most often associated with depression (also called vegetative)

1. Anorexia: loss of or decrease in appetite
2. Insomnia: lack of or diminished ability to sleep
a. Initial: difficulty falling asleep
b. Middle: difficulty sleeping through night without waking up and difficulty going back to sleep
c. Terminal: early morning awakening
3. Hypersomnia: excessive sleeping
4. Diminished libido: decreased sexual interest, drive, and performance
5. Constipation: inability or difficulty defecating

III. Motor behavior (conation): the aspect of the psyche that includes impulses, motivations, wishes, drives, instincts, and cravings, as expressed by a person's behavior or motor activity

A. Disturbances of communication

1. Echolalia: psychopathological repeating of words or phrases of one person by another; tends to be repetitive and persistent, may be spoken with mocking or staccato intonation

2. Echopraxia: pathological imitation of movements of one person by another

3. Verbigeration: meaningless repetition of specific words or phrases

4. Catatonia: motor anomalies in nonorganic disorders
a. Catalepsy: general term for an immobile position that is constantly maintained
b. Excited: agitated, purposeless motor activity, uninfluenced by external stimuli
c. Stupor: markedly slowed motor activity, often to a point of immobility and seeming unawareness of surroundings
d. Rigidity: assumption of a rigid posture, against all efforts to be moved
e. Posturing: voluntary assumption of an inappropriate or bizarre posture, generally maintained for long periods of time
f. *Cerea flexibilitas* (waxy flexibility): the person can be "molded" into a position which is then maintained. When the examiner moves the person's limb, the limb feels as if it were made of wax.

g. Negativism: motiveless resistance to all attempts to be moved or to all instructions

5. Cataplexy: temporary loss of muscle tone and weakness precipitated by a variety of emotional states

6. Stereotypy: repetitive fixed pattern of physical action or speech

7. Mannerisms: stereotyped involuntary movements

8. Automatism: automatic performance of acts representative of unconscious symbolic activity

9. Command automatism: automatic following of suggestions (also called automatic obedience)

10. Mutism: voicelessness without structural abnormalities

11. Overactivity
a. Psychomotor agitation: excessive overactivity, usually nonproductive and in response to inner tension
b. Hyperactivity (hyperkinesis): restless, aggressive, destructive activity
c. Tic: involuntary, spasmodic motor movements
d. Sleepwalking (somnambulism): motor activity during sleep
e. Compulsion: uncontrollable impulse to perform an act repetitively
i. Dipsomania: compulsion to drink alcohol
ii. Kleptomania: compulsion to steal
iii. Nymphomania: excessive and compulsive need for coitus in female
iv. Satyriasis: excessive and compulsive need for coitus in male
v. Trichotillomania: compulsion to pull out one's hair
vi. Ritual: automatic activity compulsive in nature, anxiety-reducing in origin

12. Hypoactivity (hypokinesis): decreased activity or retardation, as in psychomotor retardation; visible slowing of thought, speech, movements

13. Mimicry: simple, imitative motion activity of childhood

14. Aggression: forceful goal-directed action that may be verbal or physical; the motor counterpart of the affect of rage, anger, or hostility

IV. Thinking: goal-directed flow of ideas, symbols, and associations initiated by a problem of tasks and leading toward a reality-oriented conclusion; when a logical sequence occurs, thinking is normal. Parapraxes (lapses from logic also called "Freudian slips") are considered part of normal thinking.

A. Disturbances in form of thinking

1. Mental disorder: clinically significant behavioral or psychological syndrome, associated with distress or disability, not just an expectable response to a particular event

2. Neurosis: mental disorder in which reality testing is intact and symptoms are experienced as ego-dystonic (distressing and unacceptable); behavior does not violate gross social norms, relatively enduring or recurrent without treatment

3. Psychosis: inability to distinguish reality from fantasy; impaired reality testing, with creation of a new reality

4. Reality testing: the objective evaluation and judgment of the world outside the self

5. Formal thought disorder: disturbance in the form of thought instead of the content of thought; thinking characterized by loosened associations, neologisms, and illogical constructs; thought process is disordered, and the person is defined as psychotic

6. Illogical thinking: thinking containing erroneous conclusions or internal contradictions; is psychopathological only when it is marked, and when not due to cultural values or to intellectual deficit

7. Dereism: mental activity not concordant with logic or experience

8. Autistic thinking: thinking that gratifies unfulfilled desires but has no regard for reality; preoccupation with inner, private world; term used somewhat synonymously with dereism

9. Magical thinking: a form of dereistic thought; thinking that is similar to that of the preoperational phase in children (Piaget), in which thoughts, words, or actions assume power (for example, they can cause or prevent events)

10. Concrete thinking: literal thinking; limited use of metaphor without understanding of nuances of meaning; one-dimensional thought

11. Abstract thinking: ability to appreciate nuances of meaning; multidimensional thinking with ability to use metaphors and hypotheses appropriately

B. Specific disturbances in form of thought

1. Neologism: new words created by the patient, often from combining syllables of other words, for idiosyncratic psychological reasons

2. Word salad: incoherent mixture of words and phrases

3. Circumstantiality: indirect speech that is delayed in reaching the point, but eventually gets from original point to desired goal; characterized by an overinclusion of detail and parenthetical remarks

4. Tangentiality: inability to have goal-directed associations of thought; patient never gets from desired point to desired goal

5. Incoherence: speech that, generally, is not understandable; running together of thoughts or words with no logical or grammatical connection, resulting in disorganization

6. Perseveration: persisting response to a prior stimulus after a new stimulus has been presented, often associated with organic brain disease

7. Condensation: fusion of various concepts into one

8. Irrelevant answer: answer that is not in harmony with question asked

9. Loosening of associations: flow of thought in which ideas shift from one subject to another in a completely unrelated way; when severe, speech may be incoherent

10. Derailment: gradual or sudden deviation in train of thought without blocking; sometimes used synonymously with loosening of association

11. Flight of ideas: rapid, continuous verbalizations or plays on words produce constant shifting from one idea to another; the ideas tend to be connected and in the less severe form may be followed by a listener.

12. Clang associations: association of words similar in sound, but not in meaning; words have no logical connection, may include rhyming and punning

13. Blocking: abrupt interruption in train of thinking, before a thought or idea is finished; after brief pause, person indicates no recall of what was being said or was going to be said. (also known as thought deprivation)

14. Glossolalia: the expression of a revelatory message through unintelligible words (also known as "speaking in tongues")

C. Disturbances in speech

1. Pressure of speech: rapid speech that is increased in amount and difficult to interrupt

2. Volubility (logorrhea): copious, coherent, logical speech

3. Poverty of speech: restriction in the amount of speech used; replies may be monosyllabic

4. Poverty of content of speech: speech that is adequate in amount but conveys little information because of vagueness, emptiness, or stereotyped phrases

5. Dysprosody: loss of normal speech melody (called prosody)

6. Dysarthria: difficulty in articulation, not in word finding or in grammar

D. Aphasic disturbances (disturbances in language output)

1. Motor aphasia: disturbance of speech due to organic brain disorder in which understanding remains but ability to speak is lost (also known as Broca's nonfluent or expressive aphasia)

2. Sensory aphasia: loss of ability to comprehend the meaning of words or the use of objects (also known as Wernicke's fluent or receptive aphasia)

3. Nominal aphasia: difficulty in finding correct name for an object

4. Syntactical aphasia: inability to arrange words in proper sequence

5. Jargon aphasia: words produced are totally neologistic; nonsense words repeated with various intonations and inflections

6. Global aphasia: combination of a grossly nonfluent aphasia plus severe fluent aphasia

7. Fluent aphasia: inability to understand the spoken word; fluent, but incoherent, speech is present

E. Disturbances in content of thought

1. Poverty of content of speech: speech that gives little information due to vagueness, empty repetitions, or obscure phrases

2. Overvalued idea: unreasonable, sustained false belief maintained less firmly than delusional thinking

3. Delusion: false belief, based on incorrect inference about external reality, not consistent with patient's intelligence and cultural background, that cannot be corrected by reasoning

    a. Bizarre delusion: an absurd, totally implausible, very strange false belief (e.g., invaders from space have implanted electrodes in the patient's brain)

    b. Systematized delusion: false belief or beliefs united by a single event or theme (e.g., patient is being persecuted by the CIA, FBI, Mafia, or his boss)

    c. Mood-congruent delusion: delusions whose content is mood appropriate (e.g., a depressed patient who believes he is responsible for the destruction of the world)

    d. Mood-incongruent delusion: delusion whose content

has no association to mood or is mood-inappropriate (e.g., a depressed patient who believes he is the new Messiah)

e. Nihilistic delusion: false feeling that self, others, or the world is nonexistent or ending

f. Delusion of poverty: false belief that one is bereft, or will be, of all material possessions

g. Somatic delusion: false belief involving functioning of one's body (e.g., belief that one's brain is rotting or melting)

h. Paranoid delusions: includes persecutory delusions, as well as delusions of reference, control, and grandeur (this is to be distinguished from paranoid ideation, which is suspiciousness of less than delusional proportions)

i. Delusion of persecution: false belief that one is being harassed, cheated, or persecuted; often found in litigious patients who have a pathological tendency to take legal action because of imagined mistreatment

j. Delusion of grandeur: exaggerated conception of one's importance, power, or identity

k. Delusion of reference: false belief that the behavior of others refers to oneself; that events, objects, or other people have a particular and unusual significance, usually of a negative nature; derived from ideas of reference in which one falsely feels one is being talked about by others. This differs from an idea of reference, in which the false belief is not as firmly held as a delusion

l. Delusion of self-accusation: false feeling of remorse and guilt

m. Delusion of control: false feeling that one's will, thoughts, or feelings are being controlled by external forces

(i) Thought withdrawal: delusion that one's thoughts are being removed from one's mind by other people or forces

(ii) Thought insertion: delusion that thoughts are being implanted in one's mind by other people or forces

(iii) Thought broadcasting: delusion that one's thoughts can be heard by others, as though they are being broadcast into the air

n. Delusion of infidelity: (delusional jealousy) false belief derived from pathological jealousy that one's lover is unfaithful

o. Erotomania: delusional belief, almost exclusively in women, that a man is deeply in love with them (also known as *Clérembault's* syndrome)

p. Pseudologia fantastica: a type of lying, in which the person appears to believe in the reality of his fantasies and acts on them

4. Trend or preoccupation of thought: centering of thought content around a particular idea, associated with a strong affective tone, such as a paranoid trend or suicidal preoccupation

5. Egomania: pathological self-preoccupation

6. Monomania: preoccupation with a single object

7. Hypochondria: exaggerated concern over one's health that is not based on real organic pathology, but rather on unrealistic interpretation of physical signs or sensations as abnormal

8. Obsession: pathological persistence of an irresistible thought or feeling that cannot be eliminated from consciousness by logical effort, which is associated with anxiety

9. Compulsion: pathological need to act on an impulse which, if resisted, produces anxiety; repetitive behavior in response to an obsession or performed according to certain rules, with no true end in itself other than to prevent something from occurring in the future

10. Phobia: persistent, irrational, exaggerated, and invariably pathological dread of some specific type of stimulus or situation; results in a compelling desire to avoid the feared stimulus

a. Simple phobia circumscribed dread of a discrete object or situation (e.g., dread of spiders or snakes)

b. Social phobia: dread of public humiliation, as in fear of public speaking, performing, or eating in public

c. Acrophobia: dread of high places

d. Agoraphobia: dread of open places

e. Algophobia: dread of pain

f. Claustrophobia: dread of closed places

g. Xenophobia: dread of strangers

h. Zoophobia: dread of animals

11. Noesis: a revelation in which immense illumination occurs in association with a sense that one has been chosen to lead and command

12. Unio mystica: an oceanic feeling, one of mystic unity with an infinite power

V. Perception: process of transferring physical stimulation into psychological information; mental process by which sensory stimuli are brought to awareness

A. Disturbances associated with organic brain disease: agnosia—an inability to recognize and interpret the significance of sensory impressions

1. Anosognosia: denial of illness

2. Autotopagnosia: denial of a body part

3. Visual agnosia: inability to recognize objects or persons

4. Astereognosia: inability to recognize objects by touch

5. Prosopagnosia: inability to recognize faces

B. Disturbances associated with conversion and dissociative phenomenon: somatization of repressed material or the development of physical symptoms and distortions involving the voluntary muscles or special sense organs; not under voluntary control, and not explained by any physical disorder

1. Hysterical anesthesia: loss of sensory modalities resulting from emotional conflicts

2. Macropsia: state in which objects seem larger than they are

3. Micropsia: state in which objects seem smaller than they are (both macropsia and micropsia can also be associated with such clear organic conditions as complex partial seizures)

4. Depersonalization: a subjective sense of being unreal, strange or unfamiliar to oneself

5. Derealization: a subjective sense that the environment is strange or unreal; a feeling of changed reality

6. Fugue: taking on of a new identity with amnesia for the old and which often involves travel or wanderings to new environments

7. Multiple personality: one person who appears at different times to be in possession of an entirely different personality and character

C. Hallucinations: false sensory perceptions not associated with real external stimuli; there may or may not be a delusional interpretation of the hallucinatory experience. Hallucinations indicate a psychotic disturbance only when associated with impairment in reality testing

1. Hypnagogic hallucination: false sensory perception occurring while falling asleep

2. Hypnopompic hallucination: false perception occurring while awakening from sleep

3. Auditory hallucination: false perception of sound, usually voices, but also various noises such as music, etc.

4. Visual hallucination: false perception involving sight, consisting of both formed images, e.g., people, and unformed images, such as flashes of light

5. Olfactory hallucination: false perception in smell

6. Gustatory hallucination: false perception of taste, such as unpleasant taste due to an uncinate seizure

7. Tactile (haptic) hallucination: false perception of touch or surface sensation, as from an amputated limb (phantom limb), crawling sensation on or under the skin (formication)

8. Somatic hallucination: false sensation of things occurring in or to the body, most often visceral in origin (also known as cenesthetic hallucination)

9. Lilliputian hallucination: false perception in which objects are seen as reduced in size

10. Mood-congruent hallucination: hallucination whose content is consistent with either a depressed or manic mood (e.g., a depressed patient hears voices telling the patient he is a bad person; a manic patient hears voices telling the patient he is of inflated worth, power, knowledge, etc.)

11. Mood-incongruent hallucination: hallucination whose content is not consistent with either depressed or manic mood (e.g., in depression, hallucinations not involving such themes as guilt, deserved punishment, or inadequacy; in mania, not involving such themes as inflated worth or power)

12. Hallucinosis: hallucinations, most often auditory, which are associated with chronic alcohol abuse and occur within a clear sensorium (as opposed to DTs)

13. Synesthesia: sensations or hallucinations caused by other sensations (e.g., an auditory sensation is accompanied by or triggers a visual sensation; a sound is experienced as being seen or a visual experience is heard)

14. Trailing phenomenon: perceptual abnormality associated with hallucinogenic drugs in which moving objects are seen as a series of discrete and discontinuous images

D. Illusions: misperceptions or misinterpretations of real external sensory stimuli

VI. Memory: function by which information stored in the brain is later recalled to consciousness

A. Disturbances of memory

1. Amnesia: partial or total inability to recall past experiences, may be organic or emotional in origin

2. Paramnesia: falsification of memory by distortion of recall

a. *Fausse reconnaissance:* false recognition

b. Retrospective falsification: recollection of a true memory to which the patient adds false details

c. Confabulation: unconscious filling of gaps in memory by imagined or untrue experiences that patient believes but that have no basis in fact

d. *Déjà vu:* illusion of visual recognition in which a new situation is incorrectly regarded as a repetition of a previous memory

e. *Déjà entendu:* illusion of auditory recognition

f. *Déjà pensé:* illusion that a new thought is recognized as a thought previously felt or expressed

g. *Jamais vu:* false feeling of unfamiliarity with a real situation one has experienced

3. Hypermnesia: exaggerated degree of retention and recall

4. Eidetic images: visual memories of almost hallucinatory vividness

VII. Intelligence: the ability to understand, recall, mobilize, and constructively integrate previous learning in meeting new situations

A. Mental retardation: lack of intelligence to a degree in which there is interference with social and vocational performance: mild (I.Q. of 50 or 55 to approximately 70), moderate (I.Q. of 35 or 40 to 50 or 55), severe (I.Q. of 20 or 25 to 35 or 40), or profound (I.Q. below 20 or 25); obsolescent terms are idiot (mental age less than 3 years), imbecile (mental age of 3 to 7 years), and moron (mental age of about 8)

B. Dementia: organic and global deterioration of intellectual functioning without clouding of consciousness

C. Pseudodementia: clinical features resembling a dementia not due to organic brain dysfunction, most often due to depression

VIII. Insight: ability of the patient to understand the true cause and meaning of a situation (such as a set of symptoms)

A. Intellectual insight: understanding of the objective reality of a set of circumstances, without the ability to apply the understanding in any useful way to master the situation.

B. True insight: understanding of the objective reality of a situation coupled with the motivation and emotional impetus to master the situation

C. Impaired insight: diminished ability to understand the objective reality of a situation

IX. Judgment: ability to assess a situation correctly and act appropriately within that situation

A. Critical judgment: ability to assess, discern, and choose among different options in a situation

B. Automatic judgment: reflex performance of an action

C. Impaired judgment: diminished ability to understand a situation correctly and to act appropriately

References

Andreasen N C: The clinical assessment of thought, language, and communication disorders. I. The definition of terms and evaluation of their reliability. Arch Gen Psychiatry 36:1315, 1979.

Bender M D: *Disorders of Perception.* Charles C Thomas, Springfield, IL, 1952.

Bensen D F, Blumer D, editors: *Psychiatric Aspects of Neurological Disease,* vol 2. Grune & Stratton, New York, 1982.

Bleuler E: *Dementia Praecox: The Group of Schizophrenias.* International Universities Press, New York, 1950.

Campbell R J: *Psychiatric Dictionary,* ed 5. Oxford, New York, 1981.

Cavenar J O, Brodie, H K M: *Signs and Symptoms in Psychiatry.* J B Lippincott, Philadelphia, 1983.

Fenichel O: *Psychoanalytic Theory of Neuroses.* W W Norton, New York, 1945.

Frances A J, Hales R E: *Annual Review,* vol 5. American Psychiatric Press, Washington, DC, 1986.

Geschwind N: Aphasia. N Engl J Med *284*:654, 1971.

Hellerstein D, Frosch W, Koenigsberg H W: The clinical significance of command hallucinations. Am J Psychiatry *144*(1):219, 1987.

Solomon C M, Holzman J P S, Levin S, Gale H J: The association between eye-tracking dysfunctions and thought disorder in psychosis. Arch Gen Psychiatry *44*(1):31, 1987.

Spitzer R L, Skodol A E, Williams J B W: *Case Book Diagnostic and Statistical Manual of Mental Disorders.* American Psychiatric Association, Washington, DC, 1981.

10

Classification in Psychiatry (Including DSM–III–R)

Classification is the process by which complex phenomena are arranged into categories according to some established criteria. In psychiatry, a classification of mental disorders consists of a list of categories of specific disorders grouped into various classes on the basis of some shared characteristics.

The *reliability* of a classification of mental disorders or of a specific diagnostic category is the extent to which different users can agree on a particular diagnosis in a series of cases. *Validity* refers to the extent to which the entire classification of mental disorders and each of its specific diagnostic categories can be comprehensible, be controlled, and be communicated to others. *Predictive validity* refers to the extent to which knowledge that a person has a particular mental disorder is useful in predicting the future of that person—subsequent course of the illness, complications, response to treatment. Historically, it was largely on the basis of predictive validity that Emil Kraepelin distinguished dementia precox (which was believed to have a deteriorating course) from manic-depressive psychosis (which was believed to have a good prognosis).

DSM–III AND DSM–III–R

The third edition of the *Diagnostic and Statistical Manual of Mental Disorders* of the American Psychiatric Association (DSM-III), published in 1980, replaced previous editions as the official classification system of American psychiatry. In 1987, a revision of DSM-III, known as DSM III-R, was published; it incorporated factual changes based on data from various field trials. DSM-III-R also attempted to classify ambiguities and resolve inconsistencies that were noted to exist in DSM-III. Such changes in DSM-III-R are included in the discussion that follows. Eventually, an entirely new edition (DSM-IV) will be published, but that is not expected until sometime in the 1990s.

In DSM-III-R, for the first time, the American Psychiatric Association has issued a *cautionary statement* regarding the proper use and interpretation of the diagnostic categories in this new nosology:

The specified diagnostic criteria for each mental disorder are offered as guidelines for making diagnoses, since it has been demonstrated that the use of such criteria enhances diagnostic agreement among clinicians and investigators. The proper use of these criteria requires specialized clinical training that provides both a body of knowledge and clinical skills.

Those diagnostic criteria reflect a consensus of current formulations of evolving knowledge in our field but do not encompass all the conditions which may legitimately be the subject of treatment or research efforts.

The purpose of DSM-III-R is to provide clear descriptions of diagnostic categories in order to enable clinicians and investigators to diagnose, communicate about, study, and treat various mental disorders. It is to be understood that inclusion here, for clinical and research purposes, of a diagnostic category such as pathological gambling or pedophilia does not imply that the condition meets legal or other nonmedical criteria for what constitutes mental disease, mental disorder, or mental disability. The clinical and scientific considerations involved in the categorization of these conditions as mental disorders may not be wholly relevant to legal judgments, for example, that take into account such issues as individual responsibility, disability determination, and competency.

ICD–9

The ninth edition of the *International Classification of Diseases* (ICD-9), published by the World Health Organization, is the official classification system used in Europe and Great Britain. All DSM-III-R categories are found in ICD-9, but not all ICD-9 categories are in DSM-III-R. A clinical modification of ICD-9, known as ICD-9CM, was published in 1979 in an effort to make the two systems as compatible as possible. However, many ICD-9CM terms are not included in the DSM-III-R classification. ICD-10 is now in preparation.

Basic Features of DSM-III-R

Descriptive Approach. The approach in DSM-III-R is atheoretical with regard to etiology. Thus, DSM-III-R attempts to describe comprehensively what the manifestations of mental disorders are and only rarely attempts to account for how the disturbances come about. The general approach is descriptive in that the definitions of these disorders consist, by and large, of descriptions of the clinical features.

Diagnostic Criteria. Specified diagnostic criteria are provided for each specific mental disorder. These criteria include a list of essential features that must be present for the diagnosis to be made. Such criteria have been shown to increase the reliability of the diagnostic process between and among clinicians.

Systematic Description. DSM-III-R systematically describes each disorder in terms of its essential features and associated features, with brief comments about such factors as age at onset, course, impairment, complications, predisposing factors, prevalence, sex ratio, familial pattern, and differential diagnosis. DSM-III-R does not purport to be a textbook. No mention is made of theories of etiology, management, or treatment, nor are the controversial issues surrounding a particular diagnostic category discussed.

Multiaxial Evaluation. DSM-III-R is a multiaxial system that evaluates the patient along several variables and contains the following five axes:

Axis I. Clinical syndromes and conditions not attributable to a mental disorder

Axis II. Developmental disorders (includes mental retardation, specific developmental disorders, and pervasive developmental disorders) and personality disorders

Axis I and Axis II comprise the entire classification of mental disorders, which include 19 major classifications and more than 200 specific disorders (Table 1). According to DSM-III-R: in many instances there will be a disorder on both axes. For example, an adult may have major depression noted on Axis I and compulsive personality disorder on Axis II, or a child may have conduct disorder noted on Axis I and developmental language disorder on Axis II.

Axis III. Axis III lists any physical disorder or condition that may be present in addition to a mental disorder. The physical condition may be etiologic (e.g., kidney failure causing delirium), the result of the mental disorder (e.g., alcohol gastritis secondary to alcohol dependence), or unrelated to the mental disorder. Axis III codes are taken from the World Health Organization's *International*

Table 1
Classes or Groups of Conditions in DSM-III-R

1. Disorders usually first evident in infancy childhood or adolescence (includes DSM-III-R category of developmental disorders)
2. Organic Mental Syndromes and Disorders
3. Psychoactive Substance-Induced Organic Neural Disorders
4. Psychoactive Substance Use Disorders
5. Schizophrenia
6. Delusional Paranoid Disorders
7. Psychotic Disorder Not Elsewhere Classified
8. Mood Disorders (Previously known in DSM-III as Affective Disorders)
9. Anxiety Disorders (or Anxiety and Phobic Neuroses)
10. Somatoform Disorders
11. Dissociative Disorders (or Hysterical Neuroses, Dissociative Type)
12. Sexual Disorders
13. Sleep Disorders
14. Factitious Disorders
15. Impulse Control Disorders Not Elsewhere Classified
16. Adjustment Disorders
17. Psychological Factors Affecting Physical Condition
18. Personality Disorders
19. Conditions Not Attributable to a Mental Disorder that are a Focus of Attention or Treatment

Classification of Diseases, Injuries, and Causes of Death (ICD-9).

Axis IV. Axis IV provides a 6-point rating scale for coding the psychosocial stressors that significantly contribute to the development or exacerbation of the current disorder. There are examples for adults as well as for children and adolescents.

DSM-III-R has defined the stressors as predominantly acute events, with a duration less than 6 months (e.g., death of a spouse) or predominantly enduring, circumstances with a duration greater than 6 months (e.g., chronic marital discord). Tables 2 and 3 illustrate the 6-point psychosocial stressor scale, a score of 6 representing catastrophic stress (e.g., multiple family deaths) and 1 representing no apparent stress. The stressors are organized for adults and for children and adolescents.

The severity-of-stress rating should be based on the clinician's assessment of the stress that an average person with similar sociocultural values and circumstances would experience from the psychosocial stressors. That judgment considers the amount of change in the person's life due to the stressor, the degree to which the event is desired and under the person's control, and the number of stressors. In addition, in certain settings, it may be useful to note the specific psychosocial stressors. This information may be important in formulating a treatment plan that includes attempts to remove the psychosocial stressors or to help the person cope with them (Table 4).

Axis V. Axis V is a global assessment scale in which the clinician judges the person's highest level of functioning during the past year. Functioning is conceptualized as a composite of three major areas: social relations, occupational functioning, and psychological functioning. The scale, based on a continuum of mental health and mental illness, has been changed from a 7-point scale in DSM-III to a 90-point scale in DSM–III–R, 90 representing the highest level of functioning in all areas (Table 5).

Persons who have had a high level of functioning prior to an episode of illness generally have a better prognosis than those who had a low level of functioning. Ratings are made both for current functioning (at the time of evaluation) and for the highest level of functioning shown by the patient for at least a few months during the year preceding the current evaluation.

Summary. Each axis is used to document the presence or absence of findings. The clinician should be able to infer a great deal of information about the patient by scanning the multiaxial tree, including the presence or absence of a specific psychiatric syndrome (Axis I); whether a concomitant premorbid personality disorder is present (Axis II); the presence of a physical condition that may influence the management or prognosis of the psychiatric illness (Axis III); the life events that may be relevant to understanding precipitating factors or problems in management (Axis IV); and, finally, a global assessment of the patient's highest level of functioning prior to the onset of the illness, which provides a baseline from which to gauge severity of the illness and the prognosis (Axis V). An example of a multiaxial diagnostic schema follows:

Axis I   Delusional (Paranoid) disorder
Axis II   Paranoid personality

Table 2
Axis IV: Severity of Psychosocial Stressors Scale: Adults

Code	Term	Examples of Stressors	
		Acute Events	Enduring Circumstances
1	None	No acute events that may be relevant to the disorder	No enduring circumstances that may be relevant to the disorder
2	Mild	Broke up with boyfriend or girlfriend; started or graduated from school; child left home	Family arguments; job dissatisfaction; residence in high-crime neighborhood
3	Moderate	Marriage; marital separation; loss of job; retirement; miscarriage	Marital discord; serious financial problems; trouble with boss; being a single parent
4	Severe	Divorce; birth of first child	Unemployment; poverty
5	Extreme	Death of spouse; serious physical illness diagnosed; victim of rape	Serious chronic illness in self or child; ongoing physical or sexual abuse
6	Catastrophic	Death of child; suicide of spouse; devastating natural disaster	Captivity as hostage; concentration camp experience
0	Inadequate information, or no change in condition		

Table from DSM-III-R *Diagnostic and Statistical Manual of Mental Disorders*, ed 3, revised. (Current Classification of Mental Disorders, 1987.) Copyright American Psychiatric Association, Washington D.C., 1987. Used with permission.

Axis III   Hypertension
Axis IV   Extreme (death of spouse)
Axis V   Major impairment in work
        (patient avoids close relationships, is suspicious of coworkers, high absenteeism because of frequent headaches)

Severity of Disorder. Depending on the clinical picture, the presence or absence of signs and symptoms, and their intensity, the severity of a disorder may be mild, moderate, or severe, in partial remission, or in full remission. The following guidelines are used according to DSM-III-R:

Mild: Few, if any, symptoms in excess of those required to make the diagnosis and symptoms result in only minor impairment in occupational functioning or in usual social activities or relationships with others.

Moderate: Symptoms or functional impairment between "mild" and "severe."

Severe: Several symptoms in excess of those required to make the diagnosis and symptoms markedly interfere with occupational functioning or with usual social activities or relationships with others.

In partial remission or *residual state:* The full criteria for the disorder were previously met, but currently only some of the symptoms or signs of the illness are present. *In partial remission* should be used when there is the expectation that the person will completely recover (or have a complete remission) within the next few years, as, for example, in the case of a major depressive episode. *Residual state* should be used when there is little expectation of a complete remission or recovery within the next few

years, as, for example, in the case of autistic disorder or attention-deficit hyperactivity disorder. (*Residual state* should not be used with schizophrenia, since by tradition there is a specific residual type of schizophrenia.) In some cases the distinction between *in partial remission* and *residual state* will be difficult to make.

In full remission: There are no longer any symptoms or signs of the disorder. The differentiation of *in full remission* from recovered (no current mental disorder) requires consideration of the length of time since the last period of disturbance, the total duration of the disturbance, and the need for continued evaluation or prophylactic treatment.

CLASSIFICATION OF MENTAL DISORDERS

Table 6 presents the DSM-III-R classification of mental disorders (Axis I and II). Table 7 presents the ICD-9 classification of mental disorders. The reader is referred to the specific section of this text where each disorder is discussed separately and in depth.

Several terms do not appear in DSM-III-R as part of official nomenclature, for example, psychosis, neurosis, and psychosomatic. Nevertheless, they have important applications to the field of psychiatry and are in common use among clinicians.

Psychosis

Although the traditional meaning of the term "psychotic" emphasized loss of reality testing and impairment of mental functioning—manifested by delusions, hallucina-

Table 3
Axis IV: Severity of Psychosocial Stressors Scale: Children and Adolescents

Code	Term	Examples of Stressors	
		Acute Events	Enduring Circumstances
1	None	No acute events that may be relevant to the disorder	No enduring circumstances that may be relevant to the disorder
2	Mild	Broke up with boyfriend or girlfriend; change of school	Overcrowded living quarters; family arguments
3	Moderate	Expelled from school; birth of sibling	Chronic disabling illness in parent; chronic parental discord
4	Severe	Divorce of parents; unwanted pregnancy; arrest	Harsh or rejecting parents; chronic life-threatening illness in parent; multiple foster home placements
5	Extreme	Sexual or physical abuse; death of a parent	Recurrent sexual or physical abuse
6	Catastrophic	Death of both parents	Chronic life-threatening illness
0	Inadequate information, or no change in condition		

Table from DSM-III-R Diagnostic and Statistical Manual of Mental Disorders, ed 3, revised. (Current Classification of Mental Disorders, 1987.) Copyright American Psychiatric Association, Washington, D.C., 1987. Used with permission.

Table 4
Types of Psychosocial Stressors

To ascertain etiologically significant psychosocial stressors, the following areas may be considered:

Conjugal (marital and nonmarital): e.g., engagement, marriage, discord, separation, death of spouse.

Parenting: e.g., becoming a parent, friction with child, illness of child.

Other interpersonal: problems with one's friends, neighbors, associates, or nonconjugal family members, e.g., illness of best friend, discordant relationship with boss.

Occupational: includes work, school, homemaking, e.g., unemployment, retirement, school problems.

Living circumstances: e.g., change in residence, threat to personal safety, immigration.

Financial: e.g., inadequate finances, change in financial status.

Legal: e.g., arrest, imprisonment, lawsuit, or trial.

Developmental: phases of the life cycle, e.g., puberty, transition to adult status, menopause, "becoming 50."

Physical illness or injury: e.g., illness, accident, surgery, abortion. (Note: A physical disorder is listed on Axis III whenever it is related to the development or management of an Axis I or II disorder. A physical disorder can also be a psychosocial stressor if its impact is due to its meaning to the individual, in which case it would be listed on both Axis III and Axis IV.)

Other psychosocial stressors: e.g., natural or man-made disaster, persecution, unwanted pregnancy, out-of-wedlock birth, rape.

Family factors (children and adolescents): In addition to the above, for children and adolescents the following stressors may be considered: cold, hostile, intrusive, abusive, conflictual, or confusingly inconsistent relationship between parents or toward child; physical or mental illness in a family member; lack of parental guidance or excessively harsh or inconsistent parental control; insufficient, excessive, or confusing social or cognitive stimulation; anomalous family situation, e.g., complex or inconsistent parental custody and visitation arrangements; foster family; institutional rearing; loss of nuclear family members.

Table from DSM-III-R Diagnostic and Statistical Manual of Mental Disorders, ed 3, revised. (Current Classification of Mental Disorders, 1987.) Copyright American Psychiatric Association, Washington, D.C., 1987. Used with permission.

tions, confusion, and impaired memory—two other meanings have evolved during the past 50 years. In the most common psychiatric use of the term, psychotic became synonymous with severe impairment of social and personal functioning characterized by social withdrawal and inability to perform the usual household and occupational roles. The other use of the term specifies degree of ego regression as the criterion for psychotic illness. As a consequence of those multiple meanings, the term has lost its precision in current clinical and research practice.

According to the glossary of the American Psychiatric Association, the term psychotic refers to gross impairment in reality testing. It may be used to describe the behavior of an individual at a

Table 5
Axis V: Global Assessment of Functioning Scale (GAF Scale)

Consider psychological, social, and occupational functioning on a hypothetical continuum of mental health-illness. Do not include impairment in functioning due to physical (or environmental) limitations.

Note: Use intermediate codes when appropriate, e.g., 45, 68, 72.

Code	
90	**Absent or minimal symptoms** (e.g., mild anxiety before an exam), **good functioning in all areas, interested and involved in a wide range of activities, socially effective, generally satisfied with life, no more than**
81	**everyday problems or concerns** (e.g., an occasional argument with family members).
80	**If symptoms are present, they are transient and expectable reactions to psychosocial stressors** (e.g., difficulty concentrating after family argument); **no more than slight impairment in social, occupational, or**
71	**school functioning** (e.g., temporarily falling behind in school work).
70	**Some mild symptoms** (e.g., depressed mood and mild insomnia) **OR some difficulty in social, occupational, or school functioning** (e.g., occasional truancy, or theft within the household), **but generally functioning pretty**
61	**well, has some meaningful interpersonal relationships.**
60	**Moderate symptoms** (e.g., flat affect and circumstantial speech, occasional panic attacks) **OR moderate**
51	**difficulty in social, occupational, or school functioning** (e.g., few friends, conflicts with co-workers).
50	**Serious symptoms** (e.g., suicidal ideation, severe obsessional rituals, frequent shoplifting) **OR any serious**
41	**impairment in social, occupational, or school functioning** (e.g., no friends, unable to keep a job).
40	**Some impairment in reality testing or communication** (e.g., speech is at times illogical, obscure, or irrelevant) **OR major impairment in several areas, such as work or school, family relations, judgment, thinking, or mood** (e.g., depressed man avoids friends, neglects family, and is unable to work; child frequently beats up
31	younger children, is defiant at home, and is failing at school).
30	**Behavior is considerably influenced by delusions or hallucinations OR serious impairment in communication or judgment** (e.g., sometimes incoherent, acts grossly inappropriately, suicidal preoccupation) **OR inability**
21	**to function in almost all areas** (e.g., stays in bed all day, no job, home, or friends).
20	**Some danger of hurting self or others** (e.g., suicide attempts without clear expectation of death, frequently violent, manic excitement) **OR occasionally fails to maintain minimal personal hygiene** (e.g., smears feces)
11	**OR gross impairment in communication** (e.g., largely incoherent or mute).
10	**Persistent danger of severely hurting self or others** (e.g., recurrent violence) **OR persistent inability to**
1	**maintain minimal personal hygiene OR serious suicidal act with clear expectation of death.**

Table from DSM-III-R Diagnostic and Statistical Manual of Mental Disorders, ed 3, revised. (Current Classification of Mental Disorders, 1987.) Copyright American Psychiatric Association, Washington D.C., 1987. Used with permission.

given time, or a mental disorder in which at some time during its course all persons with the disorder have grossly impaired reality testing. When there is gross impairment in reality testing, the person incorrectly evaluates the accuracy of his or her perceptions and thoughts and makes incorrect inferences about external reality, even in the face of contrary evidence. The term psychotic does not apply to minor distortions of reality that involve matters of relative judgment. For example, a depressed person who underestimates his achievements is not described as psychotic, whereas one who believes he caused a natural catastrophe is so described.

Direct evidence of psychotic behavior is the presence of either delusions or hallucinations without insight into their pathological nature. The term psychotic is sometimes appropriate when behavior is so grossly disorganized that a reasonable inference can be made that reality testing is disturbed. Examples include markedly incoherent speech without apparent awareness by the person that the speech is not understandable, and the agitated, inattentive, and disoriented behavior seen in alcohol withdrawal delirium. . . . It should also be noted that a person with a nonpsychotic mental disorder may exhibit psychotic behavior, though rarely. For example, a person with obsessive-compulsive disorder may at times come to believe in the reality of the danger of being contaminated by shaking hands with strangers. In DSM-III-R the psychotic disorders include pervasive developmental disorders, schizophrenic

and delusional (paranoid) disorders, psychotic disorders not elsewhere classified, some organic mental disorders, and some mood (affective) disorders.

Neurosis

A neurosis is a chronic or recurrent, nonpsychotic disorder that is characterized mainly by anxiety, which is experienced or expressed directly or altered through defense mechanisms; it appears as a symptom, such as obsession, compulsion, phobia, or sexual dysfunction, among others. According to DSM-III, a neurotic disorder is defined as:

A mental disorder in which the predominant disturbance is a symptom or group of symptoms that is distressing to the individual and is recognized by him or her as unacceptable and alien (egodystonic); reality testing is grossly intact. Behavior does not actively violate gross social norms (though it may be quite disabling). The disturbance is relatively enduring or recurrent without treatment, and is not limited to a transitory reaction to stressors. There is no demonstrable organic etiology or factor.

In DSM-III-R there is no overall diagnostic class of "neuroses"; however, the following DSM-III-R diagnostic categories are considered neurosis by many clinicians and

Table 6
DSM-III-R Classification: Axes I and II Categories and Codes

All official DSM-III-R codes are included in ICD-9-CM. Codes followed by a * are used for more than one DSM-III-R diagnosis or subtype in order to maintain compatibility with ICD-9-CM.

A long dash following a diagnostic term indicates the need for a fifth digit subtype or other qualifying term.

The term *specify* following the name of some diagnostic categories indicates qualifying terms that clinicians may wish to add in parentheses after the name of the disorder.

NOS = Not Otherwise Specified

The current severity of a disorder may be specified after the diagnosis as:

mild
moderate
severe

currently
meets
diagnostic
criteria

in partial remission (or residual state)
in complete remission

DISORDERS USUALLY FIRST EVIDENT IN INFANCY, CHILDHOOD, OR ADOLESCENCE

> **DEVELOPMENTAL DISORDERS**
> Note: These are coded on Axis II.
>
> **Mental Retardation**
> 317.00 Mild mental retardation
> 318.00 Moderate mental retardation
> 318.10 Severe mental retardation
> 318.20 Profound mental retardation
> 319.00 Unspecified mental retardation
>
> **Pervasive Developmental Disorders**
> 299.00 Autistic disorder
> *Specify* if childhood onset
> 299.80 Pervasive developmental disorder NOS
>
> **Specific Developmental Disorders**
> Academic skills disorders
> 315.10 Developmental arithmetic disorder
> 315.80 Developmental expressive writing disorder
> 315.00 Developmental reading disorder
> Language and speech disorders
> 315.39 Developmental articulation disorder
> 315.31* Developmental expressive language disorder
> 315.31* Developmental receptive language disorder
> Motor skills disorder
> 315.40 Developmental coordination disorder
> 315.90* Specific developmental disorder NOS
>
> **Other Developmental Disorders**
> 315.90* Developmental disorder NOS

Disruptive Behavior Disorders
314.01 Attention-deficit hyperactivity disorder
Conduct disorder
312.20 group type

312.00 solitary aggressive type
312.90 undifferentiated type
313.81 Oppositional defiant disorder

Anxiety Disorders of Childhood or Adolescence
309.21 Separation anxiety disorder
313.21 Avoidant disorder of childhood or adolescence
313.00 Overanxious disorder

Eating Disorders
307.10 Anorexia nervosa
307.51 Bulimia nervosa
307.52 Pica
307.53 Rumination disorder of infancy
307.50 Eating disorder NOS

Gender Identity Disorders
302.60 Gender identity disorder of childhood
302.50 Transsexualism
Specify sexual history: asexual, homosexual, heterosexual, unspecified
302.85* Gender identity disorder of adolescence or adulthood, nontranssexual type
Specify sexual history: asexual, homosexual, heterosexual, unspecified
302.85* Gender identity disorder NOS

Tic Disorders
307.23 Tourette's disorder
307.22 Chronic motor or vocal tic disorder
307.21 Transient tic disorder
Specify: single episode or recurrent
307.20 Tic disorder NOS

Elimination Disorders
307.70 Functional encopresis
Specify: primary or secondary type
307.60 Functional enuresis
Specify: primary or secondary type
Specify: nocturnal only, diurnal only, nocturnal and diurnal

Speech Disorders Not Elsewhere Classified
307.00* Cluttering
307.00* Stuttering

Other Disorders of Infancy, Childhood, or Adolescence
313.23 Elective mutism
313.82 Identity disorder
313.89 Reactive attachment disorder of infancy or early childhood
307.30 Stereotype/habit disorder
314.00 Undifferentiated attention-deficit disorder

ORGANIC MENTAL DISORDERS

Dementias Arising in the Senium and Presenium
Primary degenerative dementia of the Alzheimer type, senile onset
290.30 with delirium
290.20 with delusions

Table 6 *continued*

290.21	with depression
290.00*	uncomplicated
	(Note: code 331.00 Alzheimer's disease on Axis III)

Code in fifth digit:
1 = with delirium, 2 = with delusions, 3= with depression, 0* = uncomplicated

290.1x	Primary degenerative dementia of the Alzheimer type, presenile onset, ____
	(Note: code 331.00 Alzheimer's disease on Axis III)
290.4x	Multi-infarct dementia, ____
290.00*	Senile dementia NOS
	Specify etiology on Axis III if known
290.10*	Presenile dementia NOS
	Specify etiology on Axis III if known (e.g., Pick's disease, Jakob-Creutzfeldt disease)

Psychoactive Substance–Induced Organic Mental Disorders

Alcohol
303.00	intoxication
291.40	idiosyncratic intoxication
291.80	uncomplicated alcohol withdrawal
291.00	withdrawal delirium
291.30	hallucinosis
291.10	amnestic disorder
291.20	dementia associated with alcoholism

Amphetamine or similarly acting sympathomimetic
305.70*	intoxication
292.00*	withdrawal
292.81*	delirium
292.11*	delusional disorder

Caffeine
305.90*	intoxication

Cannabis
305.20*	intoxication
292.11*	delusional disorder

Cocaine
305.60*	intoxication
292.00*	withdrawal
292.81*	delirium
292.11*	delusional disorder

Hallucinogen
305.30*	hallucinosis
292.11*	delusional disorder
292.84*	mood disorder
292.89*	posthallucinogen perception disorder

Inhalant
305.90*	intoxication

Nicotine
292.00*	withdrawal

Opioid
305.50*	intoxication
292.00*	withdrawal

Phencyclidine (PCP) or similarly acting arylcyclohexylamine
305.90*	intoxication
292.81*	delirium
292.11*	delusional disorder
292.84*	mood disorder
292.90*	organic mental disorder NOS

Sedative, hypnotic, or anxiolytic
305.40*	intoxication
292.00*	uncomplicated sedative, hypnotic, or anxiolytic withdrawal
292.00*	withdrawal delirium
292.83*	amnestic disorder

Other or unspecified psychoactive substance
305.90*	intoxication
292.00*	withdrawal
292.81*	delirium
292.82*	dementia
292.83*	amnestic disorder
292.11*	delusional disorder
292.12	hallucinosis
292.84*	mood disorder
292.89*	anxiety disorder
292.80*	personality disorder
292.90*	organic mental disorder NOS

Organic Mental Disorders associated with Axis III physical disorders or conditions, or whose etiology is unknown
293.00	Delirium
294.10	Dementia
294.00	Amnestic disorder
293.81	Organic delusional disorder
293.82	Organic hallucinosis
293.83	Organic mood disorder
	Specify: manic, depressed, mixed
294.80*	Organic anxiety disorder
310.10	Organic personality disorder
	Specify if explosive type
294.80*	Organic mental disorder NOS

PSYCHOACTIVE SUBSTANCE USE DISORDERS

Alcohol
303.90	dependence
305.00	abuse

Amphetamine or similarly acting sympathomimetic
304.40	dependence
305.70*	abuse

Cannabis
304.30	dependence
305.20*	abuse

Cocaine
304.20	dependence
305.60*	abuse

Hallucinogen
304.50*	dependence
305.30*	abuse

Inhalant
304.60	dependence
305.90*	abuse

Table 6 *continued*

	Nicotine
304.10	dependence
	Opioid
304.00	dependence
305.50*	abuse
	Phencyclidine (PCP) or similarly acting arylcyclohexylamine
304.50*	dependence
305.90*	abuse
	Sedative, hypnotic, or anxiolytic
304.10	dependence
305.40*	abuse
304.90*	Polysubstance dependence
304.90*	Psychoactive substance dependence
305.90*	Psychoactive substance abuse

SCHIZOPHRENIA

Code in fifth digit; 1 = subchronic, 2 = chronic, 3= subchronic with acute exacerbation, 4 = chronic with acute exacerbation, 5 = in remission, 0 = unspecified

	Schizophrenia
295.2x	catatonic, _____
295.1x	disorganized, _____
295.3x	paranoid, _____
	Specify if stable type
295.9x	undiffereniated, _____
295.6x	residual, _____
	Specify if late onset

DELUSIONAL (PARANOID) DISORDER

297.10	Delusional (Paranoid) disorder
	Specify type: erotomanic
	grandiose
	jealous
	persecutory
	somatic
	unspecified

PSYCHOTIC DISORDER NOT ELSEWHERE CLASSIFIED

298.80	Brief reactive psychosis
295.40	Schizophreniform disorder
	Specify: without good prognostic features or with good prognostic features
295.70	Schizoaffective disorder
	S*pecify:* bipolar type or depressive type
297.30	Induced psychotic disorder
298.90	Psychotic disorder NOS (Atypical psychosis)

MOOD DISORDERS

Code current state of Major Depression and Bipolar Disorder in fifth digit:

1 = mild
2 = moderate
3 = severe, without psychotic features
4 = with psychotic features (*specify* mood-congruent or mood-incongruent)
5 = in partial remission
6 = in full remission
0 = unspecified

For major depressive episodes, *specify* if chronic and *specify* if melancholic type.

For Bipolar Disorder, Bipolar Disorder NOS, Recurrent Major Depression and Depressive Disorder NOS, *specify* if seasonal pattern.

Bipolar Disorders

	Bipolar disorder
296.6x	mixed, _____
296.4x	manic, _____
296.5x	depressed, _____
301.13	Cyclothymia
296.70	Bipolar disorder NOS

Depressive Disorders

	Major Depression
296.2x	single episode, _____
296.3x	recurrent, _____
300.40	Dysthymia (or Depressive neurosis)
	Specify: primary or secondary type
	Specify: early or late onset
311.00	Depressive disorder NOS

ANXIETY DISORDERS (or Anxiety and Phobic Neuroses)

	Panic disorder
300.21	with agoraphobia
	Specify current severity of agoraphobic avoidance
	Specify current severity of panic attacks
300.01	without agoraphobia
	Specify current severity of panic attacks
300.22	Agoraphobia without history of panic disorder
	Specify with or without limited symptom attacks
300.23	Social phobia
	Specify if generalized type
300.29	Simple phobia
300.30	Obsessive compulsive disorder (or Obsessive compulsive neurosis)
309.89	Post-traumatic stress disorder
	Specify if delayed onset
300.02	Generalized anxiety disorder
300.00	Anxiety disorder NOS

SOMATOFORM DISORDERS

300.70*	Body dysmorphic disorder
300.11	Conversion disorder (or Hysterical neurosis, conversion type)
	Specify: single episode or recurrent
300.70*	Hypochondriasis (or Hypochondriacal neurosis)
300.81	Somatization disorder
307.80	Somatoform pain disorder
300.70*	Undifferentiated somatoform pain disorder
300.70*	Somatoform disorder NOS

DISSOCIATIVE DISORDERS (or Hysterical Neuroses, Dissociative Type)

300.14	Multiple personality disorder
300.13	Psychogenic fugue
300.12	Psychogenic amnesia
300.60	Depersonalization disorder (or depersonalization neurosis)
300.15	Dissociative disorder NOS

Table 6 *continued*

SEXUAL DISORDERS

Paraphilias
302.40	Exhibitionism
302.81	Fetishism
302.89	Frotteurism
302.20	Pedophilia
	Specify: same sex, opposite sex, same and opposite sex
	Specify if limited to incest
	Specify: exclusive type or nonexclusive type
302.83	Sexual masochism
302.84	Sexual sadism
302.30	Transvestic fetishism
302.82	Voyeurism
302.90*	Paraphilia NOS

Sexual Dysfunctions
Specify: psychogenic only, or psychogenic and biogenic (Note: If biogenic only, code on Axis III)
Specify: lifelong or acquired
Specify: generalized or situational

	Sexual desire disorders
302.71	Hypoactive sexual desire disorder
302.79	Sexual aversion disorder
	Sexual arousal disorders
302.72*	Female sexual arousal disorder
302.72*	Male erectile disorder
	Orgasm disorders
302.73	Inhibited female orgasm
302.74	Inhibited male orgasm
302.75	Premature ejaculation
	Sexual pain disorders
302.76	Dyspareunia
306.51	Vaginismus
302.70	Sexual dysfunction NOS

Other Sexual Disorders
302.90*	Sexual disorder NOS

SLEEP DISORDERS

Dyssomnias
	Insomnia disorder
307.42*	related to another mental disorder (nonorganic)
780.50*	related to known organic factor
307.42*	Primary insomnia
	Hypersomnia disorder
307.44	related to another mental disorder (nonorganic)
780.50*	related to known organic factor
780.54*	Primary hypersomnia
307.45	Sleep-wake schedule disorder
	Specify: advanced or delayed phase type, disorganized type, frequently changing type
	Other dyssomnias
307.40*	Dyssomnia NOS

Parasomnias
307.47	Dream anxiety disorder (nightmare disorder)
307.46*	Sleep terror disorder
307.46*	Sleepwalking disorder
307.40*	Parasomnia NOS

FACTITIOUS DISORDERS
	Factitious disorder
301.51	with physical symptoms
300.16	with psychological symptoms
300.19	Factitious disorder NOS

IMPULSE CONTROL DISORDERS NOT ELSEWHERE CLASSIFIED
312.34	Intermittent explosive disorder
312.32	Kleptomania
312.31	Pathological gambling
312.33	Pyromania
312.39*	Trichotillomania
312.39*	Impulse control disorder NOS

ADJUSTMENT DISORDER
	Adjustment disorder
309.24	with anxious mood
309.00	with depressed mood
309.30	with disturbance of conduct
309.40	with mixed disturbance of emotions and conduct
309.28	with mixed emotional features
309.82	with physical conditions
309.83	with withdrawal
309.23	with work (or academic) inhibition
309.90	Adjustment disorder NOS

PSYCHOLOGICAL FACTORS AFFECTING PHYSICAL CONDITION
316.00	Psychological factors affecting physical condition
	Specify physical condition on Axis III

PERSONALITY DISORDERS
Note: These are coded on Axis II.

Cluster A
301.00	Paranoid
301.20	Schizoid
301.22	Schizotypal

Cluster B
301.70	Antisocial
301.83	Borderline
301.50	Histrionic
301.81	Narcissistic

Cluster C
301.82	Avoidant
301.60	Dependent
301.40	Obsessive compulsive
301.84	Passive aggressive
301.90	Personality disorder NOS

V CODES FOR CONDITIONS NOT ATTRIBUTABLE TO A MENTAL DISORDER THAT ARE A FOCUS OF ATTENTION OR TREATMENT
V62.30	Academic problem
V71.01	Adult antisocial behavior

V40.00	Borderline intellectual functional (Note: This is coded on Axis II.)

Table 6 continued

			ADDITIONAL CODES	
V71.02	Childhood or adolescent antisocial behavior		300.90	Unspecified mental disorder (nonpsychotic)
V65.20	Malingering		V71.09*	No diagnosis or condition on Axis I
V61.10	Marital problem		799.90*	Diagnosis or condition deferred on Axis I
V15.81	Noncompliance with medical treatment			
V62.20	Occupational problem			
V61.20	Parent-child problem			
V62.81	Other interpersonal problem		V71.09*	No diagnosis or condition on Axis II
V61.80	Other specified family circumstances		799.90*	Diagnosis or condition deferred on Axis II
V62.89	Phase of life problem or other life circumstance problem			
V62.82	Uncomplicated bereavement			

Table from DSM-III-R Diagnostic and Statistical Manual of Mental Disorders, ed 3, revised. (Current Classification of Mental Disorders, 1987.) Copyright American Psychiatric Association, Washington D.C., 1987. Used with permission.

the reader will note that DSM-III-R uses the term neurosis in parentheses for some of these conditions.

Anxiety Disorders (or Anxiety and Phobic Neuroses). These include agoraphobia without history of panic disorder, social phobia, and simple phobia; panic disorder (with or without agoraphobia), generalized anxiety disorder, and obsessive compulsive disorder (or obsessive compulsive neurosis); and posttraumatic stress disorder.

Somatoform Disorder. These disorders include somatization disorder, conversion disorder (hysterical neurosis, conversion type), somatoform pain disorder, hypochondriasis (or hypochondriacal neurosis), body dysmorphic disorder, and undifferentiated somatoform disorder.

Dissociative Disorders (Hysterical Neuroses, Dissociative Type). These disorders include psychogenic amnesia, psychogenic fugue, multiple personality, depersonalization disorder (or depersonalization neurosis), and dissociative disorder not otherwise specified.

Sexual Disorders. This broad category includes paraphilias, and sexual dysfunction. In common use, the categories have been considered neurotic disorders.

Dysthymic Disorder. This disorder, also known as depressive neurosis, is now classified in DSM-III-R as a type of mood disorder.

In summary, the term "neurosis" encompasses a broad range of disorders of different signs and symptoms. As such, it has lost any degree of precision except to signify that the person's gross reality testing and personality organization are intact. A neurosis, however, can be and usually is sufficient to impair the person's functioning in a variety of areas.

Psychosomatic

The term psychosomatic expresses the interrelationship between the mind (psyche) and body (soma) and refers to those physical conditions that are either caused or influenced by psychological factors. In DSM-III-R, this term is replaced by the category "psychological factors affecting physical conditions," with the physical condition having either a demonstrable organic pathology (e.g., rheumatoid arthritis) or a known pathophysiological process (e.g., vomiting).

NEW AND CONTROVERSIAL CATEGORIES

DSM-III-R contains three new categories (discussed below) that are considered to be controversial for a variety of reasons. Not all psychiatrists agree that they exist as discrete psychological disorders; for those who believe that they exist, there is lack of consensus as to what are the essential diagnostic features of each of the disorders. In addition, certain groups argue that the new categories reflect lingering antifeminist cultural biases that may be promulgated by assigning diagnostic labels with a high potential for misapplication and abuse. The DSM-III-R will probably undergo revision as data regarding the diagnostic validity and reliability of these three disorders accumulate.

Late Luteal Phase Dysphoric Disorder (LLPDD)

This condition occurs in women and is associated with the luteal phase of the menstrual cycle that occurs in the week prior to the onset of menses. Essential features include affective lability, irritability, anger, and signs and symptoms of depression (e.g., feelings of worthlessness, loss of energy, appetite change, sleep disorders). Some women may develop suicidal ideation. Physical symptoms (e.g., headache, musculoskeletal pain, and edema) may occur premenstrually. The prevalence of the disorder is unknown. It has been reported to occur at any age after menarche, but most frequently in women over 30. See Chapter 26, which discusses psychological factors affecting physical condition, for a further discussion of this syndrome.

Self-Defeating Personality Disorder

In this condition persons deliberately place themselves in situations in which they will suffer, be hurt, be disappointed, or be mistreated, and subsequently feel humiliated or guilty.

Sadistic Personality Disorder

In this condition the person behaves in a cruel and aggressive way (including the use of physical violence) toward others. The person takes pleasure in being sadistic and is often fascinated by violence and methods of torture.

Table 7
ICD-9 Classification of Mental Disorders

ORGANIC PSYCHOTIC CONDITIONS
Senile and pre-senile organic psychotic conditions
290.0 Senile dementia, simple type
290.1 Pre-senile dementia
290.2 Senile dementia, depressed or paranoid type
290.3 Senile dementia with acute confusional state
290.4 Arteriosclerotic dementia
290.8 Other
290.9 Unspecified

Alcoholic psychoses
291.0 Delirium tremens
291.1 Korasakov's psychosis, alcoholic
291.2 Other alcoholic dementia
291.3 Other alcoholic hallucinosis
291.4 Pathological drunkenness
291.5 Alcoholic jealousy
291.8 Other
291.9 Unspecified

Drug psychoses
292.0 Drug withdrawal syndrome
292.1 Paranoid and/or hallucinatory states induced by drugs
292.2 Pathological drug intoxication
292.8 Other
292.9 Unspecified

Transient organic psychotic conditions
293.0 Acute confusional state
293.1 Subacute confusional state
293.8 Other
293.9 Unspecified

Other organic psychotic conditions (chronic)
294.0 Korsakov's psychosis (non-alcoholic)
294.1 Dementia in conditions classified elsewhere
294.8 Other
294.9 Unspecified

OTHER PSYCHOSES
Schizophrenic psychoses
295.0 Simple type
295.1 Hebephrenic type
295.2 Catatonic type
295.3 Paranoid type
295.4 Acute schizophrenic episode
295.5 Latent schizophrenia
295.6 Residual schizophrenia
295.7 Schizo-affective type
295.8 Other
295.9 Unspecified

Affective psychoses
296.0 Manic-depressive psychosis, manic type
296.1 Manic-depressive psychosis, depressed type
296.2 Manic-depressive psychosis, circular type but currently manic
296.3 Manic-depressive psychosis, circular type but currently depressed
296.4 Manic-depressive psychosis, circular type, mixed
296.5 Manic-depressive psychosis, circular type, current condition not specified
296.6 Manic-depressive psychosis, other and unspecified
296.8 Other
296.9 Unspecified

Paranoid states
297.0 Paranoid state, simple
297.1 Paranoia
297.2 Paraphrenia
297.3 Induced psychosis
297.8 Other
297.9 Unspecified

Other nonorganic psychoses
298.0 Depressive type
298.1 Excitative type
298.2 Reactive confusion
298.3 Acute paranoid reaction
298.4 Psychogenic paranoid psychosis
298.8 Other and unspecified reactive psychosis
298.9 Unspecified psychosis

Psychoses with origin specific to childhood
299.0 Infantile autism
299.1 Disintegrative psychosis
299.8 Other
299.9 Unspecified

NEUROTIC DISORDERS, PERSONALITY DISORDERS, AND THER NONPSYCHOTIC MENTAL DISORDERS
Neurotic disorders
300.0 Anxiety states
300.1 Hysteria
300.2 Phobic state
300.3 Obsessive-compulsive disorder
300.4 Neurotic depression
300.5 Neurasthenia
300.6 Depersonalization syndrome
300.7 Hypochondriasis
300.8 Other
300.9 Unspecified

Personality disorders
301.0 Paranoid
301.1 Affective
301.2 Schizoid
301.3 Explosive
301.4 Anankastic
301.5 Hysterical
301.6 Asthenic
301.7 With predominantly sociopathic or asocial manifestations
301.8 Other
301.9 Unspecified

Sexual deviations and disorders
302.0 Homosexuality
302.1 Bestiality
302.2 Paedophilia
302.3 Transvestism
302.4 Exhibitionism
302.5 Transsexualism
302.6 Disorders of psychosexual identity
302.7 Frigidity and impotence
302.8 Other
302.9 Unspecified

Table 7 *continued*

303. Alcohol dependence

Drug dependence
304.0 Morphine type
304.1 Barbiturate type
304.2 Cocaine
304.3 Cannabis
304.4 Amphetamine type and other psychostimulants
304.5 Hallucinogens
304.6 Other
304.7 Combinations of morphine type drug with any other
304.8 Combinations excluding morphine type drug
304.9 Unspecified

Nondependent abuse of drugs
305.0 Alcohol
305.1 Tobacco
305.2 Cannabis
305.3 Hallucinogens
305.4 Barbiturates and tranquilizers
305.5 Morphine type
305.6 Cocaine type
305.7 Amphetamine type
305.8 Antidepressants
305.9 Other, mixed or unspecified

Physical conditions arising from mental factors
306.0 Musculoskeletal
306.1 Respiratory
306.2 Cardiovascuar
306.3 Skin
306.4 Gastrointestinal
306.5 Genitourinary
306.6 Endocrine
306.7 Organs of special sense
306.8 Other
306.9 Unspecified

Special symptoms or syndromes not elsewhere classified
307.0 Stammering and stuttering
307.1 Anorexia nervosa
307.2 Tics
307.3 Stereotyped-repetitive movements
307.4 Specific disorders of sleep
307.5 Other disorders of eating
307.6 Enuresis
307.7 Encopresis
307.8 Psychalgia
306.9 Other and unspecified

Acute reaction to stress
308.0 Predominant disturbances of emotions
308.1 Predominant disturbances of consciousness
308.2 Predominant psychomotor disturbance
308.3 Other
308.4 Mixed
308.9 Unspecified

Adjustment reaction
309.0 Brief depressive reaction

309.1 Prolonged depressive reaction
309.2 With predominant disturbances of other emotions
309.3 With predominant disturbances of conduct
309.4 With mixed disturbances of emotions and conduct
309.8 Other
309.9 Unspecified

Specific nonpsychotic mental disorders following organic brain damage
310.0 Frontal lobe syndrcme
310.1 Cognitive or personality change of other type
310.2 Postconcussional syndrome
310.8 Other
310.9 Unspecified

311. Depressive disorder, not elsewhere classified

Disturbance of conduct not elsewhere classified
312.0 Unsocialized disturbance of conduct
312.1 Socialized disturbance of conduct
312.2 Compulsive conduct disorder
312.3 Mixed disturbance of conduct and emotions
312.8 Other
312.9 Unspecified

Disturbance of emotions specific to childhood and adolescence
313.0 With anxiety and fearfulness
313.1 With misery and unhappiness
313.2 With sensitivity, shyness and social withdrawal
313.3 Relationship problems
313.8 Other or mixed
313.9 Unspecified

Hyperkinetic syndrome of childhood
314.0 Simple disturbance of activity and attention
314.1 Hyperkinesis with developmental delay
314.2 Hyperkinetic conduct disorder
314.8 Other
314.9 Unspecified

Specific delays in development
315.0 Specific reading retardation
315.1 Specific arithmetical retardation
315.2 Other specific learning difficulties
315.3 Developmental speech or language disorder
315.4 Specific motor retardatfion
315.5 Mixed development disorder
315.8 Other
315.9 Unspecified

316. Psychic factors associated with diseases classified elsewhere

317. Mild mental retardation

Other specified mental retardation
318.0 Moderate mental retardation
318.1 Severe mental retardation
318.2 Profound mental retardation

319. Unspecified mental retardation

---

*From World Health Organization: *Manual of the International Classification of Diseases, Injuries, and Causes of Death,* ed 9, revised. World Health Organization, Geneva, 1978. Used with permission.

(For a further discussion on self-defeating and sadistic personality disorders see Chapter 27.)

References

American Psychiatric Association: *Diagnostic and Statistical Manual of Mental Disorders,* ed 3-R. American Psychiatric Association, Washington, DC, 1987.

Chodoff P: DSM-III and psychotherapy. Am J Psychiatry *143*:187, 1986.

Kendell R E: *The Role of Diagnosis in Psychiatry.* Blackwell, Oxford, 1975.

Mezzich J E: International experience with DSM-III. J Nervous Mental Disorders *173*:12, 1985.

Rounsaville B J, Kosten T R, Williams J B W, Spitzer R L: A field trial of DSM-III-R psychoactive substance dependence disorders. Am J Psych *144*:351, 1987.

Schwartz A, Wiggins O P: Typifications. The first step for clinical diagnosis in psychiatry. J Nervous Mental Disease *175*:65, 1987.

Shrout P E, Spitzer R L, Fleiss J L: Quantification of agreement in psychiatric diagnosis revisited. Arch Gen Psychiatry *44*:100, 1987.

Spitzer R L, Skodol A E, Gibbon M, Williams J B W: *Casebook: Diagnostic and Statistical Manual of Mental Disorders.* American Psychiatric Association, Washington, DC, 1981.

Spitzer R L, Williams J B W: *Instruction Manual for the Structured Clinical Interview for DSM-III (SCID) New York.* Biometrics Research Department, State Psychiatric Institute, New York, 1985.

Strauss J S: A comprehensive approach to psychiatric diagnosis. Am J Psychiatry *132*:1193, 1975.

Strauss J S, Helmchen H: Review paper on multiaxial diagnosis. Paper presented at the World Health Organization Conference on Diagnosis and Classification of Mental Disorders, Alcohol, and Drug-Related Problems. Copenhagen, Denmark, 1982.

World Health Organization: *International Classification of Diseases,* rev 9. World Health Organization, Geneva, 1977.

World Psychiatric Association: *Diagnostic Criteria for Schizophrenic and Affective Psychoses.* American Psychiatric Press, Washington, DC, 1983.

Zimmerman M, Ohohl B, Coryell W, Stangl D: The prognostic validity of DSM-III Axis IV in depressed inpatients. Am J Psychiatry *144*(1):102, 1987.

11

Organic Mental Syndromes and Disorders

Organic mental syndromes and disorders are a class of conditions caused directly by abnormalities of brain structure or by alterations of brain neurochemistry or neurophysiology. In some cases it is impossible to identify the specific underlying abnormality in brain structure or function that gives rise to the syndrome. In these instances, the organic basis for the clinical abnormality is inferred from characteristic clinical findings. In DSM-III-R, the term "disorder" is used when an organic mental syndrome is associated with an Axis III disorder or condition, and the term "syndrome" is used to refer to a set of psychological or behavioral signs and symptoms without reference to etiology. According to DSM-III-R, the essential feature of all these disorders is a psychological or behavioral abnormality associated with transient or permanent dysfunction of the brain. The underlying cerebral disease or disorder may be primary—that is, originating in the brain—or secondary to some systemic disease. The resulting psychopathological manifestations reflect destruction or metabolic derangement of brain structures subserving cognitive functions, emotions, and motivation of behavior.

Cognitive loss is generally considered to be the hallmark of organic disorder. Such loss is marked by impairment of four major areas: orientation, memory, intellectual functions (e.g., comprehension, calculation, learning), and judgment. Cognitive impairment may be accompanied by anxiety, depression, irritability, and shame. Paranoia, euphoria, apathy, and decreased control over sexual, aggressive, and acquisitive impulses may also accompany cognitive loss.

CLASSIFICATION

According to DSM-III-R the organic mental syndromes are delirium, dementia, amnestic syndrome, organic delusional syndrome, organic hallucinosis, organic mood syndrome, organic anxiety syndrome, organic personality syndrome, intoxication, withdrawal, and organic mental syndrome not otherwise specified (NOS, a residual category). If the etiology is known (e.g., delirium due to pneumonia) the condition is coded on Axis III.

In DSM-III-R the organic mental disorders include dementias arising in the senium and presenium, psychoactive substance–induced organic mental disorders, and organic mental disorders associated with Axis III physical disorders or conditions or whose etiology is unknown. In the category of dementias arising in the senium or presenium, the etiology or the pathophysiologic process involves aging. DSM-III-R lists three types of dementias: primary degenerative dementia of the Alzheimer type, senile onset; primary degenerative dementia of the Alzheimer type, presenile onset; and multi-infarct dementia.

DELIRIUM

Definition

Delirium is an organic mental syndrome characterized by acute onset and fluctuating course of impaired cognitive functioning resulting from widespread cerebral nervous tissue dysfunction. The patient's ability to receive, process, store, and recall information is markedly impaired. Delirium is usually transient and reversible when the cause is determined and treated. Its total duration is brief.

Epidemiology

Delirium is the organic psychiatric syndrome encountered most often by psychiatrists who are called to consult on patients in general medical and surgical wards. About 10 percent of all hospital inpatients manifest some degree of delirium. The incidence varies in different studies and on different hospital services. For example, delirium occurs in 30 percent of patients in surgical intensive care and in coronary intensive care units. About 20 percent of severely burned patients become delirious. Delirium most commonly occurs in the aged and in children, and pre-existing brain damage or a history of delirium seems to increase the risk of developing the syndrome.

Etiology

The etiology of delirium is multifactorial—a combination of individual, situational, and pharmacologic variables. Patients with organic brain lesions are especially liable to develop delirium, as are patients with alcohol or drug addiction. Patients who have had a prior episode of delirium are likely to have a recurrent episode under the same condition. The cause of *postoperative delirium* includes the stress of surgery, postoperative pain, insomnia, pain medication, electrolyte imbalance, infection, fever, and blood loss. *Black-patch delirium*, a particular type of delirium following cataract surgery, results from the disorientation caused by covering the eyes. A pinhole in the patch that allows light to enter reduces the syndrome markedly.

Psychiatric patients being treated with psychotropic agents are at risk of developing delirium due to overmedication (such as an anticholinergic delirium), as are the elderly, who are susceptible to drug side effects. According to some

Table 1
Causes of Delirium

Intracranial causes
  Epilepsy and postictal states
  Brain trauma (especially concussion)
  Infections
    Meningitis
    Encephalitis
  Subarachnoid hemorrhage
Extracranial causes
  Drugs (ingestion or withdrawal) and poisons
    Sedatives (including alcohol) and hypnotics
    Tranquilizers
    Other drugs
      Anticholinergic agents
      Anticonvulsants
      Antihypertensive agents
      Antiparkinsonian agents
      Cardiac glycosides
      Cimetidine
      Disulfiram
      Insulin
      Opiates
      Phencyclidine
      Salicylates
      Steroids
    Poisons
      Carbon monoxide
      Heavy metals and other industrial poisons
  Endocrine dysfunction (hypo- or hyperfunction)
    Pituitary
    Pancreas
    Adrenal
    Parathyroid
    Thyroid
  Diseases of nonendocrine organs
    Liver
      Hepatic encephalopathy
    Kidney and urinary tract
      Uremic encephalopathy
    Lung
      Carbon dioxide narcosis
      Hypoxia
    Cardiovascular system
      Cardiac failure
      Arrhythmias
      Hypotension
  Deficiency diseases
    Thiamine deficiency
  Systemic infections with fever and sepsis
  Electrolyte imbalance of any cause
  Postoperative states

Table by Wells C E: Organic syndromes: Delirium. In *Comprehensive Textbook of Psychiatry*, ed 4, H I Kaplan and B J Sadock, editors, p 844. Williams & Wilkins, Baltimore, 1985.

studies, patients who are most fearful of medical and surgical procedures are more likely to become delirious than patients who are less frightened.

Table 1 outlines many of the causes of delirium. It should be noted that certain nonpsychoactive drugs, such as the frequently used cimetidine, an antiulcer agent, may also produce delirium.

Clinical Features

Although the onset of delirium is usually acute, prodromal symptoms (e.g., daytime restlessness, anxiety, fearfulness, or hypersensitivity to light or sounds) may occur. The patient is usually confused, disoriented, and unable to test reality. There is an inability to distinguish between dreams, illusions, and true hallucinations, or between sleep and wakefulness with a disturbance resulting in the sleep-wake cycle. The patient is easily distracted by irrelevant stimuli. The ability to think coherently is reduced, and thought processes often become slowed, disorganized, and more concrete. Reasoning and problem solving may become difficult or impossible. Recall of what transpires during a delirium once it is over is characteristically spotty, and the patient may refer to it as a bad dream or a nightmare that is remembered only vaguely (Table 2).

As a rule, orientation to time and place is impaired. According to DSM-III-R, disorientation to time may be the first symptom to appear in mild delirium. Except for the most severe cases, orientation to person is intact; that is, the patient is aware of his or her own identity. Attempts to compensate for basic cognitive deficits may cause the patient to misidentify persons in the environment. Perceptual disturbances are common, including illusions and hallucinations. These disturbances are most often visual, but they may occur in all sensory modalities. Accompanying the disturbances is often a belief of delusional proportion of the reality of the experience, and there is an emotional and behavioral response appropriate to the content of the disturbance. Vivid dreams and nightmares are also common, and may merge with hallucinations.

Cognitive impairment in delirium tends to fluctuate unpredictably. Diurnal variability is a clinical sign of delirium. Delirium is predictably more severe and incapacitating during the night and early morning hours, an observation that has led to delirious patients being called "sundowners." Some patients, in fact, may appear delirious only at night and regain lucidity during the day. So-called lucid intervals, during which patients are more attentive, rational, and in better contact with their surroundings, may appear at any time and last for minutes to hours.

Psychomotor behavior is usually abnormal. The patient is either hypoactive and lethargic or hyperactive to the point of exhaustion and may unexpectedly and abruptly shift from a relatively quiet state to a state of agitation, and vice versa. Autonomic dysfunction may also occur: pallor, flushing, sweating, cardiac irregularities, nausea, vomiting, and hyperthermia may be observed in the delirious patient. The most commonly observed emotions are fear and anxiety. If fear is intense and the result of frightening illusions and hallucinations, the patient may make determined attempts to escape possible injury to himself or herself or to others.

Table 2
Diagnostic Criteria for Delirium

A. Reduced ability to maintain attention to external stimuli (e.g., questions must be repeated because attention wanders) and to appropriately shift attention to new external stimuli (e.g., perseverates answer to a previous question).

B. Disorganized thinking, as indicated by rambling, irrelevant, or incoherent speech.

C. At least two of the following:
(1) reduced level of consciousness (e.g., difficulty keeping awake during examination)
(2) perceptual disturbances: misinterpretations, illusions, or hallucinations
(3) disturbance of sleep-wake cycle with insomnia or daytime sleepiness
(4) increased or decreased psychomotor activity
(5) disorientation to time, place, or person
(6) memory impairment (e.g., inability to learn new material, such as the names of several unrelated objects after 5 minutes, or to remember past events, such as history of current episode of illness)

D. Clinical features develop over a short period of time (usually hours to days) and tend to fluctuate over the course of a day.

E. Either (1) or (2):
(1) evidence from the history, physical examination, or laboratory tests of a specific organic factor (or factors) judged to be etiologically related to the disturbance
(2) in the absence of such evidence, an etiologic organic factor can be presumed if the disturbance cannot be accounted for by any nonorganic mental disorder (e.g., manic episode accounting for agitation and sleep disturbance)

Table from *DSM-III-R Diagnostic and Statistical Manual of Mental Disorders*, ed 3, revised. (Current Classification of Mental Disorders, 1987.) Copyright American Psychiatric Association, Washington, D.C., 1987. Used with permission.

A deeply depressed patient may attempt suicide, but a delirious patient is much more likely to sustain an injury as a result of a wild flight.

Diagnosis

Delirium is usually diagnosed at the bedside and is characterized by the sudden onset of symptoms. Diurnal fluctuations are characteristic. The presence of a known physical illness or a history of head trauma, alcoholism, or drug addiction increases the likelihood of the diagnosis. Multiple cognitive deficits in the mental status examination and clouding of consciousness are characteristic.

Course and Prognosis

Delirium is reversible if the underlying cause is diagnosed and treated in a timely manner. Untreated delirium may clear spontaneously, or it may progress to dementia or to another organic brain syndrome.

Differential Diagnosis

Delirium needs to be distinguished from other organic brain syndromes, especially dementia (Table 3). Dementia usually has an insidious onset, and although both conditions show cognitive impairment, the changes in dementia are more fixed. Also, although impaired, the patient with dementia is alert. Occasionally, delirium may occur in a patient suffering from dementia, a condition known as *beclouded dementia*. According to DSM-III-R, one cannot diagnose dementia in the presence of significant delirium because the symptoms of delirium interfere with the proper assessment of dementia. Both diagnoses are given only when there is a definite history of pre-existing dementia. When the diagnosis is in question, it is recommended that a provisional diagnosis of delirium be made, so that a more rigorous therapeutic approach will be made. Patients with factitious disorder attempt to simulate the symptoms of delirium; however, careful observation will usually reveal that the symptoms are under voluntary control, the patient often showing inconsistencies on tests of mental status. A normal electroencephalogram can help to make the diagnosis, because a person with a delirium shows diffuse slowing of background activity on EEG.

Schizophrenia is characterized by hallucinations or delusions that are more constant and better organized than those of delirium. Schizophrenic patients usually experience no change in level of consciousness, and orientation is also intact. Brief reactive psychosis and schizophreniform disorder show disorganized speech and loosening of associations, but the global cognitive impairment of delirium is lacking. Patients with dissociative disorders may appear disoriented and show purposeless wandering, but such episodes are usually self-limited, and memory disturbances are spotty and temporary.

Treatment

A cardinal rule in the treatment of delirium is to identify the cause and to apply appropriate medical or surgical therapeutic techniques. Laboratory tests should be obtained as indicated. In addition to treating the cause, the management of delirium involves general and symptomatic measures aimed at the relief of distress and the prevention of complications such as accidents of trauma. Proper nutritional, electrolyte, and fluid balance must be maintained. Management also depends to some extent on the setting in which the delirium occurs, on the age of the affected person, and on the overall medical and neurological status.

Optimal sensory, social, and nursing environment should be provided. If sensory isolation is playing a role in the delirium, the patient will benefit from a dimmed light at night, frequent visits by staff and family, and explanation and reassurance about procedures being performed. Placing a television set in a patient's room and calling the patient by name help maintain orientation.

An agitated, restless, fearful, or belligerent patient needs to be sedated to prevent complications and accidents. No single psychotropic drug is recommended for all cases of delirium. As a general rule, haloperidol (Haldol) is the drug of choice. Depending on the patient's age, weight, and physical condition, the initial dose may range from 2 to 10

Table 3
Clinical Differentiation of Delirium and Dementia

	Delirium	Dementia
Onset	Acute	Usually insidious; if acute, preceded by coma or delirium
Duration	Usually less than 1 month	At least 1 month, usually much longer
Orientation	Faulty, at least for a time; tendency to mistake unfamiliar for familiar place, person	May be correct in mild cases
Thinking	Disorganized	Impoverished
Memory	Recent impaired	Both recent and remote impaired
Attention	Invariably disturbed, hard to direct or sustain	May be intact
Awareness	Always reduced, tends to fluctuate during daytime and be worse at night	Usually intact
Alertness	Increased or decreased	Normal or decreased
Perception	Misperceptions often present	Misperceptions often absent
Sleep-wake cycle	Always disrupted	Usually normal for age

After Lipowski Z J: *Delirium: Acute Brain Failure in Man.* Charles C Thomas, Springfield, IL. 1979.

mg intramuscularly, to be repeated hourly if the patient remains agitated. As soon as the patient is calm, oral medication in liquid concentrate or tablet form should begin. Two daily oral doses should suffice, two thirds of the dose being given at bedtime. In order to achieve the same therapeutic effect, the oral dose should be about 1.5 times higher than the parenteral dose. The effective total daily dose of haloperidol (Haldol) may range from 10 to 60 mg for most delirious patients. The patient's insomnia is best treated with small doses of a short-acting benzodiazepine, such as triazolam (Halcion).

DEMENTIA

Definition

Dementia is characterized by loss of cognitive and intellectual abilities that is severe enough to impair social or occupational performance. The full clinical picture consists of impairment of memory, abstract thinking, and judgment, with some degree of personality change. The disorder may be progressive, static, or reversible, and results from widespread cerebral damage or dysfunction. An underlying organic cause is always assumed, although in some cases it may be impossible to determine a specific organic factor. In these cases where a specific factor has not been established, a thorough search for an organic etiology must nonetheless be made, and all nonorganic diagnoses must be ruled out. The reversibility of a dementia is related to the underlying pathology and to the availability and application of effective treatment.

Epidemiology

Dementia occurs most often in old age. One million Americans over age 65 (5 percent of the aged population) have a significant degree of dementia and are unable to care for themselves. Another 2 million (10 per cent of the aged) have mild dementia, and about 60 percent of persons in nursing homes have some dementia. The prevalence of dementia increases with age; it is five times more common in persons 80 years and older than in those 70 and younger. However, according to DSM-III-R, the diagnosis of dementia may be made at any time after the I.Q. is fairly stable, usually by the age of 3 or 4. Thus, according to DSM-III-R, a child of age 4 or above who develops a chronic neurologic disorder that interferes with already acquired functions to the degree of significant intellectual and adaptive functioning would be diagnosed as both mentally retarded and demented.

Because the number of elderly is increasing (by the year 2030 it is estimated that 20 percent of the population will be over age 65), dementia is a major public health problem. The annual cost of caring for patients with chronic dementia is estimated to be about 15 billion dollars.

Etiology

Most cases of dementia do not suggest a specific etiology. The most common cause of dementia is primary degenerative dementia of the Alzheimer's type (about 65 percent of all cases). The next most common etiological factor is multi-infarct dementia (10 percent of all cases). The alarming increase in acquired immune deficiency syndrome (AIDS) has led to the recognition of an increasing number of dementias related to human immunodeficiency virus (HIV). About 15 percent of all dementia cases are reversible if the physician initiates timely treatment, before irreversible damage has taken place. Table 4 lists the various causes of dementia and indicates the most treatable factors.

Clinical Features

Defects in orientation, memory, perception, intellectual function, reasoning, and judgment are characteristic features of dementia. Affective and behavioral changes, such

Table 4
Diseases That Cause Dementia

Parenchymatous diseases of the central nervous system
   Alzheimer's disease (primary degenerative dementia)
   Pick's disease (primary degenerative dementia)
   Huntington's disease
   Parkinson's disease*
   Multiple sclerosis
Systemic disorders
   Endocrine and metabolic disorders
     Thyroid disease*
     Parathyroid disease*
     Pituitary-adrenal disorders*
     Post-hypoglycemic states
   Liver disease
     Chronic progressive hepatic encephalopathy*
   Urinary tract disease
     Chronic uremic encephalopathy*
     Progressive uremic encephalopathy (dialysis dementia)*
   Cardiovascular disease
     Cerebral hypoxia or anoxia*
     Multi-infarct dementia*
     Cardiac arrhythmias*
     Inflammatory diseases of blood vessels*
   Pulmonary disease
     Respiratory encephalopathy*
Deficiency states
   Cyanocobalamin deficiency*
   Folic acid deficiency*
Drugs and toxins*
Intracranial tumors* and brain trauma*
Infectious processes
   Creutzfeldt-Jakob disease
   Cryptococcal meningitis*
   Neurosyphilis*
   TB and fungal meningitis*
     Viral encephalitis
   Human immunodeficiency Virus (HIV)–related disorders
     (e.g. AIDS and AIDS related complex [ARC])
Miscellaneous disorders
   Hepatolenticular degeneration*
   Hydrocephalic dementia*
   Sarcoidosis*
   Normal pressure hydrocephalus*

*Conditions calling for specific therapeutic intervention.
Adapted from Wells C E: Organic syndromes: dementia. In *Comprehensive Textbook of Psychiatry*, ed 4, H I Kaplan and B J Sadock, editors, p 855. Williams & Wilkins, Baltimore, 1985.

as defective control of impulses or lability of mood, are frequent, as are accentuations or alterations of premorbid personality traits.

In mild or early cases of dementia, there is difficulty in sustaining mental performance, with the early appearance of fatigue and a tendency for the patient to fail when a task is novel, complex, or requires shifts in problem-solving strategy. As the disorder progresses, failures to perform become increasingly more frequent and spread to simple everyday tasks, so that the patient is rendered incapable of taking care of basic needs.

Memory disturbance is formally tested by demonstrating difficulty in learning new information (short-term memory loss) and in recalling personal data or commonly known facts (long-term memory loss). Memory impairment is typically an early and prominent feature. According to DSM-III-R, in mild dementia there is moderate memory loss, more marked for recent events, such as forgetting telephone numbers, conversations, and events of the day. In more severe cases, only highly learned material is retained, and new information is rapidly forgotten. In the most advanced stages, the person may forget the names of close relatives, his or her own occupation, or even his or her own name. Memory impairment is partly responsible for faulty orientation in space and time. The patient with advanced dementia who displays spatial disorientation tends to get lost in familiar surroundings. Impaired orientation for time may appear early and always precedes disorientation for place and person. Level of consciousness, however, remains stable. Language may be affected by some dementias. DSM-III-R states that language may be vague, stereotyped, imprecise, and circumstantial. There may be evidence of aphasia, such as difficulty naming objects. Severely demented people actually may be mute. DSM-III-R describes a disturbance in so-called constructional ability, which can be tested by having the person copy three-dimensional figures, assemble blocks, or arrange sticks in specific designs. Agnosias and apraxias may also be present.

The patient also exhibits a reduced ability to apply what Kurt Goldstein called the *abstract attitude*. There is difficulty in generalizing from a single instance, in forming concepts, and in grasping similarities and differences between concepts. Further, the ability to solve problems, to reason logically, and to make sound judgments is somewhat defective. Goldstein also described a *catastrophic reaction*, which is marked by agitation secondary to the subjective awareness of one's intellectual deficits under stressful circumstances. Patients usually attempt to compensate for defects by using strategies to avoid demonstrating failures in intellectual performance, such as changing the subject, making jokes, or otherwise diverting the interviewer. Lack of judgment and impulse control are commonly found, particularly in dementias that primarily affect the frontal lobes. Examples given in DSM-III-R of these impairments include coarse language, inappropriate jokes, neglect of personal appearance and hygiene, and a general disregard for the conventional rules of social conduct.

Sundowner Syndrome. This syndrome is characterized by drowsiness, confusion, ataxia, and falling. It occurs in the aged who are overly sedated and in demented patients who react adversely to even a small dose of a psychoactive drug. The syndrome also occurs in demented persons when external stimuli, such as light and interpersonal orienting cues are diminished.

Diagnosis

Clinical diagnosis of dementia is based on the history derived from the patient and any available informants and on the mental status examination. Evidence of change in the patient's accustomed performance and behavior at home or in the workplace is sought. Behavioral or personality change in a person known to suffer from some form of cerebral pathology, or even in one not known to be physically ill, should raise the question of dementia, especially if the patient is more than 40 years old and lacks a positive psychiatric history.

Complaints by the patient about intellectual impairment and forgetfulness should be noted, as should any evidence of evasion, denial, or rationalization aimed at concealing cognitive deficits. Excessive orderliness, social withdrawal, or a tendency to relate events in minute detail can be characteristic. Sudden outbursts of anger or sarcasm may occur. The patient's appearance and behavior should be noted. A dull, apathetic, or vacuous facial expression and manner, a lability of emotions, sloppy grooming, uninhibited remarks, or silly jokes suggest the presence of dementia, especially when coupled with memory impairment. According to DSM-III-R, paranoid ideation may at times be very marked and result in false accusations and verbal or physical attacks. These accusations can lead a person whom DSM-III-R calls "habitually jealous" to develop a delusion of marital infidelity when demented, and actually assault the spouse. The clinical diagnosis of dementia depends on whether the patient fulfills the criteria specified in DSM-III-R (Table 5).

Differential Diagnosis. Dementia must be distinguished from other organic brain syndromes and from non-organic mental disorders.

Delirium. The distinction between delirium and dementia may be difficult and, at times, impossible to make. Delirium is distinguished by rapid onset, brief duration, fluctuation of cognitive impairment during the course of day, nocturnal exacerbation of symptoms, marked disturbance of the sleep-wake cycle, and prominent disturbances of attention and perception. Hallucinations, especially visual ones, and transient delusions are more common in delirium than in dementia. An organic mental disorder lasting longer than a few months is more likely to represent dementia than delirium (Table 3).

Mood disorders. A major diagnostic problem concerns the differentiation of dementia from a mood disorder, especially depression. A depressive disorder frequently accompanies dementia and may be one of its presenting features. *Pseudodementia* or, as DSM-III-R also refers to it, the dementia syndrome of depression, refers to a major depressive disorder featuring cognitive dysfunction that resembles dementia (Table 6).

According to DSM-III-R, abnormalities of mood in dementia are less frequent and when present, less pervasive than in depression. Cognitive defects in depression usually occur at about the same time as the depression itself, and the patient expresses concern about the memory defect. Symptoms usually progress more rapidly than in true dementia. In dementia, however, depression usually follows the patient's intellectual deterioration, which the patient then rationalizes or denies. Additionally, in pseudodementia there may be a history of previous affective illness. DSM-III-R states that in the dementia syndrome of depression, the depression unmasks an underlying structural abnormality in the central nervous system, resulting in the clinical features of dementia. DSM-III-R also states that in the absence of a specific organic etiologic factor, if the symptoms of depression are at least as prominent as those suggesting dementia, it is best to diagnose a major depressive episode, and to assume that the symptoms suggesting dementia are secondary to the depression.

Factitious illness. Rarely, persons who attempt to simulate memory loss, as in factitious illness, do so in an erratic and inconsistent manner. In dementia, memory for time and place is lost before memory for person, and recent memory is lost before remote memory.

Schizophrenia. Schizophrenia is an illness associated with a clear sensorium. Schizophrenia, especially when chronic, may be associated with some degree of intellectual deterioration. DSM-III-R states that the absence of identifiable brain pathology helps rule out the additional diagnosis of dementia.

Normal aging. Normal aging is accompanied by a reduction in the speed of mental processes and by some difficulty committing new material to memory. However, such changes do not interfere with the person's ordinary social or occupational life, as they do in dementia.

Course and Prognosis

Once dementia has been diagnosed on clinical grounds (with or without the aid of neuropsychological tests), a determination of its cause and the possibility of treatment should be made. About 10 percent of dementias are treatable. Most cases, however, are progressive and incurable.

The onset of dementia may be sudden, resulting from head trauma, cardiac arrest with cerebral hypoxia, or encephalitis. More often, however, the onset is insidious, as in primary degenerative dementia of the Alzheimer type, cerebrovascular disease, or hypothyroidism. Dementia resulting from brain tumors, subdural hematomas, and metabolic disorders may also have an insidious onset.

The syndrome may gradually recede over a period of weeks, months, or even years, in response to treatment or as a result of natural healing processes when the underlying disorder can be treated. Dementia secondary to hypothyroidism, subdural hematoma, normal-pressure hydrocephalus, or tertiary neurosyphilis has the potential to be reversed. It may progress relentlessly and steadily (e.g., primary degenerative dementia of the Alzheimer type), in an incremental fashion (e.g., multi-infarct dementia), or it may remain relatively stationary after a single acute insult (e.g., head trauma). This variability of the onset, course, and prognosis of dementia must be emphasized, since the term dementia no longer connotes progressive and irreversible intellectual deterioration. Psychosocial factors influence the degree and severity of dementia in many cases. For example, the greater the premorbid intelligence and education, the better the patient's ability to compensate for intellectual deficits. Patients who have a rapid onset of dementia utilize fewer defenses than patients who experience insidious onset. Anxiety and depression may intensify and aggravate symptoms. As mentioned, a condition known as *pseudodementia* occurs in depressed elderly patients who complain of impaired memory but are in fact suffering from a depressive disorder. When the depression is treated, the cognitive defects disappear.

The earliest symptoms of dementia are manifold and subtle and may escape the attention of people in the patient's environment. Alcohol is poorly tolerated by demented persons and may precipitate grossly disinhibited behavior. As dementia progresses or is temporarily severe, the symptoms tend to become more conspicuous, and new

Table 5
Diagnostic Criteria for Dementia

A. Demonstrable evidence of impairment in short- and long-term memory. Impairment in short-term memory (inability to learn new information) may be indicated by inability to remember three objects after 5 minutes. Long-term memory impairment (inability to remember information that was known in the past) may be indicated by inability to remember past personal information (e.g., what happened yesterday, birthplace, occupation) or facts of common knowledge (e.g., past Presidents, well-known dates).

B. At least one of the following:
  (1) impairment in abstract thinking, as indicated by inability to find similarities and differences between related words, difficulty in defining words and concepts, and other similar tasks
  (2) impaired judgment, as indicated by inability to make reasonable plans to deal with interpersonal, family, and job-related problems and issues
  (3) other disturbances of higher cortical function, such as aphasia (disorder of language), apraxia (inability to carry out motor activities despite intact comprehension and motor function), agnosia (failure to recognize or identify objects despite intact sensory function), and "constructional difficulty" (e.g., inability to copy three-dimensional figures, assemble blocks, or arrange sticks in specific designs)
  (4) personality change, i.e., alteration or accentuation of premorbid traits

C. The disturbance in A and B significantly interferes with work or usual social activities or relationships with others.
D. Not occurring exclusively during the course of Delirium.
E. Either (1) or (2):
  (1) there is evidence from the history, physical examination, or laboratory tests of a specific organic factor (or factors) judged to be etiologically related to the disturbance
  (2) in the absence of such evidence, an etiologic organic factor can be presumed if the disturbance cannot be accounted for by any nonorganic mental disorder (e.g., Major Depression accounting for cognitive impairment)

Criteria for severity of Dementia:

Mild: Although work or social activities are significantly impaired, the capacity for independent living remains, with adequate personal hygiene and relatively intact judgment.

Moderate: Independent living is hazardous, and some degree of supervision is necessary.

Severe: Activities of daily living are so impaired that continual supervision is required (e.g., unable to maintain minimal personal hygiene; largely incoherent or mute.)

Table from DSM-III-R *Diagnostic and Statistical Manual of Mental Disorders,* ed 3, revised. (Current Classification of Mental Disorders, 1987.) Copyright American Psychiatric Association, Washington D.C., 1987. Used with permission.

Table 6
Differentiation of Dementia from Depressive Pseudodementia

	Dementia	Pseudodementia
Onset	Intellectual deficits antedate depression	Depressive symptoms antedate cognitive deficits
Presentation of symptoms	Patient minimizes or denies cognitive deficits, tries to conceal them by circumstantiality, perseveration, changing topic of conversation	Patient complains vocally of memory impairment and poor intellectual performance, exaggerates and dwells on these deficits
Appearance and behavior	Often neglected, sloppy; manner facetious or apathetic and indifferent; catastrophic reaction may be evoked; emotional expression often labile and superficial	Facial expression sad, worried; manner retarded or agitated, never facetious or euphoric; bemoans or ridicules own impaired performance but no true catastrophic reaction
Response to questions	Often evasive, angry, or sarcastic when pressed for answers, or tries hard to answer correctly but just misses	Often slow, "I don't know" type of answer
Intellectual performance	Usually globally impaired and consistently poor	Often confined to memory impairment; inconsistent; if globally impaired, it is so because patient refuses to make effort
Sodium amobarbital interview	All cognitive deficits accentuated	Performance improved

Table by Z J Lipowski, M.D.

ones may appear. At this stage, the family or the employer is liable to become alarmed, but the patient is likely to be oblivious to his deterioration. The patient may display insomnia with agitated and psychotic behavior. He may get lost in familiar surroundings and be picked up wandering helplessly in the streets. In the end, the patient becomes an empty shell of his former self—profoundly disoriented, incoherent, amnesic, and incontinent of urine and feces.

Treatment

Dementia is regarded as a treatable syndrome because in some cases the dysfunctional brain tissue retains the capacity for recovery if treatment is timely. A complete medical history, physical examination, and laboratory tests, including appropriate brain imaging, should be accomplished as soon as the diagnosis is suspected. If the patient is suffering from a treatable cause of dementia, therapy will be directed toward treating the underlying disorder. For example, the dementia that accompanies hypothyroidism can be treated with thyroid replacement; but if hormone replacement is delayed too long, recovery may be incomplete.

Symptomatic or general treatment of dementia is used in conjunction with disease-specific treatment. Such symptomatic treatment measures include the maintenance of a nutritious diet, proper exercise, recreational and activity therapy, attention to visual or auditory problems, and treatment of associated medical problems such as urinary tract infection, decubitus ulcers, and cardiopulmonary dysfunction.

Psychosocial treatment involves giving support and advice to the patient and family. Demented patients do best in quiet, familiar surroundings with adequate but familiar distractions. New and complex situations are often disruptive.

Pharmacotherapy of dementia is indicated for symptoms of agitation, impulsiveness, aggression, anxiety, depression, paranoid ideation, insomnia, and night wandering. Anxiety is best treated with small doses of a benzodiazepine. For depression, tricyclics may be used, especially those with fewer anticholinergic side effects to which the aged are susceptible. A therapeutic trial with an antidepressant or ECT (if not contraindicated) may help to distinguish pseudodementia from true dementia: if the disorder is in fact a major depressive episode, the cognitive impairments usually resolve as mood improves. The antipsychotic agents are generally used to treat paranoid and other psychotic symptoms, as well as to control potentially harmful behavior, such as hyperactivity and assaultiveness. For insomnia, a shorter-acting benzodiazepine, such as triazolam, is of use. Patients with dementia are liable to develop delirium from any of the psychotropic agents, so the clinician should be alert for an idiosyncratic drug reaction (e.g., exacerbation of symptoms).

AMNESTIC SYNDROME

Definition

An impairment of memory is the single or predominant cognitive defect in the amnestic syndrome. The memory pathology is of two types: retrograde amnesia (pathological loss of memories established before the onset of the illness) and anterograde amnesia (inability to establish new memories following the onset of the illness).

Epidemiology

There are no adequate studies on the incidence or prevalence of this disorder. In the absence of epidemiologic data, no definite statement about the frequency of the various etiologic factors can be given. However, amnestic syndrome is most likely encountered in persons with chronic alcoholism. The syndrome is generally felt to be relatively uncommon.

Etiology

A number of organic pathological factors and conditions can give rise to the amnestic syndrome, which results from any pathologic process that causes bilateral damage to such diencephalic and medial temporal structures as the mamillary bodies, hippocampal complex, and fornix. The most common cause in this country is thiamine deficiency associated with chronic alcoholism. Other causes include brain trauma, cerebral hypoxia, tumors, and degenerative diseases. The factors and disorders known to cause the amnestic syndrome are listed in Table 7.

Clinical Features

The core feature of the amnestic syndrome is the impairment of memory. Short-term and recent memory (a few minutes to a few days) is impaired. The patient cannot remember what he had for breakfast or lunch or the name of the hospital or his doctor. The deficit in recent memory accounts for the anterograde amnesia. Memory for overlearned information or events from the remote past, such as childhood experiences, is good; but memory for events from the less remote past (over the past decade or longer) is impaired, which accounts for retrograde amnesia. Immediate memory (tested by asking the patient to repeat six numbers) remains intact.

Lack of insight into memory deficits is frequently prominent, and the patient tends to minimize, rationalize, or even explicitly deny them. Minor deficits in perception and concept formation may be found in alcoholic patients, but generally the sensorium is relatively clear. A significant degree of amnesia, however, can result in disorientation. Lack of initiative, emotional blandness, and apathy are common, though the patient is responsive to the environment. Because immediate memory is intact, the patient is able to recognize surroundings or communications addressed to him, but they are soon forgotten owing to his impaired forward memory span. Confabulation, in which the patient fills in memory gaps with false information, is a common characteristic, and is most often seen in the amnestic syndrome associated with alcoholism (Korsakoff's psychosis). Confabulation tends to disappear with time.

Diagnosis

The diagnosis of amnestic syndrome rests on finding its essential features, particularly short- and long-term memory

Table 7
Causes of Amnestic Syndrome

Thiamine deficiency (Wernicke-Korsakoff's syndrome) usually due to alcoholism

Head trauma with damage of the diencephalic or temporal regions; postconcussive states; whiplash injury

Brain tumor involving the floor and the walls of the third ventricle or both hippocampal formations

Subarachnoid hemorrhage

Intoxication: carbon monoxide, isoniazid, arsenic, lead

Vascular disorders: bilateral hippocampal infarction due to thrombosis or embolism occluding posterior cerebral arteries or their inferior temporal branches

Intracranial infections: herpes simplex encephalitis, tuberculous meningitis

Cerebral anoxia: after unsuccessful hanging attempt, cardiac arrest, inadequate aeration or prolonged hypotension during general anesthesia

Degenerative cerebral diseases: Alzheimer's disease, senile dementia

Bilateral temporal lobectomy with bilateral hippocampal lesions

Surgery for ruptured aneurysm of the anterior communicating artery

Electroshock treatment

Epilepsy

Transient global amnesia

Table by Z J Lipowski, M.D.

impairment. The DSM-III-R diagnostic criteria for amnestic syndrome are listed in Table 8.

Course and Prognosis

The course and prognosis of the amnestic syndrome depends on the cause of the case in question. The onset in most cases tends to be relatively sudden. The syndrome may be transient or persistent, and its outcome may be a complete or partial recovery of memory function or an irreversible or even progressive memory defect. Generally, the course is a chronic one. Transient amnestic syndrome with full recovery is common in temporal lobe epilepsy, vascular insufficiency, electroconvulsive therapy, intake of such drugs as benzodiazepines or barbiturates, and cardiac arrest. Permanent amnestic syndrome of some degree of severity may follow head trauma, carbon monoxide poisoning, subarachnoid hemorrhage, cerebral infarction, and herpes simplex encephalitis.

Differential Diagnosis

Wernicke's Syndrome. The amnestic syndrome associated with chronic alcoholism (Korsakoff's psychosis) should be differentiated from Wernicke's syndrome, an encephalopathy that develops acutely in patients with a history of many years of alcohol abuse. Wernicke's syndrome is marked by delirium, ataxia of gait, nystagmus, and ophthalmoplegia and is believed to be caused by a lack

Table 8
Diagnostic Criteria for Amnestic Syndrome

A. Demonstrable evidence of impairment in both short- and long-term memory; with regard to long-term memory, very remote events are remembered better than more recent events. Impairment in short-term memory (inability to learn new information) may be indicated by inability to remember three objects after 5 minutes. Long-term memory impairment (inability to remember information that was known in the past) may be indicated by inability to remember past personal information (e.g., what happened yesterday, birthplace, occupation) or facts of common knowledge (e.g., past Presidents, well-known dates).

B. Not occurring exclusively during the course of delirium, and does not meet the criteria for dementia (i.e., no impairment in abstract thinking or judgment, no other disturbances of higher cortical function, and no personality change).

C. There is evidence from the history, physical examination, or laboratory tests of a specific organic factor (or factors) judged to be etiologically related to the disturbance.

Table from DSM-III-R Diagnostic and Statistical Manual of Mental Disorders, ed 3, revised. (Current Classification of Mental Disorders, 1987.) Copyright American Psychiatric Association, Washington, D.C., 1987. Used with permission.

of thiamine. Brain autopsies show characteristic lesions of the mamillary bodies. Although the delirium clears up within a month or so, the amnestic syndrome either accompanies or follows untreated Wernicke's syndrome in about 85 percent of cases.

Other Disorders. In dementia and delirium, amnesia is only one component of global intellectual and cognitive dysfunction. The development of a slowly progressive amnestic syndrome should suggest a brain tumor, Alzheimer's disease, or another dementia. Psychogenic amnesia is characterized by the sudden onset of retrograde amnesia for personally significant memories; it is usually accompanied by a loss of sense of personal identity, of which the patient may or may not be aware. There is usually evidence of a subjectively stressful or conflict-arousing precipitating event. Anterograde amnesia is rarely psychogenic. Psychogenic amnesia may be precipitated by head trauma, an epileptic seizure, or acute alcohol intoxication. In the psychogenic memory disorders, however, the patient's responses are typically inconsistent, and there is usually an intact memory for personally neutral information. A sodium amobarbital interview may help distinguish amnestic syndrome from psychogenic amnesia by revealing the motivation for the psychogenic amnesia. The patient who has factitious disorder with psychological symptoms gets inconsistent results on memory testing and has no organic problem. These findings coupled with evidence of primary or secondary gain on the part of the patient should suggest a factitious disorder.

Treatment

Treatment of the amnestic syndrome must first be directed at its underlying cause (e.g., brain tumor). It is particularly important to try to prevent the development of

Wernicke's encephalopathy in the alcoholic patient with high doses of thiamine and other vitamins. Once encephalopathy has developed, it must be treated vigorously to prevent or minimize the amnestic syndrome that is likely to follow. In addition, the patient should receive other B-complex vitamins. Once the amnestic syndrome has become fixed, supportive measures (e.g., structured environment, pharmacotherapy for anxiety or agitation) are helpful. Drugs to enhance memory have not been effective.

ORGANIC HALLUCINOSIS

Definition

Organic hallucinosis is characterized by prominent recurrent or persistent hallucinations in a state of full wakefulness that can be attributed to some specific organic factor.

Epidemiology

Relevant epidemiologic data about organic hallucinosis is lacking. However, it is most likely encountered in a setting of chronic alcoholism and hallucinogen or other drug abuse.

Etiology

Psychoactive drug abuse, as with hallucinogens or through prolonged use of alcohol, is the most common cause of organic hallucinosis. Physical conditions such as brain tumor, particularly of the occipital or temporal areas of the brain, should be considered. Sensory deprivation, as in blindness or deafness, may also cause the syndrome. Conditions associated with hallucinosis are listed in Table 9.

Table 9
Causative Factors in Organic Hallucinosis

Substance abuse
  Alcohol (acute alcoholic hallucinosis)
  Hallucinogens: LSD, psilocybin, mescaline, morning glory
    seed
  Cocaine
Drug toxicity: levodopa, bromocriptine, amantadine, ephedrine, pentazocine, propranolol, methylphenidated
Space-occupying lesions of the brain:
  Neoplasm: craniopharyngioma, chromophobe adenoma, meningioma of the olfactory groove, temporal lobe tumors
  Aneurysm
  Abscess
Temporal arteritis
Migraine
Hypothyroidism
Neurosyphilis
Huntington's chorea
Cerebrovascular disease
Disease of sense organs: bilateral cataracts, glaucoma, otosclerosis

Table by Z J Lipowski, M.D.

Clinical Features

Hallucinations may occur in one or more sensory modalities. Tactile or haptic hallucinations (e.g., bugs crawling on the skin) are characteristic of cocainism; auditory hallucinations are common in alcoholic hallucinosis; visual hallucinations are usually associated with psychoactive substance abuse; and olfactory hallucinations occur in temporal lobe epilepsy. Auditory hallucinations may occur in deaf people; visual hallucinations may occur in people who are blind owing to cataracts. Auditory hallucinations are the most common type. Hallucinations are either recurrent or persistent. They are experienced in a state of full wakefulness and alertness, and there is no significant change in the patient's cognitive functions. Visual hallucinosis often takes the form of scenes involving diminutive (Lilliputian) human figures or various small animals. Rare musical hallucinosis typically features religious songs. A patient with hallucinosis may act on the hallucinations, which they believe to be true. In alcoholic hallucinosis, there are typically threatening, critical, or insulting voices of people speaking about the patient in the third person. They may tell the patient to harm either himself or others; such patients are dangerous and are at significant risk for suicide or homicide. The patient may or may not believe that the hallucinations are real. Delusional convictions of their reality, however, are not the major features of this syndrome and are limited to the content of the hallucinations and to the belief in the hallucinations as being real.

Hallucinosis is diagnosed on the basis of the patient's history and on the presence of persistent or recurrent hallucinations. The sensorium is clear. When a patient develops hallucinations an organic cause should be sought. Visual hallucinations should raise the question of a focal cerebral lesion, hallucinogen abuse, side effects of drug therapy, migraine, or temporal arteritis. Auditory hallucinations should prompt an inquiry about alcohol abuse. Diagnostic criteria for this syndrome are presented in Table 10.

Course and Prognosis

The course and the prognosis depend on the underlying pathology. The onset is usually acute, and the average duration is days or weeks, or, as in the case of ingested hallucinogens, only a few hours. In some patients, hallucinosis becomes chronic, as with untreated cataracts or deafness secondary to otosclerosis. Some cases of acute hallucinosis progress to delirium.

Table 10
Diagnostic Criteria for Organic Hallucinosis

A. Prominent persistent or recurrent hallucinations.
B. There is evidence from the history, physical examination, or laboratory tests of a specific organic factor (or factors) judged to be etiologically related to the disturbance.
C. Not occurring exclusively during the course of Delirium.

Table from DSM-III-R *Diagnostic and Statistical Manual of Mental Disorders,* ed 3, revised. (Current Classification of Mental Disorders, 1987.) Copyright American Psychiatric Association, Washington, D.C., 1987. Used with permission.

Differential Diagnosis

Organic hallucinosis needs to be distinguished from delirium, in which there is a clouded sensorium, and from dementia, in which there are major intellectual deficits. Delusions that occur in organic hallucinosis are related to the hallucinations and are not prominent. In organic delusional syndrome the delusions are predominant and are usually well-systematized. If both prominent delusions and prominent hallucinations coexist, DSM-III-R states that both organic delusional syndrome and organic hallucinosis may be diagnosed. It may be difficult to differentiate hallucinations from confabulations at times, but memory impairment is absent in hallucinosis and present in confabulatory states. Hypnagogic and hypnopompic hallucinations occur only upon falling asleep or on awakening.

Epilepsy, especially the temporal lobe type, may be accompanied by either auditory or visual hallucinations. Such hallucinations are usually part of an ictus (or attack), are accompanied by other ictal phenomena, are paroxysmal, and occur in a setting of reduced awareness. Alcoholic hallucinosis is differentiated from delirium tremens (DTs) by the presence of a clear sensorium in hallucinosis. The hallucinations of DTs are usually visual rather than auditory and are usually most prominent at night. Schizophrenia and mood disorders may present with hallucinations, but within the context of the clear overriding diagnosis, and with no specific organic factor demonstrated.

Treatment

Treatment depends on the underlying condition. If the cause is temporary, the anxious or agitated patient will respond to the reassurance that he is suffering from what is likely to be a temporary mental disorder. It is best to hospitalize a markedly fearful and delusional patient. Antipsychotic medication (e.g., haloperidol) often relieves hallucinatory phenomenon, and antianxiety agents (e.g., diazepam) are useful for agitation.

ORGANIC DELUSIONAL SYNDROME

Definition

Organic delusional syndrome is characterized by the presence of prominent delusions in a state of full wakefulness and alertness that can be attributed to some clearly defined organic factor.

Epidemiology

There are few epidemiologic studies of incidence or prevalence of the disorder. The delusional syndrome that accompanies complex partial seizures is more common in women than in men.

Etiology

Drugs are the most common cause of the disorder. A variety of chemical substances, especially amphetamine, cannabis, hallucinogens, and cocaine, may induce the syn-

drome. The syndrome often (but not always) lifts after the toxic agent has been withdrawn or the physical illness has subsided. Lesions involving the temporal lobe and other cerebral lesions, especially of the right hemisphere and parietal lobe, are associated with delusions. According to DSM-III-R, some people with temporal lobe epilepsy have an interictal organic delusional syndrome that can look very much like schizophrenia. DSM-III-R also describes a paranoid organic delusional syndrome which has been reported in some cases of Huntington's chorea.

Clinical Features and Diagnosis

The essential feature of the organic delusional syndrome is the presence of delusions in a state of full wakefulness. There is no change in the level of consciousness although mild cognitive impairment may be observed. The delusions may be systematized or fragmentary, and their content may vary; that is, there may be delusions of persecution, grandiosity, and jealousy, among others. Persecutory delusions, however, are the most common. A diagnosis of the syndrome involves finding evidence of an organic factor antedating the onset of the syndrome that is judged to be etiologically significant. The person may appear confused, dishevelled, or eccentric. Speech may be tangential or even incoherent, and hyperactivity as well as apathy may be observed. An associated dysphoric mood is felt to be common. The diagnostic criteria are listed in Table 11.

Course and Prognosis

The course and the prognosis depend to some extent on the underlying cause. Amphetamine psychosis is usually self-limited with delusions abating after 7 to 10 days. Flashbacks may be triggered by the use of even small amounts of amphetamines. Epileptic patients may have delusional experiences for many years. Their delusions, however, may be phasic and paradoxically vary inversely with seizure frequency; that is, the greater the frequency of seizures, the fewer the number of delusional experiences.

Differential Diagnosis

The major differential diagnosis is between organic delusional syndrome and paranoid schizophrenia. For example, amphetamine abuse may lead to a highly systematized paranoid delusional condition, that appears identical to the active phase of schizophrenia. In contrast to paranoid schizophrenia, however, hallucinations in organic delu-

Table 11
Diagnostic Criteria for Organic Delusional Syndrome

A. Prominent delusions.
B. There is evidence from the history, physical examination, or laboratory tests of a specific organic factor (or factors) judged to be etiologically related to the disturbance.
C. Not occurring exclusively during the course of Delirium.

Table from DSM-III-R *Diagnostic and Statistical Manual of Mental Disorders*, ed 3, revised. (Current Classification of Mental Disorders, 1987.) Copyright American Psychiatric Association, Washington, D.C., 1987. Used with permission.

sional syndrome are more often visual than auditory. The affect is also more appropriate, and the thought processes are better preserved. A history of a specific organic factor known to produce delusional psychoses also helps in distinguishing the organic delusional syndrome from the nonorganic psychotic disorders. According to DSM-III-R, the first appearance of a delusion occuring after the age of 35, when there is no history of schizophrenia or delusional disorder, necessitates a work-up for organic delusional syndrome. Clearly, if there is concern about a possible organic factor in a person with a history of a nonorganic psychosis, the work-up must still be done.

Delirium is associated with a change in the level of consciousness. Dementia shows significant impairment of intellectual capacities. Organic hallucinosis shows persistent and prominent hallucinations. Organic anxiety shows neither hallucinations nor delusions. Organic mood disorder shows predominant symptoms of a mood disorder, and any delusions or hallucinations present are related in content to the mood disturbance.

Treatment

Management of the syndrome depends on its underlying cause, which should be identified and treated. Otherwise, symptomatic treatment follows the general guidelines applicable to schizophrenic and delusional disorders—neuroleptics, supportive environment or hospitalization, and psychotherapy

ORGANIC MOOD SYNDROME

Definition

Previously called organic affective syndrome, organic mood syndrome is characterized by either a depressive or a manic mood that is attributed to a clearly defined organic factor.

Etiology

Medications, especially antihypertensives, are probably the most frequent cause. Drugs such as reserpine and methyldopa (both antihypertensive agents) can precipitate a depression by depleting serotonin in over 10 percent of persons who take these drugs. A number of somatic disorders have been implicated in the causes of mood changes: endocrine disorders, especially Cushing's syndrome, and cerebral disorders of various causes (e.g., brain tumors, encephalitis, epilepsy). Structural damage to the brain, similar to that which occurs with hemispheric strokes, is a common cause of the syndrome. Conditions associated with organic depressive or manic features are listed in Table 12.

Clinical Features and Diagnosis

Disturbances of mood resembling those observed in depressive or manic states are the predominant and essential clinical features. To make the diagnosis, an organic cause should be noted in the history that antedates the onset of symptoms and is known to be associated with the disorder. The syndrome may vary in severity from mild to severe or

Table 12
Conditions Associated with Organic Mood Syndrome

Drugs: reserpine, corticosteroids, methyldopa, levedopa, cycloserine, ethionamide, oral contraceptive amphetamines, hallucinogens

Endocrine diseases: hypothyroidism, Cushing's syndrome, Addison's disease, hyperparathyroidism

Infectious diseases: influenza, infectious mononucleosis, infectious hepatitis, viral pneumonia

Pernicious anemia

Carcinoma of the pancreas

Brain tumor

Systemic lupus erythematosus

Parkinsonism

Carcinoid syndrome

Neurosyphilis

Table by Z J Lipowski, M.D.

psychotic and may be indistinguishable from manic and depressive episodes that are not attributable to a specific organic factor. Delusions, hallucinations, and other associated features of bipolar disorders may also be present in the organic mood disorders; mild cognitive impairment may be observed. Table 13 lists the criteria for organic mood disorder.

Course and Prognosis

The onset may be acute or insidious, and the course varies, depending on the underlying cause. The removal of the cause does not necessarily result in the patient's prompt recovery from the mood disorder; it may persist for weeks or months after the successful treatment of the underlying physical condition or the withdrawal of the implicated toxic agent. It has been reported that 10 percent of patients with depressed mood secondary to Cushing's syndrome attempt suicide.

Differential Diagnosis

The major differential is between organic and nonorganic (functional) mood disorder. Functional illness is usually accompanied by a family history of depression or mania,

Table 13
Diagnostic Criteria for Organic Mood Syndrome

A. Prominent and persistent depressed, elevated, or expansive mood.
B. There is evidence from the history, physical examination, or laboratory tests of a specific organic factor (or factors) judged to be etiologically related to the disturbance.
C. Not occurring exclusively during the course of Delirium.
Specify: manic, depressed, or mixed.

Table from DSM-III-R *Diagnostic and Statistical Manual of Mental Disorders*, ed 3, revised. (Current Classification of Mental Disorders, 1987.) Copyright American Psychiatric Association, Washington, D.C., 1987. Used with permission.

recurrent cycles of depression or mania, and the absence of a specific organic etiologic factor. Drugs may trigger an underlying mood disorder in a patient who is biologically vulnerable, and according to DSM-III-R, this would not be an organic mood disorder. For instance, antidepressants may trigger manic episodes in patients with underlying bipolar illness. A history of previous mood disorder in the patient or in relatives suggests the psychoactive substance merely triggered an existing underlying disorder; the absence of such a history suggests a true organic mood syndrome.

Treatment

Management of the syndrome involves determining the etiology and treating the underlying disorder. Psychopharmacologic treatment may be indicated and should follow the guidelines applicable to the treatment of depression or mania, with due regard to the coexisting physical condition. Psychotherapy is utilized as an adjunct to the other treatments.

ORGANIC PERSONALITY SYNDROME

Definition

Organic personality syndrome is characterized by a marked change in personality style or traits from a previous level of functioning. There must be evidence of an organic factor antedating the onset of the personality changes that is judged to be causally significant.

Etiology

Structural damage to the brain is usually the cause of the syndrome, head trauma being probably the most important cause. Cerebral lesions, particularly of the temporal or frontal lobe, are other significant causes. The conditions most often associated with the syndrome are listed in Table 14.

Clinical Features and Diagnosis

A change in personality from previous patterns of behavior or an exacerbation of previous personality characteristics is notable. Impaired control of the expression of emotions and impulses is a cardinal feature. Emotions are characteristically labile and shallow, though euphoria or apathy may be prominent. The euphoria may mimic hypomania, but true elation is absent, and the patient may admit to not really feeling happy. There is a hollow and silly ring to the patient's excitement and facile jocularity, particularly if the frontal lobe is involved. Also associated with damage to the frontal lobes, the so-called frontal lobe syndrome, is prominent indifference and apathy, characterized by no concern for events in the immediate environment. Temper outbursts with little or no provocation may occur, especially after alcohol ingestion, and may result in violent behavior. The expression of impulses may be manifested by inappropriate jokes, coarse manner, improper sexual advances, and antisocial conduct resulting in conflicts with the law, such as assaults on others, sexual mis-

Table 14
Conditions Associated with Organic Personality Syndrome

Head trauma
Subarachnoid hemorrhage and other vascular accidents
Space-occupying lesions of the brain: neoplasm, aneurysm, abcess, granuloma
Temporal lobe epilepsy
Postencephalitic parkinsonism
Huntington's chorea
Multiple sclerosis
Endocrine disorders
Chronic poisoning: manganese, mercury
Drugs: cannabis, LSD, steroids, etc.
Neurosyphilis
Arteritis, as in systemic lupus erythematosus

Table by Z J Lipowski, M.D.

demeanors, and shoplifting. Foresight and the ability to anticipate the social or legal consequences of one's actions are typically diminished. People with temporal lobe epilepsy characteristically demonstrate humorlessness, hypergraphia, hyperreligiosity, and marked aggressiveness during seizures.

Patients with organic personality syndrome have a clear sensorium. Mild disorders of cognitive function often coexist but do not amount to intellectual deterioration. Patients tend to be inattentive, which may account for disorders of recent memory. With some prodding, however, the patient is likely to recall what he claims to have forgotten. The diagnosis should be suspected in patients who show a marked change in behavior or personality involving emotional lability and impaired impulse control, who have no history of psychiatric illness, and whose personality change occurs abruptly or over a relatively brief period of time. See Table 15 for the DSM-III-R features.

Course and Prognosis

Both the course and the prognosis of organic personality syndrome depend on its cause. If the result of structural damage to the brain, it will tend to persist. The syndrome may follow a period of coma and delirium in cases of head trauma or vascular accident and may be permanent. Organic personality syndrome may evolve into dementia in cases of brain tumor, multiple sclerosis, or Huntington's disease. Personality changes produced by chronic intoxication, medical illness, or drug therapy (e.g., levodopa for parkinsonism) may be reversed if the underlying cause is treated. Some patients require custodial care or, at least, close supervision in order to meet their basic needs, avoid repeated conflicts with the law, and protect them and their families from the hostility of others and destitution resulting from impulsive and ill-considered actions.

Differential Diagnosis

Dementia involves global deterioration in intellectual and behavioral capacities, of which personality change

Table 15
Diagnostic Criteria for Organic Personality Syndrome

A. A persistent personality disturbance, either lifelong or representing a change or accentuation of a previously characteristic trait, involving at least one of the following:
   (1) affective instability (e.g., marked shifts from normal mood to depression, irritability, or anxiety)
   (2) recurrent outbursts of aggression or rage that are grossly out of proportion to any precipitating psychosocial stressors
   (3) markedly impaired social judgment (e.g., sexual indiscretions)
   (4) marked apathy and indifference
   (5) suspiciousness or paranoid ideation

B. There is evidence from the history, physical examination, or laboratory tests of a specific organic factor (or factors) judged to be etiologically related to the disturbance.

C. This diagnosis is not given to a child or adolescent if the clinical picture is limited to the features that characterize Attention-deficit Hyperactivity Disorder.

D. Not occurring exclusively during the course of Delirium, and does not meet the criteria for Dementia.

Specify explosive type if outbursts of aggression or rage are the predominant feature.

Table from DSM-III-R *Diagnostic and Statistical Manual of Mental Disorders*, ed 3, revised. (Current Classification of Mental Disorders, 1987.) Copyright American Psychiatric Association, Washington, D.C., 1987. Used with permission.

is just one category. A personality change may herald an organic mental syndrome that will eventually evolve into dementia. In these cases, as the deterioration begins to encompass significant memory and cognitive deficits, the diagnosis is changed from organic personality syndrome to dementia. In differentiating the specific syndrome from other disorders in which personality change may occur, such as schizophrenia, delusional disorders, mood disorder, and impulse disorders, the most important factor is the presence in organic personality syndrome of a specific organic etiologic factor.

Treatment

Management of the organic personality syndrome involves treatment of the underlying organic condition, if the condition is indeed treatable. Psychopharmacologic treatment of specific symptoms may be indicated in some cases (e.g., imipramine for depression).

The patient may need counseling to help avoid difficulties at work or to prevent social embarrassment. As a rule, the patient's family needs emotional support and concrete advice on how to help minimize the patient's undesirable conduct. Alcohol should be avoided. Social engagements should be curtailed if the patient has a tendency to act in a grossly offensive manner.

ORGANIC ANXIETY SYNDROME

This category is new to DSM-III-R. Organic anxiety syndrome is characterized by prominent, recurrent, panic attacks, or generalized anxiety that are attributable to some clearly defined organic factor. Cognitive functioning may be adversely affected as a secondary phenomenon.

Etiology

A variety of general central nervous system stimulants can cause massive anxiety. A broad class of sympathomimetic drugs, such as epinephrine, norepinephrine, amphetamine, caffeine, and cocaine are included in this group. Other drugs, such as atropine and scopolamine, can cause excitement due to idiosyncrasy or to administration of the drug to persons in pain. Hyperthyroidism, hypothyroidism, hypoparathyroidism, and Vitamin B_{12} deficiency are other causes of organic anxiety syndrome. Pheochromocytoma produces epinephrine, which can cause paroxysmal anxiety attacks. Certain lesions of the brain or postencephalitic states have produced obsessive-compulsive symptoms as sequelae. Some medical conditions such as cardiac arrhythmia, can produce physiologic symptoms of panic. Hypoglycemia can also mimic anxiety. Autonomic nervous system imbalance and mitral value prolapse have been associated with anxiety. A list of disorders associated with anxiety is found in Table 16.

Clinical Features and Diagnosis

In general, according to DSM-III-R, the clinical features of this syndrome are similar to those of panic disorder or generalized anxiety. The presence of chronic or paroxysmal anxiety associated with physical disease known to produce anxiety should lead the clinician to suspect an organic etiology. Paroxysmal bouts of hypertension suggest pheochromocytoma, and in such cases, elevated urinary catecholamines are found. A history of chronic low-level drug use, especially of sympathomimetics, may produce chronic anxiety and aid in the diagnosis. As a result of anxiety the patient may perform poorly on cognitive tests of comprehension, calculation, and memory. Such changes are reversible if the anxiety is diminished. A general medical work-up may reveal diabetes, adrenal tumor, thyroid disease, or neurological conditions that may be accompanied by or present with anxiety as a sign or symptom (Table 17). Some patients with complex partial seizures have extreme anxiety or episodes of fear as the only manifestation. There have also been reports of compulsive behavior following prolonged use of phenmetrazine (Preludin), cocaine, and amphetamines.

Course and Prognosis

The unremitting experience of anxiety can be extremely disabling, interfering with every aspect of functioning—social, occupational, and psychological. A sudden change in behavior may prompt the person to seek medical or psychiatric help more quickly than when onset is insidious. The treatment and removal of the cause should help diminish the anxiety in most cases (e.g., cessation of intake of sympathomimetics). In some cases the cause of the anxiety may not abate after the illness is cured (e.g., postencephalitic anxiety). In those instances, attempts to manage the

Table 16
Disorders Associated with Anxiety

Neurological disorders
    Cerebral neoplasms
    Cerebral trauma and postconcussive
        syndromes
    Cerebrovascular disease
    Subarachnoid hemorrhage
    Migraine
    Encephalitis
    Cerebral syphilis
    Multiple sclerosis
    Wilson's disease
    Huntington's disease
    Epilepsy
 	
Systemic conditions
    Hypoxia
        Cardiovascular disease
        Cardiac arrhythmias
        Pulmonary insufficiency
        Anemia
 	
Endocrine disturbances
    Pituitary dysfunction
    Thyroid dysfunction
    Parathyroid dysfunction
    Adrenal dysfunction
    Pheochromocytoma
    Virilization disorders of females
 	
Inflammatory disorders
    Lupus erythematosus
    Rheumatoid arthritis
    Polyarteritis nodosa
    Temporal arteritis
 	
Deficiency states
    Vitamin B_{12} deficiency
    Pellagra
	Miscellaneous conditions
	    Hypoglycemia
	    Carcinoid syndrome
	    Systemic malignancies
	    Premenstrual syndrome
	    Febrile illnesses and chronic infections
	    Porphyria
	    Infectious mononucleosis
	    Posthepatitis syndrome
	    Uremia
	
	Toxic conditions
	    Alcohol and drug withdrawal
	    Amphetamines
	    Sympathomimetic agents
	    Vasopressor agents
	    Caffeine and caffeine withdrawal
	    Penicillin
	    Sulfonamides
	    Cannabis
	    Mercury
	    Arsenic
	    Phosphorus
	    Organophosphates
	    Carbon disulfide
	    Benzene
	    Aspirin intolerance
	
	Idiopathic psychiatric disorders
	    Depression
	    Mania
	    Schizophrenia
	    Anxiety disorders
	    Generalized anxiety
	    Panic attacks
	    Phobic disorders
	    Posttraumatic stress disorder

Data from Hall (1980) and Jefferson and Marshall (1981); Table from Cummings J: *Clinical Neuropsychiatry*, p 214. Grune & Stratton, Orlando, 1985.

symptoms through medication, environmental modification, or social support systems are necessary. The prognosis for reversing cognitive changes is excellent if the offending anxiety symptoms are removed. The least favorable prognosis is for conditions with associated obsessive-compulsive features. Even though the causative agent is removed, a habit pattern of obsessive-compulsive behavior may be fixed in the personality. In such cases, specific intervention, such as behavior modification techniques, may be desirable. Some patients medicate themselves with antianxiety agents or alcohol, thus producing a secondary drug dependence.

Differential Diagnosis

Anxiety as a symptom is associated with many psychiatric disorders. To diagnose organic anxiety syndrome, both predominant anxiety and a specific etiologic organic factor must be present. To ascertain the degree to which an organic factor is truly etiologic, it is necessary to know how closely related the organic factor and the anxiety are, the age of onset (for most anxiety disorders, before age 35), and

the family history of organic factors (such as hyperthyroidism) that cause organic anxiety syndrome.

Treatment

Management of the organic anxiety syndrome requires treatment of the underlying organic condition. Specific symptoms such as phobias, panic, or generalized anxiety can be treated with the appropriate psychopharmacologic agent. Obsessive-compulsive symptoms have been treated successfully with antidepressants in some cases. The patient who has become alcohol dependent must be treated accordingly. In some cases of very severe disabilities (e.g., postencephalitic obsessive-compulsive states) that have not responded to other treatments, psychosurgery has been used successfully.

INTOXICATION AND WITHDRAWAL

DSM-III-R lists and discusses intoxication and withdrawal as organic mental syndromes. The definition of

Table 17
Diagnostic Criteria for Organic Anxiety Syndrome

A. Prominent, recurrent, panic attacks

B. There is evidence from the history, physical examination, or laboratory tests of a specific organic factor (or factors) judged to be etiologically related to the disturbance.

C. Not occurring exclusively during the course of Delirium.

Table from DSM-III-R *Diagnostic and Statistical Manual of Mental Disorders,* **ed 3, revised. (Current Classification of Mental Disorders, 1987.) Copyright American Psychiatric Association, Washington, D.C., 1987. Used with permission.**

intoxication in DSM-III-R is maladaptive behavior and a substance-specific syndrome secondary to recent ingestion of a psychoactive substance. Withdrawal is defined as substance-specific syndrome following cessation of or reduction in a regularly used psychoactive substance. In this book, intoxication and withdrawal are discussed in Chapter 13 under psychoactive substance–induced organic mental disorder.

DEMENTIAS ARISING IN THE SENIUM AND PRESENIUM

This class of mental disorders consists of a single category called *primary degenerative dementia.* The category is subdivided according to the age of onset to maintain continuity with ICD as follows: primary degenerative dementia of the Alzheimer type, senile onset (after age 65) and primary degenerative dementia of the Alzheimer type, presenile onset (age 65 and under). Dementia associated with Alzheimer's disease formerly was called senile dementia, and Pick's disease was called presenile dementia. The distinction no longer applies because almost all dementias occurring in the senium and presenium are caused by Alzheimer's disease, and the differentiation between the two disorders can be made only by histopathologic examination, not on clinical grounds.

Primary Degenerative Dementia (PDD) of the Alzheimer Type

Definition. Primary degenerative dementia of the Alzheimer type is a clinical disorder in an elderly patient characterized by a severe loss of intellectual function for which no other cause is found. It is progressive and insidious. Pick's disease has also traditionally been considered a primary degenerative dementia, but it is felt to be extremely rare with no adequate guidelines that distinguish between it and the Alzheimer type, and with no specific treatment for either disorder. In DSM-III-R, Pick's disease would be classified with Creutzfeldt-Jakob disease, under presenile dementia not otherwise specified. DSM-III-R distinguishes Alzheimer's disease itself as a physical disorder, coded on Axis III, and differentiates it from primary degenerative dementia of the Alzheimer type, coded on Axis I.

Epidemiology. About 5 percent of persons over age 65 have dementia, and of this group, about 65 percent of all cases are thought to be primary degenerative dementia of the Alzheimer type. Prevalence increases with age. PDD of the Alzheimer type occurs slightly more frequently in women than in men.

Etiology. The etiology of Alzheimer's disease remains unknown. Genetic factors are presumed to play a role because evidence of one or more relatives with the same disorder is not uncommon. In one study, 40 percent of cases had a family history of the disease. A high concordance rate has been found in twins. Several families have been reported with apparent autosomal-dominant transmission. Also, most patients with Down's syndrome who survive into their third decade develop Alzheimer's disease; and recently, an anomaly on gene 21 was found in Alzheimer's patients, the same gene that is damaged in Down's syndrome.

Aluminum toxicity or metabolism may be an etiologic factor, since high levels of aluminum have been found in the brains of patients who died from the disease. In addition, an unusually small amount of acetylcholine has been found in the brains of Alzheimer's patients. A reduction in brain choline acetyltransferase, the enzyme needed to synthesize acetylcholine, has been proposed to account for that finding. Abnormalities in peptide neurotransmitters also have been noted.

A viral etiology has been postulated since some degenerative brain diseases, such as Creutzfeldt-Jakob, are transmitted in that way. But there is no evidence to support a viral etiology for Alzheimer's disease. Finally, there have been reports of reduced immunoglobins in Alzheimer's disease, which may point to a defect in the autoimmune process. In summary, none of the above theories is bolstered by strong scientific evidence, although there is no question that genetic factors are important.

Pathology. Pathological findings in Alzheimer's disease include diffuse atrophy of the brain with flattened cortical sulci and enlarged cerebral ventricles. Microscopically, senile plaques, neurofibrillary tangles, and granulovacuolar degeneration of neurons are present. In Pick's disease, usually the frontal and temporal lobes are most seriously affected, and the neurofibrillary changes and senile plaques that characterize Alzheimer's disease are absent.

Clinical Features and Course. PDD of the Alzheimer type may begin at any age, but is much more common later in life. Fifty percent of patients are stricken between ages 65 and 70. It begins insidiously, the patient showing impaired memory or subtle personality changes that usually are first noticed by the family, rather than by the patient. The classical features of dementia eventually appear, such as disturbances of orientation, memory, calculation, and judgment (Table 18).

Previous personality traits become accentuated or exaggerated and patients may become depressed, paranoid, and withdrawn. Obsessive thoughts or compulsive rituals are not unusual. Defects in judgment may account for inappropriate behavior such as exhibitionism.

These symptoms are generally associated with some slowing and rigidity of movement and often with a slow shuffling gait. The late phase of the illness shows severe neurologic defects with associated aphasia and agnosia. Grand mal seizures have been reported in up to 75 percent of cases. Such patients are totally unable to care for themselves and require institutionalization. It is not possible to

Table 18
Diagnostic Criteria for Primary Degenerative Dementia of the Alzheimer Type

A. Dementia

B. Insidious onset with a generally progressive deteriorating course.

C. Exclusion of all other specific causes of dementia by history, physical examination, and laboratory tests.

Table from DSM-III-R *Diagnostic and Statistical Manual of Mental Disorders,* ed 3, revised. (Current Classification of Mental Disorders, 1987.) Copyright American Psychiatric Association, Washington, D.C., 1987. Used with permission.

differentiate Pick's disease from Alzheimer's disease on clinical grounds. However, it has been suggested that focal neurologic signs may be more prominent in Pick's disorder than in Alzheimer's disease. A postmortem neuropathologic examination is the only method whereby the diagnosis can be confirmed. With senile onset, both disorders progress to severe dementia, and death intervenes usually between 2 and 5 years after the diagnosis has been made. According to DSM-III-R, if the clinical picture is complicated by the presence of significant depressive features, delusions, or superimposed delirium, these additional features should be noted with a specific DSM-III-R code.

Differential Diagnosis. PDD of the Alzheimer type is distinguished from normal aging by clear evidence of progressive and significant deterioration of intellectual, social, or occupational functioning. Clearly, specific and potentially reversible causes of dementia, such as subdural hematoma, cerebral neoplasm, vitamin B_{12} deficiency, and hypothyroidism, need to be ruled out by history, physical exam, and lab tests. Multi-infarct dementia is distinguished from PDD of the Alzheimer type by its more variable and classically step-wise deteriorating course and by the presence of focal neurologic signs and symptoms of vascular disease. Older people with a major depressive episode may have pseudodementia, which has been discussed in the section on the differential diagnosis of dementia.

Treatment. There is no specific treatment for PDD of the Alzheimer's type. Experimental drugs have been tried with mixed results, the latest being tetrahydroaminoacridine (THA), which influences acetylcholine metabolism. Ultimately, all patients require institutionalization or 24-hour custodial care owing to the severe psychological and physical deterioration that accompanies the disorder. Maintenance of physical health, supportive environment, and symptomatic psychopharmacologic treatment are indicated. Particular attention must be given to caretakers and family members who must deal with frustration, grief, and psychological burnout as they care for the patient over a long period of time.

MULTI-INFARCT DEMENTIA

Definition

Multi-infarct dementia (MID) is characterized by a decremental or patchy deterioration in cognitive functioning due to significant cerebrovascular disease.

Epidemiology

The disorder is most prevalent between ages 60 and 70, although it may begin in middle age, and is generally earlier than that of PDD of the Alzheimer type. MID occurs more frequently in men than in women. Hypertension predisposes a person to the disease. MID accounts for about 15 percent of all cases of dementia in the elderly.

Etiology

Vascular disease is assumed to be present and responsible for the dementia and the focal neurologic signs. The disorder affects small- and medium-size cerebral vessels, which undergo infarction and produce multiple parenchymal lesions spread over wide areas of the brain. Cerebral infarcts may result from damage in situ of a particular vessel or by thromboemboli originating in the heart or vessels outside the brain. Carotid bruits, funduscopic abnormalities, or an enlarged heart may be present. Hypertension is commonly associated with MID and may indicate a genetic contribution to the disorder.

Clinical Features and Course

A variety of symptoms occur in MID: headaches, dizziness, faintness, weakness, focal neurological symptoms, memory impairment, sleep disturbance, and personality changes such as emotional lability and hypochondriasis. Pseudobulbar palsy, dysarthria, and dysphagia are very common. The DSM-III-R diagnostic criteria for MID are listed in Table 19.

The onset of MID is usually sudden and the course is progressive, although the clinical picture may appear to stabilize for a period of time before worsening again. There is decremental and fluctuating deterioration in cognitive functioning that, early in the course, leaves some functions unaffected. Seizures occur in about 20 percent of cases.

Table 19
Diagnostic Criteria for Multi-Infarct Dementia

A. Dementia

B. Stepwise deteriorating course with "patchy" distribution of deficits (i.e., affecting some functions, but not others) early in the course.

C. Focal neurologic signs and symptoms (e.g., exaggeration of deep tendon reflexes, extensor plantar response, pseudobulbar palsy, gait abnormalities, weakness of an extremity, etc.).

D. Evidence from history, physical examination, or laboratory tests of significant cerebrovascular disease (recorded on Axis III) that is judged to be etiologically related to the disturbance.

Table from DSM-III-R *Diagnostic and Statistical Manual of Mental Disorders,* ed 3, revised. (Current Classification of Mental Disorders, 1987.) Copyright American Psychiatric Association, Washington, D.C., 1987. Used with permission.

Differential Diagnosis

MID must be differentiated from a single stroke, transient ischemic attacks (TIA), and from PDD of the Alzheimer type. A single stroke in general does not cause dementia. MID is due to multiple strokes that occur from time to time.

TIAs are brief episodes of focal neurological dysfunction lasting less than 24 hours (usually 5 to 15 minutes). Although a variety of mechanisms may be responsible, these episodes are frequently the result of microembolization from a proximal extracranial arterial lesion that produces transient brain ischemia and resolves without significant pathological alteration of the parenchymal tissue.

The clinican should distinguish episodes involving the vertebrobasilar system from those involving the carotid arterial system. In general, symptoms of vertebrobasilar disease reflect a transient functional disturbance in either the brain stem or the occipital lobe; carotid distribution symptoms reflect unilateral retinal or hemispheric abnormality. Anticoagulant therapy, antiplatelet agglutinating drugs such as acetylsalicyclic acid (aspirin), and extra- and intracranial reconstructive vascular surgery have been reported to be effective in reducing the risk of infarction in patients with TIAs.

About one third of untreated patients with transient ischemic attacks later develop a brain infarction. Since nearly half of the patients with TIAs who later develop infarction do so within a few weeks after the transient episodes, prompt recognition and treatment are crucial to the prevention of a major cerebrovascular accident.

MID is distinguished from PDD of the Alzheimer type by the typical decremental deterioration of the patient (as opposed to the continuous progression observed in PDD). Patients with MID are also more likely to show focal neurological signs and symptoms, presumably as a result of ischemic areas of the brain. Hypertension and evidence of cerebrovascular disease are also more common in MID than in PDD. It is possible for MID and PDD of the Alzheimer type to coexist. If clinical features of both are present, both diagnoses should be made.

Treatment

Once the diagnosis of MID is made, contributing risk factors should be identified and treated as early as possible in order to prevent further progression. These factors include hypertension, hyperlipidemia, heart disease, diabetes, and alcoholism. Control of hypertension prevents stroke in these patients. Cessation of smoking improves their cerebral perfusion and cognitive functioning.

The general principles of management of dementia apply: maintenance of overall physical health, stable supportive environment, and drug therapy of symptoms. The clinician may prescribe benzodiazepines for insomnia and anxiety, antidepressants for depression, and antipsychotic drugs for delusions or hallucinations; however, the clinician should be aware of possible idiosyncratic drug effects in the elderly (e.g., paradoxical excitement, confusion, or increased sedation).

OTHER CONDITIONS

A variety of other disorders have dementia as a presenting symptom or associated feature of the disease. These are dementias associated with an organic factor that arise before (presenile) or after (senile) the age of 65 and which cannot be classified as a specific dementia. Some disorders have known etiology such as infarction and disorders of inborn errors of metabolism; others are idiopathic. At times, delirium or mental confusion is the only sign present, which may progress to irreversible dementia if the underlying condition is not diagnosed and treated. According to DSM-III-R, these conditions are classified as either senile dementia not otherwise specified (NOS) or presenile dementia NOS (Tables 20 and 21).

Parkinsonism

Parkinsonism is a progressive disorder that generally begins in late adult life. The annual prevalence in the Western hemisphere has been reported to be about 200 per 100,000 people. In most cases, the etiology is unknown. There is a loss of cells in the substantia nigra, a decrease in dopamine, and a degeneration of dopaminergic tracts. Often, the first characteristic sign is a loss of associated movements, with a peculiar immobility of the patient. Tremor may become apparent later; it is most prominent at rest or on assuming a posture and is a characteristic pill-rolling tremor. As in most extrapyramidal disorders, the tremor becomes more prominent with tension and disappears with sleep. In some patients, tremor never becomes an important part of the illness; in others, it may be the most prominent symptom.

Physical examination reveals an impairment of fine movements and a peculiar, cogwheel kind of rigidity that is most apparent in the neck and in the upper extremities. Sucking reflexes, positive

Table 20
Diagnostic Criteria for Presenile Dementia Not Otherwise Specified

Dementias associated with an organic factor and arising before age 65 that cannot be classified as a specific Dementia (e.g., Primary Degenerative Dementia of the Alzheimer Type, Presenile Onset)

Table from DSM-III-R *Diagnostic and Statistical Manual of Mental Disorders,* ed 3, revised. (Current Classification of Mental Disorders, 1987.) Copyright American Psychiatric Association, Washington, D.C., 1987. Used with permission.

Table 21
Diagnostic Criteria for Senile Dementia Not Otherwise Specified

Dementias associated with an organic factor and arising after age 65 that cannot be classified as a specific Dementia (e.g., as Primary Degenerative Dementia of the Alzheimer Type, Senile Onset, or Dementia Associated with Alcoholism)

Table from DSM-III-R *Diagnostic and Statistical Manual of Mental Disorders,* ed 3, revised. (Current Classification of Mental Disorders, 1987.) Copyright American Psychiatric Association, Washington, D.C., 1987. Used with permission.

Babinski signs, and other evidence of pyramidal tract involvement are common.

Intellectual impairment is a common component of parkinsonism. Recent studies estimating that 40 to 80 percent of patients with parkinsonism eventually develop dementia. Dementia is initially mild, and the patients are able to continue their ordinary activities. However, the dementia tends to increase with the duration and severity of the disease and may prevent patients from working at their usual occupation.

Depression is associated with parkinsonism, in one third to one half of all cases; a trial of antidepressant medication is indicated in these patients. Regardless of therapy, the course of parkinsonism is gradually progressive. Some patients may have long periods in which the illness appears to show no real progression; others may be completely disabled within a few years of onset.

The treatment for Parkinson's is L–dopa (levodopa), a metabolic precursor of dopamine since dopamine itself does not cross the blood–brain barrier. L–dopa is often combined with carbidopa, a dopa decarboxylase inhibitor that aids L–dopa in reaching the brain. Amantadine hydrochloride (Symmetrel) has also proved useful; it acts synergistically with L–dopa. Recently, implanted tissue from the medulla of the adrenal gland into the brain has produced dopamine, eliminating the symptoms of the disease in some cases.

Huntington's Chorea

In 1872, Huntington described a hereditary disorder, characterized by choreiform movements and dementia that began in adult life. Huntington's chorea is rare; it is estimated that there are about 6 cases per 100,000 persons in the Western hemisphere. The disorder is inherited in an autosomal-dominant pattern with good penetrance. The disorder leads to atrophy of the brain with extensive degeneration of the basal ganglia, particularly the caudate nucleus.

The onset is usually insidious; it is often heralded by a personality change that interferes with the patient's ability to adapt to his environment. The disease may begin at any age, but is most common in late middle life. Both sexes are affected in equal numbers. When choreiform movements are first noted, they are frequently misinterpreted as inconsequential habit spasms or tics. As a result, the disease is frequently not recognized for several years, especially if the family history is not known. The diagnosis depends on recognition of the progressive choreiform movements and dementia in a patient with a family history of the disorder. Eventually, the choreiform movements or the dementia makes chronic hospitalization necessary. The clinical course is one of gradual progression, with death occurring 15 to 20 years after the onset of the disease. Suicide is not unusual in patients with this disorder.

The only satisfactory treatment at present is prevention of the transmission of the responsible genes. Some symptomatic relief of the movement disorder and the psychotic symptoms may be achieved by a neuroleptic such as haloperidol (Haldol). Now that a genetic marker for Huntington's disease has been found, it is questionable whether affected persons should have children.

Creutzfeldt-Jakob Disease

Creutzfeldt-Jakob disease is a rare degenerative brain disease caused by a slow virus infection. A progressive dementia occurs, accompanied by ataxia, extrapyramidal signs, choreoathetosis, and dysarthria. The disease is most common in adults in their 50s,

and usually death occurs within 2 years after the diagnosis is made. Males and females are affected equally. No means of treatment is known. CT scans show cerebellar and cortical atrophy, and EEG changes in the later stages are characteristic and confirmatory.

Kuru

Kuru is a progressive dementia accompanied by extrapyramidal signs. It is found among natives of New Guinea who practice cannibalistic rites. In eating the brains of infected individuals, the natives take in the slow virus that produces this fatal disease.

General Paresis

This disorder is a chronic dementia and psychosis caused by the tertiary form of syphilis that affects the brain. Symptoms include dementia, a manic syndrome with euphoria and grandiose delusions, and neurological signs (e.g., Argyll-Robertson pupil). Depression and delusions of persecution may also occur. There are prominent abnormalities in the cerebrospinal fluid, and there is generally a positive Wasserman reaction. The disease appears 10 to 15 years after the primary Treponema infection, and affects approximately 5 percent of patients who have neurosyphilis. Since the advent of penicillin, general paresis is rarely seen.

Normal-Pressure Hydrocephalus

Normal-pressure hydrocephalus is a treatable type of dementia in patients with enlarged ventricles and normal cerebrospinal fluid pressure. However, the disorder appears to be relatively uncommon and only a few cases of dementia are caused by this disorder. The clinical features are a progressive dementia that occurs, for the most part, in adults in middle or late life. An associated gait disturbance occurs, and urinary incontinence is present. When diagnosed, the treatment of choice is shunting the cerebrospinal fluid from the ventricular space to either the atrium or the peritoneal space. Reversal of dementia and associated signs is sometimes dramatic after treatment.

Multiple Sclerosis

Multiple sclerosis is characterized by diffuse multifocal lesions in the white matter of the central nervous system and a course characterized by exacerbations and remissions. The cause is unknown, but studies have been focused on slow viral infections and disturbances in the immune system.

It has been estimated that the prevalence of multiple sclerosis in the Western hemisphere is 50 patients per 100,000 people. The disease is much more frequent in cold and temperate climates than in the tropics and subtropics. It is more common in women than in men and is predominantly a disease of young adults. The onset in the vast majority of patients is between the ages of 20 and 40 years. Initially, neurologic symptoms often include weakness, ataxia, diffuse sensory and motor abnormalities and vision changes. As a result of the central nervous system lesions, symptoms suggesting a psychiatric disorder are so frequent that they create a diagnostic problem. Mental disturbances are present in at least 50 percent of patients with multiple sclerosis. Early signs may mimic a conversion disorder. Often, there is a change in emotional tone, which is usually reported as being euphoric, although mood instability is diagnosed just as often. Less often, signs and symptoms of an acute psychosis may be associated with the neurologic symptoms. Impairment of cognition often occurs as the disease progresses, and this impairment may lead to dementia or an amnestic syndrome in some cases. CT scans show patchy degenerative areas of cerebral white matter. Cerebrospinal fluid findings, especially elevation of gamma globulins, help to confirm the diagnosis.

Amyotrophic Lateral Sclerosis

Amyotrophic lateral sclerosis (ALS) is a progressive, noninherited, asymmetrical muscle atrophy. It begins in adult life and progresses over months or years to involve all the striated muscles except the cardiac and ocular muscles. In addition to muscle atrophy, patients have signs of pyramidal tract involvement. The illness is rare, occurring in about 1.6 persons per 100,000 a year. A few of these patients have concomitant dementia. The disease progresses rapidly, and death generally occurs within 4 years of onset.

Systemic Lupus Erythematosus (SLE)

SLE is an inflammatory connective tissue disease of unknown etiology that occurs primarily in young adult females. Drugs such as methyldopa and chlorpromazine may have a causative role in a minority of cases. Abnormalities in mental function have been reported in 15 to 50 percent of patients. The patient may have an acute psychosis with disorientation, confusion, inattention, delusions, and hallucinations or a chronic progressive dementia with a general deterioration of intellectual function and memory.

Transient Global Amnesia

The patient with transient global amnesia abruptly loses his ability to recall recent events or to record new memories. Events of the distant past are readily recalled. Although the patient is often aware of some disturbance in function during the episode, he may still perform highly complex mental and physical acts. Episodes last from 6 to 24 hours. Recovery is usually complete, with few recurrences. The disorder is thought to result from a temporary physiological alteration of the brain. Transient global amnesia is most likely caused by ischemia involving midline limbic structures, but it may also be an epileptiform phenomenon.

Intracranial Neoplasms

Psychiatric symptoms are often the earliest (and occasionally, the only) symptoms of an intracranial tumor. They may take the form of dementia or of a particular organic mental syndrome. They may precede the more obvious motor or sensory manifestations of brain tumor by weeks or even months. The mental symptoms of patients who have brain tumors vary, not only among patients but in the same patient from hour to hour. Computed tomographic (CT) scans are the major means of ruling out a neoplasm in the work-up of dementia.

Clinical Symptoms and Course. The patient with a brain tumor suffers a relentless progression of symptoms. The classic neurological symptoms are headache and impaired motor or sensory function. Even when these disturbances are present, they may be initially obscured by the patient's mental symptoms and may be detected only after careful interrogation and examination. Certain focal brain lesions produce specific intellectual deficits, although most patients with a brain tumor have simultaneous evidence of more generally impaired intellectual function. The following areas are affected:

Cognition. Impaired intellectual function often accompanies the presence of a brain tumor, regardless of its type or location.

Language skills. Disorders of language function may be severe, particularly if tumor growth is rapid. In fact, defects of language function often obscure all other mental symptoms.

Memory. Loss of memory is a frequent symptom of brain tumors. Patients with brain tumors may present with Korsakoff's syndrome, retaining no memory of events that occurred since the illness began. Events of the immediate past, even painful ones, are lost. Old memories, however, are retained, and the patient is unaware of his loss of recent memory.

Perception. Prominent perceptual defects are often associated with behavioral disorders, especially when the patient needs to integrate tactile, auditory, and visual perceptions.

Awareness. Alterations of consciousness are common late symptoms of increased intracranial pressure due to a brain tumor. Tumors arising in the upper part of the brain stem may produce a unique symptom called akinetic mutism or coma vigil. The patient appears asleep but ready to be aroused.

Response to cerebral loss. Most mental symptoms in patients with brain tumors result from the patient's response to the cerebral destruction. If the patient only gradually becomes aware of the destruction, the earliest psychiatric symptom is often irritability. Later, the patient usually becomes anxious and depressed. He may finally respond to his progressive cerebral impairment by denial of even the most flagrant loss, with a resultant disappearance of his anxiety and depression.

Metabolic and Endocrine Disorders

Metabolic encephalopathy is a common cause of organic brain dysfunction and capable of producing alterations in mental processes, behavior, and neurological function. This diagnosis should be considered whenever recent and rapid changes in behavior, thinking, and consciousness have occurred. The earliest signals are likely to be impairment of memory, particularly recent memory, and orientation. Some patients become agitated, anxious, and hyperactive; others become quiet, withdrawn, and inactive. As metabolic encephalopathies progress, confusion or delirium gives way to decreased responsiveness, to stupor, and, eventually, to coma.

Hepatic Encephalopathy. This brain dysfunction is due to severe impairment of liver function from acute or chronic liver disease or the shunting of portal vein blood into the systemic circulation. Hepatic encephalopathy may present with disturbances of consciousness, mental changes, asterixis, hyperventilation, and electroencephalographic abnormalities. Disturbances of consciousness can vary from apathy and drowsiness to coma. The changes in memory, intellect, and personality are nonspecific. Death is likely in severe cases.

Uremic Encephalopathy. Acute or chronic failure of normal renal function leads to serious systemic metabolic changes, and uremia may be the most frequent metabolic cause of organic mental syndromes. Neurological dysfunction—particularly alterations in memory, orientation, and consciousness—is a common accompaniment. Restlessness, crawling sensations of the limbs, twitching of muscles singly or in groups, and persistent hiccups can be distressing and exhausting to the patient. In severe uremia, generalized convulsions can occur, at times in rapid succession, increasing the risk of death. Intravenously administered diazepam may be an effective treatment, but the use of barbiturates or even anesthetics may be required for seizure control. When episodes of uremia are short lived, especially in younger patients, the organic mental syndrome is more likely to be reversible, but older people with recurrent and chronic uremia often develop irreversible damage. During rapid renal dialysis in the presence of very high blood urea levels, a dialysis dysequilibrium syndrome has been seen, with headache, confusion, alterations in consciousness, and convulsions.

Hypoglycemic Encephalopathy. Excessive or inappropriate administration of insulin and hyperinsulinism caused by a functioning benign adenoma of islet cells of the pancreas, are the most likely causes of hypoglycemic encephalopathy. Hypoglycemic episodes are likely to occur in the early morning hours or after exercise. Premonitory symptoms, which do not occur in every patient, include nausea, sweating, tachycardia, and feelings of hunger, apprehension, and restlessness. With progressive impairment, disorientation, confusion, hallucinations, pallor, and extreme restlessness or agitation develop. Diplopia, grand mal or focal seizures, myoclonic jerks, and hyperreflexia with clonus and Babinski's responses can be other features. Stupor and then coma may follow quickly. Prolonged coma can be followed by a residual and persistent dementia. An occasional patient has no signs or symptoms preceding convulsions.

Diabetic Ketoacidosis. The condition begins with feelings of weakness, early fatigability and listlessness, and increasing polyuria and polydipsia. Headache and sometimes nausea and vomiting appear. Depending on the severity of the diabetes and the presence of infection, the situation worsens in a matter of hours to several days. Patients with diabetes mellitus have an increased likelihood of developing a chronic dementia associated with general arteriosclerosis.

Diabetic coma is a medical emergency. In any unconscious patient who is known or suspected to be diabetic, the differential diagnosis of hypoglycemic coma and diabetic coma must be made. Hypoglycemia as a cause of the coma can be virtually excluded if the patient does not regain consciousness within a few minutes after the intravenous administration of 25 ml of a 50-percent glucose solution.

Diabetic coma without ketoacidosis (nonketotic hyperglycemic coma) may occur, particularly in older persons with adult-onset diabetes mellitus, and it may be the first manifestation of that disease. The principles of treatment include adequate fluid and electrolyte replacement, insulin, and the management of any associated infection or underlying disease.

Acute intermittent porphyria. This disorder is inherited as an autosomal-dominant trait, and its symptoms are most apt to begin after puberty or in the third or fourth decade of life. Women are affected more often than men. An inborn error of metabolism exists in the regulation of the liver enzyme, δ-aminolevulinic acid synthetase, which is important to pyrrole metabolism. The use of barbiturates for any reason is absolutely contraindicated in a person with acute intermittent porphyria and in anyone who has a relative with the disease. Barbiturates precipitate or aggravate the attacks of acute porphyria.

Symptoms of nervousness and emotional instability are frequently present for a long while. Recurrent abdominal pains, often colicky in nature, are common and sometimes lead to an unnecessary abdominal operation before accurate diagnosis is made. Neurological symptoms are also common and may become so severe that death results. Peripheral neuropathy involving one or all of the limbs and cranial nerve signs—such as optic atrophy, facial palsy, ophthalmoplegia, and dysphagia—may be seen. Confusion, delirium, convulsions, and coma can develop during acute attacks.

As yet, there is no satisfactory or specific treatment for acute intermittent porphyria. During acute episodes, only careful symptomatic measures can be used. Antipsychotic medications may be safely used and can provide significant relief from psychiatric symptoms.

Endocrine Disorders. Changes in personality, mental functions, and memory, as well as neurological abnormalities, frequently occur in endocrine disorders and may become prominent in some instances. Correction of the underlying endocrine problem usually reverses these changes.

Thyroid disorders produce hyper- or hypothyroidism. A sensation of easy fatigability and generalized weakness is felt by most hyperthyroid patients. Insomnia, weight loss in spite of increased appetite, tremulousness, palpitations, and increased perspiration are all common changes. Prominent mental disturbances may develop in a few patients, with impairment of memory, orientation, and judgment; manic excitement, and schizophreniform symptoms, such as delusions and hallucinations.

Treatment of hyperthyroidism in most adults consists of the administration of radioactive iodine. Antithyroid agents and surgical thyroidectomy are useful in certain patients. Mental symptoms can be expected to improve with adequate treatment of the hyperthyroidism, but for the occasional patient with severe mental symptoms, hospitalization is necessary.

Hypothyroidism (myxedema) arises because of a deficiency of thyroid hormone. Easy fatigability, feelings of weakness and sleepiness, increased sensitivity to cold, reduced sweating with dryness and thickening of the skin, brittle and thinning hair, and puffy facies are all common manifestations of myxedema. There is evidence of hypochromic anemia, diffuse slowing on the EEG, and reduced or absent T waves on a low-voltage EKG. In some patients, changes in personality, memory, and intellectual function are prominent, which may simulate major psychiatric or organic brain disease. Cerebellar gait ataxia is a feature of some cases. Congenital hypothyroidism produces mental retardation (cretinism), and is potentially treatable if discovered and managed promptly.

Parathyroid dysfunction produces derangements of calcium metabolism. Excessive secretion of parathyroid hormone from a parathyroid adenoma or hyperplasia causes hypercalcemia. Common complaints are lassitude, weakness, increased irritability, and anxiety. Some patients display frank disorders of personality and mental function, such as agitation, paranoid thinking, depression, psychotic reactions, confusion, and stupor. Neuromuscular excitability, which depends on a proper calcium ion concentration, is reduced, and muscle weakness may appear.

Lowered serum calcium levels in hypoparathyroidism lead to increased neuromuscular excitability, with transient paresthesias, muscle cramping and twitching, overt tetany with spontaneous carpopedal muscle spasms, and convulsive seizures. Such mental symptoms as confusion, agitation, drowsiness, hallucinations, and depression may also develop.

Adrenal disorders cause changes in the normal secretion of hormones from the adrenal cortex and produce significant neurological and psychological changes. Patients with chronic adrenocortical insufficiency (Addison's disease), which is most frequently the result of adrenocortical atrophy or granulomatous invasion due to tuberculous or fungal infection, exhibit mild mental symptoms such as apathy, easy fatigability, irritability, and depression. Occasionally psychotic reaction or confusion develops. Cortisone or one of its synthetic derivatives is effective in correcting such abnormalities.

Excessive quantities of cortisol produced endogenously by an adrenocortical tumor or hyperplasia (Cushing's syndrome) lead to an organic mood disorder of agitated depression with risk of suicide. Decreased concentration and memory defects may also be present. Psychotic reactions, with schizophreniform symptoms, are seen in a small number of patients. Administration of high doses of exogenous corticosteroids, on the other hand, more typically leads to an organic mood disorder similar to mania. Severe depression may follow the sudden termination of steroid therapy.

Nutritional Disorders

Beriberi. Thiamine (vitamin B_1) is required in the formation of the coenzyme thiamine pyrophosphate, which is essential in the intermediary metabolism of carbohydrate. Thiamine deficiency leads to beriberi, characterized chiefly by cardiovascular and neurological changes, and also Wernicke-Korsakoff's syndrome, which is most often associated with chronic alcoholism.

This disorder occurs primarily in Asia and in areas of famine or poverty; historically, it was an important disease in prisoner of war camps in Asia during World War II. Subacute or chronic onset is most common, but it occasionally runs a more rapid, acute course. Such mental disturbances as apathy, depression, irritability, nervousness, and poor concentration are frequently seen. However, Wernicke-Korsakoff's syndrome is difficult to exclude when more severe changes in memory and intellectual function occur.

Pellagra. Dietary insufficiency of niacin (nicotinic acid) and its precursor, tryptophan, is associated with pellagra, a nutritional deficiency disease of global importance. Nervous system involvement includes headaches, insomnia, apathy, confusional states, delusions, and, eventually, dementia. Cerebellar ataxia can be seen, as well as skin and GI involvement. Peripheral neuropathy is also a frequent feature, but it is probably a manifestation of other associated vitamin deficiencies, particularly thiamine deficiency. Traditionally, pellagra was described by five words beginning with the letter D—dermatitis, diarrhea, delirium, dementia, and death.

The response of the pellagra patient to treatment with nicotinic acid is rapid; significant improvement in confusion, abdominal symptoms, and painful swollen tongue are evident in the first 24 hours. However, dementia from prolonged illness may improve slowly and incompletely. If a peripheral neuropathy is present, administration of supplemental thiamine is important.

Vitamin B_{12} Deficiency. This state arises because of the failure of the gastric mucosal cells to secrete a specific substance, intrinsic factor, required for the normal absorption of dietary vitamin B_{12} from the ileum. The deficiency state is characterized by the development of a chronic macrocytic megaloblastic anemia (pernicious anemia) and neurological manifestations due to degenerative changes in the peripheral nerves, the spinal cord, and the brain. About 80 percent of patients develop neurological changes; these changes are commonly associated with the megaloblastic anemia, but they occasionally precede the onset of hematological abnormalities.

Mental changes such as apathy, depression, irritability, and moodiness are common. In a few patients, encephalopathy with associated confusion, delusions, hallucinations, dementia, and sometimes with paranoid features, are prominent manifestations which have been called megaloblastic madness. Presumably, they are related to cerebral involvement with patchy areas of demyelination and degeneration. The neurological manifestations of vitamin

B_{12} deficiency can be completely and rapidly arrested by the early and continued administration of parenteral vitamin B_{12} therapy.

PSYCHOACTIVE SUBSTANCE–INDUCED ORGANIC MENTAL DISORDERS

In DSM-III-R, the organic mental disorders caused by drugs with psychoactive properties are grouped together under the overall classification of psychoactive substance–induced organic mental disorders. A great variety of psychoactive substances can induce organic mental disorders; including sedatives, hypnotics, anxiolytics, opioids, cocaine, amphetamines, and similarly acting sympathomimetics, phencyclidine and similarly acting arylcyclohexylamines, hallucinogens, cannabis, caffeine, nicotine, and inhalants with psychoactive properties. Each drug can produce one of the syndromes already discussed: delirium, dementia, amnestic syndrome, delusional syndrome, hallucinosis, mood syndrome, anxiety syndrome, and personality syndrome. In addition, psychoactive substances can produce intoxication and withdrawal syndromes; however, there is a controversy about whether these syndromes are specific to a particular substance. For example, there is little reason to believe that delirium caused by alcohol withdrawal, barbiturate withdrawal, amphetamines, and phencyclidine can be distinguished from one another with any certainty on clinical grounds alone.

From both a conceptual and a nosological standpoint, it is best for the clinician to aim first for syndrome recognition and second for identification of the specific cause of the syndrome. Only in this way can a reasonable and useful differential diagnosis be constructed. The various organic mental disorders associated with psychoactive substances are covered in Chapter 13, Psychoactive Substance Use Disorders.

EPILEPSY

Introduction

Psychiatric problems are common in patients with epilepsy and, so, constitute an important mental health problem. It is the most common chronic neurological disease, having a prevalence of approximately 1 percent in the general population. Thirty to 50 percent of all epileptic subjects have significant psychiatric difficulties. Although the incidence of psychosis is high in epilepsy, personality disturbances are the most frequently encountered psychiatric problems.

Definition

The term epilepsy refers to a chronic condition of recurrent or repeated seizures. A seizure is a transient, paroxysmal, pathophysiological disturbance of cerebral function caused by a spontaneous, excessive discharge of cortical neurons. The clinical manifestation of seizures depends on the site of origin and on the pattern and spread of the discharge in the brain. A seizures may be abnormal movements or an arrest of movement, a disorder of sensation or perception, a disturbance of behavior, or an impairment of consciousness. Almost any acquired or genetic pathological process involving the brain may cause epilepsy.

Classification

Seizures are broadly characterized as partial seizures (caused by a focal lesion) and generalized seizures (caused by diffuse brain dysfunction). See Table 22 for an outline of the various types. The psychiatric manifestations of epilepsy are divided (below) into those associated with the seizure itself and those occurring between seizures (interictally).

Clinical Manifestations. Changes in mental function following generalized tonic-clonic convulsions (Figure 1) seldom present diagnostic problems when the convulsion itself has been witnessed. The postictal state is manifested by slow; gradual recovery of consciousness and cognition from the level of coma that usually characterizes the immediate postictal condition. The period required for full recovery varies from a few minutes to many hours. The clinical picture is that of a gradually clearing delirium.

Far less frequent and less well recognized are the transient episodes of psychiatric dysfunction that occur with petit mal epilepsy or with focal seizures that arise in a limited area of the brain, especially in the temporal lobes.

Table 22
Outline of the International Classifications of Epileptic Seizures

I. Partial seizures (seizures beginning locally)
  A. Partial seizures with elementary symptoms (generally without impairment of consciousness)
    1. With motor symptoms
    2. With sensory symptoms
    3. With autonomic symptoms
    4. Compound forms
  B. Partial seizures with complex symptoms (generally with impairment of consciousness; temporal lobe or psychomotor seizures)
    1. With impairment of consciousness only
    2. With cognitive symptoms
    3. With affective symptoms
    4. With psychosensory symptoms
    5. With psychomotor symptoms (automatisms)
    6. Compound forms
  C. Partial seizures secondarily generalized
II. Generalized seizures (bilaterally symmetric and without local onset)
  A. Absences (petit mal)
  B. Myoclonus
  C. Infantile spasms
  D. Clonic seizures
  E. Tonic seizures
  F. Tonic-clonic seizures (grand mal)
  G. Atonic seizures
  H. Akinetic seizures
III. Unilateral seizures
IV. Unclassified seizures (because of incomplete data)

Modified from Gastaut H: Clinical and electroencephalographical classification of epileptic seizures. Epilepsia *11:*102, 1970.

The epileptic nature of these episodes may go unrecognized, because the characteristic motor or sensory manifestations of epilepsy may be absent or so slight that they do not arouse the physician's suspicion. A functional psychiatric disorder is especially likely to be suspected when the patient suffers from what has been called subclinical status epilepticus; that is, when the epileptic discharge persists for long periods, even many hours, without producing the characteristic movements of epilepsy.

Petit mal (or absence) epilepsy usually begins in childhood, between the ages of 5 and 7, and ceases by puberty. Absence seizures produce a brief disruption of consciousness during which the patient suddenly loses contact with the environment, without true loss of consciousness or convulsive movements. The EEG produces a characteristic pattern of 3-per-second spike-and-wave activity (Figure 2). Petit mal epilepsy may have its onset in adulthood; when it does, the clinical picture may be very different. The classic absence pattern may not occur; in its place may be sudden, recurrent psychotic episodes or deliria which appear and disappear abruptly. The EEG pattern of 3-per-second spike-and-wave activity is present. In the adult pattern, a history of fainting or falling spells may be elicited. Complex partial seizures of temporal lobe origin are discussed below.

Difficult diagnostic problems arise in distinguishing an organic mental disorder of epileptic origin from a psychiatric disorder, when the clinical manifestations of epilepsy are more floridly emotional or psychotic, and when changes in level of consciousness and cognition are not so readily apparent. In these instances, the episodes may not even be recognized as organic in origin, much less as epileptic, for they may be manifested by hallucinations, delusions, severe agitation and hyperactivity, profound depression, transient aphasia or muteness, and catatonic states, effectively mimicking many functional psychiatric disorders.

Such episodic psychiatric dysfunction should always be suspected to be epileptic in origin when it occurs in patients in whom epilepsy has been diagnosed previously. The diagnosis is confirmed if the EEG during the episode reveals continuous or nearly continuous epileptic discharges. It is often impossible to obtain an EEG during the episode, however; in such cases the diagnosis is substantially confirmed if the episodes disappear or are greatly reduced in number and severity with more careful regulation of anticonvulsant medications.

The diagnosis is clearly much more difficult in patients who are not known to have epilepsy. In these cases, four clinical features should suggest to the physician the possibility of epilepsy: the abrupt onset of psychosis in a person previously regarded as psychologically healthy, the abrupt onset of delirium that cannot be accounted for by more common causes, a history of similar episodes with abrupt and spontaneous onset and remission, and a history of previous fainting or falling spells that were unexplained. Correct diagnosis is especially important, because treatment with appropriate anticonvulsant medications may prevent the individual episodes.

Episodic violence has been a problem in some patients with epilepsy especially of temporal lobe origin. The question has arisen, whether this violence is a manifestation of the seizure itself (an epileptic automatism) or of interictal

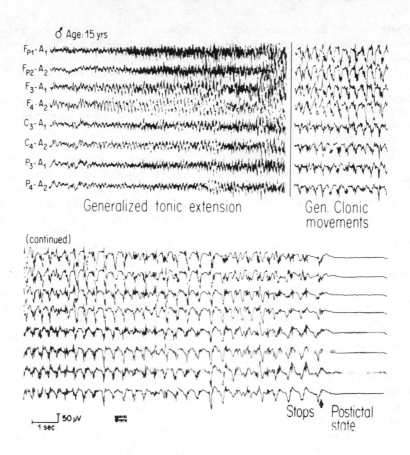

Figure 1 *EEG recording during generalized tonic-clonic seizure, showing rhythmic sharp waves and muscle artifact during tonic phase, spike-and-wave discharges during clonic phase, and attenuation of activity during postictal state. (Courtesy Barbara F Westmoreland, MD.)* From Wollo C E: Other organic brain syndromes. In *Comprehensive Textbook of Psychiatry*, ed 4, H I Kaplan and B J Sadock, editors, p 879. Williams & Wilkins, Baltimore, 1985.

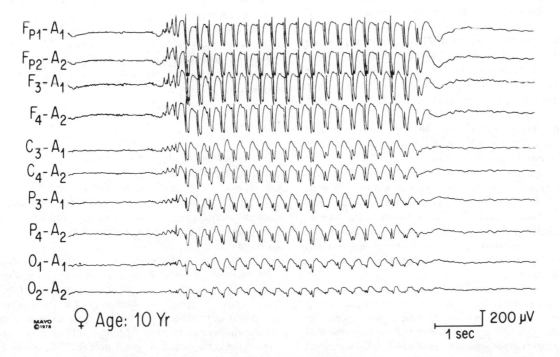

Figure 2 *Generalized-Hz spike-and-wave discharge in a 10-year-old patient with absence seizures.* (Courtesy Barbara F Westmoreland, MD.). From Wells C E: Other organic brain syndromes. In *Comprehensive Textbook of Psychiatry*, ed 4, H I Kaplan and B J Sadock, editors, p 880. Williams & Wilkins, Baltimore, 1985.

psychopathology. To date, most of the evidence points to the extreme rarity of violence as an ictal phenomenon. Only in very rare cases should violence of an epileptic patient be attributed to the seizure itself.

Interictal manifestations

Psychoses. Interictal psychotic states are encountered more often than ictal psychoses but less often than the interictal personality disturbances (discussed below). Psychoses that resemble schizophrenia have been described, and evidence has accumulated that the psychoses are more frequent in patients with epilepsy of temporal lobe origin than in patients with epilepsy that is nonfocal in origin or that arises from foci outside the temporal lobe.

These chronic schizophreniform psychoses may come on acutely, subacutely, or insidiously. They usually occur only after the subjects have suffered from complex partial seizures of temporal lobe origin for many years, so that the duration of the epilepsy has come to be regarded as an important factor in the causation. Personality changes often precede the appearance of psychosis.

These psychoses are manifested most prominently by paranoid delusions and hallucinations (especially auditory hallucinations) in the presence of a clear consciousness. Affective flattening may occur, but patients are often described as remaining warm and appropriate in affect. Although thought disorders of a schizophrenic variety are commonly reported, thought disorders of an organic type, such as poor conceptualization or circumstantiality, are more frequent. The relationship between these psychoses and seizure frequency is unclear. In some patients, worsening of the psychosis has been observed when good seizure control has been achieved, but this deterioration is not inevitable. Response to treatment with antipsychotic medications is variable and unpredictable.

In most patients, these psychoses differ from classic schizophrenia in several important respects. Affect and personality are often less disturbed than in many chronic schizophrenics, and the incidence of schizophrenia in family members is considerably lower than in the families of patients with true schizophrenia. Several observations point to the overriding importance of organic factors in the causation of these psychoses. They generally appear only after the patient has suffered from epilepsy for many years. They are much more common in epilepsy that originates in the dominant temporal lobe, especially when the epileptic foci involve the deep mesial temporal structures of the dominant hemisphere. When these patients are followed over time, they come to resemble patients with chronic organic brain disorders much more than patients with chronic schizophrenia; that is, cognitive losses overshadow abnormalities in thought processes.

Affective psychoses or mood disorders, such as depression, mania, and manic-depressive illness, are seen less often than the schizophreniform psychoses. In contrast to them, however, affective psychoses tend to be episodic and to occur more often when the epileptic foci affect the temporal lobe of the nondominant cerebral hemisphere. The importance of the mood disorders in epilepsy may be attested to by the increased incidence of attempted suicide in persons with epilepsy.

Personality disturbances. Personality disturbances are the most frequent psychiatric abnormality reported in epileptic subjects and are especially likely to occur in patients with epilepsy of temporal lobe origin. Although the homogeneity and specificity of these personality changes in people with complex partial seizures of temporal lobe origin (temporal lobe epilepsy) remain debatable, the specific features reported to make up this syndrome generally include changes in sexual behavior, a quality usually called viscosity, religiosity, and a heightened experience of emotions.

Changes in sexual behavior may be manifested by hypersexuality; deviations in sexual interest such as fetishism or transvestism; or hyposexuality, but the last is by far the most common. This hyposexuality is manifested both by a lack of interest in sexual matters and by reduced sexual arousal. Patients whose complex partial seizures begin before puberty may fail to develop normal levels of sexuality, a circumstance that may not greatly distress the affected person. For patients whose complex partial seizures lead to hyposexuality after they have developed a normal level of sexuality, however, the problem may be severely troubling. Unilateral temporal lobectomy, when it is successful in controlling seizures, sometimes provides striking improvement of hyposexuality. This procedure is rarely performed.

Perhaps the most difficult of these personality changes to describe is viscosity ("stickiness"). This change is apt to be most noticeable in the patient's conversation, which is likely to be slow, serious, ponderous, pedantic, overly replete with detail, swollen with nonessentials and often circumstantial. The listener grows bored, wonders if the speaker will ever reach the point, and wants to escape, but the speaker offers no opportunity for courteous and successful disengagement; hence the term viscosity. The same quality may be seen in the patient's writing and drawings, and hypergraphia has been considered by some to be a cardinal manifestation of this syndrome. The tendency to verbosity, circumstantiality, and overinclusiveness that is apparent in speech is mirrored in writing. Some patients are able, with much effort, to improve their style of communication when these difficulties are pointed out to them by a sympathetic counselor, but many cannot accept the criticism or do not perceive it as a problem. Religiosity may be striking and may be manifested not only by increased attention to and participation in overtly religious activities but also by unusual concern for moral and ethical issues, preoccupation with right and wrong, and heightened interest in global and philosophical concerns.

The syndrome in its complete form is relatively rare, even in those with complex partial seizures of temporal lobe origin. Many patients are not affected by personality disturbances; others suffer from a variety of disturbances that differ strikingly from the syndrome delineated above.

Treatment

Anticonvulsant drugs are necessary to control most patients' seizures. Currently, the most commonly used anticonvulsant agents are phenobarbital, phenytoin, carbamazepine, primidone, ethosuximide, trimethadione, diazepam, clonazepam, and most recently, sodium valproate. The drugs of choice for the various types of seizures are listed in Table 23.

The personality disturbances associated with temporal lobe epilepsy sometimes respond well to psychotherapy, anticonvulsant medications, or a combination of both. Carbamazepine (Tegretol) is often helpful in controlling the symptoms of irritability and the outbursts of aggression, as are the antipsychotic drugs. Although antipsychotic medications have certain epileptogenic potential, in practice they seldom result in increased frequency of seizures in treated epileptic patients.

Table 23
Drugs of Choice for Various Types of Seizures

Generalized tonic-clonic (grand mal) seizures:
  Phenobarbital
  Phenytoin (Dilantin)
  Carbamazepine (Tegretol)
Absence (petit mal) seizures:
  Ethosuximide (Zarontin)
  Sodium valproate (Depakene)
  Trimethadione (Tridione)
Simple partial (focal) seizures:
  Phenobarbital
  Phenytoin (Dilantin)
Complex partial (temporal lobe) seizures:
  Phenytoin (Dilantin)
  Carbamazepine (Tegretol)
  Primidone (Mysoline)

Myoclonic, atonic, akinetic, and atypical absence seizures:
  Clonazepam (Clonopin)
  Diazepam (Valium)
Infantile spasms:
  Adrenocorticotropic hormone
  Corticosteroids
Status epilepticus:
  Diazepam (Valium)
  Phenobarbital
  Amobarbital (Amytal)
  Phenytoin (Dilantin)
  Paraldehyde
  Anesthetic agent

References

Davis K L, Hollander E, Davidson M, Davis B M, Mohs R C, Horvath T B: Induction of depression with oxotremorine in patients with Alzheimer's disease. Am J Psychiatry 144(4):468, 1987.

Lazarus L W, Newton N, Cohler B, Lesser J, Schweon C: Frequency and presentation of depressive symptoms in patients with primary degenerative dementia. Am J Psychiatry 144(1):41, 1987.

McEroy J P, McCue M, Spring B, Mohs R C, Lavor P W, Farr R M: Effects of amentadine and tribexyphenidyl on memory in elderly normal volunteers. Am J Psychiatry 144(5):573, 1987.

Myers B A: The mini mental state in those with developmental disabilities. J Nervous Mental Dis 175(2):85, 1987.

Saravay S M, Marke J, Steinberg M D, Rabiner C J: "Doom anxiety" and delirium in lidocaine toxicity. Am J Psychiatry 144:159, 1987.

Wolkowitz O M, Weingartner H, Thompson K, Richar D, Paul S M, Homer D W: Diazepam induced amnesia: A neuropharmacological model of an "organic amnestic syndrome." Am J Psychiatry 144(1):25, 1987.

12

Psychiatric Aspects of Acquired Immune Deficiency Syndrome (AIDS)

DEFINITION

AIDS is a disease transmitted by a slow retrovirus. The virus, previously called human T cell lymphotropic virus Type III (HTLV–III) or lymphadenopathy-associated virus (LAV), is now referred to as human immunodeficiency virus (HIV). The virus selectively infects and destroys T helper–inducer (T_4) lymphocytes, thus disrupting the cell-mediated immune response and allowing opportunistic infections and neoplasms (e.g., lymphoma, Kaposi's sarcoma) to develop. The virus also directly attacks the central nervous system causing dementia, myelopathy, and neuropathy, as well as personality changes, depression, and psychosis. The virus has been identified in blood, semen, tears, saliva, and cerebrospinal fluid.

EPIDEMIOLOGY

According to the World Health Organization, as of 1986, about 100,000 persons worldwide have AIDS, and as many as 10 million are infected with the virus. By the end of 1991, the U.S. Surgeon General estimates that more than 250,000 persons in the United States will have the disease and over 180,000 will have died from it. As of January 1987, over 28,000 people in the United States had been diagnosed as having AIDS, and about 16,000 had succumbed.

The virus is transmitted from person to person via body fluids such as semen and blood, and through intravenous (IV) use of contaminated syringes and needles. In the United States, the high-risk groups—homosexual men, bisexual men, and IV drug users—account for most of the cases. Homosexual men make up 70 to 80 percent of reported cases. Heterosexual transmission currently accounts for 1 percent of new cases, mainly through male-to-female transmission. Most infected women are IV drug abusers and prostitutes. Newborns are infected via placental transmission from infected mothers. Recipients of HIV–contaminated blood transfusions (including hemophiliacs) are also at risk for developing the disease. This risk group makes up 2 percent of all cases. The virus is not transmitted through casual contact. Family members and health workers have not contracted AIDS, except in very rare cases where there has been exposure to contaminated blood. Other risk groups include Haitians and Central Africans (6 percent of U.S. AIDS patients).

SERUM TESTING

The serum test used to detect HIV is known as the enzyme-linked immunosorbent assay (ELISA). About 1 to 2 million Americans are seropositive for HIV and are considered carriers of the disease. In a 1985 survey of military recruits, all of whom are tested for AIDS virus, 1.7 percent were positive for HIV.

HIV false-positives occur in about 1 percent of cases. If an ELISA result is suspected of being incorrect, then the serum can be subjected to a Western blot test, which is more accurate. A person should not be notified immediately of a positive ELISA test before a confirmatory test, such as the Western blot, is conducted. Blood banks currently must exclude sera that are ELISA positive. Donor notification has important ramifications both to the person involved and to the society at large. In some states, such as Colorado, Minnesota, and South Carolina, the names and addresses of antibody-positive persons are reported to public health authorities.

CLINICAL SIGNS AND SYMPTOMS

Infected persons are seropositive; that is, antibodies to HIV are detectable in serum. The incubation period—the interval between infection and seropositivity—can be from months to years. At least 35 percent of patients who are seropositive will develop AIDS.

AIDS is diagnosed when an opportunistic infection occurs in an immunosuppressed person who is HIV-positive. The most common infections include pneumocystis carinii pneumonia (63 percent of patients), toxoplasmosis, cryptococcal meningitis, candida albicans (which presents as a hairy leukoplakia of the tongue), cytomegalovirus, herpes simplex, cryptosporidium (which presents as diarrhea), and tuberculosis. Kaposi's sarcoma is a common cancer that occurs in about 40 percent of these patients, who usually die within 2 or 3 years of being diagnosed. The presenting signs and symptoms of the illness depend on the stage of the disease and on which organ systems are affected (most often the lungs and the central nervous system though any organ system is vulnerable). A general wasting away of the body occurs, known as emaciation disorder.

A syndrome called AIDS–related complex (ARC) has been described in patients who do not have an opportunistic infection. Such patients are seropositive and present with weight loss, fever, night sweats, generalized lymphadenopathy, chronic fatigue, and depression. About 25 to 50 percent of ARC patients develop AIDS within 3 years. Others may continue with the symptoms, undergo a course characterized by remissions or exacerbations, or become symptom free. Because they remain seropositive, they are considered carriers of the disease.

CNS Infections

CNS infections with HIV lead to a subacute encephalopathy, referred to as AIDS dementia complex or AIDS encephalopathy. Forgetfulness, difficulty concentrating, mild confusion, withdrawal or agitation, and depressed mood are common complaints that may occur in the absence of any other symptoms. These may progress to frank dementia, confusion, poor judgment, impulsive behavior, and psychosis. Some degree of dementia has been reported in about 60 percent of patients with AIDS.

Cerebral atrophy, ventricular enlargement (both observable with CT), and vacuolization of white matter occur. The multinucleated giant cells of the brain are involved in over 95 percent of cases (Figure 1). Eighty percent of postmortem studies show neuropathological signs. Multiple small nodules of inflammatory cells in the cerebral gray matter have been noted, especially in the basal ganglia and thalamus. Vacuolar myelopathy of the spinal cord is also found, particularly in the posterior and lateral columns at the thoracic levels. Cerebral lymphomas have been reported as well.

Psychiatric Signs and Symptoms

About 10 percent of patients present with neurological or psychiatric symptoms, and as the disease progresses, up to 60 percent of patients will develop a neuropsychiatric syndrome.

Signs of subacute encephalitis include general fatigue, lethargy, and headache that can progress to a dementia, delirium, or another organic mental syndrome, such as a mood disorder or a personality syndrome. Aphasia, cognitive impairment, memory defects, and impaired judgment are most common. Patients are aware of their diminishing mental functioning and may show signs of frustration, anxiety, or even a catastrophic reaction as they attempt to deal with tasks beyond their capacity. Delusions and hallucinations occur in the early stages, which may progress to global dementia, seizures, coma, and death. The course may be fulminating or progressive over a number of years. Every type of regressed psychotic behavior has been described, including fecal smearing, suicide, and homicide.

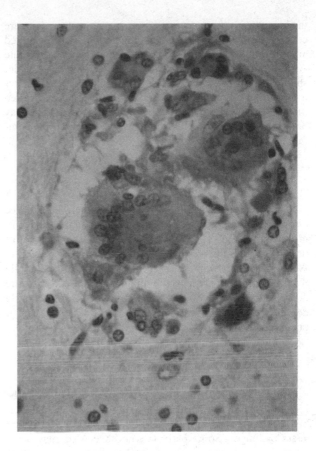

Figure 1. *Abnormal cell masses contain the AIDS virus.* Multinucleated giant cells in brain tissue from an AIDS patient. These fused clumps of cells contain the AIDS retrovirus (courtesy of Anthony Faust). Figure from Barnes D M: AIDS–related brain damage unexplained. Science *232*:1092, 1986.

The psychiatric symptoms of ARC are usually reactions to the general malaise, fatigue, night sweats, and lymphadenopathy. Patients become anxious, fearful, and depressed over their condition. AIDS may remain undiagnosed unless the physician knows the patient to be at high risk.

AIDS IN CHILDREN

Mothers transmit the virus to fetuses. Several hundred children have been diagnosed as having AIDS, although the actual number of children who are seropositive may be much larger nationwide. As with adults, children are subject to opportunistic infections and usually die by the age of 2, although some children reach puberty.

Fetal transmission usually occurs in the first trimester. Newborn infants with AIDS are reported to have characteristic AIDS facies. Seropositive mothers may elect to have an abortion rather than risk having a baby with AIDS.

Afflicted children may require special schooling, especially if they are neurologically impaired. Others may be treated in pediatric units during the day and permitted to return to the parental home at night. The majority of children with AIDS come from single-parent homes or have inadequate mothers, so foster care placement or day care centers are necessary. AIDS is apparently not transmitted among family members, so there is no reason to segregate AIDS children on that basis. Similarly, children, if able, should be permitted to attend school without fear of their transmitting the disease to others. However, other children may pose a threat if they have a contagious disease that may be transmitted to an AIDS child with a compromised immune system.

DIAGNOSIS

The diagnosis of AIDS is made when there is evidence of opportunistic infections or neoplasms in an immunocompromised host who is HIV-positive, typically a member of one of the high-risk groups. The clinician should be alert to AIDS in patients who do not meet those criteria, especially if vague somatic or flu-like complaints persist and there are neurologic and psychiatric complaints (e.g., chronic mild depression). The serum should be tested for HIV, and if positive, the diagnosis of AIDS or ARC is confirmed.

COURSE AND PROGNOSIS

Once diagnosed, the disease is currently thought to be invariably fatal; the average life span for an AIDS patient is between 6 months and 1 year. Some patients have lived 5 years or longer. Some patients who have ARC may never go on to develop the complete AIDS syndrome, and others may undergo remission.

TREATMENT

No treatment has yet proved effective against AIDS. The specific opportunistic infection is treated with the appropriate antibacterial agents, and precautions are taken to prevent further infections. The ultimate goal of treatment is to restore immunocompetence and to clear the body of opportunistic infections. Currently, drugs that block reverse transcriptase (e.g., azothymidine [AZT]) are being clinically tested and have improved longevity and the quality of life of many AIDS victims. Since these drugs only block the production of new viruses, however, their long-term efficacy is doubtful. Other tested drugs include suramin, ribavarin, ansamycin, and interferon. Vaccines, although under development, are not expected to be available for at least a decade. Chemotherapy and radiotherapy administered for Kaposi's sarcoma do not affect the basic pathology of immunosuppression.

When CNS involvement occurs, especially symptoms of an organic mental disorder, such as anxiety, psychosis, or depression, appropriate psychotropic medications are indicated. Antipsychotics (e.g., trifluoperazine [Stelazine], haloperidol [Haldol]) in small doses may be useful in controlling agitation. Antidepressants, particularly those with few anticholinergic side effects, are of benefit in treating depression. If brain damage is present, drugs with anticholinergic effect must be used cautiously to prevent an atropine psychosis. Some clinicians have had positive results treating depressed AIDS patients with small doses of amphetamine. Benzodiazepines are often useful for anxiety or insomnia, though they may exacerbate cognitive symptoms. Small doses of sedating neuroleptics (e.g., 25 mg of thioridazine [Mellaril]) or an antihistamine may then be used. Lithium may be useful in individuals with manic symptoms, but renal function and lithium concentrations must be carefully monitored if there is renal impairment from the illness. Suicidal depression is common in advanced cases; antidepressant medication and close supervision of the patient, including psychiatric hospitalization with suicidal precautions, may be necessary. Approximately 60 percent of AIDS patients develop some type of organic brain syndrome, and the usual measures of medical, environmental, and social support should be instituted in those situations.

Psychotherapy

Once diagnosed, most AIDS patients react with overwhelming anxiety, especially when they become aware of the fatal outcome. If a sense of hoplessness develops, the patient is likely to develop a suicidal depression; however, if the patient can be reassured that he will not be abandoned by his family and friends and that every effort will be made to deal with his medical and psychiatric complications, including pain relief, a sense of despair can be converted into one of acceptance or even hope. Some patients use denial as a defense. That can be healthy provided it does not interfere with obtaining proper medical treatment.

The role of psychotherapy, both individual and group, is important. The psychiatrist can help patients deal with feelings of guilt regarding behavior that contributed to developing AIDS that are disapproved of by other segments of society. Many AIDS patients feel that they are being punished for a deviant life style. Difficult health care decisions (e.g., whether to participate in an experimental drug trial) as well as terminal care and life support systems should be explored. In addition, all infected individuals must be educated concerning safe sexual practices (e.g., the use of condoms and the avoidance of anal sex). Treatment of homosexuals and bisexuals with AIDS often involves helping the patient "come out" to his family and dealing with the possible issues of rejection, guilt, shame, and anger. Involvement of a homosexual patient's lover in couples therapy is warranted in many cases.

Treatment of intravenous drug users involves discussing the patient's continued use of intravenous drugs. The possible ill effects of drug abuse on a patient's health needs to be weighed against the effect of adding drug withdrawal to an AIDS patient's existing problems. Educating patients about the danger of sharing contaminated needles is of utmost importance.

A subgroup of patients termed the "worried well" is comprised of persons in high-risk groups who, although they are seronegative and disease free, develop anxiety or an obsession about contracting the virus or AIDS. Some such patients are reassured by a negative ELISA. Others, however, obsess about the possible long incubation period and cannot be reassured; they can have an underlying somatoform disorder. Supportive or insight-oriented psychotherapy is indicated in these cases. Often, there are unconscious feelings of guilt about forbidden sexual activities, and patients punish themselves with obsessive thoughts or fantasies. ARC patients especially benefit from group therapy composed of similar patients, as do persons who are at risk on the basis of past sexual activity or current practices.

Institutional care

AIDS patients in hospitals must deal with staff whose attitudes about the illness range from altruistic acceptance to prejudicial rejection. A significant number of medical and nonmedical staff have a high degree of anxiety about contracting AIDS from patients under their care, in spite of the fact that AIDS cannot be spread by casual contact or fomites. Health care workers who have occasionally pricked their skin by accident while taking blood from AIDS patients have rarely come down with the disease and rarely become seropositive. In addition, there have always been persons who resent or are anxious about working with homosexuals and drug addicts. Those health care workers must be identified and allowed to withdraw from caring for AIDS patients if they cannot master such feelings. Finally, staff require support services, such as education in grief therapy, if they are to maintain their effectiveness and avoid professional burnout, which is not uncommon among those who work with chronically and terminally ill persons.

References

Binder R: AIDS antibody tests on inpatient psychiatric units. Am J Psychiatry *144*(2):176, 1987.

Cohen M, Weisman H W: A biopsychosocial approach to AIDS. Psychosomatics *27*:245, 1986.

Curran J W, Morgan W M, Hardy A M: The epidemiology of AIDS: Current status and future prospects. Science *229*:1352, 1985.

DeVita V T, Hellman S, Rosenberg S A, editors: *AIDS: Etiology, Diagnosis, Treatment, and Prevention.* J B Lippincott, Philadelphia, 1985.

Dilley J W, Shelp E E, Batki S L: Psychiatric and ethical issues in the care of patients with AIDS. Psychosomatics, *27*:562, 1986.

Faulstich M E: Psychiatric aspects of AIDS. Am J Psychiatry *144*(5):551, 1987.

Johnson R T, McArthur J C: AIDS and the brain. Trends Neurosci *9*:91, 1986.

Navia B A, Choo E S, Petito C K: The AIDS dementia complex: II Neuropathology. Ann Neurol *19*:525, 1986.

Navia B A, Jordan B D, Price R W: The AIDS dementia complex: I Clinical features. Ann Neurol *19*:517, 1986.

Nichols S E, Ostrow D G, editors: *Psychiatric Implications of Acquired Immune Deficiency Syndrome.* American Psychiatric Press, Washington, DC, 1984.

Runden J R: Three cases of AIDS-related psychiatric disorders. Am J Psychiatry *143*:777, 1986.

Stoler M N, Eskin T A, Benn S, Angerer R C, Angerer L M: Human T-cell lymphotrophic virus type III infection of the central nervous system. JAMA, *256*:2360, 1986.

13

Psychoactive Substance Use Disorders

13.1
Overview

In this chapter psychoactive substance use disorders are discussed together with the organic mental disorders that may be associated with them. In DSM-III-R, the organic mental disorders caused by drugs with psychoactive properties are grouped together under the overall classification of psychoactive substance–induced organic mental disorders. A great variety of psychoactive substances can induce organic mental disorders, including sedatives, hypnotics, anxiolytics, opioids, cocaine, amphetamines and similarly acting sympathomimetics, phencyclidine and similarly acting arylcyclohexylamines, hallucinogens, cannabis, caffeine, nicotine, and inhalants with psychoactive properties. Each drug can produce one or more of the syndromes already discussed: delirium, dementia, amnestic syndrome, delusional syndrome, hallucinosis, mood syndrome, anxiety syndrome, and personality syndrome. In addition, psychoactive substances can produce intoxication and withdrawal syndromes (Tables 1 and 2); but there is controversy about whether these syndromes are specific to a particular substance. For example, there is little reason to believe that the delirium caused by alcohol withdrawal, barbiturate withdrawal, amphetamines, or phencyclidine can be distinguished from each other with any certainty on clinical grounds alone. From both a conceptual and a nosological standpoint, it is best for the clinician to aim first for syndrome recognition and second for identification of the specific cause of the syndrome. Only in this way can a reasonable and serviceable differential diagnosis be constructed.

DSM-III-R differentiates psychoactive substance–induced organic mental disorders from psychoactive substance–use disorders; the former refers to the direct acute or chronic effects of psychoactive substances on the nervous system; the latter, to maladaptive behavior associated with regular use of psychoactive substances. According to DSM-III-R, the two diagnoses usually coexist.

A psychoactive substance is defined as one which when taken into the body can alter consciousness or state of mind. Such compounds in the form of therapeutic drugs, liquids, potions, and plants, among others have been used since antiquity. In the United States such substances are (1) legal, although controlled or taxed by the government (e.g., alcohol, tobacco), (2) legal and prescribed by physicians (e.g., diazepam, barbiturates), or (3) illegal (e.g., marijuana, heroin). Some drugs may be prescribed in certain states only on special governmental forms (e.g. state triplicate prescriptions for amphetamines). All psychoactive substances are subject to abuse, misuse, and psychological or physical dependence.

About 1.4 billion prescriptions for more than 10,000 different chemical substances are written in the United States each year. About 20 percent of them are for psychoactive or mood altering drugs, such as tranquilizers, sedatives, stimulants, sleeping pills, and analgesics. Fifty percent of all patients who suffer from chronic pain take between one and five pain relievers, and 25 percent of this group develop physical dependence on one of those drugs.

EPIDEMIOLOGY

A 1985 survey found that use of illicit drugs (e.g., cocaine, heroin, marijuana) is far more prevalent among the young adult population (ages 18 to 25 years) than among other age groups. For example, only 6 percent of adults over 26 years of age reported having used marijuana or

Table 1
Diagnostic Criteria for Intoxication

A. Development of a substance-specific syndrome due to recent ingestion of a psychoactive substance. (**Note:** More than one substance may produce similar or identical syndromes.)

B. Maladaptive behavior during the waking state due to the effect of the substance on the central nervous system (e.g., belligerence, impaired judgment, impaired social or occupational functioning).

C. The clinical picture does not correspond to any of the other specific Organic Mental Syndromes, such as Delirium, Organic Delusional Syndrome, Organic Hallucinosis, Organic Mood Syndrome, or Organic Anxiety Syndrome.

Table from DSM-III-R *Diagnostic and Statistical Manual of Mental Disorders,* ed 3, revised. (Current Classification of Mental Disorders, 1987.) Copyright American Psychiatric Association, Washington, D.C., 1987. Used with permission.

Table 2
Diagnostic Criteria for Withdrawal

A. Development of a substance-specific syndrome that follows the cessation of, or reduction in, intake of a psychoactive substance that the person previously used regularly.

B. The clinical picture does not correspond to any of the other specific Organic Mental Syndromes, such as Delirium, Organic Delusional Syndrome, Organic Hallucinosis, Organic Mood Syndrome, or Organic Anxiety Syndrome.

Table from DSM-III-R *Diagnostic and Statistical Manual of Mental Disorders,* ed 3, revised. (Current Classification of Mental Disorders, 1987.) Copyright American Psychiatric Association, Washington, D.C., 1987. Used with permission.

cocaine in the past 30 days, compared to 22 percent of those between 18 and 25 years old. These figures may change as the population ages. Although drug use by females is increasing faster than drug use by males, lifetime use of illicit drugs remains far more common among urban males than among females, a ratio of about 3 to 1.

DEFINITION OF TERMS

In 1964, the World Health Organization concluded that the term "addiction" was no longer a scientific term and recommended substituting the term "drug dependence." In spite of that, the word "addiction" continues to appear in both the medical and lay literature and is used to refer to (1) psychological dependence on a substance that produces drug-seeking behavior, (2) an inability to stop using the drug because of a physical dependence on the drug and tolerance to its effects, and (3) deterioration of physical and mental health as a result of continued substance abuse. In DSM-III-R, the term "psychoactive substance use disorder" involves two major areas:

A. Pattern of pathological use: inability to reduce or stop use; intoxication throughout the day; use of the offending substance nearly every day for at least a month; episodes of overdose or intoxication so that mental functioning is impaired.

B. Impairment in physical, social, or occupational functioning due to use of the substance (e.g., fights, loss of friends, absence from work, loss of job, or legal difficulties).

Tolerance is defined as the need for markedly increased amounts of the substance to achieve the desired effect that results from repeated use of a drug. Tolerance that develops to one drug as a result of exposure to another drug is called *cross-tolerance. Dispositional tolerance,* sometimes known as metabolic tolerance refers to the drug being metabolized at a faster rate than it is ingested; therefore, a constant intake does not produce the desired (euphoric) response. People vary widely in the amount of substance, in particular alcohol, they can tolerate independent of their experience with the substance. Some people cannot drink more than a small amount without distressing symptoms, while others seem to be able to drink large amounts with few bad effects. This capacity appears to be inborn, not one

developed from exposure. Difference in tolerance for alcohol also applies to certain racial groups. Many Asians develop uncomfortable symptoms after taking only small amounts of alcohol.

Dependence on a drug may be physical, psychological, or both. *Psychological dependence,* also referred to as habituation, is characterized by a continuous or intermittent craving for the substance in order to avoid a dysphoric state. *Physical dependence* is characterized by a need to take the substance to prevent the occurrence of a withdrawal or abstinence syndrome.

Drug abuse and drug misuse are defined differently. *Abuse* usually refers to the person's illicit use of a substance, whereas *misuse* usually refers to a physician's prescribing a drug in a medically unacceptable way.

Table 3
Diagnostic Criteria for Psychoactive Substance Dependence

A. At least three of the following:

(1) substance often taken in larger amounts or over a longer period than the person intended

(2) persistent desire or one or more unsuccessful efforts to cut down or control substance use

(3) a great deal of time spent in activities necessary to get the substance (e.g., theft), taking the substance (e.g., chain smoking), or recovering from its effects

(4) frequent intoxication or withdrawal symptoms when expected to fulfill major role obligations at work, school, or home (e.g., does not go to work because hung over, goes to school or work "high," intoxicated while taking care of his or her children), or when substance use is physically hazardous (e.g., drives when intoxicated)

(5) important social, occupational, or recreational activities given up or reduced because of substance use

(6) continued substance use despite knowledge of having a persistent or recurrent social, psychological, or physical problem that is caused or exacerbated by the use of the substance (e.g., keeps using heroin despite family arguments about it, cocaine-induced depression, or having an ulcer made worse by drinking)

(7) marked tolerance: need for markedly increased amounts of the substance (i.e., at least a 50% increase) in order to achieve intoxication or desired effect, or markedly diminished effect with continued use of the same amount

Note: The following items may not apply to cannabis, hallucinogens, or phencyclidine (PCP):

(8) characteristic withdrawal symptoms (see specific withdrawal syndromes under Psychoactive Substance–Induced Organic Mental Disorders)

(9) substance often taken to relieve or avoid withdrawal symptoms

B. Some symptoms of the disturbance have persisted for at least 1 month, or have occurred repeatedly over a longer period of time.

Table from DSM-III-R *Diagnostic and Statistical Manual of Mental Disorders,* ed 3, revised. (Current Classification of Mental Disorders, 1987.) Copyright American Psychiatric Association, Washington, D.C., 1987. Used with permission.

CLASSIFICATION

In DSM-III-R, psychoactive substance use disorders are divided into psychoactive substance dependence or psychoactive substance abuse disorders. The criteria for psychoactive substance dependence are presented in Table 3. Table 4 contains the criteria for psychoactive substance abuse, the residual category for those cases in which

Table 4
Diagnostic Criteria for Psychoactive Substance Abuse

A. A maladaptive pattern of psychoactive substance use indicated by at least one of the following:
   (1) continued use despite knowledge of having a persistent or recurrent social, occupational, psychological, or physical problem that is caused or exacerbated by use of the psychoactive substance
   (2) recurrent use in situations in which use is physically hazardous (e.g., driving while intoxicated)
B. Some symptoms of the disturbance have persisted for at least 1 month, or have occurred repeatedly over a longer period of time.
C. Never met the criteria for Psychoactive Substance Dependence for this substance.

Table from DSM-III-R *Diagnostic and Statistical Manual of Mental Disorders,* ed 3, revised. (Current Classification of Mental Disorders, 1987.) Copyright American Psychiatric Association, Washington, D.C., 1987. Used with permission.

Table 5
Diagnostic Criteria for Severity of Psychoactive Substance Dependence

Mild: Few, if any, symptoms in excess of those required to make the diagnosis, and the symptoms result in no more than mild impairment in occupational functioning or in usual social activities or relationships with others.

Moderate: Symptoms or functional impairment between "mild" and "severe."

Severe: Many symptoms in excess of those required to make the diagnosis, and the symptoms markedly interfere with occupational functioning or with usual social activities or relationships with others.[1]

In Partial Remission: During the past 6 months, some use of the substance and some symptoms of dependence.

In Full Remission: During the past 6 months, either no use of the substance, or use of the substance and no symptoms of dependence.

[1]Because of the availability of cigarettes and other nicotine-containing substances and the absence of a clinically significant nicotine intoxication syndrome, impairment in occupational or social functioning is not necessary for a rating of severe Nicotine Dependence.
Table from DSM-III-R *Diagnostic and Statistical Manual of Mental Disorders,* ed 3, revised. (Current Classification of Mental Disorders, 1987.) Copyright American Psychiatric Association, Washington, D.C., 1987. Used with permission.

Table 6
Diagnostic Criteria for Polysubstance Dependence

This category should be used when, for a period of at least 6 months, the person has repeatedly used at least three categories of psychoactive substances (not including nicotine and caffeine), but no single psychoactive substance has predominated. During this period the criteria have been met for dependence on psychoactive substances as a group, but not for any specific substance.

Table from DSM-III-R *Diagnostic and Statistical Manual of Mental Disorders,* ed 3, revised. (Current Classification of Mental Disorders, 1987.) Copyright American Psychiatric Association, Washington, D.C., 1987. Used with permission.

pathologic drug use exists but all the criteria for drug dependence are not met. According to DSM-III-R, the diagnosis of an abuse disorder is most likely in people who have just recently started using psychoactive substances and to involve substances less likely to be associated with marked withdrawal symptoms, such as cannabis or hallucinogens.

Dependence may vary from person to person or from time to time in one person. It can be classified as mild, moderate, or severe and in as being full or partial remission (Table 5). Some individuals use several categories of drugs and are clearly drug dependent. However, it is sometimes not possible to know if they were dependent on any one specific class of drugs. In DSM-III-R, this condition is called *polysubstance dependence* (Table 6).

DSM-III-R also describes two additional substance dependence–related diagnoses: psychoactive substance dependence not otherwise specified and psychoactive substance abuse not otherwise specified. These are residual categories for disorders in which there is dependence or abuse, respectively, on a psychoactive substance that cannot be classified in any of the previous categories (e.g., anticholinergics), or for use as an initial diagnosis in cases of dependence or abuse in which the specific substance is not yet known.

References

Grinspoon L: *Marihuana Reconsidered,* ed 2. Harvard University Press, Cambridge, MA, 1977.
Grinspoon L, Bakalar J B: *Cocaine: A Drug and Its Social Evolution.* Basic Books, New York, 1977.
Grinspoon L, Bakalar J B: *Psychedelic Drugs Reconsidered.* Basic Books, New York, 1979.
Institute of Medicine: *Marihuana and Health.* National Academy Press, Washington, DC, 1982.
Petersen L C, Stillman R C, editors: *Phencyclidine (PCP) Abuse: An Appraisal,* NIDA Research Monograph 21. US Government Printing Office, Washington, DC, 1978.
Shulgin A T, Nichols D E: Characterization of three new psychotomimetics, In *The Pharmacology of Hallucinogens,* R C Stilman, R E Willette, editors. New York, Pergamon Press, New York, 1978.
Strassman R: Adverse reactions to psychedelic drugs: A review of the literature. J Nervous Mental Dis *172:*577–595, 1984.
Szara S I, Ludford J P, editors: *Benzodiazepines: A Review of Research Results, 1980,* NIDA Research Monograph 33. US Government Printing Office, Washington, DC, 1980.
Wesson D R, Smith D E: *Barbiturates: Their Use, Misuse, and Abuse.* Human Sciences Press, New York, 1977.

13.2 ————

Alcoholism

DEFINITION

There is no specific diagnostic category known as alcoholism in the revised edition of DSM-III-R. Alcoholism is classified under the general term of psychoactive substance use disorder and the specific syndromes that relate to alcoholism (e.g., alcohol dependence and abuse, alcohol-induced organic mental disorders). However, the term "alcoholism" is in common use and can be defined as a disease marked by the chronic, excessive use of alcohol that produces psychological, interpersonal, and medical problems.

According to DSM-III-R, alcohol dependence is characterized by any one of these three major patterns of pathological alcohol use: (1) the need for daily use of large amounts of alcohol for adequate functioning, (2) regular heavy drinking limited to weekends, and (3) long periods of sobriety interspersed with binges of heavy alcohol intake lasting for weeks or months. These patterns encompass behaviors such as (1) the inability to cut down or stop drinking; (2) the repeated efforts to control or reduce excessive drinking by "going on the wagon" (periods of temporary abstinence) or restricting drinking to certain times of the day; (3) binges (remaining intoxicated throughout the day for at least 2 days); (4) the occasional consumption of a fifth of spirits (or its equivalent in wine or beer); (5) amnesic periods for events occurring while intoxicated (blackouts); (6) the continuation of drinking despite a serious physical disorder that the individual knows is exacerbated by alcohol use; and (7) drinking of nonbeverage alcohol (e.g., fuel, commercial products containing alcohol). In addition, alcoholics show impaired social or occupational functioning due to alcohol use, such as violence while intoxicated, absence from work, loss of job, legal difficulties (e.g., arrest for intoxicated behavior, traffic accidents while intoxicated), and arguments or difficulties with family or friends because of excessive alcohol use. According to DSM-III-R, some researchers have divided alcoholism into different patterns of drinking, which they call "species." One example of this is the species called "gamma alcoholism," which is felt to be common in the United States and is representative of the alcoholism seen in people who are active Alcoholics Anonymous (AA) members. Gamma alcoholism refers to "control" problems; such alcoholics are unable to stop drinking once they start. If the drinking ends as a result of ill health or lack of money, they are capable of abstaining for varying degrees of time. In another species of alcoholism, more common in Europe, the alcoholic must drink a certain amount each day but is unaware of a lack of control. The alcoholism may not be discovered until the person must stop drinking and develops withdrawal symptoms.

EPIDEMIOLOGY

Alcohol is the major psychoactive drug used worldwide. In the United States, there are an estimated 13 million people who are diagnosed as alcoholics. DSM-III-R reports that according to one community study, approximately 13 percent of adults had alcohol abuse or dependence at some point in their life. Following heart disease and cancer, alcoholism is the third largest health problem in the United States today. According to DSM-III-R, about 35 percent of American adults abstain, 55 percent drink fewer than three alcoholic drinks a week, and only 11 percent drink an average of 1 ounce or more of alcohol a day.

Drinking patterns vary by age and by sex. For both men and women, the prevalence of drinking is highest and abstention is lowest in the 21- to 34-year age range. Young white males drink more than any other group in this country. Among persons 65 years and older, abstainers exceed drinkers in both sexes, and only 7 percent of men and 2 percent of women in this age group are considered heavy drinkers (defined as one who drinks almost every day and becomes intoxicated several times a month). More men use alcohol (20 percent) than women (8 percent).

A small percentage of the population consumes most of the alcohol. Seventy percent of the drinking population consumes 20 percent of the total; 30 percent of the drinkers consumes 80 percent; and 10 percent of the drinkers, 50 percent. The lifelong expectancy rate for alcoholism among men is 3 to 5 percent; the rate for women is about 1 percent. Expectancy rates are about the same in Germany, Sweden, Denmark, and England and higher in Portugal, Spain, Italy, France, and Russia.

In the United States, blacks in urban ghettos appear to have a particularly high rate of alcohol-related problems; it is not known whether the risk among rural blacks is comparable. Consumption varies markedly in different geographic areas. In the United States, consumption is greatest in the Northeast and lowest in the South. American Indians and Eskimos have high rates of alcoholism.

Alcohol problems are correlated with a history of school difficulty. High school dropouts and individuals with a record of frequent truancy and delinquency appear to be at particularly high risk for alcoholism. No systematic studies have explored the relationship between occupation and alcoholism, but cirrhosis data suggest that persons in certain occupations are more likely to develop alcoholism. Waiters, bartenders, longshoremen, musicians, authors, and reporters have relatively high cirrhosis rates; accountants, mail carriers, and carpenters have relatively low rates. Alcoholism is associated with at least 50 percent of traffic fatalities, 50 percent of homicides, 25 percent of suicides, and 30,000 deaths from alcohol-related diseases. Alcoholics reduce their life expectancy by about 10 years; alcohol leads all drugs in disease-related deaths. Alcoholism affects about 52 million spouses and children.

Males and females seem to have different histories of alcoholism. The onset in males is usually in the late teens or 20s, has an insidious course, and is often not recognized as dependence until the 30s. In men, symptoms of alcohol dependence rarely occur for the first time after age 45. If first symptoms do occur at this age, DSM-III-R requires that mood disorder or organic mental disorder be ruled out. Studies that have looked at female alcoholics indicate that the course is more varied in women than in men. The onset in women is generally later, and spontaneous remission (which, if it occurs, will occur in men generally in the 50s and 60s) is felt to be less likely.

ETIOLOGY

There appears to be a strong genetic factor in alcoholism. Alcohol dependence tends to run in families. Children of alcoholics become alcoholic about four times more often than children of nonalcoholics, even when they are not raised by their biological parents. Sons of alcoholics are more vulnerable to alcoholism than are daughters. In a 30-year longitudinal Swedish study of adopted male children who eventually became alcoholics, about 25 percent had biological fathers who were also alcoholics. Another Swedish study found that monozygotic twins had about twice the concordance rate for alcoholism as dizygotic twins of the same sex. Interestingly, studies report a higher concordance rate for alcoholism among dizygotic twins than among nontwin siblings.

Childhood History

A childhood history of attention-deficit hyperactivity disorder or conduct disorder or both increases a child's risk of becoming alcoholic, particularly if there is alcoholism in the family. Personality disorders, in particular antisocial personality disorder, predispose to the development of substance use disorder.

Psychoanalytic

Alcohol is extremely effective in alleviating anxiety, and many persons use alcohol for this reason. Psychoanalytic theory posits that persons with harsh superegos who are self-punitive turn to alcohol as a way of diminishing their unconscious stress. A common psychoanalytic aphorism is that the superego is soluble in alcohol. Some alcoholics are fixated at the oral stage of development and relieve frustration by taking in substances by mouth. The alcoholic personality is described as shy, isolated, impatient, irritable, anxious, hypersensitive, and sexually repressed. Alcoholics may have an enhanced need for power but feel inadequate to achieve their goals. Alcohol gives them a sense of release and of power as well as feelings of achievement.

Cultural Factors

Some cultures are more restrained than others about alcohol consumption. For example, Jews, Asians, and conservative Protestants use alcohol less frequently than do liberal Protestants and Catholics. Social and cultural factors need to be taken into account when evaluating a person's risk for alcoholism.

Biological

Alcohol influences a variety of neurotransmitters (e.g., serotonin, dopamine, and GABA), and some products of metabolism bind to opiate receptors. The biological theory holds that cellular neuroadaptation occurs, which makes the body dependent on alcohol to maintain homeostasis.

Learning Theory

Learning theory suggests that alcohol results in a temporary reduction of fear and conflict, which strengthens the drive to drink. The release of anxiety arising from the first drinking experience is the source of reinforcement in alcoholism.

PHYSIOLOGICAL EFFECTS OF ALCOHOL

Ingested alcohol first gets into the bloodstream in very small amounts through the oral mucous membranes and lungs. It is then absorbed from the alimentary tract and carried by the blood to the brain and other organs. The speed with which alcohol enters the bloodstream depends on many factors: the amount and type of food in the stomach, the type of beverage consumed and its alcohol concentration, the circumstances under which it is being drunk, and the drinker's constitutional state.

Absorption

Foods in the stomach, especially mixed meals, slow alcohol absorption. Drinking water with alcohol increases absorption: the same is true for carbonated beverages (carbon dioxide). Champagnes and highballs are well known for causing rapid and heightened effects.

The body has certain protective devices against being inundated by alcohol. For example, unlike other foodstuffs, alcohol can be absorbed into the blood stream directly from the stomach. If the concentration of alcohol becomes too high in the stomach, mucus is then secreted, and the pyloric valve closes. This action slows absorption and prevents the alcohol from passing into the small intestine, where no significant restraints to absorption exist. Thus, a large amount of alcohol can remain unabsorbed for hours. Further, the pylorospasm often results in nausea and vomiting.

Once alcohol is absorbed into the bloodstream, it is distributed to all the tissues of the body. Since it is uniformly dissolved in the water of the body, those tissues containing a high proportion of water receive a high concentration of alcohol. The intoxicating effects are greater when the blood alcohol rises rapidly than when it is being destroyed or oxidized and falling. For this reason, the rate of absorption has a direct bearing on the intoxicating responses.

Metabolism

Immediately after absorption, destruction and elimination begin. The kidneys and lungs excrete about one tenth of the total alcohol ingested unchanged; the rest undergoes oxidation. The rate of oxidation of alcohol is fairly constant and is independent of the body's energy requirements. The average person oxidizes three fourths of an ounce of 40 percent alcohol (80 proof) an hour. If the person sips alcohol at this rate, he or she does not accumulate alcohol in the body or become intoxicated.

Alcohol's oxidation provides heat and work energy. However, because excessive consumers receive so many calories from their alcohol intake, they tend to neglect other food sources and may ignore nutritional needs. Vitamin-deficiency diseases and other nutritional disorders (e.g., pellegra, beriberi) may result. Moreover, alcohol stimulates the release of ACTH from the pituitary, thus raising blood cortisol levels.

Effects on the Brain

Alcohol is a central nervous system (CNS) depressant, similar to other anesthetics. At a level of 0.05 percent alcohol in the blood, thought, judgment, and restraint are loosened and sometimes disrupted. At a concentration of 0.10 percent, voluntary motor actions usually become perceptibly clumsy. At 0.20 percent, the function of the entire motor area of the brain is measurably depressed; the parts of the brain that control emotional behavior may be affected. At 0.30 percent, a person is commonly confused or may become stuporous. At 0.40 to 0.50 percent, a person is in a coma. At higher levels, the primitive centers of the brain that control breathing and heart rate are affected, and death ensues. Death is usually secondary to direct respiratory depression or by aspiration of vomitus. Alcohol decreases REM sleep and causes insomnia. In most states, legal intoxication ranges from 0.10 to 0.15 percent blood alcohol level.

Blackouts. Alcohol produces amnesia (blackouts). These periods of amnesia can be particularly distressing because people may fear that they have unknowingly harmed someone or behaved imprudently while intoxicated. The amnesia is anterograde. During a blackout, people have relatively intact remote and immediate memory. However, people experience a specific short-term memory deficit in which they are unable to recall events that happened in the previous five or ten minutes. Because their other intellectual faculties are well-preserved, they can perform complicated tasks and appear normal to the casual observer. Present evidence suggests that alcoholic blackouts represent an impaired consolidation of new information.

Other Physiological Effects

Alcohol affects the liver, the main site for alcohol catabolism. A reversible fatty infiltration of the liver is thought to occur with heavy consumption of alcohol. What relation, if any, this infiltration plays in the production of liver cirrhosis is not yet known. Acute intoxication may be associated with hypoglycemia that, when unrecognized, may be responsible for some of the sudden deaths of intoxicated persons.

Chronic heavy drinking is associated with gastritis, achlorhydria, and gastric ulcers. Occasionally, maladies of the small intestine, pancreatitis, and pancreatic insufficiency are associated with alcoholism. Heavy alcohol intake may interfere with the normal processes of food digestion and absorption. As a result, the food that is consumed is inadequately digested. Alcohol abuse also appears to inhibit the capacity of the intestine to absorb various nutrients, including vitamins and amino acids. Muscle weakness is a side effect of alcoholism. Alcohol has been shown to affect the hearts of even nonalcoholic persons, increasing the resting cardiac output, heart rate, and myocardial oxygen consumption. Chronic excessive use can cause cardiomyopathy.

Drug Interactions

The interaction between alcohol and other drugs can be dangerous, even fatal. Certain drugs, such as alcohol and phenobarbital, are metabolized by the liver; the prolonged use of these drugs may lead to an acceleration of their metabolism. When the alcoholic person is sober, this accelerated metabolism makes him unusually tolerant to many other drugs, such as sedatives and tranquilizers, but when the alcoholic is intoxicated, these other drugs compete with the alcohol for the same detoxification mechanism, and potentially toxic blood levels can accumulate.

The effects of alcohol and other CNS depressants are usually synergistic. Sedatives and hypnotics as well as drugs that relieve pain, motion sickness, head cold, and allergy symptoms, must be used with caution by alcoholic persons. Narcotics depress the sensory areas of the cerebral cortex, resulting in relief of pain, sedation, apathy, drowsiness, and sleep. High doses can result in respiratory failure and death. Increasing doses of sedative-hypnotic drugs, such as chloral hydrate and benzodiazepines, especially when combined with alcohol, produce a range of effects from sedation to motor and intellectual impairment, progressing to stupor, coma, and death. Since tranquilizers and other psychotropics can potentiate the effects of alcohol, patients should be instructed about the dangers of combining CNS depressants and alcohol, particularly when driving or operating machinery.

ALCOHOL-INDUCED ORGANIC MENTAL DISORDERS

Alcohol Intoxication

Intoxication is characterized by maladaptive behavior (e.g., impaired judgment, belligerence) following the recent ingestion of alcohol. Signs of intoxication include ataxia, nystagmus, slurred speech, flushing of the face, irritability, and impaired attention. Some persons become talkative and gregarious; others become withdrawn and sullen. In some there is a lability of mood with intermittent episodes of laughing and crying. At equivalent blood alcohol levels the signs of intoxication are more marked when the level is increasing than when it is decreasing. In addition, short-term tolerance to alcohol occurs so that a person may seem less intoxicated after many hours of drinking than after only a few hours. If the alcohol ingested was less than would cause most people to become intoxicated, DSM-III-R states that the diagnosis of alcohol idiosyncratic intoxication may be the more accurate one.

Medical complications of intoxication include those that result from falls, such as subdural hematomas and fractures. A telltale sign of chronic bouts of intoxication are facial hematomas, particularly about the eyes, a result of falls while drunk. In cold climates, hypothermia and death may occur because the intoxicated person is exposed to the elements. Alcohol intoxication may also possibly predispose to infections, secondary to a suppression of the

Table 1
Diagnostic Criteria for Alcohol Intoxication

A. Recent ingestion of alcohol (with no evidence suggesting that the amount was insufficient to cause intoxication in most people).

B. Maladaptive behavior changes (e.g., disinhibition of sexual or aggressive impulses, mood lability, impaired judgment, impaired social or occupational functioning)

C. At least one of the following signs:
   (1) slurred speech
   (2) incoordination
   (3) unsteady gait
   (4) nystagmus
   (5) flushed face

D. Not due to any physical or other mental disorder.

Table from DSM-III-R *Diagnostic and Statistical Manual of Mental Disorders,* ed 3, revised. (Current Classification of Mental Disorders, 1987.) Copyright American Psychiatric Association, Washington, D.C., 1987. Used with permission.

immune system. The DSM-III-R criteria for alcohol intoxication are listed in Table 1.

Alcohol Idiosyncratic Intoxication

This condition, also known as "pathological intoxication," is characterized by the sudden onset of marked behavioral changes after the consumption of a small amount of alcohol. The person is confused, disoriented, and may experience illusions, transitory delusions, and visual hallucinations. There is greatly increased psychomotor activity. The person may display impulsive aggressive behavior and be dangerous to others or depression, with suicidal ideas and attempts. The disorder, which usually lasts for a few hours, terminates in a prolonged period of sleep; the person is unable to recall the episode. The cause of the condition is unknown but is more common in persons with high levels of anxiety; the alcohol may cause sufficient disorganization and loss of control to release aggressive impulses. It has also been suggested that brain damage, particularly encephalitic or traumatic, predisposes people to intolerance for alcohol, leading to abnormal behavior after taking a small amount. Other predisposing factors include advancing age, taking sedative-hypnotic drugs, or feeling fatigued. The behavior tends to be atypical of the person when not under the influence; for example, a quiet, shy person after one weak drink becomes belligerent and aggressive.

Treatment involves protecting the patient from harming himself and others. Physical restraint may be necessary, but is difficult because of the abrupt onset of the condition. Once the patient has been restrained, an injection of a neuroleptic such as haloperidol (Haldol) is useful in controlling assaultiveness.

The condition must be differentiated from other causes of abrupt behavior change, such as temporal lobe seizures and interictal phenomena. In fact, several persons with this disorder have been reported to show temporal lobe spiking on EEG after small amounts of alcohol. The DSM-III-R characteristics of alcohol idiosyncratic intoxication are listed in Table 2.

Table 2
Diagnostic Criteria for Alcohol Idiosyncratic Intoxication

A. Maladaptive behavioral changes (e.g., aggressive or assaultive behavior, occurring within minutes of ingesting an amount of alcohol insufficient to induce intoxication in most people.)

B. The behavior is atypical of the person when not drinking.

C. Not due to any physical or other mental disorder.

Table from DSM-III-R *Diagnostic and Statistical Manual of Mental Disorders,* ed 3, revised. (Current Classification of Mental Disorders, 1987.) Copyright American Psychiatric Association, Washington, D.C., 1987. Used with permission.

Uncomplicated Alcohol Withdrawal and Alcohol Withdrawal Delirium

Alcohol withdrawal is a syndrome that follows the cessation of or reduction in prolonged or heavy drinking. Within hours, a variety of signs and symptoms develop, including tremors, hyperreflexia, tachycardia, hypertension, general malaise, and nausea or vomiting. Major motor seizures may occur, particularly in people with a preexisting history of seizure disorder. Patients may have transient, poorly formed hallucinations, illusions or vivid nightmares, and sleep is usually disturbed (Table 3). Conditions that may predispose to or aggravate the syndrome include fatigue, malnutrition, physical illness, and depression. Treatment is symptomatic, with bed rest and hydration. A cross-dependent drug, such as a benzodiazepine, can be of value in controlling the overactivity of the sympathetic nervous system and is used until symptoms subside. Other drugs used to treat alcohol withdrawal include clonidine, propranolol, and carbamazepine, but they are not generally as effective as benzodiazepines.

Table 3
Diagnostic Criteria for Uncomplicated Alcohol Withdrawal

A. Cessation of prolonged (several days or longer) heavy ingestion of alcohol or reduction in the amount of alcohol ingested, followed within several hours by coarse tremor of hands, tongue, or eyelids, and at least one of the following:

   (1) nausea or vomiting
   (2) malaise or weakness
   (3) autonomic hyperactivity (e.g., tachycardia, sweating, elevated blood pressure)
   (4) anxiety
   (5) depressed mood or irritability
   (6) transient hallucinations or illusions
   (7) headache
   (8) insomnia

B. Not due to any physical or other mental disorder, such as Alcohol Withdrawal Delirium

Table from DSM-III-R *Diagnostic and Statistical Manual of Mental Disorders,* ed 3, revised. (Current Classification of Mental Disorders, 1987.) Copyright American Psychiatric Association, Washington, D.C., 1987. Used with permission.

Patients with uncomplicated alcohol withdrawal should be carefully monitored to prevent progression to alcohol withdrawal delirium, the most severe form of the withdrawal syndrome, also known as delirium tremens (DTs). The essential feature of this syndrome is delirium that occurs within 1 week after the person stops drinking actively or reduces his intake. Additional features include (1) autonomic hyperactivity, such as tachycardia, sweating, and elevated blood pressure; (2) a severe disturbance in sensorium manifested by disorientation and clouding of consciousness; (3) perceptual distortions, which are most frequently visual or tactile hallucinations; and (4) fluctuating levels of psychomotor activity ranging from hyperexcitability to lethargy. Delusions and agitated behavior are commonly present. Fever is common. Grand mal seizures are a common occurrence in withdrawal, although they usually precede the onset of the delirium (Table 4).

The delirious patient is a danger to self and to others because of the unpredictability of behavior. The patient may be assaultive or suicidal or may be acting on the hallucinations or delusional thoughts as if they were genuine dangers. Untreated, DTs has a mortality rate of 20 percent, usually as a result of intercurrent medical illness (e.g., pneumonia, renal disease, hepatic insufficiency, or heart failure).

Approximately 5 percent of alcoholics who are hospitalized develop DTs. Since the syndrome most commonly develops on the third hospital day, a patient admitted for an unrelated condition may unexpectedly develop an episode of delirium, which is the first sign of previously undiagnosed alcoholism. DTs usually begins in the patient's 30s or 40s after 5 to 15 years of heavy drinking, typically of the binge type. Physical illness predisposes to this syndrome; a person in good physical health rarely develops DTs during alcohol withdrawal.

Treatment. The best way to deal with DTs is to prevent it. Patients withdrawing from alcohol who exhibit any withdrawal phenomena should receive a benzodiazepine, such as 25 milligrams to 50 mg of chlordiazepoxide hydrochloride (Librium) every 2 to 4 hours, until they seem to be out of danger. Once the delirium appears, however, doses of 50 mg to 100 mg of chlordiazepoxide should be given every 4 hours orally (or intramuscularly if the patient cannot retain oral medication). A high-calorie, high-carbohydrate diet supplemented by multivitamins is important. Patients with DTs should never be physically restrained as they may fight the restraints to exhaustion. When patients are disorderly and uncontrollable, a seclusion room can be used. Dehydration can be corrected with fluids by mouth or intravenously. Anorexia, vomiting, and diarrhea often occur during withdrawal. Diaphoresis and fever may also contribute to volume depletion. Phenothiazines should be avoided because they tend to reduce seizure thresholds and introduce the possibility of hepatitis superimposed upon pre-existing impaired hepatic functioning.

The need for warm, supportive psychotherapy in the treatment of DTs must be emphasized. Patients are often bewildered, frightened, and anxious because of their tumultuous symptoms. Skillful verbal support is imperative.

The emergence of focal neurological symptoms, lateralizing seizures, increased intracranial pressure, skull fracture, or other indications of central nervous system pathology calls for further neurological investigation and treatment. It is now generally believed that anticonvulsant medication is not useful in preventing or treating alcohol withdrawal convulsions; the use of chlordiazepoxide or diazepam is generally effective.

Alcohol Hallucinosis

The essential feature of alcohol hallucinosis is an organic hallucinosis, either visual or auditory, usually beginning within 48 hours after cessation of drinking and persisting after a person has recovered from the symptoms of alcohol withdrawal. The hallucinations are not part of alcohol withdrawal delirium. For most people they are unpleasant, perhaps taking the form of voices or unformed sounds such as buzzing. The disorder can occur at any age; however the person must have been drinking to excess long enough to become alcohol dependent (Table 5). In some cases, the hallucinations last for several weeks; in other cases, for several months; and in still other cases, they seem to be permanent. The condition is considered rare.

The typical case of alcohol hallucinosis differs from schizophrenia by its temporal relation to alcohol withdrawal, its short-lived course, and the absence of a history of schizophrenia. The disorder is four times as common in men as in women. Alcohol hallucinosis is usually described as a condition manifested primarily by auditory hallucinations, sometimes accompanied by delusions, in the absence of symptoms of an affective disorder or organic mental

Table 4
Diagnostic Criteria for Alcohol Withdrawal Delirium

A. Delirium developing after cessation of heavy alcohol ingestion or a reduction in the amount of alcohol ingested (usually within 1 week).

B. Marked autonomic hyperactivity (e.g., tachycardia, sweating).

C. Not due to any physical or other mental disorder.

Table from DSM-III-R *Diagnostic and Statistical Manual of Mental Disorders,* ed 3, revised. (Current Classification of Mental Disorders, 1987.) Copyright American Psychiatric Association, Washington, D.C., 1987. Used with permission.

Table 5
Diagnostic Criteria for Alcohol Hallucinosis

A. Organic Hallucinosis with vivid and persistent hallucinations (auditory or visual) developing shortly (usually within 48 hours) after cessation of or reduction in heavy ingestion of alcohol in a person who apparently has Alcohol Dependence.

B. No Delirium as in Alcohol Withdrawal Delirium.

C. Not due to any physical or other mental disorder.

Table from DSM-III-R *Diagnostic and Statistical Manual of Mental Disorders,* ed 3, revised. (Current Classification of Mental Disorders, 1987.) Copyright American Psychiatric Association, Washington, D.C., 1987. Used with permission.

disorder. Alcoholic hallucinosis is differentiated from DTs by the absence of a clear sensorium in delirium tremens.

The treatment for alcohol hallucinosis is much like that for DTs—benzodiazepines, adequate nutrition, and fluids if necessary. When that regimen fails, and in chronic cases, antipsychotics may be used.

Alcohol Amnestic Disorder (Korsakoff's Syndrome) and Alcoholic Encephalopathy (Wernicke's Syndrome)

The essential feature of alcohol amnestic disorder is a disturbance in short-term, but not immediate, memory due to the prolonged heavy use of alcohol. Other complications of alcoholism, such as cerebellar signs, peripheral neuropathy, and cirrhosis, may be present. Since the disorder usually occurs in persons who have been drinking heavily for many years, it rarely occurs before the age of 35 years (Table 6).

The irreversible memory deficit known as Korsakoff's syndrome or alcohol amnestic disorder often follows an acute episode of Wernicke's syndrome, also called alcoholic encephalopathy, a neurological disease manifested by ataxia, ophthalmoplegia (particularly involving the sixth cranial nerve), nystagmus, and confusion. Alcoholic encephalopathy may clear spontaneously in a few days or weeks. It can also progress into the alcohol amnestic disorder, in which the patient has an irreversible short-term memory impairment in the presence of a clear sensorium. The early acute stage of Wernicke's syndrome responds rapidly to large doses of parenteral thiamine, which is believed to be effective in preventing the progression into the alcohol amnestic disorder. However, once the disorder is established, the course is chronic and impairment is always severe. Lifelong custodial care is often required.

Wernicke's encephalopathy and alcohol amnestic disorder—the two are sometimes combined in the term "Wernicke-Korsakoff's syndrome"—are believed to be caused by thiamine deficiency. Therefore, malnutrition can be considered a predisposing factor. Heavy alcohol ingestion produces a malabsorption syndrome. The prevalence is unknown, but the condition is apparently rare and may have become more rare in recent years because of the almost routine administration of thiamine during detoxification. Although the syndrome is usually irreversible, various degrees of recovery have been reported with a daily regimen of 50 mg to 100 mg of thiamine hydrochloride.

Dementia Associated with Alcoholism

The essential feature of dementia associated with alcoholism is a dementia that persists at least 3 weeks after cessation of prolonged alcohol use and for which all other causes of dementia have been ruled out. Other complications of alcoholism such as cerebellar signs, peripheral neuropathy, and cirrhosis may be present. Since the disorder occurs in persons who have been drinking heavily for many years, the disorder rarely occurs before the age of 35 years (Table 7).

By definition, there is always some impairment in social or occupational functioning. In mild cases cognitive deficits may be demonstrable only by neuropsychological testing.

Table 6
Diagnostic Criteria for Alcohol Amnestic Disorder

A. Amnestic Syndrome following prolonged, heavy ingestion of alcohol.

B. Not due to any physical or other mental disorder.

Table from DSM-III-R *Diagnostic and Statistical Manual of Mental Disorders,* ed 3, revised. (Current Classification of Mental Disorders, 1987.) Copyright American Psychiatric Association, Washington, D.C., 1987. Used with permission.

Table 7
Diagnostic Criteria for Dementia Associated with alcoholism

A. Dementia following prolonged, heavy ingestion of alcohol and persisting at least 3 weeks after cessation of alcohol ingestion

B. Exclusion, by history, physical examination, and laboratory tests, of all causes of Dementia other than prolonged heavy use of alcohol

Table from DSM-III-R *Diagnostic and Statistical Manual of Mental Disorders,* ed 3, revised. (Current Classification of Mental Disorders, 1987.) Copyright American Psychiatric Association, Washington, D.C., 1987. Used with permission.

More rarely, when impairment is severe, the patient becomes totally oblivious to his surroundings and requires constant care. It is not yet known whether dementia associated with alcoholism is the primary effect of alcohol or its metabolites on the brain or an indirect consequence of the malnutrition, frequent head injury, and liver disease that occur with chronic alcoholism.

FETAL ALCOHOL SYNDROME

Studies of infants with neonatal abnormalities revealed that many of the mothers were alcoholics. Mental retardation, growth deficiencies, craniofacial and midline defects, limb malformation, cardiac defects, and delayed motor development are some of the disabling consequences of fetal alcohol syndrome.

The risk of an alcoholic woman's having a defective child is perhaps as high as 35 percent. Although the precise mechanism of the damage to the fetus is unknown, the damage seems to be the result of exposure in utero to ethanol or its metabolites. Alcohol may also cause hormone imbalances that increase the risk of abnormalities.

TREATMENT OF ALCOHOLISM

A major issue in the treatment of alcoholism is the question of abstinence: Must the person never again have alcohol or can the drinking be controlled? In general, controlled drinking (e.g., one drink per weekend) carries a high risk of relapse. Groups, such as Alcoholics Anonymous, as well as most experts are proponents of the abstinence approach and believe that there is no such condition as a "recovered alcoholic."

Most alcoholic patients come to treatment as a result of

pressure from a spouse or employer or fear that continued drinking will have a fatal outcome. Those patients who are persuaded, encouraged or even coerced into treatment by persons who are meaningful to them (e.g., spouse or children) are more apt to remain in treatment and have a better prognosis than those who are not so pressured. The best prognosis is for those persons who come to a psychiatrist voluntarily because they conclude that they are alcoholic and need help; but such persons are extremely rare.

Psychotherapy

Psychotherapy is useful when it focuses on the reasons for the alcoholic's desire to be intoxicated, such as higher tolerance for frustration, reduction of anxiety, and so on. The drinking itself—past, present, and future consequences—must be given firm emphasis. Involving an interested and cooperative spouse in conjoint therapy is often beneficial to the psychotherapeutic process.

Medication

Two groups of drugs are useful in the treatment of alcoholism: the deterrent drug (disulfiram) and psychotropic drugs

Disulfiram. Disulfiram (Antabuse) competitively inhibits the enzyme aldehyde dehydrogenase, so that even a single drink usually causes a toxic reaction due to acetaldehyde accumulation in the blood. Administration of the drug should not begin until 24 hours have elapsed since the patient's last drink. The patient must be in good health, highly motivated, and cooperative. The physician must warn the patient about the consequences of ingesting alcohol while on the drug or for as long as 2 weeks thereafter. Those who drink while taking the 250 mg daily dose of disulfiram experience flushing and feelings of heat in the face, sclera, upper limbs, and chest. They may become pale, hypotensive, nauseated, and experience serious malaise. There may also be dizziness, blurred vision, palpitations, air hunger, and numbness of the extremities. The most serious potential consequence is severe hypotension. Patients may also have a response to alcohol ingested in such substances as sauces or vinegars, or even to inhaled alcohol vapors from aftershave lotions. The syndrome, once elicited, typically lasts some 30 to 60 minutes, but can persist longer. With doses above 250 mg, toxic psychoses can occur, with memory impairment and confusion. The drug can also exacerbate psychotic symptoms in schizophrenic patients.

Psychotropics. Antianxiety agents and antidepressants are useful during various stages of treatment. In the initial stage of abstinence, anxiety, restlessness, and insomnia may be prominent features; they can be controlled by one of the antianxiety agents, such as diazepam or chlordiazepoxide, which may have to be prescribed for weeks or even months. Under controlled conditions, the risk of the alcoholic becoming addicted to an antianxiety agent is remote. Antidepressants are useful for those patients who are clinically depressed while abstinent. Lithium has also been used with some success. An experimental drug known as Ro 15-451B blocks the effects of alcohol and is currently being tested at the National Institutes of Mental Health (NIMH.) Rats given the drug do not become intoxicated or, if previously intoxicated, become sober within 3 minutes of ingesting the compound.

Behavior Therapy

Behavior therapy teaches the alcoholic other ways to reduce anxiety. Relaxation training, assertiveness training, self-control skills, and new strategies to master the environment are emphasized.

A number of operant conditioning programs have been described which condition alcoholics to modify their drinking behavior or stop. The reinforcers have included monetary rewards, an opportunity to live in an enriched inpatient environment, and access to pleasurable social interactions. Trials of aversive conditioning—apomorphine and emetine to induce vomiting, electrical stimulation to produce pain—were consistently successful only in very highly motivated persons and are no longer widely used in the treatment of alcoholism.

Alcoholics Anonymous (A.A.)

A.A. is a voluntary, supportive fellowship of hundreds of thousands of alcoholics that was founded in 1935 by two alcoholics, a stockbroker and a surgeon. Physicians should refer an alcoholic to A.A. as part of a multiple treatment approach. Frequently, patients who object when A.A. is initially suggested later derive much benefit from the organization and become enthusiastic participants. Its members make a public admission of their alcoholism, and abstinence is the rule.

Al-Anon. This organization for the spouses of alcoholics is structured along the same lines as Alcoholics Anonymous. The aims of Al-Anon are through group support to assist the efforts of the spouses to regain self-esteem, to refrain from feeling responsible for the spouse's drinking, and to develop a rewarding life for themselves and their families. Alateen is directed to children of alcoholics, so that they may better understand their parents' alcoholism.

Halfway Houses

The discharge of an alcoholic patient from the hospital often poses serious placement problems. Home or other familiar environments may be counterproductive, unsupportive, or too unstructured. The halfway house is an important treatment resource which provides emotional support, counseling and progressive entry into society.

References

Donovan J M: An etiological model of alcoholism. Am J Psychiatry *143*:1, 1986

Fawcett J, Clark D C, Aagesen C A, Pisani V D, Tilkin J M, Sellers D, McGuire M, Gibbons R D: A double-blind, placebo-controlled trial of lithium carbonate therapy for alcoholism. Arch Gen Psych *44*:248, 1986.

Fuller R K, Branchey L, Brightwell D R: Disulfuram treatment of alcoholism: A Veterans Administration cooperative study. JAMA, *256*:1449, 1986.

Galanter M, editor: *Recent Developments in Alcoholism*, vol 3. Plenum Press, New York, 1985.

Goodwin D W: *Alcoholism: The Facts.* Oxford, New York, 1981.

Goodwin D W: Genetic component of alcoholism. Annual Rev Med *32*:93, 1981.

Goodwin D W: Drug therapy of alcoholism. In *Psychopharmacology*, D G Grahame-Smith, H Hippius, G Winokur, editors, vol 1, p 295. Excerpta Medica, Amsterdam, 1982.

Goodwin D W: Alcoholism and genetics. Arch Gen Psychiatry *42*:171, 1985.

Jellinek E M: *The Disease Concept of Alcoholism*. College and University Press, New Haven, 1960.

Ritchie M J: The aliphatic alcohols. In *The Pharmacological Basis of Therapeutics*, A G Gilman, L S Goodman, A Gilman, editors, ed 7, p 372. Macmillan, New York, 1985.

Ryback R S, Eckardt M J, Felsher B: Biochemical and hematological correlates of alcoholism and liver disease. JAMA *248*:2261, 1982.

Westermeyer J: *A Clinical Guide to Alcohol and Drug Problems*. Praeger, New York, 1986.

13.3 ————

Sedative-Hypnotics, and Anxiolytic Substance Use Disorder

A sedative is a drug that reduces activity and induces calmness; a hypnotic induces drowsiness and sleep. These drugs are also known as minor tranquilizers, antianxiety agents, or anxiolytic agents. All sedatives can induce sleep, and all hypnotics can cause sedation if doses are increased or decreased, respectively. Sedative-hypnotics and anxiolytics are also used to raise the convulsive threshold, to increase muscle relaxation, and to induce general anesthesia (although they possess no analgesic qualities themselves). All sedative-hypnotics and anxiolytics are cross-tolerant with one another and with alcohol. All are capable of producing both physical and psychological dependence as well as typical withdrawal syndromes. Addicted persons can die from withdrawal. Overdose can be fatal.

BARBITURATES

The first barbiturate, barbital (Veronal), was introduced in 1903, followed by another long-acting (12 to 24 hours) drug, phenobarbital. Still later, the intermediate-range (6 to 12 hours) barbiturates, such as amobarbital (Amytal), and the short-acting (3 to 6 hours), frequently abused pentobarbital (Nembutal) and secobarbital (Seconal) were introduced. Barbiturates are used mainly as sedatives, hypnotics, tranquilizers, anticonvulsants, and to induce anesthetia. Because they are legitimately manufactured in large quantities and are readily available in numerous forms, barbiturates are the target of illicit activity. The black market meets its needs by diverting shipments from manufacturers and by robbing drug warehouses; the drugs are then often cut with sugar and other substances. The three major barbiturates common on the black market are secobarbital (reds, red devils, seggys, downers), pentobarbital (yellow jackets, yellows, nembies), and a combination of secobarbital and amobarbital (reds and blues, rainbows, double-trouble, tooies). Pentobarbital, secobarbital, and amobarbital are now under the same federal legal controls as morphine. Both licit and illicit use of barbiturates seems to be declining.

Patterns of Abuse

Chronic Intoxication. Barbiturate abuse and dependence are now recognized as major health problems. Abusers fall into one of three major patterns. The first pattern, chronic intoxication, occurs mainly in middle-aged, middle-class people who obtain the drug from the family physician as a prescription for insomnia or anxiety. Now that the number of refills is limited by law, these abusers may visit many physicians, obtaining a prescription from each. Their drug dependence may go unnoticed for months or even years, or until their work begins to suffer or they show physical signs, such as slurred speech.

Episodic Intoxication. Users in this category are generally teens or young adults who take barbiturates to produce a "high," a sense of euphoria or well-being. Personality, set (expectations), and setting determine whether the effect is sedation or euphoria.

Intravenous Barbiturate Use. The third, most dangerous pattern is intravenous barbiturate use. Users are mainly young adults intimately involved in the illegal-drug subculture. Their drug experience typically has been extensive, ranging from pill popping to intravenous heroin and methamphetamine. They often use barbiturates because the habit is less expensive to maintain than a heroin habit. The "rush" is described as a pleasant, warm, drowsy feeling. Like amphetamine abusers ("speed freaks") these barbiturate abusers tend to be irresponsible, violent, and disruptive. The physical dangers of injection include acquired immune deficiency syndrome (AIDS; through the sharing of needles), cellulitis, vascular complications from accidental injection into an artery, infections, and allergic reactions to contaminants. Barbiturates are also used by heroin addicts to boost the effects of weak heroin; by alcoholics to enhance the intoxication or relieve the symptoms of alcohol withdrawal; and by speed freaks, as a sedative to help avoid paranoia and agitation.

Adverse Effects

Mild barbiturate intoxication, acute or chronic, resembles alcohol intoxication. Symptoms include sluggishness, incoordination, difficulty in thinking, poor memory, slowness of speech and comprehension, faulty judgment, disinhibition of sexual or aggressive impulses, narrowed range of attention, emotional lability, and exaggeration of basic personality traits (Table 1). The sluggishness usually wears off after a few hours, but judgment may remain impaired, mood distorted, and motor skills impaired for as long as 10 to 22 hours. Other symptoms are hostility, quarrelsomeness, moroseness, and, occasionally, paranoid ideation and suicidal tendencies. Neurological effects include nystagmus, diplopia, strabismus, ataxic gait, positive Romberg's sign, hypotonia, dysmetria, and decreased superficial reflexes. The diagnosis of barbiturate intoxication, based on these signs and symptoms, may be confirmed by a number of laboratory tests.

All patterns of use present dangers to health. Acute intoxication can produce death from suicide, accident, or unintentional overdose. Barbiturates in home medicine cabinets are second only to aspirin as a cause of fatal drug

Table 1
Diagnostic Criteria for Sedative, Hypnotic, or Anxiolytic Intoxication

A. Recent use of a sedative, hypnotic, or anxiolytic.

B. Maladaptive behavioral changes (e.g., disinhibition of sexual or aggressive impulses, mood lability, impaired judgment, impaired social or occupational functioning).

C. At least one of the following signs:
   (1) slurred speech
   (2) incoordination
   (3) unsteady gait
   (4) impairment in attention or memory

D. Not due to any physical or other mental disorder.

Note: When the differential diagnosis must be made without a clear-cut history or toxicologic analysis of body fluids, it may be qualified as "Provisional."

Table from DSM-III-R *Diagnostic and Statistical Manual of Mental Disorders,* ed 3, revised. (Current Classification of Mental Disorders, 1987.) Copyright American Psychiatric Association, Washington, D.C., 1987. Used with permission.

overdose in children. Barbiturates are also second to alcohol as a cause of lethal accidents, and they are the drugs most commonly taken with suicidal intent. The effects of alcohol and barbiturates are additive, and the combination is especially dangerous. Barbiturate-induced death follows a sequence of deep coma, respiratory arrest, and cardiovascular failure. The lethal dose varies with the route of administration, excitability of the central nervous system, and acquired tolerance. For the most commonly abused barbiturates the ratio of lethal to effective dose can be as low as 3 to 1 or as high as 50 to 1.

Treatment

Barbiturate overdose patients who are awake should be kept from slipping into unconsciousness and, if necessary, vomiting should be induced and activated charcoal administered, to delay gastric absorption. Airways should be kept clear and vital signs watched until there is no danger of coma. If the patient is comatose, a life-threatening emergency exists. It is then necessary to clear the airway, establish an intravenous fluid system, monitor vital signs, insert an endotracheal tube to maintain an airway, and perform gastric lavage with fluid containing activated charcoal. Nursing care in an intensive care unit should follow.

Tolerance and Withdrawal

Like many other drugs, barbiturates produce pharmacodynamic or CNS tolerance. They also produce metabolic tolerance and reduce the effectiveness of a number of other drugs, especially anticoagulants and tricyclic antidepressants. There is cross-tolerance with alcohol.

A withdrawal reaction occurs when the drug has become necessary to maintain homeostasis. This usually requires at least several weeks or more at doses well above the recommended therapeutic level. The barbiturate withdrawal reaction ranges from mild symptoms, such as anxiety, weak-

Table 2
Diagnostic Criteria for Uncomplicated Sedative, Hypnotic, or Anxiolytic Withdrawal

A. Cessation of prolonged (several weeks or more) moderate or heavy use of a sedative, hypnotic, or anxiolytic, or reduction in the amount of substance used, followed by at least three of the following:
   (1) nausea or vomiting
   (2) malaise or weakness
   (3) autonomic hyperactivity, e.g., tachycardia, sweating
   (4) anxiety or irritability
   (5) orthostatic hypotension
   (6) coarse tremor of hands, tongue, and eyelids
   (7) marked insomnia
   (8) grand mal seizures

B. Not due to any physical or other mental disorder, such as Sedative, Hypnotic, or Anxiolytic Withdrawal Delirium.

Note: When the differential diagnosis must be made without a clear-cut history or toxicologic analysis of body fluids, it may be qualified as "Provisional."

Table from DSM-III-R *Diagnostic and Statistical Manual of Mental Disorders,* ed 3, revised. (Current Classification of Mental Disorders, 1987.) Copyright American Psychiatric Association, Washington, D.C., 1987. Used with permission.

ness, sweating, and insomnia, to seizures, delirium, and cardiovascular collapse leading to death (Tables 2 and 3). At its worst, it is the most severe of the drug abstinence syndromes. Pentobarbital or secobarbital users with 400 mg per day habits show only mild withdrawal symptoms. Users taking 800 mg per day experience orthostatic hypotension, weakness, tremor, anxiety, and considerable discomfort; about 75 percent have convulsions. Users of even higher doses may suffer from apprehension, anorexia, confusion, delirium, hallucinations, and psychoses, as well as convulsions resembling grand mal epilepsy. The psychosis is clinically indistinguishable from that of alcoholic delirium tremens: its main features are agitation, delusions, and hallucinations that are usually visual but sometimes tactile or auditory. Fever may be present. Most of the symptoms appear in the first 3 days of abstinence, and seizures generally occur on the second or third day, when the symptoms are worst. If seizures do occur, they always precede the development of delirium. The syndrome rarely occurs more than a week after abstinence. Psychosis, if it develops, starts on the third to the eighth day. The various symptoms generally run their course within 2 to 3 days but may last as long as 2 weeks. The first episode of the syndrome usually occurs after 5 to 15 years of heavy drug use. An amnestic syndrome may occur as the result of sedative, hypnotic, or anxiolytic abuse. DSM-III-R states that the onset appears to be in the 20s, and the course is variable, having the potential for full recovery (Table 4).

Dependent users often take an average daily dose of 1.5g of a short-acting barbiturate, and some have been reported to take as much as 2.5 g per day for months. The lethal dose is not much greater for the chronic abuser than it is for the neophyte, so eventually tolerance develops to the point where withdrawal in a hospital becomes necessary to prevent accidental death from overdose. To avoid sudden death

Table 3

Diagnostic Criteria for Sedative, Hypnotic, or Anxiolytic Withdrawal Delirium

---

A. Delirium developing after the cessation of heavy use of a sedative, hypnotic, or anxiolytic, or a reduction in the amount of substance used (usually within 1 week).

B. Autonomic hyperactivity (e.g., tachycardia, sweating).

C. Not due to any physical or other mental disorder.

Note: When the differential diagnosis must be made without a clear-cut history or toxicologic analysis of body fluids, it may be qualified as "Provisional."

Table from DSM-III-R *Diagnostic and Statistical Manual of Mental Disorders,* ed 3, revised. (Current Classification of Mental Disorders, 1987.) Copyright American Psychiatric Association, Washington, D.C., 1987. Used with permission.

Table 4

Diagnostic Criteria for Sedative, Hypnotic, or Anxiolytic Amnestic Disorder

---

A. Amnestic Syndrome following prolonged heavy use of a sedative, hypnotic, or anxiolytic.

B. Not due to any physical or other mental disorder.

Note: When the differential diagnosis must be made without a clear-cut history or toxicologic analysis of body fluids, it may be qualified as "Provisional."

Table from DSM-III-R *Diagnostic and Statistical Manual of Mental Disorders,* ed 3, revised. (Current Classification of Mental Disorders, 1987.) Copyright American Psychiatric Association, Washington, D.C., 1987. Used with permission.

during the withdrawal process, treatment must be very conservative. First, barbiturates must be withheld from a comatose or grossly intoxicated patient until these symptoms clear. Meanwhile, the size of the habitual dose must be determined. Because the patient is not a reliable source for this information, often underestimating the dosage, family and pharmacists should be consulted for confirmation. The dose level must then be clinically verified; for example, a test dose of 200 mg pentobarbital may be given by mouth on an empty stomach and repeated every hour while the withdrawal syndrome is still evident. When a level has been attained at which mild intoxication and sedation occur, the patient should be stabilized on that dosage for 1 or 2 days. Then the dose can be gradually reduced (by no more than 10 percent per day). During this process, the patient may begin to exhibit withdrawal symptoms; in that case, the daily decrement should be halved.

Phenobarbital may be substituted in the withdrawal procedure for the more commonly abused short-acting barbiturates. The effects of phenobarbital last longer, and because there is less fluctuation of barbiturate blood levels this drug does not produce observable toxic signs or a serious overdose. An adequate dose is 30 mg of phenobarbital for every 100 mg of the short-acting substance. The user should be maintained for at least 2 days at this level before the dosage is reduced further. The regimen is somewhat analogous to the substitution of methadone for heroin.

After withdrawal is complete the patient must overcome the desire to start taking the drug again. Although it has been suggested that nonbarbiturate sedative-hypnotics be substituted for barbiturates as a preventive therapeutic measure, this too often results in replacing one drug dependence with another. If a user is to remain drug-free, follow-up treatment, usually with psychiatric help and resort to community resources, is vital. Otherwise the patient will almost certainly return to barbiturates or to a drug with similar hazards because it is a proven means of adjusting to problems such as tension, anxiety, feelings of inadequacy, or a personality disorder.

METHAQUALONE

Methaqualone (Quaalude) is a nonbarbiturate sedative-hypnotic used mostly by young people who believe that it heightens the sexual experience. There is no accepted medical use and it is no longer manufactured in the U.S. Most methaqualone is now manufactured here in illicit laboratories or smuggled into the United States. Users take one or two standard tablets (300 to 600 mg) to get high. Street names include "mandrakes" (from the British preparation Mandrax) and "soapers" (from the brand name Sopor). "Luding out" means taking methaqualone with alcohol, usually wine.

Adverse Effects

Undesirable effects are dryness of the mouth, headache, urticaria, dizziness, diarrhea, chills, tremors, hangover, paresthesia, menstrual disturbance, epistaxis, and depersonalization. Overdose may result in restlessness, delirium, hypertonia, muscle spasms leading to convulsions, and death. Unlike barbiturates, methaqualone rarely causes severe cardiovascular and respiratory depression, and most fatalities result from combining methaqualone with alcohol. Treatment consists mainly of supportive measures to maintain vital functions. If a patient who is still conscious recently ingested the drug, gastric lavage is indicated.

BENZODIAZEPINES

The benzodiazepines include about 20 drugs, such as diazepam (Valium), flurazepam (Dalmane), oxazepam (Serax), and chlordiazepoxide (Librium). They are used mainly to treat anxiety, but also as sedatives, muscle relaxants, anticonvulsants, and anesthetics, and in the treatment of alcohol withdrawal. Introduced in the 1960s, benzodiazepines soon became some of the most popular prescription drugs in the United States. About 15 percent of persons in this country have had a benzodiazepine prescribed by a physician; however, a recent substantial decline in medical use suggests that physicians are becoming more cautious about them. All benzodiazepines are classified in category IV of controlled substances by Drug Enforcement Agency (DEA) regulations. Diazepam is frequently taken by cocaine addicts to minimize the withdrawal reaction following cocaine intoxication and is taken by opioid addicts to enhance euphoria. The abuse incidence is unknown but probably overestimated.

Adverse Effects

Unlike barbiturates, benzodiazepines do not cause microsomal enzyme induction or REM sleep suppression, and they have a high margin of safety. Benzodiazepines produce little respiratory depression, and the ratio of lethal to effective dose is very high; it is estimated at 200 to 1 or more. Very large amounts (more than 2 g) taken in suicide attempts produce drowsiness, lethargy, ataxia, and sometimes confusion. They depress vital signs somewhat, but do not cause permanent damage. The adverse effects of lower doses include drowsiness, unsteadiness, and weakness. Some benzodiazepines have a disinhibiting effect, which may cause hostile or aggressive behavior in people susceptible to frustration. Benzodiazepines produce less euphoria than other tranquilizing drugs, so the risk of dependence and abuse is relatively low. But both tolerance and withdrawal symptoms can develop. The withdrawal reaction is most likely to occur at cessation of doses in the 40 mg per day range but it can occur at therapeutic doses (as low as 10 or 20 mg per day), if the drug has been used for a month or more. The onset of withdrawal usually occurs within 2 or 3 days after cessation of use, but with longer-acting drugs, such as diazepam, the latency before onset may be 5 or 6 days. Symptoms include anxiety, numbness in the extremities, dysphoria, intolerance for bright lights and loud noises, nausea, sweating, muscle twitching, and sometimes convulsions (generally at doses of 100 mg per day or more). Withdrawal is not usually accompanied by craving for the drug. Because benzodiazepines are eliminated from the body slowly, symptoms may continue to develop for several weeks. To prevent seizures and other problems, withdrawal is accomplished by gradual reduction of the dose. Rare side effects of benzodiazepines include blood dyscrasias such as agranulocytosis and possibly fetal malformations, although evidence for this side effect is controversial. Benzodiazepines never cause extrapyramidal side effects or tardive dyskinesia.

LEGAL ISSUES

Recently, attempts have been made by state and federal agencies to further restrict the distribution of benzodiazepines by requiring special reporting forms. For example, through the use of New York State triplicate prescription forms, the names of doctors and patients are kept on file in a data bank. Presumably such measures are taken to stem the tide of abuse. But most abuse is the result of the illicit manufacture, sale, and diversion of these drugs, particularly to cocaine and opioid addicts, and not from physicians' prescriptions or legitimate pharmaceutical companies. To attempt to curtail the use of these drugs, which have unquestionable and invaluable therapeutic benefits, is an example of increasing governmental interference in the practice of medicine and in the confidential relationship between doctor and patient. The authors believe that such restrictions will do little to curb cocaine, opioid or benzodiazepine abuse.

References

Bergman H, Borg S, Holm L: Neuropsychological impairment and the exclusive abuse of sedatives or hypnotics. Am J Psychiatry *137*:215, 1980.

Busto U, Sellers E M, Naranjo C A, Cappe H H, Sanchez-Craig M, Sykora K: Withdrawal reaction after long-term therapeutic use of benzodiazepines. N Engl J Med, *315*:854, 1986.

Harvey S C: Hypnotics and sedatives. In *The Pharmacological Basis of Therapeutics*, A G Gilman, L S Goodman, A Gilman, editors, ed 7, p 339. Macmillan, New York, 1985.

Kales A, Bixler E O, Ton T L: Chronic hypnotic drug use: Ineffective drug withdrawal, insomnia, and dependence. JAMA 227:513, 1974.

Medelson W B: *The Use and Misuse of Sleeping Pills: A Clinical Guide*. Plenum Medical Book Co, New York, 1980.

Richels K: Benzodiazepines: Use and misuse. In *Anxiety: New Research and Changing Concepts*, D F Klein, J G Rabkin, editors. Raven Press, New York, 1981.

Shader R I, Caine E D, Meyer R E: Treatment of dependence on barbiturates and sedative-hypnotics. In *Manual of Psychiatric Therapeutics*, R I Shader, editor. Little Brown, Boston, 1975.

Szara S I, Ludford J P, editors: *Benzodiazepines: A Review of Research Results*, NIDA Research Monograph 33. US Government Printing Office, Washington, DC, 1980.

Wesson D R, Smith D E: *Barbiturates: Their Use, Misuse, and Abuse*. Human Sciences Press, New York, 1977.

Wikler A: Diagnosis and treatment of drug dependence of the barbiturate type. Am J Psychiatry *125*:759, 1968.

13.4 ————
Opioid Dependence

Opioids are a class of drugs that produce physical and psychological dependence. The basic substance, opium, is obtained from the juice of opium poppy, *Papaver somniferum*. There are about 20 distinct alkaloids derived from opium, the best-known being morphine. Semisynthetic opioid alkaloids occur naturally in opium or can be manufactured from morphine, including heroin (diacetyl morphine), codeine, and hydromorphine (Dilaudid). Synthetic opioids made in the laboratory include meperidine (Demerol), methadone, and propoxyphene (Darvon). Opioid antagonists, synthetic compounds that block the action of opium, include nalorphine, levallorphan, naloxone, and apomorphine. Mixed agents with both agonist and antagonist properties include pentazocine (Talwin), butorphanol, and buprenorphine.

EPIDEMIOLOGY

Heroin is the most widely abused opiate. Epidemics of heroin abuse occurred in the United States during the mid-1960s, the mid-1970s, and the early 1980s. Psychiatric epidemiologic studies conducted from 1981 to 1983 found that 0.7 percent of the adult population had met DSM-III diagnostic criteria for opioid abuse or dependence at some time in their lives. It is smuggled into the United States primarily from the Middle and Far East, where the opium poppy is a major cash crop. There are an estimated 400,000 to 600,000 heroin addicts in this country. It has been estimated that almost half of all opioid addicts in the US live in New York City. Male addicts outnumber female addicts in a ratio of 3 to 1; most are in their early to mid-30s and started using drugs in their late teens or early 20s. Heroin addicts may spend $200 or more per day to support their habit, most of that money being obtained by crime.

A variety of risk factors have been associated with heroin abuse. Intravenous drug abuse contributes to hepatitis B viral infection and more recently to acquired immune deficiency syndrome (AIDS). Intravenous drug abusers make up a major group at risk for AIDS and are a source of contamination to the general population through coital transmission. There is no permissible medical use for heroin in the United States.

MECHANISM OF ACTION

Opioids exert their effect by attaching to specific neural binding sites known as opioid receptors. Antagonists (e.g., naltrexone) block opioid receptor binding sites and reverse or prevent the opioid effects. In 1974, an endogenous factor with opiate-like actions was identified as a pentapeptide, enkephalin, several forms of which were isolated from the brain and named endorphins. Endorphins are involved in neural transmission and serve to suppress pain. They are released naturally in the body when a person is physically hurt and account in part for the absence of pain during acute injury states. Heroin is more potent and more lipid soluble than morphine; it crosses the blood-brain barrier in less time and produces a more rapid onset of action than morphine. Codeine, 3-methoxymorphine, occurs naturally (0.5 percent) in opium. After absorption, it is transformed to some degree into morphine and binds to the same neuroanatomical sites. Synthetic opioids, such as methadone, meperidine, and pentazocine (Talwin), also bind to opioid receptors.

Tolerance and Dependence

Changes in the number of opioid receptors may occur as the result of continuous exposure to opioids and can produce dependence on the drug. Intracellular changes in calcium, cyclic AMP, and adenyl nucleotides also result from chronic exposure. When the drug is displaced from its receptor (by an antagonist) or is unavailable (as in abstinence), a withdrawal syndrome occurs. Tolerance probably develops in humans within the first four doses, but some period of continuous receptor binding is required for the withdrawal syndrome to occur. Withdrawal responses are more intense and more readily detectable when the opioid is rapidly removed from its receptor, as by an opioid antagonist. Chronic use may also induce supersensitivity of the dopaminergic, cholinergic, and serotonergic systems. The activity of adrenergic neurons in the locus ceruleus decreases. Rebound hyperactivity of those systems occurs with abstinence. Clonidine, an adrenergic agonist, inhibits the activity of neurons in the locus ceruleus, which may explain its ability to block the withdrawal syndrome. Because of the above mentioned changes, the term

"neuroadaptation" has been proposed to describe physical dependence.

ETIOLOGY

The causes of heroin addiction are multiple. Low socioeconomic group affiliation carries greater risk; however, opioid addiction has spread to upper socioeconomic groups, especially to physicians, who are disproportionately affected. Drug availability and the previous use of other psychoactive substances, such as alcohol and marijuana, predispose a person to heroin abuse. Illicit drugs are more available in urban than in rural areas. More than 50 percent of urban heroin users belong to single-parent or divorced families; alcoholism and drug abuse are common among the families of drug abusers. Neonatal addiction is a significant problem; approximately three fourths of infants born to addicted mothers experience the withdrawal syndrome. Close to 90 percent of opioid addicts have a diagnosed psychiatric disorder, most often depression. Alcoholism, antisocial personality, and anxiety are the next most common disorders. Suicidal ideation is frequent; in one study, 13 percent of heroin addicts had made at least one suicide attempt.

CLINICAL EFFECTS

The clinical effects of morphine may be used as the model for all opioids. Analgesia, drowsiness, mood changes, and mental clouding follow ingestion of small amounts of the drug (5 to 10 mg). The analgesic effects peak about 20 minutes after intravenous injection or 1 hour after subcutaneous injection and last 4 to 6 hours, depending on the type of opioid, the dose, and the previous history of drug-taking. Other manifestations are a feeling of warmth, heaviness of the extremities, and dry mouth. The face, particularly the nose, may itch and become flushed (this effect may occur from a release of histamine). Some patients experience euphoria, which may last 10 to 30 minutes. Among the intravenous users, an immediate high, described as being akin to an orgasm (called a "rush") is reported when the drug reaches the brain a few minutes after injection. That is followed by sedation (known as "nodding off" by users). Morphine analgesia is selective. The threshold of a nerve ending to noxious stimuli is not altered, nor is the conduction of nerve impulses affected. Rather, perception of pain is altered so that the patient becomes indifferent to it. For many people, the effect of taking an opioid for the first time is dysphoric rather than euphoric, and nausea and vomiting may result.

Morphine is a respiratory depressant because of its direct effect on the brain stem respiratory center; in humans, death from overdose is nearly always due to respiratory arrest. Changes in blood pressure, heart rate, and cerebral circulation may also occur but are not as prominent. Idiosyncratic responses such as allergic reactions, anaphylactic shock, and pulmonary edema account for cases of sudden death. The depressant effects of morphine and other opioids may be enhanced by phenothiazines and monoamine oxidase inhibitors. Fatalities have been reported in patients receiving antidepressants especially monoamine oxidase inhibitors (MAOIs) who were also given Demerol. Other effects of morphine include pupillary constriction, smooth muscle contraction (including ureters and bile ducts), and constipation.

Heroin, pharmacologically similar to morphine, induces analgesia, drowsiness, and changes in mood. The pleasurable and euphoric actions of heroin are about twice as potent as those of morphine. Although the manufacture, sale, and possession of heroin is illegal in the United States, because of its excellent analgesic and euphoric effects, attempts have been made to make heroin available to pain-ridden terminal cancer patients. Many people, including legislators, favor a change in the law, but such legislation has been repeatedly voted down by the US Congress.

Tolerance to opioids develops in terminally ill patients, who may require 200 to 300 mg of morphine per day to manage pain. Tolerance to the respiratory depressant effects does not develop, however, which places such patients at risk if their needs for opiates are met. Many patients suffer unnecessary pain before they die because physicians are unwilling to prescribe such large doses or because of restrictive legislation.

Intoxication and Overdose

Opioid intoxication occurs after the recurrent use of an opioid and is characterized by altered mood, psychomotor retardation, drowsiness, slurred speech, and impaired memory or attention (Table 1). An overdose is life-threatening and is characterized by marked unresponsiveness, coma, slow respiration, hypothermia, hypotension, shock, and bradycardia. Death is usually from respiratory arrest. Needle tracks in the arms, legs, ankles, groin (or even the dorsal vein of the penis) of an unconscious patient should alert the

Table 1
Diagnostic Criteria for Opioid Intoxication

A. Recent use of an opioid.

B. Maladaptive behavioral changes (e.g., initial euphoria followed by apathy, dysphoria, psychomotor retardation, impaired judgment, impaired social or occupational functioning).

C. Pupillary constriction (or pupillary dilation due to anoxia from severe overdose) and at least one of the following signs:
   (1) drowsiness
   (2) slurred speech
   (3) impairment in attention or memory

D. Not due to any physical or other mental disorder.

Note: When the differential diagnosis must be made without a clear-cut history, testing with an opioid antagonist, or toxicologic analysis of body fluids, it may be qualified as "Provisional."

Table from DSM-III-R *Diagnostic and Statistical Manual of Mental Disorders,* ed 3, revised. (Current Classification of Mental Disorders, 1987.) Copyright American Psychiatric Association, Washington, D.C., 1987. Used with permission.

physician to the possibility of narcotic overdose. The triad of coma, pinpoint pupils, and respiratory depression suggest opioid overdose.

MPTP-Induced Parkinsonism. In 1976, after ingesting a synthetic opioid contaminated with MPTP (N-methyl-4-phenyl-1,2,3,6 tetrahydropyridine), a number of persons developed a syndrome of irreversible parkinsonism. The mechanism for the neurotoxic effect is as follows: MPTP is converted into MPP^+ by the enzyme monoamine oxidase and then is taken up by dopaminergic neurons. Because MPP^+ binds to melanin in substantia nigra neurons, MPP^+ is concentrated in these neurons and eventually kills the cells. Positron emission tomographic (PET) studies of persons who ingested MPTP but who remained asymptomatic have actually shown a decrease in the number of dopamine binding sites in the substantia nigra.

TREATMENT OF OVERDOSE

Opioid overdose is a medical emergency. The patient's respiration is severely depressed, and he or she may be semicomatose or comatose or in shock. The first task is to ensure that there is an open airway and that vital signs are maintained. An opioid antagonist naloxone (Narcan) is administered, 0.4 mg intravenously, which can be repeated four to five times within the first 30 to 45 minutes. The patient generally becomes more responsive, but because naloxone has only a short duration of action, the patient may relapse into a semicomatose state in 4 or 5 hours; therefore, careful observation is imperative. Grand mal seizures occur with meperidine overdose and are prevented by naloxone. Antagonists must be used carefully because they can precipitate a severe withdrawal reaction. Other narcotic antagonists include nalorphine and levallorphan.

WITHDRAWAL

Morphine and heroin addicts may take hundreds of milligrams of heroin; as much as 5,000 mg of morphine has been taken by tolerant addicts. In nontolerant persons, death from overdose may occur with 60 mg of morphine. The morphine and heroin withdrawal syndrome begins within 6 to 8 hours after the last dose, usually after a 1- to 2-week period of continuous use or the administration of a narcotic antagonist. It reaches its peak intensity during the second or third day and subsides during the next 7 to 10 days. However, some symptoms may persist for 6 months or longer (Table 2). The withdrawal syndrome from meperidine (Demerol), begins more quickly, reaches a peak within 8 to 12 hours, and is complete in 4 to 5 days. Methadone withdrawal usually begins 1 to 3 days after the last dose, and is complete in 10 to 14 days. The general rule is that substances with shorter durations of action tend to produce shorter, more intense withdrawal syndromes, and substances that have longer durations of action produce prolonged but milder withdrawal syndromes. An exception to the rule, narcotic antagonist–precipitated withdrawal following long-acting substance addiction can be very severe. The withdrawal syndrome consists of severe muscle

Table 2
Opioid Withdrawal Symptoms

Behavioral	Physical
Anxiety	Sweating
Craving for opioids	Fever
Insomnia	Rhinorrhea
Anorexia	Mydriasis
Agitation	Piloerection
Possible violence	Nausea and vomiting
	Cardiovascular instability: hypertension, tachycardia
	Abdominal cramping
	Grand mal seizures with meperidine

cramps and bone aches, profuse diarrhea, abdominal cramps, rhinorrhea, lacrimation, piloerection or goose-flesh (from whence comes the name "cold turkey" for the abstinence syndrome), yawning, fever, pupillary dilation, hypertension, tachycardia, and temperature dysregulation, including fever. An addict seldom dies from withdrawal, unless there is a severe pre-existing physical illness such as cardiac disease. Residual effects of insomnia, bradycardia, changes in temperature, and a craving for opioids may persist for months after withdrawal. At any time during the abstinence syndrome, a single injection of morphine or heroin will eliminate all symptoms. The DSM-III-R signs of opioid withdrawal are listed in Table 3. Associated features include restlessness, irritability, depression, tremor, weakness, nausea, and vomiting. All of the symptoms described resemble the clinical picture of influenza. An abstinence syndrome may be precipitated by the administration of an antagonist. The symptoms may begin within 60 seconds after such an intravenous injection and peak in about 1 hour. It is relatively uncommon for opioid craving to occur in the context of analgesic administration for pain from physical disorders or associated with surgery. The full withdrawal syndrome including intense craving for opioids usually occurs only secondary to abrupt cessation of use in opioid-dependent persons.

Treatment of Opioid Withdrawal

Methadone. Methadone is a synthetic opioid that can be taken orally and that substitutes for heroin. It is given to addicts in place of their usual drug of abuse and suppresses withdrawal symptoms. The action of methadone is such that 20 to 80 mg per day (although doses up to 120 mg per day have been used) is sufficient to stabilize the patient. It has a duration of action exceeding 24 hours. Methadone maintenance is continued until the patient can be withdrawn from methadone, which is itself addicting. Patients are detoxified from methadone more easily than from heroin, although a similar abstinence syndrome occurs with methadone. Usually clonidine (0.1 to 0.3 mg, three to four times per day) is given during the detoxification period.

Levo-α-acetylmethadol (LAMM) is a longer-acting opioid than methadone. In contrast to the daily methadone treatment, LAMM can be administered in doses of 30 to 80 mg, three times a week.

Methadone maintenance has several advantages: it frees the addict from dependence on injectable heroin (invariably taken with contaminated needles); it is legal; it causes minimal euphoria, and rarely causes drowsiness or depression when taken chronically; and it allows the person to engage in gainful employment instead of criminal activity. The disadvantage is that the patient remains addicted to a narcotic.

The pregnant addict. Although opioid withdrawal is almost never fatal for the otherwise healthy adult, opioid withdrawal is hazardous to the fetus and can lead to miscarriage or fetal death. Maintaining the pregnant addict on low doses of methadone (10 to 40 mg per day) may be the least hazardous course to follow. At this dosage, neonatal withdrawal is usually mild and can be managed with low doses of paregoric. If the pregnancy begins while the patient is on high doses of methadone, dosage should be reduced quite slowly (e.g., 1 mg every 3 days) and fetal movements should be monitored. If withdrawal is necessary or desired it is accomplished with least hazard during the second trimester.

Opioid Antagonists. Opioid antagonists block or antagonize the effects of opioids, preventing them from acting. Unlike methadone, they do not in themselves exert narcotic effects, nor are they addicting. The antagonists include the following drugs: naloxone (Narcan) which is used in the treatment of opioid overdose because it reverses the effects of narcotics; and naltrexone, which is the longest-acting (72 hours) antagonist. The theory behind the use of antagonists for opioid addiction is that the blocking of drug effects, particularly euphoria, discourages addicts from drug-seeking behavior and thus deconditions them to opioids. The major weakness of the antagonist model is the lack of any mechanism compelling addicts to continue to take the antagonist.

Therapeutic Community. The therapeutic community is a residence composed of members who all share the same problem of drug abuse. Abstinence is the rule, and in order to be admitted to such a community, the person requires a high level of motivation. The goal is to effect a complete change of life style, including abstinence from drugs; the development of personal honesty, responsibility, and useful social skills; and the elimination of antisocial attitudes and criminal behavior.

The staff of most therapeutic communities is made up of

Table 3
Diagnostic Criteria for Opioid Withdrawal

A. Cessation of prolonged (several weeks or more) moderate or heavy use of an opioid, or reduction in the amount of opioid used (or administration of an opioid antagonist after a brief period of use), followed by at least three of the following:
(1) craving for an opioid
(2) nausea or vomiting
(3) muscle aches
(4) lacrimation or rhinorrhea
(5) pupillary dilation, piloerection, or sweating
(6) diarrhea
(7) yawning
(8) fever
(9) insomnia

B. Not due to any physical or other mental disorder.

Table from DSM-III-R *Diagnostic and Statistical Manual of Mental Disorders,* ed 3, revised. (Current Classification of Mental Disorders, 1987.) Copyright American Psychiatric Association, Washington, D.C., 1987. Used with permission.

former addicts who often put the prospective candidate through a rigorous screening process to test motivation. Self help through the use of confrontational groups and isolation from the outside world and from friends associated with the drug life are emphasized. The prototypical community for addicts is Phoenix House, where patients live for long periods (usually 12 to 18 months) while receiving treatment. They are allowed to return to their old environment only when they have demonstrated their ability to handle increased responsibility in the center. Therapeutic communities are effective, but they require large staffs and extensive facilities. Moreover, dropout rates are high; as many as 75 percent of those who enter therapeutic communities leave within the first month.

References

Cooper J R, Altman F, Brown B S: *Research on the Treatment of Narcotic Addiction: State of the Art,* NIDH Research Monograph 83. US Government Printing Office, Washington, DC, 1985.
Dole V P, Nyswander M E L: Methadone maintenance treatment: A ten-year perspective. JAMA 235:2117, 1976.
Jaffe J H, Martin W R: Opioid Analgesics and Antagonists. In *The Pharmacological Basis of Therapeutics,* A G Gilman, L S Goodman, A Gilman, editors, ed 7, p491. Macmillan, New York, 1985.
Kosten T R, Rounsaville B J, Kleber J D: A 2.5-year follow-up of cocaine use among treated opioid addicts. Arch Gen Psychiatry 44(3):281, 1987.
Kozel N J, Adams E H: Epidemiology of drug abuse: An overview. Science 234:970, 1986.
Meyer R E, Mirin S M: *The Heroin Stimulus: Implications for a Theory of Addiction.* Plenum, New York, 1979.
Resnick R B, Schuyten-Resnick E, Washton A M: Assessment of narcotic antagonists in the treatment of opioid dependence. Ann Rev Pharmacol Toxicol 20:463, 1980.
Sells S B: Treatment effectiveness. In *Handbook on Drug Abuse,* R L Dupont, A Goldstein, J O'Donnell, editors. US Government Printing Office, Washington, DC, 1979.
Woody G E, McLellan A T, Luborsky L, O'Brien C: Twelve-month follow-up of psychotherapy for opiate dependence. Am J Psychiatry 144:590, 1987.

13.5 _____
Cocaine

HISTORY

Cocaine (snow, coke, girl, lady) is an alkaloid derived from the shrub *Erythroxylon coca,* a plant indigenous to Bolivia and Peru, where its leaves are chewed by peasants for their stimulating effect. Cocaine was isolated in 1860, and after 1884 became the first effective local anesthetic, the only purpose for which it is still used in medicine. In the 1880s and 1890s, cocaine was used therapeutically in a variety of ways. In 1914, cocaine was subjected to the same laws as morphine and heroin and since then has been legally classified with the narcotics.

EPIDEMIOLOGY

In the past decade, the prevalence of cocaine use has increased. There are over 20 million persons who have used the drug, of which 4 million are considered to be chronic abusers. In a 1985 survey 6.7 percent of high school seniors had used cocaine and 25 percent of young adults reported some experience with it. Increases have been noted in nonfatal emergencies associated with cocaine, and there were over 550 cocaine-related deaths in 1985, mainly from heart attacks in relatively healthy persons. Previously considered to be a drug of the affluent, cocaine is now more available and cheaper. Crack, a form of freebase cocaine, is marketed at $10 for a 65- to 100-mg dose (in contrast to $100 for 1 g of cocaine powder).

PHARMACOLOGY

Cocaine stimulates the dopaminergic system, causing massive dopamine release and inhibiting serotonin reuptake. The euphoria produced by the drug is intense. Psychological dependence may occur after a single dose. The effects of cocaine are shorter than amphetamine, usually lasting 30 minutes to an hour after intravenous or intranasal use. The acute depletion of serotonin contributes to depression and suicidal ideation after the drug wears off in acute and chronic users.

METHODS OF USE

Street cocaine varies greatly in purity. It is usually cut with sugar, procaine, amphetamine, or other substances. It is rarely taken by mouth, because the effect is regarded as too mild to warrant the expense. There are three widespread methods of ingestion: inhaling (snorting), subcutaneous or intravenous injection, and freebasing. Freebasers take street cocaine hydrochloride and chemically extract pure cocaine alkaloid (the free base), which produces a strong effect when smoked in a pipe or, occasionally, in a cigarette.

Crack is extremely potent, can be produced cheaply by the freebase method, and has contributed to the increase in abuse. Inhaling is the most common and least dangerous method; however, it does not provide the ecstatic rush of smoking or injection. The occasional use of cocaine is hazardous because of the high abuse potential as well as danger from cardiac arrest; however, nonproblematic cocaine use has been described in which the drug is used for recreational purposes and the user does not become dependent.

CLINICAL EFFECTS

The central nervous system effects of cocaine are similar to those of amphetamine—elation, euphoria, heightened self-esteem, and improved performance of mental and physical tasks. The peripheral sympathomimetic effect of vasoconstriction and the analgesic effect account for its being the anesthetic of choice for many surgical procedures of the eye, ear, nose, and throat.

Cocaine Intoxication

Clinical effects pass easily into cocaine intoxication characterized by extreme agitation, irritability, impaired judgment, impulsive sexual behavior, aggression, increased psychomotor activity, and manic excitement (Table 1). Tachycardia, hypertension, and mydriasis occur. The course of cocaine intoxication is usually self-limited, full recovery occurring within 48 hours. As the drug effects wear off, the person experiences marked dysphoria and agitation, which is relieved by taking more cocaine; thus, a vicious cycle of use, dysphoria, and more use is perpetuated until toxic effects occur. The dysphoric mood (or "crash") is associated with anxiety, irritability, and fatigue. When the crash extends beyond 24 hours after the last use of cocaine, it becomes cocaine withdrawal. As an alternative, the person may use alcohol, sedatives, or such antianxiety agents as diazepam (usually obtained illicitly) to alleviate the dysphoric response. (In high doses, cocaine can induce seizures, depression of the medullary centers, and death from cardiac or respiratory arrest. Syncope or chest pain may occur.) Death from a combination of opioids and cocaine taken intravenously (a "speedball") is more common than death from cocaine alone.

Cocaine Psychosis

Cases of psychosis are not uncommon in habitual intravenous abusers and freebasers; cocaine psychosis is apparently qualitatively similar to amphetamine psychosis. Cocaine intoxication with high doses may lead to transient ideas of reference, paranoid ideation, increased libido, tinnitus, and bizarre behavior, such as sorting objects into pairs. Delirium with disorientation and violent behavior may occur (Table 2). Perceptual disturbances and persecutory trends with overt paranoid delusions (commonly delusions of jealousy) are associated with prolonged use and classified as cocaine delusional disorder (Table 3). Homicidal impulses may be carried out. Tactile or haptic hallucinations have been described, in which the person believes that bugs are crawling just beneath the skin (also known as formication).

Chronic use is associated with a runny or clogged nose and is often self-treated with nasal decongestant sprays. Noses may also become inflamed, swollen, or ulcerated; heavy users occasionally develop perforated septa. Freebasing may damage the surface of the lungs, and injection involves the usual dangers of infection and embolism as well as an increased risk of contracting acquired immune deficiency syndrome (AIDS) through the practice of sharing needles.

Along with amphetamines, cocaine is the drug most eagerly self-administered by experimental animals under restraint; they will kill themselves with voluntary injections. Few human beings use cocaine in that manner, but craving

Table 1
Diagnostic Criteria for Cocaine Intoxication

A. Recent use of cocaine.

B. Maladaptive behavioral changes (e.g., euphoria, fighting, grandiosity, hypervigilance, psychomotor agitation, impaired judgment, impaired social or occupational functioning).

C. At least two of the following signs within 1 hour of using cocaine:
   (1) tachycardia
   (2) pupillary dilation
   (3) elevated blood pressure
   (4) perspiration or chills
   (5) nausea or vomiting
   (6) visual or tactile hallucinations

D. Not due to any physical or other mental disorder.

Table from DSM-III-R *Diagnostic and Statistical Manual of Mental Disorders,* ed 3, revised. (Current Classification of Mental Disorders, 1987.) Copyright American Psychiatric Association, Washington, D.C., 1987. Used with permission.

Table 2
Diagnostic Criteria for Cocaine Delirium

A. Delirium developing within 24 hours of use of cocaine.

B. Not due to any physical or other mental disorder.

Table from DSM-III-R *Diagnostic and Statistical Manual of Mental Disorders,* ed 3, revised. (Current Classification of Mental Disorders, 1987.) Copyright American Psychiatric Association, Washington, D.C., 1987. Used with permission.

Table 3
Diagnostic Criteria for Cocaine Delusional Disorder

A. Organic Delusional Syndrome developing shortly after use of cocaine.

B. Rapidly developing persecutory delusions are the predominant clinical feature.

C. Not due to any physical or other mental disorder.

Table from DSM-III-R *Diagnostic and Statistical Manual of Mental Disorders,* ed 3, revised. (Current Classification of Mental Disorders, 1987.) Copyright American Psychiatric Association, Washington, D.C., 1987. Used with permission.

often becomes a serious problem for people who have constant access to the drug, especially for freebasers and intravenous abusers. The financial, physical, and psychological costs of compulsive cocaine abuse can be devastating.

DIAGNOSIS

Cocaine abuse should be suspected if a person shows a change in personality characterized by irritability, disturbed concentration, compulsive behavior, perceptual changes, severe insomnia, and weight loss. (Surveys have shown that after-hours night clubs are a common meeting ground for cocaine abusers.) If other signs are present, a pattern of frequenting such clubs as well as the recent acquisition of debt (to support the expensive cocaine habit) should arouse suspicion. Cocaine users will often excuse themselves from social situations frequently (every 30 minutes) to snort or inject the drug privately.

COCAINE WITHDRAWAL

DSM-III-R describes cocaine withdrawal as consisting of symptoms that reach a peak in 2 to 4 days, but with certain symptoms such as depression and irritability potentially persisting for weeks. Abrupt cocaine withdrawal by a chronic user may produce a severe craving for the drug and drug-seeking behavior; however, there are no definite physiologic signs of withdrawal (Table 4). Some persons do become hypersomnolent and complain of fatigue, anhedonia, depression, suicidal ideas, and general malaise. These symptoms clear up within a few weeks or months. An underlying emotional disorder may then surface, which may include a dependence on alcohol or benzodiazepines if those substances were used to manage the crash after each bout of cocaine abuse. DSM-III-R states that a coexisting depressive disorder should be considered if a depressive syndrome persists for several weeks.

TREATMENT

For acute cocaine overdose, the recommended treatment is administration of oxygen (under pressure if necessary) with the patient's head down in the Trendelenburg position, muscle relaxants if required to accomplish this, and if there are convulsions, intravenous short-acting barbiturates (25 to 50 mg of sodium pentothal) or diazepam (5 to 10 mg). For anxiety with hypertension and tachycardia, 10 to 30 mg of intravenous or intramuscular diazepam is of use. An alternative for this purpose that seems to be a specific antagonist of cocaine's sympathomimetic effects is the β-adrenergic blocker propranolol (Inderal), 1 mg injected in-

Table 4
Diagnostic Criteria for Cocaine Withdrawal

A. Cessation of prolonged (several days or longer) heavy use of cocaine, or reduction in the amount of cocaine used, followed by dysphoric mood (e.g., depression, irritability, anxiety) and at least one of the following, persisting more than 24 hours after cessation of substance use:
   (1) fatigue
   (2) insomnia or hypersomnia
   (3) psychomotor agitation

B. Not due to any physical or other mental disorder, such as Cocaine Delusional Disorder.

Table from DSM-III-R *Diagnostic and Statistical Manual of Mental Disorders,* ed 3, revised. (Current Classification of Mental Disorders, 1987.) Copyright American Psychiatric Association, Washington, D.C., 1987. **Used with permission.**

travenously every minute, for up to 8 minutes. However, propranolol should not be regarded as a protection against lethal doses of cocaine or as a treatment for severe overdose. Hospitalization is useful to keep the cocaine abuser away from the drug, to provide group counseling, and to monitor antipsychotic or antianxiety agents carefully. Outpatient treatment has been attempted using substitution therapy with amphetamine or methylphenidate in conjunction with individual or group therapy, but such treatment is not as effective as hospitalization. A recent method is sleep therapy with lorazepam (Halcion), the rationale being to prevent the patient from experiencing withdrawal signs. In some cases, imipramine or desipramine has been used successfully to maintain abstinence. Other drugs used in a similar way include lithium, bromocriptine, and monoamine oxidase inhibitors.

References

Byck R, editor: *Cocaine Papers: Sigmund Freud.* Stonehill Publishing Co, New York, 1974.

Dackis C A, Gold M S: New concepts in cocaine addiction: The dopamine depletion hypothesis. Neurosci Biobehav Rev *9:*469, 1985.

Gawin F H, Kleber H D: Cocaine abuse treatment. Arch Gen Psychiatry *41:*903, 1984.

Grabowski J, editor: *Cocaine: Pharmacology, Effects, and Treatment of Abuse,* NIDA Research Monograph 50. US Government Printing Office, Washington, DC, 1984.

Grinspoon L, Bakalar J B: *Cocaine: A Drug and Its Social Evolution.* Basic Books, New York, 1977.

Kozel N J, Adams E M: *Cocaine Use in America: Epidemiology and Clinical Perspectives,* NIDH Monograph 62. US Government Printing Office, Washington, DC, 1985.

Siegel R K: *Changing Patterns of Cocaine Use: Longitudinal Observation, Consequences and Treatment,* NIDA Monograph 13. US Government Printing Office, Washington, DC, 1977.

Siegel R K: Cocaine smoking. N Engl J Med, *300:*373, 1979.

Van Dyke C, Byck R: Cocaine. Sci American *246:*128, 1982.

Washton A M, Gold M S, Pottash A C: Survey of 500 callers to a national cocaine helpline. Psychosomatics, *25:*771, 1984.

13.6 ——————
Central Nervous System Stimulants

AMPHETAMINES

History

Amphetamines and amphetamine congeners comprise a large group of central stimulant drugs. Among the best known are dextroamphetamine (Dexedrine), methamphetamine (Methedrine), and methylphenidate (Ritalin). Racemic amphetamine sulfate (Benzedrine) was first synthesized in 1887, but it was not introduced as a pharmaceutical until 1932. At this time, the Benzedrine inhaler became available by nonprescription, over-the-counter sales in drug stores as a treatment for nasal congestion and asthma. In late 1937 the new drug was introduced in tablet form to treat narcolepsy and postencephalitic parkinsonism. It was also recommended to treat depression and to heighten energy. Soon amphetamine was receiving much sensational publicity, with numerous references to brain, pep, and superman pills. Amphetamine abuse reached epidemic proportions in the 1970s. By then the annual legal U.S. production reached more than 10 billion 5-mg tablets. There was also considerable growth in both illicit laboratory synthesis of amphetamines and black market diversion of legitimately produced drugs, which is still the major source of illicit drugs. Attempts were made to restrict and regulate the prescribing practices of physicians in an effort to stem abuse. Some of these restrictions, however, have limited the availability of these drugs for legitimate therapeutic applications. Amphetamine abuse is not uncommon among professional athletes and long-distance truck drivers, who use the drug to decrease fatigue and to increase energy.

Clinical Effects

Amphetamine is readily absorbed orally and has a rapid onset of action. Abusers often use the drug intravenously. It acts mainly by releasing serotonin from presynaptic terminals and by inhibiting its uptake. In the average person, a dose of 5 mg produces an increased sense of well-being, improves performance on written, verbal, and performance tasks, decreases fatigue, induces anorexia, and elevates the pain threshold.

These effects account for its therapeutic use in conditions such as attention-deficit hyperactivity disorder of children and adults, narcolepsy, obesity, mild depression, as well as for augmentation of tricyclic antidepressants and analgesics. Only the first three disorders mentioned above are currently listed as recommended indications by the Food and Drug Administration (FDA) however, more and more reports are appearing in the literature about the positive effects of these drugs when used judiciously in selected cases. In medically ill depressed patients, for example, amphetamine in dose range of 2.5 to 30 mg per day was found to be of use in alleviating depressive symptomatology. Response is more rapid than with tricyclic antidepressants, which may require a 2-week delay before a clinical response is seen. In therapeutic doses there are generally no dangerous side effects, such as the orthostatic hypotension or anticholinergic complications encountered with TCAs. In patients who are refractory to tricyclic antidepressants, the addition of amphetamine has also been found to be helpful. And in severe or chronic pain, amphetamine combined with analgesics enhances the pain-killing effects. The drug has also been used successfully to counteract the fatigue that accompanies chronic wasting diseases such as multiple sclerosis. Tolerance develops to the appetite suppressant effects of the drug more quickly than to fatigue reduction. Currently, there is an enormous amount of pressure on the medical profession from regulatory agencies, such as the FDA and DEA, and various state agencies, such as the New York State Department of Health, that have seriously curtailed the prescribing of amphetamines and other psychoactive drugs. Some of that pressure is exerted through the use of triplicate drug prescriptions, which affects the confidentiality of the doctor-patient relationship.

As the dose increases as a result of abuse or misuse, adverse effects eventually occur. Tolerance develops, and some abusers may take 1 g of amphetamine per day. In persons not used to the drug, death may occur with doses of 120 mg.

Adverse Effects

Physical Effects. Both the physical and psychological effects begin within 1 hour after administration and may occur within a few seconds. There are numerous adverse physical effects of both acute amphetamine intoxication and chronic use (Table 1). The physical signs and symptoms include flushing, pallor, cyanosis, fever, headache, tachycardia and palpitations, serious cardiac problems, markedly elevated blood pressure, hemorrhage or other vascular acci-

Table 1
Diagnostic Criteria for Amphetamine or Similarly Acting Sympathomimetic Intoxication

A. Recent use of amphetamine or a similarly acting sympathomimetic.

B. Maladaptive behavioral changes (e.g., fighting, grandiosity, hypervigilance, psychomotor agitation, impaired judgment, impaired social or occupational functioning).

C. At least two of the following signs within one hour of use:

    (1) tachycardia
    (2) pupillary dilation
    (3) elevated blood pressure
    (4) perspiration or chills
    (5) nausea or vomiting

D. Not due to any physical or other mental disorder.

Table from DSM-III-R *Diagnostic and Statistical Manual of Mental Disorders,* ed 3, revised. (Current Classification of Mental Disorders, 1987.) Copyright American Psychiatric Association, Washington, D.C., 1987. Used with permission.

dents, nausea, vomiting, bruxism (teeth grinding), difficulty in breathing, tremor, ataxia, loss of sensory abilities, twitching, tetany, convulsions, loss of consciousness, and coma. Death from overdose is usually associated with hyperpyrexia, convulsions, and cardiovascular shock. Intravenous abuse produces other serious physical reactions, including serum hepatitis, lung abscess, endocarditis, and necrotizing angiitis. Some studies have shown a change in brain neurochemistry after chronic use.

Psychological Effects. The psychological effects include restlessness, dysphoria, logorrhea, insomnia, irritability, hostility, tension, confusion, anxiety, panic, and, in some cases, psychosis (Table 2). When amphetamine is taken intravenously there is a characteristic "rush" of well-being and euphoria. Intoxication with high doses can lead to transient ideas of reference, paranoid ideation, increased libido, tinnitus, hearing one's name being called, and formication (tactile sensation of bugs crawling on the skin). Stereotyped movements may occur. Delirium with episodes of violence may also be seen (Table 3). The symptoms of amphetamine delusional disorder may resemble those of paranoid schizophrenia, with predominately and rapidly developing persecutory delusions; however, the predominance of visual hallucinations, appropriate affect, at times confusion and incoherence, hyperactivity, hypersexuality, or absence of thought disorder helps to distinguish amphetamine psychosis from schizophrenia. With amphetamines, distortions of body image and misperceptions of people's faces may occur. At times, a strictly clinical differentiation is all but impossible. The most reliable methods of diagnosis are specific laboratory tests that detect amphetamine in urine,

however, these tests are ineffective if more than 48 hours have elapsed since the last dose of amphetamine. In the absence of a reliable history, urinalysis, or obvious physical signs, amphetamine delusional disorder is often recognized only in retrospect, when the symptoms disappear—generally within days or, at most, weeks after the drug has been withdrawn. However, delusions, suspiciousness, tendencies toward misinterpretation, and ideas of reference may persist for months. The course of the intoxication, on the other hand, is usually self-limited, with full recovery within 48 hours. A letdown or "crash" occurs when the immediate effects of high doses have diminished. A debilitating cycle of runs (heavy use for several days to a week) and crashes is a common pattern of amphetamine abuse. The physical and psychological symptoms of the crash include anxiety, tremulousness, dysphoric mood, lethargy, fatigue, nightmares (from greatly increased REM sleep), headache, profuse sweating, muscle cramps, stomach cramps, and insatiable hunger. Loss of self-control may lead to violent acting out of aggressive impulses. According to DSM-III-R, when the crash extends beyond 24 hours after the last use of the substance, the condition is reclassified as amphetamine or similarly acting sympathomimetic withdrawal (Table 4). Withdrawal symptoms peak usually in 2 to 4 days. The most characteristic and dangerous symptom is a depression, suicidal at times, which peaks 48 to 72 hours after the last dose of amphetamine but which may persist for several weeks.

Treatment

Because amphetamine intoxication and delusional disorder are generally self-limiting, treatment usually requires supportive measures. Elimination of the drug may be facilitated by acidifying the urine with ammonium chloride. Antipsychotics, either a phenothiazine or haloperidol, may be prescribed for the first few days. In the absence of psychosis, diazepam is useful for agitation and hyperactivity. The withdrawal depression may be treated with tricyclic antidepressants; here symptomatic treatment may require

Table 2
Diagnostic Criteria for Amphetamine or Similarly Acting Sympathomimetic Delusional Disorder

A. Organic Delusional Syndrome developing shortly after use of amphetamine or a similarly acting sympathomimetic.

B. Rapidly developing persecutory delusions are the predominant clinical feature.

C. Not due to any physical or other mental disorder.

Table from DSM-III-R *Diagnostic and Statistical Manual of Mental Disorders,* ed 3, revised. (Current Classification of Mental Disorders, 1987.) Copyright American Psychiatric Association, Washington, D.C., 1987. Used with permission.

Table 3
Diagnostic Criteria for Amphetamine or Similarly Acting Sympathomimetic Delirium

A. Delirium developing within 24 hours of use of amphetamine or a similarly acting sympathomimetic.

B. Not due to any physical or other mental disorder.

Table from DSM-III-R *Diagnostic and Statistical Manual of Mental Disorders,* ed 3, revised. (Current Classification of Mental Disorders, 1987.) Copyright American Psychiatric Association, Washington, D.C., 1987. Used with permission.

Table 4
Diagnostic Criteria for Amphetamine or Similarly Acting Sympathomimetic Withdrawal

A. Cessation of prolonged (several days or longer) heavy use of amphetamine or a similarly acting sympathomimetic, or reduction in the amount of substance used, followed by dysphoric mood (e.g., depression, irritability, anxiety) and at least one of the following, persisting more than 24 hours after cessation of substance use:

(1) fatigue
(2) insomnia or hypersomnia
(3) psychomotor agitation

B. Not due to any physical or other mental disorder, such as Amphetamine or Similarly Acting Sympathomimetic Delusional Disorder.

Table from DSM-III-R *Diagnostic and Statistical Manual of Mental Disorders,* ed 3, revised. (Current Classification of Mental Disorders, 1987.) Copyright American Psychiatric Association, Washington, D.C., 1987. Used with permission.

weeks, a month, or even longer. The physician should establish a therapeutic alliance to deal with the underlying depression, personality disorder, or both; however, because many of these patients are heavily dependent on the drug, psychotherapy may be especially difficult.

AMPHETAMINE LOOK-ALIKES

Look-alikes are a mixture of three stimulant drugs—caffeine, ephedrine, and propanolamine (PPA)—which, until recently, were sold legally over the counter in the form of tablets designed to resemble, but not duplicate, the appearance of prescription amphetamines. Ephedrine and PPA are still marketed as nasal decongestants, and PPA as an appetite suppressant. Either drug can be dangerous to people suffering from high blood pressure or diabetes and may cause a toxic psychosis after long-term use at high doses. PPA has a relatively narrow safety margin; as little as three or four times the amount in an average tablet can produce a hypertensive crisis.

References

AMA Council on Scientific Affairs: Clinical aspects of amphetamine abuse. JAMA *240*:2317, 1978.

Angrist B, Sothananthan G, Wilk S, Geshon S: Amphetamine psychosis: behavioral or biochemical aspects. J Psychiat Res *11*:13, 1974.

Chiarello R J, Cole J O: The use of psychostimulants in general psychiatry. Arch Gen Psych *44*:286, 1987.

Grinspoon L, Hedblom P: *The Speed Culture: Amphetamine Use and Abuse in America*. Harvard University Press, Cambridge, MA, 1975.

Kalant O J: *The Amphetamine: Toxicity and Addiction*. Charles C Thomas, Springfield, IL, 1966.

Milkman J, Frosch W A: On the preferential abuse of heroin and amphetamines. J Nerv Ment Dis *156*:242, 1973.

McLellon A T, Woody G E, O'Brien C P: Development of psychiatric illness in drug abusers. N Engl J Med *201*:1310, 1979.

Morgan J P: Amphetamine. In *Substance Abuse: Clinical Problems and Perspectives*. p 167, J H Lowinson, P Ruiz, editors. Williams & Wilkins, Baltimore, 1981.

Rapoport J L, Buchsbaum M S, Zahn T P, Weinbarter H, Ludlow C, Mikkelsen E J: Dextroamphetamine: Cognitive and behavioral effects in normal prepubertal boys. Science *199*:560, 1978.

Woods S W, Tesar G E, Murray G B, Cassem N H: Psychostimulant treatment of depressive disorders secondary to medical illness. J Clin Psychiat *47*:12, 1986.

13.7 ————

Hallucinogens and Arylcyclohexylamines

Hallucinogens (also called psychedelics and psychotomimetics) are a class of drugs that produce psychosis-like symptoms including hallucinations, loss of contact with reality, oneiroid states, and other dramatic changes in thinking and feeling. Psychedelic drugs are said to expand or heighten consciousness. Hallucinogens are an ill-defined category of over 100 natural and synthetic drugs. The two best known natural psychedelics are psilocybin, found in mushrooms, and mescaline, found in the peyote cactus.

Synthetic psychedelics include lysergic acid diethylamide (LSD) and dipropyltryptamine (DPT).

Phencyclidine (PCP) and related arylcyclohexylamines are synthetic drugs that in DSM-III-R are classified separately from true psychedelics. Pharmacologically they are known as dissociative anesthetics, but their clinical effects may be indistinguishable from those of psychedelics.

PHARMACOLOGY

Hallucinogens produce such sympathomimetic effects as tremors, tachycardia, hypertension, sweating, blurring of vision, tremors, and mydriasis. They affect the catecholamine system, dopamine, acetylcholine, serotonin, and GABA. There may be specific receptor sites in the brain for some of these drugs, especially PCP and 3, 4-methylenedioxymethamphetamine (MDMA, also known as Ecstasy). LSD has an inhibitory effect on the serotonin-producing neurons of the dorsal raphe, which may account for the hallucinations. In animal models, a single dose of MDMA can reduce striatal serotonin for days.

Humans develop tolerance for the effects of LSD. After 3 or 4 days of use, psychedelic effects are no longer produced; however, they return after several days of abstinence. Tolerance to PCP does not occur. Physical dependency to psychedelics has not been reported, but many persons become psychologically dependent and use the drugs repeatedly for their "mind-expanding experiences."

LSD

The synthetic drug lysergic acid diethylamide (LSD) is related to psychoactive alkaloids found in morning glory seeds, known as lysergic acid amides. Its effects are typical of those of all hallucinogens. Other psychedelic drugs are the natural substances harmine, harmaline, ibogaine, dimethyltryptamine (DMT) and a large number of synthetic drugs with a tryptamine or methoxylated amphetamine structure. A few of these drugs are diethyltryptamine (DET), dipropyltryptamine (DPT), 5-methoxy-3,4-methylenedioxyamphetamine (MMDA), and 2, 5-dimethoxy-4-methylamphetamine (DOM, also known as STP). The average effective dose varies considerably; for example, it is 75 μg of LSD, 3 μg of DOM, 6 μg of psilocybin, 50 μg of DMT, 100 μg of MDA, and 200 μg of mescaline.

Clinical Effects

There are some differences in quality and duration of the subjective effects of these drugs, but LSD produces the widest range of effects and can be taken as a prototype. Onset of effects is usually within an hour of ingestion. For LSD, the effects last from 8 to 12 hours. For other hallucinogens the duration may range from an hour to a day or several days. Physical symptoms include mydriasis, tachycardia, palpitations, diaphoresis, blurred vision, and tremors. The psychological reaction varies with personality, expectations, and setting more than do reactions to other psychoactive drugs, but LSD almost always produces profound alterations in perception, mood, and thinking. Usually, the user realizes that the perceptual alterations are due to the drug. At other times, the person is convinced that he or she is going crazy and fears never regaining sanity. When the user develops a delusional conviction that the disturbed perceptions correspond to reality, DSM-III-R classifies this as hallucinogen delusional disorder. Perceptions become unusually brilliant and intense: colors and textures seem richer, contours sharpened, music more emotionally profound, and smells and tastes heightened. Synesthesia is common; colors may be heard or sounds seen. Changes in body image and alterations of time and space perception also occur. Hallucinations are usually visual, often of geometric forms and figures, but auditory and tactile hallucinations are sometimes experienced. Emotions become unusually intense and may change abruptly and often; two seemingly incompatible feelings may be experienced at one time. Suggestibility is greatly heightened, and sensitivity to nonverbal cues is increased. Exaggerated empathy with or detachment from other people may arise. Other features that often appear are seeming awareness of internal organs, recovery of lost early memories, release of unconscious material in symbolic form, and regression and apparent reliving of past events, including birth. Introspective reflection and feelings of religious and philosophical insight are common. The sense of self is greatly changed, sometimes to the point of depersonalization, merging with the external world, separation of self from body, or total dissolution of the ego in mystical ecstasy. Some drugs, such as MDMA, cause less disorientation and perceptual distortion than LSD.

People sometimes maintain that a single psychedelic experience or a few such experiences have given them increased creative capacity, new psychological insight, relief from neurotic and psychosomatic symptoms, or a desirable change in personality. For many years, especially from 1950 to the mid-1960s, psychiatrists showed great interest in LSD and related drugs as possible drug models of schizophrenia and as therapeutic agents for a wide variety of disorders. Since 1966, it has become impossible to obtain the drugs legally for therapeutic purposes. However, there are renewed attempts to investigate these drugs, especially in light of the recent advances in neurochemistry. Currently MDMA is being used on an experimental basis as an adjunct to psychotherapy.

Adverse Effects

The most common adverse effect of LSD and related drugs is a "bad trip," which resembles the acute panic reaction to cannabis but can be more severe and occasionally produces true psychotic symptoms. The bad trip generally ends when the immediate effects of the drug wear off—in the case of LSD, generally within 8 to 12 hours. However, the course of a bad trip is variable, and occasionally a protracted psychotic episode that is difficult to distinguish from a nonorganic psychotic disorder may ensue. The best treatment is protection, companionship, and reassurance, although occasionally tranquilizers may be required—diazepam, chloral hydrate, or haloperidol in extreme cases. The use of phenothiazine antipsychotics is not recommended, owing to the possible synergistic anticholinergic and CNS-depressant effects. [DSM-III-R lists four disorders associated with hallucinogen use: hallucinogen hallucinosis, delusional disorder, mood disorder, and posthallucinogen perception disorder (Tables 1 through 4).]

Table 1
Diagnostic Criteria for Hallucinogen Hallucinosis

A. Recent use of a hallucinogen.

B. Maladaptive behavioral changes (e.g., marked anxiety or depression, ideas of reference, fear of losing one's mind, paranoid ideation, impaired judgment, impaired social or occupational functioning).

C. Perceptual changes occurring in a state of full wakefulness and alertness (e.g., subjective intensification of perceptions, depersonalization, derealization, illusions, hallucinations, synesthesias).

D. At least two of the following signs:
(1) pupillary dilation
(2) tachycardia
(3) sweating
(4) palpitations
(5) blurring of vision
(6) tremors
(7) incoordination

E. Not due to any physical or other mental disorder.

Table from DSM-III-R, *Diagnostic and Statistical Manual of Mental Disorders*, ed 3, revised. (Current Classification of Mental Disorders, 1987.) Copyright American Psychiatric Association, Washington, D.C., 1987. Used with permission.

Table 2
Diagnostic Criteria for Hallucinogen Delusional Disorder

A. Organic Delusional Syndrome developing shortly after hallucinogen use.

B. Not due to any physical or other mental disorder, such as Schizophrenia.

Table from DSM-III-R, *Diagnostic and Statistical Manual of Mental Disorders*, ed 3, revised. (Current Classification of Mental Disorders, 1987.) Copyright American Psychiatric Association, Washington, D.C., 1987. Used with permission.

Flashback. Another common effect of hallucinogenic drugs is the flashback, a spontaneous transitory recurrence of drug-induced experience that occurs when the subject has taken no drug recently. Most flashbacks are episodes of visual distortion, geometric hallucinations, hallucinations of sounds or voices, false perceptions of movement in peripheral fields, flashes of color, trails of images from moving objects, positive afterimages and halos, macropsia and micropsia, time expansion, physical symptoms, or relived intense emotion lasting usually a few seconds to a few minutes, but sometimes longer. More rarely, paresthesias and echos occur. The flashback is often triggered by emerging from a dark room or by use of cannabis. Sometimes the person can bring flashbacks on voluntarily. Probably about a quarter of all psychedelic drug users have experienced some form of flashback. In DSM-III-R the diagnosis of posthallucinogen perception disorder is made if these flashback symptoms cause marked distress. Most often, even in the presence of distinct perceptual disturbance, the person has insight into the pathologic nature of the disturbance. Approximately 50 percent of those with this perception disorder experience a remission within months; others continue to have symptoms for years. Suicidal behavior, major depression, and panic disorder are complications. There are no significant personal-

Table 3
Diagnostic Criteria for Hallucinogen Mood Disorder

A. Organic Mood Syndrome developing shortly after halluci-nogen use (usually within 1 or 2 weeks), and persisting more than 24 hours after cessation of such use.

B. Not due to any physical or other mental disorder.

Table from DSM-III-R, *Diagnostic and Statistical Manual of Mental Disorders,* ed 3, revised. (Current Classification of Mental Disorders, 1987.) Copyright American Psychiatric Association, Washington, D.C., 1987. Used with permission.

Table 4
Diagnostic Criteria for Posthallucinogen Perception Disorder

A. The reexperiencing, following cessation of use of a hallu-cinogen, of one or more of the perceptual symptoms that were experienced while intoxicated with the hallucinogen (e.g., geometric hallucinations, false perceptions of movement in the peripheral visual fields, flashes of color, intensified colors, trails of images from moving objects, positive afterimages, halos around objects, macropsia, and micropsia).

B. The disturbance in A causes marked distress.

C. Other causes of the symptoms, such as anatomic lesions and infections of the brain, Delirium, Dementia, sensory (visual) epilepsies, Schizophrenia, entoptic imagery, and hypnopompic hallucinations, have been ruled out.

Table from DSM-III-R, *Diagnostic and Statistical Manual of Mental Disorders,* ed 3, revised. (Current Classification of Mental Disorders, 1987.) Copyright American Psychiatric Association, Washington, D.C., 1987. Used with permission.

ity differences on objective tests between those persons who have flashback and those who do not. Flashbacks are more likely to occur in people who are under stress or at a time of diminished ego control, such as when fatigued or ill. Most people can be reassured that the experience will pass, but in cases of extreme agitation or panic, a neuroleptic or an anxiolytic may be necessary. Flashbacks have lasted 24 to 48 hours, and some persist even longer.

Flashbacks may also be experienced in posttraumatic stress disorder. This disorder is associated with a severe, identifiable stressor such as a flood or accident, and there is no relation to previous psychedelic drug experiences. The reliving of the stress in flashback form usually occurs shortly after the event, although it can be delayed for months or even years.

Prolonged Adverse Reactions. These reactions to LSD present the same variety of symptoms as bad trips and flashbacks. They have been classified as mood disorders and delusional disorders; often they resemble prolonged and more or less attenuated bad trips. Most of these adverse reactions end after 24 to 48 hours, but sometimes they last weeks or even months. Psychedelic drugs are capable of magnifying and bringing into consciousness almost any internal conflict, so there is no typical prolonged adverse reaction to LSD, as there is a typical amphetamine delusional disorder. Instead, many different mood, neurotic, and psychotic symptoms may appear, depending on individual forms of vul-nerability. This lack of specificity makes it difficult to distinguish between LSD reactions and unrelated pathological processes, es-

pecially when some time passes between the drug trip and the onset of the disturbance.

The most likely candidates for adverse reactions are persons with schizoid and prepsychotic personalities, an unstable ego bal-ance, and a great deal of anxiety. Such persons cannot cope with the perceptual changes, body-image distortions, and symbolic, unconscious material produced by the drug trip. There is a very high rate of previous mental instability in persons hospitalized for LSD reactions. In the late 1960s a number of adverse reactions occurred because LSD was being promoted as a self-prescribed psychotherapy for emotional crises in the lives of seriously dis-turbed people. Because that is happening less today, prolonged adverse reactions are rarely seen now.

The treatment for prolonged reactions to psychedelic drugs is the same as the treatment for similar symptoms not produced by drugs: an appropriate form of psychotherapy and, if necessary, minor tranquilizers or antidepressants. Antipsychotics used in the past carry a greater risk and are recommended only when the hallucinogen-induced episode is protracted suggesting that a nonorganic psychosis may be present.

Other Aspects

Long-term psychedelic drug use is not very common. There is no physical addiction, and although psychological dependence occurs, it is rare because each LSD experience is different and there is no reliable euphoria. Tolerance to these drugs develops quickly but also disappears rapidly after 2 or 3 days. There is no clear evidence of drastic personality change or chronic psychosis pro-duced by long-term LSD use in users not otherwise predisposed to these conditions. It is likely, however, that some heavy psychedelic drug users, like other heavy drug users, suffer from chronic anxi-ety, depression, or feelings of inadequacy. In these cases, the drug abuse is a symptom rather than the central problem.

A persistent issue has been the question of whether halluci-nogens cause gene damage and birth defects. Available evidence suggests that LSD produces no chromosome damage in reproduc-tive cells of a kind that is likely to cause birth defects; the same is true of other psychedelic drugs to the extent that they have been tested. There is also no evidence of teratogenicity at normal doses in humans. Nevertheless, all drugs should be avoided if possible during pregnancy, especially in the early stages when the embryo is most vulnerable.

VOLATILE SOLVENTS

Among abused volatile solvents are gasoline, varnish remover, lighter fluid, airplane glue, rubber cement, clean-ing fluid, and aerosols (especially spray paints). The active ingredients include toluene, acetone, benzene, and halogen-ated hydrocarbons. Since these substances are legal, cheap, and accessible, they are used mostly by the young (ages 6 to 16 years) and the poor, who inhale them from a tube, a can, a plastic bag, or a rag held over the nose. Intoxication often comes on within 5 minutes, and it usually lasts 15 to 30 minutes. Neither volatile solvents nor psychedelics, can be detected in urine. Solvents produce a central depressant effect (the initial effects being disinhibitory and the later effects, inhibitory) characterized by euphoria, excitement, a

Table 5
Diagnostic Criteria for Inhalant Intoxication

A. Recent use of an inhalant.

B. Maladaptive behavioral changes (e.g., belligerence, assaultiveness, apathy, impaired judgment, impaired social or occupational functioning).

C. At least two of the following signs:
    (1) dizziness
    (2) nystagmus
    (3) incoordination
    (4) slurred speech
    (5) unsteady gait
    (6) lethargy
    (7) depressed reflexes
    (8) psychomotor retardation
    (9) tremor
    (10) generalized muscle weakness
    (11) blurred vision or diplopia
    (12) stupor or coma
    (13) euphoria

D. Not due to any physical or other mental disorder.

Table from DSM-III-R, *Diagnostic and Statistical Manual of Mental Disorders*, ed 3, revised. (Current Classification of Mental Disorders, 1987.) Copyright American Psychiatric Association, Washington, D.C., 1987. Used with permission.

floating sensation, dizziness, slurred speech, ataxia, and a sense of heightened power. Solvents may cause inhalant intoxication, consisting of apathy, diminished social and occupational function, and impaired judgment leading to impulsive and aggressive behavior; there may also be amnesia for the period of intoxication. Other acute effects are nausea, anorexia, nystagmus, depressed reflexes, diplopia, and, with high doses, stupor and even unconsciousness (Table 5). Deaths may be caused by central respiratory depression, asphyxiation, or accident. Inhalants often leave visible external evidence, such as a rash around the nose and mouth, breath odors, and residue on the face, hands, and clothing. Irritation of the eyes is common, as well as of the throat, lungs, and nose.

It is not yet clear whether there is a withdrawal reaction, but substantial tolerance develops after repeated sniffing. A serious risk is irreversible damage to the liver, kidney, and other organs from benzene and halogenated hydrocarbons. Peripheral neuritis has also been reported. Permanent neuromuscular and brain damage must be considered a possibility, particularly because inhalants often contain high concentrations of copper, zinc, and heavy metals. There are some reports of brain atrophy and chronic motor impairment in toluene users.

According to DSM-III-R, excluded from the classification of inhalant intoxication are anesthetic gases (e.g., nitrous oxide, ether), and short-acting vasodilators such as the amyl- and butylnitrites. These substances are excluded because the intoxication associated with them is different clinically from inhalant intoxication and they are generally used by a population who are quite different from those who abuse inhalants. Use of these, or other substances, would in DSM-III-R be classified under other or unspecified psychoactive substance organic mental disorder.

PHENCYCLIDINE (PCP)

History

Phencyclidine, 1-(1-phenylcyclohexy 1) piperidine was first investigated for its properties as an intravenous surgical anesthetic and as a general preoperative and postoperative analgesic. Because of a severe emergence syndrome characterized by disorientation, agitation, and delirium, the drug is now available for veterinary use only. PCP first appeared in San Francisco, in 1967, as a street drug known as the "peace pill." Widespread use began in the 1970s and continues today. Although it may be taken orally, intravenously, or by sniffing, it is usually sprinkled onto a parsley or marijuana cigarette and smoked, as this is the best means of self-titration. Street names include angel dust, crystal, peace, peace weed, super grass, super weed, hog, rocket fuel, and horse trancks.

By-products of PCP

Phencyclidine is relatively cheap and easy to synthesize in the garage laboratory. This provides a powerful incentive for street chemists, whose illicit products are not always pure PCP. One very common contaminant is 1-piperidinocyclo-hexanecarbonitrile (PCC), a by-product of illicit syntheis, that on decomposition releases hydrogen cyanide in small amounts. Another of its degradation products, piperidine, has a strong fishy odor. There are about 30 chemical analogues of PCP, some of which have appeared on the illicit market. Another related drug is ketamine (Ketalar), a short acting anesthetic with psychoactive properties similar to those of phencyclidine.

Psychological Effects

There is great variation in the amount of PCP from cigarette to cigarette; 1 g may be used to make as few as four or as many as several dozen cigarettes. This variability, together with the extreme uncertainty of PCP content in street samples, makes it difficult to predict the effect, which also depends on the setting and the user's previous experience. Onset may occur within 5 minutes. Less than 5 mg of phencyclidine is considered a low dose, and doses above 10 mg are considered high. Convulsions, coma, and possible death are associated generally with doses of 20 mg or more. Experienced users report that the effects of 2 to 3 mg of smoked PCP are felt within 5 minutes and plateau within half an hour. Users are frequently uncommunicative, appear oblivious, and report active fantasy production. They experience "speedy" feelings, euphoria, bodily warmth, tingling, peaceful floating sensations, and, occasionally, feelings of depersonalization, isolation, and estrangement. Sometimes there are auditory and visual hallucinations. There are often striking alterations of body image, distortions of space and time perception, and delusions. There may be intensification of dependency feelings as well as confusion and disorganization of thought. The user may be sympathetic, sociable, and talkative at one moment, hostile and negative at another. Anxiety is also sometimes reported; it is often the most prominent presenting symptom in an adverse reaction. Sometimes observed are head-rolling movements, stroking, grimacing, muscle rigidity on stimulation, repeated episodes of vomiting, and repetitive, chanting speech. The high lasts 3 to 6 hours and sometimes

Table 6

Diagnostic Criteria for Phencyclidine (PCP) or Similarly Acting Arylcyclohexylamine Intoxication

A. Recent use of phencyclidine or a similarly acting arylcyclohexylamine.

B. Maladaptive behavioral changes (e.g., belligerence, assaultiveness, impulsiveness, unpredictability, psychomotor agitation, impaired judgment, impaired social or occupational functioning).

C. Within an hour (less when smoked, insufflated ["snorted"], or used intravenously), at least two of the following signs:
   (1) vertical or horizontal nystagmus
   (2) increased blood pressure or heart rate
   (3) numbness or diminished responsiveness to pain
   (4) ataxia
   (5) dysarthria
   (6) muscle rigidity
   (7) seizures
   (8) hyperacusis

D. Not due to any physical or other mental disorder (e.g., Phencyclidine (PCP) or Similarly Acting Arylcyclohexylamine Delirium.

Table from DSM-III-R, *Diagnostic and Statistical Manual of Mental Disorders,* ed 3, revised. (Current Classification of Mental Disorders, 1987.) Copyright American Psychiatric Association, Washington, D.C., 1987. Used with permission.

gives way to a mild depression in which the user may become irritable, somewhat paranoid, and occasionally belligerent, irrationally assaultive, suicidal, or homicidal (Table 6). Effects can last for several days. Users sometimes find that it takes 24 to 48 hours to recover completely from the high; laboratory tests show that PCP may remain in the blood and urine for more than a week.

Adverse Effects

Mild cases of adverse phencyclidine reaction or overdose usually do not come to medical attention. When they do, they are often treated in the outpatient department. Low-dose symptoms are quite variable and may range from mild euphoria and restlessness to increasing levels of anxiety, fear, confusion, and agitation. These patients may exhibit difficulty in communication, a blank, staring expression, disordered thinking, depression, and occasionally violent, self-destructive behavior. If the symptoms are not severe and if one can be certain that enough time has elapsed so that all PCP has been absorbed (in those cases where the drug is ingested), the patient may be monitored for an hour or so in the outpatient department and, if the symptoms improve, released to family or friends. Even at low doses, however, symptoms on the more disturbed end of this continuum may worsen, requiring that the person be hospitalized.

Chronic Use. As with the other effects of phencyclidine intoxication, neurological and physiological symptoms are dose related. Among the common symptoms seen in Emergency Rooms are hypertension, increased pulse rate, and nystagmus (horizontal, vertical, or both). At low doses, there may be dysarthria, gross ataxia, and muscle rigidity, particularly of the face and neck.

Increased deep tendon reflexes and diminished response to pain are commonly observed. Higher doses may lead to hyperthermia, agitated and repetitive movement, athetosis or clonic jerking of the extremities, and occasionally opisthotonic posturing. Involuntary isometric muscle activity can lead to acute rhabdomyolysis, myoglobinuria, and kidney failure. With even larger doses patients may be drowsy, stuporous with eyes open, comatose, and, in some instances, responsive only to noxious stimuli. Clonic movements and muscle rigidity may sometimes precede generalized seizure activity, and status epilepticus has been reported. Cheyne-Stokes breathing has also been observed; respiratory arrest can occur and can be fatal. Vomiting, probably of central origin, may occur; hypersalivation and diaphoresis are occasional symptoms, and ptosis, usually bilateral, has been observed.

Although some patients may be brought to psychiatric attention within hours of ingesting PCP, it is not at all uncommon for 2 to 3 days to elapse before psychiatric help is sought. The long interval between drug ingestion and appearance at the clinic usually reflects the attempts of friends to deal with the psychosis through "talking down"; persons who lose consciousness appear earlier than those who remain conscious. While most recover completely within a day or 2, some remain psychotic for as long as 2 weeks. Patients who are first seen in coma often manifest disorientation, hallucinations, confusion, and difficulty in communication upon regaining consciousness. These symptoms may also be seen in noncomatose patients, but they appear to be less severe. A PCP psychotic patient also commonly manifests the following symptoms: staring into space, echolalia, posturing, sleep disturbance, paranoid ideation, depression, and a behavior disorder. Sometimes, the behavioral disturbance is quite severe; it may include public masturbation, stripping off clothes, violence, urinary incontinence, crying, and inappropriate laughing. Frequently, there is amnesia for the entire period of the psychosis. See Tables 7 through 10 for different organic mental disorders associated with PCP use.

Some observers believe that PCP psychosis is seriously underdiagnosed because toxic symptoms indicating the presence of a drug are often not obvious, and the most commonly used tests for PCP in blood and urine are unreliable.

Treatment

Depending on the patient's status at the time of admission, the differential diagnosis may include sedative or narcotic overdose, psychosis as a consequence of the use of psychedelic drugs, and brief reactive psychosis. Laboratory analysis may be helpful in establishing the diagnosis, particularly in the many cases where the drug history is unreliable or unattainable. Treatment of acute PCP intoxication can have potentially severe complications and often must be

Table 7

Diagnostic Criteria for Phencylidine (PCP) or Similarly Acting Arylcyclohexylamine Delirium

A. Delirium developing shortly after use of phencyclidine or a similarly acting arylcyclohexylamine.

B. Not due to any physical or other mental disorder.

Table from DSM-III-R, *Diagnostic and Statistical Manual of Mental Disorders,* ed 3, revised. (Current Classification of Mental Disorders, 1987.) Copyright American Psychiatric Association, Washington, D.C., 1987. Used with permission.

Table 8
Diagnostic Criteria for Phencyclindine (PCP) or Similarly Acting Arylcyclohexylamine Mood Disorder

A. Organic Mood Syndrome developing shortly after use of phencyclidine or a similarly acting arylcyclohexylamine (usually within 1 or 2 weeks) and persisting more than 24 hours after cessation of substance use.

B. Not due to any physical or other mental disorder.

Table from DSM-III-R, *Diagnostic and Statistical Manual of Mental Disorders*, ed 3, revised. (Current Classification of Mental Disorders, 1987.) Copyright American Psychiatric Association, Washington, D.C., 1987. Used with permission.

Table 9
Diagnostic Criteria for Phencyclidine (PCP) or Similarly Acting Arylcyclohexylamine Delusional Disorder

A. Organic Delusional Syndrome developing shortly after use of phencyclidine or a similarly acting arylcyclohexylamine, or emerging up to a week after an overdose.

B. Not due to any physical or other mental disorder, such as Schizophrenia.

Table from DSM-III-R, *Diagnostic and Statistical Manual of Mental Disorders*, ed 3, revised. (Current Classification of Mental Disorders, 1987.) Copyright American Psychiatric Association, Washington, D.C., 1987. Used with permission.

Table 10
Diagnostic Criteria for Phencyclidine (PCP) or Similarly Acting Arylcyclohexylamine Organic Mental Disorder not Otherwise Specified

A. Recent use of phencyclidine or a similarly acting arylcyclohexylamine.

B. The resulting illness involves features of several Organic Mental Syndromes or a progression from one Organic Mental Syndrome to another (e.g., initially there is Delirium, followed by an Organic Delusional Syndrome).

C. Not due to any physical or other mental disorder.

Table from DSM-III-R, *Diagnostic and Statistical Manual of Mental Disorders*, ed 3, revised. (Current Classification of Mental Disorders, 1987.) Copyright American Psychiatric Association, Washington, D.C., 1987. Used with permission.

considered a psychiatric emergency. Unconscious patients must be carefully monitored, particularly those who are toxic with PCP, because the excessive secretions may interfere with already compromised respiration. In an alert patient who has recently taken PCP, gastric lavage presents a risk of inducing laryngeal spasm and aspiration of emesis. Muscle spasm and seizures are best treated with diazepam. The environment should afford minimal sensory stimulation; reassurance or talking down is generally useless. Ideally, one person stays with the patient in a quiet, dark room. Four-point restraint is dangerous, because it may lead to rhadomyolysis; total body immobilization may occasionally be necessary. Diazepam is often effective in reducing agitation, but a patient with severe behavioral disturbance may require short-term antipsychotic medication; some clinicians recommend haloperidol rather than a phenothiazine

because PCP is somewhat anticholinergic, and because illegal drugs are often contaminated with belladonna alkaloids. A hypotensive drug, such as phentolamine, may occasionally be needed. Ammonium chloride at the acute stage and ascorbic acid or cranberry juice later on are used to acidify the urine and promote elimination of the drug.

PCP intoxication can lead to death due to hyperpyrexia and other autonomic instability. Intravenous benzodiazepines are an effective treatment for such patients.

Long-Term Effects

The street term "crystallized" is sometimes applied to chronic PCP users who seem to suffer from dulled thinking and reflexes, loss of memory and impulse control, depression, lethargy, and difficulty in concentrating. There is no clear evidence of permanent brain damage, but neurologic and cognitive dysfunction has been reported in chronic users even after 2 to 3 weeks of abstinence. Tolerance and a withdrawal reaction consisting of lethargy, depression, and craving have been reported.

References

Claridge G: Animal models of schizophrenia: The case for LSD-25. Schizophr Bull *4*:186, 1978.

Cohen S: Lysergic acid diethylamide: Side effects and complications. J Nerv Ment Dis *130*:30, 1960.

Domino E F, editor: *PCP (Phencyclidine): Historical and Current Perspectives*. NPP Books, Ann Arbor, 1981.

Fauman M A, Fauman B J: *The Psychiatric Aspects of Chronic Phencyclidine Use: A Study of Chronic PCP Users*, NIDA Research Monograph 21. U.S. Government Printing Office, Washington, DC, 1978.

Grinspoon L, Bakalar J B: *Psychedelic Drugs Reconsidered*. Basic Books, New York, 1979.

Luisada P V: Phencyclidine. In *Substance Abuse: Clinical Problems and Perspectives*, p 209. J M Lowinson, R Ruiz, editors. Williams & Wilkins, Baltimore, 1981.

Petersen L C, Stillman R C, editors: *Phencyclidine (PCP) Abuse: An Appraisal*, NIDA Research Monograph 21. US Government Printing Office, Washington, DC, 1978.

Stillman R C, Willette R E, editors: *The Pharmacology of Hallucinogens*. Pergamon Press, New York, 1978.

Strassman R J: Adverse reactions to psychedelic drugs: A review of the literature. J Nerv Ment Dis *172*:577, 1984.

Vardy M, Kay S: LSD psychosis or LSD-induced schizophrenia? Arch Gen Psychiatry *40*:877, 1983.

13.8 _____
Marijuana

HISTORY

Known for thousands of years as a medicine and intoxicant, marijuana was widely used in the 19th century as an analgesic, anticonvulsant, and hypnotic. Recently, interest has developed in using it to treat glaucoma and the nausea produced by cancer chemotherapy; it may also have antineoplastic and antibiotic properties. One of marijuana's nonpsychoactive constituents, cannabidiol, may also prove useful as an anticonvulsant, yet marijuana has been valued throughout history mainly as a euphoriant.

EPIDEMIOLOGY

Over 40 million Americans have used marijuana at some time in their lives, and about 10 million use the drug regularly. Throughout the world, about 200 million people are regular users. A 1985 survey showed that 5 percent of high school seniors use the drug regularly. It is the most widely abused illegal drug in the country. Marijuana is known as a gateway drug because it leads to use of other drugs, particularly cocaine.

PREPARATIONS

Drug preparations from the hemp plant, *Cannabis sativa*, vary widely in quality and potency. The plant's resin contains the active substances. The drug can be taken as a drink or in foods, but in this country it is usually smoked, either in a pipe or in a cigarette called a "joint." Preparations of the drug come in three grades, identified by Indian names. The cheapest and least potent grade, called *bhang,* is derived from the cut tops of uncultivated plants and has a low resin content. Much of the marijuana smoked in the United States is of this grade. *Ganja,* the second grade, is obtained from the flowering tops and leaves of carefully selected cultivated plants, and it has a higher quality and quantity of resin than bhang. More cannabis of this strength is now available in the United States. The third and highest grade, called *charas* in India, is made largely from the resin itself, obtained from the tops of mature plants; only this version is properly called "hashish." Marijuana is also known as grass, pot, Mary Jane, tea, and weed.

Many derivatives of cannabinol have been prepared. The active constituents of the resin are various isomers of tetrahydrocannabinol; the most important as an intoxicant is Δ-9-tetrahydrocannabinol (THC). The metabolite 11-hydroxy THC is more active than the parent compound.

CLINICAL EFFECTS

Psychological effects of cannabis (a general term for the psychoactive products of the plant) include euphoria, oneiroid states, calmness, and drowsiness. DSM-III-R classifies this disorder as cannabis intoxication (Table 1). Intoxication occurs almost immediately after smoking marijuana, peaks within 30 minutes and lasts for 2 to 4 hours. The effects from ingestion continue for 5 to 12 hours. The intoxication heightens sensitivity to external stimuli, reveals details that would ordinarily be overlooked, makes colors seem brighter and richer, and subjectively enhances the appreciation of art and music. Time seems to slow down, and more seems to happen in each moment. There is an increase in appetite as well as conjunctival injection, tachycardia, and dry mouth.

Curiously, there is often a splitting of consciousness; while they are experiencing the high, the smokers are at the same time objective observers of their own intoxication. They may have paranoid thoughts, yet at the same time, laugh at them. Depersonalization and derealization may occur. This ability to retain objectivity may explain why many experienced users manage to behave in a perfectly

Table 1
Diagnostic Criteria for Cannabis Intoxication

A. Recent use of cannabis.

B. Maladaptive behavioral changes (e.g., euphoria, anxiety, suspiciousness or paranoid ideation, sensation of slowed time, impaired judgment, social withdrawal).

C. At least two of the following signs developing within 2 hours of cannabis use:
   (1) conjunctival injection
   (2) increased appetite
   (3) dry mouth
   (4) tachycardia

D. Not due to any physical or other mental disorder.

Table from DSM-III-R, *Diagnostic and Statistical Manual of Mental Disorders,* ed 3, revised. (Current Classification of Mental Disorders, 1987.) Copyright American Psychiatric Association, Washington, D.C., 1987. Used with permission.

sober fashion in public even when they are highly intoxicated.

Marijuana, which with very high blood levels acts as a hallucinogen, produces some of the same effects as lysergic acid diethylamide (LSD) and LSD–type substances: distorted perception of body parts, spatial and temporal distortion, increased sensitivity to sound, synesthesia, heightened suggestibility, and a deeper sense of awareness. Marijuana can also cause anxiety and paranoid reactions. The agonizingly nightmarish reactions that even the experienced LSD user may endure, however, rarely seem to afflict the experienced marijuana smoker, who is using a far less potent drug and has much closer and more continuous control over its effects. Marijuana lacks the powerful consciousness-altering qualities of LSD, mescaline, and psilocybin; therefore it is doubtful whether the average doses of marijuana used in this country can ever produce true hallucinations. Cannabis tends to sedate, whereas LSD and the LSD–type drugs often induce wakefulness and even restlessness. Unlike LSD, marijuana does not dilate the pupils or raise blood pressure, reflexes, and body temperature. Tolerance rapidly develops with LSD–type drugs, but it develops much more slowly, if at all, with marijuana. Adverse reactions from cannabis intoxication are more likely to occur in persons with rigid personalities or a history of psychosis or in potentially threatening circumstances.

Cannabis Dependence

There are some indications of tolerance and a mild withdrawal reaction after frequent use of high doses. However, there is no clinical evidence that withdrawal symptoms, or a need to increase the dose, present any serious problem to users. Craving or difficulty in withdrawal can occur as part of a pattern of pathological use. An abstinence syndrome of sleep disturbances, nausea, vomiting, tremors, and sweating has been observed.

Chronic Use

Chronic heavy use has been said to cause an *amotivational syndrome* characterized by the person's unwillingness to persist at a task, be it school, work, or any activity that requires prolonged attention or tenacity. Such persons become apathetic and anergic, usually gain weight, and have been described as slothful. Reports by many investigators, particularly in Egypt and in parts of the Orient, indicate that long-term users of the potent versions of cannabis are passive, unproductive, and lacking in ambition. This finding suggests that chronic use of the drug in its stronger forms may have debilitating effects, as does prolonged heavy drinking. Chronic marijuana use may cause various syndromes, which are described below.

Psychoses. Hemp insanity or cannabis psychosis has been reported mainly in India, Egypt, and Morocco—more often in the late 19th and early 20th centuries than today. It is described as a prolonged psychosis caused mainly by chronic heavy use of the drug. This phenomenon, however, has not been reported among marijuana smokers in the United States. Several studies of large sample populations of marijuana users have found no evidence of a cannabis psychosis produced de novo in well integrated, stable persons.

Cannabis Delirium. Cannabis may precipitate delirium characterized by clouding of consciousness, restlessness, confusion, bewilderment, disorientation, oneiroid thinking, apprehension, fear, illusions, and hallucinations. Toxic delirium generally requires a rather large ingested dose of cannabis; the reaction is very rare when cannabis is smoked. This may be because the active substances are not absorbed fast enough, or perhaps in the process of smoking, the cannabinol derivatives most likely to precipitate this syndrome are modified in some way as yet unknown. In DSM-III-R, there is also a classification of an organic delusional syndrome called cannabis delusional disorder (Table 2) which is characterized by persecutory delusions developing shortly after use. Associated features are listed as marked anxiety, lability, depersonalization, and possible amnesia for the episode. The delusional disorder is rare and remits within a day, but may persist for a few days.

Anxiety. Cannabis users may also suffer short-lived, acute anxiety states, sometimes accompanied by paranoid thoughts. The anxiety may become so intense as to be called panic. Although uncommon, panic is probably the most frequent adverse reaction to the moderate use of smoked marijuana. The sufferer may believe that body-image distortions mean illness or possible death or may interpret psychological changes induced by the drug as an indication of loss of sanity. Rarely, the panic becomes incapacitating; it usually lasts for a relatively short time. Simple reassurance is the best treatment. The likelihood of panic varies directly with the dose and inversely with the user's experience; thus, the most vulnerable persons are the inexperienced users who inadvertently, because they lack familiarity with the drug, take a large dose that produces perceptual and somatic changes for which they are unprepared.

Flashback. One rather rare reaction to cannabis is the flashback, a spontaneous recurrence of drug symptoms when not intoxicated. Some reports suggest that this effect may occur in marijuana users even without prior use of any other drug. In general, however, flashbacks seem to arise only when people use more powerful hallucinogenic or psychedelic drugs and then smoke marijuana at a later time. When the flashbacks follow a history of hallucinogen use, they would be classified under posthallucinogen perception disorder.

Physical Effects. The main physical effects are reddening of the conjunctiva and a dose-related increase in heart rate. The ratio of lethal to effective dose is estimated to be in the range of

Table 2
Diagnostic Criteria for Cannabis Delusional Disorder

A. Organic Delusional Syndrome developing shortly after cannabis use.

B. Not due to any physical or other mental disorder.

Table from DSM-III-R, *Diagnostic and Statistical Manual of Mental Disorders*, ed 3, revised. (Current Classification of Mental Disorders, 1987.) Copyright American Psychiatric Association, Washington, D.C., 1987. Used with permission.

20,000 to 1 to 40,000 to 1. There is no adequately documented case of a fatality in a human being.

A great deal of recent research on cannabis has been concerned with possible adverse physical effects of chronic use. There have been studies of cerebral atrophy, seizure susceptibility, chromosome damage and birth defects, impairment of immune response, and effects on testosterone and the menstrual cycle. Results generally have been contradictory and inconclusive. Nevertheless, irregular menstrual cycles and decreased testosterone have been reported with chronic use. Clinical observation of marijuana users, including recent studies of long-term users in the Caribbean and Greece, shows no evidence of disease or organic pathology attributable to any of these causes.

The only well documented adverse effects of chronic marijuana use are produced in the lungs. Mild airway constriction and emphysema are reported in studies of both animals and human beings. Marijuana smoke also contains many of the same carcinogenic hydrocarbons as tobacco smoke. Chronic respiratory disease and lung cancer have to be considered as dangers for long-term heavy users.

THC has been used successfully to combat nausea associated with anticancer drugs; its use for that purpose is approved by the FDA. There are no other medical uses except for some reports of reduced intraocular pressure in glaucoma patients.

TREATMENT

There is no specific treatment for cannabis abuse. If the person uses the substance for anxiety reduction or for the alleviation of depression, an antianxiety agent or an antidepressant should be considered as substitution therapy. For an acute anxiety reaction to the drug, diazepam is useful.

Educating persons about the amotivational syndrome and the possible complications may dissuade some from using the drug in the first place. There is a strong movement to legalize marijuana in this country that has met with limited success.

References

Council on Scientific Affairs: Marijuana: Its health hazards and therapeutic potentials. JAMA *246*:1823, 1981.
Grinspoon L: Marijuana. Sci Am *221*:17, 1969.
Grinspoon L: Effects of marijuana. Hosp Commun Psychiatry *34*:307, 1983.
Jones R T: Cannabis and health. Ann Rev Med *34*:247, 1983.
Relmon A, editor: *Marijuana and Health*. Institute of Medicine, National Academy Press, Washington, DC, 1982.
Schwartz R H, Hawks R L: Toward optimal laboratory use: Laboratory detection of marijuana use. JAMA *254*:788, 1985.
Teitel B: Observations on marijuana withdrawal. Am J Psychiatry *134*:587, 1977.
Weller R A: Marijuana. Med Aspects Human Sexuality *19*:92, 1985.
Weller R A, Halikas J A: Change in effects from marijuana: A five-to-six year study. J Clin Psychiatry *43*:362, 1983.

13.9 _____

Caffeine and Nicotine (Tobacco) Dependence

CAFFEINE

Caffeine is in use throughout the world and is present in a great variety of forms—coffee, tea, cola drinks, cocoa, chocolate, and over-the-counter (OTC) cold preparations (Table 1). About 30 percent of adult Americans use coffee. Children are exposed to caffeine in certain soft drinks and in chocolate.

Clinical Effects

A rough guide to calculating caffeine intake is as follows: 100 to 150 mg of caffeine per cup of coffee; tea is about half as strong; a glass of cola is about one third as strong. Most prescription drugs and OTC medications containing caffeine are one third to one half the strength of a cup of coffee. Two exceptions to this are migraine medications and OTC stimulants that contain 100 mg per tablet. The clinical effects of an acute dose of caffeine (50 to 100 mg) include increased alertness, sense of well-being, and improved

Table 1
Some Common Sources of Caffeine

Source	Approximate Amounts of Caffeine per Unit*
Beverages	
Brewed coffee	80–140 mg per cup
Instant coffee	66–100 mg per cup
Tea (leaf)	30–75 mg per cup
Tea (bagged)	42–100 mg per cup
Decaffeinated coffee	2–4 mg per cup
Cola drinks	25–55 mg per glass
Cocoa	5–50 mg per cup
Prescription medications	
A.P.C.s (aspirin, phen- acetin, caffeine)	32 mg per tablet
Cafergot	100 mg per tablet
Darvon compound	32 mg per tablet
Fiorinal	40 mg per tablet
Migral	50 mg per tablet
Over-the-counter analgesics	
Anacin, aspirin compound, Bromo-Seltzer	32 mg per tablet
Cope, Easy-Mens, Empirin compound, Midol	32 mg per tablet
Vanquish	32 mg per tablet
Excedrin	60 mg per tablet
Pre-Mens	66 mg per tablet
Many over-the-counter cold preparations	30 mg per tablet
Many over-the-counter stimulants	100–200 mg per tablet
Small chocolate bar	25 mg per bar

*Cup = 5–6 ounces; cola drinks = 8–12 ounces.

verbal and motor performance. It is because of these effects that persons become psychologically dependent on caffeine. In addition, caffeine produces diuresis, cardiac muscle stimulation, increased peristalsis, gastric acid secretion, and blood pressure elevation.

Tolerance. Chronic users develop tolerance to the effects of caffeine. The average adult American consumes more than 500 mg of caffeine a day, but usually in the markedly diluted form of brewed coffee. The plasma half-life varies from 3 to 10 hours; peak plasma concentrations occur at about 30 minutes after absorption. Caffeine intake over 500 mg increases the risk of developing intoxication; however, some persons can consume 2 to 3 g per day without complaints.

Neuropharmacology. Caffeine causes various pharmacological changes in the nervous system, including sensitization of dopamine receptors, antagonism of adenosine receptors, and antagonism of benzodiazepine receptors. In addition, a noncaffeine component of coffee (not found in tea or cocoa) has been reported to have opiate receptor–antagonist activity.

Caffeine Intoxication

Signs of caffeine intoxication include anxiety, psychomotor agitation and restlessness, irritability, and such psychophysiological complaints as muscle twitching, flushed face, nausea, diuresis, gastrointestinal complaints, and insomnia (Table 2). Intoxication can occur with daily doses of as little as 250 mg of caffeine, but most people require much larger doses. At levels of more than 1 g per day, there may be rambling flow of thought and speech, cardiac arrhythmia, inexhaustibility, and agitation. Tinnitus and flashes of light have been reported. With doses of 10 g or higher, grand mal seizures and respiratory failure can lead to death. Caffeine can produce peptic ulcer and hematemesis, as well as marked hypotension and circulatory failure.

Caffeine Withdrawal

In about 25 percent of persons, the primary sign of abrupt cessation of caffeine intake is a withdrawal headache characterized by a steady or throbbing pain that is relieved by caffeine. The headache usually appears 15 to 18 hours after the last dose. Lethargy, irritability, anhedonia, and depression may also occur. The higher the daily intake, the greater the likelihood that depression will appear as a withdrawal sign.

Chronic Use

Chronic caffeine use stimulates gastric hyperacidity, which can aggravate ulcer disease and can lead to the development of cardiac arrhythmias. Some studies have demonstrated that the elimination of caffeine produces improvement in women with fibrocystic disease. Chronic excessive users have been misdiagnosed as suffering from generalized anxiety disorder and have been treated unnecessarily with antianxiety agents.

Diagnosis and Treatment

Caffeine intoxication or withdrawal is diagnosed on the basis of a detailed history to confirm significant caffeine intake. The patient's report should include caffeine sources other than coffee in addition to signs and symptoms of anxiety, in the case of intoxica-

Table 2
Diagnostic Criteria for Caffeine Intoxication

A. Recent consumption of caffeine, usually in excess of 250 mg.

B. At least five of the following signs:

   (1) restlessness
   (2) nervousness
   (3) excitement
   (4) insomnia
   (5) flushed face
   (6) diuresis
   (7) gastrointestinal disturbance
   (8) muscle twitching
   (9) rambling flow of thought and speech
   (10) tachycardia or cardiac arrhythmia
   (11) periods of inexhaustibility
   (12) psychomotor agitation

C. Not due to any physical or other mental disorder, such as an Anxiety Disorder.

Table from DSM-III-R, *Diagnostic and Statistical Manual of Mental Disorders,* ed 3, revised. (Current Classification of Mental Disorders, 1987.) Copyright American Psychiatric Association, Washington, D.C., 1987. Used with permission.

tion, and headache or lethargy in the case of withdrawal. The clinician needs to rule out general anxiety disorders, mood disorder, sleep disorder, and thyroid disease, all of which may coexist.

Treatment consists of abstinence, which can be accomplished if the person is highly motivated. Anxiolytics are not indicated except in rare cases, and simple analgesics, such as aspirin, may be used to treat headache. Water and decaffeinated coffee and soft drinks can be substituted for caffeinated beverages. Withdrawal usually takes 4 to 5 days.

NICOTINE

Nicotine is used worldwide and is consumed by about 30 percent of the American population in the form of cigarettes. Although the overall percentage of smoking adults has decreased, the percentage of female, teenage, and black smokers is rising. Cigarette smoking has been implicated in a variety of illnesses, primarily lung cancer, emphysema, and cardiovascular disease. There has been an increase in the use of chewing tobacco and snuff among some segments of the population, primarily teenagers, and both have been implicated in oropharyngeal cancer. There is no doubt that cigarettes and cigarette smoke inflict physical damage on the nicotine addict.

Pharmacology of Nicotine

Nicotine is highly toxic, and an overdose of 60 mg is fatal. The average cigarette contains 0.5 mg of nicotine. The physiological effects of nicotine include (1) vasoconstriction of peripheral blood vessels, (2) increased peristalsis, (3) increased catecholamine output with norepinephrine and epinephrine release, (4) stimulation of the hypothalamic pleasure center, which may account for the habitual use of the drug, (5) decreased metabolic rate, (6) REM sleep changes, and (7) tremor. Women who smoke are reported to have low-birth-weight babies. An occasional case of nicotine poisoning may be seen, consisting of excessive salivation, abdominal pain, vomiting, tachycardia, mental confusion, and headache.

Nicotine Dependence

Dependence on nicotine develops quickly. After smoking just one cigarette, approximately 85 percent of persons continue to smoke. The average smoker uses 20 to 30 cigarettes per day. Dependence is also reinforced by psychosocial factors. For example, among adolescent girls, smoking is associated with being rebellious or with peer group pressure to smoke. For adults, smoking is often associated with pleasurable events, such as parties, dinners, and sex. Other reinforcers include smoking paraphernalia and advertising. Smokers differ from nonsmokers psychosocially: they are more often divorced or separated, impulsive, less educated, extroverted, hostile, and more apt to drink alcohol.

Nicotine Withdrawal

The nicotine withdrawal syndrome develops within 90 to 120 minutes after the last cigarette smoked and peaks within the first 24 hours after cessation. It lasts for several weeks or months in some persons. The major symptom is an intense craving for a cigarette associated with tension and irritability. The person feels generally frustrated or angry, restless, anxious, has difficulty concentrating, and is drowsy, but has difficulty sleeping. Decreased heart rate and blood pressure, reduced motor performance, increased muscle contractions, and slow EEG rhythms also occur. Increased appetite and weight gain occur in most persons after they stop smoking. Some former smokers report that their craving for a cigarette remains intense even after 10 to 20 years, although they have no other signs of the withdrawal syndrome (Table 3). Mild symptoms of withdrawal may occur after switching to low tar or nicotine cigarettes, and after stopping the use of chewing tobacco or nicotine gum.

Treatment

The relapse rate for smokers who attempt to stop is as high as 80 percent within the first 2 years of abstinence. No treatment has proven superior to another. Most smoking-cessation programs report a success rate of only 20 percent. Other treatments include

Table 3
Diagnostic Criteria for Nicotine Withdrawal

A. Daily use of nicotine for at least several weeks.

B. Abrupt cessation of nicotine use, or reduction in the amount of nicotine used, followed within 24 hours by at least four of the following signs:

   (1) craving for nicotine
   (2) irritability, frustration, or anger
   (3) anxiety
   (4) difficulty concentrating
   (5) restlessness
   (6) decreased heart rate
   (7) increased appetite or weight gain

Table from DSM-III-R, *Diagnostic and Statistical Manual of Mental Disorders,* ed 3, revised. (Current Classification of Mental Disorders, 1987.) Copyright American Psychiatric Association, Washington, D.C., 1987. Used with permission.

hypnosis, aversive therapy, acupuncture, lobeline chewing gum (a congener of nicotine), and nicotine nasal sprays. Persons who successfully discontinue smoking are more likely to have been encouraged by someone close to them (such as a spouse or children), to have been fearful of the ill effects of smoking, and to have joined a support group of ex-smokers. Encouragement from a nonsmoking physician is also highly correlated with abstinence. The judicious use of benzodiazepines during the acute withdrawal stage may be of help.

A summary of some of the major points of this chapter is given in Tables 4 and 5.

Table 4
Psychoactive Drugs Associated with Organic Mental Disorders

Drug	Behavioral Effects	Physical Effects	Lab Findings	Treatment
Opioids: opium, morphine, heroin, meperidine (Demerol), methadone, pentazocine (Talwin)	Euphoria, drowsiness, anorexia, decreased sex drive, hypoactivity, change in personality	Miosis, pruritus, nausea, bradycardia, constipation, needle tracks in arms, legs, groin	Detected in blood up to 24 hours after last dose	For gradual withdrawal: methadone 5–10 mg every 6 hr for 24 hr, then decrease dose for 10 days. For overdose: naloxone (Narcan) 0.4 mg IM every 20 minutes for 3 doses, keep airway open; give O$_2$
Amphetamine and other sympathomimetics including cocaine	Alertness, loquaciousness, euphoria, hyperactive, irritability, aggressiveness, agitation, paranoid trends, impotence, visual and tactile hallucinations	Mydriasis, tremor, halitosis, dry mouth, tachycardia, hypertension, weight loss, arrhythmias, fever, convulsions, perforated nasal septum (with cocaine)	Detected in blood and urine	For agitation: diazepam (Valium) IM or PO 5–10 mg every 3 hr; for tachyarrhythmias: propanolol (Inderal) 10–20 mg PO q every 4 hr; vitamin CO .5 gm qid PO may increase urinary excretion by acidifying urine
Central nervous system depressants: barbiturates, methaqualone (illegal to make in U.S.), meprobamate, benzodiazepines, glutethimide (Doriden)	Drowsiness, confusion, inattentiveness	Diaphoresis, ataxis hypotension, seizures, delirium, miosis	Detected in blood	For barbiturates: Substitute 30 mg liquid phenobarbital for every 100 mg barbiturates abused and give in divided doses every 6 hr and then decrease by 20% every other day; may also substitute diazepam (Valium) for barbiturate abused. Give 10 mg every 2–4 hr for 24 hr and then reduce dose; for benzodiazepines; gradual reduction of Valium every other day over 10-day period
Other inhalants: nitrous oxide	Euphoria, drowsiness, ataxia, confusion	Analgesia, respiratory depression, hypotension	None	Hypoxia is treated with O$_2$ inhalation
Alcohol	Poor judgment, loquaciousness, mood change, aggression, impaired attention, amnesia	Nystagmus, flushed face, ataxia, slurred speech	Blood level between 100 and 200 mg/dl	For delirium: diazepam (Valium) 5–10 mg IM or PO every 3 hr, IM vitamin B complex, hydration; for hallucinosis: haloperidol (Haldol) 1–4 mg every 6 hr IM or PO

(continued)

Table 4 *continued*

Drug	Behavioral Effects	Physical Effects	Lab Findings	Treatment
Hallucinogens: LSD (D-lysergic acid diethylamide), psilocybin (mushrooms), mescaline (peyote), DET (diethyltriptamine), DMT (dimethyltriptamine), DOM or STP (dimethoxymethylamphetamine), MDA (methylene dioxyamphetamine)	8–12 hour duration with flashback after abstinence, visual hallucinations, paranoid ideation, false sense of achievement and strength, suicidal or homicidal tendencies, depersonalization, derealization	Mydriasis, ataxia, hyperemic conjunctiva, tachycardia, hypertension	None	Emotional support ("talking down"); for mild agitation: diazepam (Valium) 10 mg IM or PO every 2 hr for 4 doses; for severe agitation: haloperidol (Haldol) 1–5 mg IM and repeat every 6 hr prn. May have to continue Haldol 1–2 mg per day PO for weeks to prevent flashback syndrome. Phenothiazines may be used only with LSD. Caution: phenothiazines can produce *fatal* results if used with other hallucinogens (DET, DMT, etc.) especially if they are adulterated with strychnine or belladonna alkaloids.
Phencyclidine (PCP)	8–12 hour duration, hallucinations, paranoid ideation, labile mood, loose associations (may mimic schizophrenia), catatonia, violent behavior, convulsions	Nystagmus, mydriasis, ataxia, tachycardia, hypertension	Detected in urine up to 5 days after ingestion	Phenothiazines contraindicated for first week after ingestion; for violent delusions: haloperidol (Haldol) 1–4 mg IM or PO every 2–4 hr until patient is calm
Volatile hydrocarbons and petroleum derivatives: glue, benzene, gasoline, varnish thinner, lighter fluid, aerosols	Euphoria, clouded sensorium, slurred speech, ataxia, hallucinations in 50% of cases, psychoses, permanent brain damage if used daily over 6 mo	Odor on breath, tachycardia with possible ventricular fibrillation, possible damage of brain, liver, kidneys, myocardium	Relevant to determine tissue damage (SGOT)	For agitation: haloperidol (Haldol) 1–5 mg every 6 hr until calm; avoid epinephrine because of myocardial sensitization
Belladonna alkaloids (found in over-the-counter medications and morning glory seeds): strammonium, homatropine, atropine, scopalomine, hyoscyamine	Hot skin, erythema, weakness, thirst, blurred vision, confusion, excitement, delirium, stupor, coma (anticholinergic delirium)	Dry mouth and throat, mydriasis, twitching, dysphagia, light sensitivity, pyrexia, hypertension followed by shock, urinary retention	None	Antidote is physostigmine (Antilirium) 2 mg IV every 20 min; IV should be controlled at no more than 1 mg/min; watch for copious salivary secretion because of anticholinesterase activity. Propranolol for tachyarrhythmias

Modified from *Desk Reference on Drug Misuse and Abuse,* **New York State Medical Society, New York, 1984.**

Table 5
Organic Mental Syndromes Associated with Psychoactive Substances

	Intoxication	Withdrawal	Delirium	Withdrawal Delirium	Delusional Disorder	Mood Disorder	Other Syndromes
Alcohol	X	X		X			[1]
Amphetamine and related substances	X	X	X		X		
Caffeine	X						
Cannabis	X				X		
Cocaine	X	X	X		X		
Hallucinogen	X (hallucinosis)				X	X	[2]
Inhalant	X						
Nicotine		X					
Opioid	X	X					
Phencyclidine (PCP) and related substances	X		X		X	X	[3]
Sedative, hypnotic, or anxiolytic	X	X		X			[4]

[1]Alcohol idiosyncratic Intoxication, Alcohol Hallucinosis, Alcohol Amnestic Disorder, Dementia Associated with Alcoholism
[2]Posthallucinogen Perception Disorder
[3]Phencyclidine (PCP) or Similarly Acting Arylcyclohexylamine Organic Mental Disorder NOS
[4]Sedative, Hypnotic or Anxiolytic Amnestic Disorder
Table from DSM-III-R, *Diagnostic and Statistical Manual of Mental Disorders*, ed 3, revised. (Current Classification of Mental Disorders, 1987.) Copyright American Psychiatric Association, Washington, D.C., 1987. Used with permission.

References

Bellet S, Roman L, DeCastro O, Kim K D, Kershbaum A: Effect of coffee ingestion on catecholamine release. Metabolism 18:288, 1969.

Boulenger J P, Uhde T W: Caffeine consumption and anxiety: Preliminary results of a survey comparing patients with anxiety disorders and normal controls. Psychopharmacol Bull 18:53, 1982.

Dreisbach R H, Pfeiffer C: Caffeine-withdrawal headache. J Lab Clin Med 28:1212, 1943.

Greden J F: Anxiety or caffeinism: A diagnostic dilemma. Am J Psychiatry 131:1089, 1974.

Greden J F: Caffeinism and caffeine withdrawal. In *Substance Abuse: Clinical Problems and Perspectives*, J H Lowinson, P Ruiz, editors, p 274. Williams & Wilkins, Baltimore, 1981.

Hughes J R, Gust S W, Pechacek T F: Prevalence of tobacco dependence and withdrawal. Am J Psych 144:205, 1987.

Jaffe J H, Kanzler M: Nicotine: Tobacco use, abuse and dependence. In *Substance Abuse: Clinical Problems and Perspectives*. J H Levinson, C Ruiz, editors, p256. Williams & Wilkins, Baltimore, 1981.

Krasnagor NA, editor: *The Behavioral Aspects of Smoking*, NIDA Research Monograph 26. US Government Printing Office, Washington, DC, 1979.

Russell M A H: Cigarette smoking: Natural history of a dependence disorder. Br J Med Psychol 44:1, 1971.

United States Public Health Service: *Smoking and Health: Report and Advisory Committee to the Surgeon General of the Public Health Service*. U.S. Government Printing Office, Washington, D C, 1964.

Weiss B, Laties V G: Enhancement of human performance by caffeine and the amphetamines. Pharmacol Rev 14:1, 1962.

14

Schizophrenia

Schizophrenia, which afflicts approximately 1 percent of the population, usually begins before age 25 and persists throughout life. Schizophrenia affects people of all social classes. Both patients and their families often suffer from poor care and social ostracism because of widespread ignorance about schizophrenia. Each year, only $14 per patient is spent on schizophrenia research in the United States (cf. $300 per patient on cancer research). This is a particularly lopsided "investment" because the financial cost of schizophrenia to society is greater than that of all cancers combined.

Although schizophrenia is discussed as if it were a single disease, it quite likely includes a variety of disorders that present with somewhat similar behavioral symptoms; it probably comprises a group of disorders with heterogeneous etiologies, and it definitely includes patients whose clinical presentations, treatment responses, and courses of illness are varied. Physicians should appreciate that the diagnosis of schizophrenia is based entirely on the psychiatric history and mental status examination. There is no laboratory test for schizophrenia.

HISTORY

The two key people in the history of schizophrenia were Emil Kraepelin (German, 1856–1926) and Eugen Bleuler (Swiss, 1857–1939). At least three important figures preceded Kraeplin and Bleuler. Benedict Morel (1809–1873), a Belgian psychiatrist, used the term démence précoce for deteriorated patients whose illness began in adolescence; Karl Kahlbaum (1828–1899) described the symptoms of catatonia; and Ewold Hecker (1843–1909) wrote about the extremely bizarre behavior of hebephrenia.

Kraepelin organized the seriously mentally ill patients by three diagnostic groups: dementia praecox, manic-depressive psychosis, and paranoia. Kraepelin's description of dementia precox emphasized a chronic deteriorating course, in addition to including such clinical phenomena as hallucinations and delusions. Kraepelin reported that approximately 4 percent of his patients had complete recoveries and 13 percent had significant remissions. The term "manic-depressive psychosis" identified patients who experienced episodes of illness separated by virtually complete remissions. Patients diagnosed as having paranoia had as their major symptom persistent persecutory delusions.

Bleuler coined the term "schizophrenia," which means split mindedness, in reference to the theoretical schism between thought, emotion, and behavior. Unfortunately, this term historically has caused confusion with split personality (now called "multiple personality disorder"), a completely different disorder from schizophrenia. Bleuler's definition of schizophrenia differed from Kraepelin's dementia praecox in two major ways. First, Bleuler did not feel that deterioration was a necessary symptom of the disorder. Second, Bleuler divided the symptoms into fundamental (primary) and accessory (secondary) symptoms. The most important fundamental symptom was a thought disorder characterized by associational disturbances, particularly looseness. The other fundamental symptoms were affective disturbances, autism, and ambivalence. (Bleuler's so-called four As consist of associations, affect, autism, and ambivalence.) Accessory symptoms included hallucinations and delusions. Both Bleuler and Kraepelin assumed that there was an underlying biological basis for this disorder.

Four modern psychiatrists who theorized about schizophrenia were Adolf Meyer, Harry Stack Sullivan, Gabriel Langfeldt, and Kurt Schneider. Meyer, the founder of psychobiology, believed that schizophrenia and other mental disorders were reactions to a variety of life stresses so he called the syndrome a "schizophrenic reaction." Sullivan, the founder of the interpersonal psychoanalytic school, emphasized social isolation as both a cause and a symptom of schizophrenia.

Gabriel Langfeldt, unlike Bleuler, derived his criteria from empirical experience, rather than a theoretical formulation. Langfeldt divided the disorder into true schizophrenia and schizophreniform psychosis (see Section 16.2). The diagnosis of true schizophrenia rests on the findings of depersonalization, autism, emotional blunting, insidious onset, and feelings of derealization and unreality. True schizophrenia is often referred to as nuclear schizophrenia, process schizophrenia, or nonremitting schizophrenia.

Kurt Schneider described a number of so-called first-rank symptoms of schizophrenia that he considered in no way specific for the disease but of great pragmatic value in making a diagnosis. Schneider's first-rank symptoms include the hearing of one's thoughts spoken aloud, auditory hallucinations that comment on the patient's behavior, somatic hallucinations, the experience of having one's thoughts controlled, the spreading of one's thoughts to others, delusions, and the experience of having one's actions controlled or influenced from the outside.

Schizophrenia, Schneider pointed out, also can be diagnosed exclusively on the basis of second-rank symptoms, along with an otherwise typical clinical appearance. Second-rank symptoms include other forms of hallucination, perplexity, depressive and euphoric disorders of affect, and emotional blunting.

Schneider did not mean these symptoms to be rigidly applied, and he warned the clinician that the diagnosis should be made in certain patients, even though they failed to show first-rank symptoms. Unfortunately, this warning is frequently ignored, and the absence of such symptoms in a single interview is taken as evidence that the person is free of a schizophrenic disorder.

EPIDEMIOLOGY

Incidence and Prevalence

Epidemiological studies of schizophrenia are confounded by the lack of objective diagnostic methods, the difficulty of identifying all cases in a particular community and of identifying an actual date of onset, and the variety of age groups that must be studied to obtain complete data. The rates for the age group 15 years and over range from 0.30 to 1.20 per 1,000. Pooled studies show an incidence of approximately 1 per 1,000 population. Approximately 200,000 new cases are diagnosed each year in the United States, with approximately 2 million worldwide.

The variation in prevalence rates from studies around the world is much higher than the variation in incidence rates. In the United States, the lifetime prevalence is about 1 percent; that is, about 2 million Americans suffer from schizophrenia. Approximately .025 to .05 percent of the total population is treated for schizophrenia in any one year; two thirds of these patients require hospitalization.

Age, Sex, and Race

The peak age of onset for men is between age 15 and 25 and for women, between 25 and 35. It is possible that the age differential reflects societal biases about behavior of the two sexes rather than actual differences in age of onset. Onset of schizophrenia before age 10 or after age 50 is extremely rare. Approximately 90 percent of patients in treatment for schizophrenia are between 15 and 54 years old. There is no difference in the prevalence of schizophrenia between males and females. Although some older studies reported a higher prevalence among blacks, these findings are thought to represent biased application of diagnostic standards rather than actual racial differences.

Reproduction Rates, Suicide, and Risk of Death

Incidence and prevalence rates of schizophrenia are affected by the reproduction and mortality rates of patients with schizophrenia. The risk of becoming schizophrenic for an individual is increased if one member of his family already suffers from the disorder. With the advent of psychoactive drugs, open-door policies, and deinstitutionalization in the state hospitals, the emphasis on rehabilitation, and community-based care for patients with schizophrenia, increased rates of marriage and fertility have been observed among schizophrenics. The number of children born to schizophrenic parents doubled from 1935 to 1955. The fertility rate currently is believed to be quite close to that of the general population.

Approximately 50 percent of patients with schizophrenia have attempted suicide and 10 percent succeeded sometime during a 20-year follow-up period. These schizophrenic persons also have an extraordinarily high mortality rate from natural causes, a phenomenon that is not explained by institution-related or treatment-related variables.

Cultural and Socioeconomic Considerations

Schizophrenia has been described in all cultures and socioeconomic classes studied. In industrialized nations there is a disproportionate number of schizophrenic patients in the lower socioeconomic classes. This observation has been explained by the "downward drift hypothesis," suggesting that affected individuals either move into lower socioeconomic classes or fail to rise out of a lower socioeconomic class because of the illness. An alternative explanation, less supported by research, is the "social causation hypothesis," proposing that stresses experienced by members of the lower socioeconomic classes contribute to the development of, or even cause, schizophrenia. The prevalence of schizophrenia has been correlated with local population density in cities with populations over 1 million. But the correlation is weaker in cities of 100,000 to 500,000 people and nonexistent in cities with fewer than 10,000 people. This effect of population density is consistent with the observation that the incidence of schizophrenia in children of either one or two schizophrenic parents is twice as high in cities than in rural communities, suggesting that social stressors may affect the development of schizophrenia in persons at risk. The problem of the homeless in large cities may be related to the deinstitutionalization of schizophrenic patients who were not adequately engaged in follow-up care. Although the exact percentage of homeless individuals who are, in fact, schizophrenic is very difficult to obtain, it is estimated that from one third to two thirds of the homeless have schizophrenia.

Immigration, industrialization, and cultural tolerance towards deviant behavior have been hypothesized to contribute to the etiology of schizophrenia. Because some studies report a higher prevalence of schizophrenia among recent immigrants, this finding has implicated abrupt cultural change as a stressor involved in the etiology of this disorder. It has been noted also that the prevalence of schizophrenia appears to rise among third-world populations as contact with technologically advanced cultures increases. Finally, it has been argued that cultures may be more or less "schizophrenogenic," depending on how mental illness is perceived, the nature of the patient role, the system of social supports, and the complexity of social communication. Schizophrenia is prognostically more benign in less developed nations where patients are reintegrated into their community and family more completely than they are in more highly civilized Western societies.

Seasonality of Birth

In the northern hemisphere, including the United States, more schizophrenic patients are born in the winter months of January to April. In the southern hemisphere, more schizophrenic patients are born in the months, July to September.

Mental Hospital Beds and Financial Cost to Society

Patterns of hospitalization for schizophrenic patients have changed over the past two decades. The duration of hospitalizations has decreased, and the number of admissions has increased. The probability of readmission within a 2-year period after discharge from the first hospitalization is about 40 to 60 percent. Schizophrenic patients occupy approximately 50 percent of mental hospital beds and account for approximately 16 percent of psychiatric patients who receive any type of treatment.

Schizophrenia is the most expensive of all mental disorders in direct treatment costs, loss of productivity, and expenditures for public assistance. It has been estimated that the annual cost of schizophrenia in the United States is about 2 percent of the gross national product. The direct delivery of psychiatric care accounts for only 20 percent of this figure; the remaining costs reflect the loss in productive capacity and costs of hospitalization.

ETIOLOGY

The etiology of schizophrenia is not known. Schizophrenia is quite likely a heterogeneous disorder, and very few of the etiological factors discussed here are exclusionary. The major model for integrating these putative etiological factors is the stress-diathesis model. It postulates that an individual may have a specific vulnerability (diathesis) that, when acted upon by some stressful environmental influence, allows the symptoms of schizophrenia to develop. In the most general stress-diathesis model, the diathesis or the stress can be biological, environmental, or both. The environmental component can be either biological (e.g., an infection) or psychological (e.g., a stressful family situation, death of a close relative). The biological basis of a diathesis can be further shaped by epigenetic influences, such as drug abuse, psychosocial stress, or trauma. Until a specific etiological factor for schizophrenia is identified, the stress-diathesis model is the most concise way to conceptualize the available data and theories.

Evidence from Biological Research

Since the discovery of the effectiveness of antipsychotic drugs in the treatment of schizophrenia, many studies have compared specific, objective biological features of schizophrenic patients with those of nonschizophrenic psychiatric patients and those of normal controls. There are two major caveats in interpreting biological abnormalities reported in schizophrenia. First, one must consider what a "biological abnormality" signifies. Such an abnormality is, at most, a correlation and rarely, if ever, can be seen as causal. Second, it is difficult to determine whether the abnormality is related to the disease process itself or to treatment, especially antipsychotic medications.

There are two other observations about the nature of the brain that need to be considered. First, the fact that pathology has been identified in one area does not mean that the primary area of pathology has been defined. For example, the hypoactive frontal lobe function in schizophrenia could be caused by hyperactive inhibitory input from some other region of the brain. Second, a single pathological process in the brain can cause a wide range of phenomena in different patients. For example, patients with Huntington's disease can present with the entire range of DSM-III-R diagnoses including no mental disorder. Conversely, a single specific abnormality in the brain can have many different etiologies. Parkinson's disease, for example, can have idiopathic, infectious, traumatic, or toxic etiologies.

Neurotransmitters. The dopamine hypothesis, the major neurotransmitter hypothesis for schizophrenia, states that there is a hyperactivity of dopaminergic systems in schizophrenia. The major support for this hypothesis is that all effective antipsychotic drugs bind to dopamine receptors. The clinical potency of antipsychotic drugs is closely correlated with their binding affinity to D2 receptors, the dopamine receptor subtype that does not stimulate adenylate cyclase. The observation that administration of amphetamine or levodopa exacerbates the symptoms of some, but not all, schizophrenic patients lends additional support to this hypothesis. However, there are three major problems with this hypothesis. First, dopamine antagonists are effective in treating *all* psychoses. Dopaminergic hyperactivity, therefore, is not uniquely associated with schizophrenia. Second, although antipsychotic drugs reach the brain very quickly to block dopamine receptors, the maximal clinical effects can take as long as 6 weeks to develop. Third, although some research has demonstrated supportive neurochemical evidence (e.g., increased dopamine metabolites), the majority of studies have not found confirmatory neurochemical data.

Of the five dopaminergic tracts in the CNS, the mesocortical and the mesolimbic tracts have received the most attention in schizophrenia. Both of these tracts have their cell bodies in the substantia nigra and the ventral tegmental area. It has been observed in animal studies that long-term neuroleptic administration causes the firing rate of some neurons in these tract to decrease. In addition, neuroleptics that have few extrapyramidal side effects do not reduce the firing rate in dopaminergic neurons of the nigrostriatal tract.

Virtually every known neurotransmitter has been studied in schizophrenia. There is some evidence that norepinephrine activity is increased in schizophrenia. This idea is supported by postmortem findings, increased CSF MHPG in some schizophrenic patients, and the fact that amphetamine, which can produce a paranoid schizophrenia–like clinical picture, acts on both dopaminergic and noradrenergic neurons. Because of its function as an inhibitory neurotransmitter, GABA may play a role in schizophrenia. Presumably, decreased GABA activity can result in hyperactivity of dopaminergic neurons. Some neurochemical evidence supports this hypothesis, and it has been observed that a small number of patients with schizophrenia improve with benzodiazepine treatment.

Neuropathology. There have been two main types of neuropathological studies of schizophrenia—studies of neurotransmitters and neurodegeneration. The neurotransmitter studies have measured neurotransmitter concentrations and receptor properties in specific areas of brains postmortem. The neurodegenerative studies have looked for areas of cell loss or abnormal histology in brain tissue.

Many postmortem neurotransmitter studies have reported increased numbers of D2 receptors in the basal ganglia and limbic system (particularly the amygdala, nucleus accumbens, and hippocampus). Although one study found both increased dopamine concentrations and increased receptor number in the left amygdala, most studies have not found increased concentrations of dopamine or its metabolites. Most studies have also been unable to distinguish changes in dopamine receptors related to schizophrenia from the increase of dopamine receptors related to antipsychotic drug treatment. There are two studies that reported increased concentrations of both norepinephrine and its metabolites in the nucleus accumbens of chronic paranoid patients. There have also been postmortem neurochemistry studies of GABA, serotonin, and several neuropeptides; however, the data are not conclusive at this time.

Neurodegenerative pathological research in schizophrenia has historically reported diverse abnormalities. However, these studies have revealed only diffuse, nonspecific abnormalities and have contributed to the misleading differentiation of organic disorders (those with identifiable pathology) from functional disorders (no identifiable brain pathology). More recent studies have not produced a single consistent structural defect; however, there is a consistent pattern of degeneration in the limbic forebrain (especially the amygdala and hippocampus) and the basal ganglia (especially substantia nigra and medial pallidum). The specific results of these studies have included increased gliosis in the periventricular diencephalon, decreased numbers of cortical neurons in prefrontal and cingulate regions, and decreased volume of the amygdala, hippocampal formation, and parahippocampal gyrus.

Brain Imaging. The majority of computed tomographic (CT) studies of the brains of schizophrenics have reported enlargement of lateral and third ventricles in 10 to 50 percent of patients and cortical atrophy in 10 to 35 percent. Controlled experiments have also revealed atrophy of the cerebellar vermis, decreased radiodensity of brain parenchyma, and reversals of the normal brain asymmetries. These results, which are not artifacts of treatment, are neither progressive nor reversible. The enlargement of the ventricles appears to be present at the time of diagnosis. These findings are objective indicators of neuronal loss. It has been suggested that schizophrenia could be subtyped on the basis of the presence or absence of CT abnormalities. A major caveat to this notion is that the difference between these two groups may be quantitative rather than qualitative, meaning that the patients with abnormal CT scans merely have more of the same pathology than the patients with normal CT scans. Other studies have correlated the presence of CT scan abnormalities with the presence of negative or deficit symptoms, neuropsychiatric impairment, increased neurological signs, more frequent extrapyramidal

symptoms from antipsychotics, poorer premorbid adjustment, increased delta activity on EEG, and (possibly) more suicide attempts. It is hoped that the more advanced technology of magnetic resonance imaging will extend these findings by imaging more specific brain regions.

Metabolic brain imaging studies of schizophrenic patients have been performed with regional cerebral blood flow (CBF) and positron emission tomography (PET). There are many complex methodological problems with both techniques, and neither has yielded consistent results in all studies. PET scan studies have reported decreased frontal lobe metabolism, decreased parietal lobe metabolism, abnormal laterality differences, and relatively high posterior metabolism. CBF studies have reported decreased resting levels of frontal blood flow, increased parietal blood flow, and decreased whole brain blood flow. More recent studies have used psychological activation procedures and have demonstrated an inability of schizophrenic patients to "turn on" their frontal lobes when performing a psychological task (Figure 1). When taken together with the CT scans, there is more evidence suggesting dysfunction of the frontal lobe than of any single other area of the brain. It should be remembered, however, that frontal lobe dysfunction can be the result of pathology in another part of the brain.

Electrophysiology. EEG studies of schizophrenics indicate a higher number of patients with abnormal records, increased sensitivity (e.g., more frequent spike activity) to activation procedures (e.g., sleep deprivation), decreased alpha activity, increased theta and delta activity, possibly more epileptiform activity, and possibly more left-sided abnormalities. Evoked potential studies have generally shown increased amplitude of early components and decreased amplitude of late components. This difference has been interpreted as an indication that although schizophrenic patients are more sensitive to sensory stimulation, they compensate for this increased sensitivity by blunting the processing of the information at higher cortical levels.

Other CNS electrophysiological investigations have included depth electrodes and quantitative EEG (QEEG). One report asserted that electrodes implanted in the limbic system of schizophrenic patients showed spiking activity that is correlated with psychotic behavior; however, no control subjects were examined. QEEG studies of schizophrenia have demonstrated increased frontal slow activity, and perhaps increased fast activity over the parietal lobes (see Figure 2). These QEEG findings have yet to be replicated.

Psychoneuroimmunology and Psychoneuroendocrinology. There has been an increased appreciation in neurology for the possibility that the etiology of some disorders (e.g., multiple sclerosis, Alzheimer's and Parkinson's disease) may involve infections (e.g., slow viruses). The data suggesting such an etiology in some cases of schizophrenia include increased numbers of physical anomalies at birth, increased rate of pregnancy and birth complications, seasonality of birth consistent with viral infections, clusters of adult cases, seasonality of hospitalizations, neuropathological changes consistent with past infections, and a variety of immunological abnormalities. Other data supporting this hypothesis, such as transmission in an animal model or identification of an infectious particle, are lacking.

Immunologic abnormalities in schizophrenia include atypical lymphocytes, decreased numbers of natural killer cells, and variable levels of immunoglobulins. These data have been interpreted

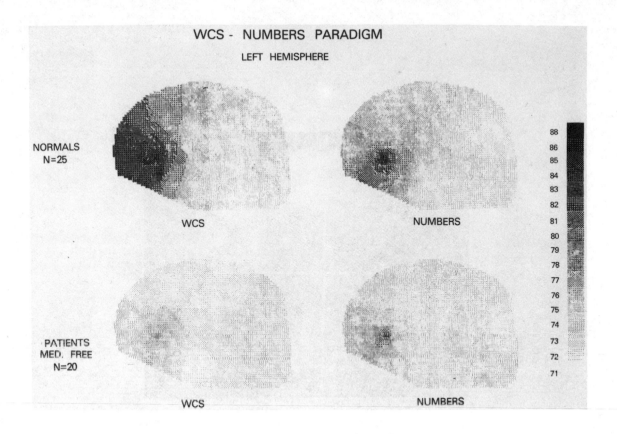

WCS - NUMBERS PARADIGM
LEFT HEMISPHERE

NORMALS N=25

WCS   NUMBERS

PATIENTS MED. FREE N=20

WCS   NUMBERS

88 86 85 84 83 82 81 80 79 78 77 76 75 74 73 72 71

Figure 1   This figure is from a study of patients with schizophrenia using cerebral blood flow (CBF). While performing the Wisconsin Card Sort Test (WCS), normals increase the blood flow to their frontal lobes above the level in a control task ("numbers"). The schizophrenic patients, as a group, failed to increase blood flow to the frontal lobes during this same task. (Supplied courtesy of Drs. K. Berman and D. Weinberger, National Institute of Mental Health, Washington, D.C.)

in several ways: an infectious agent may directly produce both the psychiatric symptoms and the immune dysfunction; an infectious agent may induce an autoimmunity against specific brain regions; a primary immune disorder may produce an autoimmune disorder of the brain.

Psychoneuroendocrine dysregulation has been reported in schizophrenia. Although most studies have suggested a normal prolactin level in schizophrenia, a few suggest that positive symptoms are correlated with decreased prolactin levels. The data have been more consistent in demonstrating decreased levels of luteinizing hormone/follicle-stimulating hormone (LH/FSH), perhaps correlated with the age of onset and the length of illness. Two additional reported abnormalities have been a blunted release of prolactin and growth hormone to gonadotropin-releasing hormone (GnRH) or thyrotropin-releasing hormone (TRH) stimulation, and a blunted release of growth hormone to apomorphine stimulation that may be correlated with the presence of negative symptoms.

A unifying theory that explains both the immune and endocrine dysfunctions is pathology (structural or neurochemical) in the hypothalamus. Hyperfunction of dopaminergic systems, for example, could explain many of the neuroendocrine findings.

Integration of Biological Theories.   Neuropsychiatric approaches to schizophrenia attempt to use biological data to locate the site of a lesion, much as neurologists used the neurological examination to locate the lesion before the CT scan was invented. The two major areas of interest are the frontal lobes and the limbic system. Involvement of the frontal lobes is supported by brain imaging studies, electrophysiology, and neuropsychological studies. Limbic involvement is supported by neuropathological and depth electrode data.

Other brain areas are also implicated. The basal ganglia are implicated by the common occurrence of psychosis in movement disorders. The hypothalamus and thalamus are implicated by the disorders of sensory processing, immune and endocrine disorders, and enlarged ventricles. The brain stem is implicated because it contains both the dopaminergic and adrenergic neuronal cell bodies as well as the reticular activating system that may be involved in the regulation of the attentional and sensory systems. The cerebellum is implicated primarily by degeneration of the vermis seen in some CT studies. The variety of possible sites for a lesion is consistent with a heterogeneous model of etiology for schizophrenia.

Electrophysiological theorists have focused on the processing of sensory information and abnormalities in laterality. Deficits in attention and sensory filtering are suggested by some of the electrophysiological data and have resulted in theories of "hypervigilance." Theories of left-hemisphere dysfunction are supported by the increased incidence of psychosis in temporal lobe epileptics with left-sided foci, the abnormalities in language seen in schizo-

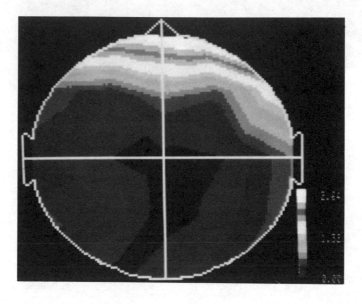

Figure 2 Computed topographic map of electrophysiologic data from a study of patients with schizophrenia. Lighter areas represent brain areas of higher power for a specific EEG frequency. (Supplied courtesy of John Morihisa, Department of Psychiatry, Georgetown University, Washington, D.C.)

phrenia, and the reported increased incidence of left-handedness in schizophrenic populations. There have also been theories that interhemispheric integration is abnormal in schizophrenia; both CT and postmortem studies have revealed increased thickness of the corpus callosum in persons with schizophrenia.

The nature of the presumed lesion is unknown. The neurochemical hypotheses suggest some relatively specific molecular abnormality, such as in the structure of some protein (e.g., an enzyme). The evidence of neuropathological damage would support an infectious, degenerative, or traumatic insult. Trauma as an etiological factor is supported by the increased incidence of prenatal (e.g., bleeding), perinatal (e.g., long labor), and neonatal (e.g., convulsions) complications in patients who later develop schizophrenia. It is not known whether such trauma is causal or represents some type of abnormality in the mother who is pregnant with a schizophrenic child. It is of note that monozygotic twins who are discordant for schizophrenia tend to be discordant for handedness, suggesting brain damage in the schizophrenic twin.

Genetic

Investigations into the population genetics of schizophrenia have produced data consistent with the hypothesis that there is a genetic basis for schizophrenia, that the genes of affected persons confer a vulnerability for schizophrenia.

The possibility exists, however, that environmental forces (both psychological and biological) could affect the expression of these genes, as well as provide a stress that could precipitate the syndrome of schizophrenia. Current approaches in genetics are directed toward identifying large pedigrees of affected individuals and investigating these families for restriction fragment length polymorphisms (RFLPs). This approach may result in the identification of a specific genetic marker for schizophrenia.

The risks among members of various groups for developing schizophrenia support a genetic hypothesis of schizophrenia (Table 1). The closer the genetic relationship of any person to an affected proband, the more likely he is to develop schizophrenia. Monozygotic twins (who share the same genetic information) have the highest concordance rate. (Virtually no genetic illness has a 100-percent concordance rate in monozygotic twins.) The studies of adopted monozygotic twins demonstrate that twins reared by adoptive parents develop schizophrenia at the same rate as their twin siblings raised by their biological parents. This finding suggests that the genetic influence outweighs that of the environment. In further support of the genetic basis is the observation that the more severe the schizophrenia, the more likely the twins are to be concordant for the disorder. One study that supports the stress-diathesis model showed that adopted monozygotic twins who later developed

Table I
Incidence of Schizophrenia in Specific Populations

Population	Incidence (%)
General Population	1.0
Nontwin sibling of a schizophrenic patient	8.0
Child with one schizophrenic parent	12.0
Dizygotic twin of a schizophrenic patient	12.0
Child of two schizophrenic parents	40.0
Monozygotic twin of a schizophrenic patient	47.0

schizophrenia had been adopted by psychologically disordered families.

Psychosocial

Patients with schizophrenia seem to have a significant, albeit unidentified, biologically based vulnerability. Nevertheless psychosocial factors are considered significant and are a major area of research and study that affects the development, expression, and course of the disorder.

Theories Regarding the Individual

Psychoanalytic theories. According to psychoanalytic theory, a crucial defect in schizophrenia is a disturbance in ego organization, which affects the interpretation of reality and the control of inner drives (e.g., sex and aggression). These disturbances occur as a consequence of distortions in the reciprocal relationship between the infant and the mother. As described by Margaret Mahler, the child is unable to separate and progress beyond the closeness and complete dependence that characterizes the mother-child relationship in the oral phase of development. The schizophrenic person never achieves object constancy, which is characterized by a sense of secure identity and which results from a close attachment to the mother during infancy. Paul Federn concluded that the fundamental disturbance in schizophrenia is the patient's early inability to achieve self-object differentiation. Some psychoanalysts hypothesize that the defect in rudimentary ego functions permits intense hostility and aggression to distort the mother-infant relationship, leading to a personality organization that is vulnerable to stress. The onset of symptoms during adolescence occurs at a time when the individual requires a strong ego to deal with increased internal drives, separation, identity tasks, intense external stimulation, and need to function independently.

Freud believed that schizophrenic patients regress to a phase of primary narcissism and ego disintegration. The concept of ego disintegration refers to a return to the time when the ego was not yet established or had just begun to be established. The person is unable to develop a mature ego capable of interpreting reality.

Current psychoanalytic theory postulates that the various symptoms of schizophrenia have symbolic meaning for the individual patient. For example, fantasies of the world coming to an end indicate a perception that the person's internal world has broken down; feelings of grandeur reflect reactivated narcissism, in which the person believes that he is omnipotent; hallucinations are substitutes for the patient's inability to deal with objective reality and represent his inner wishes or fears; and delusions, similar to hallucinations, are regressive, restitutive attempts to create a new reality or to express hidden fears or impulses.

Harry Stack Sullivan concluded from his clinical investigations that some schizophrenic patients had been made anxious as infants by their anxious mothers which caused the disintegration of ego function seen in the disorder.

Learning theory. According to learning theorists, as children, patients with schizophrenia learn irrational reactions and ways of thinking by imitating parents who may have their own significant emotional problems. Deficiency in social skills account for poor interpersonal relationships.

Theories regarding the family. There is no controlled evidence that a specific family pattern plays an etiological role in the development of schizophrenia; however, there have been at least three major theories in the past 30 years. (1) Gregory Bateson described a family situation called the "double bind," in which a child is put into a situation where he has to make a choice between two alternatives, both of which will produce confusion and are unbearable. (2) Theodore Lidz described two abnormal patterns of family behavior. In one type of family, there is a prominent "schism" between the parents (one parent gets overly close to the child of the opposite sex), and in the other, there is a "skewed" relationship with one parent (a power struggle in which one parent is dominant). (3) Lyman Wynne described families in which emotional expression is suppressed by the consistent use of a "pseudomutual" or "pseudohostile" verbal communication and all members relate to one another in a characteristic way unique to that family.

Social. Some theorists have suggested that industrialization and urbanization are involved in the etiology of schizophrenia. Although there has been some data to support such theories, these stresses are now thought to have their major effects on the development and course of the illness.

CLINICAL SIGNS AND SYMPTOMS

There are three key issues regarding the clinical signs and symptoms of schizophrenia. First, no clinical sign or symptom is pathognomonic for schizophrenia; every sign or symptom seen in schizophrenia can be seen in other psychiatric and neurologic disorders. This observation is contrary to the often heard clinical opinion that certain symptoms are diagnostic of schizophrenia. Therefore, it is not possible to diagnose schizophrenia simply by a mental status examination; past history is essential for the diagnosis of schizophrenia. Second, the symptoms of an individual patient change with time. For example, a patient may have intermittent hallucinations and a varying ability to perform adequately in social situations. Third, it is absolutely necessary to take into account the educational level, intellectual ability, and cultural and subcultural membership of the patient. An impaired ability to understand abstract concepts, for example, may reflect the patient's education or intelligence. Various religious organizations or cults may have customs that seem strange to those outside that organization, but are considered perfectly normal to those within the cultural setting.

Premorbid Symptoms

An arbitrary line for each individual patient divides the premorbid or prepsychotic personality from the prodromal phase of the illness. The typical, but not invariable, history is that of a schizoid or schizotypal personality—quiet, passive, with few friends as a child, daydreaming, introverted, and shut in as an adolescent and adult. The child is often reported to have been especially obedient and never in any mischief. The preschizophrenic adolescent may have no close friends and few dates. He may avoid competitive sports but enjoy watching movies and television and listening to music, to the exclusion of more social activities.

Although the onset of illness is often defined at either the time of diagnosis or first hospitalization, symptoms of the illness often develop slowly over months or years. The person may begin complaining of somatic symptoms, such as headache, back and muscle pain, weakness, or digestive problems. The initial diagnosis may be malingering or a somatization disorder. Family and friends may eventually notice that the person has changed, and is no longer functioning well in occupational, social, and personal activities. During this stage the patient may begin to feel anxious or perplexed and may develop an interest in abstract ideas, philosophy, the occult, or religious matters. DSM-III-R includes markedly peculiar behavior, abnormal affect, unusual speech, bizarre ideas, and strange perceptual experiences among the prodromal signs.

The Mental Status Examination in Schizophrenia

General Description. The patient may be quite talkative and may exhibit bizarre postures, and behavior may be quite agitated or violent and apparently in response to hallucinations. Catatonic excitement is the term used to describe a state of particularly intense but disorganized activity. This behavior contrasts dramatically with catatonic stupor, often referred to merely as catatonia, in which the patient seems completely lifeless and may exhibit symptoms such as muteness, negativism, or automatic obedience. Waxy flexibility used to be a common symptom in catatonia, but now it is quite rare. Many patients have a less extreme presentation of marked social withdrawal and egocentricity, lack of spontaneous speech or movement, and an absence of goal-directed behavior. Other obvious behaviors may include an odd clumsiness or stiffness in body movements, deterioration of social habits (e.g., very poor grooming, obvious failure to bathe, smearing of feces), odd tics, stereotypies or mannerisms, or, in some cases, echopraxia.

Some clinicians report a "precox feeling" that describes an intuitive experience of their inability to establish an emotional rapport with the patient. Although this experience is not uncommon for clinicians to experience, there is no data to indicate that it is a valid or reliable criterion in the diagnosis of schizophrenia.

Mood, Feelings, and Affect. The two most common affective presentations of schizophrenia are reduced emotional responsiveness or even anhedonia, or overly active and inappropriate emotions of extreme rage, happiness, or anxiety. The presentation of a flat or blunted affect can represent either symptoms of the illness itself or the par-

kinsonian side effects of antipsychotic medications. The patient may describe exultant feelings of omnipotence, religious ecstasy, terror at the disintegration of his soul, or paralyzing anxiety about the destruction of the universe. Other feeling tones include perplexity, terror, a sense of isolation and overwhelming ambivalence.

Perceptual Disturbances. Hallucinations may occur in any of the five sensory modalities. Auditory hallucinations are the most common in schizophrenic patients; they may complain of hearing one or more voices, which may be threatening, obscene, accusatory, or insulting. Visual hallucinations occur less frequently, but they are not rare. Tactile, olfactory, and gustatory hallucinations do occur, but their presence should cause the clinician to investigate carefully and rule out organic causes. Schizophrenic patients may experience cenesthetic hallucinations (sensations of altered states in body organs without plausible explanation such as a burning sensation in the brain, a pushing sensation in the blood vessel, or a cutting sensation in the bone marrow). Illusions may also occur in schizophrenia and the differentiation of hallucination and illusions is often quite difficult.

Thought Process. Nonperceptual disorders of thought may be divided into disorders of content, form, and process. Disorders of content reflect ideas, beliefs, and interpretations of stimuli. Delusions are the most obvious example of a disorder of content. Delusions can be quite varied in schizophrenia—persecutory, grandiose, religious, or somatic. The patient may have the belief that some outside entity is controlling his thoughts or behavior, or, conversely, that he is controlling outside events in some extraordinary fashion (e.g., causing the sun to rise and set, preventing earthquakes). The patient may have an intense and consuming preoccupation with esoteric, abstract, symbolic, psychological, or philosophical ideas. The patient may also be quite concerned about allegedly life-threatening but completely bizarre and implausible somatic conditions.

The phrase "loss of ego boundaries" describes the patient's lack of a clear sense of where his own body, mind, and influence end and where those of other animate and inanimate objects begin. For example, the patient may have ideas of reference that other people, the television, or the newspapers are making reference to him. Other symptoms include the sense that he has fused with outside objects (e.g., a tree, another person) or that he has disintegrated. Given this state of mind, some schizophrenic patients may have doubts as to what sex they are or what their sexual orientation is. These symptoms, however, should not be confused with transvestism, transsexuality, or homosexuality.

Disorders of the form of thought are objectively observable in the spoken and written language of the patient. These disorders include looseness of associations, derailment, incoherence, tangentiality, circumstantiality, neologisms, echolalia, verbigeration, word salad, and mutism. Although looseness of associations was once described as pathognomonic for schizophrenia, this symptom is seen frequently in mania. To distinguish between looseness of associations and tangentiality can be difficult for even the most experienced clinician.

Disorders in process of thought refer to how ideas and

language are formulated. The examiner infers a disorder from what and how the patient speaks, writes, or draws. It may also be possible to assess the patient's thought process by observing his behavior, especially in carrying out discrete tasks that the clinician might see in occupational therapy. Disorders of thought process include flight of ideas, thought blocking, impaired attention, poverty of thought and content of speech, poor memory, poor abstraction abilities, perseveration, idiosyncratic association (e.g., identical predicates, clang associations), overinclusion, illogical ideas, vagueness, and circumstantiality.

A newer and clinically useful system for describing the thought disorders of schizophrenic patients is to divide them into negative and positive symptoms—sometimes referred to as deficit and productive symptoms, respectively. The deficit symptoms include affective flattening or blunting, poverty of speech or speech content, blocking, poor grooming, lack of motivation, anhedonia, social withdrawal, cognitive defects, and attentional deficits. Positive symptoms include loose associations, hallucinations, bizarre behavior, and increased speech.

Impulse Control, Suicide, and Homicide. Patients with schizophrenia may be quite agitated and have little impulse control when acutely ill. They also have decreased social sensitivity, so they may appear impulsive when, for example, they grab another patient's cigarettes, change television channels abruptly, or throw food on the floor. Some of the apparently impulsive behavior, including suicide or homicide attempts, may be in response to hallucinations commanding the patient to act.

Fifty percent of schizophrenic patients attempt suicide, and 10 percent succeed. Suicide may be precipitated by feelings of absolute emptiness, depression, wanting escape from the mental torture, or by auditory hallucinations that command the patient to kill himself. Risk factors for suicide are as follows: the patient's awareness of his illness, a college education, a young male, a large number of exacerbations and remissions, a change in the course of disease, an improvement from a relapse, depression, dependence on the hospital, overly high ambitions, prior suicide attempts early in the course of illness, and living alone.

It is currently believed that homicide is not more common in schizophrenic patients than it is in the general population. A schizophrenic patient is driven to homicide often for very unpredictable and bizarre reasons based on hallucinations or delusions. Furthermore, some schizophrenic patients display dangerous behavior in the hospital such as violence toward others. These problems are related to the severity of psychosis, history of prior violence, and inadequate or low serum concentrations of antipsychotic drugs.

Orientation. Schizophrenic patients are usually oriented to person, time, and place. Lack of such orientation should prompt an investigation for an organic brain problem. Some schizophrenic patients, however, may give incorrect or bizarre answers to such questions—for example, "I am Christ; this is heaven; and it is 35 A.D."

Memory. Memory, as tested in the mental status examination, is usually intact. It may be impossible, however, to get a patient to attend closely enough to the memory tests to assess this ability adequately.

Judgment and Insight. Classically, the schizophrenic patient has very little insight into his illness, at least as evidenced by his ability to talk about the disease process or his emotional reaction to it. The judgment of the patient is variable in schizophrenia and is best assessed from both the patient's behavior in the interview and outside sources of information.

Reliability. Although a particular schizophrenic patient may be a completely reliable historian, the nature of the illness requires that the examiner verify important information through additional sources.

Neurological Findings

The neurologic findings in schizophrenia are subtle. Some research has shown that the presence of neurologic signs and symptoms correlates with increased severity of illness, affective blunting, and a poor prognosis. Minor neurological symptoms, also called "soft signs," are nonlocalizing neurologic findings that include agraphesthesia, glabellar reflex, grasp reflex, and dysdiadochokinesia. They are seen in groups of schizophrenic patients more often than in normals or in patients with other psychiatric disorders. Schizophrenic patients also have disorders of motor behavior, as evidenced by tics and stereotypies, grimacing, impaired fine motor skills, and abnormal motor tone.

There are two major abnormalities of the eyes in schizophrenia. First, schizophrenic patients have an increased rate of blinking, thought to reflect hyperdopaminergic CNS activity. Second, they have abnormal rapid eye movement, or saccades. Approximately 50 to 80 percent of patients have this inability to follow an object through space with smooth eye movements. Although seen in only 8 percent of normals, saccades is seen in 40 percent of first-degree relatives of schizophrenic patients and may be a neurophysiologic marker of a vulnerability for schizophrenia.

Some investigators consider the disorders of form of thought a *forme fruste* of an aphasia in schizophrenia, perhaps implicating the dominant parietal lobe. The inability of schizophrenic patients to perceive the prosody of speech or to inflect their own speech can be seen as neurologic symptoms of the nondominant parietal lobe. Other parietal-like symptoms in schizophrenia include the inability to carry out tasks (apraxias, which may also implicate the frontal lobes), right-left disorientation, and lack of concern about the illness.

Psychological Testing

Projective testing (e.g., the Rorschach, TAT) may indicate bizarre ideation. Personality inventories (e.g., the MMPI) are often abnormal in schizophrenia, but their contribution to diagnosis or treatment planning is quite minimal. Objective measures of neuropsychological performance, such as the Halstead-Reitan Battery or the Luria-Nebraska Battery, are also often abnormal, but they may indicate specific cognitive deficits that can be addressed in practical ways in the treatment program. These test results are consistent with bilateral frontal and temporal lobe dysfunction, including impaired attention, retention time, problem-solving ability, and intelligence. Low intelligence is often present at onset and may continue to deteriorate with the progress of the illness. In general, the findings are comparable to those of organic brain disorders.

COURSE AND PROGNOSIS

Course

The course of schizophrenia often begins with the prodromal symptoms described in the previous section. The onset of more pronounced symptoms may be acute (days) or gradual (a few months). Onset is usually in adolescence, and there may be an identified precipitating event (e.g., moving away to college, an experience with an hallucinogenic drug, death of a relative). The prodromal symptoms may be present for a year before a diagnosis is made.

The classic course of schizophrenia is one of exacerbations and relative remissions. The major distinction between schizophrenia and the mood disorders is the failure to return to baseline functioning following each relapse. There is sometimes a clinically observable postpsychotic depression following an acute episode, and a vulnerability to stress is often lifelong. Deterioration progresses for an average of 5 years, at which point most patients reach a plateau. Positive symptoms tend to become less severe with time, but the more socially debilitating negative symptoms may increase. The patient's life is characterized by aimlessness, inactivity, frequent hospitalizations, and in urban settings, homelessness and poverty.

Prognosis

Schizophrenia does not always run a deteriorating course. A variety of factors are associated with good and poor prognoses (Table 2). The range of recovery rates in the literature is 10 to 60 percent, and a reasonable estimate is that 20 to 30 percent are able to lead somewhat normal lives. Approximately 20 to 30 percent of patients continue to experience moderate symptoms, and 40 to 60 percent of patients remain significantly impaired by their illness for their entire lives. It is certainly quite clear that schizophrenic patients do much less well than patients with mood disorders, although approximately 20 to 25 percent of the latter group are also severely disturbed at long-term follow-up.

DIAGNOSIS AND SUBTYPES

DSM-III-R contains the official diagnostic guidelines for schizophrenia of the American Psychiatric Association (Table 3). Changes from DSM-III include the requirement that the major psychotic symptoms be present for at least 1 week, the inclusion of the failure of a child or adolescent to reach an expected developmental level as a criterion, and the elimination of the requirement that the illness begin before age 45.

Subtypes

There have been many efforts to subtype schizophrenia, the major clinical value of which is to identify patients with good prognoses. This differentiation, however, can be done most pragmatically by following the guidelines described in Table 2. Although some subtyping schemes have had prognostic differences in mind, others have paid more attention to differences in clinical presentations. DSM-III-R has based its subtypes mostly on clinical distinctions. There are five types: disorganized (previously called hebephrenic), catatonic, paranoid, undifferentiated, and residual which are discussed below. The DSM-III-R diagnostic criteria for subtypes are listed in Table 4.

(1) Disorganized Type (Hebephrenic). The disorganized or hebephrenic subtype is characterized by a marked regression to primitive, disinhibited, and

Table 2
Features Weighting Toward Good or Poor Prognosis in Schizophrenia

Good	Poor
Later onset	Younger onset
Obvious precipitating factors	No precipitating factors
Acute onset	Insidious onset
Good premorbid social, sexual, and work history	Poor premorbid social, sexual, and work history
Affective symptoms (especially depression)	Withdrawn, autistic behavior
Paranoid or catatonic features	Undifferentiated or disorganized features
Married	Single, divorced, or widowed
Family history of mood disorders	Family history of schizophrenia
Good support systems	Poor support systems
Undulating course	Chronic course
Positive symptoms	Negative symptoms
	Neurological signs and symptoms
	History of perinatal trauma
	No remissions in 3 years
	Many relapses

unorganized behavior. The onset is usually early, before age 25. The disorganized patient is usually active but in an aimless, nonconstructive manner. His thought disorder is pronounced, and his contact with reality is extremely poor. His personal appearance and his social behavior are dilapidated. His emotional responses are inappropriate, and he often bursts out laughing without any apparent reasons.

Incongruous grinning and grimacing are common in this type of patient, whose behavior is best described as silly or fatuous.

(2) Catatonic Type. DSM-III-R states that the essential feature of this type is marked psychomotor disturbance, which may involve stupor, negativism, rigidity, excitement, or posturing. Sometimes there is rapid alterna-

---

Table 3
Diagnostic Criteria for Schizophrenia

A. Presence of characteristic psychotic symptoms in the active phase: either (1), (2), or (3) for at least 1 week (unless the symptoms are successfully treated):

   (1) two of the following:
      (a) delusions
      (b) prominent hallucinations (throughout the day for several days or several times a week for several weeks, each hallucinatory experience not being limited to a few brief moments)
      (c) incoherence or marked loosening of associations
      (d) catatonic behavior
      (e) flat or grossly inappropriate affect
   (2) bizarre delusions involving a phenomenon that the person's culture would regard as totally implausible (e.g., thought broadcasting, being controlled by a dead person)
   (3) prominent hallucinations [as defined in (1)(b) above] of a voice with content having no apparent relation to depression or elation, or a voice keeping up a running commentary on the person's behavior or thoughts, or two or more voices conversing with each other

B. During the course of the disturbance, functioning in such areas as work, social relations, and self-care is markedly below the highest level achieved before onset of the disturbance (or, when the onset is in childhood or adolescence, failure to achieve expected level of social development).

C. Schizoaffective Disorder and Mood Disorder with Psychotic Features have been ruled out, i.e., if a Major Depressive or Manic Syndrome has ever been present during an active phase of the disturbance, the total duration of all episodes of a mood syndrome has been brief relative to the total duration of the active and residual phases of the disturbance.

D. Continuous signs of the disturbance for at least 6 months. The 6-month period must include an active phase (of at least 1 week, or less if symptoms have been successfully treated) during which there were psychotic symptoms characteristic of Schizophrenia (symptoms in A), with or without a prodromal or residual phase, as defined below.

Prodromal phase: A clear deterioration in functioning before the active phase of the disturbance that is not due to a disturbance in mood or to a Psychoactive Substance Use Disorder and that involves at least two of the symptoms listed below.

Residual phase: Following the active phase of the disturbance, persistence of at least two of the symptoms noted below, these not being due to a disturbance in mood or to a Psychoactive Substance Use Disorder.

Prodromal or Residual Symptoms:

   (1) marked social isolation or withdrawal
   (2) marked impairment in role functioning as wage-earner, student, or homemaker
   (3) markedly peculiar behavior (e.g., collecting garbage, talking to self in public, hoarding food)
   (4) marked impairment in personal hygiene and grooming
   (5) blunted or inappropriate affect
   (6) digressive, vague, overelaborate, or circumstantial speech, or poverty of speech, or poverty of content of speech
   (7) odd beliefs or magical thinking, influencing behavior and inconsistent with cultural norms (e.g., superstitiousness, belief in clairvoyance, telepathy, "sixth sense," "others can feel my feelings," overvalued ideas, ideas of reference)
   (8) unusual perceptual experiences (e.g., recurrent illusions, sensing the presence of a force or person not actually present)
   (9) marked lack of initiative, interests, or energy

Examples: Six months of prodromal symptoms with 1 week of symptoms from A; no prodromal symptoms with 6 months of symptoms from A; no prodromal symptoms with 1 week of symptoms from A and 6 months of residual symptoms.

E. It cannot be established that an organic factor initiated and maintained the disturbance.

F. If there is a history of Autistic Disorder, the additional diagnosis of Schizophrenia is made only if prominent delusions or hallucinations are also present.

Classification of course. The course of the disturbance is coded in the fifth digit:

   1-Subchronic. The time from the beginning of the disturbance, when the person first began to show signs of the disturbance (including prodromal, active, and residual phases) more or less continuously, is less than 2 years but at least 6 months.

   2-Chronic. Same as above, but more than 2 years.

Table 3 *continued*

3-Subchronic with Acute Exacerbation. Reemergence of prominent psychotic symptoms in a person with a subchronic course who has been in the residual phase of the disturbance.

4-Chronic with Acute Exacerbation. Reemergence of prominent psychotic symptoms in a person with a chronic course who has been in the residual phase of the disturbance.

5-In Remission. When a person with a history of Schizophrenia is free of all signs of the disturbance (whether or not on medication), "in Remission" should be coded. Differentiating Schizophrenia in Remission from No Mental Disorder requires consideration of overall level of functioning, length of time since the last episode of disturbance, total duration of the disturbance, and whether prophylactic treatment is being given.

0-Unspecified.

Specify late onset if the disturbance (including the prodromal phase) develops after age 45.

Table from DSM-III-R, *Diagnostic and Statistical Manual of Mental Disorders,* ed 3, revised. (Current Classification of Mental Disorders, 1987.) Copyright American Psychiatric Association, Washington, D.C., 1987. Used with permission.

Table 4
Diagnostic Criteria for Subtypes of Schizophrenia

Paranoid Type
A type of schizophrenia in which there are:

A. Preoccupation with one or more systematized delusions or with frequent auditory hallucinations related to a single theme.

B. *None* of the following: incoherence, marked loosening of associations, flat or grossly inappropriate affect, catatonic behavior, grossly disorganized behavior.

Specify stable type if criteria A and B have been met during all past and present active phases of the illness.
Catatonic Type
A type of Schizophrenia in which the clinical picture is dominated by any of the following:
    (1) catatonic stupor (marked decrease in reactivity to the environment and/or reduction in spontaneous movements and activity) or mutism
    (2) catatonic negativism (an apparently motiveless resistance to all instructions or attempts to be moved)
    (3) catatonic rigidity (maintenance of a rigid posture against efforts to be moved)
    (4) catatonic excitement (excited motor activity, apparently purposeless and not influenced by external stimuli)
    (5) catatonic posturing (voluntary assumption of inappropriate or bizarre postures)
Disorganized Type
A type of Schizophrenia in which the following criteria are met:

A. Incoherence, marked loosening of associations, or grossly disorganized behavior

B. Flat or grossly inappropriate affect

C. Does not meet the criteria for Catatonic Type
Undifferentiated Type
A type of Schizophrenia in which there are:

A. Prominent delusions, hallucinations, incoherence, or grossly disorganized behavior

B. Does not meet the criteria for Paranoid, Catatonic, or Disorganized Type
Residual Type
A type of Schizophrenia in which there are:

A. Absence of prominent delusions, hallucinations, incoherence, or grossly disorganized behavior

B. Continuing evidence of the disturbance, as indicated by two or more of the residual symptoms listed in criterion D of Schizophrenia.

Table from DSM-III-R, *Diagnostic and Statistical Manual of Mental Disorders,* ed 3, revised. (Current Classification of Mental Disorders, 1987.) Copyright American Psychiatric Association, Washington, D.C., 1987. Used with permission.

tion between the extremes of excitement and stupor. Associated features include stereotypies, mannerisms, and waxy flexibility. Mutism is particularly common.

During catatonic stupor or excitement, the person needs careful supervision to avoid hurting himself or herself or others. Medical care may be needed because of malnutrition, exhaustion, hyperpyrexia, or self-inflicted injury.

Although this type was very common several decades ago, it is now rare in Europe and North America.

(3) Paranoid Type. The paranoid type of schizophrenia is characterized mainly by the presence of delusions of persecution or grandeur. Paranoid schizophrenics are usually older than catatonic or disorganized schizophrenics when they break down; that is, they are usually in their late 20s or in their 30s. Patients who have been well up to that age have usually established a place and an identity for themselves in the community. Their ego resources are greater than those of catatonic and disorganized patients. Paranoid schizophrenics show less regression of mental faculties, emotional response, and behavior than do the other subtypes of schizophrenia.

A typical paranoid schizophrenic is tense, suspicious, guarded, and reserved. He is often hostile and aggressive. The paranoid schizophrenic usually conducts himself quite well socially. His intelligence in areas not invaded by his delusions may remain high.

(4) Undifferentiated Type. Frequently, patients who are clearly schizophrenic cannot be easily fitted into one of the other subtypes, usually because they meet the criteria for more than one subtype. Some acute, excited schizophrenic patients—diagnosed in ICD-9 as suffering from acute schizophrenic episode—and some inert, chronic patients fall into this category, for which DSM-III-R provides the designation undifferentiated.

(5) Residual Type. According to DSM-III-R this category should be used when there has been at least one episode of schizophrenia, but the clinical picture that occasioned the evaluation or admission to clinical care is without prominent psychotic symptoms, though signs of the illness persist. Emotional blunting, social withdrawal, eccentric behavior, illogical thinking, and mild loosening of associations are common. If delusions or hallucinations are present, they are not prominent, and are not accompanied by strong affect. The course of this type is either chronic or subchronic.

The following example illustrates a case of paranoid schizophrenia:

Three months after its initial contact with the patient, a 26-year-old male migratory farm worker, a community mental health team was contacted by the city police. The patient, who had been maintained in an outpatient clinic for the past few months, had suddenly appeared in a judge's chamber and demanded to be put to death because he felt he was responsible for the production of evil and violence in the world. When team members reached the jail, they found the patient agitated, easily angered, suspicious, and guarded. His speech was disorganized and often incoherent. He stated that he could not eat meat or terrible violence and evil would be unleashed on the world. He also described a plot by the California Mafia to keep him from working, and he spoke of voices that told him what to do and that "must be obeyed."

Past history included similar episodes over the previous five years, resulting in several year-long periods of inpatient hospitalization. At no time did he exhibit a full manic or depressive syndrome. Between hospitalizations the patient lived in hobo jungles, flophouses, and gospel missions; rode freight trains from town to town; and worked, picking fruit, for only a few days at a time. Since adolescence he has lived the life of a drifting loner.

Discussion

The bizarre delusions, incoherence, and chronic course with marked impairment in functioning, in the absence of an affective syndrome, leave little doubt as to the diagnosis of schizophrenia. The delusion of guilt, although often associated with major depression with psychotic features, is not sufficient, in the absence of other symptoms of a major depressive episode, to seriously raise the question of a major mood disorder.

The subtype is classified as paranoid because of the prominent persecutory delusions. The course is coded as chronic because the illness has lasted longer than two years.

[Adapted with permission from *DSM-III Case Book.* American Psychiatric Association, Washington, D.C., 1981.]

There are three subtypes in ICD-9 that are not included in DSM-III-R: paraphrenia, simple, and latent.

Paraphrenia. This term is used as a synonym for paranoid schizophrenia in ICD-9. In other systems it is used to describe a chronic downhill course with well-systematized delusions but with a well-preserved personality. Its multiple meanings render the term less useful for communication of information.

Simple. ICD-9 includes schizophrenia, simple type, which is characterized by a gradual, insidious loss of drive and ambition. The patient is usually not hallucinating or delusional, and if these symptoms do occur, they do not persist. The patient withdraws from contact with other people and often stops working. Clinicians are advised to exercise caution in making this diagnosis since this condition is not particularly responsive to medication, and the diagnostic label of schizophrenia, even if warranted, can do more harm than good to such patients.

Latent. Latent schizophrenia is diagnosed in those patients who may have marked schizoid personality and who show occasional behavioral peculiarities or thought disorders, without consistently manifesting any clearly psychotic pathology. The syndrome has been termed borderline schizophrenia in the past. It most closely resembles the DSM-III-R diagnosis of schizotypal personality disorder. Again, the clinican is wise to make a diagnosis of schizophrenia only with more significant pathology.

There are a variety of other subtypes, mostly of historical or theoretical interest. Some subtypes have obvious definitions—late-onset, childhood, and process. Late-onset schizophrenia begins after age 45 and is now included in the DSM-III-R criteria for schizophrenia. Childhood schizophrenia begins in childhood, and in DSM-III-R is simply called schizophrenia, with age of onset specified. Process schizophrenia is synonymous with poor-prognosis, deteriorating schizophrenia.

Bouffée Délirante (Acute Delusional Psychosis). This diagnostic category is used in France and is considered to be a diagnostic category in its own right, not a subtype of schizophrenia. The actual criteria are similar to those of DSM-III-R schizophrenia, but the symptoms must be present for less than 3 months, thereby approximating the DSM-III-R diagnosis of schizophreniform disorder. French psychiatrists report that about 40 percent of patients with this diagnosis are later diagnosed as having schizophrenia.

Oneiroid. In the oneiroid state, the patient feels and behaves as though in a dream. He may be deeply perplexed and not fully oriented in time and place. The oneiroid schizophrenic acknowledges everyday realities but gives priority to the world of hallucinatory experiences. Oneiroid states are usually limited in duration and might be classified as atypical psychosis in DSM-III-R. The clinician should be careful to examine the patient for an organic cause in the presence of this symptomatology.

Pseudoneurotic. These patients present predominantly with neurotic symptoms but on closer examination reveal schizophrenic abnormalities in thinking and emotional reaction. These patients are characterized by pananxiety, panphobia, panambivalence, and chaotic sexuality. Unlike patients suffering from anxiety neuroses, these patients have anxiety that is free floating and hardly ever subsides. They rarely become overtly psychotic.

DIFFERENTIAL DIAGNOSIS

There are three principal guidelines in the differential diagnosis of schizophrenia. First, the clinician should aggressively investigate the possibility of an identifiable organic etiology, especially if there are unusual or rare symptoms. Second, there should be a complete evaluation of each exacerbation of psychotic symptoms in a schizophrenic patient. The clinician should have an open mind toward the possibility of a superimposed organic cause, especially when the patient has been in remission for a long time or if there is a change in the quality of symptoms. Third, the clinician should carefully elicit and consider a family history of psychiatric and neurologic diseases.

There are a large number of neurologic and medical diseases that can have symptoms identical to those of schizophrenia (Table 5). The psychiatric manifestations of these disorders often come early in the course, before the development of other symptoms. It is generally true that patients with neurologic disorders have more insight into and more distress from their symptoms than patients with schizophrenia. The fact that so many disorders can mimic schizophrenia is consistent with the notion that schizophrenia itself is a heterogeneous disorder.

The psychiatric differential diagnosis for schizophrenia-like symptoms is also quite lengthy.

Malingering and Factitious Disorder with Psychological Symptoms. It is possible to fake the symptoms of schizophrenia since the diagnosis depends so much on the report of the patient. Patients who do, in fact, have schizophrenia may sometimes falsely complain of symptoms for secondary gain, such as increased assistance benefits or admission to a hospital.

Autistic Disorder. Autistic disorder is diagnosed when onset is after 30 months of age but before 12 years. There is an absence of delusions, hallucinations, and looseness of associations.

Mood Disorders. The differential diagnosis of schizophrenia and mood disorders can be quite difficult, but it is particularly important because of the availability of specific and effective treatments for mania and depression. DSM-III-R specifies that affective or mood symptoms in schizophrenia must be brief relative to the duration of the primary symptoms. In the absence of information other than a single mental status examination, it is usually prudent to delay a final diagnosis or to assume the presence of a mood disorder, rather than to diagnose prematurely a patient as having schizophrenia.

Schizoaffective Disorder. This diagnosis is made when a manic or depressive syndrome develops concurrently with the major symptoms of schizophrenia. In addition, delusions or hallucinations must be present for at least 2 weeks in the absence of prominent affective symptoms during some phase of the illness.

Schizophreniform Disorder and Brief Reactive Psychosis. Schizophreniform disorder is diagnosed when all the criteria for schizophrenia have been met but symptoms have been present for less than 6 months. Brief reactive psychosis is diagnosed when those symptoms have been present for less than 1 month and there is either a clear precipitating stressor or series of stressors.

Delusional Disorder. A diagnosis of delusional disorder is warranted if nonbizarre delusions have been present for at least 6 months in the absence of the other symptoms of schizophrenia or a mood disorder.

Personality Disorder. A variety of personality disorders may present with some features of schizophrenia. Personality disorders are long-standing patterns of behavior; their date of onset is less identifiable than that of schizophrenia.

Table 5
Differential Diagnosis of Schizophrenia-like Symptoms

Medical/Neurological:

Drug induced—amphetamine, hallucinogens, belladonna alkaloids, alcohol hallucinosis, barbiturate withdrawal, cocaine, PCP

Epilepsy—especially temporal lobe epilepsy

Neoplasm, stroke, or trauma—especially frontal or limbic

Other conditions—acute intermittent porphyria
vitamin B_{12} deficiency
carbon monoxide poisoning
cerebral lipoidosis
Creutzfeldt-Jakob disease
Fabry's disease
Fahr's syndrome
Hallervorden-Spatz disease
heavy metal poisoning
herpes encephalitis
homocystinuria
Huntington's disease
metachromatic leukodystrophy
neurosyphilis
normal pressure hydrocephalus
pellagra
systemic lupus erythematosus
Wernicke-Korsakoff syndrome
Wilson's disease

Psychiatric:

atypical psychosis
brief reactive psychosis
factitious disorder with psychological symptoms
infantile autism
malingering
mood disorders
normal adolescence
obsessive-compulsive disorder
paranoid disorders
personality disorders—schizotypal, schizoid, borderline, paranoid
schizoaffective disorder
schizophrenia
schizophreniform disorders

CLINICAL MANAGEMENT

Hospitalization

The primary indications for hospitalization are for diagnostic purposes, stabilization on medications, patient safety due to suicidal or homicidal ideation, or grossly disorganized or inappropriate behavior, including the inability to take care of basic needs (e.g., food, clothing, and shelter). A primary goal of hospitalization should be to establish an effective link between the patient and community support systems. Introduced in the early 1950s, antipsychotic medications have revolutionized the treatment of schizophrenia. Approximately two to four times as many patients relapse when treated with placebo rather than antipsychotics. Antipsychotics, however, treat the symptoms of the illness and are not a cure for schizophrenia. Other aspects of clinical management flow logically from a medical model of disease. Rehabilitation and adjustment implies that the specific handicaps of the patient are taken into account when planning treatment strategies. The physician also must educate the patient, and the patient's caregivers and family about schizophrenia.

Hospitalization decreases stress on a patient and helps him structure his daily activities. The length of hospitalization depends on the severity of the patient's illness and the availability of outpatient treatment facilities. Research has shown that short hospitalizations are just as effective as long-term hospitalizations and that active treatment programs with behavioral approaches are more effective than custodial insititutions or insight-oriented therapeutic communities. The hospitalization treatment plan should have a practical orientation toward issues of living situation, self-care, quality of life, employment, and social relationships. Hospitalization should be directed toward aligning the patient with aftercare facilities, including his family home, a foster family, board and care homes, and halfway houses. Day care centers and home visits can sometimes help a patient remain out of the hospital for longer periods of time, and improve the quality of the patient's daily life.

Antipsychotics

The antipsychotics (also called neuroleptics or major tranquilizers) include the phenothiazines, butyrophenones, thioxanthenes, dibenzoxazepines, and oxoindoles (see Section 31.2). There are five major guidelines for the use of antipsychotics in schizophrenia. First, the clinician should carefully define the target symptoms to be treated. Second, an antipsychotic that has worked in the past for the patient should be used again. In the absence of such information, it is important to realize that no antipsychotic has been shown to be more effective than any other, although some patients seem to respond to one and not to another. The choice of an antipsychotic is usually based on its side effect profile and how that might interfere with the life of the particular patient. Although clinical lore has it that lower potency antipsychotics (e.g., chlorpromazine, thioridazine) are more effective with agitated patients and higher potency agents (e.g., haloperidol, fluphenizine) are more effective with withdrawn patients, this idea has not been confirmed in controlled studies. Third, the minimum length of an antipsychotic trial is 4 to 6 weeks at adequate doses. If the trial is unsuccessful, an antipsychotic from another class should be tried until representative drugs from all five classes have been investigated. Fourth, polypharmacy, especially using more than one antipsychotic at a time, should be avoided. Fifth, maintenance doses of antipsychotics can usually be lower than the doses necessary for acute episodes.

Dosage.   The chlorpromazine (CPZ) milligram equivalents of various antipsychotics have been determined through clinical trials and receptor-binding studies. Acute episodes of psychosis almost always respond to 300 to 1000 CPZ equivalents of an antipsychotic. Intramuscular (IM) injections deliver peak plasma levels in approximately 30 minutes; oral medication takes 100 minutes. It may be reasonable, therefore, to give the first dose of medication IM in an emergency setting and subsequent doses, orally. Patients who fail to respond to 1500 CPZ equivalents seldom respond to so-called high-dose or megadose antipsychotics; these doses should be tried only after adequate trials at lower doses have proven unsuccessful. All antipsychotics can be given once a day, and once a day medication schedules are correlated with greater compliance than other drug schedules. Occasionally, it may be appropriate to give antipsychotics two or three times a day if the contact with the nurse is therapeutic, if the dose is coordinated with anticholinergic medications, or in an effort to minimize side effects. In general, the most common clinical mistake is to give more neuroleptic than is necessary. This occurs for two reasons. First, the commonly used high-potency neuroleptics are remarkably safe drugs, and high doses can be used with minimal immediate risk to the patient. Second, doctors and nurses in the United States have become accustomed to using higher doses and often feel inappropriately reluctant to give small doses. Research has shown, however, that lower amounts of antipsychotics generally produce the same clinical response as higher doses. Clinically, antipsychotic doses are often inappropriately raised every day or so, thereby giving the impression that it was the increase in medication that reduced the symptoms, when it actually was the passage of time on medication.

Nonresponders.   A patient should not be continued on a neuroleptic longer than 6 weeks if there is no improvement in the target symptoms with 1500 CPZ equivalents. If tests to measure plasma concentrations are available, they may indicate noncompliance or unusual metabolism resulting in dramatically low concentrations. In the case of low concentrations, high doses may be warranted, or a switch to another antipsychotic may result in adequate plasma concentrations.

Compliance.   Noncompliance with neuroleptics is a major reason for relapse. Although several studies have failed to demonstrate a difference between oral and long-acting injectable regimens, a trial of a long-acting injectable antipsychotic is warranted when noncompliance is a problem.

Maintenance.   Following recovery from an acute episode, the dose of antipsychotics can usually be carefully lowered to 100 to 500 CPZ equivalents, or about 5 mg fluphenazine decanoate biweekly. The decision to maintain a patient on antipsychotics is based on the severity of illness and the adequacy of the outpatient treatment setting. Patients who continue to have symptoms are likely to relapse if medication is discontinued. Following discontinuation of an antipsychotic, about two thirds of patients who have been in good remission for 3 to 5 years relapse within 18 months, most of them within 3 to 7 months. Patients who have good remission of symptoms on drugs and who are in responsible treatment settings may be appropriate for targeted or intermittent drug treatment. In this treatment strategy, patients are removed from antipsychotic treatment and carefully monitored. At the first sign of relapse, drugs are reinstituted for as long as is necessary to prevent the recurrence of severe symptoms.

Adverse Effects. Adverse effects are an important cause of noncompliance. The most common side effects of antipsychotics are extrapyramidal neurologic signs, weight gain, and impotence. Extrapyramidal symptoms are more common in men than in women and in younger people than in older people. Extrapyramidal symptoms usually respond to anticholinergic agents, and it is a subtle clinical decision whether to treat patients with them prophylactically. In favor of prophylaxis is the observation that an adverse experience at the onset of neuroleptic treatment correlates with future noncompliance. Against prophylactic treatment is the possibility of anticholinergic toxicity, including cognitive deficits, urinary retention, and paralytic ileus. These problems, however, are rare if modest doses are used. If anticholinergics are used, however, the clinician should attempt every 3 to 4 months to discontinue them slowly since tolerance often develops to the parkinsonian effects of neuroleptics.

The most serious side effects of antipsychotics are tardive dyskinesia and neuroleptic malignant syndrome. Tardive dyskinesia is reported to have a prevalence of 15 to 20 percent of patients treated. Most affected patients have mild symptoms, and 40 percent of patients improve if the antipsychotic is discontinued. Tardive dyskinesia is more common in women than in men and in older patients than in younger patients. Neuroleptic malignant syndrome occurs in approximately 0.5 to 1 percent of patients treated with these drugs. It is a life-threatening syndrome characterized by fever, generalized rigidity, delirium, and increased abnormal behavior. At its onset, neuroleptic malignant syndrome is often mistakenly identified as an exacerbation of the schizophrenic symptoms, and antipsychotics are erroneously increased rather than discontinued.

Other Drugs

If a patient does not respond to antipsychotic treatment alone, a physician may add lithium to the therapeutic regimen for 6 to 12 weeks and then assess whether treatment response warrants continuation of the drug. Three other drugs—propranolol, benzodiazepines, and carbamazepine—have been reported to cause improvement in a few cases of schizophrenia. In patients who do not improve with antipsychotics and lithium, or in patients who have severe tardive dyskinesia that contraindicates the use of antipsychotics, trials with these other agents may be warranted.

Other Somatic Treatments

Although much less effective than antipsychotics, electroconvulsive treatment (ECT) may be indicated for catatonic patients or for patients who for some reason cannot take neuroleptics. Patients who have been ill less than 1 year are more likely to respond.

Historical treatments for schizophrenia include insulin-induced and barbiturate-induced coma. These treatments are no longer used because of the associated hazards. Psychosurgery, particularly frontal lobotomies, were used from 1935 to 1955 for the treatment of schizophrenia. Although more sophisticated approaches to psychosurgery for schizophrenia may eventually be developed, psychosurgery is no longer considered an appropriate treatment for schizophrenia.

PSYCHOSOCIAL TREATMENTS

Although antipsychotic medications are the mainstay of treatment for schizophrenia, research has demonstrated that psychosocial interventions can augment the clinical improvement. Psychosocial modalities should be carefully integrated into the drug treatment regimen and should support it. Most schizophrenic patients benefit from the combined use of antipsychotics and psychosocial treatment.

Behavioral Therapy

Treatment planning for schizophrenia should address both the abilities and deficits of the patient. Behavioral techniques use token economies and social skills training to increase social abilities, self-sufficiency, practical skills, and interpersonal communication. Adaptive behaviors are reinforced by praise or tokens that can be redeemed for desired items (e.g., more hospital privileges, cigarettes). Consequently, the frequency of maladaptive or deviant behavior (e.g., talking loudly, talking to oneself in public, bizarre posturing) is reduced.

Family Therapy

Families tend to blame themselves for any illness or accident that happens to a family member. The problem is magnified with schizophrenia since at one time many psychiatrists counted family pathology as an etiologic factor. It may therefore be difficult to enlist the aid of families in the treatment program. Nevertheless, it has been demonstrated that specific approaches to family therapy can reduce the relapse rates of some schizophrenic patients. Families with so-called high expressed emotion can have hostile, critical, emotionally overinvolved, or intrusive interactions with the schizophrenic patient. If these behaviors are directly modified, the relapse rate for such patients may be dramatically reduced. The psychiatrist should also educate the family, support them in their difficult situation, and introduce them to family support groups for parents of schizophrenic children.

Group Therapy

Group therapy with schizophrenia generally focuses on real-life plans, problems, and relationships. Groups may be behaviorally oriented, psychodynamically or insight-oriented, or supportive. There is some doubt whether dynamic interpretation and insight therapy have much value for the typical schizophrenic patient. But group therapy is particularly effective in reducing social isolation, increasing sense of cohesiveness, and improving reality testing for patients with schizophrenia. Groups led in a supportive manner, rather than an interpretive one, appear to be more helpful for schizophrenic patients.

Social Skills Training. This process is a highly structured form of group therapy for schizophrenic patients. Social skills can be defined as those interpersonal behaviors required to attain instrumental goals necessary for community survival and independence and to establish, maintain, and deepen supportive and socially rewarding relationships. Applying behavior analysis principles to identify and remedy deficits in social behaviors, the clinician utilizes a variety of techniques (e.g., focused instructions, role modeling, feedback, and social reinforcement).

Individual Psychotherapy

Schizophrenic patients can be helped by individual psychotherapy that provides a positive treatment relationship and therapeutic alliance. The relationship between the clinician and patient is quite different from that encountered in the treatment of neurosis. In general, orthodox formal psychoanalysis has no place in the treatment of schizophrenia. Supportive psychotherapy is the type most often employed. Establishing a relationship is often a particularly difficult matter; the schizophrenic patient is desperately lonely, yet defends against closeness and trust and is likely to become suspicious, anxious, hostile, or regressed when someone attempts to draw close. Scrupulous observance of distance and privacy, simple directness, patience, sincerity, and sensitivity to social conventions are preferable to premature informality and the condescending use of first names. Exaggerated warmth or professions of friendship are out of place and are likely to be perceived as attempts at bribery, manipulation, or exploitation.

In the context of a professional relationship, however, flexibility may be essential in establishing a working alliance with the patient. At those times, the therapist may have meals with the patient, sit on the floor, go for a walk, eat at a restaurant, accept and give gifts, play table tennis, remember the patient's birthday, allow him to telephone the therapist at any hour, or just sit silently with him. The major aim is to convey that the therapist can be trusted, wants to understand the patient and will try to do so, and that the therapist has faith in the patient's potential as a human being, no matter how disturbed, hostile, or bizarre he may be at the moment. Manfred Bleuler stated that the correct therapeutic attitude toward a schizophrenic patient is to accept him as a brother, rather than watch him as a person who has become unintelligible and different from the therapist.

References

Andreasen N C, editor: Schizophrenia. In *Annual Review*, A J Frances, R E Hales, editors, vol 5. American Psychiatric Press, Washington, DC, 1986.

Davis J M, Janicak P, Chang S: Recent advances in the pharmacologic treatment of schizophrenic disorders. In *Annual Review*, L Grinspoon editor. vol 1, American Psychiatric Press, Washington, DC, 1982.

Drake R E: Suicide among schizophrenics. Compr Psychiatry 26:90, 1985.

Geer R E, Resnick S M, Alavi A, Geer R C, Caroff S, Dann R, Silver F L, Saykin A J, Chawluk J B, Kushner M, Reivich M: Regional brain function in schizophrenia. I. A positron emission tomography study. II. Repeated evaluation with positron emission tomography. Arch Gen Psychiatry 44:119, 1987.

Grebb J A, Weinberger D R, and Wyatt R J: Schizophrenia. In *Diseases of the Nervous System*, A K Asbury, G M McKhann, W I McDonald, editors, vol II. W B Saunders, Philadelphia, 1986.

Hamilton M, editor: *Fish's Clinical Psychopathology*, ed 2. Wright, Bristol, 1985.

Henn F A, Nasrallah H A, editors: *Schizophrenia as a Brain Disease*. Oxford, New York, 1982.

Kay S R, Lindenmayer J P: Outcome predictors in acute schizophrenia Prospective significance of background and clinical dimensions. J Nerv Mental Dis 175:152, 1987.

Nasrallah H A, Weinberger D R editors: The Neurology of Schizophrenia. In *Handbook of Schizophrenia*, H A Nasrallah, editor, vol 1. Elsevier, Amsterdam, 1986.

Volkow N D, Wolf A P, Von Gelder P, Brodie J O, Overall J E, Cancro R, Gomez Mont F: Phenomenological correlates of metabolic activity in 18 patients with chronic schizophrenia. Am J Psychiatry 144:151, 1987.

Wyatt R J, Cutler N R, DeLisi L: Biochemical and morphological factors in the etiology of the schizophrenic disorders. In *Psychiatry Update: American Psychiatric Association Annual Review*, L Grinspoon, editor. American Psychiatric Press, Washington, DC, 1982.

Zarcone V P, Jr, Benson K L, Berger P A: Abnormal rapid eye movement latencies in schizophrenia. Arch Gen Psychiatry 44:45, 1987.

15

Delusional (Paranoid) Disorders

By definition, the dominant symptom in delusional disorders is a delusion or delusional system that does not have an identifiable organic basis. Symptoms of a major mood disorder are absent, and the delusions lack the bizarre quality often seen in schizophrenia. Other signs and symptoms of thought disorder are minimal. The patient's affect is appropriate to the delusion, and his personality remains intact or deteriorates minimally over a prolonged period of time.

HISTORY

In 1818, Heinroth introduced the basic concept of paranoia when he described disorders of the "intellect" under the term *Verrücktheit*. In 1838, the French psychiatrist Esquirol coined the term "monomania" to characterize delusions with no associated defect in logical reasoning or general behavior. Kahlbaum, in 1863, used the term "paranoia" to describe these patients and characterized the illness as uncommon but distinct. Kraepelin, in 1921, described paraphrenia as an illness with an insidious onset and chronic course, but differentiated it from schizophrenia by the absence of hallucinations and other psychotic symptoms as well as the lack of deterioration in personality. DSM-III and other diagnostic systems have separated chronic paranoid (e.g., paranoia, paraphrenia) from acute paranoid disorders (e.g., paranoid states). Some classifications have noted that the chronic forms tend to have more systematized delusional systems than the acute forms. DSM-III-R has labeled these syndromes delusional disorders to indicate that the content of delusions is not restricted to paranoia, and that paranoia is not necessarily involved in the evolution of the disorders.

EPIDEMIOLOGY

The prevalence of delusional disorders in the United States is currently estimated to be 0.03 percent; this is in contrast to schizophrenia, 1 percent; and to mood disorders, 5 percent. Patients who present with delusions often have additional symptoms that indicate other diagnoses. It should be noted, however, that there may be an underreporting of delusional disorders since these patients rarely seek psychiatric help unless forced to do so by the family or the courts. The annual incidence of delusional disorders is from one to three new cases per 100,000 popu-

lation. This number represents approximately 4 percent of first admissions to psychiatric hospitals for nonorganic psychoses.

The mean age of onset is approximately 40 years, but the age range is from 25 to the 90s. There is a slight preponderance of female patients. Many patients are married and employed, and there may be some association with recent immigration or low socioeconomic status.

ETIOLOGY

The etiology of delusional disorder is not known. One possibility is that delusional disorder is a subtype of schizophrenia or mood disorders. However, family studies suggest that delusional disorder is a distinct clinical entity. These studies report an increased prevalence of delusional disorder and related personality traits in the relatives of delusional disorder probands. Family studies have also reported that there is neither an increased incidence of schizophrenia and mood disorders in the families of delusional disorder probands nor an increased incidence of delusional disorder in the families of schizophrenic probands. Long-term follow-up of patients diagnosed with delusional disorder found that their diagnoses are rarely revised as schizophrenia or mood disorders; hence, delusional disorder is not merely an early stage of these other disorders. Moreover, delusional disorder has a later onset than schizophrenia or mood disorders.

Biological Considerations

The neuropsychiatric approach to delusional disorders derives from the observation that delusions are a common symptom in many neurological conditions, particularly those involving the limbic system and the basal ganglia. Patients who have neurological disease tend to have complex delusions quite similar to those seen in delusional disorders when their neurological condition (e.g., tumors or trauma to the basal ganglia) is characterized by the absence of intellectual impairment. Conversely, neurologic patients with intellectual impairment (e.g., Alzheimer's disease) present more often with simple delusions. It should be remembered that the limbic system has significant reciprocal innervations with the basal ganglia, thereby creating a system that can affect mood and motivation. Thus, it has been hypothesized that discrete anatomic or molecular lesions of either the limbic system or basal ganglia, in the presence of intact cognitive functions, could provide the biological basis for delusions and delusional disorder. It is possible, for example, that reduplicative paramnesia (e.g., the delusion that a hospital room is really the patient's bedroom) stems from the patient's irrefutable and irresistible sensation of familiar surroundings. The patient then uses his intact cerebral cortex to explain the feeling of familiarity by insisting that the hospital room is, in fact, his own bedroom.

Psychodynamic Considerations

There is a strong clinical impression that many delusional disorder patients are socially isolated, have attained less than expected levels of achievement, and often have experienced cultural changes. More specific psychodynamic theories regarding the etiology and evolution of delusional symptoms have involved the concepts of hypersensitive individuals with various emotional insecurities (e.g., fears of being homosexual), as well as the ego mechanisms of reaction formation, projection, and denial. These formulations developed out of retrospective data from the psychoanalysis of patients with delusions. Although the theories may make intuitive sense, there is no prospective research data that demonstrate a causal relationship between specific psychodynamic issues and the development of delusional symptoms. Clinical experience suggests, however, that patients do benefit from psychotherapeutic treatments based on these theories.

Freud's Contributions. Freud believed that delusions, rather than being symptoms of the illness, were part of a healing process. In 1896 he described projection as the main defense mechanism in paranoia. Later, Freud read *Memoirs of My Nervous Illness,* an autobiographical account by the gifted jurist Daniel Paul Schreber. Although he never personally met Schreber, Freud theorized from his review of the autobiography how unconscious homosexual tendencies were defended against by denial and projection. Because homosexuality is consciously inadmissible to some paranoid patients, the feeling of "I love him" is denied and changed by reaction formation into "I do not love him, I hate him." This feeling is further transformed through projection into "It is not I who hate him, it is he who hates me." In a full-blown paranoid state this feeling is elaborated into "I am persecuted by him." The patient is then able to rationalize his anger by consciously hating those he perceives to hate him. Instead of being aware of passive homosexual impulses, the patient rejects the love of anyone except himself. In erotomanic delusions, the male patient changes "I love him" to "I love her," and this feeling, through projection, becomes "She loves me."

Freud also believed that unconscious homosexuality is the cause of delusions of jealousy. In an attempt to ward off threatening impulses, the patient becomes preoccupied by jealous thoughts; thus, the patient asserts, "I do not love him; she loves him." Freud believed that the man the paranoid patient suspects his wife of loving is a man to whom the patient feels sexually attracted. According to classic psychoanalytic theory, the dynamics of unconscious homosexuality are the same for a female patient as for a male patient.

Clinical evidence has not supported Freud's thesis. A significant number of delusional patients do not have demonstrable homosexual inclinations, and the majority of homosexual men do not have symptoms of paranoia or delusions.

The Paranoid Pseudocommunity. Norman Cameron described at least seven situations that favor the development of delusional disorders: (1) an increased expectation of receiving sadistic treatment; (2) situations that increase distrust and suspicion; (3) social isolation; (4) situations that increase envy and jealousy; (5) situations that lower self-esteem; (6) situations that cause a person to see his own defects in others; and (7) situations that increase the potential for rumination over probable meanings and motivations. When frustration from any combination of these conditions exceeds the limits that the individual can tolerate, the patient becomes withdrawn and anxious; he realizes that something is wrong and seeks an explanation for the problem. The crystallization of a delusional system offers a solution. Elaboration of the delusion to include imagined persons and the attribution of malevolent motivations to both real and imagined people results in the organization of the "pseudocommunity"—that is, a perceived community of plotters. This delusional entity hypothetically binds together projected fears and wishes to justify the patient's aggression and to provide a tangible target.

Other Psychodynamic Contributions. Clinical observations indicate that some paranoid patients experience a lack of trust in establishing relationships. This distrust has been hypothesized to be related to a consistently hostile family environment, often with an overcontrolling mother and a distant or sadistic father. Patients with delusional disorders primarily use the defense mechanisms of reaction formation, denial, and projection. Reaction formation is used as a defense against aggression, dependency needs, and feelings of affection. The need for dependency is transformed into staunch independence. Denial is used to avoid awareness of painful reality. Consumed with anger and hostility and unable to face responsibility for this rage, the individual projects his resentment and anger onto others. Projection is used to protect the person from recognizing unacceptable impulses in himself.

Hypersensitivity and feelings of inferiority have been hypothesized to lead, through reaction formation and projection, to delusions of superiority and grandiosity. Delusions of erotic ideas have been suggested as replacement for feelings of rejection. Other clinicians have noted that the child who is expected to perform impeccably and is undeservedly punished when he fails to do so may develop elaborate fantasies as a way of enhancing his injured self-esteem. These secret thoughts may eventually evolve into delusions. Critical and frightening delusions are often described as projections of superego criticism. The delusions of female paranoid patients, for example, often involve accusations of prostitution. As a child, the female paranoiac turned to her father for the maternal love that she was unable to receive from her mother. Incestuous desires developed. Later heterosexual encounters are an unconscious reminder of the incestuous desires of childhood; these desires are defended against by superego projection, accusing the female paranoiac of prostitution. Somatic delusions can be psychodynamically explained as a regression to the infantile narcissistic state in which the patient withdraws emotional involvement from other people and fixates on his physical self. In erotic delusions, the love can be conceptualized as projected narcissistic love used as a defense against low self-esteem and severe narcissistic injury. Delusions of grandeur may represent a regression to the omnipotent feelings of childhood in which feelings of undenied and undiminished powers predominated.

THE MENTAL STATUS EXAMINATION

General Description

The patient is usually well groomed and well dressed without evidence of gross disintegration of personality or daily activities. The patient may seem suspicious, eccentric, or hostile. Patients are sometimes quite litigious and may make this inclination quite clear to the examiner. If they attempt to engage the clinician as an ally in the delusion, the clinician should not pretend to accept the delusion since this merely further confounds reality and also sets the stage for eventual therapeutic distrust.

Mood, Feelings, and Affect

The patient's mood is consistent with the delusion. A patient with grandiose delusions is euphoric; a patient with persecutory delusions is suspicious. Whatever the nature of the delusional system, the examiner may sense some mild depressive qualities.

Perceptual Disturbances

By definition, delusional disorder patients do not have prominent or sustained hallucinations. However, a few delusional patients have rare hallucinatory experiences, virtually always auditory in nature.

Thought Processes

This area of the mental status examination contains the key pathology of the disorder—the delusion itself. In contrast to many of the delusions reported in patients with schizophrenia, the delusions in this disorder are defined as being possible, albeit highly improbable. The delusion may be persecutory, jealous, erotomanic, somatic, grandiose, or some mixture of these and other themes. The delusional system may be quite complex or rather simple. The patient usually lacks other signs of thought disorder, although some patients may seem verbose, circumstantial, or idiosyncratic in their speech when they talk about their delusions.

Impulse Control

It is very important to evaluate a patient with delusional disorder for ideation or plans to act upon his delusional material by suicide, homicide, or other violence. The incidence of these behaviors in delusional disorder patients is not known. The therapist should not hesitate to ask the patient about his suicidal, homicidal, or sexual plans and preparations for their completion. Destructive aggression is more common in patients with a history of violence. If aggressive feelings existed in the past, the patient should be asked how he managed them. If the patient is unable to control his impulses, hospitalization is mandatory. The therapist can sometimes foster the therapeutic alliance by openly discussing how hospitalization can help the patient gain additional control of his impulses.

Orientation

There is usually no abnormality in orientation in patients with delusional disorder unless there is a specific delusion concerning person, place, or time.

Memory

Memory and other cognitive processes are intact in patients with delusional disorder.

Judgment and Insight

Judgment can best be assessed by evaluating the patient's past and present behavior. Patients with delusional disorder most often have virtually no insight into their condition and are almost always brought to the hospital by the police, family members, friends, or employers.

Reliability

Patients are usually quite reliable in their information, except where it impinges upon their delusional system.

COURSE AND PROGNOSIS

At the outset of illness, there is often an identifiable event or social situation about which a modest level of suspicion is warranted. Acute onset of symptoms is thought to be more common than an insidious onset. The initial suspicions become more elaborate and eventually delusional. Approximately 50 percent of patients are recovered at long-term follow-up; another 20 percent may have a decrease in symptoms; the final 30 percent have had no change in their symptoms. It has been clinically reported that in patients with jealous delusional disorder, divorce leads to an arrest in the evolution of the delusional system, although the patient may remain delusional about the past. Remarriage may rekindle the evolution of the jealous delusional system. Persecutory, somatic, and erotic delusions have a better prognosis than grandiose and jealous delusions. The following factors correlate with a good prognosis: high levels of occupational, social, and functional adjustment; female sex; onset before age 30; acute onset; shorter duration of illness; and the presence of precipitating factors.

DIAGNOSIS AND SUBTYPES

The diagnostic guidelines for delusional disorder are listed in Table 1. The DSM-III diagnosis of shared paranoid disorder has been changed in DSM-III-R to induced psychotic disorder and is grouped with the psychotic disorders not elsewhere classified. The DSM-III diagnoses of acute paranoid disorder and atypical paranoid disorder were omitted from DSM-III-R as separate categories; such patients should be classified within the psychotic disorders not elsewhere classified.

ICD-9 groups together the *paranoid states. Simple paranoid states* are characterized by the presence of either an

Table 1
Diagnostic Criteria for Delusional Disorder

A. Nonbizarre delusion(s) (i.e., involving situations that occur in real life, such as being followed, poisoned, infected, loved at a distance, having a disease, being deceived by one's spouse or lover) of at least 1 month's duration.

B. Auditory or visual hallucinations, if present, are not prominent [as defined in Schizophrenia, A(1)*(b)*].

C. Apart from the delusion(s) or its ramifications, behavior is not obviously odd or bizarre.

D. If a Major Depressive or Manic Syndrome has been present during the delusional disturbance, the total duration of all episodes of the mood syndrome has been brief relative to the total duration of the delusional disturbance.

E. Has never met criterion A for Schizophrenia, and it cannot be established that an organic factor initiated and maintained the disturbance.

Specify type: The following types are based on the predominant delusional theme. If no single delusional theme predominates, specify as **Unspecified Type.**

Erotomanic Type
Delusional Disorder in which the predominant theme of the delusion(s) is that a person, usually of higher status, is in love with the subject.

Grandiose Type
Delusional Disorder in which the predominant theme of the delusion(s) is one of inflated worth, power, knowledge, identity, or special relationship to a deity or famous person.

Jealous Type
Delusional Disorder in which the predominant theme of the delusion(s) is that one's sexual partner is unfaithful.

Persecutory Type
Delusional Disorder in which the predominant theme of the delusion(s) is that one (or someone to whom one is close) is being malevolently treated in some way. People with this type of Delusional Disorder may repeatedly take their complaints of being mistreated to legal authorities.

Somatic Type
Delusional Disorder in which the predominant theme of the delusion(s) is that the person has some physical defect, disorder, or disease.

Unspecified Type
Delusional Disorder that does not fit any of the previous categories, e.g., persecutory and grandiose themes without a predominance of either; delusions of reference without malevolent content.

Table from DSM-III-R *Diagnostic and Statistical Manual of Mental Disorders,* ed 3, revised. (Current Classification of Mental Disorders, 1987.) Copyright American Psychiatric Association, Washington, D.C., 1987. Used with permission.

acute or chronic delusional system. *Paranoia* defines the gradual onset of chronic systematized delusions without hallucinations. The presence of hallucinations defines *paraphrenia,* and ICD-9 includes *shared paranoid disorder.*

Subtypes

DSM-III-R defines six subtypes of delusional disorder based on the content of the delusions—persecutory, jealous, erotomanic, somatic, grandiose, and unspecified. Persecutory and jealous subtypes are the most common; grandiose subtypes are also common; erotomanic and somatic subtypes are more unusual. The following are the DSM-III-R descriptions.

Erotomanic Type. The central theme of an erotic delusion is that one is loved by another. The delusion usually concerns idealized romantic love and spiritual union rather than sexual attraction. The person about whom this conviction is held is usually of higher status, such as a famous person or a superior at work, and may even be a complete stranger. Efforts to contact the object of the delusion, through telephone calls, letters, gifts, visits, and even surveillance and stalking are common, though occasionally the person keeps the delusion secret.

Whereas in clinical samples most of the cases are female, in forensic samples most are male. Some people with this disorder, particularly males, come into conflict with the law in their efforts to pursue the object of their delusion, or in a misguided effort to "rescue" him or her from some imagined danger. The prevalence of erotic delusions is such as to be a significant source of harassment to public figures. The erotomanic type has also been called *de Clerambault syndrome,* and is illustrated by the following case:

A 35-year-old married woman lived a normal suburban life with her physician husband and two children until an older couple moved in next door. The new neighbor proved to be a relatively famous writer. Following a housewarming party, the patient developed the conviction that her new neighbor was irresistibly attracted to her, and soon she became entirely preoccupied with thoughts that her neighbor loved her. The patient's delusion failed to respond to antipsychotic medication, but after several months of psychotherapy, she reluctantly agreed to move to another neighborhood. After their move, the patient's delusional belief persisted unchanged through a 4-year period of observation.

[Adapted, with permission from *DSM-III Case Book.* American Psychiatric Association, Washington, D.C., 1981.]

Grandiose Type. Grandiose delusions usually take the form of the person's being convinced that he or she possesses some great, but unrecognized, talent or insight, or has made some important discovery, which he or she may take to various governmental agencies (e.g., the Federal Bureau of Investigation or the US Patent Office). Less common is the delusion that one has a special relationship with a prominent person, in which case the actual person, if alive, is regarded as an imposter. Grandiose delusions may have a religious content, and people with these delusions can become leaders of religious cults.

Jealous Type. When delusions of jealousy are present, a person is convinced, without due cause, that his or her spouse or lover is unfaithful. Small bits of "evidence," such as disarrayed clothing or spots on the sheets, may be collected and used to justify the delusion. Almost invariably the person with the delusion confronts his or her spouse or lover and may take extraordinary steps to intervene in the imagined infidelity. These attempts may include restricting the autonomy of the spouse or lover by insisting that he or she never leave the house unaccompanied, secretly following the spouse or lover, or investigating the other "lover." The person with the delusion may physically attack the spouse or lover and, more rarely, the other "lover." When the delusions concern the fidelity of the spouse, these patients have been said to have conjugal paranoia or Othello syndrome.

Persecutory Type. This is the most common type. The persecutory delusion may be simple or elaborate, and usually involves a single theme or series of connected themes, such as being conspired against, cheated, spied on, followed, poisoned or drugged, maliciously maligned, harassed, or obstructed in the pursuit of long-term goals. Small slights may be exaggerated and become the focus of a delusional system. In certain cases the focus of the delusion is some injustice that must be remedied by legal action ("querulous paranoia"), and the affected person often engages in repeated attempts to obtain satisfaction by appeal to the courts and other government agencies. People with persecutory delusions are often resentful and angry, and may resort to violence against those they believe are hurting them.

Somatic Type. Somatic delusions occur in several forms. Most common are convictions that the person emits a foul odor from his or her skin, mouth, rectum, or vagina; that he or she has an infestation of insects on or in the skin; that he or she has an internal parasite; that certain parts of his or her body are, contrary to all evidence, misshapen and ugly; or that certain parts of his or her body (e.g., the large intestine) are not functioning. People with somatic delusions usually consult nonpsychiatric physicians for treatment of their perceived somatic conditions.

A nihilistic delusion change has been referred to as *Cotard's syndrome*. The following case illustrates a somatic delusion.

After many years of seeking treatment for a perceived heart ailment, a 38-year-old attorney filed suit against a major teaching hospital and nine physicians including the president of the local medical society. Despite repeated normal cardiovascular examinations, including stress electrocardiograms and a cardiac catheterization, the patient was convinced that he had severe heart disease and that the local medical society was conspiring to withhold evidence from him. In spite of this fixed delusion, the patient was a competent attorney and had an active practice.

[Adapted, with permission from *DSM-III Case Book*. American Psychiatric Association, Washington, D.C., 1981.]

Other Recognized Specific Delusions. Other delusions have been given specific names in the literature. In the absence of an organic explanation, patients with these delusions might be classified in DSM-III-R either as delusional disorder (unspecified type) or as psychotic disorder not elsewhere classified. *Capgras syndrome* is the delusion that familiar people have been replaced by identical impostors. *Fregoli syndrome* is the delusion that a persecutor is taking on a variety of faces, as if he were an actor. *Lycanthropy* is the delusion of being a werewolf, and *heutoscopy* is the false belief that one has a double.

DIFFERENTIAL DIAGNOSIS

There are many medical and neurological illnesses that can present with delusions (Table 2; see also Table 5—Chapter 14). As mentioned previously, the most common sites for lesions are the basal ganglia and limbic system. The medical evaluation of this presentation should include toxicology screening and routine admission lab work. Neuropsychological testing (e.g., Bender Gestalt, Wechsler Memory Scale) and, an EEG or a CT scan may be indicated at the time of initial presentation, especially if there are other signs or symptoms suggestive of cognitive impairment or electrophysiological or structural lesions. Delirium can be differentiated by the presence of a fluctuating level of consciousness or impaired cognitive abilities. Delusions early in the course of a dementing illness (e.g., Alzheimer's) may give the appearance of a delusional disorder, however, neuropsychologic testing usually detects cognitive impairment. Although alcohol abuse is an associated feature for patients with delusional disorder, delusional disorder must be distinguished from alcoholic hallucinosis or so-called alcoholic paranoia. Intoxication with sympathomimetics (including amphetamine), marijuana, or L-dopa is particularly likely to present with delusional symptomatology.

The psychiatric differential diagnosis for delusional disorder includes malingering and factitious disorder with psychological features. The nonfactitious disorders in the differential diagnosis are schizophrenia, mood disorders, psychotic disorders not elsewhere classified, and paranoid personality disorder. Delusional disorder is distinguished from schizophrenia by the absence of other schizophrenic symptoms and the nonbizarre quality of the delusion. Persecutory and jealous subtypes of delusional disorder, however, may be difficult to distinguish from some presentations of schizophrenia. The grandiose and erotomanic subtypes may resemble mania in clinical presentation; the somatic subtype may resemble depression. The absence of other signs and symptoms of mood disorders aid the clini-

Table 2
Some Neurological and Medical Conditions That Can Present With Delusions

Basal ganglia disorders—Parkinson's, Huntington's

Deficiency states—B_{12}, folate, thiamine, niacin

Delirium

Dementia—Alzheimer's, Pick's

Drug-induced—amphetamines, anticholinergics, antidepressants, antihypertensives, antituberculous drugs, antiparkinsons, cimetidine, disulfiram, hallucinogens

Endocrinopathies—adrenal, thyroid, parathyroid

Limbic System pathology—epilepsy, strokes, tumors

Systemic—hepatic encephalopathy, hypercalcemia, hypoglycemia, porphyria, uremia

cian to make the appropriate diagnosis. A clinician can reasonably consider an abnormal result on a dexamethasone suppression test to be suggestive of depression. If symptoms do not meet the guidelines for delusional disorder, schizophrenia, or mood disorder, then one of the diagnoses in psychotic disorders not elsewhere classified may be appropriate. Separating paranoid personality disorder from delusional disorder is a difficult task, that of differentiating extreme suspiciousness from a frank delusion. In general, if the clinician doubts whether the symptom is a delusion, the diagnosis of delusional disorder should not be used (Table 3).

CLINICAL MANAGEMENT

Hospitalization

The initial clinical consideration is whether the patient requires hospitalization. The possibility of suicide or homicide, severe impairment in occupational or social functioning, and the need for a diagnostic work-up are strong indications for hospitalization. If the physician is convinced that the patient is best treated in a hospital, an attempt should be made to persuade him to accept hospitalization; failing that, legal commitment may be indicated. Often, if the physician convinces the patient that hospitalization is inevitable, the patient voluntarily enters a hospital to avoid legal commitment.

Chemotherapy

In an emergency, a severely agitated patient should be given a tranquilizing drug IM. For chronic treatment, antipsychotic drugs are currently considered the drugs of choice, although adequate proof of their efficacy is lacking. Delusional disorder patients are likely to refuse medication, for they can easily incorporate the administration of drugs into their delusional system. It may be prudent for the physician not to insist on medication immediately upon hospitalization but, rather, to spend a few days establishing rapport with the patient. The physician should explain clearly potential side effects to the patient so that the patient does not later suspect that the physician lied to him or her. The

Table 3
Differential Diagnosis*

Paranoid personality disorder	Pervasive and long-standing suspiciousness of other people
Delusional disorder	Delusions

Schizophrenia	One symptom from the following:
	  Delusions of being controlled
	  Thought broadcasting
	  Thought insertion
	  Thought withdrawal
	  Fantastic or implausible delusions
	  Other delusions without persecutory or jealous content
	  Auditory hallucination in which a noise keeps up a running commentary on the patient's thoughts or behavior
	  Auditory hallucination not associated with depression or elation or limited to two words
	  Delusions of any type accompanied by hallucination of any type
	  Loosening of association combined with inappropriate affect

Manic episode	Elevated, expansive, or irritable mood with pressured speech and hyperactivity

Depressive episode	Pervasive loss of interest or pleasure combined with at least four of the following:
	  Change in weight when not dieting
	  Sleep difficulty
	  Psychomotor agitation or retardation
	  Loss of energy
	  Decrease in sex drive
	  Feelings of self-reproach or excessive guilt, either of which may be delusional
	  Indecisiveness
	  Suicidal thoughts

Organic mental disorder	Disordered memory and orientation
	  Impairment in judgment and impulse control
	  Perceptual disturbance—simple misinterpretations, illusions and hallucinations
	  Clinical features that may fluctuate rapidly

*Adapted from American Psychiatric Association: *Diagnostic and Statistical Manual of Mental Disorders*, ed 3. American Psychiatric Association, Washington, D.C., 1980.

prior history of medication response is the best guide to choosing a drug. It is often wise to start with low doses (e.g., 2 mg haloperidol) and to increase the dosage slowly. If a patient fails to respond to a drug at reasonable doses in a 6-week trial, neuroleptics from other classes should be given clinical trials. A common cause of drug failure is noncompliance, and this possibility should be carefully evaluated.

If the patient receives no benefit from antipsychotic medication, the drug should be discontinued. And in patients who do respond to antipsychotics, maintenance doses often can be quite low. There is essentially no data to suggest whether antidepressants, lithium, or carbamazepine are effective in treating delusional disorder. Clinical trials of these medications may be warranted in patients with features suggestive of mood disorders or family histories positive for such illnesses.

Psychotherapy

The essential element in effective psychotherapy is establishing a relationship in which the patient begins to trust the therapist. Individual therapy seems more effective than group therapy. Initially, the therapist should neither agree with nor challenge the patient's delusions. The physician may stimulate the patient's motivation to receive help by emphasizing a willingness to help him with his anxiety or irritability, without suggesting that the delusions be treated. The examiner, however, should not actively support the notion that the delusions represent reality.

The unwavering reliability of the therapist is essential. The therapist should be on time and make appointments as regularly as possible, the goal being to develop a solid and trusting relationship with the patient. Overgratification may actually increase the patient's hostility and suspiciousness because of the core realization that all demands cannot be met. The therapist can avoid overgratification by not extending the designated appointment period, not giving extra appointments unless absolutely necessary, and not being lenient about the fee.

The therapist should not make disparaging remarks about the patient's delusions or ideas, but can sympathetically indicate to the patient that his preoccupation with the delusion both distresses himself and interferes with a constructive life. When the patient begins to waver in his delusional belief, the therapist may increase reality testing by asking the patient to clarify his concerns. When homosexual issues are, in fact, part of the clinical picture,

the clinician should first deal with the patient's heterosexual fears rather than imply negative interpretations concerning homosexuality.

When family members are available, the clinician may decide to involve them in the treatment plan. Although the clinician has to avoid being delusionally seen as "siding with the enemy," he should attempt to enlist the family as an ally in the treatment process. Consequently, both the patient and the family need to understand that physician-patient confidentiality will be maintained, and that communications from relatives will be discussed at some point with the patient. The family may benefit from the support of the doctor and, in turn, may be more supportive of the patient.

Outcome of Therapy. Psychodynamic theories hypothesize that, through a relationship with the therapist, the patient begins to neutralize his drives and his ego is strengthened. Trust develops, defenses are reinforced, and the presenting conflict begins to resolve. The patient can learn to adjust to the delusions that remain intact. He can be taught to recognize those situations that produce and increase delusional behavior, and alternative responses to stress can be encouraged.

A good therapeutic outcome depends on the psychiatrist's ability to respond to the patient's mistrust of others and the resulting interpersonal conflicts, frustrations, and failures. The mark of successful treatment may be a satisfactory social adjustment rather than abatement of the patient's delusions.

References

Akiskal H S, Arana G W, Baldessarini R J: A clinical report of thymoleptic-responsive atypical paranoid psychoses. Am J Psychiatry *140:*1187, 1983.
Cameron N: Paranoid conditions and paranoia. In *American Handbook of Psychiatry*, S Arieti, editor, vol I, p 508. Basic Books, New York, 1959.
Cummings J L: Organic delusions: Phenomenology, anatomical correlations, and review. Br J Psychiatry *146:*184, 1985.
Kendler K S: The nosologic validity of paranoia (simple delusional disorder): A review. Arch Gen Psychiatry *37:*699, 1980.
Kendler K S: Demography of paranoid psychosis (delusional disorder): A review and comparison with schizophrenia and affective illness. Arch Gen Psychiatry *39:*890, 1982.
Kendler K S, Masteson C, Davis K: Psychiatric illness in first-degree relatives of patients with paranoid psychosis, schizophrenia, and medical illness. Br J Psychiatry *147:*524, 1985.
Retterstol N: *Paranoid and Paranoid Psychoses*. Charles C Thomas, Springfield, IL, 1966.
Winokur G: Delusional disorder (paranoia). Compr Psychiatry *18:*511, 1977.
Winokur G: Familial psychopathology in delusional disorder. Compr Psychiatry *26:*241, 1985.

16

Psychotic Disorders Not Elsewhere Classified

16.1 ───────

Schizoaffective Disorder

Patients with schizoaffective disorder have features of both schizophrenia and affective (mood) disorders, but cannot be diagnosed as having just one of the two conditions without distorting some aspect of the clinical presentation. Reflecting the changes in diagnostic criteria for schizophrenia and mood disorders, the diagnostic criteria for schizoaffective disorder have been modified by different generations.

HISTORY

Although Jacob Kasanin is recognized as having written the classic paper first describing schizoaffective disorder, there were at least two previous reports describing a similar condition. G. H. Kirby (1913) and A. Hoch (1921) both described patients with mixed features of schizophrenia and affective disorders. Because their patients did not demonstrate the deteriorating course of dementia precox, Kirby and Hoch classified them in Kraepelin's manic-depressive psychosis group. In 1933, Kasanin described a group of patients with concurrent schizophrenic and affective symptoms, a history of a precipitating stressor, an acute onset, and a family history of mood disorder in some cases. Although these patients recovered from their symptoms, Kasanin diagnosed them as having a subtype of schizophrenia. By this time, the diagnostic importance of schizophrenic symptoms, as emphasized by Bleuler, had eclipsed Kraepelin's emphasis on course of illness for differentiating schizophrenia from affective conditions. From 1933 to approximately 1970, patients whose symptoms were similar to those of Kasanin's were variously diagnosed as having schizoaffective disorder, atypical schizophrenia, good-prognosis schizophrenia, remitting schizophrenia, or cycloid psychosis—terms that emphasized a relation to the schizophrenic disorders.

Around 1970, three different sets of data caused the shift from viewing schizoaffective disorder as a schizophrenic illness to viewing it as a mood disorder. First, lithium carbonate was demonstrated to be an effective and specific treatment for bipolar as well as some schizoaffective disorders. Second, the United States-United Kingdom study,

published in 1968 by J. Cooper and his colleagues, demonstrated that the variation in the number of patients diagnosed as schizophrenic in the U.S. and the U.K. was the result of an overemphasis in the United States on the presence of psychotic symptoms as a diagnostic criterion for schizophrenia. Third, several American investigators reported a distinct cluster of manic symptoms that suggested the diagnosis of a mood disorder even though dramatic psychotic symptoms were present.

Compared to the above ideas, the current concept of schizoaffective disorder is somewhat more atheoretical and pragmatic about the relationship to schizophrenia and mood disorders. Most contemporary systems define schizoaffective disorder as an entity that includes symptoms of both disorders.

EPIDEMIOLOGY

The epidemiology of schizoaffective disorder, as currently defined, is not well explored because the frequent shifts in diagnostic practice have rendered information from earlier studies difficult to interpret. Based on available data, however, the lifetime prevalence is less than 1 percent, possibly in the range of 0.5 to 0.8 percent. In clinical practice, a preliminary diagnosis of schizoaffective disorder is frequently used when the clinician is uncertain of the diagnosis. There does not appear to be a difference in the prevalence of schizoaffective disorder between men and women.

ETIOLOGY

Although the etiology of schizoaffective disorder is unknown, there are five possible conceptual models: Schizoaffective disorder may be a subtype of schizophrenia. Schizoaffective disorder may be a subtype of mood disorders. Patients with schizoaffective disorder may have both schizophrenia and a mood disorder. Schizoaffective disorder may represent a mental illness distinct from schizophrenia and mood disorders. Patients with schizoaffective disorder may represent a heterogeneous group, some of whom have schizophrenia and some, a mood disorder. Studies designed to explore these five possibilities have examined family history, biological markers, short-term treatment response, and long-term outcome. Most of these studies have looked at schizoaffective disorder as a single group; however, some studies have separated schizoaffective disorder, depressive type from schizoaffective disorder, bipolar type.

The most reasonable conclusion from available data is that patients with schizoaffective disorder are a heterogeneous group; some having schizophrenia with prominent affective symptoms and others having a mood disorder with prominent schizophrenic symptoms. Moreover, as a group, schizoaffective patients have a better prognosis than patients with schizophrenia and a worse prognosis than patients with mood disorders. Depending somewhat on the subtype of schizoaffective disorder studied, there may be an increased prevalence of both schizophrenia and mood disorders in the relatives of the probands.

The idea that schizoaffective disorder is a subtype of schizophrenia is not supported by research; an increased prevalence of schizophrenia is not found among relatives of schizoaffective disorder (bipolar type) probands. Other investigations have demonstrated that schizoaffective patients, as a group, do not have schizophrenia-like deficits in smooth pursuit eye movements, neurological soft signs, or attentional abilities. The possibility that schizoaffective disorder is a subtype of mood disorders is not supported by the increased prevalence of schizophrenic disorders in relatives of probands with schizoaffective disorder, depressive type. However, a similarity between patients with schizoaffective disorder and patients with mood disorders is suggested by the higher prevalence of mood disorders in relatives of schizoaffective probands than in relatives of schizophrenic probands. It has also been reported that, as a group, schizoaffective patients respond to lithium and tend to have a nondeteriorating course. The view that schizoaffective disorder represents a completely different disorder is not supported by the observation that only a very small percentage of relatives of schizoaffective probands have schizoaffective disorder themselves. Finally, the hypothesis that schizoaffective patients have both schizophrenia and a mood disorder is untenable because the calculated co-occurrence of these two disorders is much lower than the incidence of schizoaffective disorder.

CLINICAL SIGNS AND SYMPTOMS

The clinical signs and symptoms seen in schizoaffective disorder include all of the signs and symptoms seen in schizophrenia, mania, and depression. The schizophrenic and affective symptoms can present together or in an alternating fashion. The psychotic symptoms can be either mood congruent or mood incongruent. The course may be one of exacerbations and remissions, a chronic deteriorating course, or some intermediate situation. Although the incidence of suicide in schizoaffective disorder is not known, it is at least the 10 percent rate of completed suicides found in schizophrenia. The following case illustrates schizoaffective disorders.

A 44-year-old mother of three teen-agers is hospitalized for treatment of depression. She gives the following history: One year previously, after a terminal argument with her lover, she became acutely psychotic. She was frightened that people were going to kill her and heard voices of friends and strangers talking about killing her, sometimes talking to each other. She heard her own thoughts broadcast aloud and was afraid that others could also hear what she was thinking. Over a three-week period she stayed in her apartment, had new locks put on the doors, kept the shades down, and avoided everyone but her immediate family. She was unable to sleep at night because the voices kept her awake, and unable to eat because of a constant "lump" in her throat. In retrospect, she cannot say whether she was depressed, denies being elated or overactive, and remembers only that she was terrified of what would happen to her. The family persuaded her to enter a hospital, where, after six weeks of treatment with Thorazine, the voices stopped. She remembers feeling "back to normal" for a week or two, but then she seemed to lose her energy and motivation to do anything. She became increasingly depressed, lost her appetite, and woke at 4:00 or 5:00 every morning and was unable to get back to sleep. She could no longer read a newspaper or watch TV because she couldn't concentrate.

The patient's condition has persisted for nine months. She has done very little except sit in her apartment, staring at the walls. Her children have managed most of the cooking, shopping, bill-paying, etc. She has continued in outpatient treatment, and was maintained on Thorazine until four months before this admission. There has been no recurrence of the psychotic symptoms since the medication was discontinued; but her depression, with all the accompanying symptoms, has persisted.

In discussing her past history, the patient is rather guarded. There is, however, no evidence of a diagnosable illness before last year. She apparently is a shy, emotionally constricted person who "has never broken any rules." She has been separated from her husband for ten years, but in that time has had two enduring relationships with boyfriends. In addition to rearing three apparently healthy and very likable children, she cared for a succession of foster children full time in the four years before her illness. She enjoyed this, and was highly valued by the agency she worked for. She has maintained close relationships with a few girl friends and with her extended family.

Discussion

During her initial period of illness this patient demonstrated such characteristic schizophrenic symptoms as bizarre delusions (people could hear what she was thinking) accompanied by auditory hallucinations (voices of friends and strangers talking to each other). There was deterioration in functioning to the point that she was unable to take care of her house. With treatment, after about nine weeks, the psychotic symptoms remitted, but she remembers being "back to normal" for only about a week. She then developed the characteristic symptoms of a major depressive episode with depressed mood, poor appetite, insomnia, lack of energy, loss of interest, and poor concentration. The depressive period has lasted for about nine months.

This case would seem to be an example of an instance in which it is impossible to make a differential diagnosis with any degree of certainty between a mood disorder and schizophrenia or schizophreniform disorder; hence, a diagnosis of schizoaffective disorder seems appropriate. This diagnosis conveys the lack of certainty and the prominence of both affective and schizophrenic-like features.

DSM-III-R Diagnosis:
Axis I: Schizoaffective Disorder

[Adapted with permission from *DSM-III Case Book*. American Psychiatric Association, Washington, D.C., 1981.]

COURSE AND PROGNOSIS

The course and prognosis of schizoaffective disorder are quite variable. As a group, patients with schizoaffective disorder have a prognosis intermediate between those of patients with schizophrenia and of patients with mood disorders. There is data to suggest that patients with schizoaffective disorder, bipolar type have a prognosis similar to that for patients with bipolar disorder, and that patients with schizoaffective disorder, depressive type have a prognosis similar to that for schizophrenia. Regardless of the subtype, the following variables weigh toward a poor prognosis: poor premorbid history; insidious onset; no precipitating factor; a predominance of psychotic symptoms, especially negative (i.e., deficit) symptoms; early onset, unremitting course; and positive family history of schizophrenia. The opposite of each of these characteristics weighs toward a better outcome. The presence of Schneiderian first-rank symptoms does not seem to predict course.

DIAGNOSIS AND SUBTYPES

The DSM-III-R diagnostic criteria for schizoaffective disorder consist of two inclusion criteria and one exclusion criterion (Table 1). The two subtypes are bipolar type (history of a manic episode), and depressive type (no history of a manic episode). The delineation of subtypes may be of particular importance in determining the prognosis of this disorder. DSM-III-R differs from DSM-III in that it contains two specific inclusion criteria. The RDC, ICD-9, and other recent diagnostic systems vary somewhat in their diagnostic criteria; however, most require the occurrence of full schizophrenic, depressive, and manic syndromes, together or in alternating fashion.

Table 1
Diagnostic Criteria for Schizoaffective Disorder

A. A disturbance during which, at some time, there is either a Major Depressive or a Manic Syndrome concurrent with symptoms that meet the A criterion of Schizophrenia

B. During an episode of the disturbance, there have been delusions or hallucinations for at least 2 weeks, but no prominent mood symptoms.

C. Schizophrenia has been ruled out (i.e., the duration of all episodes of a mood syndrome has not been brief relative to the total duration of the psychotic disturbance).

D. It cannot be established that an organic factor initiated and maintained the disturbance.

Specify: bipolar type (current or previous Manic Syndrome)
or
depressive type (no current or previous Manic Syndrome)

Table from DSM-III-R *Diagnostic and Statistical Manual of Mental Disorders*, ed 3, revised. (Current Classification of Mental Disorders, 1987.) Copyright American Psychiatric Association, Washington, D.C., 1987. Used with permission.

Differential Diagnosis

All of the organic conditions listed in the differential diagnoses for schizophrenia and mood disorders need to be considered in the differential diagnosis of schizoaffective disorder. Treatment with steroids, amphetamine and phencyclidine abuse, and some cases of temporal lobe epilepsy are particularly likely to present with concurrent schizophrenic and affective symptoms.

The psychiatric differential diagnosis also includes all of the possibilities usually considered for schizophrenia and mood disorders. In clinical practice, psychosis at the time of presentation may hinder the detection of current or past affective symptoms. Therefore, one may wish to delay making a final psychiatric diagnosis until the most acute symptoms of psychosis have been controlled. Abnormal neuroendocrine function detected by the DST or TRH stimulation test may suggest a significant affective component to the illness. This possibility has not yet been confirmed by research.

CLINICAL MANAGEMENT

The major treatment modalities for schizoaffective disorder are hospitalization, medication, and psychosocial interventions. The basic principle underlying pharmacotherapy for schizoaffective disorders is that antidepressant and anti-manic protocols should be followed if at all possible, and that antipsychotics should be used only as needed for acute control. If thymoleptic protocols are not effective in controlling the symptoms on an ongoing basis, neuroleptics may be indicated. Patients with schizoaffective disorder, bipolar type should receive trials of lithium, carbamazepine, or a combination of the two. Patients with schizoaffective disorder, depressive type should be given trials of tricyclics, monoamine oxidase inhibitors, and ECT before it is decided that a patient is unresponsive to antidepressant treatment.

References

Clayton P J: Schizoaffective disorders. J. Nerv Ment Dis *170*:646, 1982.
Clayton P J, Rodin L, Winokur G: Family history studies, III, Schizoaffective disorder, clinical and genetic factors including a one to two year follow-up. Compr Psychiatry *9*:31, 1968.
Coryell W: Schizoaffective and schizophreniform disorders. In *The Medical Basis of Psychiatry*. G Winokur, P J Clayton, editors. W B Saunders, Philadelphia, 1986.
Coryell W, Tsuang T: DSM-III schizophreniform disorder. Arch Gen Psychiatry *39*:66, 1982.
Goodwin D W, Guze S B: *Psychiatric Diagnosis*, ed 3. Oxford, New York, 1984.
Maj M: Evolution of the American concept of schizoaffective psychosis. Neuropsychobiology *11*:7, 1984.
Miller F T, Libman H: Lithium carbonate in the treatment of schizophrenia and schizoaffective disorder: Review and hypothesis. Biol Psychiatry *14*:705, 1979.
Pope H G, Lipinski J F, Cohen B M: Schizo-affective disorder: An invalid diagnosis? A comparison of schizo-affective disorder, schizophrenia, and affective disorder. Am J Psychiatry *137*:921, 1980.
Procci W R: Schizoaffective psychosis: Fact or fiction? Arch Gen Psychiatry *33*:1167, 1976.
Walker E: Attentional and neuromotor functions of schizophrenics, schizoaffectives, and patients with other affective disorders. Arch Gen Psychiatry *38*:1355, 1981.

16.2 _____

Other Psychotic Disorders

This section contains the diagnostic criteria for schizophreniform disorder, brief reactive psychosis, induced psychotic disorder, and psychotic disorder NOS (not otherwise specified; also known as atypical psychosis). Schizoaffective disorder is described in Section 16.1.

In DSM-III, induced psychotic disorder was called "shared paranoid disorder" and was listed with the other paranoid disorders. The paranoid disorders are now referred to as the delusional disorders, and shared paranoid disorder has been renamed and moved to the section describing other psychotic disorders. Information regarding induced psychotic disorder is limited because of its rarity.

Psychotic disorder NOS is called "atypical psychosis" in several diagnostic systems. This diagnosis is used for patients with psychotic symptoms who do not meet the diagnostic criteria for any other psychotic disorder. The DSM-III-R description of this disorder includes examples (Table 1).

SCHIZOPHRENIFORM DISORDER

As defined in DSM-III-R, schizophreniform disorder is identical to schizophrenia with the following exceptions: schizophreniform symptoms resolve, and there is a return to normal functioning within 6 months. Symptoms must be present for longer than 6 months to make a diagnosis of schizophrenia.

Table 1
Diagnostic Criteria for Psychotic Disorder Not Otherwise Specified (Atypical Psychosis)

Disorders in which there are psychotic symptoms (delusions, hallucinations, incoherence, marked loosening of associations, catatonic excitement or stupor, or grossly disorganized behavior) that do not meet the criteria for any other nonorganic psychotic disorder. This category should also be used for psychoses about which there is inadequate information to make a specific diagnosis. (This is preferable to "Diagnosis Deferred," and can be changed if more information becomes available.) This diagnosis is made only when it cannot be established that an organic factor initiated and maintained the disturbance.

Examples:

(1) psychoses with unusual features (e.g., persistent auditory hallucinations as the only disturbance)
(2) postpartum psychoses that do not meet the criteria for an Organic Mental Disorder, psychotic Mood Disorder, or any other psychotic disorder
(3) psychoses with confusing clinical features that make a more specific diagnosis impossible

Table from DSM-III-R, *Diagnostic and Statistical Manual of Mental Disorders*, ed 3, revised. (Current Classification of Mental Disorders, 1987.) Copyright American Psychiatric Association, Washington, D.C., 1987. Used with permission.

This definition of schizophreniform disorder is distinctly different from previous meanings attached to this diagnosis. In 1939, Gabriel Langfeldt devised the term schizophreniform to separate patients with this disorder from those with so-called true schizophrenia. Patients with schizophreniform disorder had good premorbid histories, abrupt onset of symptoms often related to a specific stress, and good prognoses. The patients with true schizophrenia, on the other hand, had more classic chronic and deteriorating courses. Between 1939 and the publication of DSM-III in 1980, various researchers and clinicians confused the meanings of the terms "schizophreniform" and "schizoaffective". The DSM-III and DSM-III-R criteria for schizophreniform disorder define a group of patients with schizophrenia-like symptoms who have a better prognosis than patients with schizophrenia. The basis for this diagnostic distinction is strictly the duration of symptoms.

Epidemiology

The incidence, prevalence, and sex ratio of DSM-III-R schizophreniform disorder have not yet been reported in the literature. Some clinicians have the impression that the disorder is more common in adolescents and in young adults, and most investigators believe that the disorder is less than half as common as schizophrenia.

Etiology

The etiology of schizophreniform disorder is not known. The few available studies strongly suggest that a heterogeneous group of patients make up this diagnosis. Some have an illness more similar to schizophrenia, whereas others have an illness more similar to the mood disorders. Several studies have shown that schizophreniform patients, as a group, have more affective symptoms (especially mania) and a better outcome than do schizophrenic patients. This relationship to the mood disorders is supported by the observation that schizophreniform patients demonstrate abnormal dexamethasone suppression and thyrotropin releasing hormone tests more often than do schizophrenic patients. Relatives of schizophreniform patients have schizophrenia less frequently than the relatives of schizophrenic patients, but more frequently than the relatives of mood disorder patients. Supportive of the notion that some schizophreniform patients have an illness that resembles schizophrenia is one study that reports a similar enlargement of cerebral ventricles in both schizophreniform and schizophrenic patients. In summary, the biological data is consistent with the hypothesis that the current diagnostic category defines a group of patients who may have illnesses similar to schizophrenia or the mood disorders.

Clinical Signs and Symptoms

The clinical signs and symptoms, as well as the mental status examination, are identical to those of schizophrenia. It is important, however, to note the patient's level of confusion or perplexity and the affect since these symptoms may be particularly important in predicting the course of the disorder.

Course and Prognosis

By definition, this disorder resolves within 6 months with a return to baseline mental functioning. The prognosis of this disorder also involves the likelihood of further schizophreniform episodes, as well as the possible future development of a schizophrenic or mood disorder. Studies have indicated that the requirement for 6 months of symptoms in schizophrenia weighs heavily toward a poor prognosis; therefore, schizophreniform patients have a better prognosis than most schizophrenic patients. In addition to the indicators of good prognosis listed in DSM-III-R (Table 2), acute onset and shorter periods of illness weigh toward a better prognosis. There is a risk of suicide during the symptomatic period and also during the period of depression that often follows the psychosis.

Diagnosis and Subtypes

DSM-III-R contains specific diagnostic criteria for schizophreniform disorder, as well as two subtypes—with and without good prognostic features (Table 2). The 6 month period must include all prodromal, active, and residual symptoms. In contrast to DSM-III criteria, there is no minimal duration of symptoms in DSM-III-R. The diagnosis of "provisional" schizophreniform disorder can be made while waiting for the symptoms to resolve. The diagnosis of schizophreniform disorder is more accurate than a diagnosis of schizophrenia when the clinician is unable to obtain a reliable history from a psychotic patient regarding the duration of his symptoms. On the other hand, a patient's anamnesis for prodromal symptoms may mislead the physician away from a correct diagnosis of schizophrenia, and a patient's anamnesis for affective symptoms may cause the physician to miss a diagnosis of mood disorder.

Table 2
Diagnostic Criteria for Schizophreniform Disorder

A. Meets criteria A and C of Schizophrenia

B. An episode of the disturbance (including prodromal, active, and residual phases) lasts less than 6 months. (When the diagnosis must be made without waiting for recovery, it should be qualified as "provisional.")

C. Does not meet the criteria for Brief Reactive Psychosis, and it cannot be established that an organic factor initiated and maintained the disturbance.

Specify: without good prognostic features or **with good prognostic features,** i.e., with at least two of the following:
(1) onset of prominent psychotic symptoms within 4 weeks of first noticeable change in usual behavior or functioning
(2) confusion, disorientation, or perplexity at the height of the psychotic episode
(3) good premorbid social and occupational functioning
(4) absence of blunted or flat affect

Table from DSM-III-R *Diagnostic and Statistical Manual of Mental Disorders,* ed 3, revised. (Current Classification of Mental Disorders, 1987.) Copyright American Psychiatric Association, Washington, D.C., 1987. Used with permission.

Differential Diagnosis

The differential diagnosis for schizophreniform disorder is identical to that for schizophrenia. Factitious disorder with psychological symptoms and organic disorders must be ruled out. Temporal lobe epilepsy, CNS tumors, strokes, infections, and drug ingestion (e.g., steroids, hallucinogens) may be associated with a relatively short-lived psychosis.

Clinical Management

It is often necessary to hospitalize a patient in order to make a diagnosis, to carry out effective clinical management, and to protect the patient from himself. Antipsychotic drugs are usually indicated to treat the psychotic symptoms, but they should be withdrawn after 3 to 6 months. Electroconvulsive therapy may be indicated for some patients, especially those with marked catatonic symptoms. Prophylactic treatment with antipsychotics is almost never indicated for schizophreniform disorder. If a patient has recurrent episodes, a trial of lithium is warranted to assess whether it would be effective in treatment and prophylaxis. Psychotherapy is usually very important for these patients who need help integrating their psychotic experience.

BRIEF REACTIVE PSYCHOSIS

The hallmarks of brief reactive psychosis are that it follows a significant stressor in the patient's life and that symptoms last less than 1 month. Brief reactive psychosis is one of the few DSM-III-R diagnoses for which a specific etiological factor (i.e., a psychosocial stressor) is identified. Patients with similar disorders have previously been labelled as having reactive, hysterical, stress, and psychogenic psychoses. The entity in French psychiatry *bouffée délirante* is quite similar to these disorders. The DSM-III-R classification of brief reactive psychosis, however, differs from these prior terms. Reactive psychosis was often used as a synonym for good-prognosis schizophrenia; brief reactive psychosis does not imply a relationship to schizophrenia. Hysterical psychosis required the absence of any evidence of premorbid thought disorder.

Epidemiology

The incidence, prevalence, and sex ratio of DSM-III-R brief reactive psychosis have not yet been definitively studied. Many clinicians believe it to be a rare disorder that occurs most often in adolescence and early adulthood. It may be more common in persons in lower socioeconomic classes and in patients with previously existing personality disorders (most commonly, histrionic, narcissistic, paranoid, schizotypal, and borderline). Individuals who have experienced previous disasters or major cultural changes may also be at higher risk.

Etiology

By definition, a significant psychosocial stressor is an etiological factor for this disorder. It is well recognized,

Table 3
Good Prognostic Features for Brief Reactive Psychosis

Good premorbid adjustment

Few premorbid schizoid traits

Severe precipitating stressor

Acute onset of symptoms

Affective symptoms

Confusion and perplexity during psychosis

Little affective blunting

Short duration of symptoms

Absence of schizophrenic relatives

however, that many of these patients have pre-existing personality disorders, which may have both biological and psychological bases. Although schizophrenia has not been found to be more common in the relatives of affected probands, there is some indication that mood disorders may be more common among these persons. Psychodynamic formulations highlight inadequate coping mechanisms and the possibility of secondary gain in these patients. It has been hypothesized that the psychosis represents a defense, wish fulfillment, or escape related to the specific stressor.

Clinical Signs and Symptoms

The clinical signs and symptoms are similar to those seen in other psychotic disorders such as schizophrenia and psychotic mood disorders. There is some indication that affective symptoms are more common than more classic schizophrenic symptoms. Emotional volatility, outlandish dress or behavior, screaming and muteness, disorientation, and impaired recent memory may be present. The patient, who may be unable initially to relate the details of the precipitating event, sometimes later relates the details in a histrionic fashion. The signs and symptoms of a pre-existing personality disorder are observable during the mental status examination.

Course and Prognosis

There are no prodromal symptoms prior to the precipitating stressor. The onset of symptoms is usually abrupt, following the stressor by as little as a few hours. The length of acute and residual symptoms is often just a few hours or days, always less than 1 month. Occasionally, there are depressive symptoms following the resolution of psychotic symptoms. Suicide is a concern during both the psychotic and postpsychotic depressive phases. There are several indicators of good prognosis (Table 3). Patients with these features are less likely to have subsequent episodes and less likely to eventually develop schizophrenic or mood disorders.

Diagnosis

The diagnostic criteria for brief reactive psychosis are listed in DSM-III-R (Table 4). The psychosocial stressor may be either a single event or a series of events, but must

Table 4
Diagnostic Criteria for Brief Reactive Psychosis

A. Presence of at least one of the following symptoms indicating impaired reality testing (not culturally sanctioned):
   (1) incoherence or marked loosening of associations
   (2) delusions
   (3) hallucinations
   (4) catatonic or disorganized behavior

B. Emotional turmoil, i.e., rapid shifts from one intense affect to another, or overwhelming perplexity or confusion

C. Appearance of the symptoms in A and B shortly after, and apparently in response to, one or more events that, singly or together, would be markedly stressful to almost anyone in similar circumstances in the person's culture.

D. Absence of the prodromal symptoms of Schizophrenia, and failure to meet the criteria for Schizotypal Personality Disorder before onset of the disturbance.

E. Duration of an episode of the disturbance of from a few hours to 1 month, with eventual full return to premorbid level of functioning. (When the diagnosis must be made without waiting for the expected recovery, it should be qualified as "provisional.")

F. Not due to a psychotic Mood Disorder (i.e., no full mood syndrome is present), and it cannot be established that an organic factor initiated and maintained the disturbance.

Table from DSM-III-R, *Diagnostic and Statistical Manual of Mental Disorders,* ed 3, revised. (Current Classification of Mental Disorders, 1987.) Copyright American Psychiatric Association, Washington, D.C., 1987. Used with permission.

be of sufficient severity to cause significant stress to any person in the same socioeconomic and cultural class. It is often necessary to obtain the history of the psychosocial stressor from a family member when the affected individual initially presents with the psychotic symptoms. There are no defined subtypes.

Differential Diagnosis

The clinician must not assume that the correct diagnosis of a briefly psychotic patient is brief reactive psychosis even when a clear precipitating factor is evident. Such a stressor could be merely coincidental or involved in another organic or psychiatric condition. Factitious disorder with psychological symptoms, malingering, and organic causes must be considered in the differential diagnosis. Drug intoxication and withdrawal can mimic this syndrome, and the patients may be unwilling to admit to the use of illegal drugs. Epilepsy and organic delirium can also present with brief psychotic periods. In addition to schizophrenia, mood disorders, and delusional disorders, other psychiatric diagnoses to be considered are multiple personality disorder and psychotic episodes associated with borderline or schizotypal personality disorders.

Clinical Management

Hospitalization may be necessary for diagnosis and clinical management of the psychosis. The support of the hospital environment may be enough to help the patient recover. Low doses of antipsychotics may be necessary in the first week of treatment but should be withdrawn as early as possible. Individual, family, and group psychotherapy should address the significance of the specific stress and bolster old coping mechanisms and encourage new ones. It should help the patient deal with the loss of self-esteem and confidence. Hypnotic medications may be useful during the first 2 to 3 weeks of the disorder.

INDUCED PSYCHOTIC DISORDER

Induced psychotic disorder occurs when the delusional system of the patient has developed out of a close relationship with another person who had a previously established, similar delusional system. This disorder was called "shared paranoid disorder" in DSM-III and in the past has also been called *folie à deux*; however, the pathogenesis and course of this disorder were found to be so different from other delusional (paranoid) disorders, that shared paranoid disorder was renamed and moved to a different section of DSM-III-R. Induced psychotic disorder is rare and most commonly involves two persons. Cases involving more than two individuals have been called folie à trois, à quatre, à cinq, etc. One case involving a family (folie à famille) involved twelve persons (folie à douze). Other names that have been used are "double insanity" and "psychosis of association."

Induced psychotic disorder was first described in 1877 by the French psychiatrists Lasègue and Falret, who called it folie à deux. There are three related clinical subtypes—*folie simultanée*, in which the patients had the same delusions at the same time coincidentally, *folie communique*, in which two persons shared aspects of their delusions with each other; and *folie imposée*, in which there is one dominant delusional person and a second more submissive person who absorbs the more dominant individual's delusions. Folie imposée is the subtype that is currently characterized in DSM-III-R as induced psychotic disorder.

Epidemiology

Induced psychotic disorder is very rare. It is more common in women than men. It may also be more common in lower than in upper socioeconomic classes; however, persons in all socioeconomic classes may be affected. Patients with physical disabilities such as stroke or deafness may also be at increased risk because of the dependency relationships that develop for such people. Over 95 percent of cases involve two members of the same family. Approximately one third of the cases involve two sisters; another one third involve husband and wife or mother and child. Two brothers, a brother and sister, and a father and child have been reported less frequently.

Etiology

The etiology of this disorder is defined as having a psychosocial basis. The key ingredients include a dyad of a more dominant and a more submissive person, a relationship that is closely knit and relatively isolated from the outside world, and mutual gain for both persons. The dominant person has an already established mental disorder with delusions as a symptom. It is hypothesized that the dominant person maintains some contact with the real world through the submissive one, who develops the induced psychotic disorder. The submissive individual, in turn, gains the acceptance of the more dominant individual whom the submissive individual may admire. This admiration for the dominant individual may lead to a hatred for that person as well. Such hatred may be turned inward by the submissive individual, producing depression and even suicide.

The recipient or passive partner in this psychotic relationship has much in common with the dominant partner because of many shared life experiences, common needs and hopes, and, most important, a deep emotional rapport with the partner.

There are almost no biological investigations of patients with this disorder. One interpretation of the observation that this disorder affects family members is that there is a genetic basis. There is a modest amount of data to suggest that there is an increased family history of schizophrenia in the relatives of affected persons.

Clinical Signs and Symptoms

The key symptom is the unquestioning acceptance of the delusions of another person. The delusions themselves are often somewhat in the realm of possibility and usually not as bizarre as is often seen in schizophrenia. The content of the delusions is often persecutory or hypochondriacal. Symptoms of a coexisting personality disorder may be present, but signs and symptoms that meet the diagnostic criteria for schizophrenia, mood disorders, or delusional disorders are absent. There may be ideation about suicide or homicide pacts, information that must be carefully elicited.

Course and Prognosis

Conventional wisdom is that separation of the passive partner with induced psychotic disorder from the dominant one usually results in a rapid and dramatic reduction of symptoms. Clinical reports vary, however, and several papers have reported recovery rates as low as 10 to 40 percent. If symptoms continue after separation, then that individual may eventually meet the diagnostic criteria for delusional disorder or schizophrenia.

Diagnosis

The diagnostic criteria for induced psychotic disorder (Table 5) include the presence of induced delusions that are similar in content to the delusions of the dominant individual. It is required that the affected individual did not have a psychotic disorder prior to the inducement of the delusional system. There are no defined subtypes.

Differential Diagnosis

Malingering, factitious disorder with psychological symptoms, and organic disorders need to be considered in the differential diagnosis of this condition. There may be a personality disorder in the affected individual. The bound-

Table 5
Diagnostic Criteria for Induced Psychotic Disorder

A. A delusion develops (in a second person) in the context of a close relationship with another person, or persons, with an already established delusion (the primary case).

B. The delusion in the second person is similar in content to that in the primary case.

C. Immediately before onset of the induced delusion, the second person did not have a psychotic disorder or the prodromal symptoms of Schizophrenia.

Table from DSM-III-R, *Diagnostic and Statistical Manual of Mental Disorders,* ed 3, revised. (Current Classification of Mental Disorders, 1987.) Copyright American Psychiatric Association, Washington, D.C., 1987. Used with permission.

ary between induced psychotic disorder and "group madness" (e.g., the Jonestown massacre in Guyana) is unclear.

Clinical Management

The recommended approach is to separate the affected individual from the source of the delusions, the dominant person. The individual with induced psychotic disorder should be supported, usually in a hospital, and observed for natural remission of the delusional symptoms. Psychotherapy with the dominant individual and other members of the family may be necessary and effective. Pharmacotherapy should be used only if necessary. Therapy may be more successful if some compensatory support is given to the patient to compensate for the loss of the dominant partner. In addition, the mental disorder of the dominant partner should be treated.

ATYPICAL PSYCHOSES

In DSM-III-R, the category of atypical psychosis subsumes a diverse group of syndromes that have such psychotic features as delusions, hallucinations, incoherence, loosening of associations, cataplexy, or other signs of disorganized behavior and that cannot be classified clearly as schizophrenia or another well delineated psychotic condition.

In general, the atypical psychoses include the rare, the exotic, and the unusual mental disorders. The classification of this group of disorders includes the following: (1) psychoses with unusual features such as a persistent auditory hallucination; (2) syndromes that occur only at a particular time (e.g., during the menses or postpartum); (3) syndromes that are restricted to a specific cultural setting, "culture-bound syndromes"; (4) syndromes that seem to belong to a well-known diagnostic entity but that show some features that cannot be reconciled with the generally accepted typical characteristics of that diagnostic category; and (5) psychoses about which there is inadequate information to make a more specific diagnosis.

Culture-Bound Syndromes

Amok. The Malayan word *amok* means to engage furiously in battle. The amok syndrome consists of a sudden, unprovoked outburst of wild rage that causes the affected person armed with a knife to run madly about (today frequently with a firearm or grenade) and to attack and maim or kill indiscriminately any persons and animals in his way until he is overpowered or kills himself. An average of ten victims are involved. This savage homicidal attack is generally preceded by a period of preoccupation, brooding, and mild depression. After the attack, the person feels exhausted, has complete amnesia for it, and often commits suicide. The Malayan natives also refer to the attack as *mata elap* (darkened eye).

Epidemiology. The condition used to be associated almost exclusively with Malayan people, where it occurred only among men; but it has also been reported occasionally in African and other tropical cultures.

Etiology. It has been theorized that a culture that imposes heavy restrictions on adolescents and adults but allows children free rein to express their aggression, may be especially prone to psychopathological reactions of the amok type. The belief in magical possession by demons and evil spirits may be another cultural factor that contributes to the development of the amok syndrome in the Malayan people. Shame and loss of face have been proposed as determining factors.

Prognosis and Treatment. The only immediate treatment consists of overpowering the amok patient and gaining complete physical control over him. The attack is usually over within a few hours. Afterward, the patient may require treatment for a chronic psychotic condition, which may have been the underlying cause.

Koro. This acute anxiety reaction is characterized by the patient's desperate fear that his penis is shrinking and may disappear into his abdomen and that he may die.

Epidemiology. The koro syndrome occurs among the people of Southeast Asia and in some areas of China, where it is known as *suk-yeong*. A corresponding disorder of women has been described, marked by complaints of shrinkage of the vulva, labia, and breasts. Occasional cases of a koro syndrome among people belonging to a Western culture have been reported.

Etiology. Koro is a psychogenic disorder resulting from the interaction of cultural, social, and psychodynamic factors in especially predisposed personalities. Culturally elaborated fears about nocturnal emission, masturbation, and sexual overindulgence seem to give rise to the condition. Probably all koro patients have been troubled by what they consider sexual excesses and by fears about their sexual identity.

Prognosis and Treatment. Patients have been treated with psychotherapy, neuroleptic drugs, and, in a few cases, electroconvulsive therapy. As with other psychiatric disorders, the prognosis is related to the premorbid personality adjustment and the associated pathology. Some cultures prescribe fellatio as a cure.

Piblokto. Occurring among the Eskimos and sometimes referred to as Arctic hysteria, piblokto is characterized by attacks lasting from 1 to 2 hours during which the patient (usually a woman) begins to scream and to tear off and destroy her clothing. While imitating the cry of some animal or bird, she may then throw herself on the snow or run wildly about on the ice, although the temperature may be well below zero. After the attack, the person appears quite normal and usually has amnesia for it. The Eskimos are reluctant to touch any afflicted person during the attack because they think that it involves evil spirits. Piblokto is almost certainly a hysterical state of dissociation. It has become much less frequent than it used to be among the Eskimos.

Wihtigo. Wihtigo or windigo psychosis is a psychiatric illness confined to the Cree, Ojibway, and Salteaux Indians of North

America. These persons believe that they may be transformed into a wihtigo, a giant monster that eats human flesh. During times of starvation, a man may develop the delusion that he has been transformed into a wihtigo, and he may actually feel and express a craving for human flesh. Because of the belief in witchcraft and in the possibility of such a transformation, symptoms concerning the alimentary tract, such as loss of appetite or nausea from trivial causes, may sometimes cause the patient to become greatly excited for fear of being transformed into a wihtigo.

OTHER ATYPICAL PSYCHOSES

These syndromes consist of one or more psychotic symptoms, usually a recurrent hallucination or single delusion (previously called monomania). Except for the particular symptom, the rest of the personality appears entirely intact.

Autoscopic Psychosis

This syndrome consists of hallucinatory experiences in which all or part of the person's own body (called a phantom) is perceived as appearing in a mirror. This spectre is usually colorless and transparent, but it is seen clearly, appears suddenly and without warning, and imitates the person's movements.

The phantoms usually appear for only a few seconds, usually at dusk. In addition to the visual perception, there may be hallucinations in the auditory and other modalities. The person usually retains a certain detached insight into the unreality of the experience and reacts with bewilderment, and often with sadness.

Epidemiology. Autoscopy is a rare phenomenon. Sex, age, heredity, and intelligence do not seem to be significantly related to its occurrence. Some persons have this experience once in a lifetime, but a few persons seem to be always close to it. An irritating neurological lesion must always be ruled out as a cause.

Etiology. The cause of the autoscopic phenomenon is not known. One theory holds that the phenomenon reflects an irritation of areas in the temporoparietal lobes; another holds that it represents the projection of specially elaborated memory traces. Occasionally, but certainly not often, the phenomenon is symptomatic of schizophrenia or depression. Some normal persons with well-developed imaginations, "visualizer" type personality structure, and narcissistic character traits may occasionally have these experiences under conditions of emotional stress.

Prognosis and Treatment. There is rarely need for special treatment of this condition as, in most cases, it is neither incapacitating nor progressive. Treatment of an accompanying neurological condition is indicated.

Capgras' Syndrome

This psychiatric syndrome was described by the French psychiatrist Capgras in 1923 as *illusion des sosies*. Its main characteristic feature is the patient's delusional conviction that other persons in his environment are not their real selves but are, instead, their own doubles who, like impostors, assume the role of the persons they impersonate and behave like them.

Epidemiology. This rare syndrome occurs somewhat more frequently in women than in men. The condition is sometimes classified as one of the delusional disorders and may occur as a manifestation of schizophrenia.

Etiology. A necessary condition for the occurrence of this syndrome is the impairment of reality testing that develops as a result of a psychotic process. Capgras explained the particular nature of this illusion as a result of feelings of strangeness combined with a paranoid tendency to distrust. The uncoupling of normally fused components of perception and recognition may have a neurophysiological cause related to parietal lobe dysfunction.

Capgras' syndrome may, on the other hand, be determined psychodynamically. The patient rejects the particular person involved and attributes bad features to him; however, he cannot allow himself to become conscious of this rejection because of guilt feelings and ambivalent attitudes. What he really feels about the person with whom he is confronted is displaced to the double, who is an impostor and, therefore, may be safely and righteously rejected.

Prognosis and Treatment. The outcome of this condition depends on the success in treating the psychosis with which it is associated. Like other psychotic manifestations, it often responds to pharmacotherapy, at least temporarily.

Cotard's Syndrome

In the 19th century, the French psychiatrist Cotard described several patients who suffered from a syndrome he referred to as *délire de négation*. Patients exhibiting this syndrome may complain of having lost not only possessions, status, and strength, but also the heart, blood, and intestines. The world beyond them may be reduced to nothingness. The full-blown syndrome may be characterized by a delusion of immortality, which may occur in combination with other megalomanic ideas.

Epidemiology. The syndrome is usually seen as a precursor to an acute schizophrenic or depressive episode. It is relatively rare and with the advent of psychopharmacotherapy is seen less frequently.

Etiology. In its pure form, the syndrome is seen in patients suffering from depression, schizophrenia and in certain brain syndromes, particularly of the senile and presenile types. The etiology is unknown. It has been classified as a nihilistic delusional disorder.

Prognosis and Treatment. The syndrome usually lasts only a few days or weeks and responds to treatment that influences the basic disorder of which it is a part. Chronic forms of the full syndrome are today almost exclusively associated with organic brain syndromes such as Alzheimer's disease.

Ganser's Syndrome

Ganser's syndrome was first described in 1898 by the German psychiatrist S. J. M. Ganser. It has been variously classified as an atypical psychosis, a factitious disorder, and most recently in DSM-III-R, as a dissociative disorder. Ganser's syndrome is a rare disorder that is observed mainly in prisoners.

Postpartum Psychosis

A postpartum psychosis is a clinical syndrome that occurs after childbirth and is characterized by delusions and severe depression. Thoughts of wanting to harm the newborn infant or oneself are not uncommon and represent a real danger.

Epidemiology.   Postpartum psychosis occurs in 1 to 2 per 1,000 deliveries. The risk of developing a postpartum disorder is increased if the patient or her mother had a previous postpartum illness or if there is a history of mood disorder. Rare cases of postpartum psychosis have been reported in fathers; but the disorder is one that is associated with women.

Etiology.   Most patients with this disorder have an underlying mental illness, most commonly a bipolar disorder and less commonly schizophrenia. A few cases result from an organic brain syndrome associated with perinatal events (e.g., infection, drug intoxication—particularly scopoloamine and Demerol used together in obstectrics and known as twilight sleep—toxemia, or blood loss. The sudden fall in estrogen and progesterone levels immediately following pregnancy may contribute to the disorder, but reports of treatment with those hormones have not been successful. Other studies involve cortisol, serotonin, thyroid hormone, calcium, and endorphins.

Psychodynamic studies of postpartum mental illness point to conflicting feelings of the mother about her mothering experience. Some women may not have wanted to become pregnant in the first place. Others may feel trapped as a result of motherhood in an unhappy marriage. Marital discord during pregnancy is associated with an increased incidence of illness. In the rare cases of postpartum disorders in fathers, the husband feels displaced by the child and competitive for the mother's love and attention.

Clinical Signs and Symptoms.   The symptoms usually occur about the third postpartum day. The patient begins to complain of insomnia, restlessness, feelings of fatigue, and shows lability of mood with bouts of tearfulness. Later symptoms include suspiciousness, evidence of confusion, incoherence, irrational statements, and obsessive concerns about the baby's health or welfare. There may be feelings of not wanting to care for the baby, not loving the baby, and, in some cases, of wanting to do harm to the baby, to self, or both. Delusional material may involve the idea that the baby is dead or defective. The birth may be denied and thoughts of being unmarried or virginal or ideas of persecution, influence, or perverse sexuality may be expressed. Hallucinations may occur with similar content and may involve voices telling the patient to kill her baby.

Diagnosis.   The main diagnostic feature of this disorder is the association with the postpartum period, most cases begin within 30 days of giving birth. Symptoms of cognitive impairment associated with mood changes, particularly depression and delusions, or hallucinations with content related to the infant or mothering are characteristic. A premorbid history of the patient's attitudes about pregnancy and conception, whether the baby was planned, attitudes of the father toward the birth, marital problems, and anticipated life-style changes may be helpful. In addition to a routine clinical psychiatric examination, a thorough neurological and medical examination is necessary to rule out an organic cause of the disorder.

Course and Prognosis.   The onset of florid psychotic symptoms is usually preceded by prodromal signs, such as insomnia, restlessness, agitation, lability of mood, and mild cognitive defects. Once the full-blown psychosis occurs, the patient may be a danger to herself or to her newborn depending on the content of her delusional system and degree of agitation. In one study, 5 percent of patients killed themselves and 4 percent killed the baby. A favorable outcome is associated with a good premorbid adaptation, the absence of depression or schizophrenia, and a supportive family network. Subsequent pregnancies are associated with an increased risk of having another episode; however most episodes occur to primiparas.

Differential Diagnosis.   Those women with a prior history of schizophrenia or mood disorders should be diagnosed as having a recurrence of those disorders, rather than an atypical psychosis. In the absence of those disorders, a diagnosis of postpartum psychosis may be made related to the stresses of pregnancy. Because of its clinical similarity to postpartum depression, hypothyroidism should always be considered. Cushing's syndrome, which may occur after a pregnancy, frequently is associated with a depressive state. Drug-induced depression is not uncommon, especially in those receiving antihypertensive, or other drugs with known central nervous system–depressant properties. Pentazocine (Talwin), a drug with psychotomimetic properties, is sometimes used in the postpartum period and has been reported to produce bizarre mental phenomena. Those patients with prominent organic mental symptoms should receive careful evaluation for infection, encephalopathy related to toxemia, and neoplasm.

Postpartum psychosis should not be confused with the so-called postpartum blues, a normal condition that occurs in up to 50 percent of women after childbirth. That syndrome is self-limited, lasts only a few days, and is characterized by tearfulness, fatigue, anxiety, and irritability that begins shortly after childbirth and lessens in severity each day postpartum.

Treatment.   Postpartum psychosis is a psychiatric emergency. Antidepressants are the treatment of choice in depressed postpartum disorders. Suicidal patients may require transfer to a psychiatric unit to prevent a suicidal attempt. For patients who suffer manic illnesses, lithium carbonate therapy, alone or in combination with an antipsychotic agent during the first 7 days, is the treatment of choice. For patients with schizophrenic-type psychoses, phenothiazines or other antipsychotic agents are indicated. These pharmacological agents are not recommended for use by mothers who are breast feeding.

It is usually advantageous for the mother to have contact with her baby if she so desires. But these visits must be closely supervised especially if the mother is preoccupied with doing harm to the infant.

Psychotherapy is indicated after the period of acute psychosis is past. Therapy is usually directed at the conflictual areas that have become evident during the period of evaluation. Therapy may involve helping the patient to accept the mothering role accentuated by the childbearing experience or to accept her angry, jealous feelings toward the child as they relate to her thwarted need to depend on her own mother. Changes in environmental factors may also be indicated. Increased support from the husband and other persons in the environment may help to reduce stress. Most studies report high rates of recovery from the acute phase of illness.

Atypical Cycloid Psychoses

This group of disorders shows some features of bipolar disorders but cannot meet the generally accepted characteristics of this diagnostic category. Three types have been described: motility psychoses (hyperkinetic or akinetic), confusional psychoses, and anxiety-blissfulness psychoses.

Motility Psychosis. In their hyperkinetic form, the motility psychoses may resemble manic or catatonic excitement. A hyperkinetic motility psychosis may be distinguished from a manic state by the presence of many abrupt gestures and expressive movements that seem to be the result of autonomous mechanisms and are apparently not responses to environmental stimuli or expressions of the patient's mood. These disorders may be differentiated from catatonic excitement by the absence of stereotyped and bizarre movements.

The akinetic form of motility psychosis seems to be identical with the typical picture of a catatonic stupor. These states are separated from typical schizophrenia mainly on the basis of their rapid and favorable course, which does not lead to any personality deterioration.

Confusional Psychosis. The excited confusional psychosis must be distinguished from some confused manic states. The difference is mainly in the greater lability of the patient's emotional state, which may be characterized by prevailing anxiety rather than euphoria. These patients are less likely to be distracted as the manic patients are, they often misidentify persons in their environment, and the incoherence of their speech seems to be independent of a flight of ideas.

Anxiety-Blissfulness Psychosis. The anxiety-blissfulness psychosis may very much resemble the clinical picture of what is generally known as agitated depression, but it may also be characterized by so much inhibition that the patient can hardly move. Periodic states of overwhelming anxiety and paranoid ideas of reference are characteristic of this condition, but self-accusation, hypochondriacal preoccupation, and other depressive symptoms, as well as hallucinations, may accompany it.

The blissful phase manifests itself most frequently in expansive behavior and grandiose ideas, which are concerned less with self-aggrandizement than with the mission of making others happy and of saving the world. In women, the dominant emotion is usually passive ecstasy, often the result of fantastic religious delusions.

Atypical Schizophrenia

A particular form of schizophrenia has been described by Gjessing and called periodic catatonia. Patients affected with this disease have periodic bouts of stuporous or excited catatonia, which Gjessing believed were related to metabolic shifts in nitrogen balance. The syndrome is rarely seen and responds well to standard antipsychotic agents and is prevented by maintainence medication.

In general, an attempt should be made to place each of the above disorders in one of the more conventional categories of mood disorders or schizophrenia if possible. Treatment is directed toward the predominant symptoms.

References

Brockington I F, Kumar R: *Motherhood and Mental Illness*. Grune & Stratton, New York, 1982.

Coryell W H, Tsuang M T: DSM–III schizophreniform disorder: Comparisons with schizophrenia and affective disorder. Arch Gen Psychiatry 39:66, 1982.

Coryell W, Tsuang M T: Outcome after 40 years in DSM–III schizophreniform disorder. Arch Gen Psychiatry 43:324, 1986.

Fogelson D I, Cohen B M, Pope H G: A study of DSM–III schizophreniform disorder. Am J Psychiatry 139:1281, 1982.

Gift T E, Strauss J S, Young Y: Hysterical psychosis: An empirical approach. Am J Psychiatry 142:345, 1985.

Lazarus A: Folie à deux: Psychosis by association or genetic determinism. Compr Psychiatry 26:129, 1985.

Stephens J H, Shaffer J W, Carpenter W T: Reactive psychoses. J Nervous Mental Dis 170:657, 1982.

Refsum H E, Astrup C: Hysteric reactive psychoses: A follow-up. Neuropsychobiol 8:172, 1982.

Targum S D: Neuroendocrine dysfunction in schizophreniform disorder: Correlation with 6-month clinical outcome. Am J Psychiatry 140:309, 1983.

Taylor M A, Abrams R: Mania and DSM–III schizophreniform disorder. J Affective Dis 6:19, 1984.

Weinberger D R, DeLisi L E, Perman G D, et al: Computed tomography and schizophreniform disorder and other acute psychiatric disorders. Arch Gen Psychiatry 39:778, 1982.

17

_____ **Mood Disorders**

Depressive and Bipolar Disorders

Mood refers to the internal emotional state of an individual; _affect,_ to the external expression of emotional content. There are pathologic conditions of mood and affect, the most serious of which are the mood disorders, depression and mania. Depression and mania were called affective disorders in DSM-III; in DSM-III-R they are grouped together as mood disorders.

Mood may be normal, elevated, or depressed. A normal individual experiences a wide range of moods and has an equally large repertoire of affective expression; he feels in control of his moods and affects. Mood disorders are a group of clinical conditions characterized by a disturbance of mood, a loss of that sense of control, and a subjective experience of great distress. Patients with elevated mood demonstrate expansiveness, flight of ideas, decreased sleep, heightened self-esteem, and grandiose ideas. Patients with depressed mood show loss of energy and interest, guilt feelings, difficulty in concentrating, loss of appetite, and thoughts of death or suicide. Others signs and symptoms include changes in activity level, cognitive abilities, speech, and vegetative functions (e.g., sleep, appetite, sexual activity, and other biological rhythms). These disorders virtually always result in impaired interpersonal, social, and occupational functioning. It is both useful and tempting to consider disorders of mood on a continuum with normal variations in mood. Patients with mood disorders, however, often report an ineffable but distinct quality to their pathologic state. The concept of a continuum, therefore, may represent the clinician's over-identification with the pathology, thus distorting his approach to mood disorder patients.

Patients who are afflicted only with major depressive episodes are said to have major depressive disorder or unipolar depression. Patients with both manic and depressive episodes or patients with manic episodes alone are said to have bipolar disorder. The terms unipolar mania and pure mania are sometimes used for bipolar patients who do not have depressive episodes. Three additional categories of mood disorders are hypomania, cyclothymia, and dysthymia. Hypomania is an episode of manic symptoms that does not meet the full DSM-III-R criteria for a manic episode. Cyclothymia and dysthymia are DSM-III-R–de-

fined disorders that represent less severe forms of bipolar disorder and major depression, respectively.

The field of psychiatry has considered unipolar depression and bipolar disorder to be two separate disorders, particularly in the last 20 years. However, reconsideration has been given more recently to the possibility that bipolar disorder is actually a more severe expression of unipolar depression. Another trend in psychiatry has been to consider depression and mania as two ends of a continuum of emotional experience. This concept is not supported by the common clinical observation that many patients have mixed states with both depressed and manic features.

HISTORY

Depression has been recorded since antiquity, and descriptions of what we now call the mood disorders can be found in many ancient documents. The Old Testament story of King Saul describes a depressive syndrome, as does the story of Ajax's suicide in Homer's _Iliad_. About 450 B.C. Hippocrates used the terms mania and melancholia to describe mental disturbances. Cornelius Celsus described melancholia in his work _De Medicina_ about 100 A.D. as a depression caused by black bile. The term continued to be used by other medical authors, including Arataeus (120–180 A.D.), Galen (129–199 A.D.), and Alexander of Tralles in the sixth century. In the middle ages, medicine remained alive in the Islamic countries and Rhazes, Avicenna; the Jewish physician Maimonides considered melancholia a discrete disease entity. Melancholia was also depicted by great artists of the time (Figure 1). In 1686, Bonet described a mental illness that he called maniaco-melancholicus.

In 1854, Jules Falret described a condition called _folie circulaire_ in which the patient experienced alternating moods of depression and mania. About the same time, another French psychiatrist Jules Baillarger described the condition _folie à double forme_ in which the patient became deeply depressed and fell into a stuporous state from which he would eventually recover. In 1882, the German psychiatrist Karl Kahlbaum, using the term "cyclothymia," described mania and depression as stages of the same illness.

Emil Kraepelin, in 1896, building on the knowledge of previous French and German psychiatrists, described a concept of manic-depressive psychosis that contained most of the criteria that psychiatrists now use to establish the diagnosis. The absence of a dementing and deteriorating

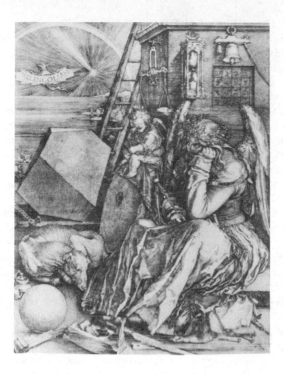

Figure 1. "Melancholia" by Albrecht Dürer, (1471-1528) showing a winged figure in the typical depressive posture surrounded by scattered rubble of a meaningless world.

course in manic-depressive psychosis differentiated it from dementia precox (schizophrenia). Kraepelin also described a type of depression that began after menopause in women and during late adulthood in men that came to be known as involutional melancholia, and has since come to be viewed as a variant form of the mood disorders.

EPIDEMIOLOGY

Incidence and Prevalence

The mood disorders, particularly unipolar depression, are among the most common psychiatric disorders of adults. The lifetime expectancy of developing unipolar depression is approximately 20 percent in women and 10 percent in men; the lifetime expectancy of developing bipolar disorder is about 1 percent in both men and women. Although most patients with bipolar disorder are eventually seen by a physician, it is estimated that only 20 to 25 percent of those who meet the criteria for major depression receive treatment.

Sex

An almost universal observation, independent of country, is the twofold greater prevalence of unipolar depression in women than in men. Though the reasons for the difference are unknown, it is not the result of socially biased diagnostic practices. The reasons may include varying stresses, childbirth, learned helplessness, and hormonal effects. In bipolar disorder, the prevalence is only very slightly higher in females (about 1.2 to 1).

Age

The onset of unipolar depression can occur from childhood through senescence, but 50 percent of patients have the onset between ages 20 and 50, the mean age being about 40. Bipolar disorder begins somewhat earlier, the range being from childhood to 50 years with a mean age of 30.

Race

The prevalence of mood disorders does not differ from race to race. However, there is a tendency for examiners to underdiagnose mood disorders and overdiagnose schizophrenia in patients who have a different racial or cultural background. White psychiatrists, for example, tend to underdiagnose mood disorders in blacks and Hispanics.

Marital Status

In general, unipolar depression occurs more often in persons who have no close interpersonal relationships or who are divorced or separated. Bipolar disorder may be more common in divorced and single individuals than among married persons; but this difference may reflect the early onset and resulting marital discord that are characteristic of the disorder.

Social and Cultural Considerations

There is no correlation between social class and unipolar depression; however, recent immigration may be positively correlated to unipolar depression. In bipolar disorder there appears to be a higher incidence among the upper socioeconomic classes, possibly because of diagnostic biases. Bipolar disorder is more common in persons who did not graduate from college than in graduates, which probably reflects the relatively early age of onset. In general, mood disorders are equally common in urban and rural areas.

ETIOLOGY

The etiology of mood disorders is unknown. As with other psychiatric disorders, the groups of patients defined by DSM-III-R undoubtedly include heterogeneous populations of patients with different illnesses. Etiologic theories of mood disorders include biological (including genetic) and psychosocial hypotheses.

Biological

Biogenic Amines. Norepinephrine and serotonin are the two neurotransmitters most implicated in the pathophysiology of mood disorders. In animal models, all effective somatic antidepressant treatments are associated with a delayed decrease in the sensitivity of postsynaptic β-adrenergic and $5HT_2$ receptors following chronic treatment. These delayed receptor changes in animal models correlate with the 1- to 3-week delay in clinical improvement usually seen in patients. It is perhaps consistent with the decrease in serotonin receptors following chronic exposure that a decrease in the number of serotonin reuptake sites (assessed by measuring the binding of 3H-imipramine) and an increased concentration of serotonin have been found at postmortem in the brains of suicides. It has also been reported that there is decreased 3H-imipramine binding to blood platelets from some depressed individuals. There is data to indicate that dopaminergic activity may be reduced in depression and increased in mania. There is also evidence for a dysregulation of acetylcholine in mood disorders. One recent study reported an increased number of muscarinic receptors on cultured skin fibroblasts from bipolar disorder patients. An enormous number of studies have reported various abnormalities in biogenic amine metabolites (e.g., 5-HIAA, HVA, MHPG) in blood, urine, and cerebrospinal fluid (CSF) from mood disorder patients. The data reported are most consistent with the hypothesis that mood disorders are associated with heterogeneous dysregulations of the biogenic amine systems.

Other Neurochemical Considerations. Although the data is not conclusive at this point, amino acid neurotransmitters (particularly GABA) and neuroactive peptides (particularly vasopressin and the endogenous opioids) have been implicated in the pathophysiology of some mood disorders. Some investigators have suggested that second messenger systems, such as adenylate cyclase, phosphatidyl inositol, or calcium regulation, may also be of etiologic relevance.

Neuroendocrine Regulation. A variety of neuroendocrine dysregulations have been reported in patients with mood disorders. Although a neuroendocrine dysregulation may be the primary etiology of mood disorders, it is best to consider neuroendocrine testing as a "window" into the brain at the present time. It is likely that neuroendocrine abnormalities reflect dysregulations in biogenic amine input to the hypothalamus.

Abnormalities of the limbic-hypothalamic-pituitary-adrenal (LHPA) axis are the most consistently reported neuroendocrine dysregulations. The finding that hypersecretion of cortisol is present in some depressed patients has been used in the dexamethasone suppression test (DST). (Dexamethasone is an exogenous steroid that suppresses the blood level of cortisol.) The DST is abnormal in approximately 50 percent of depressed patients, indicating a hyperactivity of the LHPA axis. The DST is not specific for depression, however, and may be abnormal in patients with obsessive-compulsive disorder, eating disorders, organic brain disorders (e.g., Alzheimer's disease), and other medical conditions. Some patients with mania or schizophrenia also demonstrate nonsuppression on the DST.

Other neuroendocrine markers of depression include a blunted (diminished) release of thyroid stimulating hormone (TSH) upon administration of thyroid releasing hormone (TRH), a decreased release of growth hormone to noradrenergic stimulation with clonidine, decreased nocturnal secretion of melatonin, decreased prolactin release to tryptophan administration, decreased basal levels of follicle stimulating hormone (FSH) and luteinizing hormone (LH), and decreased testosterone levels in males. A blunted response of TSH to TRH administration has been reported in mania as well.

Sleep Abnormalities. Abnormalities of sleep architecture are among the most robust biological markers of depression. The major abnormalities are a decreased REM latency (the time between falling asleep and the first REM period), which is seen in two thirds of depressed patients, an increased length of the first REM period, and an increased density of REM in the first part of sleep. There is also increased early morning awakening and discontinuity of sleep with multiple awakenings during the night.

Other Biological Data. Abnormalities in immune function have been reported in both depression and mania. It has also been hypothesized that depression is a disorder of chronobiological regulation.

Brain imaging studies of mood disorder patients have produced modest results thus far. Studies with computed tomographic (CT) scans indicate that some patients with mania or psychotic depression have enlarged cerebral ventricles. Positron emission tomographic (PET) scans have suggested reduced brain metabolism, and other studies detected reduced cerebral blood flow in depression, particularly to the basal ganglia. A single study of computed tomographic EEG in depression found abnormalities in the late components of the visual evoked responses.

Consolidation of Biological Data. Both the symptoms of the mood disorders and biological research findings support the hypothesis that mood disorders involve pathology of the limbic system, the basal ganglia, and the hypothalamus. It has been noted that neurologic disorders of the basal ganglia and limbic system (especially excitatory lesions of the nondominant hemisphere) are likely to present with depressive symptoms. The limbic system and the basal ganglia are quite intimately connected, and a major role in the production of emotions is hypothesized for the limbic system. Dysfunction of the hypothalamus is suggested by the alterations in sleep, appetite, and sexual behavior, and by the biological changes in endocrine, immunologic, and chronobiological measures. The stooped posture, motor slowness, and minor cognitive impairment seen in depression are quite similar to disorders of the basal ganglia, such as Parkinson's disease and other subcortical dementias.

Genetic

The fact that both bipolar disorder and unipolar depression run in families is also consistent with a biological etiology for mood disorders. The evidence for the heritability of bipolar disorder is stronger than that for unipolar depression. Approximately 50 percent of bipolar patients have at least one parent with a mood disorder, most often unipolar depression. If one parent has bipolar disorder, there is a 27 percent chance that any child will have a mood disorder; if both parents have bipolar disorder, there is a 50 to 75 percent chance that a child will have a mood disorder. Adoption studies have shown that the biological parents of adopted mood disordered children have an incidence of mood disorder similar to that of the parents of nonadopted mood disordered children. The incidence of mood disorders in the adoptive parents is similar to the baseline incidence of mood disorders in the general population. Twin studies have shown a concordance rate of 0.67 for bipolar disorder in monozygotic twins and 0.20 for bipolar disorder in dizygotic twins. The concordance for bipolar disorder is higher than that reported for unipolar depression. The genetic data, therefore, are consistent with the concept of a genetic basis for mood disorders.

The application of molecular genetic techniques, particularly restriction fragment length polymorphisms (RFLPs), to the study of bipolar disorder has recently led to an important discovery. A dominant gene located on the short arm of chromosome 11 has been found to confer a strong predisposition to bipolar disorder in one Amish family. This gene may be involved in the regulation of tyrosine hydroxylase, the rate-limiting enzyme for the synthesis of catecholamines. However, this particular gene was not found in other families affected by bipolar disorder. This new data is consistent with the notion that bipolar disorder represents a heterogeneous group of diseases.

Psychosocial

Life Events and Environmental Stress. Most American clinicians believe that there is a relationship between stressful life events and clinical depression. Clinical case discussions often include statements relating stress, especially from life events, to the onset of depressive episodes. In such discussions, life events are thought to play an important role in the causation of depression, as reflected by such remarks as "The depression arose in relation to . . ." and "The depression was precipitated by. . . ." Some clinicians believe that life events play the primary or principal role in depression; others are more conservative, limiting the role of life events to contributing to the onset and timing of the actual episode. The research data to support this relationship, however, is inconclusive. The most robust data indicate that the loss of a parent before age 11 and the loss of a spouse at onset of illness are correlated with major depression.

Premorbid Personality Factors. No single personality trait or type has been established as being uniquely predisposing to depression. All humans, of whatever personality pattern, can and do become depressed under appropriate circumstances; however, certain personality types—oral-dependent, obsessive-compulsive, hysterical—may be at greater risk for depression than antisocial, paranoid, and other personality types who use projection and other externalizing defense mechanisms.

Psychoanalytic Factors. Karl Abraham thought that episodes of manifest illness are precipitated by the loss of a libidinal object, eventuating in a regressive process in which the ego retreats from its mature functioning state to one in which the infantile trauma of the oral-sadistic stage of libidinal development dominates because of a fixation process in earliest childhood.

In Freud's structural theory, the ambivalent introjection of the lost object into the ego leads to the typical depressive symptoms diagnostic of a lack of energy available to the ego. The superego, unable to retaliate against the lost object externally, flails out at the psychic representation of the lost object, now internalized in the ego as an introject. When the ego overcomes or merges with the superego, there is a release of energy that was previously bound in the depressive symptoms, and as a result of denial a mania supervenes with the typical symptoms of excess.

Later analytic writers have elaborated the basic Abraham-Freud conceptualization in various ways. Although most analytic writers pay lip service to the concept that the disease has an underlying neurophysiological substrate, few attempt to conceptualize that state in any but psychological terms.

Heinz Kohut made significant contributions to the psychology of the self and the treatment of narcissistic personality disorder. Narcissistic personality disorder is one of the frequent differential diagnostic considerations in manic-depressive patients, because patients with narcissistic personality disorder frequently demonstrate transient periods of elation and depression, often with grandiosity and euphoria in one phase and self-depreciation in a succeeding phase, just as is seen in classic manic-depressive disorder.

Learned Helplessness. In experiments in which animals were repeatedly exposed to electric shocks from which they could not escape, the animals eventually "gave up" and made no attempt at all to escape future shocks. They learned that they were helpless. In humans who are depressed, one can find a similar state of helplessness. According to learned helplessness theory, depression can improve if the clinician instills in a depressed patient a sense of control and mastery of the environment. Behavioral techniques of reward and positive reinforcement are employed in such efforts.

Cognitive Theories. According to this theory common cognitive misinterpretations involve negative distortion of life experience, negative self-evaluation, pessimism, and hopelessness.

CLINICAL SIGNS AND SYMPTOMS

There are two basic symptom patterns in the mood disorders, one for depression and one for mania. The depressive episodes in bipolar disorder are identical to the depressive disorders in unipolar depression. Some cases of bipolar disorder, however, are mixed states with manic and depressive features. Also, some bipolar patients experience very brief (minutes to a few hours) episodes of depression during a manic episode.

Depressive Episodes

DSM-III-R lists many of the symptoms of depression under the criteria for major depressive episodes (Table 1) and melancholia (Table 2). A depressed mood and a loss of interest or pleasure are the key symptoms of depression. The patient may say that he feels blue, hopeless, in the dumps, or worthless. The depressed mood often has a distinct quality to the patient that differentiates it from the emotion of sadness. Patients often describe the symptom as one of agonizing emotional pain that causes them to drink excessively. Approximately two thirds of depressed patients contemplate suicide, and 10 to 15 percent complete suicide. Depressed patients sometimes complain about being unable to cry, a symptom that resolves as they improve. Depressed patients, however, sometimes appear unaware of their depression and do not complain of a mood disturbance even though they may be exhibiting withdrawal from family, friends, and activities that previously interested them.

Almost all depressed patients (97 percent) complain about reduced energy resulting in difficulty finishing tasks, school and work impairment, and decreased motivation in undertaking new projects. Approximately 80 percent of patients complain of trouble sleeping, especially early morning awakening (i.e., terminal insomnia) and multiple awakenings at night, during which they ruminate about their

Table 1
Diagnostic Criteria for Major Depressive Episode

Note: A "Major Depressive Syndrome" is defined as criterion A below.

A. At least five of the following symptoms have been present during the same two-week period and represent a change from previous functioning; at least one of the symptoms is either (1) depressed mood, or (2) loss of interest or pleasure. (Do not include symptoms that are clearly due to a physical condition, mood-incongruent delusions or hallucinations, incoherence, or marked loosening of associations.)

   (1) depressed mood (or can be irritable mood in children and adolescents) most of the day, nearly every day, as indicated either by subjective account or observation by others

   (2) markedly diminished interest or pleasure in all, or almost all, activities most of the day, nearly every day (as indicated either by subjective account or observation by others of apathy most of the time)

   (3) significant weight loss or weight gain when not dieting (e.g., more than 5% of body weight in a month), or decrease or increase in appetite nearly every day (in children, consider failure to make expected weight gains)

   (4) insomnia or hypersomnia nearly every day

   (5) psychomotor agitation or retardation nearly every day (observable by others, not merely subjective feelings of restlessness or being slowed down)

   (6) fatigue or loss of energy nearly every day

   (7) feelings of worthlessness or excessive or inappropriate guilt (which may be delusional) nearly every day (not merely self-reproach or guilt about being sick)

   (8) diminished ability to think or concentrate, or indecisiveness, nearly every day (either by subjective account or as observed by others)

   (9) recurrent thoughts of death (not just fear of dying), recurrent suicidal ideation without a specific plan, or a suicide attempt or a specific plan for committing suicide

B. (1) It cannot be established that an organic factor initiated and maintained the disturbance

   (2) The disturbance is not a normal reaction to the death of a loved one (Uncomplicated Bereavement)

   Note: Morbid preoccupation with worthlessness, suicidal ideation, marked functional impairment or psychomotor retardation, or prolonged duration suggest bereavement complicated by Major Depression.

C. At no time during the disturbance have there been delusions or hallucinations for as long as two weeks in the absence of prominent mood symptoms (i.e., before the mood symptoms developed or after they have remitted).

D. Not superimposed on Schizophrenia, Schizophreniform Disorder, Delusional Disorder, or Psychotic Disorder NOS.

Table from DSM-III-R, *Diagnostic and Statistical Manual of Mental Disorders,* ed 3, revised. (Current Classification of Mental Disorders, 1987.) Copyright American Psychiatric Association, Washington, D.C., 1987. Used with permission.

problems. Many patients have decreased appetite and weight loss. Some patients, however, have increased appetite, weight gain, and increased sleep. The various changes in food intake and rest can aggravate coexisting medical illnesses, such as diabetes, hypertension, chronic obstructive lung disease, and heart disease. Other vegetative symptoms include abnormal menses and decreased interest and performance in sexual activities. Sexual problems can sometimes lead to such inappropriate referrals as marital counseling or sex therapy if the clinician fails to recognize the underlying depressive disorder.

Anxiety (including panic attacks), alcohol abuse, and somatic complaints (e.g., constipation, headaches) often complicate the treatment of depression. Approximately 50 percent of patients describe a diurnal variation in their symptoms, with a increased severity in the morning and a lessening of symptoms by evening. Cognitive symptoms include subjective reports of an inability to concentrate (84 percent of patients) and impairments in thinking (67 percent). The individual described in the following case has been diagnosed as having this disorder:

A 50-year-old widow was transferred to a medical center from her community mental health center, to which she had been admitted three weeks previously with severe agitation, pacing, and hand-wringing, depressed mood accompanied by severe self-reproach, insomnia, and a 6–8 kg (15-pound) weight loss. She believed that her neighbors were against her, had poisoned her coffee, and had bewitched her to punish her because of her wickedness. Seven years previously, after the death of her husband, she had required hospitalization for a similar depression, with extreme guilt, agitation, insomnia, accusatory hallucinations of voices calling her a worthless person, and preoccupation with thoughts of suicide. Before being transferred, she had been treated with Dox-

Table 2
Diagnostic Criteria for Melancholia

The presence of at least five of the following:

   (1) loss of interest or pleasure in all, or almost all, activities

   (2) lack of reactivity to usually pleasurable stimuli (does not feel much better, even temporarily, when something good happens)

   (3) depression regularly worse in the morning

   (4) early morning awakening (at least two hours before usual time of awakening)

   (5) psychomotor retardation or agitation (not merely subjective complaints)

   (6) significant anorexia or weight loss (e.g., more than 5% of body weight in a month)

   (7) no significant personality disturbance before first Major Depressive Episode

   (8) one or more previous Major Depressive Episodes followed by complete, or nearly complete, recovery

   (9) previous good response to specific and adequate somatic antidepressant therapy, e.g., tricyclics, ECT, MAOI, lithium

Table from DSM-III-R, *Diagnostic and Statistical Manual of Mental Disorders,* ed 3, revised. (Current Classification of Mental Disorders, 1987.) Copyright American Psychiatric Association, Washington, D.C., 1987. Used with permission.

epin HCL, 200 mg, with only modest effect on the depression and no effect on the delusions.

Discussion

The pervasive depressed mood with the characteristic associated symptoms of the depressive syndrome (psychomotor agitation, self-reproach, insomnia, and weight loss) suggests a major depressive episode. The delusions are congruent with the depressed mood, since the content involves the theme of guilt and deserved punishment. In the absence of any specific organic factor to account for the disturbance, the diagnosis is major depression. It is further subclassified as recurrent, because of the history of a previous episode.

DSM-III-R Diagnosis:

Axis I: Major Depression, Recurrent, with Psychotic Features (Mood-congruent)

[Adapted with permission from *DSM-III Case Book*. American Psychiatric Association, Washington, D.C., 1981.]

Depression in Children and Adolescents

Excessive clinging to parents and school phobia may be symptoms of depression in children. Poor academic performance, drug abuse, antisocial behavior, sexual promiscuity, truancy, and running away may be symptoms of depression in adolescent children. See Section 44.1 on Mood Disorders for further discussion of this area of child psychiatry.

Manic Episodes

The features of a manic episode are defined in DSM-III-R (Table 3). Elevated, expansive, or irritable mood is the hallmark. The elevated mood is euphoric and often infectious in nature, sometimes causing a countertransferential denial of illness by an inexperienced clinician. Although uninvolved people may not recognize the unusual nature of the patient's mood, those who know the patient recognize it as abnormal for that person. Alternatively, the mood may be irritable, especially when the patient's overly ambitious plans are thwarted. Often, a patient exhibits a change of predominant mood from euphoria early in the course of the illness to irritability later in the process.

In addition to the criteria listed in DSM-III-R, manic patients often exhibit other symptoms. The management of manic patients on an inpatient ward can be complicated by their testing the limits of ward rules, a tendency to shift responsibility for their acts to others, exploitation of the weaknesses of others, and a tendency to divide ward staffs. Manic patients often drink alcohol excessively, perhaps in an attempt to self-medicate. The disinhibited nature of these patients is reflected in excessive use of the telephone, especially long distance calls during the early hours of the morning. Pathologic gambling, a tendency to disrobe in public places, clothing and jewelry of bright colors in unusual combinations, and an inattention to small details (e.g., forgetting to hang up the phone) are also symptomatic of this disorder. The impulsive nature of many of the patient's acts is coupled with a sense of conviction and purpose. The patient is often preoccupied by religious,

Table 3
Diagnostic Criteria for Manic Episode

Note: A "Manic Syndrome" is defined as including criteria A, B, and C below. A "Hypomanic Syndrome" is defined as including criteria A and B, but not C, i.e., no marked impairment.

A. A distinct period of abnormally and persistently elevated, expansive, or irritable mood.

B. During the period of mood disturbance, at least three of the following symptoms have persisted (four if the mood is only irritable) and have been present to a significant degree:

  (1) inflated self-esteem or grandiosity
  (2) decreased need for sleep, e.g., feels rested after only three hours of sleep
  (3) more talkative than usual or pressure to keep talking
  (4) flight of ideas or subjective experience that thoughts are racing
  (5) distractibility, i.e., attention too easily drawn to unimportant or irrelevant external stimuli
  (6) increase in goal-directed activity (either socially, at work or school, or sexually) or psychomotor agitation
  (7) excessive involvement in pleasurable activities which have a high potential for painful consequences, e.g., the person engages in unrestrained buying sprees, sexual indiscretions, or foolish business investments

C. Mood disturbance sufficiently severe to cause marked impairment in occupational functioning or in usual social activities or relationships with others, or to necessitate hospitalization to prevent harm to self or others.

D. At no time during the disturbance have there been delusions or hallucinations for as long as two weeks in the absence of prominent mood symptoms (i.e., before the mood symptoms developed or after they have remitted).

E. Not superimposed on Schizophrenia, Schizophreniform Disorder, Delusional Disorder, or Psychotic Disorder NOS.

F. It cannot be established that an organic factor initiated and maintained the disturbance. **Note:** Somatic antidepressant treatment (e.g., drugs, ECT) that apparently precipitates a mood disturbance should not be considered an etiologic organic factor.

Table from DSM-III-R, *Diagnostic and Statistical Manual of Mental Disorders*, ed 3, revised. (Current Classification of Mental Disorders, 1987.) Copyright American Psychiatric Association, Washington, D.C., 1987. Used with permission.

political, financial, sexual, or persecutory ideas that can evolve into complex delusional systems. Occasionally, these patients become quite regressed and play with their urine and feces. The following individual has been diagnosed as having bipolar disorder:

B.B., a 39-year-old Hungarian opera singer, is readmitted to a psychiatric hospital after keeping her family awake for several nights with a prayer and song marathon. She is flamboyantly dressed in a floor-length red skirt and peasant blouse, and is adorned with heavy earrings, numerous necklaces and bracelets, and medals pinned to her bosom. She speaks very rapidly and is difficult to interrupt as she talks about her intimate relationship with God. She often breaks into song, explaining that her beautiful singing voice is a special gift that God has given her to compensate for her insanity. She uses it to share the joy she feels with others who are less fortunate.

B.B. has had at least ten admissions to this hospital in the past 20 years, some because of serious suicide attempts made when she was depressed, some because she was manic, and some, in her words, "just because I was crazy." Although she does have a lovely voice, she has not been able to organize herself to work professionally during the past 15 years, and has spent much of her time at the local community mental health center. She has seen the same therapist weekly for many years and believes that he communicates with her through a local radio station, giving her instructions on how to conduct her life between therapy sessions. She also receives illuminations from Kahlil Gibran and Adele Davis, whose conversations she is able to overhear.

Discussion

There should not be much difficulty recognizing that this woman is currently in a manic episode. She has expansive mood (singing, flamboyant dress), with pressure of speech (difficult to interrupt), decreased need for sleep, and grandiosity (intimate relationship with God). In the past she has had similar episodes, as well as depressions with suicide attempts. The diagnosis of bipolar disorder is made, and would be made even in the absence of a history of depressive episodes.

The current episode is manic and has mood-congruent psychotic features (receiving illuminations from famous people). Some clinicians might interpret the delusion that she receives messages from her therapist through the local radio station as unrelated to any typical manic theme; however, this delusion also has a grandiose theme.

DSM-III-R Diagnosis:
Axis I: Bipolar Disorder, Manic, with Psychotic Features (Mood-congruent)
[Adapted with permission from *DSM-III Case Book*. American Psychiatric Association, Washington, D.C., 1981.]

Mania in Adolescents. Mania in adolescents is often misdiagnosed as sociopathy or schizophrenia. Symptoms of mania in adolescents may include psychosis, alcohol or drug abuse, suicide attempts, academic problems, philosophical broodings, obsessive-compulsive symptoms, multiple somatic complaints, marked irritability resulting in fights, and other antisocial behaviors. Although many of these symptoms can be seen in normal adolescence, severe or persistent symptoms should cause the clinician to consider bipolar disorder in the differential diagnosis.

MENTAL STATUS EXAMINATION

Depressive Episodes

General Description. Generalized psychomotor retardation is the most common symptom, although psychomotor agitation is also seen (usually in elderly patients). The classic presentation of a depressed patient is that of a stooped posture with no spontaneous movements and a downcast, averted gaze. If a depressed patient exhibits gross symptoms of psychomotor retardation, he may appear identical to a patient with catatonic schizophrenia. The

classic symptoms of psychomotor agitation that are, in fact, seen are hand wringing and hair pulling.

Mood, Affect, and Feelings. Depression is the key symptom in this disorder, although approximately one half of patients may deny depressive feelings and may not appear to the examiner as particularly depressed. These patients are often brought in by family or employers for social withdrawal and generally decreased activity.

Perceptual Disturbances. Depressed patients with delusions or hallucinations are said to have psychotic depression; the term is also used by some clinicians to describe grossly regressed depressed patients (e.g., mute, not bathing, soiling) even in the absence of delusions or hallucinations. Delusions and hallucinations that are consistent with a depressed mood are said to be mood congruent. Mood-congruent delusions include those of guilt, sinfulness, worthlessness, poverty, failure, persecution, and terminal somatic illnesses (e.g., cancer, "rotting" brain). The content of the mood-incongruent delusions or hallucinations is not consistent with the depressed mood. Mood-incongruent delusions in a depressed individual involve grandiose themes of exaggerated power, knowledge, and worth—for example, the belief that he is the Messiah. Hallucinations occur in psychotic depression but are relatively rare.

Thought Process. Depressed patients customarily have a negative view of the world and of themselves. Thought content often involves nondelusional ruminations about loss, guilt, suicide, and death. Many patients evidence a decreased rate and volume in speech, responding to questions with single words and exhibiting delayed responses to questions. The examiner may literally have to wait 2 or 3 minutes for a response to a question. Approximately 10 percent of depressed patients have marked symptoms of a thought disorder, usually thought blocking, profound poverty of content or speech, or gross circumstantiality.

Impulsiveness, Suicide, and Homicide. Approximately 10 to 15 percent of depressed patients complete suicide, and about two thirds think about it. Patients with psychotic depression may occasionally consider killing a person involved in his delusional system. However, the most severely depressed patients often lack the motivation or energy to act in an impulsive or violent way. Patients with depression are at increased risk of suicide as they begin to improve and regain the energy needed to plan and carry out a suicide (paradoxical suicide). A common clinical mistake is to give a depressed patient a large prescription for antidepressants (especially TCAs) upon discharge from the hospital.

Orientation. Most depressed patients are oriented to person, place, and time, although some may not have enough energy or interest to answer these questions during an interview.

Memory. Approximately 50 to 75 percent of depressed patients have cognitive impairment, sometimes referred to as depressive "pseudodementia." Such patients commonly complain of impaired concentration and forgetfulness.

Judgment and Insight. The patient's judgment is best assessed by reviewing his actions in the recent past and his behavior during the interview. The depressed patient's insight into his illness is often excessive in that he overly emphasizes his symptoms, his disease, and his life problems. It is very difficult to convince such patients that improvement is possible.

Reliability. All information obtained from a depressed patient overemphasizes the bad and minimizes the good. A common clinical mistake is to believe a depressed patient who states that a previous trial of antidepressant medications did not work. Such statements may be completely false and require confirmation from another source. The psychiatrist should not view the patient's misinformation as an intentional fabrication, since the admission of any hopeful information may be quite literally impossible for a person in a depressed state of mind.

Objective Rating Scales of Depression. Objective rating scales of depression can be useful in clinical practice for the documentation of clinical state in depressed patients.

Zung scale. The Zung Self-Rating Scale is a 20-item report scale. A normal score is 34 or less, and depressed, 50 or above. This scale provides a global index of the intensity of depressive symptoms including the effective expression of depression.

Raskin scale. The Raskin Severity of Depression Scale is a clinician-rated scale measuring severity of depression, as reported by the patient and as observed by the physician on a 5-point scale of three dimensions: verbal report, behavior displayed, and secondary symptom. It has a range of 3 to 13; normal is 3; depressed, 7 or above.

Hamilton depression scale. This test is a widely used depression scale with 24 items, each of which is rated 0 to 4 or 0 to 2 with a maximum range of 0 to 76. The ratings are derived from a clinical interview with the patient. Questions about feelings of guilt, suicide, sleep habits, and other symptoms of depression are evaluated by the clinician.

Manic Episodes

General Appearance. Manic patients are excited, talkative, sometimes amusing, and hyperactive. At times they are grossly psychotic and disorganized, requiring physical restraints and intramuscular tranquilizers.

Mood, Affect, and Feelings. These patients are classically euphoric, but can also be quite irritable, especially when the mania has been present for some time. They also have low frustration tolerance, which may lead to feelings of anger and hostility. Manic patients may be quite labile, switching from laughter to irritability to depression in minutes or hours with little control.

Perceptual Disturbances. Delusions are present in 75 percent of manic patients. Mood-congruent manic delusions often involve great wealth, abilities, or power. Delusions and hallucinations that are quite bizarre and not mood-congruent are also commonly seen in mania.

Thought Process. Thought content includes themes of self-confidence and self-aggrandizement. These patients cannot be interrupted while they are speaking, and they often are an intrusive nuisance to those around them. Manic patients are often quite easily distracted. The cognitive functioning of the manic state is characterized by an unrestrained and accelerated flow of ideas in which speech is often disturbed. As the mania gets more intense, formal and logical speech considerations are overthrown, and speech becomes loud, rapid, and difficult to interpret. As the activated state increases, speech becomes full of puns, jokes, rhymes, plays on words, and irrelevancies that are at first amusing; but, as the activity level increases still more, associations become loosened. The ability to concentrate fades leading to flight of ideas, word salad, and neologisms. In acute manic excitement, speech may be totally incoherent and indistinguishable from that of a schizophrenic in acute catatonic excitement.

Impulsiveness, Suicide, and Homicide. Approximately 75 percent of manic patients are assaultive or threatening. Manic patients do attempt suicide and homicide, but the incidences of these behaviors are not known. There is some indication that patients who threaten particularly important people (e.g., the President of the United States) more often have bipolar disease than schizophrenia.

Orientation and Memory. Orientation and memory are usually intact, although some manic patients may be so euphoric that they answer incorrectly. This symptom was called "delirious mania" by Kraepelin.

Judgment and Insight. Impaired judgment is a hallmark of manic patients. They may break laws regarding credit cards, sexual activities, and finances, sometimes involving their families in financial ruin. Manic patients also have very little insight into their illness.

Reliability. Manic patients are notoriously unreliable in their information. Lying and deceit are common in this disorder, often causing inexperienced clinicians to treat such patients with inappropriate disdain.

COURSE AND PROGNOSIS

Major Depressive Disorder

Course. Patients with depressive disorder usually have had no premorbid personality problems. Approximately 50 percent of them have their first episode of depression before age 40. A later onset is associated with the absence of a family history for mood disorder, sociopathy, or alcoholism. An untreated episode of depression lasts 6 to 13 months; most treated episodes last approximately 3 months. The withdrawal of antidepressants before 3 months has elapsed will almost always result in the return of symptoms. As patients become older, there is a tendency to have more frequent episodes that last longer. Over a 20-year period the mean number of episodes is five or six.

Approximately 5 to 10 percent of patients with an initial diagnosis of unipolar depression have a manic episode 6 to 10 years after the first depressive episode. The mean age for this switch is 32 years, and it often occurs after two to four depressive episodes. The depression of patients who are later rediagnosed as bipolar patients is often characterized by hypersomnia, psychomotor retardation, psychotic symptoms, a history of postpartum episodes, a family history of bipolar disorder, and a history of antidepressant-induced hypomania.

Prognosis. Major depressive disorder is fundamentally a cyclic disorder with periods of illness separated by periods of mental health. Approximately 50 to 85 percent of patients have a second depressive episode, very often in the next 4 to 6 months. The risk of recurrence is increased by coexisting dysthymia, alcohol and drug abuse, anxiety symptoms, older age at onset, and a history of more than one previous depressive episode. Approximately half of all patients are mentally healthy at long-term follow-up; about 30 percent have moderate impairment; and 20 percent have significant impairment. Men are more likely than women to experience a chronically impaired course.

Bipolar Disorder

Course. Although cyclothymia is sometimes diagnosed retrospectively in bipolar patients, no identified premorbid personality traits are associated with this disorder. However, clinicians note anecdotally an increased productivity and creativity in the premorbid histories of these patients. Bipolar disorder most often starts with depression (75 percent of the time in females, 67 percent in males). Bipolar disorder is a recurring illness. Most patients experience both depression and mania, though approximately 10 to 20 percent experience only manic episodes. The manic episodes typically have a very rapid onset (hours or days), but they may evolve over a few weeks. Early in the disorder manic episodes may be associated with precipitating events, but this is less so as the disorder progresses. An untreated manic episode lasts about 3 months; therefore, it is unwise to discontinue drugs before that time. As the illness progresses, there is a decrease in the amount of time between episodes. After approximately five episodes, however, the inter-episode interval stabilizes to about 6 to 9 months.

Prognosis. Bipolar disorder has a worse prognosis than major depressive disorder. Patients with pure manic symptoms do better; patients with depressed or mixed symptoms do worse. The presence of psychotic symptoms during manic episodes, however, does not imply a poor prognosis; approximately 7 percent of patients do not have a recurrence of symptoms; 45 percent of patients have more than one episode; and 40 percent of patients develop a chronic illness. Patients may have from 2 to 30 episodes of mania (mean, 9 episodes), but 40 percent have more than ten. On long-term follow-up, 15 percent of patients are well, 45 percent are well but have had multiple relapses, 30 percent are in partial remission, and 10 percent are chronically ill. There are chronic symptoms and evidence of social decline in one third of patients.

DIAGNOSIS AND SUBTYPES

Major Depressive Disorder

Diagnosis. For the diagnosis of a major depressive disorder, DSM-III-R requires the presence of a depressive episode (Table 1) and the absence of either a manic or an unequivocal hypomanic episode. DSM-III-R also specifies subtypes of single episode (Table 4), recurrent episodes (Table 5), or seasonal pattern (Table 6). In addition, DSM-III-R specifies the severity of illness—mild, moderate, severe without psychotic features, with psychotic features (indicating mood-congruent or mood-incongruent delusions or hallucinations), in partial remission, in full remission, chronic, and unspecified (Table 7). A diagnosis of de-

Table 4
Diagnostic Criteria for Major Depression, Single Episode

For fifth digit, use the Major Depressive Episode codes to describe current state.

A. single Major Depressive Episode

B. never had a Manic Episode or an unequivocal Hypomanic Episode

Specify if seasonal pattern

Refer to Table 1 for Depressive Criteria

Table from DSM-III-R, *Diagnostic and Statistical Manual of Mental Disorders,* ed 3, revised. (Current Classification of Mental Disorders, 1987.) Copyright American Psychiatric Association, Washington, D.C., 1987. Used with permission.

Table 5
Diagnostic Criteria for Major Depression, Recurrent

For fifth digit, use the Major Depressive Episode codes to describe current state.

A. Two or more Major Depressive Episodes, each separated by at least two months of return to more or less usual functioning. (If there has been a previous Major Depressive Episode, the current episode of depression need not meet the full criteria for a Major Depressive Episode.)

B. Has never had a Manic Episode or an unequivocal Hypomanic Episode

Specify if seasonal pattern

Refer to Table 1 for Depressive Criteria

Table from DSM-III-R, *Diagnostic and Statistical Manual of Mental Disorders,* ed 3, revised. (Current Classification of Mental Disorders, 1987.) Copyright American Psychiatric Association, Washington, D.C., 1987. Used with permission.

pressive disorder not otherwise specified (NOS) is used for disorders with depressive features that do not meet the criteria for any specific mood disorder or adjustment disorder with depressed mood. Intermittent dysthymic episodes would be an example of such a disorder (Table 8).

Subtypes. A variety of subtypes have been suggested to divide depressive patients into homogeneous groups. DSM-III-R distinguishes subtypes of depression based on the presence of symptoms of melancholia (Table 2). Patients with the melancholic subtype are particularly responsive to somatic treatment.

Other systems have been devised to identify patients with good and poor prognoses. These differentiations have included endogenous-reactive, psychotic-neurotic, and primary-secondary schemes. The endogenous-reactive continuum is a controversial division since it implies that endogenous depressions are "biological" and reactive depressions, "psychological," based primarily on the presence or absence of an identifiable precipitating stress. Other symptoms of endogenous depression include diurnal variation, delusions, psychomotor retardation, early morning awakening, and feelings of guilt; thus, it is somewhat similar to the DSM-III-R category, psychotic depression with melancholia. Symptoms of reactive depression have included initial insomnia, anxiety, emotional lability, and multiple somatic complaints. The psychotic-neurotic divi-

Table 6
Diagnostic Criteria for Seasonal Pattern

A. There has been a regular temporal relationship between the onset of an episode of Bipolar Disorder (including Bipolar Disorder NOS) or Recurrent Major Depression (including Depressive Disorder NOS) and a particular 60-day period of the year (e.g., regular appearance of depression between the beginning of October and the end of November).

Note: Do not include cases in which there is an obvious effect of seasonally related psychosocial stressors, e.g., regularly being unemployed every winter.

B. Full remissions (or a change from depression to mania or hypomania) also occurred within a particular 60-day period of the year (e.g., depression disappears from mid-February to mid-April).

C. There have been at least three episodes of mood disturbance in three separate years that demonstrated the temporal seasonal relationship defined in A and B; at least two of the years were consecutive.

D. Seasonal episodes of mood disturbance, as described above, outnumbered any nonseasonal episodes of such disturbance that may have occurred by more than three to one.

Table from DSM-III-R, *Diagnostic and Statistical Manual of Mental Disorders*, ed 3, revised. (Current Classification of Mental Disorders, 1987.) Copyright American Psychiatric Association, Washington, D.C., 1987. Used with permission.

sion separates more severely ill from less severely ill patients. Primary depression refers to what DSM-III-R calls the mood disorders, and secondary depression refers to depression that is a component of some other psychiatric or medical condition. "Double depression" refers to the condition in which a major depressive disorder is superimposed on dysthymia. A "depressive equivalent" is a symptom or syndrome that may be a *forme fruste* of a depressive episode. For example, the triad of truancy, alcohol abuse, and sexual promiscuity in a formerly well-behaved adolescent may constitute a depressive equivalent as may separation anxiety in children.

A more recently described subtype that may be of both clinical and research interest is seasonal affective disorder (SAD), characterized by depression, psychomotor slowing, hypersomnia, and hyperphagia that come on in autumn or winter and improve in spring and summer. These depressions may be associated with abnormal melatonin regulation and often respond to treatment with sleep deprivation or with light. Treatment with light (phototherapy) involves extending the photoperiod of a patient by exposing him to bright light for 2 to 6 extra hours a day.

Bipolar Disorder

Diagnosis. DSM-III-R requires the presence of a manic episode (Table 3) for the diagnosis of bipolar disorder, manic type (Table 9). If there has been a previous manic episode, however, the current episode need not meet the full criteria for a manic episode. The diagnosis of a bipolar disorder, depressed type (Table 10) requires a past history of one or more manic episodes in the presence of a

Table 7
Diagnostic Criteria for Major Depressive Episode Codes: Fifth-Digit Code Numbers and Criteria for Current State of Bipolar Disorder, Depressed or Major Depression

1-Mild: Few, if any, symptoms in excess of those required to make the diagnosis, **and** symptoms result in only minor impairment in occupational functioning or in usual social activities or relationships with others.

2-Moderate: Symptoms or functional impairment between "mild" and "severe."

3-Severe, without Psychotic Features: Several symptoms in excess of those required to make the diagnosis, **and** symptoms markedly interfere with occupational functioning or with usual social activities or relationships with others.

4-With Psychotic Features: Delusions or hallucinations. If possible, **specify** whether the psychotic features are *mood-congruent* or *mood-incongruent*.

Mood-congruent psychotic features: Delusions or hallucinations whose content is entirely consistent with the typical depressive themes of personal inadequacy, guilt, disease, death, nihilism, or deserved punishment.

Mood-incongruent psychotic features: Delusions or hallucinations whose content does *not* involve typical depressive themes of personal inadequacy, guilt, disease, death, nihilism, or deserved punishment. Included here are such symptoms as persecutory delusions (not directly related to depressive themes), thought insertion, thought broadcasting, and delusions of control.

5-In Partial Remission: Intermediate between "In Full Remission" and "Mild," **and** no previous Dysthymia. (If Major Depressive Episode was superimposed on Dysthymia, the diagnosis of Dysthymia alone is given once the full criteria for a Major Depressive Episode are no longer met.)

6-In Full Remission: During the past six months no significant signs or symptoms of the disturbance.

0-Unspecified.

Specify chronic if current episode has lasted two consecutive years without a period of 2 months or longer during which there were no significant depressive symptoms.

Specify if current episode is **Melancholic Type.**

Table from DSM-III-R, *Diagnostic and Statistical Manual of Mental Disorders*, ed 3, revised. (Current Classification of Mental Disorders, 1987.) Copyright American Psychiatric Association, Washington, D.C., 1987. Used with permission.

depressive episode (Table 3). If there has been a previous major depressive episode, however, the current episode does not need to meet the full criteria for a major depressive episode. The diagnosis of bipolar disorder, mixed type (Table 11) requires the presence of both complete manic and depressive episodes (lasting at least a full day) or the very rapid alternation of these syndromes every few days.

The severity of a manic episode is also specified in DSM-III-R: mild, moderate, severe without psychotic features, with psychotic features (indicate mood-congruent or mood-incongruent), partial remission, full remission, and unspecified (Table 12). Bipolar disorder not otherwise spec-

Table 8
Diagnostic Criteria for Depressive Disorder Not Otherwise Specified

Disorders with depressive features that do not meet the criteria for any specific Mood Disorder or Adjustment Disorder with Depressed Mood.

Examples:

(1) a Major Depressive Episode superimposed on residual Schizophrenia

(2) a recurrent, mild, depressive disturbance that does not meet the criteria for Dysthymia

(3) non-stress-related depressive episodes that do not meet the criteria for a Major Depressive Episode

Specify if seasonal pattern

Refer to Table 1 for Depressive Criteria

Table from DSM-III-R, *Diagnostic and Statistical Manual of Mental Disorders,* ed 3, revised. (Current Classification of Mental Disorders, 1987.) Copyright American Psychiatric Association, Washington, D.C., 1987. Used with permission.

Table 9
Diagnostic Criteria for Bipolar Disorder, Manic

For fifth digit, use the Manic Episode codes to describe current state.

Currently (or most recently) in a Manic Episode, (If there has been a previous Manic Episode, the current episode need not meet the full criteria for a Manic Episode.)

Specify if seasonal pattern

Refer to Table 3 for Manic Criteria

Table from DSM-III-R, *Diagnostic and Statistical Manual of Mental Disorders,* ed 3, revised. (Current Classification of Mental Disorders, 1987.) Copyright American Psychiatric Association, Washington, D.C., 1987. Used with permission.

Table 10
Diagnostic Criteria for Bipolar Disorder, Depressed

For fifth digit, use the Major Depressive Episode codes to describe current state.

A. Has had one or more Manic Episodes

B. Currently (or most recently) in a Major Depressive Episode. (If there has been a previous Major Depressive Episode, the current episode need not meet the full criteria for a Major Depressive Episode.)

Specify if seasonal pattern

Refer to Table 1 for Depressive Criteria

Table from DSM-III-R, *Diagnostic and Statistical Manual of Mental Disorders,* ed 3, Revised. (Current Classification of Mental Disorders, 1987.) Copyright American Psychiatric Association, Washington, D.C., 1987. Used with permission.

ified (NOS) is a residual category for hypomanic episodes that are not classified elsewhere in DSM-III-R (Table 13).

Subtypes. The major subtypes of bipolar disorder are depressed, manic, and mixed. One other division involves the concepts of bipolar I and bipolar II. Bipolar I is synonymous with the DSM-III-R criteria for bipolar disorder. Bipolar II refers to patients who have major depressive

Table 11
Diagnostic Criteria for Bipolar Disorder, Mixed

For fifth digit, use the Manic Episode codes to describe current state.

A. Current (or most recent) episode involves the full symptomatic picture of both Manic and Major Depressive Episodes (except for the duration requirement of two weeks for depressive symptoms), intermixed or rapidly alternating every few days. Refer to Table 1 for Depressive Criteria and to Table 3 for Manic Criteria

B. Prominent depressive symptoms lasting at least a full day.

Specify if seasonal pattern

Table from DSM-III-R, *Diagnostic and Statistical Manual of Mental Disorders,* ed 3, revised. (Current Classification of Mental Disorders, 1987.) Copyright American Psychiatric Association, Washington, D.C., 1987. Used with permission.

Table 12
Diagnostic Criteria for Manic Episode Codes: Fifth Digit Code Numbers for Severity of Current State of Bipolar Disorder, Manic or Mixed:

1-Mild: Meets minimum symptom criteria for a Manic Episode (or almost meets symptom criteria if there has been a previous Manic Episode).

2-Moderate: Extreme increase in activity or impairment in judgment.

3-Severe, without Psychotic Features: Almost continual supervision required in order to prevent physical harm to self or others.

4-With Psychotic Features: Delusions, hallucinations, or catatonic symptoms. If possible, **specify** whether the psychotic features are *mood-congruent* or *mood-incongruent.*

Mood-congruent psychotic features: Delusions or hallucinations whose content is entirely consistent with the typical manic themes of inflated worth, power, knowledge, identity, or special relationship to a deity or famous person.

Mood-incongruent psychotic features: Either (*a*) or (*b*):

(*a*) Delusions or hallucinations whose content does *not* involve the typical manic themes of inflated worth, power, knowledge, identity, or special relationship to a deity or famous person. Included are such symptoms as persecutory delusions (not directly related to grandiose ideas or themes), thought insertion, and delusions of being controlled.

(*b*) Catatonic symptoms, e.g., stupor, mutism, negativism, posturing.

5-In Partial Remission: Full criteria were previously, but are not currently, met; some signs or symptoms of the disturbance have persisted.

6-In Full Remission: Full criteria were previously met, but there have been no significant signs or symptoms of the disturbance for at least 6 months.

0-Unspecified.

Table from DSM-III-R, *Diagnostic and Statistical Manual of Mental Disorders,* ed 3, revised. (Current Classification of Mental Disorders, 1987.) Copyright American Psychiatric Association, Washington, D.C., 1987. Used with permission.

Table 13
Diagnostic Criteria for Bipolar Disorder Not Otherwise Specified

Disorders with manic or hypomanic features that do not meet the criteria for any specific Bipolar Disorder.

Examples:

(1) at least one Hypomanic Episode and at least one Major Depressive Episode, but never either a Manic Episode or Cyclothymia. Such cases have been referred to as "Bipolar II."

(2) one or more Hypomanic Episodes, but without Cyclothymia or a history of either a Manic or a Major Depressive Episode

(3) a Manic Episode superimposed on Delusional Disorder, residual Schizophrenia, or Psychotic Disorder NOS

Specify if seasonal pattern

Table from DSM-III-R, *Diagnostic and Statistical Manual of Mental Disorders*, ed 3, revised. (Current Classification of Mental Disorders, 1987.) Copyright American Psychiatric Association, Washington, D.C., 1987. Used with permission.

episodes with only hypomanic episodes. According to DSM-III-R, if such patients do not meet the criteria for cyclothymia, they are diagnosed as having bipolar disorder NOS. Bipolar II has been reported in the families of unipolar, bipolar, and bipolar II probands. It has been suggested that bipolar II patients may represent a personality disorder superimposed on a unipolar depressive disorder.

DIFFERENTIAL DIAGNOSIS

Major Depressive Disorder

Medical. Many neurologic and medical disorders and pharmacologic agents can produce symptoms of depression (Table 14). Many patients with depression first present to their general practitioners with somatic complaints. Most organic causes of depression can be detected with a comprehensive medical history, a complete physical and neurologic examination, and routine blood and urine tests.

The most common neurologic problems that manifest depressive symptoms are Parkinson's disease, dementing illnesses (including Alzheimer's disease), epilepsy, strokes, and tumors. Approximately 50 to 75 percent of patients with Parkinson's disease have marked symptoms of depression that are not correlated with degree of physical disability, age, or duration of illness but are correlated with the presence of abnormalities on neuropsychological tests. These symptoms of depression may be "masked" by the almost identical motor symptoms of Parkinson's disease. Depressive symptoms often respond to antidepressant drugs or electroconvulsive therapy (ECT).

It is usually possible to differentiate the "pseudodementia" of depression from the dementia of a disease such as Alzheimer's on clinical grounds. The cognitive symptoms in depression have a more acute onset, and other symptoms of depression, such as self-reproach, are present. A diurnal variation to the cognitive problems may be present that is not seen in primary dementias. Depressed patients with cognitive difficulties often will not try to answer questions ("I don't know"), whereas demented patients may

confabulate. In depressed patients, recent and remote memory are equally affected; in demented patients, recent memory is more affected than remote memory. Finally, depressed patients often can be coached into having better memory, an ability demented patients lack.

The interictal changes associated with temporal lobe epilepsy can mimic a depressive disorder, especially if the epileptic focus is on the right side. Depression is a common complicating feature of strokes, particularly in the 2 years following the episode. Depression is more common after anterior (than posterior) strokes and with left-sided lesions, and such depression often responds to antidepressant medications. Tumors of the diencephalic and temporal regions are particularly likely to be associated with depressive symptoms.

Failure to take a good clinical history or to consider the context of the patient's current life situation might lead to diagnostic errors. Adolescents with depression should be tested for mononucleosis. Women and men who are markedly over- or underweight should be tested for adrenal and thyroid dysfunction. Homosexuals, bisexuals, and drug users should be tested for AIDS. Elderly patients should be evaluated for viral pneumonia.

The list of drugs associated with depression is also long (Table 14). A good rule of thumb is that any drug a depressed patient is taking should be considered as a factor in the mood disorder. Cardiac drugs, antihypertensives, sedatives, hypnotics, antipsychotics, antiepileptics, antiparkinsons, analgesics, antibacterials, and antineoplastics are all commonly associated with depressive symptoms.

Psychiatric. Depression can be a feature of virtually any mental disorder listed in DSM-III-R, but the psychiatric disorders listed in Table 15 should be particularly considered in the differential diagnosis. Differentiation of syndromes is best done by following the DSM-III-R guidelines for each disorder. Perhaps the most difficult differential is between anxiety disorders (with depression) and depressive disorders (with marked anxiety). An abnormal DST, the presence of REM latency on a sleep EEG, and a negative lactate infusion test would support a diagnosis of depression. Uncomplicated bereavement is not considered a mental disorder, even though approximately one third of bereaved spouses do for a period of time meet the criteria for depressive disorder. Some patients with uncomplicated bereavement do develop major depressive disorders. However, the diagnosis is not made unless resolution of grief does not occur; the differentiation is based on severity and length of symptoms. Symptoms commonly seen in a depressive disorder that evolves from unresolved bereavement are a morbid preoccupation with worthlessness, suicidal ideation, marked functional impairment, psychomotor retardation, feeling that he or she committed an act (rather than just an omission) that caused the death, mummification (keeping the deceased's belongings exactly as they were), and a particularly severe anniversary reaction.

Bipolar Disorder (Manic Episodes)

Medical Many of the potential neurologic and medical causes of depressive symptoms also can cause manic symptoms (see asterisked items in Table 14). Many pharmacologic agents may precipitate mania (Table 16), as can antidepressant treatment or withdrawal.

Psychiatric. The major psychiatric differential diagnosis for manic symptoms includes disorders that may present with depression (Table 15). Of special consideration for manic symp-

Table 14
Neurologic, Medical, and Pharmacologic Causes of Depressive Symptoms

Neurologic
Dementias (including Alzheimer's disease)
Epilepsy*
Fahr's syndrome*
Huntington's disease*
Hydrocephalus
Infections (including HIV and neurosyphilis)*
Migraines*
Multiple sclerosis*
Narcolepsy
Neoplasms*
Parkinson's disease
Progressive supranuclear palsy
Sleep apnea
Strokes*
Trauma*
Wilson's disease*

Endocrine
Adrenal (Cushing's*, Addison's diseases)
Hyperaldosteronism
Menses-related*
Parathyroid disorders (hyper- and hypo-)
Postpartum*
Thyroid disorders (hypothyroid and "apathetic"
  hyperthyroid*)

Infectious and Inflammatory
Acquired immune deficiency syndrome (AIDS)*
Mononucleosis
Pneumonia—viral and bacterial
Rheumatoid arthritis
Sjogren's arteritis
Systemic lupus erythematosus*
Temporal arteritis
Tuberculosis

Miscellaneous Medical
Cancer (especially pancreatic and other GI)
Cardiopulmonary disease
Porphyria
Uremia (and other renal diseases)*
Vitamin deficiencies (B12, C, folate, niacin, thiamine)*

Pharmacologic (representative drugs)
Analgesics/anti-inflammatory
  Ibuprofen
  Indomethacin
  Opiates
  Phenacetin
Antibacterials/antifungals
  Ampicillin
  Clycloserine
  Ethionamide
  Griseofulvin
  Metronidazole
  Nalidixic acid
  Nitrofurantoin

Pharmacologic (continued)
  Streptomycin
  Sulfamethoxazole
  Sulfonamides
  Tetracycline
Antihypertensives/cardiac drugs
  Alphamethyldopa
  Beta blockers (propranolol)
  Bethanidine
  Clonidine
  Digitalis
  Guanethidine
  Hydralazine
  Lidocaine
  Methoserpidine
  Prazosin
  Procainamide
  Quanabenzacetate
  Rescinnamine
  Reserpine
  Veratrum
Antineoplastics
  Azathioprine (AZT)
  C-Asparaginase
  6-Azauridine
  Bleomycin
  Trimethoprim
  Vincristine
Neurologic/Psychiatric
  Amantadine
  Baclofen
  Bromocriptine
  Carbamazepine
  Levodopa
  Neuroleptics (butyrophenones, phenothiazines,
    oxyindoles)
  Phenytoin
  Sedative/hypnotics (barbiturates, benzodiazepines,
    chloral hydrate)
  Tetrabenazine
Steroids/hormones
  Corticosteroids (including ACTH)
  Danazol
  Oral contraceptives
  Prednisone
  Triamcinolone
Miscellaneous
  Acetazolamide
  Choline
  Cimetidine
  Cyproheptadine
  Diphenoxylate
  Disulfiram
  Methysergide
  Stimulants (amphetamines, fenfluramine.)

*These conditions are also associated with manic symptoms.

Table 15
Psychiatric Disorders That Commonly Have Depressive Features

Adjustment disorder with depressed mood
Alcohol abuse
Anorexia nervosa
Anxiety disorders
Bipolar disorder
Bulimia
Drug abuse
Dysthymia
Cyclothymia
Major depressive disorder
Schizoaffective disorder
Schizophrenia
Schizophreniform disorder
Somatization disorders

Table 16
Drugs Associated with Manic Symptoms

Amphetamines
Baclofen
Bromide
Bromocriptine
Captopril
Cimetidine
Cocaine
Corticosteroids (including ACTH)
Cyclosporin
Disulfiram
Hallucinogens (intoxication and flashbacks)
Hydralazine
Isoniazid
Levodopa
Methylphenidate
Metrizamide (following myelography)
Opiates
Procarbazine
Procyclidine
Yohimbine

toms, however, are the borderline, narcissistic, histrionic, and antisocial personality disorders.

A great deal has been written recently about the clinical difficulty of separating a manic episode from a schizophrenic episode. Although it is difficult, there are a few clinical guidelines. Merriment, elation, and infectiousness of mood are much more common in mania. The combination of a manic mood, rapid or pressured speech, and hyperactivity heavily weighs toward a diagnosis of mania. The onset in mania is often more rapid, being a marked change from previous behavior. One half of bipolar patients have a family history of a mood disorder. It should be noted that catatonia may be a depressive phase in a bipolar disorder. When evaluating catatonic patients, the clinician should carefully look for a past history of manic or depressive episodes, as well as a family history of mood disorders. Manic symptoms in minorities (particularly blacks and Hispanics) are often misinterpreted as schizophrenic symptoms.

CLINICAL MANAGEMENT

Treatment of mood disorders is rewarding for the psychiatrist; specific treatment is now available for both manic and depressive episodes. Because the prognosis for each individual episode is good, optimism is always warranted and welcomed by both patient and family, even if initial treatment results are not promising.

Hospitalization

The first and most critical decision the physician must make is whether to hospitalize the patient or to attempt outpatient treatment. Risk of suicide or homicide, grossly reduced ability to care for food, shelter, or clothing, and the need for diagnostic procedures are clear indications for hospitalization. A history of rapidly progressing symptoms and rupture of the usual support systems are also indications for hospitalization.

Mild depression or hypomania may be safely treated in the office if the physician evaluates the patient frequently. Clinical signs of impaired judgment, weight loss, or insomnia should be minimal. The patient's support system should be strong, neither overinvolved with nor withdrawing from the patient. Any adverse changes in symptoms, external behavior, or attitude of the support system is sufficient to warrant hospitalization.

Patients with mood disorders are often unwilling to come into a hospital voluntarily, so they may have to be committed. Depressive disorder patients are often incapable of making a decision because of their slowed thinking, negative *Weltanschauung* (worldview), and hopelessness. Manic patients often have such a complete lack of insight into their illness that hospitalization seems absolutely absurd to them.

Somatic Therapy

Drugs that treat mood disorders (thymoleptics) are the mainstay of the treatment regimen. It is imperative that the physician integrate pharmacotherapy with psychotherapeutic interventions. If a physician views mood disorders as fundamentally evolving from psychodynamic issues, his ambivalence about the use of drugs will result in poor response, noncompliance, and probably inadequate doses for too short a treatment period. Alternatively, if a physician ignores the psychosocial needs of the patient, the outcome of pharmacotherapy may be compromised. Most studies actually have demonstrated an additive treatment effect for combining optimally administered pharmacotherapy with appropriately conducted psychotherapeutic interventions.

The risk of suicide in mood disorder patients must always be borne in mind by the physician when writing prescriptions. Antidepressants are particularly lethal if taken in large amount. It is unwise to give most mood disorder patients large prescriptions when they are discharged from the hospital unless another person will monitor administration.

Depressive Episodes. Acute depression is a treatable condition in 70 to 80 percent of patients. When introducing the topic of a drug trial to the patient, the physician should emphasize that depression is a combination of biological and psychological factors, both of which benefit from drug therapy. The physician should also stress that the patient will not get addicted to antidepressants since these drugs do not give immediate gratification. The doctor should tell the patient that it may take 3 to 4 weeks for the patient to feel the antidepressant's effects; and even if there is no improvement at that time, there are many other medications to try. It is almost always good practice to explain expected side effects in detail but to emphasize that they are signs that the drug is working. Finally, it may be useful to tell the patient that his sleep and appetite will improve first, followed by a sense of returned energy; the feeling of depression, unfortunately, will be the last symptom to change.

As it is in all mental disorders, the best reason for choosing a particular drug is a past history of response to that agent in the patient or a family member. If such information is not available a heterocyclic antidepressant (HCA) trial is usually indicated. The choice of which HCA to use should be based on side effect profiles, especially the presence or absence of sedating qualities. A complete trial of an antidepressant should last an absolute minimum of 4 weeks at maximum dose, but 6 weeks is preferable. If, at that point, symptoms are still present, serum concentrations of the drug should be measured, and the HCA should be supplemented with L-triiodothyronine (T_3) and lithium for an additional 2 to 3 weeks. If a therapeutic response is still absent, a second HCA from a different class should be given a trial identical to the first one. Amphetamine, 5 to 20 mg per day, can also be added to HCA because they act synergistically. If two HCA trials fail, a trial with an monoamine oxidase inhibitor (MAOI) or electroconvulsive therapy (ECT) may be warranted. A combination of a HCA (except imipramine) and a MAOI may also be tried; however, the clinician must be careful to begin both drugs at the same time at very low doses and to raise them quite gradually. MAOIs and ECT are actually underutilized as first-line antidepressant treatments. MAOIs are at least as effective as HCAs, and tyramine-induced hypertensive reactions can be avoided by reasonable dietary precautions. Although controversial, ECT is probably the most effective antidepressant treatment and is indicated when a rapid therapeutic response is particularly desirable (e.g., high suicide risk, inanition in an elderly patient). Psychostimulants (e.g., amphetamine) may be useful as antidepressants in selected patients, including the elderly and patients with organic disorders.

Lithium should be considered as a first-line pharmacologic agent in treating depression in bipolar patients and in some depressed patients with marked periodicity to their illness. If 2 to 3 weeks on lithium is unsuccessful, an HCA and T_3 can be added to the regimen. If this fails, an MAOI and T_3 can then be tried in addition to the lithium. If these trials fail, a combined HCA and MAOI trial or ECT is warranted.

Patients with psychotic depression virtually always require an antipsychotic medication in addition to their antidepressant regimen. The antipsychotic medication may be tapered and stopped when the psychosis has subsided. Patients with seasonal affective disorder may respond to treatment with phototherapy or sleep deprivation.

Antidepressant treatment should be maintained for at least 6 months or the length of a previous episode, whichever is greater. Chronic HCA, MAOI, or lithium treatment may be indicated as prophylaxis against depression in patients with a history of recurrent serious depressions. HCAs and MAOIs should be tapered gradually over a minimum of 2 weeks or up to 2 months in cases with which care is particularly warranted. Although this issue is less critical for lithium, it is best to taper this agent over at least a week.

Manic Episodes. The drug of choice for the treatment of mania is lithium, although many agitated manic patients require antipsychotics (or perhaps IM lorazepam) at the initiation of treatment. There are reports, however, of neurotoxicity with combined administration of lithium and antipsychotics, and the clinician should watch for changes in neurologic and cognitive status. The lithium concentration should be in the 0.8 to 1.2 mEq per liter range during acute treatment. Therapeutic response usually occurs in 8 to 10 days, but a complete lithium trial should last at least 4 weeks. Noncompliance with drug regimens is a major problem with manic patients, and the physician needs to take care that it does not happen.

Although lithium is effective in most cases, a number of other drugs may be tried if lithium by itself fails to be effective. Following an unsuccessful 4-week trial of lithium an additional 2 weeks with L-tryptophan supplementation may be tried. If this regimen fails, a trial of carbamazepine is indicated. If the carbamazepine is not effective in 4 weeks, lithium should be added to the regimen. As mentioned before, ECT may be effective in the treatment of mania. Other possibly effective drugs that warrant clinical trials at this point include valproic acid, verapamil, clonidine, and clonazepam.

Pharmacotherapy for mania should be continued for 4 months or the length of a previous episode, whichever is longer. The decision to place a bipolar patient on maintenance lithium is based primarily on a past history of severe episodes. The maintenance dose of lithium should be the lowest effective dose with minimal side effects, often in the range of 0.4 to 0.8 mEq per liter. Lithium has been proven effective in reducing the number, severity, and length of manic and depressive episodes. The prophylactic effect of lithium, however, develops after the acute antimanic effects. The recurrence of manic symptoms in the first 3 months of lithium treatment does not indicate that the lithium will not provide successful prophylaxis. Minor or major episodes may occur while a patient is on lithium. These episodes should be treated with judicial doses of antidepressants for depression and antipsychotics for mania. The decision to discontinue lithium maintenance may be entertained if a patient has had no symptoms for a period equal to three cycles.

Rapid cycling is defined as the presence of at least three or four episodes per year and may even be a complication of chronic antidepressant treatment. The first step in the treatment of rapid cycling involves stopping or, at least, decreasing the dose of any antidepressant the patient is taking. Trials of levothyroxine sodium (T_4) or carbamazepine may supplement the effects of the lithium. Clorgyline, a selective MAO-A inhibitor that is not available in the United States, may be particularly effective in the treatment of rapid cycling.

Psychosocial Therapies

Psychotherapy should be integrated with drug treatment in these patients. It may also often increase compliance with drug regimens. Studies have indicated that psychotherapy in combination with antidepressants is more efficacious than either method alone. Interpersonal, cognitive, and behavior therapies have developed approaches directed specifically toward the treatment of depression. Family therapy and psychoanalytic therapy are equally applicable to both mania and depression. A reasonable goal for psychotherapy of the recovered manic patient is to help the patient undo the damage his manic behaviors may have caused and to gain some insight into his bipolar disorder.

Interpersonal Therapy. Interpersonal therapy (IPT) is short-term psychotherapy, normally consisting of 12 to 16 weekly sessions. It was developed specifically for the treatment of unipolar, nonpsychotic, ambulatory depressed patients. It is characterized by an active, therapeutic approach and an emphasis on the patient's current issues and social functioning. Intrapsychic phenomena, such as defense mechanisms or internal conflicts, are not addressed in therapy. Discrete behaviors, such as lack of assertiveness, social skills, or distorted thinking may be addressed, but only in the context of their meaning or effect on interpersonal relationships.

Cognitive Therapy. The cognitive theory of depression posits that cognitive dysfunctions are the core of depression; the signs and symptoms of depression are hypothesized to be consequences of the cognitive dysfunctions. For example, apathy and low energy are results of the individual's expectation of failure in all areas. The goal of cognitive therapy is to alleviate depression and to prevent its recurrence by helping the patient to identify and test negative cognitions, to develop alternative, more flexible and positive ways of thinking, and to rehearse new cognitive and behavioral responses.

Behavior Therapy. Several behavior therapies have been developed for the treatment of depression. Although they vary in terms of specific techniques and foci, they have certain assumptions and strategies in common. The treatment program is highly structured and generally short term. The principle of reinforcement is seen as the key element in depression. Changing behavior is considered to be the most effective way to alleviate depression. Finally, the focus is on articulation and attainment of specific goals.

Family Therapy. Family therapy is not generally viewed as a primary therapy for the treatment of depression, but it is indicated in cases where (1) the patient's depression appears to be seriously jeopardizing that person's marriage and/or family functioning or (2) an individual's depression appears to be promoted and maintained by marital and/or family interaction patterns. Family therapy examines the role of the depressed member in the overall psychological well-being of the whole family; it also examines the role of the entire family in the maintenance of the depression. Patients with mood disorders have a very high rate of divorce, and approximately 50 percent of spouses report they would not have married the patient or had children had they known that the patient was going to develop a mood disorder. Family therapy, therefore, can be a crucial and effective modality in the treatment of mood disorders.

Psychoanalytic Therapy. The psychoanalytic approach to mood disorders is based on the psychoanalytic theories for depression and mania. In general, the goal of psychoanalytic psychotherapy is to effect a change in the personality structure or character, not simply to alleviate symptoms. Improvement in interpersonal trust, intimacy, coping mechanisms, the capacity to grieve, and the ability to experience a wide range of emotions are some of the aims of psychoanalytic therapy. Treatment may often require the patient to experience heightened anxiety and distress during the course of therapy, which may continue for several years.

References

Coryek W, Andreasen N C, Endicott J, Keller M: The significance of past mania or hypomania in the course and outcome of major depression. Am J Psychiatry *144:*309, 1987.

Frank E, Kupfer D J, Jacob M, Blumenthal S J, Jarrett D B: Pregnancy-related affective episodes among women with recurrent depression. Am J Psychiatry *144:*288, 1987.

Gershon E S, Hamovit J M, Guroff J J, Nurnberger J I: Birth-cohort changes in manic and depressive disorders in relatives of bipolar and schizoaffective patients. Arch Gen Psychiatry *44:*314, 1987.

Kupfer D J, Frank E: Relapse in recurrent unipolar depression. Am J Psychiatry *144:*86, 1987.

Levinson D F, Levitt M: Schizoaffective mania reconsidered. Am J Psychiatry *144:*415, 1987.

McGlashan T H, Williams P V: Schizoaffective psychosis II. Manic, bipolar and depressive subtypes. Arch Gen Psychiatry *44:*130, 1987.

Rubin P T, Poland R E, Lesser I M, Winston R A, Blodgett A L N: Neuroendocrine aspects of primary endogenous depression. Arch Gen Psychiatry *44:*328, 1987.

Shenton M E, Solovoy M R, Holzman P: Comparative studies of thought disorders. II. Schizoaffective disorder. Arch Gen Psych *44:*13, 1987.

Solovay M R, Shenton M E, Holzman P S: Comparative studies of thought disorders. I. Mania and schizophrenia. Arch Gen Psychiatry *44:*13, 1987.

Williams P V, McGlashan T H: Schizoaffective psychosis. I. Comparative long term outcome. Arch Gen Psychiatry *44:*130, 1987.

17.2 ————

Dysthymia and Cyclothymia

Dysthymia and cyclothymia are classified as Axis I mood (affective) disorders in DSM-III-R. Dysthymia is conceptualized as being a less severe form of major depressive disorder, and cyclothymia, a less severe form of bipolar disorder; therefore, they are sometimes referred to as subaffective disorders. The classification of dysthymia and cyclothymia within the mood disorders implies that their etiology, genetic basis, prognosis, and treatment response are similar to those of major depressive disorder and bipolar disorder, respectively. This implied similarity, however, is controversial. Some psychodynamically-oriented psychiatrists believe that dysthymia and cyclothymia are more accurately conceptualized as the result of incompletely resolved issues in a person's psychodynamic development.

DYSTHYMIA

Dysthymia is characterized by chronic, nonpsychotic signs and symptoms of depression that meet specific diagnostic criteria, but do not meet the diagnostic criteria for major depressive disorder. Dysthymia means "ill-humored," and these patients are often introverted, morose, and self-deprecating. Dysthymic disorder does not include patients who have episodic, rather than chronic, periods of mild depression. Such syndromes of episodic dysthymia are classified as a depressive disorder NOS (not otherwise specified) in DSM-III-R.

The diagnosis of dysthymia has gone by a variety of names in the past. Although each of the terms has its own history and connotations, they describe overlapping groups of patients. Dysthymia implies a temperamental dysphoria, that is, an inborn tendency to experience a specific mood. In contrast, neurotic depression (also called depressive neurosis), implies a maladaptive, repetitive pattern of thinking and behavior resulting in depression. Patients described as having a depressive neurosis are often anxious, obsessive, and prone to somatization. Characterological depression implies a dysphoric mood that is integral to a person's character. The term "hypochondriacal" depression is sometimes used to refer to a condition characterized by multiple somatic complaints. Such patients may more appropriately be diagnosed as having either somatization disorder or dysthymia.

Epidemiology

Since the DSM-III-R diagnostic guidelines for dysthymia are relatively new, there is no epidemiologic data for the disorder. However, both clinical impression and research data suggest that dysthymia is a relatively common condition. The lifetime prevalence is thought to be about 45 per 1,000, and the incidence in psychiatric outpatients is about 10 percent. Females are more often affected than males.

Etiology

Biological. Some patients with dysthymia have a positive family history for mood disorders, decreased REM latency, and a positive therapeutic response to antidepressants. They truly would seem to have a subaffective syndrome that shares a genetic and pathophysiologic basis with major depressive disorder. One study, however, has reported that the dexamethasone suppression test and the thyrotropin releasing hormone test are not abnormal in dysthymic patients as a group. Nevertheless, a patient with dysthymia who has abnormalities on neuroendocrine tests is a reasonable candidate for a therapeutic trial of antidepressants.

Psychosocial. DSM-III-R defines a subtype of dysthymia with onset before age 21. In contrast to the theories that suggest that early-onset dysthymia represents the expression of an inborn temperament, psychodynamic theories suggest that dysthymia results from faulty personality and ego development culminating in difficulty adapting to adolescence and young adulthood. Karl Abraham suggested that the conflicts of depression center around oral- and anal-sadistic traits. Anal traits include excessive orderliness, guilt, and concern for others; they are postulated to be a defense against preoccupation with anal matters and with

disorganization, hostility, and self-preoccupation. A major defense used is reaction formation. Low self-esteem, anhedonia and introversion are often associated with the depressive character.

In *Mourning and Melancholia,* Freud asserted that a vulnerability to depression could be caused by an interpersonal disappointment very early in life, which leads to ambivalent love relationships as an adult, and that real or threatened losses in adult life then trigger depression. Persons prone to depression are orally dependent and require constant narcissistic gratification. If deprived of such love, affection, and care, they become clinically depressed. When these persons experience a real loss, they internalize or introject the lost object and turn their anger upon it and thus upon themselves.

The cognitive theory of depression holds that there is a disparity between one's actual and one's fantasized and idealized situation, which leads to a diminished self-esteem and a sense of helplessness. One recent study of dysthymic persons reported increased neurotic features, both extra- and intrapunitive tendencies, and decreased self-esteem.

Clinical Signs and Symptoms

The clinical signs and symptoms are specified in DSM-III-R (Table 1). The specifics of the mental status examination are similar to those for a major depressive disorder. Dysthymic persons can have symptoms of depression almost as severe as those for a major depressive disorder; however, the duration of these symptoms may be insufficient to warrant a diagnosis of a major depressive episode. Dysthymia is conceptualized as a chronic disorder, not an episodic disorder with extended asymptomatic periods. Nevertheless, dysthymic persons can have temporal variations in the severity of their symptoms. The major symptom is a depressed mood, characterized by feeling sad, blue, down in the dumps, or low, and by a lack of interest in usual activities. Patients with dysthymia may often be sarcastic, nihilistic, brooding, demanding, and complaining. They can be very tense and rigid and quite resistant to therapeutic interventions even though they may come regularly to appointments. As a result, the clinician may feel angry toward the patient and may even disregard the patient's complaints. By definition, dysthymic patients do not have any psychotic symptoms.

Associated symptoms include changes in appetite and sleep patterns, low self-esteem, loss of energy, psychomotor retardation, decreased sexual drive, and obsessive preoccupation with health matters. Patients may complain that they have difficulty concentrating and may report that their school or work performance is suffering. Pessimism, hopelessness, and helplessness may result in dysthymic patients being seen as masochistic. If the pessimism is directed outward, however, the patient may rant against the world and complain that he has been poorly treated by relatives, children, parents, colleagues, and the "system."

Impairment in social functioning is sometimes the reason the patient seeks psychiatric help. Dysthymic patients may have marital problems resulting from an inability to sustain emotional intimacy or from sexual dysfunction

Table 1
Diagnostic Criteria for Dysthymia

A. Depressed mood (or can be irritable mood in children and adolescents) for most of the day, more days than not, as indicated either by subjective account or observation by others, for at least 2 years (1 year for children and adolescents).

B. Presence, while depressed, of at least two of the following:

(1) poor appetite or overeating
(2) insomnia or hypersomnia
(3) low energy or fatigue
(4) low self-esteem
(5) poor concentration or difficulty making decisions
(6) feelings of hopelessness

C. During a 2-year period (1-year for children and adolescents) of the disturbance, never without the symptoms in A for more than 2 months at a time.

D. No evidence of an unequivocal Major Depressive Episode during the first 2 years (1 year for children and adolescents) of the disturbance.

Note: There may have been a previous Major Depressive Episode, provided there was a full remission (no significant signs or symptoms for 6 months) before development of the Dysthymia. In addition, after these 2 years (1 year in children or adolescents) of Dysthymia, there may be superimposed episodes of Major Depression, in which case both diagnoses are given.

E. Has never had a Manic Episode (p. 293) or an unequivocal Hypomanic Episode (see p. 299).

F. Not superimposed on a chronic psychotic disorder, such as Schizophrenia or Delusional Disorder.

G. It cannot be established that an organic factor initiated and maintained the disturbance (e.g., prolonged administration of an antihypertensive medication).

Specify primary or secondary type:

Primary type: the mood disturbance is not related to a pre-existing, chronic, nonmood, Axis I or Axis III disorder, e.g., Anorexia Nervosa, Somatization Disorder, a Psychoactive Substance Dependence Disorder, an Anxiety Disorder, or rheumatoid arthritis.

Secondary type: the mood disturbance is apparently related to a pre-existing, chronic, nonmood, Axis I or Axis III disorder.

Specify early onset or late onset:

Early onset: onset of the disturbance before age 21

Late onset: onset of the disturbance at age 21 or later

Table from DSM-III-R, *Diagnostic and Statistical Manual of Mental Disorders,* ed 3, revised. (Current Classification of Mental Disorders, 1987.) Copyright American Psychiatric Association, Washington, D.C., 1987. Used with permission.

(e.g., impotence). Because of social withdrawal and difficulty concentrating, patients' performance at work may suffer. They may miss many work days and social occasions due to physical illness. Consequently, divorce, unemployment, and school failure are common problems for these patients. A clinical case example is as follows:

A 28-year-old junior executive was referred by a senior psychoanalyst for "supportive" treatment. She had obtained a master's degree in business administration and moved to California a year and a half earlier to begin work in a large firm. She complained of being "depressed" about everything: her job, her husband, and her prospects for the future.

She had had extensive psychotherapy previously. She had seen an "analyst" twice a week for three years while in college, and a "behaviorist" for a year and a half while in graduate school. Her complaints were of persistent feelings of depressed mood, inferiority, and pessimism, which she claims to have had since she was 16 or 17 years old. Although she did reasonably well in college, she consistently ruminated about those students who were "genuinely intelligent." She dated during college and graduate school, but claimed that she would never go after a guy she thought was "special," always feeling inferior and intimidated. Whenever she saw or met such a man, she acted stiff and aloof, or actually walked away as quickly as possible, only to berate herself afterward and then fantasize about him for many months. She claimed that her therapy had helped, although she still could not remember a time when she didn't feel somewhat depressed.

Just after graduation, she married the man she was going out with at the time. She thought of him as reasonably desirable, though not "special," and married him primarily because she felt she "needed a husband" for companionship. Shortly after their marriage, the couple started to bicker. She was very critical of his clothes, his job, and his parents; and he, in turn, found her rejecting, controlling, and moody. She began to feel that she had made a mistake in marrying him.

Recently she has also been having difficulties at work. She is assigned the most menial tasks at the firm and is never given an assignment of importance or responsibility. She admits that she frequently does a "slipshod" job of what is given her, never does more than is required, and never demonstrates any assertiveness or initiative to her supervisors. She feels that she will never go very far in her profession because she does not have the right "connections" and neither does her husband, yet she dreams of money, status, and power.

Her social life with her husband involves several other couples. The man in these couples is usually a friend of her husband's. She is sure that the women find her uninteresting and unimpressive, and that the people who seem to like her are probably no better off than she.

Under the burden of her dissatisfaction with her marriage, her job, and her social life, feeling tired and uninterested in "life," she now enters treatment for the third time.

DSM-III-R Diagnosis:
Axis I: Dysthymic Disorder

Discussion

This woman's marriage and occupational functioning are severely affected by her chronically depressed mood, low self-esteem, and pessimism. Although she now complains also of loss of interest and energy, it is unlikely that this represents a significant change from her usual condition. Since her depression is not severe enough to meet the criteria for a major depressive episode, and the mood disturbance and associated symptoms have persisted for more than two years, the diagnosis of dysthymic disorder is made.

[Adapted with permission from *DSM-III Case Book.* American Psychiatric Association, Washington, D.C., 1981.]

Alcohol and Drug Abuse. Alcohol and drug abuse can present a diagnostic dilemma to the clinician. Not only can dysthymia result in alcohol and drug abuse, but alcohol and drug abuse can result in symptoms that are indistinguishable from those of dysthymia. However, treatment of a primary dysthymia may result in the disappearance of the drug dependency syndrome.

Course and Prognosis

The course and prognosis of dysthymia varies somewhat with the specific subtype of this disorder. The prognosis of secondary dysthymia depends on the course of the primary disorder. In contrast, early onset, primary dysthymia may be so chronic that the patient accepts the symptoms as part of his very nature. Early onset primary dysthymia, especially with a positive family history for mood disorder, may eventually evolve into a major mood disorder. Studies of patients diagnosed as having depressive neurosis indicate that approximately 20 percent develop major depressive disorder, 15 percent develop major depressive episodes with hypomanic episodes (e.g., bipolar II disorder), and less than 5 percent develop bipolar disorder. In addition to a family history of mood disorder, a positive therapeutic response to antidepressants increases the possibility that a major mood disorder will develop in the future. Late onset, primary dysthymia can have a variable onset, prognosis, and course.

Suicide. Suicide is a risk in most psychiatric disorders, but the relationship between dysthymia and depression make suicide a particular concern in this disorder. Information concerning previous suicide attempts, family history of suicide, and suicidal ideation should be elicited from the patient to assess his suicidal potential. Treatment of these patients with psychopharmacological agents should include an awareness that these drugs could be used in overdose attempts.

Diagnosis and Subtypes

The diagnosis of dysthymia is made on the basis of specific inclusion and exclusion criteria in DSM-III-R (Table 1). The symptoms of criterion A must be present for at least 2 years (1 year in children and adolescents) without an asymptomatic period of longer than 2 months. Although a major depressive disorder may not be present during the first 2 years of dysthymic symptoms, dysthymia can be diagnosed if a prior major depressive episode has been in full remission for 6 months prior to the development of dysthymic symptoms. If a major depressive episode follows 2 years or more of dysthymic symptoms, then the patient is given both diagnoses. The concurrent appearance of both dysthymia and major depressive disorder has been called "double depression" by some clinicians. Such patients are likely to have more frequent and severe depressive episodes than are depressive disorder patients who do not have a diagnosis of dysthymia. Exclusion criteria are a past history of a manic or hypomanic episode, psychotic symptoms, or the presence of residual schizophrenia. If the dysthymic symptoms are sustained by a specific organic factor or drug, then a diagnosis of dysthymia is excluded. Primary and secondary subtypes, and early and late onset are also specifically defined (Table 1).

DSM-III-R encourages the use of multiple diagnoses if appropriate. Secondary dysthymia may be diagnosed along with other

Table 2
Differential Diagnosis for Dysthymic Symptoms

Organic etiology
   Medical illness (e.g., cancer, cardiac disorder)
   Prescription drug treatment
   Drug dependency syndrome
Major depressive disorder
Bipolar disorder, depressed or mixed type
Cyclothymia
Generalized anxiety disorder
Anorexia nervosa
Bulimia
Obsessive-compulsive disorder
Ego-dystonic homosexuality
Personality disorders
   Borderline
   Dependent
   Histrionic
Somatization disorder

Axis I disorders or Axis III (i.e., medical) disorders. Primary dysthymia can be diagnosed with an Axis II personality disorder when the dysthymia is secondary to an underlying personality disorder.

Differential Diagnosis

Symptoms identical to those of dysthymia may be present in several organic and idiopathic disorders. When a patient presents with a dysthymic symptom pattern, especially if the symptoms have not been present for 2 years, all of the diagnoses listed in Table 2 should be considered.

Treatment

Hospitalization is usually not indicated for dysthymic patients; however, the presence of particularly severe symptoms, marked social or professional incapacitation and suicidal ideation are all indications for hospitalization. Although many clinicians believe that dysthymia often is not responsive to psychopharmacologic treatment, a history of unsuccessful treatment by psychotherapy alone, the presence of severe symptoms, a family history of mood disorder, decreased REM latency on a sleep EEG, and abnormal neuroendocrine tests should encourage the clinician to attempt a trial of drug therapy. Heterocyclic antidepressants (possibly with lithium or T3 supplementation) are usually the drugs of first choice. Monoamine oxidase inhibitors (MAOIs) may be the drugs of first choice in the presence of hypersomnia, hyperphagia, marked anxiety, and multiple somatic complaints—a syndrome sometimes referred to as atypical depression or hysteroid dysphoria. A trial of lithium alone may be warranted if trials of heterocyclics and MAOIs are unsuccessful. The use of sympathomimetics, such as amphetamine (5 to 15 mg per day), for this condition may be of benefit in selected cases when prescribed judiciously so as to avoid problems of abuse.

Individual insight-oriented psychotherapy is the most common treatment modality for dysthymia and many clinicians believe this to be the treatment of choice; however, psychotherapy is sometimes combined with medication. This psychotherapeutic approach attempts to relate the development and maintenance of depressive symptoms and maladaptive personality features to unresolved conflicts from early childhood. Insight into depressive equivalents, such as substance abuse, or into childhood disappointments as antecedents to adult depression can be gained through treatment. Ambivalent current relationships with parents, friends, and others in the patient's current life are examined. How the patient tries to gratify an excessive need for outside approval to counter low self-esteem and a harsh superego is an important goal in such insight-oriented therapies.

Other individual therapies for dysthymia include interpersonal, cognitive, and behavior therapy.

Interpersonal Therapy of Depression (IPT). The patient's current interpersonal experiences and ways of coping with stress are examined with the goal of reducing depressive symptoms and improving self-esteem. IPT consists of about 15 weekly sessions and can be combined with antidepressant medication.

Behavior Therapy. Behavior therapy of depression is based upon the theory that depression is caused by a loss of positive reinforcement as a result of separation, death, or sudden environmental change. The various treatment methods focus on specific goals to increase activity, to provide pleasant experiences, and to teach patients how to relax. The alteration of personal behavior in depressed patients is believed to be the most effective way to change the associated depressed thoughts and feelings. Behavior therapy is often used to treat the "learned helplessness" of some of these patients, who seem to meet every life challenge with a sense of impotence. There is considerable overlap among behavioral approaches.

Cognitive Therapy. Cognitive therapy is a technique in which the patient is taught new ways of thinking and behaving to replace faulty negative attitudes about himself, the world, and the future. It is a short-term therapy program oriented toward current problems and their resolution. See Section 30.8 for an expanded discussion of this approach.

Family therapy may help both patient and family deal with the symptoms of this disorder, especially in cases where a biologically based, subaffective syndrome seems to be present. Group therapy may help withdrawn patients learn new ways to overcome their interpersonal problems in social situations.

CYCLOTHYMIA

Cyclothymia is generally considered to be a less severe form of bipolar disorder. The conceptualization of cyclothymia as a disorder of inborn temperament with a strong biological basis is somewhat less controversial than the parallel view for dysthymia. Some psychiatrists, however, see certain cyclothymic patients as having a disorder resulting primarily from chaotic object relations early in life.

This history of cyclothymia is based to some extent on the observations of Kraepelin, and later Schneider, that one third to two thirds of patients with mood disorders exhibited personality disorders. The four types of personality disorders described by Kraepelin were depressive (i.e., gloomy), manic (i.e., cheerful and uninhibited), irritable (i.e., labile and explosive), and cyclothymic. Kraepelin described the irritable personality as the simultaneous presence of the depressive and manic personalities and the cyclothymic personality as the alternation of the manic and depressive personalities.

Epidemiology

The lifetime prevalence of cyclothymia has been reported as less than 1 percent. This figure, however, is likely to be a major underestimation because of the diagnostic criteria used, as well as the tendency for cyclothymic persons not to come to the attention of psychiatrists. Other estimates have been that cyclothymia represents 3 to 10 percent of psychiatric outpatients including many patients with interpersonal or marital difficulties. The female-to-male ratio is approximately three to two, and approximately 50 to 75 percent of cases have an onset between ages 15 and 25.

Etiology

Biologic. A considerable amount of research data supports the hypothesis that cyclothymia is a subaffective disorder related to bipolar disorder. Approximately 30 percent of cyclothymic patients have positive family histories for bipolar disorder; this rate is similar to that for patients with bipolar disorder. Moreover, the pedigrees of families with bipolar disorder often contain generations of bipolar disorder "linked" by a generation with cyclothymia. Conversely, the prevalence of cyclothymia in the relatives of bipolar patients is much higher than the prevalence of cyclothymia either in relatives of patients with other psychiatric disorders or in mentally healthy individuals. The observations that approximately one third of patients with cyclothymic disorder subsequently develop major mood disorders, that they are particularly sensitive to antidepressant-induced hypomania, and that approximately 60 percent of them respond clinically to lithium add further support to the conceptualization of cyclothymia as a mild or attenuated form of bipolar disorder.

Some patients may have hyperactivity of the cortisol axis as demonstrated by nonsuppression on the dexamethasone suppression test. The reasons for the presence of a less severe form of cyclothymia may be fewer or less penetrant pathological genes, the presence of compensating genes, or more favorable epigenetic factors.

Psychosocial. In psychodynamic theories, emphasis is placed on early childhood experiences, often with the postulation of trauma and fixation during the early oral stages of infant development. Freud believed that the cyclothymic state was an attempt by the ego to overcome a harsh and punitive superego. Hypomania results when the depressed person throws off the burden of an overly harsh superego; there is no self-criticism, and all inhibitions are abolished. In hypomanic episodes, the major defense mechanism is denial—the patient keeps external reality from awareness and also avoids underlying feelings of depression.

Clinical Signs and Symptoms

Patients with cyclothymia can present with all the symptoms of bipolar disorder in depressed, manic, and mixed states (Table 3). The details of the mental status examination are similar to those described for depressive and manic episodes in the previous section. The symptoms can often be almost as severe as in bipolar disorder, but may not be of sufficient duration to meet the criteria for that disorder. Approximately one half of cyclothymic patients have depression as their major symptom, and these patients are most likely to seek psychiatric help while depressed. Some cyclothymic patients have primarily hypomanic symptoms and are less likely to consult a psychiatrist than the primarily depressed patients. Rarely, patients suffer from equally long episodes of mania and depression. Almost all cyclothymic patients have periods of mixed symptoms with marked irritability. Most cyclothymic patients seen by psychiatrists have not succeeded in their professional and social lives because of this disorder. Other cyclothymic patients, however, have become high achievers who have worked especially long hours, requiring little sleep. The ability of some individuals to control more successfully the symptoms of this disorder depends on multiple individual, social, and cultural differences. In general, cyclothymia is an impediment to happiness and success.

The life of most cyclothymic patients is very difficult. The cycles of cyclothymia tend to be much shorter than they are in bipolar disorder. The changes in mood are irregular and abrupt, sometimes occurring within hours. Occasional periods of normal mood and the unpredictable nature of the mood changes cause the patient a great deal of stress. He often feels "out of control" of his moods. In irritable, mixed

Table 3
Diagnostic Criteria for Cyclothymia

A. For at least 2 years (1 year for children and adolescents), presence of numerous Hypomanic Episodes (all of the criteria for a Manic Episode, except criterion C that indicates marked impairment) and numerous periods with depressed mood or loss of interest or pleasure that did not meet criterion A of Major Depressive Episode.

B. During a 2-year period (1 year in children and adolescents) of the disturbance, never without hypomanic or depressive symptoms for more than 2 months at a time

C. No clear evidence of a Major Depressive Episode or Manic Episode during the first 2 years of the disturbance (1 year in children and adolescents)

   Note: After this minimum period of Cyclothymia, there may be superimposed Manic or Major Depressive Episodes, in which case the additional diagnosis of Bipolar Disorder or Bipolar Disorder NOS should be given.

D. Not superimposed on a chronic psychotic disorder, such as Schizophrenia or Delusional Disorder

E. It cannot be established that an organic factor initiated and maintained the disturbance (e.g., repeated intoxication from drugs or alcohol).

Table from DSM-III-R, *Diagnostic and Statistical Manual of Mental Disorders*, ed 3, revised. (Current Classification of Mental Disorders, 1987.) Copyright American Psychiatric Association, Washington, D.C., 1987. Used with permission.

periods, he may become involved in unprovoked disagreements with friends, family, and co-workers.

Although many patients seek psychiatric help for depression, their problems are often related to the chaos that their manic episodes have caused. It is important for the clinician to consider a diagnosis of cyclothymia when a patient presents with what may seem like sociopathic behavioral problems. Marital difficulties and instability of relationships are common complaints because cyclothymic patients are often promiscuous and irritable while in manic or mixed states. Although there are anecdotal reports of increased productivity and creativity while hypomanic, most clinicians report that their patients become disorganized and ineffective in work or school during these periods. Alcohol and drug abuse are very common in cyclothymic patients, who use these agents either to self-medicate (e.g., alcohol, benzodiazepines, marijuana) or to achieve even further stimulation (e.g., cocaine, amphetamine, hallucinogens) when they are manic. Approximately 5 to 10 percent of cyclothymic patients develop drug dependency disorders. Cyclothymic individuals often have a history of multiple geographic moves, past involvements in different religious cults, and dilettantism. The following is a case example of a cyclothymic disorder:

A 29-year-old car salesman was referred by his current girl friend, a psychiatric nurse, who suspected he had an affective disorder, even though the patient was reluctant to admit that he might be a "moody" person. According to him, since the age of 14 he has experienced repeated alternating cycles that he terms "good times and bad times." During a "bad" period, usually lasting four to seven days, he oversleeps 10–14 hours daily, lacks energy, confidence, and motivation—"just vegetating," as he puts it. Often he abruptly shifts, characteristically upon waking up in the morning, to a three-to-four-day stretch of overconfidence, heightened social awareness, promiscuity, and sharpened thinking—"things would flash in my mind." At such times he indulges in alcohol to enhance the experience, but also to help him sleep. Occasionally the "good" periods last seven to ten days, but culminate in irritable and hostile outbursts, which often herald the transition back to another period of "bad" days. He admits to frequent use of marijuana, which he claims helps him "adjust" to daily routines.

In school, A's and B's alternated with C's and D's, with the result that the patient was considered a bright student whose performance was mediocre overall because of "unstable motivation." As a car salesman his performance has also been uneven, with "good days" canceling out the "bad days"; yet even during his "good days" he is sometimes perilously argumentative with customers and loses sales that appeared sure. Although considered a charming man in many social circles, he alienates friends when he is hostile and irritable. He typically accumulates social obligations during the "bad" days and takes care of them all at once on the first day of a "good" period.

Discussion

This patient has had numerous periods during the last two years in which he had some symptoms characteristic of both the depressive and the manic syndromes. Characteristic of the "good days" are overconfidence, heightened social awareness, promiscuity, and sharpened thinking. Although these periods come close to meeting the criteria for a manic episode they are not sufficiently severe to justify a diagnosis of bipolar disorder. Similarly, the "bad days," characterized by oversleeping and lack of energy, confidence, and motivation, are not of sufficient severity and duration to meet the criteria for a major depressive episode. Moreover, the brief cycles follow each other with intermittent irregularity on a chronic basis. Therefore, the appropriate diagnosis is cyclothymic disorder.

DSM-III-R Diagnosis:
Axis I: Cyclothymic Disorder

[Adapted with permission from *DSM-III Case Book*. American Psychiatric Association, Washington, D.C. 1981.]

Course and Prognosis

Cyclothymia most often has an insidious onset in the late teens and early 20s. Retrospectively, cyclothymic patients are often described as having been sensitive, hyperactive, or moody as young children. The presence of cyclothymia during late adolescence and early adulthood may cause very disruptive relationships with family and friends and may result in poor performance in school and work. The reactions of patients to such a disorder in life vary; patients with more adaptive coping strategies or ego defenses have better outcomes. Approximately 40 to 50 percent of cyclothymic patients treated with antidepressants experience hypomanic or manic episodes. About one third of cyclothymic patients develop a major mood disorder, usually bipolar II disorder, that is, major depressive episodes with hypomanic periods.

Diagnosis

DSM-III-R contains specific inclusion and exclusion criteria for cyclothymia (Table 3). A 2-year period of abnormally elevated, expansive, or irritable mood with numerous periods of depressed mood is required, with no asymptomatic period lasting longer than 2 months. The symptoms must not meet the criteria for either a major depressive or manic episode. By definition, no psychotic features are present. Nor may the symptoms be sustained by a specific organic factor or substance. There are no subtypes of cyclothymia specified in DSM-III-R.

Differential Diagnosis

Organic brain disorders (e.g., seizures) and drug abuse (e.g., cocaine, amphetamines, steroids) need to be ruled out as causes for cyclothymic presentation. Borderline, antisocial, histrionic, and narcissistic personality disorders should also be considered in the differential diagnosis. A pattern of chaotic behavior and unstable relationships that may appear to meet the criteria for borderline personality disorder may actually be a case of cyclothymia that would respond to lithium treatment. Attention deficit disorder with hyperactivity can be very hard to differentiate from cyclothymia in children and adolescents. A trial of stimulants will help most patients with attention-deficit hyperactivity disorder and exacerbate the symptoms of most patients with cyclothymia.

Clinical Management

Although individual psychotherapy alone is generally not considered adequate treatment for cyclothymia, it is often very useful in helping patients to be more aware of their mood swings and the consequences of their acts on others in the environment. Because of the chronic nature of their mental disorder, patients often require lifelong treatment. Family and group therapy may be supportive, educational, and therapeutic for these patients and those in their support systems.

Lithium is also used in the treatment of cyclothymic patients. Approximately 60 percent of patients respond with lithium serum levels in the 0.7 to 1.0 mEq per liter range. Treatment of cyclothymic patients who are depressed with antidepressants should be done with caution because of the possibility of inducing a hypomanic or manic episode.

References

Akiskal H S: Dysthymic disorder: Psychopathology of proposed chronic depressive subtypes. Am J Psychiatry 140:11, 1983.
Akiskal H S, Khani M K, Scott-Strauss A: Cyclothymic temperamental disorders. Psychiatr Clin North Am 2:527, 1979.
Akiskal H, Rosenthal T, Characterological depressions: Clinical and sleep EEG findings separating "subaffective dysthymias" from "character-spectrum disorders." Arch Gen Psychiatry 126:973, 1980.
Chodoff P: The depressive personality: A critical review. Arch Gen Psychiatry 27:666, 1972.
Depue R A, Kleiman R M, Davis P: The behavioral high-risk paradigm and bipolar affective disorder. VIII: Serum free cortisol in nonpatient cyclothymic subjects selected by the general behavior inventory. Am J Psychiatry 142:175, 1985.
Keller M B, Lavori P W, Endicott J: "Double depression:" Two-year follow-up. Am J Psychiatry 140:689, 1983.
Klein D N, Depue R A, Slater J F: Cyclothymia in the adolescent offspring of parents with bipolar affective disorder. J Abnormal Psychology 94:115, 1985.
Klein D N, Depue R A, Slater J F: Inventory identification of cyclothymia. IX. Validation in offspring of bipolar I patients. Arch Gen Psychiatry 43:441, 1986.
Peselow E D, Dunner D L, Fieve R R, Lautin A: Lithium prophylaxis of depression in unipolar, bipolar II, and cyclothymic patients. Am J Psychiatry 139:747, 1982.
Yerevanian B I, Akiskal H S: "Neurotic," characterological, and dysthymic depressions. Psychiatric Clin North Am 2:595, 1979.

18

Anxiety Disorders (or Anxiety and Phobic Neuroses)

18.1
Normal Anxiety

W. H. Auden called the modern era "the age of anxiety." The current complexity of civilization, the rapidity of change, and the partial relinquishment of religious and familial values are creating new conflicts and anxieties for individuals and society. Attention is now being paid to the amount, type, and effect of anxiety, as reflected in current medical practice. Indeed, anxiety is integral to psychosomatic medicine and psychiatric theory and practice. Even in patients with structural damage, anxiety due to feelings of incompetence, inadequacy, and helplessness is a prominent feature of the disturbance.

DEFINITIONS

Anxiety is a diffuse, highly unpleasant, often vague feeling of apprehension, accompanied by one or more bodily sensations—for example, an empty feeling in the pit of the stomach, tightness in the chest, pounding heart, perspiration, headache, or the sudden urge to void. Restlessness and a desire to move around are also common.

Anxiety is an alerting signal; it warns of impending danger and enables the person to take measures to deal with a threat. Fear, a similar alerting signal, is differentiated from anxiety as follows: Fear is in response to a threat that is known, external, definite, or nonconflictual in origin; anxiety is in response to a threat that is unknown, internal, vague, or conflictual in origin.

The distinction between fear and anxiety arose by accident. The early translators of Freud mistranslated angst, the German word for fear, as anxiety. Freud himself generally ignored the distinction that associates anxiety with a repressed, unconscious object and fear with a known, external object. Clearly, fear may also be due to an unconscious, repressed, internal object displaced to another "thing" in the external world. For example, a boy may be afraid of dogs because he is actually afraid of his father and unconsciously associates his father with dogs. As another example, a child may be vaguely apprehensive about leaving his home because he has experienced sexual excitement while witnessing dogs mating in the street and now unconsciously links dogs with his guilt-laden sexual feelings.

PSYCHOLOGICAL FEATURES OF ANXIETY AND FEAR

According to psychoanalytic formulations, the separation of fear and anxiety is psychologically justifiable. The emotion caused by a rapidly approaching car as one crosses a street differs from the vague discomfort one may experience when one meets new people in a strange setting. The main psychological difference between the two emotional responses is in their acuteness or chronicity; Darwin maintained that the word "fear" is derived from what is sudden and dangerous. Duration also seems to be vital in the neurophysiological phenomena of anxiety and fear. In 1896, Charles Darwin gave the following psychophysiological description of acute fear merging into terror.

Fear is often preceded by astonishment, and is so far akin to it, that both lead to the senses of sight and learning being instantly aroused. In both cases the eyes and mouth are widely opened, and the eyebrows raised. The frightened man at first stands like a statue motionless and breathless, or crouches down as if instinctively to escape observation. The heart beats quickly and violently, so that it palpitates or knocks against the ribs; but it is very doubtful whether it then works more efficiently than usual, so as to send a greater supply of blood to all parts of the body; for the skin instantly becomes pale, as during incipient faintness. This paleness of the surface, however, is probably in large part, or exclusively, due to the vasomotor centre being affected in such a manner as to cause the contraction of the small arteries of the skin. That the skin is much affected under the sense of great fear, we see in the marvelous and inexplicable manner in which perspiration immediately exudes from it. This exudation is all the more remarkable, as the surface is then cold, and hence the term a cold sweat; whereas, the sudorific glands are properly excited into action when the surface is heated. The hairs also on the skin stand erect; and the superficial muscles shiver. In connection with the disturbed action of the heart, the breathing is hurried. The salivary glands act imperfectly; the mouth becomes dry, and is often opened and shut.

I have also noticed that under slight fear there is a strong tendency to yawn. One of the best-marked symptoms is the trembling of all the muscles of the body; and this is often first seen in the lips. From this cause, and from the dryness of the mouth, the voice becomes husky or indistinct, or may altogether fail. . . .

As fear increases into an agony of terror, we behold, as under all violent emotions, diversified results. The heart beats wildly or may fail to act and faintness ensues; there is a deathlike pallor; the breathing is labored; the wings of the nostrils are widely dilated; 'there is a gasping and convulsive motion of the lips, a tremor on the hollow cheek, a gulping and catching of the throat; the uncovered and protruding eyeballs are fixed on the object of terror; or they may roll restlessly from side to side. The pupils are said to be enormously dilated. All the muscles of the body may become rigid, or may be thrown into convulsive movements. The hands are alternately clenched and opened, often with a twitching movement. The arms may be protruded, as if to avert some dreadful danger, or may be thrown wildly over the head . . . In other cases there is a sudden and uncontrollable tendency to headlong flight; and so strong is this, that the boldest soldiers may be seized with a sudden panic.

Individual patterns of anxiety vary widely. Some patients have cardiovascular symptoms, such as palpitation and sweating; some have gastrointestinal symptoms, such as nausea, vomiting, feeling of emptiness, butterflies in the stomach, gas pains, or even diarrhea; some have urinary frequency; and some have shallow breathing and tightness in the chest. All of the above are visceral reactions. However, in some patients, muscle tension prevails, and they complain of muscle tightness or of spasm, headache, and wry neck.

STRESS AND ANXIETY

Whether an event is perceived as stressful depends on the nature of the event as well as on the resources, the defenses, and the coping mechanisms of the person. These all involve the ego, a collective abstraction that refers to the processes by which a person perceives, thinks, and acts on external events or internal drives. If a person's ego is functioning properly, he will be in adaptive balance with both his external and internal worlds; if it is not functioning properly and the imbalance continues long enough, he will develop chronic anxiety. The time required to establish a psychoneurosis varies widely among human beings.

Whether the imbalance is external, between the pressures of the outside world and the patient's ego, or internal, between his impulses (e.g., aggressive, sexual, or dependent) and his conscience, the imbalance produces a conflict. Conflicts caused by external events are usually termed "interpersonal," whereas those caused by internal events are called "intrapsychic" or "intrapersonal." A combination of the two is possible, as in the case of the underling who has an excessively demanding or critical boss and who must control his impulse to hit the boss on the head for fear of losing his job. Interpersonal and intrapsychic conflicts are, in fact, usually combined since human beings are social animals and their main conflicts are with other people.

Conflict seems to be another essential ingredient of anxiety; but its absence is not a requisite for fear, as conflict is present in a special type of fear called phobia. In the genesis of experimental neurosis, conflict is a necessity. Conflict also exists when sexual arousal is prevented or interfered with so that a strong excitation cannot be discharged or when an attack of rage is not executed due to an inhibition of movement.

The cause of chronic anxiety can be summarized in the following way. Repeated attacks of fear—or a single attack in exceptional cases, as in persons with a post-traumatic stress disorder or in those with certain phobias—provide the chronic stress to produce intense and long-lasting autonomic neuroendocrine reactivity, accompanied at the psychological level by conflict. This pattern results in chronic anxiety.

Levels of Anxiety

All emotions, including anxiety, exist at three levels. In ascending order, there is a neuroendocrine level, a motor-visceral level, and, finally, a level of conscious awareness. Generally, the person who is anxious is conscious of only a disagreeable feeling and rarely feels intense discomfort; he is usually not aware of the cause of his anxiety.

The disagreeable feeling has two components: (1) the awareness of the physiologic sensations (palpitation, sweating, butterflies in the stomach, tightness in the chest, shaking knees, quavering voice), and (2) the awareness of being nervous or frightened. The anxiety may be increased by a feeling of shame—"Others will recognize that I am frightened." Many persons are astonished to find that others are not cognizant of their anxiety, or, if they are, do not appreciate its intensity.

In addition to the motor and visceral effects of anxiety, its effects on thinking, perception, and learning should not be overlooked. The brain is a central integrating mechanism, but it is also an end organ. Anxiety tends to produce confusion and distortions of perception, not only of time and space but of people and the meaning of events. These distortions can interfere with learning by lowering concentration, reducing recall, and impairing the ability to relate one item to another (association).

An important aspect of emotional thinking, including anxious or fearful thinking, is its selectivity. An anxious person is apt to select certain items in his environment and overlook others in his effort to prove that he is justified in considering the situation frightening and in responding accordingly or, conversely, that his anxiety is misplaced and unnecessary. If he falsely justifies his fear, his anxieties will be augmented by the selective response, setting up a vicious circle of anxiety, distorted perception, increased anxiety. If, on the other hand, he falsely reassures himself by selective thinking, appropriate anxieties may be reduced, and he may then fail to take the necessary precautions.

Selective perception and thinking may affect not only the inclusion and the exclusion of events, people, and things, but also the meaning of words and actions. Selective attention thus becomes an instrumental factor in prejudice, which, *a priori,* determines the meaning of an event before it happens or stereotypically assigns a person or action to a certain class or group on the basis of a shared attribute.

Adaptive Functions of Anxiety

As an alerting signal, anxiety can be considered to be basically the same emotion as fear. It warns of an external or internal threat; it has life-saving qualities. At a lower level, anxiety warns of threats of bodily damage, pain, helplessness, possible punishment, or frustration of social or bodily needs; of separation from loved ones; of a menace to one's success or status; and ultimately of threats to one's unity or wholeness. In this way it prompts the organism to take the necessary steps to prevent the threat or at least to lessen its consequences. A few examples of warding off threats in daily life include getting down to the hard work of preparing for an examination; dodging a ball thrown at one's head; sneaking into the dormitory after curfew to prevent punishment; and, running to catch the last commuter train. Anxiety prevents damage by alerting the person to carry out certain acts that forestall the danger.

Table 1
Defense Mechanisms

Denial. A mechanism in which the existence of unpleasant realities is disavowed. The term refers to a keeping out of conscious awareness any aspects of external reality that, if acknowledged, would produce anxiety.

Displacement. A mechanism by which the emotional component of an unacceptable idea or object is transferred to a more acceptable one.

Dissociation. A mechanism involving the segregation of any group of mental or behavioral processes from the rest of the person's psychic activity. It may entail the separation of an idea from its accompanying emotional tone, as seen in dissociative disorders.

Identification. A mechanism by which a person patterns himself after another person; in the process, the self is more or less permanently altered.

Identification with the Aggressor. A process by which a person incorporates within himself the mental image of a person who represents a source of frustration from the outside world. A primitive defense, it operates in the interest and service of the developing ego. The classic example of this defense occurs toward the end of the oedipal stage, when a boy, whose main source of love and gratification is his mother, identifies with his father. The father represents the source of frustration, being the powerful rival for the mother; the child cannot master or run away from his father, so he is obliged to identify with him.

Incorporation. A mechanism in which the psychic representation to another person or aspects of another person are assimilated into oneself through a figurative process of symbolic oral ingestion. It represents a special form of introjection and is the earliest mechanism of identification.

Intellectualization. A mechanism in which reasoning or logic is used in an attempt to avoid confrontation with an objectionable impulse and thus defends against anxiety. It is also known as brooding compulsion and thinking compulsion.

Introjection. The unconscious, symbolic internalization of a psychic representation of a hated or loved external object with the goal of establishing closeness to and constant presence of the object. It is considered an immature defense mechanism. In the case of a loved object, anxiety consequent to separation or tension arising out of ambivalence toward the object is diminished; in the case of a feared or hated object, internalization of its malicious or aggressive characteristics serves to avoid anxiety by symbolically putting those characteristics under one's own control.

Isolation. In psychoanalysis, a mechanism involving the separation of an idea or memory from its attached feeling tone. Unacceptable ideational content is thereby rendered free of its disturbing or unpleasant emotional charge.

Projection. Unconscious mechanism in which a person attributes to another those generally unconscious ideas, thoughts, feelings, and impulses that are in himself undesirable or unacceptable. Projection protects the person from anxiety arising from an inner conflict. By externalizing whatever is unacceptable, the person deals with it as a situation apart from himself.

Rationalization. A mechanism in which irrational or unacceptable behavior, motives, or feelings are logically justified or made consciously tolerable by plausible means.

Regression. A mechanism in which a person undergoes a partial or total return to earlier patterns of adaptation. Regression is observed in many psychiatric conditions, particularly schizophrenia.

Repression. A mechanism in which unacceptable mental contents are banished or kept out of consciousness. A term introduced by Freud, it is important in both normal psychological development and in neurotic and psychotic symptom formation. Freud recognized two kinds of repression. (1) repression proper—the repressed material was once in the conscious domain; (2) primal repression—the repressed material was never in the conscious realm.

Sublimation. A mechanism in which the energy associated with unacceptable impulses or drives is diverted into personally and socially acceptable channels. Unlike other defense mechanisms, sublimation offers some minimal gratification of the instinctual drive or impulse.

Substitution. A mechanism in which a person replaces an unacceptable wish, drive, emotion, or goal with one that is more acceptable.

Suppression. Conscious act of controlling and inhibiting an unacceptable impulse, emotion, or idea. Suppression is differentiated from repression in that repression is an unconscious process.

Symbolization. A mechanism by which one idea or object comes to stand for another because of some common aspect or quality in both. Symbolization is based on similarity and association. The symbols formed protect the person from the anxiety that may be attached to the original idea or object.

Undoing. A mechanism by which a person symbolically acts out in reverse something unacceptable that has already been done or against which the ego must defend itself. A primitive defense mechanism, undoing is a form of magical action. Repetitive in nature, it is commonly observed in obsessive-compulsive disorder.

Since it is clearly to one's advantage to respond with anxiety in certain threatening situations, one can speak of normal anxiety in contrast to abnormal or pathological anxiety. Anxiety is normal for the infant who is threatened by separation from parents or by loss of love, for the child on his first day in school, for the adolescent on his first date, for the adult when he contemplates old age and death, and for anyone who is faced with illness. Anxiety is a normal accompaniment of growth, of change, of experiencing something new and untried, and of finding one's own identity and meaning in life. Pathological anxiety, on the other hand, is an inappropriate response to a given stimulus by virtue of either its intensity or duration.

Anxiety usually leads to action designed to remove or reduce a threat. This action may be constructive, in which case a person utilizes coping mechanisms if the action is mainly conscious or deliberate (such as studying for an examination) or defense mechanisms if behavior is largely determined by unconscious forces (such as repressing or pushing out of awareness a threatening impulse or idea).

A mechanism of defense can be adaptive or nonadaptive, depending on the consequences. Repression is used many times in the course of a person's life to achieve harmony with environment and self. Only if symptoms of pathological behavior result can repression or any other defense mechanism be considered abnormal. A summary of common defense mechanisms is listed in Table 1.

References

Engel G L, Ferris E D, Logan M: Hyperventilation: Analysis of clinical symptomatology. Ann Intern Med 27:683, 1947.
Group for the Advancement of Psychiatry (GAP): *Pharmacotherapy and Psychotherapy: Paradoxes, Problems and Progress.* Mental Health Materials Center, New York, 1975.
Klein D, Rabkin J: *Anxiety: New Research and Changing Concepts.* Raven Press, New York, 1981.
Marks I, Lader M: Anxiety states (anxiety neurosis): A review. J Nerv Ment Dis 156:3, 1973.
Noyes R, Anderson J, Clancy J, Crouse R, Slymen D, Ghoneim M, Hinrichs V: Diazepam and propranolol in panic disorder and agoraphobia. Arch Gen Psychiatry 41:287, 1984.
Pasnau R, editor: *Diagnosis and Treatment of Anxiety Disorders.* American Psychiatric Press, Washington, DC, 1983.
Von Korff M, Shapiro S, Burke J D, Teitelbaum M, Skinner E A, German P, Turner R W, Klein L, Burns B: Anxiety and depression in a primary care clinic. Arch Gen Psychiatry 44:152, 1987.

18.2 ————
Pathological Anxiety

When evaluating a patient, the clinician must distinguish between normal and pathological levels of anxiety. Patients with normal anxiety can be treated with reassurance and if needed, brief psychotherapy. On a practical level, pathological anxiety is differentiated from normal anxiety by the fact that a patient, his family and friends, and the clinician think that pathological anxiety is present. Such an assessment is based on the patient's reported internal state, his behavior, and his ability to function. Patients with pathological anxiety require complete neuropsychiatric evaluations and individually tailored treatment. The clinician must be aware that anxiety can be a component of many medical conditions, as well as other psychiatric disorders.

DSM-III-R ANXIETY DISORDERS

Disorders of pathological anxiety can be classified as organic anxiety syndromes, adjustment disorder with anxious mood, or anxiety disorders. DSM-III-R defines various types of anxiety disorders: panic disorders, phobias (agoraphobia, social, and simple), obsessive-compulsive disorder, post-traumatic stress disorder, and generalized anxiety disorder. There is also a diagnosis of anxiety disorder not otherwise specified (NOS) for disorders involving prominent anxiety or phobic avoidance that are not classifiable as a specific anxiety disorder or as an adjustment disorder with anxious mood. It is estimated that the lifetime prevalence of the anxiety disorders in the United States is between 10 and 15 percent. This group of disorders is classified together because anxiety is theorized to be the fundamental symptom in all of these syndromes. However, the fact that these disorders are differentially responsive to pharmacotherapy already suggests that the DSM-III-R anxiety disorders represent a quite heterogeneous group of diseases.

ETIOLOGIC THEORIES OF ANXIETY

Except for the organic mental disorders, DSM-III-R attempts to be an atheoretical document; that is, it avoids identifying the etiologic bases of mental disorders. Four major schools of thought—psychoanalytic, behavioral, existential, and biological—have contributed important theories regarding the causes of anxiety, each of which has both conceptual and practical usefulness in treating patients with anxiety disorders.

Psychoanalysis

The evolution of the theories of Sigmund Freud regarding anxiety can be traced from his 1895 paper *Obsessions and Phobias,* to his later paper, *Studies in Hysteria,* and finally to his 1926 paper, *Inhibitions, Symptoms, and Anxiety.* In this last paper, Freud proposes that anxiety is a signal to the ego that an unacceptable drive is pressing for conscious representation and discharge. As a signal, anxiety arouses the ego to take defensive action against the pressures from within. If anxiety rises above the low level of intensity characteristic of its function as a signal, it may emerge with all the fury of a panic attack. Ideally, the use of repression alone should result in a restoration of psychological equilibrium without symptom formation, since effective repression completely contains the drives and their associated affects and fantasies by rendering them unconscious. If repression is unsuccessful as a defense, other defense mechanisms (e.g., conversion, displacement, regression) may result in symptom formation, thus producing the picture of a classic neurotic disorder (e.g., hysteria, phobia, obsessive-compulsive neurosis). The classification in DSM-III-R of the psychoanalytically defined neurotic disorders attempts to maintain an atheoretical stance (Table 1). Thus, rather than classifying all of the classic neurotic disorders as anxiety disorders, as might be suggested by the psychoanalytic model, it classifies each disorder according to its primary symptoms.

Within psychoanalytic theory, anxiety is seen as falling into four major categories, depending on the nature of the feared consequences: superego anxiety, castration anxiety, separation anxiety, and id or impulse anxiety. These varieties of anxiety are believed to develop at various points along the continuum of early growth and development. Id or impulse anxiety is seen as being related to the primitive, diffuse discomfort of the infant when he feels himself overwhelmed with needs and stimuli over which his helpless state provides him no control. Separation anxiety refers back to the stage of the somewhat older but still preoedipal child, who fears the loss of love or even abandonment by his parents if he fails to control and direct his impulses in conformity with their standards and demands. The fantasies of castration that characterize the oedipal child, particularly in relation to his developing sexual impulses, are reflected in the castration anxiety of the adult. Superego anxiety is the direct result of the final development of the superego that marks the passing of the Oedipus complex and the advent of the prepubertal period of latency.

There are differences of opinion in psychoanalysis about the sources and nature of anxiety. Otto Rank, for example, traced the genesis of all anxiety back to the processes associated with the trauma of birth. Harry Stack Sullivan placed emphasis on the early relationship between mother and child and the importance of the transmission of the mother's anxiety to her infant. Regardless of the particular school of psychoanalysis, however, treatment of anxiety disorders within this model usually involves long-term, insight-oriented psychotherapy or psychoanalysis directed toward the formation of a transference that then allows the reworking of the developmental problem and the resolution of the neurotic symptoms.

Behavioral Theories

The behavioral or learning theories of anxiety have spawned some of the most effective treatments for anxiety disorders. Behavioral theories suggest that anxiety is a conditioned response to specific environmental stimuli. In a model of classical conditioning, a person who does not have any food allergies may, for example, become very sick after eating shellfish at a restaurant. Subsequent exposures to shellfish may cause that person to feel sick. Conceivably, through generalization, such a person might come to distrust all food that he has not prepared himself. As an alternative etiological possibility, a person may learn to have an internal response of anxiety by imitating the anxiety responses of his parents (social learning theory). In either case, treatment is usually with some form of desensitization by repeated exposure to the anxiogenic stimulus, coupled with cognitive psychotherapeutic approaches.

Existential Theories

Existential theories of anxiety provide excellent models for generalized anxiety disorder in which there is no specifically identifiable stimulus for a chronically anxious feeling. The central concept of existential theory is that a person becomes aware of a profound "nothingness" in his life, which may be even more profoundly discomforting than an acceptance of his inevitable death. Anxiety is the person's response to this vast void of existence and meaning. It has been suggested that existential concerns have increased since the development of nuclear weapons.

Biological Theories

Biological theories are based on objective measures that compare brain function in patients with anxiety disorders to that of normal persons. Whether the biological measures are primary or secondary to the anxious affect is currently an unanswerable question. It is also not known whether biological changes in patients with anxiety disorders represent overstimulation of an otherwise normal system, or whether the data represent a uniquely pathological function. It is possible, however, that certain individuals are more susceptible to the development of an anxiety disorder on the basis of a biologically based sensitivity to the development of this affect.

Autonomic Nervous System. Stimulation of the autonomic nervous system (ANS) causes certain cardiovascular, muscular, gastrointestinal, and respiratory symptoms (Table 2). These peripheral manifestations of anxiety are neither peculiar to anxiety states nor necessarily correlated with the subjective experience of anxiety. In the first third of the 20th century Walter Cannon demonstrated that cats exposed to barking dogs exhibited behavioral and physiologic signs of fear that were associated with the adrenal release of epinephrine. The James Lange theory hypothesized that subjective anxiety was a response to these peripheral phe-

Table 1
Comparison of Psychoanalytic Neuroses with Classification of Neuroses in DSM-III-R

Neurosis (Classical)	DSM-III-R Classification
Anxiety	Generalized Anxiety Disorder
Phobic	Agoraphobia, Simple and Social Phobic Disorders
Obsessive-Compulsive	Obsessive-Compulsive Disorder
Depressive	Dysthymia
Hysterical (conversion)	Conversion Disorder
Hysterical (dissociative)	Depersonalization Disorder
Hypochondriacal	Hypochondriasis
Paraphilic	Sexual Disorders

nomena. It is now generally thought that central nervous system anxiety precedes the peripheral manifestations of anxiety, except where there is a specific peripheral cause (e.g., pheochromocytoma). Many anxiety disorder patients, especially those with panic disorders, have an ANS that exhibits increased sympathetic tone, adapts more slowly to repeated stimuli, and responds excessively to moderate stimuli.

Neurotransmitters. Much of the basic neuroscience information about anxiety comes from animal experiments involving behavioral paradigms and psychoactive agents. One such animal model of anxiety is the conflict test in which the animal is simultaneously presented with positive (e.g., food) and negative (e.g., electric shock) stimuli. Anxiolytic drugs (e.g., benzodiazepine) tend to facilitate the adaptation of the animal to this situation, whereas other drugs (e.g., amphetamine) further disrupt the behavioral responses of the animal. The three major neurotransmitters associated with anxiety on the basis of such studies are norepinephrine, γ-aminobutyric acid (GABA), and serotonin.

Norepinephrine. The locus ceruleus in the rostral pons contains the cell bodies for most of the noradrenergic neurons in the brain. These neurons project to the cerebral cortex, limbic system, brain stem, and spinal cord. The locus ceruleus receives sensory input regarding pain and potentially dangerous situations and projects to all the brain areas that might be activated during escape from such situations. In experiments with monkeys, stimulation of the locus ceruleus produces a fear response, and ablation of it decreases this response.

Data defining a pathological role for norepinephrine in human anxiety is inconsistent. Drugs affecting norepinephrine (e.g., tricyclics and MAOIs) are effective in treating several of the anxiety disorders. Some studies have reported increased norepinephrine metabolites (e.g., MHPG) in urine; others have not. It is clear, however, that the administration of isoproterenol (a β-adrenergic agonist) and yohimbine (an α2-adrenergic antagonist) cause anxiety in humans, and that clonidine (an α2-adrenergic agonist) can reduce anxiety in some situations. Research is currently under way to identify unique β-adrenergic and α2-adrenergic receptor pathology in specific anxiety disorders.

GABA. GABA is the principal neurotransmitter that mediates presynaptic inhibition in the CNS. GABAergic neurons synapse onto presynaptic terminals and cause a reduction in the amount of neurotransmitter released by those terminals. The GABA receptor complex consists of a GABA binding site, a site that binds benzodiazepines, and a chloride channel. Stimulation of the GABA receptor causes chloride ions to flow into the neuron, thereby hyperpolarizing and inhibiting that neuron. Benzodiazepines increase the affinity of GABA for its binding site, causing more chloride to enter the neuron.

The efficacy of benzodiazepines in treating anxiety implicates GABA in the pathophysiology of this disorder. Benzodiazepine binding sites are found throughout the brain, but are particularly concentrated in the hippocampal formation and prefrontal cortex, as well as in the amygdala, hypothalamus, and thalamus.

Other anxiolytic substances may affect the GABA receptor complex. The anxiolytic effects of barbiturates are thought to result from their binding to the chloride channel and increasing the amount of time the ion channel is open. Ethanol, phenytoin, and valproate also may act on the GABA receptor complex. It has been hypothesized that there are endogenous ligands for the benzodiazepine binding site that may either increase or decrease anxiety. β-carboline-3-carboxy acid ethyl ester (β-CCE) has been identified in human urine and rat brain. This molecule binds to the benzodiazepine binding site and has been called an "active antagonist" because it actually causes anxiety and seizures. Ro-15-1788 is a recently developed benzodiazepine receptor antagonist that blocks the effects of benzodiazepines but does not itself cause effects opposite to those of benzodiazepines. Other possible endogenous ligands include purines, nicotinamide, tryptophan, and endogenous peptides (e.g., GABA-modulin and diazepam-binding inhibitor (DBI)).

Serotonin. The serotonergic neurons of the raphe nuclei in the rostral brain stem project to the cerebral cortex, the limbic system (especially the amygdala and the hippocampus), and the hypothalamus. Administration of serotonin to animals is associated with signs suggestive of anxiety. The data is much less compelling in human studies, although the efficacy of antidepressant treatment in panic disorders may be associated with serotonergic effects. The reduced number of imipramine binding sites (which label serotonin reuptake sites) seen in the post-mortem brain tissue of suicides may suggest a role in anxiety and depression for serotonin.

Other neurotransmitters. Increased dopaminergic activity may be associated with anxiety, but it appears not to be specifically related to anxiety disorders. Psychotropic drugs that block dopamine receptors are not effective in treating anxiety disorders, although they do reduce the anxiety associated with psychosis. It has been suggested that the endogenous opioids may interact with α2-adrenergic binding sites and, so, may be involved in anxiety. Treatment of anxiety patients with opioid agonists and antagonists has not yet demonstrated effectiveness. The anxiety-like withdrawal symptoms of heroin addicts, however, are reduced by clonidine, an α2-adrenergic agonist. Other neurotransmitters implicated in anxiety include histamine, acetylcholine, and adenosine. Adenosine receptors, in fact, may be the site of action for the anxiogenic effects of caffeine.

Aplysia. A neurotransmitter model for anxiety has been proposed based on the study of *Aplysia*, a sea snail that reacts to danger by moving away, withdrawing into its shell, and decreasing its feeding behavior. These behaviors can be classically conditioned so that the snail responds to a neutral stimulus as if it were a dangerous stimulus. The snail can also be sensitized by random shocks so that it exhibits a flight response in the absence of real danger. Parallels have been drawn between the classically con-

Table 2
Peripheral Manifestations of Anxiety

Diarrhea
Dizziness, light-headedness
Hyperhidrosis
Hyperreflexia
Hypertension
Palpitations
Pupillary mydriasis
Restlessness (e.g., pacing)
Syncope
Tachycardia
Tingling in the extremities
Tremors
Upset stomach ("butterflies")
Urinary frequency, hesitancy, urgency

ditioned model and human phobic anxiety. The classically conditioned Aplysia demonstrates measurable changes in presynaptic facilitation, resulting in release of increased amounts of neurotransmitter. Although the sea snail is a simple animal, this work illustrates an experimental approach to complex neurochemical processes potentially involved in anxiety.

Neuroanatomic Considerations. The locus ceruleus and raphe nuclei were mentioned above in discussions of norepinephrine and serotonin, respectively, and both brain areas are potential sites of pathology in anxiety disorders. It should be remembered, however, that in the intact human brain each of these anatomic areas is involved in more than one function.

Limbic system. The limbic system receives input from the locus ceruleus and raphe nuclei. It also contains a very high concentration of benzodiazepine binding sites. Ablation of the limbic system and temporal cortex results in reduced levels of fear and aggression; stimulation of this area results in the expression of these behaviors. Two areas of the limbic system have received special attention in the literature. It has been hypothesized that the septohippocampal pathway takes a dominant role in physiological functioning in anxiety states; increased activity in this pathway leads to anxiety. The cingulate gyrus has been implicated by a variety of research evidence in obsessive-compulsive disorder.

Cerebral cortex. The frontal cerebral cortex is connected with the parahippocampal region, the cingulate gyrus, and the hypothalamus; therefore, it could be important in the production of anxiety. The temporal cerebral cortex has been implicated as a pathophysiologic site in anxiety. This association is based on the similarity in clinical presentation and electrophysiology between some patients with temporal lobe epilepsy and patients with obsessive-compulsive disorder.

References

Braestrup C, Nielsen M: Anxiety. Lancet *2:*1030, 1982.

Cameron O G, Thyer B A, Neese R M: Symptom profiles of patients with DSM–III anxiety disorders. Am J Psychiatry *142:*1132, 1986.

Curtis G C, Thyer B A, Rainey J M, editors: Anxiety disorders. Psychiatr Clin North Am *8:*1, 1985.

Darwin C: *The Expression of the Emotions in Man and Animals.* Appleton, New York, 1886.

Freud S: *The Problem of Anxiety.* W W Norton, New York, 1936.

Freud S: Inhibitions, symptoms, and anxiety. In *Standard Edition of the Complete Psychological Work of Sigmund Freud,* vol 20. Hogarth Press, London, 1959.

Gray J A: *The Neuropsychology of Anxiety.* Oxford, New York, 1982.

Hoehn-Saric R: Neurotransmitters of anxiety. Arch Gen Psychiatry *39:*735, 1982.

Kandel E R: From metapsychology to molecular biology: Explorations into the nature of anxiety. Am J Psychiatry *140:*1277, 1983.

18.3 _____
Panic Disorder and Agoraphobia

The hallmark symptom of panic disorder is spontaneous, episodic, and intense periods of anxiety, usually lasting less than an hour. Such panic attacks commonly occur twice weekly in affected individuals, although they may occur more or less often. Patients with panic disorder may also develop agoraphobia, the fear of being alone in public places, especially in situations from which a rapid exit would be difficult. It has been estimated that at least two thirds of patients with agoraphobia also have panic attacks, and some clinicians believe that panic attacks are an etiological factor in virtually all agoraphobic patients. Agoraphobia is often the most disabling of the phobic disorders. DSM-III-R contains diagnostic criteria for panic disorder with agoraphobia, panic disorder without agoraphobia, and agoraphobia without a history of panic disorder.

HISTORY

Until the publication of DSM-III in 1980, panic disorders and generalized anxiety disorder were combined into one disorder called "anxiety neurosis," and all phobic disorders were combined as "phobic neurosis." The division of the anxiety disorders in DSM-III was based on observations that specific syndromes had different natural courses, family histories, and, perhaps most importantly, responses to treatments. Specifically, patients with panic disorder had discrete episodes of intense anxiety, whereas patients with generalized anxiety disorder experienced chronic anxiety. Moreover, it was noted that panic disorder was quite responsive to treatment with tricyclic antidepressants and monoamine oxidase inhibitors, whereas generalized anxiety seemed much less responsive to these drugs. There is recent evidence, however, that generalized anxiety disorder may be responsive to tricyclic antidepressants. The term "agoraphobia" was coined in 1871 to describe patients who seemed afraid to venture into public places unaccompanied by friends or relatives. The word is derived from Greek and means "fear of the marketplace." The concurrence of agoraphobia and panic attacks was noted by Sigmund Freud in 1885. The importance of this observation was rediscovered when it was demonstrated that tricyclic antidepressant treatment of many patients with panic attacks and agoraphobia often resulted in amelioration of both symptom complexes. It is now hypothesized that many patients develop agoraphobia as a result of classical conditioning after experiencing a panic attack in a public place (e.g., a crowded supermarket).

EPIDEMIOLOGY

The epidemiologic data on panic disorder and agoraphobia is somewhat confused since many studies did not adequately define whether they were investigating patients with one or both of these disorders. Nevertheless, panic disorder is thought to have a lifetime prevalence of approximately 2 percent of the population, although some estimates are as high as 5 percent. Patients with panic disorder may comprise as many as 15 percent of patients who consult cardiologists, 27 percent of those who consult general practitioners with psychiatric symptoms, and anywhere from 5 to 25 percent of patients in outpatient psychiatric practices. The sex distribution for panic disorder without agoraphobia is thought to be about equal; the female-to-male ratio is two to one for patients with panic disorder with agoraphobia. Panic disorder most commonly develops in young adulthood, the mean age of presentation being about 25, but either disorder can develop at virtually any age.

Agoraphobia is estimated to have a lifetime prevalence of 0.6 percent. At least two thirds of agoraphobic patients actually have panic disorder with agoraphobia. The onset of agoraphobia is in the middle to late second decade and is more common among females than males. In many cases, the onset of agoraphobia is reported to follow a traumatic event.

ETIOLOGY

Biological Theories

The search for biological factors in the etiology of panic disorder was encouraged by the successful treatment of this disorder with antidepressants. A specific biological basis for agoraphobia has not been proposed as yet. The three major areas of biological interest in panic disorder have been the lactate infusion test, brain imaging studies, and the observation that panic disorder and mitral value prolapse often coexist in patients. In addition, the autonomic nervous systems of some panic disorder patients have been reported to exhibit increased sympathetic tone, to adapt more slowly to repeated stimuli, and to respond excessively to moderate stimuli. Neuroendocrine investigations have generally found no abnormality in dexamethasone suppression in panic disorder, but have reported a blunted growth hormone response to clonidine stimulation, as well as a decreased prolactin and thyrotropin stimulating hormone response to infusions of thyrotropin releasing hormone.

Lactate Infusions. As previously noted, patients with anxiety disorder had poor exercise tolerance and produced more lactic acid, sometimes resulting in postexercise panic attacks. Research now indicates that infusions of sodium lactate bring on panic attacks in 70 percent of panic disorder patients and only in 5 percent of normals. Although increased serum concentrations of lactate or decreased concentrations of calcium were initially thought to be the chemical basis of this response, it now seems as if lactate infusions induce an abnormal increase of norepinephrine in susceptible individuals. Inhalation of CO_2 by susceptible persons also bring on anxiety, panic, and mitral valve prolapse. Although the mechanisms for this response are not known, it has been shown that CO_2 inhalation increases the firing rate of neurons in the locus ceruleus.

Brain Imaging. One cerebral blood flow study demonstrated increased blood flow in the right (nondominant) parahippocampal area of panic disorder patients who had positive lactate infusion tests. These patients also had increased whole brain metabolism. These results were not present in panic disorder patients with negative lactate infusions or in normal subjects. This evidence is consistent with the neuroanatomic and neurochemical data in that the parahippocampal region contains both the input (entorhinal cortex) and output (subiculum) tracts of the hippocampus. The laterality difference is supported by one cerebral blood flow study of normal subjects infused with a benzodiazepine. The subjects showed decreased blood flow only on the right side following lactate infusion, particularly in the frontal area. One positron emission tomography (PET) study in normal subjects has shown that a small degree of anxiety results in increased frontal metabolic activity, but that increases in anxiety result in decreased metabolic activity. This finding may eventually prove to be a remarkable physiologic correlate to the U-shaped anxiety-performance curve.

Mitral Valve Prolapse. Mitral valve prolapse is a heterogeneous syndrome consisting of prolapse of one of the mitral valve leaflets, resulting in a midsystolic click on cardiac auscultation. Mitral valve prolapse is commonly seen in connective tissue diseases such as Marfan's and Ehlers-Danlos syndrome. It is present in as many as 50 percent of patients with panic disorder, but only 5 percent of the general population. Although mitral valve prolapse is asymptomatic in approximately 20 percent of patients, the cardiac and respiratory symptoms that are usually associated with it are quite similar to those seen in panic disorder. Mitral valve prolapse and panic disorder seem to have a genetic component, and both are more common in women than in men. The presence of a midsystolic click on physical examination of a patient with panic disorder should prompt the psychiatrist to order an electrocardiogram, and perhaps a phonocardiogram and echocardiogram. Since most psychiatrists do not perform physical examinations in outpatient or office practice such validation requires close cooperation with an internist. Because thyrotoxicosis is associated with both mitral valve prolapse and panic disorder, the presence of these two disorders should prompt the clinician to be particularly careful to assess the thyroid status of the patient. Mitral valve prolapse or the occasionally coexisting ventricular ectopic foci seen on electrocardiogram are not contraindications to treatment with antidepressants. Imipramine, in fact, may be of benefit in treating such cardiac disorders. Nevertheless, consultation with a cardiologist and more frequent electrocardiograms are indicated when treating a mitral valve prolapse patient with antidepressants. The basis and significance of the association between mitral valve prolapse and panic disorder is unknown. The following case illustrates this association:

A 38-year-old professional began to experience sudden attacks of rapid heart beat and pounding chest that were transiently disabling, lasting for seconds to minutes. He was forced to interrupt business meetings, often abruptly leaving the conference room. Episodes increased in frequency to several times a day. Following each episode, he would feel washed out and jittery for the interval between attacks. The distress began to occur in traffic as well, and he found himself avoiding bridges, tunnels, and traffic bottlenecks, at great inconvenience.

He sought consultation from his internist, who identified on cardiac auscultation a midsystolic click and systolic murmur. Two-dimensional echocardiography confirmed the presence of MVP. Therapy was initiated with propranolol, which was increased to 160 mg a day. He noted that he was slightly less jittery and suffered less from the symptoms; nevertheless, the attacks persisted. He began to feel demoralized and, for the first time in his career, was absent from work. Furthermore, he found that the medication was unpleasant because it impaired his energy level and alertness. He discontinued the drug. After reading about agoraphobia in a newsletter, he attended a psychopharmacology unit evaluation where the diagnosis of panic disorder was proposed. Medication treatment with imipramine—25 mg given just before sleep—was initiated, but he was unable to tolerate the onset of imipramine effect with increased jitteriness, sweating, and grogginess. He was switched to phenelzine 15 mg twice a day.

In two weeks, the patient reported complete remission of all his symptoms. Eight months later, he discontinued treatment without relapse.

Genetics

There is very strong evidence for a genetic basis to panic disorder. Approximately 15 to 17 percent of first-degree relatives of patients with panic disorder are affected. The concordance rate for monozygotic twins is 80 to 90 percent, as compared with 10 to 15 percent for dizygotic twins. The genetic basis for agoraphobia is less certain, although several reports suggest that as many as 20 percent of first-degree relatives of agoraphobic patients may have agoraphobia.

Psychosocial Theories

Psychoanalytic theories conceptualize panic attacks as resulting from an unsuccessful defense against anxiety-provoking impulses. What was previously a less severe signal anxiety becomes an overwhelming feeling of apprehension complete with somatic symptoms. Regarding agoraphobia, psychoanalytic theories emphasize the occurrence of loss of a parent in childhood and separation anxiety. The phobia of being alone in public places symbolizes this childhood anxiety of being abandoned. Defense mechanisms used are repression, displacement, avoidance and symbolization, among others. Perhaps traumatic separations during childhood affect the child's developing nervous system in such a manner that he becomes more susceptible to such anxieties in adulthood. In the section that follows on social and simple phobias the psychodynamics of phobic formation are discussed at greater length.

Behavioral theorists postulate that anxiety is a learned response—either from modeling parental behavior or through the process of classical conditioning. According to behavioral theories, panic attacks and agoraphobia develop simultaneously or agoraphobia may even precede the development of panic attacks; however, this sequence contrasts with what most clinicians have observed.

CLINICAL SIGNS AND SYMPTOMS

Panic Attacks

The first panic attack is often completely spontaneous, although panic attacks occasionally follow excitement, physical exertion, sexual activity, or moderate emotional trauma. The onset of the attack often begins with a 10-minute period of rapidly increasing symptoms. The major mental symptoms are extreme fear and a sense of impending death and doom, and the patient may not be able to name the source of his fear. The patient may feel quite confused and have trouble concentrating. Physical signs often include tachycardia, palpitations, dyspnea, and sweating. The patient will often try to leave whatever situation he is in to seek help. The attack generally lasts 20 to 30 minutes and rarely more than an hour. A formal mental status examination during a panic attack may also demonstrate rumination, difficulty speaking (e.g., stammering), and impaired memory. The patient may also experience depression or depersonalization during an attack. The symptoms may disappear quickly or gradually. Between attacks, the patient may have anticipatory anxiety about having another attack. The differentiation between anticipatory anxiety and generalized anxiety disorder can be somewhat difficult, although a panic disorder patient with anticipatory anxiety should be able to name the focus of his anxiety.

Somatic concerns regarding death from a cardiac or respiratory problem may be the major focus of a patient's attention during a panic attack. The patient may believe that the palpitations and pain in his chest indicate that he is about to die from a heart attack. As many as 20 percent of these patients actually have syncopal episodes during a panic attack. It is not uncommon for such patients to present to emergency rooms as young (20s), physically healthy individuals who, nevertheless, insist that they are about to die from a heart attack. Rather than immediately considering such patients "hypochondriacs," the emergency room physician should consider a diagnosis of panic disorder. Hyperventilation may produce respiratory alkalosis and additional symptoms. The age-old treatment of breathing into a paper bag sometimes helps in this situation.

An agoraphobic patient rigidly avoids situations in which it would be difficult to obtain help. An agoraphobic patient prefers to be accompanied by a friend or family member in such places as busy streets, crowded stores, closed-in spaces (e.g., tunnels, bridges, elevators), and closed-in transportation vehicles (e.g., subways, buses, airplanes). The patient may begin to insist that he be accompanied every time he leaves the house. This behavior may result in marital discord, which may be misdiagnosed as the primary problem. More severely affected patients may simply refuse to leave the house. Patients with panic disorder and agoraphobia, particularly before a correct diagnosis is made, may be terrified that they are "going crazy." The following case describes a patient with agoraphobia:

A 28-year-old housewife presented with the complaint that she was afraid she would no longer be able to care for her three young children. Over the past year she has had recurrent episodes of "nervousness," light-headedness, rapid breathing, trembling, and dizziness, during which things around her suddenly feel strange and unreal.

Formerly active and outgoing, over the past six months the patient has become afraid to leave home unless in the company of her husband or mother. She now avoids supermarkets and department stores and states that any crowded place makes her uneasy. When unable to avoid such situations, she tries to get near the doorways and always checks for windows and exits. Last summer the family did not go on their usual country vacation because the patient told her husband, "I wouldn't feel safe so far away; it would make me a nervous wreck." Neither she nor her family can understand what is happening to her. Recently she has wanted her mother to stay with her when the children are at home as she worries about what would happen if an accident occurred and she, immobilized by one of her nervous episodes, were unable to help them.

Discussion

Clearly this woman has had recurrent panic attacks, characterized by light-headedness, rapid breathing, trembling, dizziness, and derealization (things around her feel unreal). If she had been seen six months ago, the diagnosis of panic disorder might have been made. Now, however, she has developed a common complication of panic disorder: because she associates her panic attacks with various places where they might have occurred, she now has a fear of leaving her home and avoids being in public places (supermarkets and department stores) from which escape might be difficult or help not available in case of sudden incapacitation (she tries to get near the doorways and always checks for windows and exits). The increasing constriction of her activities and the domination of her life by these fears indicate the diagnosis of agoraphobia.

Since, as is usually the case with agoraphobia, there is a history of panic attacks, the full diagnosis is agoraphobia with panic attacks.

DSM-III Diagnosis:

Axis I: Agoraphobia with Panic Attacks

[Adapted with permission from *DSM-III Case Book.* American Psychiatric Association, Washington, D.C., 1981.]

COURSE AND PROGNOSIS

Panic Disorder

Following the first one or two panic attacks, a patient may be relatively unconcerned about his condition; however, the symptoms soon become a major concern. The patient may attempt to keep the panic attacks secret, thereby causing his family and friends concern about unexplained changes in his behavior. The frequency and severity of panic attacks may fluctuate. The frequency of such attacks is often as many as one to two per week (though they can happen several times a day or as few as once a year). Excessive intake of caffeine may exacerbate the symptoms. Approximately 50 percent of patients with panic disorder have recovered at long-term follow-up; approximately 20 percent remain unchanged. The effects of pharmacologic treatment on these figures has not been established as yet. Depression may complicate the symptom picture in as many as 70 percent of patients. Although these patients do not tend to talk about suicidal ideation, they are, in fact, at increased risk of committing suicide. Alcohol and other drug dependence occurs in approximately one fifth of patients, and obsessive-compulsive disorder may also develop. Performance in school and work, and family interactions may suffer from the symptoms of this disorder. Patients with good premorbid function and a briefer duration of symptoms tend to have a better prognosis.

Agoraphobia

Most cases of agoraphobia are thought to be due to panic disorder. If the panic disorder is treated, the agoraphobia often improves with time. For a more rapid and more complete reduction of agoraphobia, however, behavioral therapy is sometimes indicated. Agoraphobia without panic attacks can often be quite incapacitating and chronic. Depression and alcoholism often complicate the symptom picture.

DIAGNOSIS AND SUBTYPES

Panic Disorder

DSM-III-R contains the specific diagnostic criteria for panic disorder (Table 1) and two major subtypes—with and without agoraphobia (Tables 2 and 3). The diagnosis of panic disorder requires that a specific organic etiology be ruled out; however, the presence of mitral valve prolapse does not exclude the diagnosis of panic disorder. Minor subtyping includes the specification of the severity of the

Table 1
Diagnostic Criteria for Panic Disorder

A. At some time during the disturbance, one or more panic attacks (discrete periods of intense fear or discomfort) have occurred that were (1) unexpected, i.e., did not occur immediately before or on exposure to a situation that almost always caused anxiety, and (2) not triggered by situations in which the person was the focus of others' attention.

B. Either four attacks, as defined in criterion A, have occurred within a 4-week period, or one or more attacks have been followed by a period of at least a month of persistent fear of having another attack.

C. At least four of the following symptoms developed during at least one of the attacks:

   (1) shortness of breath (dyspnea) or smothering sensations
   (2) dizziness, unsteady feelings, or faintness
   (3) palpitations or accelerated heart rate (tachycardia)
   (4) trembling or shaking
   (5) sweating
   (6) choking
   (7) nausea or abdominal distress
   (8) depersonalization or derealization
   (9) numbness or tingling sensations (parestheslas)
  (10) flushes (hot flashes) or chills
  (11) chest pain or discomfort
  (12) fear of dying
  (13) fear of going crazy or of doing something uncontrolled

Note: Attacks involving four or more symptoms are panic attacks; attacks involving fewer than four symptoms are limited symptom attacks (see Agoraphobia without History of Panic Disorder).

D. During at least some of the attacks, at least four of the C symptoms developed suddenly and increased in intensity within 10 minutes of the beginning of the first C symptom noticed in the attack.

E. It cannot be established that an organic factor initiated and maintained the disturbance, e.g., Amphetamine or Caffeine Intoxication, hyperthyroidism.

Note: Mitral valve prolapse may be an associated condition, but does not preclude a diagnosis of Panic Disorder.

Table from DSM-III-R, *Diagnostic and Statistical Manual of Mental Disorders,* ed 3, revised. (Current Classification of Mental Disorders, 1987.) Copyright American Psychiatric Association, Washington, D.C., 1987. Used with permission.

panic attacks and agoraphobia. It is important to note that there is no exclusion criteria for other psychiatric disorders; therefore, a patient may have a diagnosis of both panic disorder and another Axis I disorder such as depression or schizophrenia.

Agoraphobia

The DSM-III-R criteria for agoraphobia specify two subtypes (Table 4). One subtype is agoraphobia without panic attacks, and the other is agoraphobia with limited panic attacks that are not thought to be etiologically related to the agoraphobia.

Table 2
Diagnostic Criteria for Panic Disorder with Agoraphobia

A. Meets the criteria for Panic Disorder.

B. Agoraphobia: Fear of being in places or situations from which escape might be difficult (or embarrassing) or in which help might not be available in the event of a panic attack. (Include cases in which persistent avoidance behavior originated during an active phase of Panic Disorder, even if the person does not attribute the avoidance behavior to fear of having a panic attack.) As a result of this fear, the person either restricts travel or needs a companion when away from home, or else endures agoraphobic situations despite intense anxiety. Common agoraphobic situations include being outside the home alone, being in a crowd or standing in a line, being on a bridge, and traveling in a bus, train, or car.

Specify current severity of agoraphobic avoidance:

Mild: Some avoidance (or endurance with distress), but relatively normal life-style (e.g., travels unaccompanied when necessary, such as to work or to shop; otherwise avoids traveling alone).

Moderate: Avoidance results in constricted life style (e.g., the person is able to leave the house alone, but not to go more than a few miles unaccompanied).

Severe: Avoidance results in being nearly or completely housebound or unable to leave the house unaccompanied.

In Partial Remission: No current agoraphobic avoidance, but some agoraphobic avoidance during the past 6 months.

In Full Remission: No current agoraphobic avoidance and none during the past 6 months.

Specify current severity of panic attacks:

Mild: During the past month, either all attacks have been limited symptom attacks (i.e., fewer than four symptoms), or there has been no more than one panic attack.

Moderate: During the past month attacks have been intermediate between "mild" and "severe."

Severe: During the past month, there have been at least eight panic attacks.

In Partial Remission: The condition has been intermediate between "In Full Remission" and "Mild."

In Full Remission: During the past 6 months, there have been no panic or limited symptom attacks.

Table from DSM-III-R, *Diagnostic and Statistical Manual of Mental Disorders,* ed 3, revised. (Current Classification of Mental Disorders, 1987.) Copyright American Psychiatric Association, Washington, D.C., 1987. Used with permission.

Differential Diagnosis

The organic differential diagnosis for panic disorder, as well as for other anxiety disorders, is lengthy (Table 5). The psychiatric differential diagnosis includes malingering, factitious disorder, hypochondriasis, depersonalization, social and simple phobias, post-traumatic stress disorder, depression, and schizophrenia. The organic differential diagnosis for agoraphobia without panic attacks includes all of the disorders that may cause anxiety or depression. The

Table 3
Diagnostic Criteria for Panic Disorder Without Agoraphobia

A. Meets the criteria for Panic Disorder.

B. Absence of Agoraphobia, as defined above.

Specify current severity of panic attacks, as defined above.

Table from DSM-III-R, *Diagnostic and Statistical Manual of Mental Disorders,* ed 3, revised. (Current Classification of Mental Disorders, 1987.) Copyright American Psychiatric Association, Washington, D.C., 1987. Used with permission.

Table 4
Diagnostic Criteria for Agoraphobia Without History of Panic Disorder

A. Agoraphobia: Fear of being in places or situations from which escape might be difficult (or embarrassing) or in which help might not be available in the event of suddenly developing a symptom(s) that could be incapacitating or extremely embarrassing. Examples include: dizziness or falling, depersonalization or derealization, loss of bladder or bowel control, vomiting, or cardiac distress. As a result of this fear, the person either restricts travel or needs a companion when away from home, or else endures agoraphobic situations despite intense anxiety. Common agoraphobic situations include being outside the home alone, being in a crowd or standing in a line, being on a bridge, and traveling in a bus, train, or car.

B. Has never met the criteria for Panic Disorder.

Specify with or without limited symptom attacks

Table from DSM-III-R, *Diagnostic and Statistical Manual of Mental Disorders,* ed 3, revised. (Current Classification of Mental Disorders, 1987.) Copyright American Psychiatric Association, Washington, D.C., 1987. Used with permission.

psychiatric differential diagnosis includes major depression, schizophrenia, paranoid personality disorder, avoidant personality disorder, and dependent personality disorder.

CLINICAL MANAGEMENT

Pharmacologic Therapy

The principal treatment of panic disorder is pharmacologic—tricyclic antidepressants and monoamine oxidase inhibitors (MAOIs). Imipramine has been the most frequently utilized drug, although there are also several reports that desipramine is as effective and has fewer side effects. There are also many reports that phenelzine, an MAOI, is effective. Other tricyclics and MAOIs may be effective; propranolol and alprazolam may be tried in individuals who are either not responsive to tricyclics and phenelzine or who cannot tolerate these drugs because of adverse effects. Buspirone, a new anxiolytic drug, is not effective in the treatment of panic disorder. These tricyclics and MAOIs should be used in the same manner in which they are used for treating depression; however, it may be advisable to increase the dose about half as quickly in these

Table 5
Organic Differential Diagnosis for Anxiety Disorders

Cardiovascular
Anemia
Angina
Congestive heart failure
Hyperactive β-adrenergic state
Hypertension
Mitral valve prolapse
Myocardial infarction
Paradoxical atrial tachycardia

Pulmonary
Asthma
Hyperventilation
Pulmonary embolus

Neurologic
Cerebrovascular accident
Epilepsy
Huntington's disease
Infection
Meniere's disease
Migraine
Multiple sclerosis
Transient ischemic attack
Tumor
Wilson's disease

Endocrine
Addison's disease
Carcinoid
Cushing's syndrome
Diabetes
Hyperthyroid
Hypoglycemia
Hypoparathyroid
Menopausal
Pheochromocytoma
Premenstrual

Drug intoxications
Amphetamine
Amyl nitrite
Anticholinergics
Cocaine
Hallucinogens
Marijuana
Nicotine
Theophylline

Drug withdrawal
Alcohol
Antihypertensives
Opiates
Sedative hypnotics

Other
Anaphylaxis
B_{12} deficiency
Electrolyte disturbances
Heavy metal poisoning
Systemic infections
Systemic lupus erythematosus
Temporal arteritis
Uremia

anxiety disorder patients because of a higher incidence of adverse effects. The full maximum dose of these drugs, however, may be required to obtain relief from the panic symptoms. It may take 2 to 4 weeks for panic attacks to decrease with treatment. The clinician should obtain blood levels of antidepressants if the patient is not responsive to maximal doses. Following recovery, patients should be maintained on the drug for 6 to 12 months, after which time an attempt may be made to taper the drug slowly. If symptoms return, the drug treatment should be reinstituted. No conclusive data are available on whether antidepressant treatment is effective in agoraphobia without panic attacks. If the agoraphobia is particularly disabling, however, a trial of drug therapy in coordination with behavioral approaches would seem warranted.

Behavior Therapy

Even if panic attacks are completely removed by pharmacologic treatment, the patient may continue to have agoraphobic symptoms or anticipatory anxiety. These symptoms are often most responsive to behavioral desensitization involving increased exposure to the real or imagined phobic situation. When a patient is committed to improvement of symptoms, this repeated exposure to the phobic stimulus frequently results in a desensitization to the stimulus. Behavioral approaches also often involve cognitive exercises to deal with the anxiety, as well as formal muscle relaxation or meditation exercises.

Family Therapy

The family of a patient with panic disorder and agoraphobia may have become quite disrupted during the course of the illness. Family therapy directed toward education and support are often quite beneficial.

Insight-Oriented Psychotherapy

Insight-oriented psychotherapy is of benefit in the treatment of panic disorder or agoraphobia. Treatment focuses on helping the patient understand the unconscious meaning of the anxiety, the symbolism of the avoided situation, the need to repress impulses, and the secondary gain of the symptoms. A restriction of early infantile and oedipal conflicts occurs which correlates with the resolution of current stresses.

References

Breier A, Charney D S, Heninger G R: The diagnostic validity of anxiety disorders and their relationship to depressive illness. Am J Psychiatry *142*:787, 1985.
Breier A, Charney D S, Heninger G R: Agoraphobia with panic attacks: Development, diagnostic stability, and course of illness. Arch Gen Psychiatry *43*:1029, 1986.
Katon W, Vitaliano P P, Russo J, Jones M, Anderson K: Panic disorder. Spectrum of severity and somatization. J Nervous Mental Dis. *175*:12, 1987.
Klein D F, Ross D C, Cohen: Panic and avoidance in agoraphobia. Arch Gen Psychiatry *44*:377, 1987.
Lader M H: Assessment methods and the differential diagnosis of anxiety. J Clin Psychopharmacol *1*:342, 1981.
Liberthson R, Sheehan D C, King M E, et al: The prevalence of mitral valve prolapse in patients with panic disorders. Am J Psychiatry *143*:511, 1986.

Liebowitz M R, Gorman J M, Fyer A, et al.: Possible mechanisms for lactate's induction of panic. Am J Psychiatry *143*:495, 1986.

Marks I, Lader M: Anxiety states (anxiety neurosis): A review. J Nerv Ment Dis *156*:3, 1973.

Matuzas W, Al-Sadir J, Uhlenhuth E H, Glass R M: Mitral valve prolapse and thyroid abnormalities in patients with panic attacks. Am J Psychiatry *144*:493, 1987.

Noyes R, Crowe R R, Harris E L, et al.: Relationship between panic disorder and agoraphobia; A family study. Arch Gen Psychiatry *43*:227, 1986.

Raskin M, Peeke H V S, Dickman W, et al.: Panic and generalized anxiety disorder. Arch Gen Psychiatry *39*:687, 1982.

Reiman E M, Raichle M E, Robins E: The application of positron emission tomography to the study of panic disorder. Am J Psychiatry *143*:469, 1986.

Roth W T, Telch M J, Taylor C B, et al.: Autonomic characterization of agoraphobia with panic attacks. Biol Psychiatry *21*:1133, 1986.

Woods S, Charney D S, McPherson C A, Gradman A H, Heninger G R: Situational panic attacks. Arch Gen Psychiatry *44*:365, 1987.

18.4 ————
Social and Simple Phobias

A phobia is an irrational fear resulting in conscious avoidance of a specific feared object, activity, or situation. The fear and behavior are ego dystonic to the patient, who consciously realizes that the fear is unfounded and irrational. DSM-III-R defines social phobia as the fear of humiliation or embarrassment in public places. It differs from agoraphobia, in which the patient is not overly concerned with the reaction of other people to his behavior. Social phobias include phobias about eating in restaurants, urinating in public restrooms, public speaking, and public musical performance. Simple phobia is a residual category that includes specific phobias not covered in agoraphobia or social phobia. A classic example of a simple phobia is an irrational and overly intense belief about the danger of spiders.

EPIDEMIOLOGY

Social phobia is less common than simple phobia. Social phobias affect 3 to 5 percent of the population. Males and females are approximately equally represented. The onset is usually in the early to late teens, although it can begin at any age. The 6-month prevalence of simple phobia varies from 5 to 12 percent in different studies. Females are more often affected than males. The following objects and situations are listed in descending frequency of appearance in simple phobia: animals, storms, heights, illness, injury, and death.

HISTORY AND ETIOLOGY

The history of phobias and the theories about their etiology are so entwined that they can be discussed together. There is no significant information about the role of biological factors in the etiology of social and simple phobias. Some biological theorists have proposed that phobic patients have a specific inability to habituate to certain situations. However, some evidence points to a genetic component in that the relatives of phobic probands are more likely to have phobias themselves.

Psychoanalytic Theories

Freud presented a formulation of phobic neurosis, which in essence has remained the analytic explanation of social and simple phobias. Freud hypothesized that the major function of anxiety is to signal the ego that a forbidden unconscious drive is pushing for conscious expression, thus alerting the ego to strengthen and marshal its defenses against the threatening instinctual force. Freud viewed the phobic disorder—or "anxiety hysteria," as he continued to call it—as a result of conflicts centered on an unresolved childhood oedipal situation. Since the sex drive continues to have a strong incestuous coloring in the adult, sexual arousal tends to kindle anxiety that is characteristically a fear of castration. When repression fails to be entirely successful, it is necessary for the ego to call on auxiliary defenses. In phobic patients, the defense primarily involves the use of displacement; that is, the sexual conflict is displaced from the person who evokes the conflict to a seemingly unimportant, irrelevant object or situation, which then has the power to arouse the entire constellation of affects, including signal anxiety. It can often be plausibly suggested that the phobic object or situation has a direct associative connection with the primary source of the conflict and thus has come to symbolize it (the defense mechanism of symbolization). Furthermore, the situation or object is usually such that the patient is able to keep out of its way and, by this additional defense mechanism of avoidance, escape suffering from serious anxiety. Freud first discussed this theoretical formulation of phobia formation, which attributes the phobia to the use of the ego defense mechanisms of displacement and avoidance against incestuous oedipal genital drives and castration anxiety, in his famous case history of "Little Hans," a 5-year-old boy who had a fear of horses.

Although it was originally thought that phobias resulted from castration anxiety, more recent theorists have suggested that other types of anxiety may be involved. In agoraphobia, for example, separation anxiety clearly plays a leading role, and in erythrophobia (which can be manifested as a fear of blushing), the element of shame implies the involvement of superego anxiety. It is perhaps closer to clinical observation to view the anxiety associated with phobias as having a variety of sources and colorings.

Counterphobic Attitude. Otto Fenichel called attention to the fact that phobic anxiety can be hidden behind attitudes and behavior patterns that represent a denial, either that the dreaded object or situation is dangerous or that one is afraid of it. Basic to this phenomenon is a reversal of the situation in which one is the passive victim of external circumstances, to a position of attempting actively to confront and master what one fears. The counterphobic person seeks out situations of danger and rushes enthusiastically toward them. The devotee of dangerous sports such as parachute jumping and rock climbing, for example, may be exhibiting counterphobic behavior. Such patterns may be secondary to neurotic phobic anxieties, or may be used as a normal means of dealing with a realistically dangerous situation. The play of children may contain counterphobic elements, such as the common game of playing doctor and giving to their doll the shot they received earlier in the day in the pediatrician's office. This pattern of behavior may involve the related defense mechanism of identification with the aggressor.

Behavioral Theories

In 1920, John B. Watson wrote an article called *Conditioned Emotional Reactions* in which he recounted his experiences with Little Albert, an infant with a phobia of rats and rabbits. Unlike Freud's Little Hans, who developed symptoms in the natural course of his maturation, Little Albert's difficulties were the direct result of the scientific experiments of two psychologists, who used techniques that had successfully induced conditioned responses in laboratory animals.

Watson's formulation invokes the traditional Pavlovian stimulus-response model of the conditioned reflex to account for the initial creation of the phobia. That is, anxiety is aroused by a naturally frightening stimulus that occurs in contiguity with a second inherently neutral stimulus. As a result of the contiguity, especially when the two stimuli are paired on several successive occasions, the originally neutral stimulus takes on the capacity to arouse anxiety by itself. The neutral stimulus, therefore, becomes a conditioned stimulus for anxiety production.

In the classical stimulus-response theory, the conditioned stimulus is seen as gradually losing its potency to arouse a response if it is not reinforced by a periodic repetition of the unconditioned stimulus. In the phobic symptom, this attenuation of the response to the phobic (i.e., conditioned) stimulus does not occur, yet the symptom may last for years without any apparent external reinforcement. In the more recently formulated operant conditioning theory, however, a model is provided for explaining that phenomenon. In the newer theory, anxiety is viewed as a drive that motivates the organism to do what it can to obviate the painful affect. In the course of its random behavior, the animal soon learns that certain actions enable it to avoid the stimulus for anxiety. These avoidance patterns remain stable for long periods of time as a result of the reinforcement they receive from their capacity to diminish anxiety. This model is readily applicable to phobias in that avoidance of the anxiety-provoking object or situation plays a central part. Such avoidance behavior becomes fixed as a stable symptom because of its effectiveness in protecting the patient from the phobic anxiety.

Learning theory has a particular relevance to phobic disorders and provides simple and intelligible explanations of many aspects of phobic symptoms. Critics contend, however, that it deals more with surface mechanisms of symptom formation and is perhaps less useful than psychoanalytic theories in providing an understanding of some of the more complex underlying psychic processes involved.

CLINICAL SIGNS AND SYMPTOMS

Phobias are characterized by the arousal of severe anxiety when the patient is exposed to a specific phobic situation or object. Both mental and somatic symptoms of anxiety are present. The somatic symptom of blushing is said to be more common in social phobias. In an attempt to prevent the development of anxiety, the patient does everything in his power to avoid the situation that stimulates his phobic response. The patient's daily activities may be hindered to some degree, depending on how easy it is to avoid the phobic situation. Alcohol and drug dependence and major depressive disorder can be complicating associated features in phobic disorders. The following illustrates a case of social phobia:

A 21-year-old pre-law student was called in by her advisor for a discussion of her performance. Although she did very well on tests, she was totally unable to participate in classroom discussions. She had managed with a succession of excuses to avoid all formal presentations well into her junior year, but her avoidance was finally catching up with her, as professors began to lower her grades. She admitted with great embarrassment that she was terrified of speaking before others and had on more than one occasion left her classroom in a state of panic, fearful that she would be called upon to speak. At such times she was short of breath, sweaty, was conscious of her heart racing, and felt faint.

She explained to her advisor that she felt that she had an unpleasant accent and was not as articulate as her fellow students. She was convinced that they would find her "dumb" and think she was a "fool" for trying to become a lawyer.

Discussion

This patient's avoidance of speaking in the classroom is due to an excessive fear of humiliation, a common example of a social phobia. Since her panic attacks apparently occur only when she is exposed to the phobic stimulus, the additional diagnosis of panic disorder is not made; and since there is no evidence of avoidance of interpersonal relationships in general, the diagnosis of avoidant personality disorder is not appropriate.

DSM-III-R Diagnosis:
Axis I: Social Phobia

[Adapted with permission from *DSM-III Case Book*. American Psychiatric Association, Washington, D.C. 1981.]

The major finding on the mental status examination is the presence of an irrational and ego-dystonic fear of a specific situation, activity, or object. The patient is also able to describe how he avoids contact with the phobic situation. Depression is commonly observable on the mental status examination.

COURSE AND PROGNOSIS

Most patients are able to live relatively normal lives in spite of their phobic disorder because the phobic object or situation is easily avoidable. For example, fear of horses is not a problem for a city dweller. The onset of social phobias is often gradual and occasionally follows a precipitating psychosocial stressor. Social phobias may have a chronic course, although there is some evidence that they decrease after middle age. Simple phobias that begin in childhood usually remit spontaneously; however some simple phobias may be chronic. Rigorous studies of the outcome of phobic disorders are not available.

DIAGNOSIS AND SUBTYPES

The DSM-III-R diagnostic criteria (Table 1) for social phobia require that the primary fear not be related to another Axis I or Axis III disorder and that the condition interfere with the life of the patient. The generalized subtype of social phobia describes a patient who is phobic of most social situations.

The DSM-III-R diagnostic criteria for simple phobia (Table 2) define a residual category that covers phobias not included in agoraphobia or social phobia. The diagnostic guidelines also indicate that the phobic stimulus cannot be related to the obsessional component of obsessive-compulsive disorder. Impairment in occupational or social functioning is required as well.

DIFFERENTIAL DIAGNOSIS

The most common organic differential diagnosis of phobic disorder is intoxication with hallucinogens, sympathomimetics,

Table 1
Diagnostic Criteria for Social Phobia

A. A persistent fear of one or more situations (the social phobic situations) in which the person is exposed to possible scrutiny by others and fears that he or she may do something or act in a way that will be humiliating or embarrassing. Examples include: being unable to continue talking while speaking in public, choking on food when eating in front of others, being unable to urinate in a public lavatory, hand-trembling when writing in the presence of others, and saying foolish things or not being able to answer questions in social situations.

B. If an Axis III or another Axis I disorder is present, the fear in A is unrelated to it, e.g., the fear is not of having a panic attack (Panic Disorder), stuttering (Stuttering), trembling (Parkinson's disease), or exhibiting abnormal eating behavior (Anorexia Nervosa or Bulimia Nervosa).

C. During some phase of the disturbance, exposure to the specific phobic stimulus (or stimuli) almost invariably provokes an immediate anxiety response.

D. The phobic situation(s) is avoided, or is endured with intense anxiety.

E. The avoidant behavior interferes with occupational functioning or with usual social activities or relationships with others, or there is marked distress about having the fear.

F. The person recognizes that his or her fear is excessive or unreasonable.

G. If the person is under 18, the disturbance does not meet the criteria for Avoidant Disorder of Childhood or Adolescence.

Specify generalized type if the phobic situation includes most social situations, and also consider the additional diagnosis of Avoidant Personality Disorder.

Table from DSM-III-R *Diagnostic and Statistical Manual of Mental Disorders,* ed 3, revised. (Current Classification of Mental Disorders, 1987.) Copyright American Psychiatric Association, Washington, D.C., 1987. Used with permission.

Table 2
Diagnostic Criteria for Simple Phobia

A. A persistent fear of a circumscribed stimulus (object or situation) other than fear of having a panic attack (as in Panic Disorder) or of humiliation or embarrassment in certain social situations (as in Social Phobia).

 Note: Do not include fears that are part of Panic Disorder with Agoraphobia or Agoraphobia without History of Panic Disorder.

B. During some phase of the disturbance, exposure to the specific phobic stimulus (or stimuli) almost invariably provokes an immediate anxiety response.

C. The object or situation is avoided, or endured with intense anxiety.

D. The fear or the avoidant behavior significantly interferes with the person's normal routine or with usual social activities or relationships with others, or there is marked distress about having the fear.

E. The person recognizes that his or her fear is excessive or unreasonable.

F. The phobic stimulus is unrelated to the content of the obsessions of Obsessive Compulsive Disorder or the trauma of Post-traumatic Stress Disorder.

Table from DSM-III-R *Diagnostic and Statistical Manual of Mental Disorders,* ed 3, revised. (Current Classification of Mental Disorders, 1987.) Copyright American Psychiatric Association, Washington, D.C., 1987. Used with permission.

and other abused drugs. Most organic disorders do not cause isolated symptoms of phobia in the absence of other psychiatric or neurologic symptoms. Nevertheless, it is possible for a small cerebral tumor or cerebrovascular accident to produce such a symptom complex. The clinician should be especially careful to consider unusual organic causes whenever atypical symptoms are present.

The psychiatric differential diagnosis of social phobia includes depression, schizophrenia, and schizoid and avoidant personality disorders. It has been suggested that social phobia and alcohol dependence may coexist more often than has been appreciated; therefore, phobic disorder should also be considered in the differential diagnosis of alcohol abuse. The psychiatric differential diagnosis of simple phobia should include schizophrenia, major depression, obsessive-compulsive disorder, paranoid personality disorder, and avoidant personality disorder.

The differentiation of a phobia from a delusion of schizophrenia is based primarily on three clinical observations. First, the phobic patient is very aware of the irrational nature of his feelings and avoidant behavior. Second, the nature of the phobia lacks the bizarre quality that can be seen in schizophrenics, who may have phobias. Third, the other symptoms of schizophrenia are not present in phobic patients.

The differentiation of a phobia from obsessive-compulsive disorder sometimes can be difficult. For example, the common phobia of knives or other dangerous objects often rests on the patient's fantasy that he will actively hurt someone else. The patient is able to control his anxiety by avoiding such objects. The differentiation between these two conditions, however, is of less clinical relevance at this time since the treatments for both disorders are similar.

CLINICAL MANAGEMENT

Pharmacological Therapy

There is reasonable preliminary evidence that phenelzine may be of use in treating social phobia. Other potentially useful drugs include propranolol and tricyclic anti-depressants. The social phobia of stage fright in musicians and other performers has been particularly effectively treated with β-adrenergic antagonists such as propranolol. The evidence supporting the use of these drugs in treating simple phobia is less extensive, but therapeutic drug trials in connection with behavior therapy may be warranted in severe cases.

Insight-Oriented Psychotherapy

Early in the development of psychoanalysis and the dynamically oriented psychotherapies, it was believed that these methods were the treatment of choice for phobic neurosis, which then was thought to stem from oedipal-genital conflicts. Soon, however, therapists recognized that, despite progress in uncovering and analyzing unconscious conflicts, patients frequently failed to lose their phobic symptoms. Moreover, by continuing to avoid the phobic situation, patients excluded a significant degree of anxiety and its related associations from the analytic process. Both Freud and his pupil Sandor Ferenczi had recognized that, if progress in analyzing the symptoms was to be made, therapists had to go beyond their merely analytic roles and actively urge phobic patients to seek out the phobic situation and experience the anxiety and resultant insight. There has since been general agreement among psychiatrists that a measure of activity on the part of the therapist is often required to successfully treat phobic anxiety. The decision to apply the techniques of psychodynamic insight therapy should be based not on the presence of the phobic symptom alone, but on positive indications from the patient's ego structure and life patterns for the use of this method of treatment. Insight therapy enables the patient to understand the origin of the phobia, the phenomenon of secondary gain, the role of resistance, and enables him to develop healthier ways of dealing with anxiety provoking stimuli.

Behavior Therapy

The most studied and most effective treatment for phobias is probably behavior therapy. The keys to successful treatment are (1) the patient's commitment to treatment, (2) clearly identified problems and objectives, and (3) available alternative strategies for coping with the feelings. A variety of behavioral treatment techniques have been employed, the most common being systematic desensitization, a method pioneered by Joseph Wolpe. In this method, the patient is exposed serially to a predetermined list of anxiety-provoking stimuli graded in a hierarchy from the least to the most frightening. Through the use of tranquilizing drugs, hypnosis, and instruction in muscle relaxation, patients are taught how to induce in themselves both mental and physical repose. Once they have mastered the techniques, patients are instructed to employ them to induce relaxation in the face of each anxiety-provoking stimulus. As they become desensitized to each stimulus in the scale, the patients move up to the next stimulus until, ultimately, what previously produced the most anxiety is no longer capable of eliciting the painful affect.

Other behavioral techniques that have more recently been employed involve intensive exposure to the phobic stimulus either through imagery or desensitization *in vivo*. In imaginal flooding, patients are exposed to the phobic stimulus for as long as they can tolerate the fear until they reach a point at which they can no longer feel it. Flooding (also known as implosion) *in vivo* requires patients to experience similar anxiety through and exposure to the actual phobic stimulus.

Other Theapeutic Modalities

Hypnosis, supportive therapy, and family therapy may be of use in the treatment of phobic disorders. Hypnosis is used to enhance the therapist's suggestion that the phobic objection is not dangerous, and it can be taught to the patient as a method of relaxation when confronted with the phobic object. Supportive psychotherapy and family therapy are often useful in helping the patient actively confront the phobic object during treatment. Not only can family therapy enlist the aid of the family in treating the patient, but it may help the family to understand the nature of the patient's problem.

References

Aimes P L, Gelder M G, Shaw P M: Social phobia. A comparative clinical study. Br J Psychiatry *142*:174, 1983.

Freud S: Analysis of a phobia of a five-year-old boy. In S Freud: *The Standard Edition of the Complete Psychological Works of Sigmund Freud,* vol 10, p5. Hogarth Press, London, 1955.

Gorman J M, Liebowitz M R, Fyer A J: Treatment of social phobia with atenolol. J Clin Psychopharm *5*:298, 1985.

James I M, Pearson R M, Griffith D N W: Effect of oxaprenolol on stage fright in musicians. Lancet *134*:952, 1977.

Liebowitz M R, Fyer A J, Gorman J M: Social phobia. Review of a neglected anxiety disorder. Arch Gen Psychiatry *42*:729, 1985.

Liebowitz M R, Fyer A J, Gorman J M: Phenelzine in social phobia. J Clin Psychopharm *6*:93, 1986.

Marks I M: The classification of phobic disorders. Br J Psychiatry *116*:377, 1970.

Marks I M, Gelder M G: Different ages of onset in varieties of phobia. Am J Psychiatry *123*:218, 1966.

Mullaney J A, Trippett C J: Alcohol dependence and phobias: Clinical description and relevance. Br J Psychiatry *135*:563, 1979.

Nemiah J: A psychoanalytic view of phobias. Am J Psychoanalysis *41*:115, 1981.

Torgersen S: Genetic factors in anxiety disorders. Arch Gen Psychiatry *40*:1085, 1983.

18.5 _____

Obsessive-Compulsive Disorder

An obsession is a recurrent and intrusive mental event, which can be a thought, a feeling, an idea, or a sensation. A compulsion is a conscious, standardized, recurrent behavior, such as counting, checking, or avoiding. According to DSM-III-R, the essential feature of this disorder is recurrent obsessions or compulsions sufficiently severe to cause marked distress, to be time consuming, or to significantly interfere with the person's normal routine, occupational functioning, or with usual social activities or relationships with others. A patient with obsessive-compulsive disorder realizes the irrationality of this obsession and experiences both the obsession and the compulsion as ego dystonic. A patient with obsessive-compulsive disorder may have an obsession, a compulsion, or both. Although the compulsive act may be carried out in an attempt to reduce the anxiety associated with the obsession, this is not always the result. The compulsive act sometimes may not alter the patient's anxiety, or may even increase it.

EPIDEMIOLOGY

Obsessive-compulsive disorder is a rare syndrome with a prevalence of 0.05 percent in the general population. More recent studies, however, suggest that it may be more common than was previously appreciated. The secretive nature of affected patients may have contributed to an underestimation of its occurrence. Obsessive-compulsive disorder may represent as much as 1 percent of patients in psychiatric treatment. The disorder begins most often in adolescence and early adulthood and affects males and females equally. Patients with obsessive-compulsive disorder tend to have an above average intelligence, and approximately one third have at least a college education.

ETIOLOGY

Biological Factors

A variety of biological abnormalities have been reported in groups of obsessive-compulsive patients. Two observations stimulated the search for a biological etiology for this disorder. First, it was noted by investigators that patients with obsessive-compulsive disorder commonly had a history of traumatic births, suggesting the possibility of a role for brain trauma in the etiology. It was also noted that some patients with temporal lobe epilepsy had symptoms identical to those seen in idiopathic obsessive-compulsive disorder. One positron emission tomographic (PET) study of obsessive-compulsive disorder patients, however, reported increased metabolic activity in the left orbital gyrus and in both left and right caudate nuclei. Although this biological evidence is not conclusive, it has been hypothesized that the cingulate gyrus, in particular, might be involved in the pathophysiology of this disorder.

The major biological abnormalities seen in this disorder have been reported from EEG, sleep EEG, neuroendocrine, and computed tomographic (CT) studies. There is a higher incidence of nonspecific EEG abnormalities in obsessive-compulsive patients. It has been hypothesized that these abnormalities may be located more in the left hemisphere, a hypothesis that is supported by the observation that there is a higher incidence of left-handedness in these patients. Sleep EEG studies have demonstrated abnormalities similar to those seen in depression, such as decreased REM latency. Neuroendocrine studies have also found some similarities to depression, such as nonsuppression on the dexamethasone suppression test in about one third of these patients and decreased growth hormone secretion with clonidine infusions. Finally, there are somewhat controversial reports that the more severely ill obsessive-compulsive patients may have enlarged ventricles that are detectable on CT.

Genetics

The genetic studies of obsessive-compulsive disorder have been limited by its rarity. However, there does seem to be a heritable basis for at least some cases. There is an incidence of 3 to 7 percent of the disorder in first-degree relatives, compared with only 0.5 percent in relatives of patients with other anxiety disorders.

Psychosocial Factors

Personality Factors. Obsessive-compulsive disorder is not a severe form of compulsive personality disorder. The majority of obsessive-compulsive disorder patients do not have premorbid compulsive symptoms; therefore, such traits are neither necessary nor sufficient for the development of the obsessive-compulsive disorder. Approximately 15 to 35 percent of patients have had premorbid obsessional traits, as compared with 50 percent of psychiatric patients without obsessive-compulsive disorder who have such traits.

Psychodynamic Factors. Freud described three major psychological defense mechanisms that determine the form and the quality of obsessive-compulsive symptoms and character traits: isolation, undoing, and reaction formation.

Isolation. Isolation is a defense mechanism that protects a person from anxiety-provoking affects and impulses. Under ordinary circumstances, a person experiences in consciousness both the affect and the imagery of an emotion-laden idea, whether it be a fantasy or the memory of an event. When isolation occurs, the affect and the impulse of which it is a derivative are separated from the ideational component and pushed out of consciousness. If isolation is completely successful, the impulse and its associated affect are totally repressed, and the patient is consciously aware only of the affectless idea that is related to it.

Undoing. Owing to the constant threat that the impulse may escape the primary defense of isolation and break free, further secondary defensive operations are required to combat it and to quiet the anxiety that the imminent eruption of the impulse into consciousness arouses.

The compulsive act constitutes the surface manifestation of a defensive operation aimed at reducing anxiety and at controlling the underlying impulse that has not been sufficiently contained by isolation. A particularly important secondary defensive operation of this sort is the mechanism of undoing. As the word suggests, it refers to a compulsive act that is performed in an attempt to prevent or undo the consequences that the patient irrationally anticipates from a frightening obsessional thought or impulse.

Reaction formation. Both isolation and undoing are defensive maneuvers that are intimately involved in the production of clinical symptoms. Reaction formation results in the formation of character traits rather than symptoms. As the term implies, reaction formation involves manifest patterns of behavior and consciously experienced attitudes that are exactly the opposite of the underlying impulses. Often these patterns seem to an observer to be highly exaggerated, and at times quite inappropriate.

Other Psychogenic Factors. One of the striking features of patients with obsessive-compulsive disorder is the degree to which they are preoccupied with aggression or cleanliness, either overtly in the content of their symptoms or in the associations that lie behind them. This and other observations have led to the proposition that the psychogenesis of the obsessive-compulsive disorder lies in disturbances in normal growth and development related to the anal-sadistic phase.

Ambivalence. Ambivalence is the direct result of a change in the characteristics of the impulse life. It is an important feature of the normal child during the anal-sadistic developmental phase— that is, he feels both love and murderous hate toward the same object sometimes seemingly simultaneously. One finds the obsessive-compulsive patient often consciously experiencing both love and hate toward his object. This conflict of opposing emotions may be seen in the doing-undoing patterns of behavior, and the paralyzing doubt in the face of choices that are frequently found in persons with this emotional disorder.

Magical thinking. In the phenomenon of magical thinking, the regression uncovers earlier modes of thought, rather than impulses—that is, ego functions, as well as id functions, are affected by regression. Inherent in magical thinking is the phenomenon of the omnipotence of thought. The person feels that, merely by thinking about an event in the external world, he can cause that event to occur without intermediate physical actions. This feeling makes having an aggressive thought frightening to obsessive-compulsive patients.

In summary, the psychoanalytic theory of obsessive-compulsive disorder ascribes the appearance of symptoms to a defensive regression of the psychic apparatus to the preoedipal anal-sadistic phase, with the consequent emergence of earlier modes of functioning of the ego, superego, and id. These factors, along with the use of specific ego defenses—isolation, undoing, reaction formation— combine to produce the clinical symptoms of obsessions, compulsions, and compulsive acts. Many of these conclusions are illustrated in Freud's classical case on the *Rat Man.*

Learning Theory. According to learning theory, obsessions represent a conditioned stimulus to anxiety. Because of an association with an unconditioned anxiety-provoking stimulus, the originally neutral obsessional thought gains the capacity to arouse anxiety; that is, a new mode of behavior has been learned. The compulsion is established in a different way. The person discovers that a certain action reduces the anxiety attached to the obsessional thought. The relief brought about when the anxiety, which operates as a negative drive state, is thus reduced by the performance of the compulsive act, reinforces this act. Gradually, because of its usefulness in reducing a painful secondary drive (the anxiety), the act becomes fixed into a learned pattern of behavior. Learning theory provides useful concepts for explaining certain aspects of the obsessive-compulsive phenomena, for example, the anxiety-provoking capacity of ideas that are not necessarily frightening in themselves, and the establishment of compulsive patterns of behavior.

CLINICAL SIGNS AND SYMPTOMS

Obsessions and compulsions have certain features in common: (1) An idea or an impulse intrudes itself insistently and persistently into the person's conscious awareness. (2) A feeling of anxious dread accompanies the central manifestation and frequently leads the person to take countermeasures against the initial idea or impulse. (3) The obsession or compulsion is ego alien; that is, it is experienced as being foreign to the person's experience of himself as a psychological being. (4) No matter how vivid and compelling the obsession or compulsion, the person recognizes it as absurd and irrational. (5) The person suffering from obsessions and compulsions feels a strong desire to resist them. However, approximately one half of patients offer little resistance to the compulsion. Approximately 80 percent of patients feel that the compulsion is irrational and silly.

There are four major symptom patterns in obsessive-compulsive disorder. The most common is an obsession of contamination followed by washing. The feared object is often hard to avoid (e.g., feces, urine), and the compulsion involves washing and cleansing. Such patients may literally rub the skin off of their hands from excessive hand washing. The second most common pattern is an obsession of doubt followed by a compulsion of checking. The obsession often implies some danger or violence (e.g., forgetting to turn off the stove). The checking may involve multiple trips back into the house to check the stove. Such patients have an obsessional self-doubt, as if they always feel guilty for having forgotten or committed something. Other descriptive terms for various compulsions are avoiding, repeating, completeness, and meticulousness. Patients with both obsessions and compulsions comprise 75 percent of the total. A less common form of obsessive-compulsive disorder is one with merely intrusive obsessional thoughts without a compulsion. Such obsessions are usually repetitive thoughts of some sexual or aggressive act that is reprehensible to the individual. Finally, there is obsessional slowness, in which the obsession and compulsion seem to be united into the very slow carrying out of daily behaviors. Such patients can take literally hours to eat a meal or shave their face. Although it is possible to delineate somewhat separate clinical pictures, it is also true that the symptoms of an individual patient may overlap these types and change in character with time.

The other major finding on mental status examination in obsessive-compulsive patients is depression or symptoms of dysthymia. Such symptoms are present in approximately 50 percent of patients. Some obsessive-compulsive patients do have character traits suggestive of compulsive disorder, but this is not true in the majority of cases. There is a higher than average celibacy rate in these patients, especially in men. There is also a higher incidence of marital discord.

COURSE AND PROGNOSIS

Over 50 percent of these patients experience onset of symptoms before 24 years of age, and over 80 percent before age 35. The mean age of onset is 20 years. Approximately 50 to 70 percent of patients have the onset of symptoms following a stressful event, such as a pregnancy, a sexual problem, or a death of a relative. There is an acute onset in over half of the cases. Because many patients manage to keep their symptoms secret, there is often a delay of 5 to 10 years before the patients comes to psychiatric attention, and the mean age of first hospitalization is 30 years. The course is usually chronic. Symptoms fluctuate in some patients and remain quite constant in others.

It has been reported that approximately 20 to 30 percent of these patients have significant improvement in their symptoms, and 40 to 50 percent have moderate improvement. It has been variously reported that 20 to 40 percent of patients either remain ill or even have a worsening of their symptoms. Approximately one third of these patients develop major depression, and suicide is a risk for all of these patients. Various reports suggest that they are at a minimally increased risk of developing schizophrenia. A poorer prognosis is suggested by yielding (rather than resisting) to compulsions, childhood onset, bizarre compulsions, and the need for hospitalization. A better prognosis is suggested by good social and occupational adjustment, the absence of compulsions in the presence of obsessions, the presence of a precipitating event, and an episodic nature to the symptoms. The actual obsessional content does not seem to be related to prognosis.

DIAGNOSIS AND DIFFERENTIAL DIAGNOSIS

The DSM-III-R diagnostic criteria for obsessive-compulsive disorder require the presence of either obsessions or compulsions (Table 1). The criteria also require that the symptoms cause distress and interfere with social and occupational functioning. DSM-III-R defines no subtypes for obsessive-compulsive disorder.

The DSM-III-R diagnostic requirement of personal distress and functional impairment differentiates obsessive-compulsive disorder from ordinary or mildly excessive thoughts and habits. The major neurologic disorders to consider in the differential diagnosis are Tourette's syndrome, other tic disorders, and temporal lobe epilepsy. The major psychiatric considerations are schizophrenia, depression (with obsessive thoughts), phobic disorders, and compulsive personality disorder. Obsessive-compulsive disorder can usually be distinguished from schizophrenia by the absence of other schizophrenic symptoms, the less bizarre nature of the symptoms, and the patient's insight into his disorder. Depression with obsessive thoughts is distinguished by the presence of depressive symptoms that

Table 1
Diagnostic Criteria for Obsessive-Compulsive Disorder

A. Either obsessions or compulsions:
   Obsessions: (1), (2), (3), and (4):
   (1) Recurrent and persistent ideas, thoughts, impulses, or images that are experienced, at least initially, as intrusive and senseless (e.g., a parent's having repeated impulses to kill a loved child, a religious person's having recurrent blasphemous thoughts).
   (2) The person attempts to ignore or suppress such thoughts or impulses or to neutralize them with some other thought or action.
   (3) The person recognizes that the obsessions are the product of his or her own mind, not imposed from without (as in thought insertion).
   (4) If another Axis I disorder is present, the content of the obsession is unrelated to it (e.g., the ideas, thoughts, impulses, or images are not about food in the presence of an Eating Disorder, about drugs in the presence of a Psychoactive Substance Use Disorder, or guilty thoughts in the presence of a Major Depression).
   Compulsions: (1), (2), and (3):
   (1) Repetitive, purposeful, and intentional behaviors that are performed in response to an obsession, or according to certain rules or in a stereotyped fashion
   (2) The behavior is designed to neutralize or to prevent discomfort or some dreaded event or situation; however, either the activity is not connected in a realistic way with what it is designed to neutralize or prevent, or it is clearly excessive.
   (3) The person recognizes that his or her behavior is excessive or unreasonable (this may not be true for young children; it may no longer be true for people whose obsessions have evolved into overvalued ideas).

B. The obsessions or compulsions cause marked distress, are time-consuming (take more than an hour a day), or significantly interfere with the person's normal routine, occupational functioning, or usual social activities or relationships with others.

Table from DSM-III-R *Diagnostic and Statistical Manual of Mental Disorders,* ed 3, revised. (Current Classification of Mental Disorders, 1987.) Copyright American Psychiatric Association, Washington, D.C., 1987. Used with permission.

meet the DSM-III-R criteria for major depression. Phobias can be somewhat difficult to distinguish from obsessive-compulsive disorder; however, obsessive-compulsive disorder patients are usually much less successful at avoiding the feared object than are phobic patients.

CLINICAL MANAGEMENT

Pharmacotherapy

Clomipramine (Anafranil) appears to be the most effective pharmacological treatment for obsessive-compulsive disorder. The drug is not available in the United States, but is available in Canada and occasionally through special investigative protocols. The effects of clomipramine may be delayed for as long as 2 months, and it is most effective when specific compulsions are present. Other tricyclics and phenelzine have also been reported to be effective, although some clinicians believe they are much less useful than clomipramine. Phenelzine may be indicated, however, if an obsessive-compulsive disorder patient describes panic attacks as one of his symptoms. Treatment should continue for 6 to 12 months before an attempt is made to stop the medication. Many patients relapse when medication is discontinued.

Psychotherapy

Obsessive-compulsive patients do respond to the psychotherapeutic maneuvers of the psychiatrist. However, in the absence of adequate studies of psychotherapy in obsessive-compulsive disorder, it is hard to make any valid generalizations about its effectiveness. Individual analysts have seen striking and lasting changes for the better in patients with obsessional personality disorders, especially when they are able to come to terms with the aggressive impulses lying behind their character traits. Likewise, analysts and dynamically oriented psychiatrists have observed marked symptomatic improvement in their patients in the course of analysis or prolonged insight psychotherapy.

Supportive psychotherapy undoubtedly has its place, especially for that group of obsessive-compulsive patients who, despite symptoms of varying degrees of severity, are able to work and make a social adjustment. The continuous and regular contact with an interested, sympathetic, and encouraging professional person may make it possible for the patient to continue to function by virtue of that help, without which he would become completely incapacitated by his symptoms. Occasionally, when obsessional rituals and anxiety reach an intolerable intensity, it is necessary to hospitalize the patient until the shelter of an institution and the removal from external environmental stresses bring about a lessening of the symptoms to a more tolerable level. Nor must it be forgotten that the patient's family is often driven to the verge of despair by the patient's behavior. Any psychotherapeutic endeavors must include attention to family members through the provision of emotional support, reassurance, explanation, and advice on how to manage and respond to the patient.

Behavior Therapy

Behavior therapy is successful in 60 to 75 percent of patients. Desensitization, thought stopping, flooding, implosion therapy, and aversive conditioning have all been utilized in these patients. It is important that the patient be truly committed to improvement. Some behavioral therapists use response prevention in which the patient is sometimes forcibly prevented from carrying out the compulsion.

Other Therapies

Family therapy is often very useful in supporting the family, helping reduce marital discord resulting from the disorder, and building a treatment alliance with the un-

affected family members for the good of the patient. Finally, for very seriously impaired patients who have not responded to any other treatment modality, bimedial leukotomies that produce lesions in the thalamofrontal connections have been reported to be effective.

References

Akhtar S, Wig N N, Varma N N: A phenomenological analysis of symptoms in obsessive-compulsive neurosis. Br J Psychiatry *127*:342, 1975.

Baxter L R Jr, Phelps M E, Mazziotta J C, Guze B H, Schwartz J M, Selin C E: Local cerebral glucose metabolic rates in obsessive-compulsive disorder. Arch Gen Psychiatry *44*:211, 1987.

Cobb J: Behavior therapy in phobic and obsessional disorders. Psychiatr Devel *4*:351, 1983.

Insel T R, Murphy D L, Cohen R M: Obsessive-compulsive disorder: A double-blind trial of clomipramine and clorgyline. Arch Gen Psych *40*:605, 1983.

Jenike M A: Obsessive compulsive disorder. Compr Psychiatry *24*:99, 1983.

Jenike M A: Obsessive-compulsive disorder: A question of a neurologic lesion. Compr Psychiatry *25*:298, 1984.

Rasmussen S A, Tsuang M T: Clinical characteristics and family history in DSM-III obsessive-compulsive disorder. Am J Psychiatry *143*:317, 1986.

Salzman L, Thaler F H: Obsessive-compulsive disorders: A review of the literature. Am J Psychiatry *138*:286, 1981.

Stern R S, Cobb J P: Phenomenology of obsessive-compulsive neurosis. Br J Psychiatry *132*:233, 1978.

Tippin J and Henn F A: Modified leukotomy in the treatment of intractable obsessional neurosis. Am J Psychiatry *139*:1601, 1982.

18.6 _____
Post-Traumatic Stress Disorder

Post-traumatic stress disorder develops in persons who have experienced emotional or physical stress that would be extremely traumatic for virtually any person. Such traumas include combat experience, natural catastrophes, assault, rape, and disasters such as building fires. The three major features are the re-experiencing of the trauma through dreams and waking thoughts; emotional numbing to other life experiences, including relationships; and associated symptoms of autonomic instability, depression, and cognitive difficulties, such as poor concentration.

HISTORY

A syndrome very similar to what is now called post-traumatic stress disorder was noted in soldiers during the American Civil War. It was then called "soldier's heart" because of the presence of autonomic cardiac symptoms. DaCosta wrote a paper, *On Irritable Heart*, in 1871, describing such soldiers. In World War I, the syndrome was called "shell shock" and was hypothesized to result from brain trauma from the explosion of shells. Post-traumatic stress disorder was seen in World War II in the survivors of Nazi concentration camps and in the survivors of the United States' atomic bombings of Japan. In 1941, the survivors of a fire in a crowded nightclub in Boston, the Coconut Grove, showed increased nervousness, fatigue, and nightmares. In all these situations, the appearance of the syndrome was correlated with the severity of the stressor—the most severe stresses (e.g., concentration camp) resulted in the appearance of the syndrome in over 75 percent of the victims. DSM-I included a diagnosis of gross stress reaction, which was dropped from DSM-II. The reintroduction of post-traumatic stress disorder in DSM-III was the result of the description of this syndrome in veterans of the Vietnam War, as described in the following case:

The patient is a 26-year-old married Vietnam veteran recently laid off from a job that he had held for 3 years. He was admitted to the hospital for severe symptoms of anxiety, which began after he was laid off work and found himself at home watching reports of the fall of South Vietnam on television.

He described himself as well-adjusted and outgoing prior to his service in Vietnam. Although initially he found killing to be repulsive, he gradually learned to tolerate it and to rationalize it. He had several experiences that he found particularly painful and troubling. One of these experiences occurred when he was ambushed by a Vietnamese guerrilla; the veteran's gun jammed, and he was forced to kill his enemy by bludgeoning him over the head. Many years later, he could still hear "the gook's" screams. Another extremely painful incident occurred when his closest friend was killed by mortar fire. Because they were lying side by side, the friend's blood was splattered all over the patient.

Although the patient had some difficulty adjusting during the first year after his return from Vietnam, he eventually settled down. He was making plans to return to college at the time he was laid off. At home, with time on his hands and watching the fall of Vietnam on television, he began to experience unwanted intrusive recollections of his own Vietnam experiences. In particular, he was troubled by the memories of the "gook" he had killed and the death of his friend. He found himself ruminating about all the people who were killed or injured and wondering what the purpose of it all had been. He began to experience nightmares, during which he relived the moments when he himself was almost injured. During one nightmare he dove for cover out of his bed and sustained a hairline fracture of the humerus. Another time, he was riding his bike on a path through tall grass and weeds, which suddenly reminded him of the terrain in Vietnam, prompting him to dive off the bike for cover and sustain several lacerations when he hit the ground. He also became increasingly irritated with his wife and was admitted to the hospital because of her concern about his behavior. He was treated with diazepam and psychotherapy, during which he was encouraged to ventilate and abreact. He responded well to this treatment and was discharged after three weeks. On six-month follow-up, he was essentially symptom-free and had returned to college.

EPIDEMIOLOGY

The epidemiology of post-traumatic stress disorder naturally varies with the occurrence of disasters and traumatic situations affecting large numbers of people. After a devastating disaster, 50 to 80 percent of the survivors may develop the syndrome. The prevalence of post-traumatic stress disorder in the general population is 0.5 percent for men and 1.2 percent for women; children can also develop the disorder. The trauma for men is usually combat experience, and the severity of the syndrome is related to the degree of the trauma. The trauma for women is most often assault or rape. Though post-traumatic stress disorder can appear at any age, owing to the nature of precipitating situations, it is most prevalent in young adults.

ETIOLOGY

The major factors in the etiology of this disorder are the stressor, the social environment of the stressor and the victim, and the character traits of the victim, and his biological vulnerability. The more severe the stressor, the more people will develop the syndrome and the more severe the disorder will be. When the trauma is comparatively mild—for example, an auto accident without fatalities—fewer of those involved develop post-traumatic stress disorder. Being part of a group who live through a disaster sometimes enables a person to deal better with the trauma because others share the experience. On the other hand, survivor guilt sometimes complicates the management of post-traumatic stress.

In general, the very young and the very old have more difficulty coping with traumatic events than those whose trauma occurs in midlife. For example, about 80 percent of young children who sustain a burn injury show symptoms of post-traumatic stress disorder 1 or 2 years after the initial injury. On the other hand, only 30 percent of adults who suffer such injury have a post-traumatic stress disorder after 1 year. Presumably, young children have not yet developed adequate coping mechanisms to deal with the physical and emotional insults of the trauma. Likewise, older people, when compared with younger adults, are likely to have more rigid coping mechanisms and to be less able to muster a flexible approach to dealing with the effects of the trauma. Furthermore, the effects of the trauma may be exacerbated by physical disabilities characteristic of late life, particularly disabilities of the nervous and cardiovascular systems, such as reduced cerebral blood flow, failing vision, palpitations, and arrhythmias. Preexisting psychiatric disability, whether a personality disorder or a more serious condition, also increases the impact of particular stressors.

The availability of social supports may also influence the development, severity, and duration of post-traumatic stress disorder. In general, patients who have a good network of social supports are less likely to develop the disorder or to experience it in its most severe forms. The disorder is more likely to occur in those who are single, divorced, widowed, economically handicapped, or socially deprived.

Biological Theories

Biologically oriented theorists have proposed that patients who develop post-traumatic stress disorder were premorbidly prone to excessive autonomic reactions to stress. Patients with post-traumatic stress disorder show increased release of catecholamine while reexperiencing the trauma. Sleep EEG studies of these patients suggest some similarities with major depressive disorder, as indicated by decreased REM latency and stage 4 sleep. One recent hypothesis posits a release of endogenous opioids caused by reliving the trauma and suggests that intervening symptoms may be the result of an endogenous opioid withdrawal syndrome.

Psychodynamic Theories

The psychoanalytic view of post-traumatic stress disorder is that the trauma reactivates unresolved conflicts from early childhood, including emotional traumas of childhood that had been unconscious. The revival of the childhood trauma results in regression and the use of the defense mechanisms of repression, denial, and undoing. There is a repetition by the ego to relive and thereby master and reduce anxiety. The victim also receives secondary gain from the external world, common forms being monetary compensation, increased attention or sympathy, and the satisfaction of dependency needs. These serve to reinforce the disorder and its persistence. A cognitive view of post-traumatic stress disorder suggests that the brain is trying to process the massive amount of information that the trauma provoked by alternating periods of acknowledging and blocking the event.

CLINICAL SIGNS AND SYMPTOMS

The specific clinical signs and symptoms of the episodes of re-experiencing and numbing are described in DSM-III-R (Table 1). The mental status examination often demonstrates feelings of guilt, rejection, and humiliation. The patient may also describe dissociative states and panic attacks. Illusions and hallucinations may be present. Cogni-

Table 1
Diagnostic Criteria for Post-traumatic Stress Disorder

A. The person has experienced an event that is outside the range of usual human experience and that would be markedly distressing to almost anyone (e.g., serious threat to one's life or physical integrity; serious threat or harm to one's children, spouse, or other close relatives and friends; sudden destruction of one's home or community; or seeing another person who has recently been, or is being, seriously injured or killed as the result of an accident or physical violence).

B. The traumatic event is persistently reexperienced in at least one of the following ways:
(1) Recurrent and intrusive distressing recollections of the event (in young children, repetitive play in which themes or aspects of the trauma are expressed)
(2) Recurrent distressing dreams of the event
(3) Sudden acting or feeling as if the traumatic event were recurring (includes a sense of reliving the experience, illusions, hallucinations, and dissociative [flashback] episodes, even those that occur upon awakening or when intoxicated)
(4) Intense psychological distress at exposure to events that symbolize or resemble an aspect of the traumatic event, including anniversaries of the trauma

C. Persistent avoidance of stimuli associated with the trauma or numbing of general responsiveness (not present before the trauma), as indicated by at least three of the following:
(1) Efforts to avoid thoughts or feelings associated with the trauma
(2) Efforts to avoid activities or situations that arouse recollections of the trauma

(3) Inability to recall an important aspect of the trauma (psychogenic amnesia)
(4) Markedly diminished interest in significant activities (in young children, loss of recently acquired developmental skills such as toilet training or language skills)
(5) Feeling of detachment or estrangement from others
(6) Restricted range of affect (e.g., unable to have loving feelings)
(7) Sense of a foreshortened future (e.g., does not expect to have a career, marriage, children, or a long life)

D. Persistent symptoms of increased arousal (not present before the trauma), as indicated by at least two of the following:
(1) Difficulty falling or staying asleep
(2) Irritability or outbursts of anger
(3) Difficulty concentrating
(4) Hypervigilance
(5) Exaggerated startle response
(6) Physiologic reactivity upon exposure to events that symbolize or resemble an aspect of the traumatic event (e.g., a woman who was raped in an elevator breaks out in a sweat when entering any elevator)

E. Duration of the disturbance (symptoms in B, C, and D) of at least one month.

Specify delayed onset if the onset of symptoms was at least 6 months after the trauma.

Table from DSM-III-R *Diagnostic and Statistical Manual of Mental Disorders*, ed 3, revised. (Current Classification of Mental Disorders, 1987.) Copyright American Psychiatric Association, Washington, D.C., 1987. Used with permission.

tive testing may reveal that the patient has impairments of memory and attention. Associated symptoms are aggression, violence, poor impulse control, and alcohol and drug dependence. Patients have elevated Sc, D, F, and Ps scores on the MMPI, and the Rorschach often includes aggressive and violent material.

COURSE AND PROGNOSIS

The full syndrome of post-traumatic stress usually develops some time after the trauma. The delay can be as little as 1 week or as long as 30 years. Symptoms can fluctuate over time and may be more intense during periods of stress. Approximately 30 percent of patients recover, 40 percent have mild symptoms, 20 percent have moderate symptoms, and 10 percent remain unchanged or become worse. A good prognosis is predicted by rapid onset of symptoms, shorter duration of symptoms (less than 6 months), good premorbid functioning, strong social supports, and the absence of any other psychiatric or medical problems.

DIAGNOSIS, SUBTYPES, AND DIFFERENTIAL DIAGNOSIS

The specific criteria for diagnosis are included in DSM-III-R (Table 1). A subtype of delayed onset is diagnosed if the onset of symptoms occurs more than 6 months after the traumatic event.

A major consideration in the diagnosis of post-traumatic stress disorder is the possibility that the patient also has incurred a head injury during the trauma. Other organic considerations that can both cause and exacerbate the symptoms are alcohol and drug dependencies. The psychiatric differential diagnosis includes factitious disorder, malingering, adjustment reaction, borderline personality disorder, schizophrenia, depression, panic disorder, and generalized anxiety disorder. One of the most common problems concerns the misdiagnosis of post-traumatic disorder as one of these other syndromes, resulting in inappropriate treatment of the condition. It is particularly important to consider posttraumatic stress disorder in patients who have pain disorders, substance abuse, other anxiety disorders, or mood disorders.

CLINICAL MANAGEMENT

Pharmacotherapy

Tricyclic antidepressants, especially amitriptyline and imipramine, and phenelzine are the drugs most often used. They are particularly indicated when depression or panic disorder–like symptoms are present. Increasing numbers of clinicians report therapeutic success with clonidine, and there are a few reports suggesting that propranolol may be an effective treatment. Antipsychotic medications may be necessary for brief periods during treatment if behavior is particularly agitated.

Psychotherapy

Many clinicians advocate time-limited psychotherapy for the victims of trauma. Such therapy usually takes a cognitive approach and also provides support and security. The short-term nature of the psychotherapy minimizes the risk of dependency and chronicity. Issues of suspicion, paranoia, and trust, however, often adversely affect compliance. In this disorder, the therapist should overcome the patient's denial of the traumatic event, encourage him to relax, and remove him from the source of the stress. The patient should be encouraged to sleep, using medication if necessary. Support from the environment (e.g., friends and relatives) should be provided. The patient should be encouraged to review and abreact emotional feelings associated with the traumatic event and plan for future recovery.

Group therapy and family therapy have been reported to be effective in treating these patients. Group therapy has been particularly successful with Vietnam veterans. Family therapy often helps sustain a marriage through periods of exacerbated symptoms. Hospitalization may be necessary when symptoms are particularly severe or there is a risk of suicide or other violence.

References

Bleich A, Siegel B, Garb R: Post-traumatic stress disorder following combat exposure: Clinical features and psychopharmacological treatment. Br J Psychiatry 149:365, 1986.

Breslau N, Davis G C: Post-traumatic stress disorder: The etiologic specificity of wartime stressors. Am J Psychiatry 144(5):578, 1987.

Brett E A, Ostroff R: Imagery and post-traumatic stress disorder: An overview. Am J Psychiatry 142:417, 1985.

Hogben G L, Cornfield R B: Treatment of traumatic war neurosis with phenelzine. Arch Gen Psychiatry 38:440, 1981.

Horowitz M J: Stress response syndromes: Character style and brief psychotherapy. Arch Gen Psychiatry 31:768, 1974.

Horowitz M J: Stress Response Syndromes. Jason Aronson, 1976.

Kinzie J D, Fredrickson R H, Ben R: Post-traumatic stress disorder among survivors of Cambodian concentration camps. Am J Psychiatry 141:645, 1984.

Kolb L C: A neuropsychological hypothesis explaining post-traumatic stress disorders. Am J Psychiatry 144:8, 1987.

Kolk B, Greenberg M, Boyd H: Inescapable shock, neurotransmitters, and addiction to trauma: Toward a psychobiology of post-traumatic stress. Biol Psychiatry 20:314, 1985.

Krupnock J L and Horowitz M J: Stress response syndromes. Arch Gen Psychiatry 38:428, 1981.

Mason J W, Giller E L, Kosten T R: Urinary free-cortisol levels in post-traumatic stress disorder patients. J Nerv Ment Dis 174:145, 1986.

Solomon Z, Weisenberg M, Zevald J S, Mikulincer M: Post-traumatic stress disorder among frontline soldiers with combat stress reaction: The 1982 Israeli experience. Am J Psychiatry 144(4):448, 1987.

18.7 ————
Generalized Anxiety Disorder

According to DSM-III-R, generalized anxiety disorder is a chronic (longer than 6 months) disorder characterized by unrealistic or excessive anxiety and worry about two or more life circumstances. Persons who have generalized anxiety disorder seem to be pathologically anxious about everything.

EPIDEMIOLOGY

Many studies have suggested that generalized anxiety disorder is present in 2 to 5 percent of the general population. However, some studies have suggested that generalized anxiety disorder is not this common and that many patients so diagnosed actually have one of the other anxiety disorders. The ratio of females to males is approximately two to one; however, the sex ratio of patients receiving inpatient treatment for this disorder is closer to one to one. The disorder most often develops in the 20s, although persons of any age can be affected. Only one third of patients who have generalized anxiety disorder actually seek psychiatric treatment. Many go to their general practitioners, cardiologists, or pulmonary specialists.

ETIOLOGY

It is presumed that noradrenergic, GABAergic, and serotonergic systems in the frontal lobe and limbic system are involved in the pathophysiology of the disorder. These patients tend to have increased sympathetic tone and both overrespond and adapt more slowly to stimuli of the autonomic nervous system. A variety of EEG abnormalities have been noted in alpha rhythm and evoked potentials. Sleep EEG studies have reported increased sleep discontinuity, decreased delta sleep, decreased stage 1 sleep, and reduced REM complement—changes that are different from those seen in depression.

There is genetic evidence that some aspects of this disorder may be inherited. Approximately 25 percent of first-degree relatives are affected, female relatives more often than males. Male relatives are more likely to have an alcohol-related disorder. Although the twin studies are controversial, some report a concordance rate of 50 percent in monozygotic twins and 15 percent in dizygotic twins.

The psychosocial theories involve the principles discussed previously about the genesis of anxiety in an individual (for a more complete overview of this topic see the Sections on Normal Anxiety and Pathological Anxiety).

CLINICAL SIGNS AND SYMPTOMS

The clinical signs and symptoms are listed in the DSM-III-R guidelines (Table 1). It has been reported that there are less severe and fewer cardiac and respiratory symptoms in generalized anxiety disorder than there are in panic disorder, but that the gastrointestinal and muscular symptoms are similar in intensity. Depression is a common feature. It is important to elicit the cause or focus of a patient's anxiety since such information is necessary for the differential diagnosis.

COURSE AND PROGNOSIS

By definition, generalized anxiety disorder is a chronic condition that may well be lifelong. As many as 25 percent of these patients go on to develop panic disorder. DSM-III-R notes that it occasionally follows a major depressive episode.

DIAGNOSIS

The diagnosis is made according to the criteria listed in DSM-III-R (Table 1). The focus of the anxiety cannot be a single item, and it cannot be related to the anticipatory anxiety seen in panic disorder or the obsession in obsessive-compulsive disorder. If a patient has a mood disorder, in order for the diagnosis of generalized anxiety disorder to be made, the symptoms of anxiety must be present in the absence of active mood disorder symptoms. There are no specific subtypes of generalized anxiety disorder.

The differential diagnosis of generalized anxiety disorder includes all medical disorders that may cause anxiety (see Table 5, in the Section Panic Disorder and Agoraphobia). It is particularly important to rule out caffeine intoxication, stimulant abuse, alcohol withdrawal, and sedative or hypnotic withdrawal. The mental status examination and history should carefully explore the diagnostic possibilities of panic disorder, phobias, and obsessive-compulsive disorder. Other diagnostic possibilities to be considered are adjustment disorder with anxious mood, depression, dysthymia, schizophrenia, somatization disorder, and depersonalization disorder. The following illustrates a case of generalized anxiety disorder:

A 27-year-old, married electrician complains of dizziness, sweating palms, heart palpitations, and ringing of the ears of more

Table 1
Diagnostic Criteria for Generalized Anxiety Disorder

A. Unrealistic or excessive anxiety and worry (apprehensive expectation) about two or more life circumstances (e.g., worry about possible misfortune to one's child who is in no danger and worry about finances for no good reason, for a period of 6 months or longer, during which the person has been bothered more days than not by these concerns. In children and adolescents, this may take the form of anxiety and worry about academic, athletic, and social performance).

B. If another Axis I disorder is present, the focus of the anxiety and worry in A is unrelated to it (e.g., the anxiety or worry is not about having a panic attack as in Panic Disorder), being embarrassed in public (as in Social Phobia), being contaminated (as in Obsessive Compulsive Disorder), or gaining weight (as in Anorexia Nervosa).

C. The disturbance does not occur only during the course of a Mood Disorder or a psychotic disorder.

D. At least six of the following 18 symptoms are often present when anxious (do not include symptoms present only during panic attacks):

Motor tension

(1) trembling, twitching, or feeling shaky
(2) muscle tension, aches, or soreness
(3) restlessness
(4) easy fatigability

Autonomic hyperactivity

(5) shortness of breath or smothering sensations
(6) palpitations or accelerated heart rate (tachycardia)
(7) sweating, or cold clammy hands
(8) dry mouth
(9) dizziness or lightheadedness
(10) nausea, diarrhea, or other abdominal distress
(11) flushes (hot flashes) or chills
(12) frequent urination
(13) trouble swallowing or "lump in throat"

Vigilance and scanning

(14) feeling keyed up or on edge
(15) exaggerated startle response
(16) difficulty concentrating or "mind going blank" because of anxiety
(17) trouble falling or staying asleep
(18) irritability

E. It cannot be established that an organic factor initiated and maintained the disturbance (e.g., hyperthyroidism, Caffeine Intoxication).

Table from DSM-III-R *Diagnostic and Statistical Manual of Mental Disorders,* ed 3, revised. (Current Classification of Mental Disorders, 1987.) Copyright American Psychiatric Association, Washington, D.C., 1987. Used with permission.

than eighteen months' duration. He has also experienced dry throat, periods of uncontrollable shaking, and a constant "edgy" and watchful feeling that often interfered with his ability to concentrate. These feelings have been present most of the time over the previous two years; they have not been limited to discrete periods.

Because of these symptoms he had seen a family practitioner, a neurologist, a neurosurgeon, a chiropractor, and an ENT specialist.

He had been placed on a hypoglycemic diet, received physiotherapy for a pinched nerve, and told he might have "an inner ear problem."

For the past two years he has had few social contacts because of his nervous symptoms. Although he has sometimes had to leave work when the symptoms became intolerable, he continues to work for the same company for which he has worked since his apprenticeship following high school graduation. He tends to hide his symptoms from his wife and children, to whom he wants to appear "perfect," and reports few problems with them as a result of his nervousness.

Discussion

Symptoms of motor tension (uncontrollable shaking), autonomic hyperactivity (dizziness, sweating palms, heart palpitations), and vigilance and scanning ("a constant 'edgy' and watchful feeling") suggest an anxiety disorder. Since the symptoms are not limited to discrete periods, as in panic disorder, and are not focused on a discrete stimulus, as in a phobic disorder, the diagnosis is generalized anxiety disorder.

Although the patient has consulted numerous physicians for his symptoms, the absence of preoccupation with fears of having a specific physical disease precludes a diagnosis of hypochondriasis.

DSM-III-R Diagnosis:
Axis I: Generalized Anxiety Disorder

[Adapted with permission from *DSM-III Case Book*. American Psychiatric Association, Washington, D.C., 1981.]

CLINICAL MANAGEMENT

Pharmacologic

The decision to prescribe an anxiolytic drug to patients with generalized anxiety disorder should rarely be made on the first visit. Because of the chronic nature of this disorder, a treatment plan must be carefully thought out.

Benzodiazepines have been the drug of choice for this disorder. In generalized anxiety disorder, these drugs can be prescribed on a *prn* basis so that the patient takes a rapidly acting benzodiazepine when he feels particularly anxious. The alternative approach is to prescribe a standing dose of benzodiazepines for a limited period of time during which psychosocial therapeutic approaches are implemented. There are several problems associated with the use of benzodiazepines in this disorder. Approximately 25 to 30 percent of patients fail to respond, and tolerance and dependence may occur. Some patients also experience impaired alertness while taking these drugs and are therefore at risk for accidents involving automobiles or machinery.

Buspirone, a nonbenzodiazepine anxiolytic, may become the drug of first choice for these patients. Although its onset of effects is delayed, it lacks many of the problems associated with benzodiazepines. It was thought previously that tricyclic antidepressants and monoamine oxidase inhibitors were ineffective in treating generalized anxiety disorder; however, there is some new evidence that this is incorrect. β-adrenergic blocking drugs, such as propranolol, have been used to treat the peripheral symptoms of anxiety, and antihistamines have been used in patients whose abuse potential for benzodiazepine treatment was particularly high.

Psychosocial

Behavioral approaches to generalized anxiety disorder involve emphasis on cognitive coping strategies, relaxation, meditation, and biofeedback.

Psychotherapy is the treatment of choice, especially when combined with antianxiety medication. Once the suitability of the patient for such therapy has been determined, the method of approach will depend on the nature of the problem underlying the anxiety. As a general rule, neurotic difficulties that involve characterological difficulties will require psychoanalysis or one of the more prolonged forms of treatment. If the psychological problem is circumscribed and is related to specific external circumstances, briefer forms of uncovering therapy may be quite effective in freeing patients from their conflicts and relieving them of their symptoms.

Most patients will experience a marked lessening of anxiety when given the opportunity to discuss their difficulties with a concerned and sympathetic physician. Frequently, after the initial hidden precipitants have been determined in the course of a few interviews, the specific supportive technique to be employed may become clear. Reassurance about unrealistic fears, encouragement to face anxiety-provoking situations, and the continued opportunity to talk regularly to the psychiatrist about their problems are all helpful to patients, even if these techniques are not definitively curative. If doctors discover external situations that are anxiety-provoking, they may be able themselves, or with the help of the patients and their families, to change the environment and thus reduce the stressful pressures. It should be remembered that a reduction in symptoms may often allow the patients to function more effectively in their daily work and relationships, which in itself provides new rewards and gratifications that are in themselves therapeutic.

References

Anderson D J, Noyes R Jr, Crowe R R: A comparison of panic disorder and generalized anxiety disorder. Am J Psychiatry *141*:572, 1984.
Barlow D H, Blanchard E B, Vermilyea J A: Generalized anxiety and generalized anxiety disorder: Description and reconceptualization. Am J Psychiatry *143*:40, 1986.
Barlow D H, Cohen A S, Waddell M T: Panic and generalized anxiety disorders: Nature and treatment. Behav Therapy *15*:431, 1984.
Buchsbaum M S, Hazlett E, Sicotte N: Topographic EEG changes with benzodiazepine administration in generalized anxiety disorder. Biol Psychiatry *20*:832, 1985.
Hoehn-Saric R: Comparison of generalized anxiety disorder with panic disorder patients. Psychopharmacol Bull *18*:104, 1982.
Kahn R J, McNair D M, Lipman R S: Imipramine and chlordiazepoxide in depressive and anxiety disorders. Arch Gen Psychiatry *43*:79, 1986.
Lipman R S: Differentiation anxiety and depression in anxiety disorders. Psychopharmacol Bull *18*:69, 1982.
Prusoff B, Klerman G L: Differentiating depressed from anxious neurotic outpatients. Arch Gen Psychiatry *30*:302, 1974.
Raskin M, Peeke H V S, Dickman W et al.: Panic and generalized anxiety disorders: Developmental antecedents and precipitants. Arch Gen Psychiatry *29*:687, 1982.
Reynolds C F, Shaw D H, Newton T F: EEG sleep in outpatients with generalized anxiety: A preliminary comparison with depressed outpatients. Psychiatric Res *8*:81, 1983.

19

Somatoform Disorders

INTRODUCTION

The somatoform disorders are characterized by physical symptoms that resemble medical disease but that exhibit no organic pathology or known pathophysiological mechanism. DSM-III-R categorizes six types of somatoform disorders: (1) somatization disorder, (2) conversion disorder, (3) somatoform pain disorder, (4) hypochondriasis, (5) body dysmorphic disorder, and (6) undifferentiated somatoform disorder. DSM-III-R also includes a seventh category, somatoform disorder not otherwise specified, for disorders that cannot be classified as any of the previous categories.

SOMATIZATION DISORDER

Definition

Somatization disorder is a chronic syndrome of multiple somatic symptoms that cannot be explained medically and is associated with psychosocial distress and medical help-seeking. The DSM-III-R diagnosis (Table 1) requires a history of several years' duration, beginning before the age of 30. The somatic symptoms must not be caused by medical disease or by medication, drugs, or alcohol; and they must be troublesome enough to cause the patient to take a medication other than aspirin, to visit a physician, or to alter his or her life-style. These diagnostic symptoms must come from among a list of symptoms, which are clustered into seven groups (Table 1). There is no requirement regarding the distribution of the symptoms among the groups.

Somatization disorder was first known as hysteria, a term first used in the 1850s to describe the syndrome as it appears today. It was also called Briquet's syndrome, after the French physician who identified patients with medical symptoms but no demonstrable medical disease.

Epidemiology

Somatization disorder probably occurs in 1 to 2 percent of all females, although some studies show lower rates. It is much more common in women than in men and is inversely related to social position, occurring more often among the less educated, the poor, and those of lower occupational status. It begins before the age of 30 and most often in the late teens.

Somatization disorder tends to run in families, occurring in 10 to 20 percent of the first-degree female relatives of somatization disorder patients. Within these families, first-degree male relatives are prone to alcoholism, drug abuse, and antisocial personality disorder. One study also reported a concordance rate of 29 percent in monozygotic twins and 10 percent in dizygotic twins.

Etiology

The etiology of somatization disorder is unknown, although its familial aggregation suggests genetic or environmental factors. Social, cultural, and ethnic factors that foster somatization in general may have an etiological role in the disorder or at least contribute to its expression. Parental teaching and parental example, as well as cultural and ethnic mores, teach some children to somatize. In addition, many patients come from unstable homes and have been physically abused.

Some studies suggest a neuropsychological basis for somatization disorder. They propose that such patients have characteristic attentional and cognitive impairments that result in the faulty perception and assessment of somatosensory input. The reported impairments include excessive distractibility, inability to habituate to repetitive stimuli, the grouping of cognitive constructs on an impressionistic basis, and partial and circumstantial associations.

Clinical Description

Patients with somatization disorder have a multitude of somatic complaints and long, complicated, medical histories. Nausea and vomiting (other than during pregnancy), difficulty swallowing, pain in the arms and legs, shortness of breath unrelated to exertion, amnesia, and complications of pregnancy and menstruation are among the most common symptoms. The belief that a person has been sickly most of his or her life is also common.

Psychological distress and interpersonal problems are prominent, with anxiety and depression being the most prevalent psychiatric conditions. Suicide threats are not infrequent, but actual suicide is rare. If suicide does occur, it is usually associated with substance abuse. Three other psychiatric disorders occur with higher than expected frequency in somatization disorder patients: antisocial personality disorder, alcohol abuse, and drug abuse. Such patients' medical histories are circumstantial, vague, im-

Table 1
Diagnostic Criteria for Somatization Disorder

A. A history of many physical complaints or a belief that one is sickly, beginning before the age of 30 and persisting for several years.

B. At least 13 symptoms from the list below. To count a symptom as significant, the following criteria must be met:
   (1) no organic pathology or pathophysiologic mechanism (e.g., a physical disorder or the effects of injury, medication, drugs, or alcohol) to account for the symptom or, when there is related organic pathology, the complaint or resulting social or occupational impairment is grossly in excess of what would be expected from the physical findings
   (2) has not occurred only during a panic attack
   (3) has caused the person to take medicine (other than over-the-counter pain medication), see a doctor, or alter life-style

Symptom list:

Gastrointestinal symptoms:

(1) **vomiting (other than during pregnancy)**
(2) abdominal pain (other than when menstruating)
(3) nausea (other than motion sickness)
(4) bloating (gassy)
(5) diarrhea
(6) intolerance of (gets sick from) several different foods

Pain symptoms:

(7) **pain in extremities**
(8) back pain
(9) joint pain
(10) pain during urination
(11) other pain (excluding headaches)

Cardiopulmonary symptoms:

(12) **shortness of breath when not exerting oneself**
(13) palpitations
(14) chest pain
(15) dizziness

Conversion or pseudoneurologic symptoms:

(16) **amnesia**
(17) **difficulty swallowing**
(18) loss of voice
(19) deafness
(20) double vision
(21) blurred vision
(22) blindness
(23) fainting or loss of consciousness
(24) seizure or convulsion
(25) trouble walking
(26) paralysis or muscle weakness
(27) urinary retention or difficulty urinating

Sexual symptoms for the major part of the person's life after opportunities for sexual activity:

(28) **burning sensation in sexual organs or rectum (other than during intercourse)**
(29) sexual indifference
(30) pain during intercourse
(31) impotence

Female reproductive symptoms judged by the person to occur more frequently or severely than in most women:

(32) **painful menstruation**
(33) irregular menstrual periods
(34) excessive menstrual bleeding
(35) vomiting throughout pregnancy

Note: The seven items in boldface may be used to screen for the disorder. The presence of two or more of these items suggests a high likelihood of the disorder.

Table from DSM-III-R *Diagnostic and Statistical Manual of Mental Disorders*, ed 3, revised. (Current Classification of Mental Disorders, 1987.) Copyright American Psychiatric Association, Washington, D.C., 1987. Used with permission.

precise, inconsistent, and disorganized. They describe their complaints in a dramatic, emotional, and exaggerated fashion, with vivid and colorful language. Such patients confuse temporal sequences and cannot clearly distinguish current symptoms from past history. They are often dressed in an exhibitionistic manner and may be coy or seductive. They are described as dependent, self-centered, hungry for admiration and praise, and manipulative.

Differential Diagnosis

The clinician must always rule out organic causes for the patient's symptoms. Medical disorders that present with nonspecific, transient abnormalities pose the greatest diagnostic difficulty: these include multiple sclerosis, systemic lupus erythematosus, acute intermittent porphyria, hyperparathyroidism, and chronic systemic infections. Moreover, the onset of many somatic symptoms late in life must be presumed to be caused by a medical illness until testing rules it out.

In addition, other disorders must be ruled out. For example, even though patients with generalized anxiety or panic disorder often complain of somatic symptoms, their anxiety or panic supersedes these symptoms. In depression, patients exhibit characteristic cognitive, behavioral, and affective symptoms, which also tend to have an episodic course. Schizophrenic patients are differentiated on the basis of somatic delusions and the characteristic thought disorder, hallucinations, and loss of reality testing.

Conversion symptoms form one of the seven subgroups in somatization disorder; therefore, multiple recurrent conversion reactions beginning before age 30 should be diagnosed as somatization disorder. The symptoms of somatization disorder are not, however, restricted to sensorimotor and neurological complaints; they cover a far broader range. According to DSM-III-R, it is possible to diagnose concurrently both somatization disorder and conversion disorder.

Hypochondriasis is distinguished from somatization disorder in that it includes the conviction and fear of disease as well as bodily preoccupation, and it usually begins after age 30. Somatoform pain patients have symptoms limited to pain but in other ways may be quite similar to individuals with somatization disorder.

Prognosis

Somatization disorder is a chronic condition that runs a fluctuating course, and so patients are rarely entirely asymptomatic. It is unusual for them to go for more than a year without some medical attention. But they do not appear to have a significantly higher mortality rate than does the general population.

Treatment

Somatization patients need a long-term, emphatic relationship with a single physician, as the more physicians are involved, the more opportunities such patients have for manipulation and for unnecessary medical interventions.

Psychotherapy is helpful to patients with somatization disorder and has been shown to decrease somatization disorder patients' personal health care expenditures by 50 percent, largely by decreasing their rates of hospitalization, but without lowering their functional status or satisfaction with medical care. In psychotherapy, patients are helped to cope with their symptoms and possibly to eliminate them.

In treating somatization disorder patients, psychotropic medications and prescription analgesics should be avoided, although some clinicians feel that antianxiety agents and antidepressants are helpful when anxiety or depression is prominent. In any case, medications must be carefully monitored because somatization disorder patients tend to use them erratically and unreliably.

CONVERSION DISORDER

Definition

In conversion disorder, there is a loss or change in bodily functioning that results from a psychological conflict or need. Such bodily symptoms cannot be explained by any known medical disorder or pathophysiological mechanism. Conversion disorder patients are not conscious of the psychological basis for their symptoms and so they cannot

Table 2
Diagnostic Criteria for Conversion Disorder

A. A loss of, or alteration in, physical functioning suggesting a physical disorder.

B. Psychological factors are judged to be etiologically related to the symptom because of a temporal relationship between a psychosocial stressor that is apparently related to a psychological conflict or need and initiation or exacerbation of the symptom.

C. The person is not conscious of intentionally producing the symptom.

D. The symptom is not a culturally sanctioned response pattern and cannot, after appropriate investigation, be explained by a known physical disorder.

E. The symptom is not limited to pain or to a disturbance in sexual functioning.

Specify: single episode or recurrent.

Table from DSM-III-R *Diagnostic and Statistical Manual of Mental Disorders,* ed 3, revised. (Current Classification of Mental Disorders, 1987.) Copyright American Psychiatric Association, Washington, D.C., 1987. Used with permission.

control them voluntarily. The DSM-III-R diagnostic criteria appear in Table 2.

Epidemiology

The incidence and prevalence of conversion disorders are unclear. In some surveys, the lifetime incidence of conversion symptoms is as high as 25 to 33 percent. The prevalence among general hospital inpatients receiving psychiatric consultations has been reported to be between 5 and 16 percent. In contrast, the prevalence of conversion reactions among patients in ongoing psychiatric treatment appears to be considerably lower. The annual incidence of conversion disorders in patients seen by general psychiatrists has been reported to be 0.01 to 0.02 percent.

Conversion disorder is between two and five times more common in women than in men and may occur at any age. It is, however, most common in adolescents and young adults, lower socioeconomic groups, rural populations, and those with less education. There is some evidence of a familial aggregation and of a tendency for conversion patients to be the youngest children in their families.

Etiology

According to psychoanalytic theory, conversion is caused by the repression of unconscious intrapsychic conflict and converting the anxiety into a physical symptom. The conflict occurs between an instinctual impulse (e.g., aggressive or sexual) and the prohibitions against its expression. The symptoms allow partial expression of the forbidden wish or urge but disguise it sufficiently so that the patients need not consciously confront their unacceptable impulses. That is, the conversion symptom has a symbolic relationship to the unconscious conflict.

The conversion symptoms also enable the patients to communicate that they need special consideration and special treatment. Such symptoms thus may function as a nonverbal means of controlling or manipulating others.

Some clinicians believe that conversion disorder has a neuropsychological basis, as some conversion patients appear to have a disturbance in their central nervous system arousal. It has been theorized that their symptoms are caused by an excessive cortical arousal that sets off negative feedback loops between the cerebral cortex and the brain stem's reticular formation. Elevated levels of corticofugal output, in turn, inhibit afferent sensorimotor impulses, thus diminishing the awareness of bodily sensation that in some conversion disorder patients could explain the observed sensory deficits. In some conversion disorder patients, neuropsychological tests reveal subtle cerebral impairments in verbal communication and memory, affective incongruity, suggestibility, vigilance, and attention.

Clinical Description

Sensory Symptoms. In conversion disorder, anesthesia and paresthesia are common, especially of the extremities. All sensory modalities are involved, and the distribution of the disturbance is inconsistent with that of either central or peripheral neurological disease. Thus, one sees the characteristic stocking-and-glove anesthesia of the hands or feet or the hemianesthesia of the body beginning precisely along the midline.

Conversion symptoms may involve the organs of special sense, producing deafness, blindness, and tunnel vision. These symptoms may be unilateral or bilateral. Neurological evaluation, however, reveals intact sensory pathways. In conversion blindness, for example, patients walk around without collisions or self-injury; their pupils react to light; and their cortical evoked potentials are normal. Anosmia, vomiting, and pseudocyesis (false pregnancy) are other conversion symptoms.

Motor Symptoms. Motor symptoms include abnormal movements, gait disturbance, weaknesses, and paralyses. Gross rhythmical tremors, as well as choreiform tics and jerks, may be present. These movements generally worsen when attention is called to them. A common gait disturbance is a wildly ataxic, staggering gait accompanied by gross, irregular, jerky truncal movements and thrashing and waving arms (also known as astasia-abasia). But these patients rarely fall, and if they do, they are generally not injured. Convulsive-like movements are also sometimes seen.

Other common motor disturbances are paralysis and paresis, involving one, two, or all four limbs, although the distribution of the involved muscles does not conform to neural pathways. Reflexes remain normal; there are no fasciculations or muscle atrophy (except after long-standing conversion paralysis); and electromyography is normal.

The Presence of Organic Disease. One of the major problems in diagnosing conversion disorder is the difficulty in ruling out a medical disorder. Concomitant organic disease is common in hospitalized patients with conversion symptoms, and evidence of current or prior neurological disorder or of systemic disease affecting the brain has been reported in between 18 and 64 percent of such patients.

Other Associated Features. The absence of a medical etiology is necessary, but not sufficient, for the diagnosis of conversion disorder. A psychological etiology should also be established. DSM-III-R requires the identification of a psychological etiology, as evidenced by a temporal relationship between the symptom and a significant psychosocial stress or by the presence of secondary gain.

Primary gain. Patients achieve primary gain by keeping internal conflicts outside their awareness. The symptom then has symbolic value in that it represents the unconscious psychological conflict.

Secondary gain. Secondary gain refers to the tangible advantages and benefits that accrue to people as a result of their becoming sick, such as being excused from obligations and difficult life situations, receiving support and assistance that might not otherwise be forthcoming, and controlling other people's behavior.

La Belle indifférence. La belle indifférence refers to the patient's inappropriately cavalier attitude toward a serious symptom. That is, the patient seems unconcerned about what appears to be a major impairment. This bland indifference, however, may be lacking in some conversion patients and is also seen in some seriously ill medical patients who develop a stoic attitude.

Identification. Conversion patients may unconsciously model their symptoms on those of someone important to them. For example, a parent or a person who has recently died may serve as a model for the conversion disorder. It is common during the bereaved's pathological grief reaction to develop the symptoms of the deceased.

Differential Diagnosis

Neurological disorders (e.g., dementia and other degenerative diseases), brain tumors, and basal ganglia disease must be ruled out. For instance, weakness may be confused with myasthenia gravis, polymyositis, acquired myopathies, or multiple sclerosis. Optic neuritis may be misdiagnosed as conversion blindness. Signs and symptoms that are inconsistent with anatomic distributions and known pathophysiological mechanisms or that vary from one examination to another are more likely to be caused by conversion disorder than by medical disease. A thorough medical and neurological work-up is thus essential to all cases. If the symptoms can be resolved by suggestion, hypnosis, or intravenous amobarbital (Amytal), the symptoms are probably psychogenic.

Conversion symptoms occur in schizophrenia and in depressive disorder. Schizophrenia, with its dissolution of reality testing and illogical thinking, generally can be distinguished. Depression usually can be separated from conversion disorder because it is more pervasive and lasts longer.

Sensorimotor symptoms occur in somatization disorder as well. But somatization disorder is a more chronic illness, beginning early in life and including symptoms in many other organ systems. DSM-III-R permits both diagnoses concurrently, and patients with repetitive conversion disorder often also meet the criteria for somatization disorder. In hypochondriasis, there is no actual loss or distortion of function. The somatic complaints are more chronic and are not limited to neurologic symptoms, and the characteristic hypochondriacal attitudes and beliefs are present. If the patient's symptoms are limited to pain, then psychogenic pain disorder can be diagnosed. The patient whose complaints are limited to sexual function is diagnosed as having a sexual dysfunction rather than a conversion disorder.

In both malingering and factitious disorders, the symptoms are under conscious, voluntary control. The malingerer's history is usually more inconsistent and contradictory than is the conversion patient's history, and his or her fraudulent behavior is clearly goal directed.

Prognosis

Individual conversion symptoms are generally of short duration, starting and stopping abruptly. About 25 percent of patients develop another conversion symptom during the succeeding 1 to 6 years. There is generally only one symptom during a single conversion episode. Subsequent episodes may involve either the same or a different symptom. Patients with long histories of conversion symptoms and those with many secondary gains do poorly.

Treatment

A thorough medical work-up is essential. If no medical causes are found, the patients can be told that nothing is wrong, that the symptom will eventually subside, and that a psychological approach to managing the problem is indicated. Telling such patients that their symptoms are imaginary will often make things worse rather than better. Psychodynamic approaches include psychoanalysis and insight-oriented psychotherapy, in which patients explore intrapsychic conflict and the symbolism of the conversion symptom. Hypnosis, anxiolytics (for those patients who are unusually anxious), and behavioral relaxation exercises are effective in some cases. An amobarbital (Amytal) interview may be necessary to obtain more history, especially when there has been a specific traumatic event, to help the patient reexperience the traumatic event and to suggest that the symptom will disappear. Briefer and more directive forms of short-term, psychotherapy have also been used to treat conversion disorder. The longer that such patients have been in the sick role and the more that they have regressed, the more difficult the treatment will be.

SOMATOFORM PAIN DISORDER

Definition

In somatoform pain disorder (previously called psychogenic or idiopathic pain disorder in DSM-III), the predominant disturbance is severe and prolonged pain for which there is no medical explanation (Table 3).

Somatoform pain patients do not constitute a uniform or internally cohesive group but, instead, are a collection of heterogenous subgroups of pain, such as low back pain, headache, atypical facial pain, and chronic pelvic pain. The patients' pain may be posttraumatic, neuropathic, neurologic, iatrogenic, or musculoskeletal; some patients may have other major psychiatric disorders, whereas others may have none.

Causes of somatoform pain are presumed to be psychological, even though evidence for them may not be readily apparent in each case. DSM-III-R requires that there be 6 months of preoccupation with pain and that either there be no organic pathology to account for the pain or the pain grossly exceeds whatever demonstrable pathology is present.

Epidemiology

The symptom of pain is perhaps the most frequent complaint in medical practice. Intractable pain syndromes are also common. In 1980, more than $10 billion were spent on disability payments to patients with chronic pain problems. Low back pain alone has disabled an estimated 7 million Americans and accounts for more than 8 million physician office visits yearly.

Somatoform pain disorder is diagnosed two times more frequently in women than in men. The peak age of onset is in the fourth and fifth decades, as the tolerance of pain declines with age. It is also more common among people in blue-collar occupations.

Etiology

Psychodynamics. Pain has unconscious meanings, which originate in infantile and childhood experiences. It is a method of obtaining love, a punishment for wrongdoing,

Table 3
Diagnostic Criteria for Somatoform Pain Disorder

A. Preoccupation with pain for at least six months.
B. Either (1) or (2):
  (1) appropriate evaluation uncovers no organic pathology or pathophysiologic mechanism (e.g., a physical disorder or the effects of injury) to account for the pain
  (2) when there is related organic pathology, the complaint of pain or resulting social or occupational impairment is grossly in excess of what would be expected from the physical findings

Table from DSM-III-R *Diagnostic and Statistical Manual of Mental Disorders*, ed 3, revised. (Current Classification of Mental Disorders, 1987.) Copyright American Psychiatric Association, Washington, D.C., 1987. Used with permission.

and a way of expiating guilt and of atoning for an innate sense of badness. Among the defense mechanisms used are displacement, substitution, and repression. Identification plays a role when the patient takes on the role of an ambivalent love object who also had pain such as a parent. The defense of symbolization is used when the pain represents a nonarticulated affective equivalent.

Learning Theory. Pain behaviors are reinforced when rewarded and are inhibited when ignored or punished. For example, pain symptoms may become more intense when followed by the solicitous and attentive behavior of others, monetary gain, or the successful avoidance of distasteful activities.

Interpersonal. Intractable pain has been conceptualized as a means for manipulation and gaining advantage in interpersonal relationships (e.g., to ensure the devotion of a family member or to stabilize a fragile marriage). Such secondary gain is most important to these patients.

Neurological. The cerebral cortex can inhibit the firing of afferent pain fibers. Serotonin is probably the main neurotransmitter in the descending inhibitory pathways, and endorphins also probably play a role in the central modulation of pain. Endorphin deficiency seems to correlate with the augmentation of incoming sensory stimuli.

Clinical Description

The predominant feature of somatoform pain disorder is a preoccupation with severe and continuous pain of at least 6 months' duration that has no adequate medical explanation. The pain is often inconsistent with the anatomic distribution of the nervous system, but it may sometimes closely mimic the pain distribution of a known disease.

Somatoform pain disorder patients often have long histories of medical and surgical care, visiting many doctors and requesting many medications. They may be especially insistent in their desire for surgery. Indeed, they are completely preoccupied with their pain, citing it as the source of all their misery. Such patients often deny any emotional dysphoria and maintain that the rest of their lives is blissful. They may also have a frequent history of drug abuse or alcoholism.

Major depression is present in about 25 to 50 percent of somatoform pain patients, and dysthymia or depressive symptoms are reported in 60 to 100 percent of these patients. Some investigators believe that chronic pain is almost always a variant of depressive disorder, that it is a masked or somatized form of depression. The most prominent depressive symptoms in such pain patients are anergia, anhedonia, decreased libido, insomnia, and irritability. Diurnal variation, weight loss, and psychomotor retardation appear to be less common.

Differential Diagnosis

Pathologic pain can be difficult to distinguish from psychogenic pain, especially because they are not mutually exclusive. Pathologic pain fluctuates in intensity and is highly sensitive to emotional, cognitive, attentional, and situational influences. Pain that does not vary and is insensitive to any of these factors is more likely to be psychogenic. If the pain does not wax and wane and is not even temporarily relieved by distraction or analgesics, then the clinician can suspect an important psychogenic component.

Pain is among the symptoms of somatization disorder, and both diagnoses may be given if the patient meets the criteria for both disorders. Somatization disorder, however, includes many other physical symptoms, begins before the age of 30, and is rare in men. Hypochondriacs may complain of pain, and their bodily preoccupation and disease conviction are present in somatoform pain patients as well. Hypochondriacs, however, have many symptoms, and their clinical picture fluctuates over time. Conversion disorder is generally short-lived, whereas somatoform pain is chronic; moreover, pain is not, by definition, a conversion symptom. Malingerers consciously provide a false symptom report, and their complaints are connected to a clearly recognizable goal. The differential diagnosis can be difficult because chronic pain patients often receive disability compensation or a litigation award. They are not, however, pretending to be in pain. For example, muscle contraction (tension) headaches have a pathophysiologic mechanism to account for the pain and so are not diagnosed as a somatoform pain disorder.

Prognosis

By definition, somatoform pain lasts for at least 6 months. The pain generally begins abruptly and increases in severity over the next few weeks or months. The prognoses of the various somatoform pain syndromes are not clear, but in general, they are chronic, very disturbing, and disabling. Psychogenic pain may sometimes subside with treatment, after the elimination of external reinforcement or after the successful therapy of associated psychopathology. But more often, it persists for years. The patients with the poorest prognoses, with or without treatment, have preexisting characterological problems, especially pronounced passivity; are involved in litigation or receive financial compensation; use addictive drugs; or have long histories of pain.

Treatment

Treatment aims to rehabilitate the patients rather than cure the pain. It may be useful to discuss the issue of psychologic etiology with the patients early in treatment, telling them frankly that psychological factors are important to the cause and consequence of both pathogenic and psychogenic chronic pain and that treatment must take them into account. However, it must be emphasized at the same time that the patients' pain is "real."

Medical Interventions. Analgesic medications are not helpful for most chronic psychogenic pain. In addition, drug abuse and addiction are often major problems for somatoform pain patients.

Sedatives and antianxiety agents are not especially beneficial and often become problems in themselves because of their frequent abuse, misuse, and side effects. Antidepressants, such as amitryptiline (Elavil), imipramine (Tofranil), and doxepin (Sinequan), are more useful. Whether antidepressants reduce pain via their antidepressant action or exert an independent, direct, analgesic effect (possibly by stimulating the efferent inhibitory pain pathways) remains controversial.

Biofeedback can be moderately helpful, particularly in migraine, myofascial pain, and muscle tension states, such as tension headaches. Hypnosis, transcutaneous nerve stimulation, and dorsal column stimulation have also been used. Nerve blocks and surgical ablative procedures are ineffective for most patients, with pain returning after 6 to 18 months.

Pain Control Programs. It may sometimes be necessary to remove the patients from their usual setting and place them in a comprehensive, inpatient pain control program. These multidisciplinary pain units use many different modalities, such as cognitive, behavioral, and group therapies. They provide extensive patient education, teach relaxation techniques, emphasize improved physical conditioning through physical therapy and exercise, and offer vocational evaluation and rehabilitation. Concurrent psychiatric disorders are diagnosed and treated, and patients addicted to analgesics and hypnotics are detoxified. Inpatient treatment programs generally report encouraging results.

HYPOCHONDRIASIS

Definition

Hypochondriasis is an excessive concern about disease and a preoccupation with one's health. Hypochondriasis is an unrealistic interpretation of physical symptoms and sensations, leading to a preoccupation with the fear or belief of having a serious disease, even though there is no medical disease to account for the physical signs or sensations. This fear or conviction of disease is disabling and persists despite appropriate reassurance (Table 4).

Epidemiology

In general medical practice, hypochondriasis is present in 3 to 14 percent of patients. The prevalence in the general population is unknown. Hypochondriasis is found approximately equally in men and women, but perhaps somewhat more often in men. The peak incidence is thought to occur during the fourth or fifth decades; however, all age groups are affected, particularly adolescents and those over age 60. There is also some evidence of an increased prevalence of

Table 4
Diagnostic Criteria for Hypochondriasis

A. Preoccupation with the fear of having, or the belief that one has, a serious disease, based on the person's interpretation of physical signs or sensations as evidence of physical illness.

B. Appropriate physical evaluation does not support the diagnosis of any physical disorder that can account for the physical signs or sensations or the person's unwarranted interpretation of them, **and** the symptoms in A are not just symptoms of panic attacks.

C. The fear of having, or belief that one has, a disease persists despite medical reassurance.

D. Duration of the disturbance is at least six months.

E. The belief in A is not of delusional intensity, as in Delusional Disorder, Somatic Type (i.e., the person can acknowledge the possibility that his or her fear of having, or belief that he or she has, a serious disease is unfounded).

Table from DSM-III-R *Diagnostic and Statistical Manual of Mental Disorders*, ed 3, revised. (Current Classification of Mental Disorders, 1987.) Copyright American Psychiatric Association, Washington, D.C., 1987. Used with permission.

hypochondriasis among identical twins and other first-degree relatives.

Etiology

Hypochondriasis has a psychodynamic origin. Aggressive and hostile wishes toward others are transferred (repression and displacement) into physical complaints. Hypochondriacs' anger originates in past disappointments, rejections, and losses but is expressed in the present by soliciting other people's help and concern and then rejecting them as ineffective. Hypochondriasis has also been viewed as a defense against guilt, a sense of innate badness, an expression of low self-esteem, and a sign of excessive self-concern. Pain and somatic suffering thus become a means of atonement and expiation (undoing) and can be experienced as deserved punishment for past wrongdoing (either real or imaginary) and the sense that one is wicked and sinful.

Hypochondriasis may have a sociocultural origin. It has been viewed as a request for admission to the sick role made by a person who is facing seemingly insurmountable and insolvable problems. The sick role offers a way out because the sick patient is allowed to avoid noxious obligations and to postpone unwelcome challenges and is excused from onerous duties.

There is some evidence suggesting that hypochondriacs augment and amplify somatic sensations, in that they have lower thresholds for, and a lower tolerance of, physical discomfort. For example, what a normal individual perceives as abdominal pressure, the hypochondriac experiences as abdominal pain. There may also be a faulty cognitive scheme in which the hypochondriac focuses on bodily sensations, misinterprets them, and becomes alarmed by them.

A medical disorder can predispose a patient to hypochondriasis in two ways. First, transient hypochon-

driacal reactions often follow a severe or life-threatening illness (e.g., during recuperation after a myocardial infarction). Second, primary hypochondriacs seem to have had more childhood medical illnesses and more extensive medical histories.

Clinical Description

Hypochondriacs complain of many symptoms involving multiple organ systems and many anatomical locations. The most common complaints are pain and symptoms regarding the gastrointestinal and cardiovascular systems.

Hypochondriacs also believe that they have a serious disease that has not yet been detected, and they cannot be persuaded to the contrary. This conviction persists despite negative laboratory results, a benign course over time, and appropriate reassurance from the physician. But this belief is not so fixed that it is a delusion, nor is it culturally unacceptable.

Transient hypochondriacal reactions occur after major stresses, most commonly the death or serious illness of someone important to the patient or a serious and perhaps life-threatening illness that has been resolved but leaves the patient temporarily hypochondriacal in its wake. Such hypochondriacal states lasting less than 6 months should be diagnosed as somatoform disorder not otherwise specified. Transient hypochondriacal responses to external stress generally remit when the stress is resolved, but they can become chronic if reinforced by people in the patient's social system or by health professionals.

Differential Diagnosis

As with all somatoform disorders, hypochondriasis must be differentiated from organic diseases, especially diffuse illnesses that affect many organ systems (e.g., endocrine disease or connective tissue disease).

Depression is diagnosed if the hypochondriacal symptoms have an episodic course similar to that of recurrent depression or if they appear for the first time in elderly patients who were never before hypochondriacal. Other depressive symptoms, such as hopelessness, suicidal ideas, and low self-esteem, are also present.

Hypochondriacal symptoms are also common in generalized anxiety disorder and panic disorder. According to DSM-III-R, hypochondriasis cannot be diagnosed if the symptoms occur only during panic attacks. Indeed, anxiety disorder patients are often alarmed about their health, have prominent somatic symptoms, and manifest extreme bodily vigilance and disease fears. But for such patients, the hypochondriasis is not the predominant disturbance but is, rather, a feature of a more pervasive disorder.

Hypochondriacal concerns and frank somatic delusions occur in schizophrenia, other psychotic states, and organic brain syndromes. Hypochondriacs' disease conviction is not delusional, and they can entertain, if only briefly, the possibility that they do not have the particular disease they dread. In contrast, somatic delusions are static and unchanging, whereas hypochondriacal symptoms fluctuate over time. In addition, schizophrenics' somatic delusions tend to be bizarre, idiosyncratic, and out of keeping with their cultural milieu.

Some obsessions and phobias may resemble hypochondriasis, but in these cases, the patients know that their symptoms are irrational, excessive, or unrealistic.

The relationship of hypochondriasis to the other somatoform disorders is somewhat unclear. It is possible to diagnose hypochondriasis along with any other somatoform disorder. Somatization disorder does not include disease conviction, disease fear, or bodily preoccupation, and it begins before age 30. The somatization disorder patient is more often female and is more likely to have a hysterical cognitive and interpersonal style, as compared with the more obsessional hypochondriac. These two conditions may, however, overlap significantly. Conversion disorder is acute and transient, involving a single neurological symptom at a time, whereas hypochondriasis is chronic and involves several symptoms in multiple sites and organ systems. If *la belle indifférence* is present in conversion disorder, it will contrast markedly with the hypochondriac's anguish. Somatoform pain disorder is chronic, as is hypochondriasis, but the symptoms are limited to pain. Body dysmorphic disorder patients wish to appear normal but believe that others notice that they are not, whereas hypochondriacs wish to draw attention to themselves and proclaim loudly that they are not normal.

Hypochondriasis is distinguished from factitious disorder with physical symptoms and from malingering in that hypochondriacs actually experience and do not simulate the symptoms they report.

Prognosis

On long-term follow-up, one quarter of hypochondriacs do poorly, and about two thirds run chronic, fluctuating courses. Most hypochondriacal children, however, have been found to have recovered by late adolescence or early adulthood. Treatment helps a significant proportion of patients. Favorable prognostic features include the concurrent presence of anxiety or depression, acute onset, the absence of personality disorder, higher socioeconomic status, younger age, and the absence of organic disease.

Treatment

Hypochondriacs are usually resistant to psychiatric treatment. Some hypochondriacs will accept psychiatric treatment if it takes place in a medical setting and focuses on stress reduction and education in coping with chronic illness. Among such patients, group psychotherapy has been reported to be the modality of choice, in part because it provides the social support and social interaction that these patients need. Individual, insight-oriented, traditional psychotherapy for primary hypochondriasis is generally not successful.

Frequent physical examinations are useful to reassure the patients that they are not being abandoned by their doctors and that their complaints are being taken seriously. Invasive diagnostic and therapeutic procedures, however, should be undertaken only on the basis of objective evidence. When possible, it is best to refrain from treating equivocal or incidental findings.

Pharmacotherapy alleviates hypochondriacal symptoms only when there is an underlying drug-sensitive condition, such as an anxiety disorder or a major depression. When hypochondriasis is secondary to some other primary psychiatric disorder, that entity must be treated in its own right. When hypochondriasis is a transient situational reaction, patients must be helped to cope with the stress without reinforcing their illness behavior and their use of the sick role as solutions to the problem.

BODY DYSMORPHIC DISORDER

Definition

Patients with body dysmorphic disorder (also known as dysmorphophobia) believe that they are physically misshapen or defective in some way, although their appearance is objectively unremarkable. Such patients do not hold this belief with the conviction of a delusion, however (Table 5). According to DSM-III-R, body dysmorphic disorder can be diagnosed as long as anorexia nervosa is absent.

Epidemiology

The average ages of patients with body dysmorphic disorder is 30 years. The sex distribution is unclear.

Etiology

The etiology of body dysmorphic disorder is unknown. Some patients' beliefs are based on another more pervasive psychiatric disorder, such as schizophrenia, mood disorder, or severe personality disorder. Psychodynamically, some persons invest a particular body part with a high level of unconscious meaning that can be traced to an event during an earlier stage of psychosexual development. Important defense mechanisms are repression, dissociation, distortion, symbolization and projection.

Clinical Description

Body dysmorphic disorder patients imagine some defect in their appearance, most commonly in regard to their face,

---

Table 5
Diagnostic Criteria for Body Dysmorphic Disorder

A. Preoccupation with some imagined defect in appearance in a normal-appearing person. If a slight physical anomaly is present, the person's concern is grossly excessive.

B. The belief in the defect is not of delusional intensity, as in Delusional Disorder, Somatic Type (i.e., the person can acknowledge the possibility that he or she may be exaggerating the extent of the defect or that there may be no defect at all).

C. Occurrence not exclusively during the course of Anorexia Nervosa or Transsexualism.

Table from DSM-III-R *Diagnostic and Statistical Manual of Mental Disorders,* ed 3, revised. (Current Classification of Mental Disorders, 1987.) Copyright American Psychiatric Association, Washington, D.C., 1987. Used with permission.

nose, hair, breasts, or genitals. The patients' anguish is intensified in social situations. Secondary symptoms include depression, insomnia, and severe anxiety. Such persons are normal in appearance, although if they do have a slight physical anomaly, their concern is excessive.

Differential Diagnosis

Another underlying primary psychiatric disorder, most commonly schizophrenia, a mood disorder, or an organic brain syndrome (such as that accompanying temporal lobe epilepsy) must be ruled out. Distortions of body image occur in anorexia nervosa, transsexualism, and some specific types of brain damage, and body dysmorphic disorder should not be diagnosed if these conditions are present.

Prognosis

The onset of body dysmorphic disorder is insidious, the concern about one's appearance developing gradually. Indeed, patients often brood about their imagined defect for several years before consulting a physician.

Treatment

Despite intense suffering, these patients tend to refuse psychiatric treatment outright. If another underlying psychiatric disorder is present, that condition should be treated first. Some persons persist in seeking plastic surgery to correct what they perceive as a deformity and so an essential part of a surgeon's diagnostic task—often with the help of a psychiatric consultant—is to identify those with legitimate indications. Pimozide (Orap) is sometimes effective in suppressing the symptoms of body dysmorphic disorder. Most patients retain some concern about their problem, but its intensity is blunted enough to allow them to lead more normal lives. Long-term treatment is necessary, as relapses after discontinuing medication are common. Recent case reports suggest that antidepressants and monoamine oxidase inhibitors may be effective for some patients.

UNDIFFERENTIATED SOMATOFORM DISORDER

DSM-III-R contains one new somatoform disorder, termed undifferentiated somatoform disorder. This diagnosis requires 6 months of multiple physical symptoms without an adequate medical explanation. The symptoms must occur outside the course of any other major psychiatric disorder. The classification of undifferentiated somatoform disorder was created because of the common finding that although cases meeting the full criteria for somatization disorder are relatively rare, many cases of chronic multiple "functional" symptoms are otherwise similar to somatization disorder and do not meet the criteria for any other somatoform disorder (Table 6). These include general fatigue, anorexia, or vague gastrointestinal or urinary symptoms.

Table 6
Diagnostic Criteria for Undifferentiated Somatoform Disorder

A. One or more physical complaints, e.g., fatigue, loss of appetite, gastrointestinal or urinary complaints.

B. Either (1) or (2):
   (1) appropriate evaluation uncovers no organic pathology or pathophysiologic mechanism (e.g., a physical disorder or the effects of injury, medication, drugs, or alcohol) to account for the physical complaints
   (2) when there is related organic pathology, the physical complaints or resulting social or occupational impairment is grossly in excess of what would be expected from the physical findings

C. Duration of the disturbance is at least six months.

D. Occurrence not exclusively during the course of another Somatoform Disorder, a Sexual Dysfunction, a Mood Disorder, an Anxiety Disorder, a Sleep Disorder, or a psychotic disorder.

Table from DSM-III-R *Diagnostic and Statistical Manual of Mental Disorders,* ed 3, revised. (Current Classification of Mental Disorders, 1987.) Copyright American Psychiatric Association, Washington, D.C., 1987. Used with permission.

Table 7
Diagnostic Criteria for Somatoform Disorder Not Otherwise Specified

Disorders with somatoform symptoms that do not meet the criteria for any specific Somatoform Disorder or Adjustment Disorder with Physical Complaints.

Examples:
   (1) an illness involving nonpsychotic hypochondriacal symptoms of less than six months' duration
   (2) an illness involving non-stress-related physical complaints of less than six months' duration

Table from DSM-III-R *Diagnostic and Statistical Manual of Mental Disorders,* ed 3, revised. (Current Classification of Mental Disorders, 1987.) Copyright American Psychiatric Association, Washington, D.C., 1987. Used with permission.

SOMATOFORM DISORDER NOT OTHERWISE SPECIFIED

Somatoform disorder not otherwise specified is a residual category for hypochondriacal symptoms of less than 6 months' duration or for an illness with a single complaint (e.g., malaise, emitting a bad smell). (See Table 7 for the DSM-III-R criteria for this disorder.) For example, patients who fear that they have a symptom of AIDS, although they had no exposure to a putative carrier, can be classified as being in this category.

References

Barsky A J, Klerman G L: Overview: Hypochondriasis, bodily complaints, and somatic styles. Am J Psychiatry *140*:273, 1983.
Engel G: Psychogenic pain and the pain-prone patient. Am J Med *26*:899, 1959.
Ford C V: *The Somatizing Disorders. Illness as a Way of Life.* Elsevier Biomedical, New York, 1983.

Kellner R: Functional somatic symptoms and hypochondriasis. Arch Gen Psychiat *42*:821, 1985.

Lazare A: Current concepts in psychiatry: Conversion symptoms. N Engl J Med *305*:745, 1981.

Smith G R, Monson R A: Patients with multiple unexplained symptoms: Their characteristics, functional health, and health care utilization. Arch Int Med *146*:69, 1986.

Smith G R, Monson R A, Ray D C: Psychiatric consultation in somatization disorder: A randomized controlled study. N Engl J Med *314*:1407, 1986.

Sternbach R: *Pain Patients: Traits and Treatment*. Academic Press, New York, 1974.

Swartz M, Hughes D, Blazen D, George L. Somatization disorder in the community. A study of diagnostic concordance among three diagnostic systems. J Nervous and Mental Disease *175*:26, 1987.

Torgersen S: Genetics of somatoform disorders. Arch Gen Psychiatry *43*:502, 1986.

Weintraub M I: *Hysterical Conversion Reactions: A Clinical Guide to Diagnosis and Treatment*. Spectrum Publications, New York, 1983.

20

Dissociative Disorders

According to DSM-III-R, the dissociative disorders are a group of syndromes characterized by a sudden, temporary alteration in the normally integrated functions of consciousness, identity, or motor behavior, so that some part of these functions is lost. In the past, they were known as hysterical neuroses of the dissociative type.

There are five major types of dissociative disorders: psychogenic amnesia, psychogenic fugue, multiple personality, depersonalization disorder, and dissociative disorder not otherwise specified.

PSYCHOGENIC AMNESIA

Definition

Psychogenic amnesia is defined as a sudden inability to recall important personal information already stored in memory. The inability is such that it cannot be explained by ordinary forgetfulness. The capacity to learn new information is retained. Psychogenic amnesia occurs in the absence of underlying brain disease.

Epidemiology

Psychogenic amnesia is the most common type of dissociative disorder. It is more common during periods of war or during natural disasters. The disorder occurs most often in adolescents and young adults and is more common in women than in men.

Etiology

Although some episodes of amnesia occur spontaneously, a careful history usually reveals some precipitating emotional trauma charged with painful emotions and psychological conflict, for example, natural disaster in which a patient may have witnessed severe injuries or feared for his own life. Fantasized or actual expression of an impulse (sexual or aggressive) with which the patient is unable to deal may also act as a precipitant. Amnesia may follow an extramarital affair which the patient finds morally reprehensible. At times, amnesia follows a physical head trauma that is so slight that it does not seem severe enough to have physiologic significance. In some cases, electroconvulsive therapy produces psychogenic amnesia.

Defense Mechanisms. The major defense mechanism in this disorder is dissociation: the person alters consciousness as a way of dealing with an emotional conflict or an external stressor. Secondary defenses include repression (disturbing impulses are blocked from consciousness) and denial (some aspect of external reality is ignored by the conscious mind). Similar defenses are used in the other dissociative disorders.

Clinical Features

The disorder usually begins abruptly, and the patient is usually aware that he has lost his memory. Some patients are upset about the memory loss but others appear to be unconcerned or indifferent. Amnestic patients are usually alert before and after the amnesia occurs. A few patients, however, report a slight clouding of consciousness during the period immediately surrounding the amnestic period.

The amnesia may take one of several forms: (1) *localized amnesia*, the most common type, is characterized by a loss of memory for the events of a short period of time (a few hours to a few days); (2) *generalized amnesia*, the loss of memory for a whole lifetime of experience; (3) *selective* (also known as *systematized*) *amnesia*, failure to recall some, but not all, events during a short period of time; and (4) *continuous amnesia*, characterized by forgetting each successive event as it occurs, although the patient is clearly alert and aware of what is happening in the environment at the time.

Amnesia may have a primary or secondary gain. The patient who is amnestic for the birth of a dead baby achieves primary gain by protecting herself from painful emotions. An example of secondary gain is a soldier who develops sudden amnesia and is removed from combat areas as a result. The DSM-III-R diagnostic criteria for psychogenic amnesia are presented in Table 1.

Differential Diagnosis

The differential diagnosis includes organic mental disorders in which there is a memory disturbance, especially transient global amnesia (TGA). TGA, however, is not related to stress; the memory loss is concentrated on recent rather than remote events, and there is rarely a loss of personal identity. Full return of memory is rare in most organic mental disorders; when it does occur, it does so very gradually. TGA is most common in patients over 65 with underlying vascular disease. In substance-induced intoxication there may be "blackouts," with inability to remember events that occurred during the intoxicated state. In alcohol amnestic disorder, short-term memory loss occurs; that is, events can be remembered immediately after they occur, but the memory fades after a few minutes. This

Table 1
Diagnostic Criteria for Psychogenic Amnesia

A. The predominant disturbance is an episode of sudden inability to recall important personal information that is too extensive to be explained by ordinary forgetfulness.

B. The disturbance is not due to Multiple Personality Disorder or to an Organic Mental Disorder (e.g., blackouts during Alcohol Intoxication).

Table from DSM-III-R Diagnostic and Statistical Manual of Mental Disorders, *ed 3, revised. (Current Classification of Mental Disorders, 1987.) Copyright American Psychiatric Association, Washington, D.C., 1987. Used with permission.*

disorder, also known as Korsakoff's syndrome, is associated with prolonged alcohol abuse. In postconcussion amnesia, the memory disturbance follows head trauma and is often retrograde (as opposed to the anterograde disturbance of psychogenic amnestics) and usually, does not extend beyond 1 week. Hypnosis or amytal interview can often be used to distinguish between the retrograde and anterograde disturbance. Prompt return of memory strongly suggests a psychogenic etiology. Epilepsy leads to sudden memory impairment associated with motor and EEG abnormalities. A history of an aura, head trauma, or incontinence assists in the diagnosis. Malingering, in this case a deliberate attempt to mimic amnesia, may be difficult to confirm. Any possible secondary gain should increase suspicion; information may be gained by questioning the patient while under hypnosis or during an amytal interview.

Course and Prognosis

Amnesia usually terminates very abruptly, and recovery is generally complete with few recurrences. In some cases, especially if there is secondary gain, the condition may last a long time. It is important to restore the lost memories to consciousness as soon as possible; otherwise, the repressed memory may form a nucleus in the unconscious mind for the production of future amnesic episodes.

Treatment

The use of intermediate and short-acting barbiturates, such as thiopental and sodium amobarbital (Amytal) given intravenously, may be used in the treatment to help the patient recover his memory. Hypnosis can be used primarily as a means of relaxing the patient enough to recall what has been forgotten. The patient is placed in a somnolent state at which point mental inhibitions are diminished, the repressed material emerges into consciousness, and is then recalled. Once the lost memories have been retrieved, psychotherapy is generally recommended to help the patient deal with the associated emotions.

PSYCHOGENIC FUGUE

Definition

Fugue is defined as sudden unexpected wandering, often far from home, and an inability to remember one's former life or identity. The person may take on an entirely new identity and a new occupation.

Epidemiology

The disorder is rare and, like psychogenic amnesia, occurs most often during wartime, following natural disasters, or as a result of personal crises with intense conflict.

Etiology

Although it is believed that heavy alcohol abuse may predispose an individual to the disorder, the etiology is believed to be basically psychological. The essential motivating factor appears to be a desire to withdraw from emotionally painful experiences. Patients with mood disorders and certain personality disorders (e.g., borderline, histrionic, and schizoid) are predisposed to fugue states.

Clinical Features

There are several typical features of psychogenic fugue. The patient wanders, in a purposeful way, usually far from home and often for days at a time. During this period, he has complete amnesia for his past life and associations but, unlike the patient with psychogenic amnesia, he is unaware that he has forgotten anything. It is only when he suddenly returns to his former self that he recalls the time antedating the onset of the fugue, but then he remains amnesic for the period of the fugue itself. The patient in a psychogenic fugue does not seem to others to be behaving in an extraordinary way, nor does he give evidence of acting out any specific memory of a traumatic event. On the contrary, the fugue patient leads a quiet, prosaic, somewhat reclusive existence, works at simple occupations, lives modestly, and in general does nothing to draw attention to himself. The DSM-III-R criteria for psychogenic fugue are listed in Table 2.

Differential Diagnosis

Differential diagnosis includes organic mental disorder, although the wandering that occurs in organic conditions is usually not the same complex or socially adaptive type seen in psychogenic fugue. Temporal lobe epilepsy may involve episodes of travel but a new identity is not assumed, and the episodes are generally not precipitated by psychological stress. Psychogenic amnesia presents with a loss of memory as the result of psychologic stress, but there are no episodes of purposeful travel or of a new identity. Malingering may

Table 2
Diagnostic Criteria for Psychogenic Fugue

A. The predominant disturbance is sudden, unexpected travel away from home or one's customary place of work, with inability to recall one's past.

B. Assumption of a new identity (partial or complete).

C. The disturbance is not due to Multiple Personality Disorder or to an Organic Mental Disorder (e.g., partial complex seizures in temporal lobe epilepsy).

Table from DSM-III-R Diagnostic and Statistical Manual of Mental Disorders, *ed 3, revised. (Current Classification of Mental Disorders, 1987.) Copyright American Psychiatric Association, Washington, D.C., 1987. Used with permission.*

be very difficult to distinguish from psychogenic fugue. Any evidence of clear secondary gain should raise suspicions. Hypnosis and amytal interviews are often useful in clarifying the picture.

Course and Prognosis

A fugue is usually brief—hours to days. Less commonly, a fugue may last many months and involve very extensive travel covering thousands of miles. Generally, recovery is spontaneous and rapid. Recurrences are rare.

Treatment

Outside of supportive care no treatment is usually required. If the fugue is particularly prolonged, psychotherapy may facilitate recall of the past identity; techniques such as hypnosis or amytal interviews may be useful.

MULTIPLE PERSONALITY DISORDER (MPD)

Definition

This disorder is characterized by a person's having two or more distinct and separate personalities each of which determines the nature of his behavior and attitudes during the period when it is dominant. The original or host personality is usually amnestic for the other personalities.

Epidemiology

Recent reports suggest that this disorder is not nearly as rare as it has been thought to be. It is most common in late adolescence and young adult life and is much more frequent in women than men. Several studies have demonstrated that the disorder is more common in first-degree biological relatives of people with the disorder than in the general population. There has been a great deal of interest in multiple personality, and its incidence is being reappraised. There are over 350 case reports in the literature.

Etiology

It is believed that severe sexual, physical, or psychological abuse in childhood predisposes a person to this condition. In some studies, a history of sexual abuse was reported in 80 percent of cases. Epilepsy was found in 25 percent of cases in another study. One study of regional cerebral blood flow revealed temporal hyperperfusion in one of the subpersonalities but not in the main personality.

Clinical Features

The transition from one personality to another is sudden, often dramatic. There is generally amnesia during each personality state for the existence of the others and for the events that took place when another personality was dominant. Sometimes, however, one personality state is not bound by such amnesia and retains complete awareness of the existence, qualities, and activities of the other personalities. At other times, personalities are aware of some

or all of the others to varying degrees, and may experience the others as friends, companions, or adversaries. In classic cases, each personality has a fully integrated, highly complex set of associated memories with characteristic attitudes, personal relationships, and behavior patterns. Most often the personalities have proper names; occasionally one or more is given the name of its function, for example "the Protector." On examination, the patient generally shows nothing unusual in his mental status, other than a possible amnesia for periods of varying duration; others are unable to tell from a single, casual encounter that the patient at times leads other lives. Only prolonged contact that affords the opportunity to observe the sudden discontinuities in mental functioning and personality presentation provides this information. See Table 3 for the DSM-III-R diagnostic criteria for this disorder.

The first appearance of the secondary personality or personalities may be spontaneous, or it may emerge in relation to what seems to be a precipitant (including hypnosis or amobarbital interview). The personalities may be of the opposite sex, of different races and ages, and from a different family than the family of origin. The most common subordinate personality is childlike. Often the different personalities are quite disparate, and may even be opposites. In the same person, one of the personalities may be very extroverted, even sexually promiscuous, while others may be introverted, withdrawn, and sexually inhibited. According to DSM-III-R, studies have indicated that different personalities may have different physiologic characteristics (e.g., different eyeglass prescriptions) and different responses on psychological testing (e.g., different I.Q.s).

Differential Diagnosis

The differential diagnosis of multiple personality includes psychogenic fugue and psychogenic amnesia. Both of these dissociative disorders, however, lack the shifts in identity and the awareness of the original identity that are seen in multiple personality. Schizophrenic disorders may be confused with multiple personality only because schizophrenics may be delusional and believe they have many separate identities or report hearing other personalities' voices. In schizophrenia, a formal thought disorder, chronic social deterioration, and other signs are present. Malingering presents a particularly difficult diagnostic problem. Clear secondary gain raises suspicion, while amytal interviews and hypnosis are useful in resolving the diagnosis.

Table 3
Diagnostic Criteria for Multiple Personality Disorder

A. The existence within the person of two or more distinct personalities or personality states (each with its own relatively enduring pattern of perceiving, relating to, and thinking about the environment and self).

B. At least two of these personalities or personality states recurrently take full control of the person's behavior.

Table from DSM-III-R *Diagnostic and Statistical Manual of Mental Disorders,* ed 3, revised. (Current Classification of Mental Disorders, 1987.) Copyright American Psychiatric Association, Washington, D.C., 1987. Used with permission.

Borderline personality disorder may coexist with multiple personality disorder, but often the alteration of personalities is mistakenly interpreted as nothing more than the irritability of mood and self-image that are characteristic of borderline personalities.

Course and Prognosis

The earlier the onset of multiple personality, the worse the prognosis. One or more of the different personalities may function relatively well while others function quite marginally. The level of impairment ranges from moderate to severe, determining variables being the number, type, and chronicity of the various subpersonalities. This disorder is considered the most severe and chronic of the dissociative disorders and recovery generally is incomplete. To compound the diagnostic challenge, individual personalities may have their own separate mental disorders of which—mood, personality, and other dissociative disorders are the most common.

Treatment

Since this condition has been thought to be rare, it is difficult to make definitive generalizations about treatment approaches. However, the treatment that is recognized as achieving some success is intensive insight-oriented psychotherapy. The goal is to provide insight into the conflicts underlying the psychological need for the various personalities, to recall and abreact any precipitating trauma, and to integrate the different personalities into one. Hypnosis and amytal interviews can elicit data and foster abreaction. Pharmacologic therapy has not been very successful; however, if the main personality is depressed or anxious, antidepressant and antianxiety agents can be tried as adjuncts to psychotherapy.

DEPERSONALIZATION DISORDER

Definition

Depersonalization disorder is characterized by a persistent or recurrent alteration in the perception of the self to the extent that the feeling of one's own reality is temporarily lost. In DSM-III-R it is described as the experience of feeling mechanical, being in a dream, or feeling detached from one's body (Table 4). All of these feelings are ego dystonic, and the person maintains intact reality testing.

Some clinicians distinguish between depersonalization and derealization. Depersonalization is the feeling that one's body or one's personal self is strange and unreal; derealization is the perception of objects in the external world as being strange and unreal. Strictly speaking, the distinction provides a more accurate description of each phenomenon than would be achieved by grouping them together under the rubric of depersonalization.

Epidemiology

As an occasional isolated experience in the life of any person, depersonalization is a common phenomenon and is

Table 4
Diagnostic Criteria for Depersonalization Disorder

A. Persistent or recurrent experiences of depersonalization as indicated by either (1) or (2):
  (1) an experience of feeling detached from, and as if one is an outside observer of, one's mental processes or body
  (2) an experience of feeling like an automation or as if in a dream
B. During the depersonalization experience, reality testing remains intact.
C. The depersonalization is sufficiently severe and persistent to cause marked distress.
D. The depersonalization experience is the predominant disturbance and is not a symptom of another disorder, such as Schizophrenia, Panic Disorder, or Agoraphobia without History of Panic Disorder but with limited symptom attacks of depersonalization, or temporal lobe epilepsy.

Table from DSM-III-R *Diagnostic and Statistical Manual of Mental Disorders*, ed 3, revised. (Current Classification of Mental Disorders, 1987.) Copyright American Psychiatric Association, Washington, D.C., 1987. Used with permission.

not necessarily pathological. Studies of incidence indicate that transient depersonalization may occur in as many as 70 percent of a given population, with no significant difference in incidence between men and women. It is a frequent event in children as they develop the capacity for self-awareness, and adults often undergo a temporary sense of unreality when they travel to new and strange places.

Information about the epidemiology of depersonalization of pathological proportions is scanty. In a few recent studies, depersonalization has been found to occur in women at least twice as frequently as in men, and is rarely found in persons over 40 years of age.

Etiology

Depersonalization disorder may be caused by psychological, neurologic, or systemic disease. Experiences of depersonalization have been associated with epilepsy, brain tumors, the use of psychotomimetic drugs, sensory deprivation, and emotional trauma. Depersonalization phenomena have been caused by electrical stimulation of the cortex of the temporal lobes during neurosurgery. Systemic causes include endocrine disorders of the thyroid and pancreas. Anxiety and depression are predisposing factors, as is severe stress such as one experiences in combat or in an auto accident. Depersonalization is frequently a symptom in association with anxiety states, depression, and schizophrenia; it is apparently rare as a pure syndrome.

Clinical Features

The central characteristic of depersonalization is the quality of unreality and estrangement that is attached to conscious experience. Inner mental processes and external events go on seemingly exactly as before, but they "feel" different and no longer seem to have any relation or significance to the person. Parts of the body or the entire physical being may seem foreign, as may mental operations and accustomed behavior. Hemidepersonalization, the patient's feeling that half of the body is unreal or does not exist, may be related to contralateral parietal lobe disease. Anxiety often accompanies the disorder, and many patients complain of distortion in their sense of time and space. Particularly common is the sensation of a change in the patient's body; for instance, the patient may feel that his extremities are bigger or smaller than usual.

An occasional and particularly curious phenomenon is that of doubling; the patient feels that his point of conscious "I-ness" is outside his body, often a few feet overhead, from where he actually observes himself, as if he were a totally separate person. Sometimes the patient believes he is in two different places at the same time, a condition known as *reduplicative paramnesia* or *double orientation*. Most patients are aware of the disturbances in their sense of reality, which is considered one of the salient characteristics of the syndrome. Psychodynamically, there seems to be a heightening of the psychic energy invested in the self-observing ego, the mental function on which the capacity for insight rests.

Differential Diagnosis

Depersonalization may occur as a symptom in numerous other psychiatric syndromes. The common occurrence of depersonalization in patients with depression and schizophrenia should alert the clinician to the possibility that the patient who initially complains of feelings of unreality and estrangement is actually suffering from one of these more common disorders. A carefully taken history and the mental status examination should in most cases disclose the characteristic features of these two illnesses. Because psychotomimetic drugs often induce long-lasting changes in the experience of the reality of self and environment, it is important to inquire about the use of these substances. The presence of other clinical phenomena in patients complaining of unreality should usually take precedence in determining the diagnosis; in general, the label "depersonalization disorder" is reserved for those conditions in which depersonalization constitutes the main and predominating symptom.

The fact that depersonalization phenomena may result from gross disturbances in brain function underlines the necessity for a careful neurologic evaluation, especially when the depersonalization is not accompanied by other more common and obvious psychiatric symptoms. In particular, the possibility of brain tumor or epilepsy should be considered. The experience of depersonalization may be the earliest presenting symptom of a neurologic disorder; therefore, patients complaining of depersonalization phenomena should be followed carefully.

Course and Prognosis

In the large majority of patients, the symptoms first appear suddenly; only a few patients report gradual onset. The disorder starts most often between the ages of 15 and 30 years, but it has been seen in patients as young as 10 years of age; it occurs less frequently after age 30 and almost never in the later decades of life. A few follow-up studies indicate that in more than half the cases, depersonalization

tends to be a long-lasting, chronic condition. In many patients, the symptoms run a steady course without significant fluctuation of intensity; but, they may occur episodically, interspersed with symptom-free intervals. Little is known about precipitating factors, although the disorder has been observed to begin during a period of relaxation after a person has experienced fatiguing psychological stress. The disorder is sometimes ushered in by an attack of acute anxiety that is frequently accompanied by hyperventilation.

Treatment

Little attention has been given to the treatment of patients with depersonalization disorder. At this time there is not sufficient data upon which a specific pharmacologic regimen might be based. However the anxiety usually responds to an antianxiety agent. Any underlying disorder (e.g., schizophrenia) can also be treated pharmacologically. Psychotherapeutic approaches are equally untested. As in all patients with neurotic symptoms, the decision to use psychoanalysis or insight-oriented psychotherapy is determined not by the presence of the symptom itself, but by a variety of positive indications derived from an assessment of the patient's personality, human relationships, and life situation.

DISSOCIATIVE DISORDER NOT OTHERWISE SPECIFIED

This is a residual category for disorders in which the predominant feature is a dissociative symptom that does not meet the criteria for one of the specific dissociative disorders described above (Table 5). According to DSM-III-R, it includes such entities as follows.

(1) *Ganser's Syndrome.* Ganser's syndrome is the voluntary production of severe psychiatric symptomatology, sometimes described as the giving of approximate answers or "talking past the point" (e.g., when asked to multiply four times five, the patient might answer "twenty-one"). This syndrome may occur in persons with other mental disorders such as schizophrenia, depression, toxic states, paresis, alcoholism and factitious disorder. The psychological symptoms generally represent the patient's sense of mental illness rather than any recognized diagnostic category. The syndrome is commonly associated with such dissociative phenomena as amnesia, fugue, perceptual disturbances, and conversion symptoms. Ganser's syndrome is apparently more common in men and in prisoners, although prevalence data and familial patterns are unestablished. A major predisposing factor is the existence of a severe personality disorder. Differential diagnosis may be extremely difficult. Unless the patient is able to admit the factitious nature of the presenting symptoms or unless there is conclusive evidence from objective psychological tests that the symptoms are false, it may be impossible to determine whether the patient has a true major disorder. The disorder may be recognized by its pan-symptomatic nature or by the fact that symptoms are often worse when the patient believes that he is being watched. Recovery from the syndrome is sudden; the patient claims amnesia for the

Table 5
Diagnostic Criteria for Dissociative Disorder Not Otherwise Specified

Disorders in which the predominant feature is a dissociative symptom (i.e., a disturbance or alteration in the normally integrative functions of identity, memory, or consciousness) that does not meet the criteria for a specific Dissociative Disorder

Examples:

(1) Ganser's syndrome: the giving of "approximate answers" to questions, commonly associated with other symptoms such as amnesia, disorientation, perceptual disturbances, fugue, and conversion symptoms

(2) cases in which there is more than one personality state capable of assuming executive control of the individual, but not more than one personality state is sufficiently distinct to meet the full criteria for Multiple Personality Disorder, or cases in which a second personality never assumes complete executive control

(3) trance states (i.e., altered states of consciousness with markedly diminished or selectively focused responsiveness to environmental stimuli). In children this may occur following physical abuse or trauma

(4) derealization unaccompanied by depersonalization

(5) dissociated states that may occur in people who have been subjected to periods of prolonged and intense coercive persuasion (e.g., brainwashing, thought reform, or indoctrination while the captive of terrorists or cultists)

(6) cases in which sudden, unexpected travel and organized, purposeful behavior with inability to recall one's past are not accompanied by the assumption of a new identity, partial or complete

Table from DSM-III-R *Diagnostic and Statistical Manual of Mental Disorders,* ed 3, revised. (Current Classification of Mental Disorders, 1987.) Copyright American Psychiatric Association, Washington, D.C., 1987. Used with permission.

events. Ganser's syndrome was previously classified as a factitious disorder.

(2) *Variants of Multiple Personality Disorder.* Variants do occur; an example would be a case in which there is more than one entity capable of assuming executive control of the individual but only one entity sufficiently complex and integrated to meet the full criteria for multiple personality disorder. Another is a case in which a second personality never assumes complete executive control.

(3) *Trance States.* Trance states are altered states of consciousness with diminished responsivity to environmental stimuli. Children may exhibit repeated amnestic periods or trance-like states following physical abuse or trauma. Possession and trance states are curious and imperfectly understood forms of dissociation. A common example of a trance state is that of the medium who presides over a spiritual seance. Typically, the medium enters a dissociative state, during which time a person from the so-called spirit world takes over much of his conscious awareness and influences his thoughts and speech.

The phenomena associated with automatic writing and crystal gazing are curious but less common manifestations of possession or trance states. In automatic writing, the dissociation affects only the arm and hand that write the message, which often discloses mental contents of which the writer is unaware. Crystal gazing, however, results in a trance state in which visual hallucinations are prominent.

Phenomena related to trance states include highway hypnosis and the similar mental states experienced by airplane pilots. In both, the monotony of moving at high speeds through environments that provide little in the way of distractions to the operator of the vehicle leads to a fixation on a single object—for example, a dial on the instrument panel or the never-ending horizon of a road running straight ahead for miles. A trance-like state of consciousness results in which visual hallucinations may occur and in which the danger of a serious accident is always present. Possibly in the same order of phenomena are the hallucinations and dissociated mental states in patients who have been confined to respirators for long periods of time without adequate environmental distractions.

The religions of many cultures have recognized the fact that the practice of concentration may lead to a variety of dissociative phenomena, such as hallucinations, paralyses, and other sensory disturbances. On occasion, hypnosis may precipitate a self-limited, but sometimes prolonged, trance state.

(4) *Derealization Unaccompanied by Depersonalization.*

(5) *Dissociated States.* Certain degrees of dissociation may occur in persons who have been subjected to periods of prolonged and intense coercive persuasion (e.g., brainwashing, thought reform, or indoctrination while being held captive by terrorists or cultists). Whether these are truly dissociative states is open to question since some evidence, especially in victims of Nazi concentration camps, indicates that such persons are often alexithymic, which results from massive regression rather than from dissociation.

Patients suffering from somnambulism behave in a strange manner that resembles the behavior of someone in a dissociative state. In somnambulism, the patient exhibits an altered state of conscious awareness of his surroundings; he often has vivid hallucinatory recollections of an emotionally traumatic event in the past of which there is no memory during the usual waking state. The patient is out of contact with the environment, appears preoccupied with a private world, and stares into space if the eyes are open. He may appear emotionally upset, speak excitedly in words and sentences that are frequently hard to understand, or engage in a pattern of seemingly meaningful activities that is repeated every time an episode occurs. There is amnesia for the somnambulistic episode once it has ended.

Although amnesia for a period of immediate past experience is found in patients with somnabulism and with localized or general amnesia, the state of consciousness during the period for which they are amnesic differs in character. Somnambulistic patients seem out of touch with their environment and appear as in a dream. Amnestic patients, on the other hand, usually give no indication to observers that there is anything amiss and seem entirely alert both before and after the amnesia occurs.

In DSM-III-R somnabulism is classified as a sleep disorder and is termed "sleepwalking disorder," one of the parasomnias.

References

Braun B, editor: Multiple personality. Psychiatric Clin North Am 7:1, 1984.

Braun B, editor: *Treatment of the Multiple Personality Disorder*. American Psychiatric Press, Washington, D C, 1986.

Confer W N, Ables B S: *Multiple Personality: Etiology, Diagnoses, and Treatment*. Human Sciences Press, New York, 1983.

Dysken M W: Clinical usefulness of sodium amobarbital interviewing. Arch Gen Psychiatry 36:789, 1979.

Kiersch T A: Amnesia: A clinical study of ninety-eight cases. Am J Psychiatry 119:57, 1962.

Kluft R, editor: *Childhood Antecedents of Multiple Personality*. American Psychiatric Press, Washington, D C, 1985.

Kluft R P: First-rank symptoms as a diagnostic clue to multiple personality disorder. Am J Psychiatry 144:293, 1987.

Lehman L S: Depersonalization. Am J Psychiatry 131:1221, 1974.

Lowenstein R, Hamilton J, Alogna S, Reid N, DeVries M: Experimental sampling in the study of multiple personality disorder. Am J Psychiatry 144:19, 1987.

Nemiah J: Dissociative amnesia: A clinical and theoretical reconsideration. In *Functional Disorders of Memory*. J Kihlstrom, editor, p 303. Lawrence Erlbaum Associates, Hillsdale, NJ, 1979.

Prince M: *Dissociation of Personality*. Longmans, Green and Co, New York, 1906.

21

—————— # Human Sexuality

21.1 ——————
Normal Sexuality

Human sexual behavior is so diverse and its interrelations with almost every facet of life so complex that a comprehensive understanding of it is extremely difficult. Understanding has been further complicated by age-old prejudices, myths, superstitions, half truths, and erroneous theories. Since the delineation of what is normal in human sexual behavior is beset with difficulties, clinical experience suggests that no delineation should be drawn too rigidly or too narrowly. From a clinical standpoint, sexual behavior may be considered normal even when it does not involve either exclusively monogamous heterosexual intercourse or the use of stimulation techniques confined to the primary sexual organs, or when it does not culminate in the achievement of mutually satisfactory orgasm. Sexual behavior that deviates widely from such delimited standards may not be designated pathological unless the behavior is also compulsive, exclusive, destructive, or accompanied by much anxiety and guilt. Thus, sex outside of marriage, masturbation, and various forms of sexual stimulation involving other than the primary sexual organs may still fall within normal limits, depending on the total context.

PSYCHOSEXUALITY

A person's sexuality is so closely entwined with his total personality—affecting his concept of himself, his relations with others, and his general patterns of behavior—that it is virtually impossible to speak of sexuality as a separate entity. The term "psychosexual" is therefore used to imply personality development and functioning as these are affected by one's sexuality. It is clearly not limited to sexual feelings and behavior alone, nor is it synonymous with libido in the broad Freudian sense.

In Freud's view all pleasurable impulses and activities are *ultimately* sexual and should be so designated from the start. This generalization has led to endless misinterpretations of Freudian sexual concepts by the laity and to confusion of one motivation with another by psychiatrists. For example, some oral activities are directed toward obtaining food, whereas others are directed toward achieving sexual gratification. Just because both are pleasure-seeking behavior and both use the same organ,

they are not, as Freud contended, necessarily sexual. Labeling all pleasure-seeking behavior "sexual" precludes clarification of motivation. On the other hand, a person may use sexual activities for gratification of nonsexual needs, such as dependent, aggressive, or status needs. Although sexual and nonsexual impulses may jointly motivate behavior, the analysis of behavior depends on understanding underlying individual motivations and their interactions.

SEXUAL LEARNING IN CHILDHOOD

Not until Freud described the impact of a child's experience on his character as an adult did the world recognize the universality of sexual activity and sexual learning in children. This concept has had greater effect on treatment and on education than any of the other sexual theories Freud propounded.

Most of the sexual learning experiences in childhood occur without thought on the part of the parent, but the consciousness of sex usually determines the degree of vigor of play, the frequency of father-child and mother-child contacts, the tolerance for aggression, the reinforcement or extinction of activity or passivity and of intellectual, aesthetic, or athletic interests in the child.

It is clear from direct observation of children in various situations that genital play in infants is part of the normal pattern of development. According to Harlow, interaction with mothers and peers is necessary for the development of effective adult heterosexual contacts in monkeys, a finding that has relevance to the normal socialization of children. There is a critical period in development beyond which the infant may be immune or resistant to certain types of stimulation but during which time he is particularly susceptible to such stimuli. The detailed relation of critical periods to psychosexual development has yet to be established; presumably Freud's stages of psychosexual development—oral, anal, phallic, latent, and genital—are only gross approximations.

PSYCHOSEXUAL FACTORS

A person's sexuality is dependent on three interrelated factors: his sexual identity, his gender identity, and his sexual behavior. These factors affect his personality growth, development, and functioning, and their totality is termed "psychosexual factors." Clearly, sexuality is something more than physical sex, coital or noncoital, and something less than every aspect of behavior directed toward attaining pleasure.

Gender and Identity

Gender identity refers to a person's sense of maleness or femaleness. Sexual identity refers to biologic sexual characteristics: chromosomes, external genitalia, internal genitalia, hormonal composition, gonads, and secondary sex characteristics. In normal development, they form a cohesive pattern, so that a person has no doubt about his sex.

Modern embryologic studies have shown that all mammalian embryos—the genetically male and the genetically female—are anatomically female during the early stages of fetal life. Differentiation of the male from the female results from the action of fetal androgen; the action begins about the sixth week of embryonic life and is completed by the end of the third month. Mary Jane Sherfey contends that these observations have "demonstrated conclusively that the concept of the initial anatomical bisexuality or equipotentiality of the embryo is erroneous." Sherfey's refutation has far reaching implications for normal human sexual responsivity and alleged causes of homosexuality and sexual deviations.

By the age of 2 or 3 years, almost everyone has a firm conviction that "I am male" or "I am female." Even if maleness and femaleness develop normally, the person still has the adaptive task of developing a sense of masculinity or femininity.

According to Robert Stoller, gender identity "connotes psychological aspects of behavior related to masculinity and femininity." He considers gender social and sex biological: "Most often the two are relatively congruent, that is, males tend to be manly and females womanly." But sex and gender may develop in conflicting or even opposite ways.

Gender identity results from an almost infinite series of cues derived from experiences with family members, teachers, friends, and co-workers as well as from cultural phenomena. Physical characteristics derived from one's biological sex, such as general physique, body shape, and physical dimensions, interrelate with an intricate system of stimuli, including rewards, punishment, and parental gender labels, to establish gender identity.

The formation of gender identity is based on three factors: parental and cultural attitudes, the infant's external genitalia, and a genetic influence, which is physiologically active by the sixth week of fetal life. Whereas family, cultural, and biological influences may complicate establishment of a sense of masculinity or femininity, the standard and healthy outcome is a relatively secure sense of identification with one biological sex—a stable gender identity.

Gender Role

Related to and in part derived from gender identity is gender role behavior. This is described, in the words of John Money as "all those things that a person says or does to disclose himself or herself as having the status of boy or man, girl or woman, respectively. . . . A gender role is not established at birth but is built up cumulatively through experiences encountered and transacted through casual and unplanned learning, through explicit instruction and inculcation, and through spontaneously putting two and two together to make sometimes four and sometimes, erroneously, five." The standard and healthy outcome is a congruence of gender identity and gender role. Although biological attributes are significant, the major factor in attaining the role appropriate to one's sex is learning.

Gender role can appear to be in opposition to gender identity. A person may identify with his own sex and yet adopt the dress, hairstyle, or other characteristics of the opposite sex (as many of our present teenagers do). Or a person may identify with the opposite sex, yet for expediency adopt much of the behavior characteristic of his own sex.

SEXUAL BEHAVIOR AND RESPONSE

Masturbation

Masturbation is usually a normal precursor of object related sexual behavior. In the words of Dearborn, "No other form of sexual activity has been more frequently discussed, more roundly condemned, and more universally practiced than masturbation." Research by Alfred Kinsey into the prevalence of masturbation indicated that nearly all men and three fourths of all women masturbate sometime during their life.

Longitudinal studies of development show that sexual self-stimulation is very common in infancy and childhood. Just as the infant learns to explore the functions of his fingers and mouth, it is inevitable for him to do the same with his genitalia. At about 15 to 19 months of age, both sexes begin genital self-stimulation. Pleasurable sensations result from any gentle touch to the genital region. These sensations, coupled with the ordinary desire for exploration of one's body, produce a normal interest in masturbatory pleasure at this time. The child also develops an increased interest in the genitalia of others—parents, children, and even animals. As the youngster acquires playmates, this curiosity about his and others' genitalia motivate episodes of exhibitionism or genital exploration. Such experiences, unless blocked by guilty fear, contribute to continued pleasure from sexual stimulation.

With the approach of puberty, the upsurge of sex hormones, and the development of secondary sex characteristics, sexual curiosity is intensified and masturbation increases. The adolescent is physically capable of coitus and orgasm but is usually inhibited by social restraints. He is under the dual and often conflicting pressures of establishing his sexual identity and controlling his sexual impulses. The result is a great deal of physiologic sexual tension that demands release, and masturbation is a normal way of reducing sexual tensions. An important emotional difference between the pubescent child and the youngster of earlier years is the presence of coital fantasies accompanying masturbation in the adolescent. These fantasies are an important adjunct to the development of sexual identity, for in the comparative safety of his imagination, the adolescent learns to perform the adult sex role. This role of autoerotic activity is usually maintained into the young adult years, when it is normally replaced by coitus.

It is incorrect to assume that couples in a sexual relationship abandon masturbation entirely. When coitus is unsatisfactory or is unavailable because of illness or absence of the partner, self-stimulation often serves an adaptive purpose, combining sensual pleasure and tension release.

Moral taboos against masturbation have generated myths that masturbation causes mental illness or a decrease in sexual potency. There is no scientific evidence to support such claims. Masturbation is a psychopathological symptom only when it becomes a compulsion beyond the willful control of the person. It is then a symptom of emotional disturbance, not because it is sexual but because it is compulsive. Masturbation is almost a universal and inevitable aspect of psychosexual development, and in most cases it is adaptive.

Normal Sexual Response

Normal men and women experience a sequence of physiologic responses to sexual stimulation. In the first detailed description of these responses, Masters and Johnson observed that the physiologic process involves increasing levels of vasocongestion and myotonia (tumescence) and the subsequent release of the vascular activity and muscle tone as a result of orgasm (detumescence). The process occurs in four phases: excitement, plateau, orgasm, and resolution (Tables 1 and 2). DSM-III-R offers a somewhat different definition of these phases, and these variations are discussed following the physiologic discussion.

Stages of Sexual Response

Phase I: Excitement. This phase is brought on by psychological stimulation (fantasy or the presence of a love object), physiologic stimulation (stroking or kissing), or a combination of the two. The excitement phase is characterized by vaginal lubrication in the woman and penile erection in the man. The parasympathetic nervous system activates the process of erection. The pelvic splanchnic nerves (S2, S3, and S4) stimulate the blood vessels of the area to dilate, causing the penis to become erect. The nipples of both sexes become erect, although nipple erection is more common in women than in men. The woman's clitoris becomes hard and turgid, and her labia minora become thicker as a result of venous engorgement. The excitement phase may last several minutes to several hours.

Phase II: Plateau. With continued stimulation, the man's testes increase in size 50 percent and elevate. The woman's vaginal barrel shows a characteristic constriction along the outer third, known as the orgasmic platform. The clitoris elevates and retracts behind the symphysis pubis. As a result, the clitoris is not easily accessible. As the area is stimulated, however, traction on the labia minora and the prepuce occurs, and there is intrapreputial movement of the clitoral shaft. Breast size in the woman increases 25 percent. Continued engorgement of the penis and vagina produces specific color changes; these color changes are most marked in the labia minora, which become bright or deep red. Voluntary contractions of large muscle groups occur, rates of heartbeat and respiration increase, and blood pressure rises. The plateau stage lasts 30 seconds to several minutes.

Phase III: Orgasm. A subjective sense of ejaculatory inevitability triggers the man's orgasm. The forceful emission of semen follows. The male orgasm is also associated with four to five rhythmic spasms of the prostate, seminal vesicles, vas deferens, and urethra. In the woman, orgasm is characterized by three to fifteen involuntary contractions of the lower third of the vagina and

by strong sustained contractions of the uterus, flowing from the fundus downward to the cervix. Both men and women have involuntary contractions of the internal and external anal sphincter. These and the other contractions during orgasm occur at intervals of 0.8 second. Other manifestations include voluntary and involuntary movements of the large muscle groups, including facial grimacing and carpopedal spasm. Systolic blood pressure rises 20 mm, diastolic blood pressure rises 40 mm, and the heart rate increases up to 160 beats per minute. Orgasm lasts from 3 to 15 seconds and is associated with a slight clouding of consciousness.

The sympathetic nervous system is involved in ejaculation. Through its hypogastric plexus, the sympathetic nervous system innervates the urethral crest and the muscles of the epididymis, vas deferens, seminal vesicles, and prostate. Stimulation of the plexus causes ejaculation of seminal fluid from those glands and ducts into the urethra. That passage of fluid into the urethra provides the man with a sensation of impending climax called the stage of ejaculatory inevitability. Indeed, once the prostate contracts, ejaculation is inevitable. The ejaculate is propelled through the penis by urethral contractions. The ejaculate consists of about 1 teaspoon (2.5 ml) of fluid and contains about 120 million sperm cells.

Phase IV: Resolution. Resolution consists of the disgorgement of blood from the genitalia (detumescence), which brings the body back to its resting state. If orgasm occurs, resolution is rapid; if it does not occur, resolution may take 2 to 6 hours and be associated with irritability and discomfort. Resolution through orgasm is characterized by a subjective sense of well-being.

Refractory period. After orgasm, men have a refractory period that may last from several minutes to many hours; in that period they cannot be stimulated to further orgasm. The refractory period does not exist in women, who are capable of multiple and successive orgasms. Sexual response is a true psychophysiologic experience. Arousal is triggered by both psychological and physical stimuli, levels of tension are experienced both physiologically and emotionally, and with orgasm, there is normally a subjective perception of a peak of physical reaction and release. Psychosexual development, psychological attitudes toward sexuality, and attitudes toward one's sexual partner are directly involved with and affect the physiology of the human sexual response.

The DSM-III-R Phases of the Sexual Response Cycle. DSM-III-R consolidates the Masters and Johnson excitement and plateau phases into a single excitement phase and precedes it with an appetitive phase. The orgasm and resolution phase remain the same as originally described by Masters and Johnson.

DSM-III-R Phase I: Appetitive. This phase is distinct from any identified solely through physiology and reflects the psychiatrist's fundamental concern with motivations, drives, and personality. The phase is characterized by sexual fantasies and the desire for sexual activity.

DSM-III-R Phase II: Excitement. This phase consists of a subjective sense of sexual pleasure and accompanying physiologic changes. All the physiologic responses noted in Masters and Johnson's excitement and plateau phases are combined under this phase.

DSM-III-R Phase III: Orgasm. This phase consists of a peaking of sexual pleasure, with release of sexual tension and rhythmic contraction of the perineal muscles and pelvic reproductive organs. The phase is identical to Masters and Johnson's Phase III.

DSM-III-R Phase IV: Resolution. This phase entails a sense of general relaxation, well-being, and muscle relaxation. This phase as defined does not differ from the Masters and Johnson resolution phase.

Table 1
The Male Sexual Response Cycle*

	I. Excitement Phase (several minutes to hours)	II. Plateau Phase (30 sec to 3 min)	III. Orgasmic Phase (3–15 sec)	IV. Resolution Phase (10–15 min; if no orgasm, ½–1 day)
Skin	No change	Sexual flush: inconsistently appears; maculopapular rash originates on abdomen and spreads to anterior chest wall, face, and neck and can include shoulders and forearms	Well-developed flush	Flush disappears in reverse order of appearance; inconsistently appearing film of perspiration on soles of feet and palms of hands
Penis	Erection within 10–30 sec caused by vasocongestion of erectile bodies of corpus cavernosa of shaft. Loss of erection may occur with introduction of a sexual stimulus, loud noise	Increase in size of glans and diameter of penile shaft; inconsistent deepening of coronal and glans coloration	Ejaculation: marked by 3 to 4 contractions at 0.8 sec of vas, seminal vesicles, prostate, and urethra; followed by minor contractions with increasing intervals	Erection: partial involution in 5–10 sec with variable refractory period; full detumescence in 5–30 min
Scrotum and testes	Tightening and lifting of scrotal sac and partial elevation of testes toward perineum	50 per cent increase in size of testes over unstimulated state due to vasocongestion and flattening of testes against perineum signaling impending ejaculation	No change	Decrease to base line size due to loss of vasocongestion. Testicular and scrotal descent within 5–30 min after orgasm. Involution may take several hours if there is no orgasmic release
Cowper's glands	No change	2–3 drops of mucoid fluid that contain viable sperm	No change	No change
Other	Breasts: inconsistent nipple erection	Myotonia: semispastic contractions of facial, abdominal, and intercostal muscles. Tachycardia: up to 175 per min Blood pressure: rise in systolic 20–80 mm; in diastolic 10–40 mm Respiration: increased	Loss of voluntary muscular control Rectum: rhythmical contractions of sphincter Up to 180 beats per min 40–100 systolic; 20–50 diastolic Up to 40 respirations per min. Ejaculatory spurt: 12–20 inches at age 18 decreasing with age to seepage at 70	Return to base line state in 5–10 min

*Table prepared by Virginia A. Sadock, M.D., after Masters and Johnson data. In DSM-III-R the excitement phase and the plateau phase are combined into one phase called excitement phase.

LOVE AND INTIMACY

A precise definition of love is difficult. Rado defines love as a sustained emotional response to a known source of pleasure. Accordingly, there are many kinds of love: sexual, parental, filial, fraternal, anaclitic, and narcissistic love, as well as love for group, school, and country. A desire to maintain closeness to the love object typifies being in love. The development of sexuality and the development of the ability to love have reciprocal effects on each other.

When a person is able to give and receive love with a minumum of fear and conflict, he has the capacity to develop genuinely intimate relations with others. When involved in an intimate relationship he actively strives for the growth

Table 2
The Female Sexual Response Cycle*

	I. Excitement Phase (several minutes to hours)	II. Plateau Phase (30 sec to 3 min)	III. Orgasmic Phase (3–15 sec)	IV. Resolution Phase (10–15 min; if no orgasm, ½–1 day)
Skin	No change	Sexual flush in-constant except in fair skinned; pink mottling on abdomen, spreads to breasts, neck, face, often to arms, thighs, and buttocks—looks like measles rash	No change (flush at its peak)	Fine perspiration, mostly on flush areas; flush disappears in reverse order
Breasts	Nipple erection in two thirds of subjects Venous congestion Areolar enlargement	Flush: mottling coalesces to form a red papillary rash Size: increase one fourth over normal, especially in breasts that have not nursed Areolae: enlarge; im-pinge on nipples so they seem to dis-appear	No change (venous tree pattern stands out sharply; breasts may become tremulous)	Return to normal in reverse order of appearance in ½ hour or more
Clitoris	Glans: half of sub-jects, no change vis-ible, but with colpo-scope, enlargement always observed; half of subjects, glans di-ameter always in-creased 2-fold or more Shaft: variable in-crease in diameter; elongation occurs in only 10% of subjects	Retraction: shaft with-draws deep into swollen prepuce; just before orgasm, it is difficult to visualize; may relax and retract several times if phase II is unduly prolonged Intrapreputial move-ment with thrusting: movements syn-chronized with thrust-ing owing to traction on labia minora and prepuce	No change Shaft movements continue throughout if thrusting is main-tained	Shaft returns to nor-mal position in 5–10 sec; full de-tumescence in 5–30 min (if no orgasm, cli-toris remains en-gorged for several hours)
Labia majora	Nullipara: thin down; elevated; flatten against perineum Multipara: rapid con-gestion and edema; increases to 2 to 3 times normal size	Nullipara: totally dis-appear (may reswell if phase II unduly prolonged.) Multipara: become so enlarged and edematous, they hang like folds of a heavy curtain	No change	Nullipara: *increase* to normal size in 1–2 min or less Multipara: *decrease* to normal size in 10–15 min
Labia minora	Color change: to bright pink in nulli-para and red in multi-para Size: increase 2 to 3 times over normal; prepuce often much more; proximal por-tion firms, adding up to ¾ inch to function-al vaginal sidewalls	Color change: sud-denly turn bright red in nullipara, burgundy red in multipara, signifies onset of phase II, orgasm will then always follow within 3 min if stimulation is contin-ued Size: enlarged labia gap widely to form a vestibular funnel into vaginal orifice	Firm proximal areas contract with con-tractions of lower third	Returns to pink blotchy color in 2 min or less; total resolu-tion of color and size in 5 min (decolora-tion, clitoral return and detumescence of lower third all occur as rapidly as loss of the erection in men)

Table 2 *continued*

	I. Excitement Phase (several minutes to hours)	II. Plateau Phase (30 sec to 3 min)	III. Orgasmic Phase (3–15 sec)	IV. Resolution Phase (10–15 min; if no orgasm, ½–1 day)
Bartholin's glands	No change	A few drops of mucoid secretion form; aid in lubricating vestibule (insufficient to lubricate vagina)	No change	No change
Vagina	Vaginal transudate: appears 10–30 sec after onset of arousal; drops of clear fluid coalesce to form a well-lubricated vaginal barrel (aids in buffering acidity of vagina to neutral pH required by sperm) Color change: mucosa turns patchy purple	Copious transudate continues to form; quality of transudate generally increased only by prolonging preorgasm stimulation (increased flow occurs during premenstrual period) Color change: uniform dark purple mucosa	No change (transudate provides maximum degree of lubrication)	Some transudate collects on floor of the upper two thirds formed by its posterior wall (in supine position); ejaculate deposited in this area forming seminal pool
Upper two thirds	Balloons: dilates convulsively as uterus moves up, pulling anterior vaginal wall with it; fornices lengthen; rugae flatten	Further ballooning creates diameter of 2½–3 inches; then wall relaxes in a slow, tensionless manner	No change: fully ballooned out and motionless	Cervical descent: descends to seminal pool in 3–4 min
Lower third	Dilation of vaginal lumen to 1–1¼ in occurs; congestion of walls proceeds gradually, increasing in rate as phase II approaches	Maximum distension reached rapidly; contracts lumen of lower third and upper labia to ½ or more its diameter in phase I; contraction around penis allows thrusting traction on clitoral shaft via labia and prepuce.	3 to 15 contractions of lower third and proximal labia minora at ⅓-sec intervals	Congestion disappears in seconds (if no orgasm, congestion persists for 20–30 min)
Uterus	Ascent: moves into false pelvis late in phase I Cervix: passively elevated with uterus (no evidence of any cervical secretions during entire cycle)	Contractions: strong sustained contractions begin late in phase II; have same rhythm as contractions late in labor, lasting 2+ min. Cervix: slight swelling; patchy purple (inconstant; related to chronic cervicitis)	Contractions throughout orgasm; strongest with pregnancy and masturbation	Descent: slowly returns to normal Cervix: color and size return to normal in 4 min; patulous for 10 min
Others	Fourchette: color changes throughout cycle as in labia minora	Perineal body: spasmodic tightening with involuntary elevation of perineum Hyperventilation and carpopedal spasms; both are usually present, the latter less frequently and only in female-supine position	Irregular spasms continue Rectum: rhythmical contractions inconstant; more apt to occur with masturbation than coitus External urethral sphincter: occasional contraction, no urine loss	All reactions cease abruptly or within a few seconds

*From *The Nature and Evolution of Female Sexuality*, by Mary Jane Sherfey, Copyright 1966, 1972 by Mary Jane Sherfey. Reprinted by permission of Random House, Inc.

and happiness of the loved person. Mature heterosexual love is marked by the intimacy that is a special attribute of the relationship between a man and a woman. The quality of intimacy in a mature sexual relationship is what Rollo May calls an ability of "active receiving," wherein a person, while loving, permits himself to be loved. This capability indicates a profound awareness of love for another as well as for oneself. In such a loving relation, sex acts as a catalyst. May described the values of sexual love as an expansion of one's self-awareness, the experience of tenderness, increase of self-affirmation and pride, and sometimes, at the moment of orgasm, even loss of feelings of separateness. It is in this setting that sex and love are reciprocally enhancing and healthily fused.

The increasing equality of the sexes profoundly affects the choice of love object. A person is attracted to a potential mate for various reasons. One may be a purely physical attraction, which ordinarily establishes a transient relation. Another may be a magical desire to find the perfect lover, whose qualities will be reminiscent of the idealized qualities of one's parents or other past sources of love and affection. Other emotional reasons for choosing a mate stem from a variety of neurotic patterns in one's own personality. For example, one may take a partner to protect pride or security rather than to satisfy feelings of love. A woman who considers herself unattractive sexually may choose a mate who is passive and dependable yet sufficiently unattractive so that she does not have to compete with other women. A man who has considerable doubt about his masculinity may turn to a woman who has great sex appeal on the surface but in reality may not demand exceptional sex drive or performance. Essentially neurotic themes such as these exist in all personalities and probably in all matings. When they predominate and the couple act mainly to exchange patterns of exploitation or when interlocking complementary needs fail to bring sufficient security or happiness, discomfort and anxiety occur, and a breakdown in the relation is possible.

References

Farber, M. *Human Sexuality*. Macmillan, New York, 1985.
Freud S: General Theory of the Neuroses (1917). In S Freud: *The Standard Edition of the Complete Psychological Works of Sigmund Freud*, vol 16, p 241, Hogarth Press, London, 1974.
Harlow H F: The Nature of Love. Am Psychol, *13*:673, 1958.
Kinsey A C, Pomeroy W B, Martin C E: *Sexual Behavior in the Human Male*. W B Saunders, Philadelphia, 1948.
Kinsey A C, Pomeroy W B, Martin C E, Gebbard P H: *Sexual Behavior in the Human Female*. W B Saunders, Philadelphia, 1953.
Kirkpatrick M: *Women's Sexual Development*. Plenum, New York, 1980.
May R: *Love and Will*. W W Norton, New York, 1969.
Masters W H, Johnson V E: *Human Sexual Response*. Little, Brown & Co., Boston, 1966.
Money J, Ehrhardt A A: *Man and Woman/Boy and Girl*. Johns Hopkins University Press, Baltimore, 1972.
Sherfey M J: *The Nature and Evolution of Female Sexuality*. Random House, New York, 1972.
Stoller R J: *Sex and Gender*. Science House, New York, 1968.

21.2
Sexual Disorders

21.2a
Paraphilias

Paraphilias are characterized by specialized sexual fantasies and intense sexual urges and practices which are usually repetitive in nature and distressing to the person. The special fantasy, with its unconscious and conscious components, is the pathognomonic element, sexual arousal and orgasm being associated phenomena. The influence of the fantasy and its behavioral manifestations extend beyond the sexual sphere to pervade the person's life. Paraphilic arousal maybe transient in some persons who act out their impulses only during periods of stress or conflict.

CLASSIFICATION

The major categories of paraphilias included in DSM-III-R are pedophilia, exhibitionism, sexual sadism, sexual masochism, voyeurism, fetishism, transvestic fetishism, frotteurism, and a separate category for other paraphilias not otherwise specified (e.g., zoophilia). A given person may have multiple paraphilic disorders.

EPIDEMIOLOGY

Among legally identified cases, pedophilia is far more common than the other perversions. Ten to 20 percent of children have been molested by age 18. Because a child is the object, the act is taken more seriously, and greater effort is spent tracking down the culprit than in other paraphilias. Exhibitionists, who publicly display themselves to young children, are also commonly apprehended. Voyeurs may be apprehended, but their risk is not great. Twenty percent of adult females have been the targets of exhibitionists and voyeurs. Sexual masochism and sadism are underrepresented in any prevalence estimates. Sexual sadism usually comes to attention only in sensational cases of rape, brutality, or lust murder. The excretory perversions are scarcely reported, since any activity usually takes place between consenting adults or between prostitute and client. Fetishists ordinarily do not become entangled in the legal system. Transvestites may be arrested occasionally on disturbing-the-peace or other misdemeanors if they are obviously men dressed in women's clothes, but arrest is more common among the gender identity disorders. Zoophilia, as a true paraphilia, is rare.

As usually defined, the sexual perversions seem to be largely male conditions. In the gender identity disorders, the ratio of clinically active men to women is about two to one. Fetishism almost always occurs in men.

Over 50 percent of all paraphilias have their onset prior to age 18. Paraphiliacs frequently have three to five different paraphilias, either concomitantly or at different times in their lives. This is especially the case with exhibitionism, fetishism, masochism, sadism, transvestic fetishism, voyeurism, and zoophilia.

The occurrence of paraphilic behavior peaks between ages 15 and 25 and gradually declines; in men of 50 paraphilic acts are rare, except for those that occur in isolation or with a cooperative partner.

ETIOLOGY

Psychosocial Model

In the psychoanalytic model, a paraphiliac is a person who has failed to complete the normal developmental process toward heterosexual adjustment. What distinguishes one paraphilia from another is the method chosen by the person (usually male) to cope with the anxiety caused by the threat of (1) castration by the father and (2) separation from the mother. However bizarre its manifestation, the resulting perversion provides an outlet for the sexual and aggressive drives that would otherwise have been channeled into proper gender behavior.

Failure to resolve the oedipal crisis by identifying with the father-aggressor (for boys) or mother-aggressor (for girls) will result either in improper identification with the opposite gender parent or in an improper choice of object for libido cathexis. Regardless of current DSM-III-R classifications, according to psychoanalytic theory, homosexuality, transsexualism, and transvestic fetishism are all considered perversions since each demonstrates identification with the opposite instead of the same gender parent. For instance, a male dressing in women's clothes is believed to identify with his mother. Exhibitionism and voyeurism, however, are also seen as expressions of feminine identification since the paraphiliac must constantly examine his own or others' genitals to calm his anxiety about castration. Fetishism is an attempt to avoid anxiety by displacing libidinal impulses to inappropriate objects. The shoe fetishist unconsciously denies that women have lost their penises through castration by attaching libido to a phallic object, the shoe, that symbolizes the female penis. Both pedophiles and sexual sadists share a need to dominate and control their victims, as though to compensate for their feelings of powerlessness during the oedipal crisis. The sexual masochist overcomes his fear of injury and sense of powerlessness by demonstrating that he is impervious to harm. Although recent developments in psychoanalysis place more emphasis on treating defense mechanisms than oedipal traumas, the course of psychoanalytic therapy for the paraphiliac remains consistent with Freud's theory.

Other theories attribute the development of paraphilia to early experiences that condition or socialize the child into committing a paraphilic act. The first shared sexual experience can be important in this regard. Molestation as a child can predispose the person toward being the recipient of continued abuse as an adult or, conversely, of becoming an abuser of others. The onset of paraphilic acts can result from modeling the behavior of others who have carried out paraphilic acts, mimicking sexual behavior depicted in the media, or recalling emotionally laden events from one's past, such as one's own molestation. Learning theory suggests that since fantasizing of paraphilic interests begins at such an early age and

because personal fantasies and thoughts are not shared with others (who could block or discourge such ideas), the use and misuse of paraphilic fantasies and urges continues uninhibited until late in life. Only at this time does he begin to realize that such paraphilic interests and urges are inconsistent with societal norms. Unfortunately, by this time, the repetitive use of such fantasies has become chronic; the person's sexual thoughts and behaviors have become associated with or conditioned to paraphilic fantasies.

Organic

A number of studies have begun to identify abnormal organic findings in paraphiliacs. None has used random samples of paraphiliacs; they are, instead, extensive investigations of paraphiliacs who have been referred to large medical centers. Of those paraphiliacs evaluated at referral centers who had positive organic findings, 74 percent had abnormal hormone levels, 27 percent had hard or soft neurologic signs, 24 percent had chromosomal abnormalities, 9 percent had seizures, 9 percent had dyslexia, 4 percent had abnormal EEGs (without seizures), 4 percent had major psychiatric disorders, and 4 percent were mentally retarded. The remaining question, however, is whether these abnormalities are etiologically related to paraphilic interest or are incidental findings that bear no relevance to the development of paraphilic interests.

Psychophysiologic tests have been developed to measure penile volumetric size in response to paraphilic and nonparaphilic stimuli. This procedure may be of use in diagnosis and treatment, but is now only investigative.

PEDOPHILIA

Pedophilia involves recurrent intense sexual urge or arousal to children 13 years of age or younger that has persisted over a minimum of 6 months. The person diagnosed as a pedophile should be at least 16 years of age and at least 5 years older than the victim (Table 1). When the paraphiliac is younger than 16, clinical judgment should determine whether the diagnosis is warranted (given the maturity of the perpetrator and victim).

The vast majority of child molestations involve genital fondling or oral sex. Vaginal or anal penetration of the child is an infrequent occurrence except in cases of incest.

Table 1
Diagnostic Criteria for Pedophilia

A. Over a period of at least 6 months, recurrent intense sexual urges and sexually arousing fantasies involving sexual activity with a prepubescent child or children (generally age 13 or younger).

B. The person has acted on these urges, or is markedly distressed by them.

C. The person is at least 16 years old and at least 5 years older than the child or children in A.

Note: Do not include a late adolescent involved in an ongoing sexual relationship with a 12- or 13-year-old.

Table from DSM-III-R *Diagnostic and Statistical Manual of Mental Disorders*, ed 3, revised. (Current Classification of Mental Disorders, 1987.) Copyright American Psychiatric Association, Washington, D.C., 1987. Used with permission.

Although the majority of child victims coming to public attention are female, this finding appears to be a product of the referral process. Offenders report that when they actually touch the child, the majority (60 percent) of victims are male. This figure is in sharp contrast to nontouching victimization of children, such as window-peeping or exhibitionism, which in 99 percent of cases is perpetrated against female children. Moreover, 95 percent of pedophiles are heterosexual, and 50 percent have consumed alcohol to excess at the time of the incident. In addition to their pedophilia, a significant number of pedophiles are concomitantly or have previously been involved in exhibitionism, voyeurism, or rape.

Although not classifiable as a perversion in the true sense, incest is superficially related to pedophilia by the frequent selection of an immature child as a sex object, the subtle or overt element of coercion, and occasionally, the preferential nature of the adult-child liaison.

EXHIBITIONISM

Exhibitionism is the recurrent urge and desire to expose the genitals to a stranger or an unsuspecting person (Table 2). Sexual excitement occurs in anticipation of the exposure, and orgasm is brought about by masturbation during or after the event. In almost 100 percent of cases, exhibitionists are males exposing themselves to females.

The dynamic of the exhibitionist is to assert his masculinity by showing his penis and by watching the reaction of the victim—fright, surprise, disgust. Unconsciously, these men feel castrated and impotent. Wives of exhibitionists often substitute for the mother to whom the patient was excessively attached during childhood.

In other related perversions, the central themes involve derivatives of looking or showing. For example, in obscene phone calling, tension and arousal begin in anticipation of phoning, an unsuspecting partner is involved, the recipient of the call listens while the telephoner verbally exposes his preoccupations or induces her to talk about her sexual activity, and the conversation is accompanied by masturbation, which is often completed after the contact is interrupted.

SEXUAL SADISM

The DSM-III-R diagnostic criteria for sexual sadism are presented in Table 3. The onset is usually before the age of 18 years and most sadists are men. According to psychoanalytic theory, sadism is a defense against fears of castration—the person does to others what he fears will happen to him. Pleasure is derived from expressing the aggressive instinct. The disorder was named after the Marquis de Sade, an 18th century French author, who was repeatedly imprisoned for his violent sexual acts against women. Sexual sadism is related to rape, although the latter is more aptly considered a form of aggression. Some sadistic rapists, however, kill their victims after having sex (so-called lust murders). In most cases, these persons have an underlying schizophrenic disorder.

Table 2
Diagnostic Criteria for Exhibitionism

A. Over a period of at least 6 months, recurrent intense sexual urges and sexually arousing fantasies involving the exposure of one's genitals to an unsuspecting stranger.

B. The person has acted on these urges, or is markedly distressed by them.

Table from DSM-III-R *Diagnostic and Statistical Manual of Mental Disorders,* ed 3, revised. (Current Classification of Mental Disorders, 1987.) Copyright American Psychiatric Association, Washington, D.C., 1987. Used with permission.

Table 3
Diagnostic Criteria for Sexual Sadism

A. Over a period of at least 6 months, recurrent intense sexual urges and sexually arousing fantasies involving acts (real, not simulated) in which the psychological or physical suffering (including humiliation) of the victim is sexually exciting to the person.

B. The person has acted on these urges, or is markedly distressed by them.

Table from DSM-III-R *Diagnostic and Statistical Manual of Mental Disorders,* ed 3, revised. (Current Classification of Mental Disorders, 1987.) Copyright American Psychiatric Association, Washington, D.C., 1987. Used with permission.

SEXUAL MASOCHISM

Masochism takes its name from the activities of Leopold von Sacher-Masoch, a 19th century Austrian novelist whose characters derived sexual pleasure from being abused and dominated by women. According to DSM-III-R, there is a recurrent preoccupation with sexual urges or fantasies of being humiliated, beaten, bound, or otherwise made to suffer (Table 4). Masochistic practices are more common among men. Freud believed masochism to result from destructive fantasies turned against the self. In some cases, persons can allow themselves to experience sexual feelings only if punishment for them follows. About 30 percent of masochists also have sadistic fantasies and are known as sadomasochists. Moral masochism involves a need to suffer but is not accompanied by sexual fantasies; it is a controversial category called "self-defeating personality" in DSM-III-R.

VOYEURISM

Voyeurism is the recurrent preoccupation with fantasies or acts that involve seeking out or observing people who are naked, or are engaged in grooming or in sexual activity (Table 5). It is also known as "scoptophilia." Masturbation to orgasm usually occurs during or after the event. The first voyeuristic act usually occurs during childhood and is most common in men. Voyeurs are usually apprehended for loitering.

Table 4
Diagnostic Criteria for Sexual Masochism

A. Over a period of at least 6 months, recurrent intense sexual urges and sexually arousing fantasies involving the act (real, not simulated) of being humiliated, beaten, bound, or otherwise made to suffer.

B. The person has acted on these urges, or is markedly distressed by them.

Table from DSM-III-R *Diagnostic and Statistical Manual of Mental Disorders,* ed 3, revised. (Current Classification of Mental Disorders, 1987.) Copyright American Psychiatric Association, Washington, D.C., 1987. Used with permission.

Table 5
Diagnostic Criteria for Voyeurism

A. Over a period of at least 6 months, recurrent intense sexual urges and sexually arousing fantasies involving the act of observing an unsuspecting person who is naked, in the process of disrobing, or engaging in sexual activity.

B. The person has acted on these urges, or is markedly distressed by them.

Table from DSM-III-R *Diagnostic and Statistical Manual of Mental Disorders,* ed 3, revised. (Current Classification of Mental Disorders, 1987.) Copyright American Psychiatric Association, Washington, D.C., 1987. Used with permission.

FETISHISM

In fetishism, the sexual focus is on objects (e.g., shoes, gloves, pantyhose, or stockings) that are intimately associated with the human body (Table 6). The particular fetish is linked to someone closely involved with the patient during his childhood and has some quality associated with this loved, needed, or even traumatizing person. Usually the disorder begins by adolescence, although the fetish might have been established in childhood. Once established, this disorder tends to be chronic.

Sexual activity may be directed toward the fetish itself (e.g., masturbation with or into a shoe) or the fetish may be incorporated in sexual intercourse (e.g., with the demand that high-heeled shoes be worn). The disorder is almost exclusively male. In females, kleptomania (compulsive stealing) may produce sexual excitement. According to Freud, the fetish serves as a symbol of the phallus because the fetishist has unconscious castration fears. Learning theorists believe that the object was associated with sexual stimulation at an early age.

TRANSVESTIC FETISHISM

Transvestic fetishism or transvestism is marked by fantasized or actual dressing in female clothes for purposes of arousal and as an adjunct to masturbation or coitus (Table 7). Transvestism typically begins in childhood or early adolescence. As years pass, some individuals with trans-

Table 6
Diagnostic Criteria for Fetishism

A. Over a period of at least 6 months, recurrent intense sexual urges and sexually arousing fantasies involving the use of nonliving objects by themselves (e.g., female undergarments).

Note: The person may at other times use the nonliving object with a sexual partner.

B. The person has acted on these urges, or is markedly distressed by them.

C. The fetishes are not only articles of female clothing used in cross-dressing (Transvestic Fetishism) or devices designed for the purpose of tactile genital stimulation (e.g., vibrator).

Table from DSM-III-R *Diagnostic and Statistical Manual of Mental Disorders,* ed 3, revised. (Current Classification of Mental Disorders, 1987.) Copyright American Psychiatric Association, Washington, D.C., 1987. Used with permission.

vestism want to dress and live permanently as women. Usually, more than one article of clothing is involved; frequently, an entire wardrobe is involved. When a transvestite is cross-dressed, the appearance of femininity may be quite striking, although usually not to the degree found in transsexualism. When not dressed in women's clothes, transvestite men may be hypermasculine in appearance and occupation. Cross-dressing itself exists on a gradient from solitary, depressed, guilt-ridden dressing to ego-syntonic, sociable membership in a transvestite subculture.

The overt clinical syndrome of transvestism may begin in latency, but it is more often seen around pubescence or in adolescence. Frank dressing in women's clothes usually does not begin until mobility and relative independence from parents are fairly well established.

FROTTEURISM

This disorder is characterized by the male rubbing his penis against the buttocks or body of a fully clothed woman to achieve orgasm (Table 8). It usually occurs in crowded places, particularly subways and buses. The frotteur is extremely passive and isolated and this is often his only source of sexual gratification.

Table 7
Diagnostic Criteria for Transvestic Fetishism

A. Over a period of at least 6 months, in a heterosexual male, recurrent intense sexual urges and sexually arousing fantasies involving cross-dressing.

B. The person has acted on these urges, or is markedly distressed by them.

C. Does not meet the criteria for Gender Identity Disorder of Adolescence or Adulthood, Nontranssexual Type, or Transsexualism.

Table from DSM-III-R *Diagnostic and Statistical Manual of Mental Disorders,* ed 3, revised. (Current Classification of Mental Disorders, 1987.) Copyright American Psychiatric Association, Washington, D.C., 1987. Used with permission.

Table 8
Diagnostic Criteria for Frotteurism

A. Over a period of at least 6 months, recurrent intense sexual urges and sexually arousing fantasies involving touching and rubbing against a nonconsenting person. It is the touching, not the coercive nature of the act, that is sexually exciting.

B. The person has acted on these urges, or is markedly distressed by them.

Table from DSM-III-R *Diagnostic and Statistical Manual of Mental Disorders,* ed 3, revised. (Current Classification of Mental Disorders, 1987.) Copyright American Psychiatric Association, Washington, D.C., 1987. Used with permission.

PARAPHILIAS NOT OTHERWISE SPECIFIED

This group of atypical paraphilias is extremely varied and does not meet the criteria for any of the aforementioned categories.

Zoophilia

In zoophilia, animals—which may be trained to participate—are preferentially incorporated into arousal fantasies or sexual activities, including intercourse, masturbation, and oral-genital contact. Zoophilia as an organized perversion is rare. For a number of people, animals are the major source of relatedness, so it is not surprising that a broad variety of domestic animals are sensually or sexually used.

Sexual relations with animals may occasionally be an outgrowth of availability or convenience, especially in parts of the world where rigid convention precludes premarital sexuality or in situations of enforced isolation. Masturbation, however, is also available in such situations, so it is reasonable to suspect that some predilection for animal contact is present in opportunistic zoophilia.

Coprophilia

This is sexual pleasure associated with the desire to defecate on a partner, to be defecated upon, or to eat feces (coprophagia). A variant is the compulsive utterance of obscene words (coprolalia). These paraphilias are associated with fixation at the anal stage of psychosexual development. Similarly the use of enemas as part of sexual stimulation (klismaphilia) is related to anal fixation.

Urophilia

Also known as urolagnia, urophilia is sexual pleasure associated with the desire to urinate on a partner or to be urinated upon; it is a form of urethral eroticism. It may be associated with masturbatory techniques involving the insertion of foreign objects into the urethra for sexual stimulation in both men and women.

Oralism

Mouth-genital contact—such as cunnilingus (oral contact with the vagina), fellatio (oral contact with the penis), and analingus (oral contact with the anus)—is an activity normally associated with foreplay. Freud recognized the mucosal surfaces of the body as being erotogenic and capable of producing pleasurable sensation. When a person uses these activities as the sole source of sexual gratification and cannot or refuses to have coitus, a paraphilia exists. It is also known as *partialism,* which refers to focusing on one part of the body to the exclusion of all else.

Necrophilia

Necrophilia is the act of obtaining sexual gratification from cadavers. Most necrophiles find corpses for the exploitation of their perversion from morgues or elsewhere. Some of them have been known to rob graves. At times, the individual murders in order to satisfy his perversion. In the few cases studied, the necrophile believed that he was inflicting the most conceivable humiliation on his lifeless victim. According to Richard Krafft-Ebing, the diagnosis of psychosis is, under all circumstances, justified.

Masturbation

Masturbation is a normal activity that is common in all stages of life from infancy to old age. It was not always thought to be so. Freud believed neurasthenia to be caused by excessive masturbation. In the early 1900s, "masturbatory insanity" was a common diagnosis in hospitals for the criminally insane in the United States. It can be defined as achieving personal sexual pleasure—usually resulting in orgasm—by oneself (autoeroticism). Kinsey found it to be more prevalent in males than in females but this discrepancy may no longer exist. The frequency of masturbation varies from three to four times per week in adolescence to one to two times per week in adulthood. It is not uncommon among married people; Kinsey reported that it occured on the average of once a month.

Techniques of masturbation vary in both sexes and among individuals. Most common is direct stimulation of the clitoris or penis with the hand or fingers. Indirect stimulation may also be used, such as rubbing against a pillow or squeezing the thighs. Kinsey found that 2 percent of women are capable of achieving orgasm through fantasy alone. Men and women have been known to insert objects into the urethra to achieve orgasm, and most recently, the hand vibrator has been used as a masturbatory device by both sexes. Masturbation is abnormal when it is the only type of sexual activity preferred or performed or when it is done with such frequency as to indicate a sexual dysfunction.

Hypoxyphilia

Newly classified in DSM-III-R, hypoxyphilia refers to the desire to achieve an altered state of consciousness secondary to hypoxia while experiencing orgasm. In this disorder, the person may use a drug (e.g., a volatile nitrite or nitrous oxide) that produces hypoxia. Autoerotic asphyxiation is also associated with hypoxic states but should be classified as a form of sexual masochism.

Telephone Scatologia

More commonly known as obscene phone calls, telephone scatologia is related to voyeurism in that the person attempts to demonstrate his masculinity to a stranger.

DIAGNOSIS

In DSM-III-R, the criteria for paraphilia include the presence of the pathognomonic fantasy and its behavioral elaboration. The fantasy contains unusual sexual material that is relatively fixed and shows only minor variations. The achievement of arousal and orgasm depends on mental elaboration or behavioral playing out of the fantasy. Sexual activity is ritualized or stereotyped and makes use of degraded, reduced, or dehumanized objects.

The clinician needs to differentiate paraphilia from experimentation in which the act is done for its novel effect and not recurrently or compulsively. This activity is most likely to occur during adolescence. Some paraphilias (especially the more bizarre) are part of another disorder (e.g., schizophrenia). Organic brain syndromes may release perverse impulses.

PROGNOSIS

Poor prognosis is associated with early age of onset, high frequency of acts, no guilt or shame about the act, and alcoholism or drug abuse. The prognosis is better when there is a history of coitus in addition to the paraphilia, high motivation for change, and when the patient is self-referred rather than referred by a legal agency.

TREATMENT

Insight-oriented psychotherapy is the most common approach to treating the paraphilias. The patient has the opportunity to understand his dynamics and the events that caused the paraphilia to develop. In particular, he becomes aware of the daily events that cause him to act on his impulses (e.g., after a real or fantasized rejection). Psychotherapy also allows the person to regain self-esteem and to improve interpersonal skills and find acceptable methods for sexual gratification. Group therapy is also of use in this regard.

Behavior therapy is used to disrupt the learned paraphilic pattern. Noxious stimuli (e.g., electric shocks or bad odors) have been paired with the impulse, which then diminishes. The stimuli can be self-administered and used by the patient whenever he feels he will act on the impulse.

Drug therapy, including antipsychotic or antidepressant medication, is indicated for the treatment of schizophrenia or depression if the paraphilia is associated with those disorders. Antiandrogens, such as cyproterone acetate in Europe and medroxyprogesterone acetate (Depo-provera) in the United States, have been used experimentally in hypersexual perversions. In some carefully selected cases, there have been reports of decreases in the hypersexual behavior. Medroxyprogesterone acetate seems to be of benefit for those patients whose driven hypersexuality (e.g., virtually constant masturbation, sexual contact at every opportunity, compulsively assaultive sexuality) is out of control or dangerous.

References

Abel G G, Blanchard E B: The role of fantasy in the treatment of sexual deviation. Arch Gen Psychiatry *30:*467, 1974.

Berlin F S, Meinecke C F: Treatment of sex offenders with antiandrogenic medication: Conceptualization, review of treatment modalities, and preliminary findings. Am J Psychiatry *3:*237, 1981.

Blair C D, Lanyon R I: Exhibitionism: Etiology and treatment. Psych Bull *89:*439, 1981.

Cook M, Howells K: *Adult Sexual Interest in Children.* Academic Press, New York, 1981.

Freud S: Three essays on the theory of sexuality. In S Freud: *The Standard Edition of the Complete Works of Sigmund Freud,* vol 7, Hogarth Press, London, 1905.

Gange P: Treatment of sex offenders with medroxyprogesterone acetate. Am J Psychiatry *138:*644, 1981.

Kinsey A, Pomeroy W, Martin C E: *Sexual Behavior in the Human Male.* W B Saunders, Philadelphia, 1948.

Krafft-Ebing R: *Psychopathia Sexualis.* Stein and Day, New York, 1965.

Lief H, editor: *Sex Problems in Medical Practice.* American Medical Association, Chicago, 1981.

Levine S M, Stava L: Personality Characteristics of Sex Offenders: A Review Arch. Sexual Behav. *16:* 57, 1987

Slag, M F: Impotence in medical clinic outpatients. JAMA *249:*1736, 1983

21.2b _____

Sexual Dysfunctions and Other Sexual Disorders

Six major categories of sexual dysfunction are listed in DSM-III-R: (1) sexual desire disorders; (2) sexual arousal disorders; (3) orgasm disorders (4) sexual pain disorders; (5) sexual dysfunction not otherwise specified, and (6) other sexual disorders, a residual category for a miscellaneous group of disorders that are not classifiable in any of the previous categories.

It is useful to think of the dysfunctions as disorders related to a particular phase of the sexual response cycle. Thus, sexual drive disorders are associated with the first phase of the response cycle, known as the appetitive phase. Table 1 lists each of the DSM-III-R phases of the sexual response cycle and the sexual dysfunctions usually associated with it.

Sexual dysfunctions can be symptomatic of biological problems (biogenic), intrapsychic, or interpersonal conflicts (psychogenic), or a combination of these factors. Sexual function can be adversely affected by stress of any kind, by emotional disorders, or by ignorance of sexual function and physiology. The dysfunctions may be lifelong or develop after a period of normal functioning. The dysfunction may be generalized or situational, that is, limited to a specific partner or a certain situation, and it may be total or partial.

In considering each of the disorders, the clinician needs to rule out a physical disorder that could account for or contribute to the dysfunction. If the disorder is biogenic, it is coded on Axis III in DSM-III-R; if psychogenic, it is coded on Axis I. If both psychogenic and biogenic factors are involved (e.g., a sexual arousal disorder secondary to both diabetes and intrapsychic conflict) both codes may be

Table 1
The DSM-III-R Phases of the Sexual Response Cycle and Associated Sexual Dysfunctions

Phases	Characteristics	Dysfunction
I: Appetitive	This phase is distinct from any identified solely through physiology and reflects the patient's motivations, drives, and personality. The phase is characterized by sexual fantasies and the desire to have sex.	Hypoactive Sexual Desire Disorder; Sexual Aversion Disorder
II: Excitement	This phase consists of a subjective sense of sexual pleasure and accompanying physiological changes. All the physiological responses noted in Masters and Johnson's excitement and plateau phases are combined and occur under this phase.	Female Sexual Arousal Disorder; Male Erectile Disorder (may also occur in Stage III and Stage IV)
III: Orgasm	This phase consists of a peaking of sexual pleasure, with release of sexual tension and rhythmic contraction of the perineal muscles and pelvic reproductive organs.	Inhibited Female Orgasm (Anorgasmia); Inhibited Male Orgasm (Retarded Ejaculation) Premature Ejaculation
IV: Resolution	This phase entails a sense of general relaxation, well-being, and muscle relaxation. During this phase men are refractory to orgasm for a period of time that increases with age whereas women are capable of having multiple orgasms without a refractory period.	Postcoital Dysphoria Postcoital Headache

*DSM-III-R consolidates the Masters and Johnson excitement and plateau phases into a single excitement phase which is preceded by the appetitive phase. The orgasm and resolution phase remain the same as originally described by Masters and Johnson.

used. In some cases, a patient may suffer from more than one dysfunction (e.g., hypoactive sexual desire disorder and sexual aversion disorder).

SEXUAL DESIRE DISORDERS

Sexual desire disorders (previously called inhibited sexual desire) are divided into two classes: hypoactive sexual desire disorder, characterized by deficiency or absence of sexual fantasies and desire for sexual activity (Table 2) and sexual aversion disorder, characterized by an aversion to and avoidance of genital sexual contact with a sexual partner (Table 3). The former condition is more common than the latter; however, the true incidence of both disorders is unknown.

Masters and Johnson reported lack of desire to be one of the most common complaints among married couples, with women more affected than men. In one study, 35 percent of women (and 15 percent of men) complained of having no desire for sexual activity.

A variety of etiological factors are associated with sexual desire disorder. Patients with desire problems often use inhibition of desire in a defensive way to protect against unconscious fears about sex. Unacceptable homosexual impulse could also suppress libido or cause an aversion to heterosexual contact. Freud conceptualized low sexual desire as the result of inhibition during the phallic psychosexual phase and unresolved oedipal conflicts. Some men, fixated at the phallic stage of development, are fearful of the vagina believing they will be castrated if they approach it, a concept Freud called *vagina dentata*, because they believe unconsciously that the vagina has teeth. Hence, they avoid contact with the female genitalia entirely. Lack of desire can also be the result of chronic stress, anxiety, or depression. Drugs that depress the central nervous system or decrease testosterone production can also decrease desire. Abstinence from sex for a prolonged period sometimes results in suppression of the sexual impulse. Desire commonly decreases after major illness or surgery, particularly when body image is affected following such procedures as mastectomy, ileostomy, hysterectomy, and prostatectomy. Loss of desire may also be an expression of hostility or the sign of a deteriorating relationship.

In one study of young married couples who ceased having sexual relations for a period of 2 months, the reasons stated for this behavior were different for men and for women. The men were influenced by social factors, such as recent immigration, religion, and their wives' employment or lack thereof. The women were more influenced by their perceptions about dominance, decision making, affection, and their husbands' threats to leave home. Both men and women mentioned lack of privacy as a reason for discontinuing sexual activity. Marital discord, however, was the reason most frequently given for the cessation or inhibition of sexual activity.

In making the diagnosis, the clinician must evaluate the age, general health, and life stresses of the patient. An attempt to establish a baseline of sexual interest before the disorder began should be made. The need for sexual contact and satisfaction varies among individuals and over time in any given person. In a group of 100 couples with stable marriages, 8 percent reported having intercourse less than once a month. In another group of couples, one third reported lack of sexual relations for periods of time averaging

Table 2
Diagnostic Criteria for Hypoactive Sexual Desire Disorder

A. Persistently or recurrently deficient or absent sexual fantasies and desire for sexual activity. The judgment of deficiency or absence is made by the clinician, taking into account factors that affect sexual functioning, such as age, sex, and the context of the person's life.

B. Occurrence not exclusively during the course of another Axis I disorder (other than a Sexual Dysfunction), such as Major Depression.

Table from DSM-III-R *Diagnostic and Statistical Manual of Mental Disorders,* ed 3, revised. (Current Classification of Mental Disorders, 1987.) Copyright American Psychiatric Association, Washington, D.C., 1987. Used with permission.

Table 3
Diagnostic Criteria for Sexual Aversion Disorder

A. Persistent or recurrent extreme aversion to, and avoidance of, all or almost all, genital sexual contact with a sexual partner

B. Occurrence not exclusively during the course of another Axis I disorder (other than a Sexual Dysfunction), such as Obsessive Compulsive Disorder or Major Depression.

Table from DSM-III-R *Diagnostic and Statistical Manual of Mental Disorders,* ed 3, revised. (Current Classification of Mental Disorders, 1987.) Copyright American Psychiatric Association, Washington, D.C., 1987. Used with permission.

8 weeks. Finally, the diagnosis should not be made unless the lack of desire is a source of distress to the patient.

SEXUAL AROUSAL DISORDERS

These disorders, previously called inhibited sexual excitement, are divided by DSM-III-R into (1) male erectile disorder, characterized by the recurrent and persistent partial or complete failure to attain or maintain an erection until the completion of the sex act and (2) female sexual arousal disorder, characterized by the persistent or recurrent partial or complete failure to attain or maintain the lubrication-swelling response of sexual excitement until the completion of the sexual act. The diagnosis takes into account the focus, intensity, and duration of the sexual activity in which the patient engages (Tables 4 and 5). If sexual stimulation is inadequate in focus, intensity, or duration, the diagnosis should not be made.

Women

The prevalence of female sexual arousal disorder is generally underestimated. Women who have excitement phase dysfunction often have orgasm problems as well. In one study of relatively happily married couples, 33 percent of the women described difficulty in maintaining sexual excitement.

Many psychological factors are associated with female sexual inhibition. These conflicts may be expressed through inhibition of excitement or orgasm and are discussed under orgasmic phase dysfunctions. In some women, excitement phase disorders are associated with dyspareunia or with lack of desire.

Physiological studies of dysfunction suggest that a hormonal pattern may contribute to responsiveness in women who have excitement phase dysfunction. Masters and Johnson found normally responsive women to be particularly desirous of sex before the onset of the menses. Dysfunctional women tended to feel the greatest sexual excitement immediately following the menses or at the time of ovulation. Alterations in testosterone, estrogen, prolactin, and thyroxin levels have been implicated in excitement disorder in women.

Men

Male erectile disorder is also called erectile dysfunction or impotence. In primary impotence, the man has never been able to obtain an erection sufficient for vaginal insertion. In secondary impotence, the man has successfully achieved vaginal penetration at some time in his sexual life but is later unable to do so. In selective impotence, the man is able to have coitus in certain circumstances, but not in others; for example, a man may function effectively with a prostitute, but be impotent with his wife.

Table 4
Diagnostic Criteria for Male Erectile Disorder

A. Either (1) or (2):

   (1) persistent or recurrent partial or complete failure in a male to attain or maintain erection until completion of the sexual activity

   (2) persistent or recurrent lack of a subjective sense of sexual excitement and pleasure in a male during sexual activity

B. Occurrence not exclusively during the course of another Axis I disorder (other than a Sexual Dysfunction), such as Major Depression

Table from DSM-III-R *Diagnostic and Statistical Manual of Mental Disorders,* ed 3, revised. (Current Classification of Mental Disorders, 1987.) Copyright American Psychiatric Association, Washington, D.C., 1987. Used with permission.

Table 5
Diagnostic Criteria for Female Sexual Arousal Disorder

A. Either (1) or (2):

   (1) persistent or recurrent partial or complete failure to attain or maintain the lubrication-swelling response of sexual excitement until completion of the sexual activity

   (2) persistent or recurrent lack of a subjective sense of sexual excitement and pleasure in a female during sexual activity

B. Occurrence not exclusively during the course of another Axis I disorder (other than a Sexual Dysfunction), such as Major Depression

Table from DSM-III-R *Diagnostic and Statistical Manual of Mental Disorders,* ed 3, revised. (Current Classification of Mental Disorders, 1987.) Copyright American Psychiatric Association, Washington, D.C., 1987. Used with permission.

Secondary impotence has been reported in 10 to 20 percent of all men. Freud declared it to be a very common complaint among his patients. Among all men treated for sexual disorders, more than 50 percent have impotence as the chief complaint. Primary impotence is a rare disorder, occuring in about 1 percent of men under age 35. The incidence of impotence increases with age. Among young adults, it has been recorded in about 8 percent of the population. Kinsey reported that over 75 percent of men were impotent at age 80. Masters and Johnson report a fear of impotence in all men over 40, which the researchers believe reflects the masculine fear of loss of virility with advancing age. As it happens, however, impotence is not universal in aging men; having an available sex partner is more closely related to continuing potency than is age.

The etiology of impotence may be organic, psychological, or a combination of both. The incidence of psychological as opposed to organic impotence has been the focus of many studies. Some researchers have reported the incidence of organic impotence in a medical clinic to be as high as 75 to 85 percent. Others believe that these same populations have not had adequate psychological screening and maintain that more than 90 percent of cases of impotence have

psychological causes. The organic causes of impotence are listed in Table 6. Side effects of medication may impair sexual functioning in a variety of ways in both men and women (Table 7). Castration (removal of ovaries or testes) does not always lead to sexual dysfunction, depending on the person. Erection may still occur after castration. A reflex arc, fired when the inner thigh is stimulated, presses through the sacral cord erectile center to account for the phenomenon.

Freud described one type of impotence as caused by an inability to reconcile feelings of affection with feelings of desire toward the same woman. Such men can only function with women whom they see as degraded. Other factors that have been cited as contributing to impotence include a punitive superego, an inability to trust, feelings of inadequacy or a sense of being undesirable as a partner. There may an inability to express the sexual impulse because of fear, anxiety, anger, or moral prohibition. In an ongoing relationship, impotence may reflect difficulties between the partners, particularly if the man cannot communicate his needs or his anger in a direct and constructive way.

A good history is of primary importance in determining the etiology of the dysfunction. If a man reports having spontaneous erections at times when he does not plan to

Table 6
Diseases Implicated in Erectile Dysfunction*

Infectious and parasitic diseases
    Elephantiasis
    Mumps

Cardiovascular diseases
    Atherosclerotic disease
    Aortic aneurysm
    Leriche syndrome
    Cardiac failure

Renal and urologic disorders
    Peyronie's disease
    Chronic renal failure
    Hydrocele or varicocele

Hepatic disorders
    Cirrhosis (usually associated with alcoholism)

Pulmonary disorders
    Respiratory failure

Genetics
    Klinefelter's syndrome
    Congenital penile vascular or structural abnormalities

Nutritional disorders
    Malnutrition
    Vitamin deficiencies

Endocrine disorders
    Diabetes mellitus
    Dysfunction of the pituitary-adrenal-testis axis
    Acromegaly
    Addison's disease
    Chromophobe adenoma
    Adrenal neoplasias
    Myxedema
    Hyperthyroidism

Neurological disorders
    Multiple sclerosis
    Transverse myelitis
    Parkinson's disease
    Temporal lobe epilepsy
    Traumatic or neoplastic spinal cord disease
    Central nervous system tumors
    Amyotrophic lateral sclerosis
    Peripheral neuropathies
    General paresis
    Tabes dorsalis

Pharmacological contributants
    Alcohol and other addictive drugs (heroin, methadone, morphine, cocaine, amphetamines, and barbituates)
    Prescribed drugs (psychotropic drugs, antihypertensive drugs, estrogens, and antiandrogens)

Poisoning
    Lead (plumbism)
    Herbicides

Surgical procedures
    Perineal prostatectomy
    Abdominal-perineal colon resection
    Sympathectomy (frequently interferes with ejaculation)
    Aortoiliac surgery
    Radical cystectomy
    Retroperitoneal lymphadenectomy

Miscellaneous
    Radiation therapy
    Pelvic fracture
    Any severe systemic disease or debilitating condition

*Table by Virginia Sadock, M.D.

have intercourse, having morning erections, or having good erections with masturbation or with partners other than his usual one, then organic causes for his impotence can be considered negligible and costly diagnostic procedures can be avoided.

A number of procedures, benign and invasive, are used to help differentiate organically caused impotence from functional impotence. These procedures include the monitoring of nocturnal penile tumescence (erections that occur during sleep), normally associated with rapid eye movement; monitoring tumescence with a strain gauge; measuring blood pressure in the penis with a penile plethysmograph or an ultrasound (Doppler) flow meter, both of which assess blood flow in the internal pudendal artery; and measuring pudendal nerve latency time. Other diagnostic tests that delineate organic bases for impotence include glucose tolerance tests; plasma hormone assays; liver and thyroid function tests; prolactin, FH, and FSH determinations; and cystometric examinations. Invasive diagnostic studies include penile arteriography, infusion

Table 7
Pharmacological Agents Implicated in Male Sexual Dysfunction*

Drug	Impairs Erection	Impairs Ejaculation
Psychiatric Drugs		
Heterocyclic antidepressants†		
Imipramine (Tofranil, Geigy)	+	+
Protriptyline (Vivactil, Merck Sharpe & Dohme)	+	+
Desmethylimipramine (Pertofran, USV)	+	+
Clomipramine (Anatranil)	+	+
Amitriptyline (Elavil, Merck Sharp & Dohme)	+	+
Trazadone (Desyrel, Mead Johnson)	−	−
Monoamine oxidase inhibitors		
Tranylcypromine (Parnate, Smith Kline & French)	+	
Mebanazine (Actomal)	+	+
Phenelzine (Nardil, Parke-Davis)	+	+
Pargyline (Eutonyl, Abbott)	−	+
Isocarboxazid (Marplan, Roche)		+
Other mood-active drugs		
Lithium	+	
Amphetamines	+	+
Major tranquilizers‡		
Fluphenazine (Prolixin, Squibb)	+	
Thioridazine (Mellaril, Sandoz)	+	+
Chlorprothixene (Taractan, Roche)	−	+
Mesoridazine (Serentil, Boehringer Ingelheim)	−	+
Perphenazine (Trilafon, Schering)	−	+
Trifluoperazine (Stelazine, Smith Kline & French)	−	+
Butaperazine (Repoise)	−	+
Reserpine (Serpasil, CIBA)	+	+
Haloperidol (Haldol, McNeil Pharmaceuticals)	−	+
Minor tranquilizers§		
Chlordiazepoxide (Librium, Roche)	−	+
Antihypertensive Drugs		
Clonidine (Catapres, Boehringer Ingelheim)	+	
Debrisoquin (Declinax)	−	+
Methyldopa (Aldomet, Merck Sharp & Dohme)	+	+
Spironolactone (Aldactone, Searle)	+	−
Hydrochlorthiazide (Apresoline, CIBA)	+	−
Arramethidine (Ismelin, CIBA)	+	+
Commonly Abused Drugs		
Alcohol	+	+
Barbiturates	+	+
Cannabis	+	−
Cocaine	+	+
Heroin	+	+
Methadone	+	−
Morphine	+	+

Table 7 *continued*

Drug	Impairs Erection	Impairs Ejaculation
Miscellaneous Drugs		
Antiparkinsonian agents	+	+
Clofibrate (Atromid-S, Ayerst)	+	−
Digoxin	+	−
Glutethimide (Doriden, UVS)	+	+
Indomethacin (Indocin, Merck Sharp & Dohme)	+	−
Phentolamine (Regitine, CIBA)	−	+
Propranolol (Inderal, Ayerst)	+	−

*Table by Virginia Sadock, M.D. The effects of drugs on the sexual function of the female have not been extensively evaluated, but women appear to be less vulnerable to pharmacologically induced sexual dysfunction than are men. Oral contraceptives are reported to decrease libido in some women and phenelzine (Nardil, Parke-Davis) impairs the orgasmic response in some women. Both increase and decrease in libido have been reported with psychoactive agents. It is difficult to separate those effects from the underlying condition or from improvement of the condition. Sexual dysfunction associated with the use of a drug disappears when the drug is discontinued.

†The incidence of erectile dysfunction associated with the use of tricyclic antidepressants is low.

‡Impairment of sexual function is not a common complication of the use of major tranquilizers. Trazadone (Desyrel, Mead Johnson) has been reported to produce priapism. Monoamine oxidase inhibitors have been reported to impair the orgasmic response in women. Priapism has occasionally occurred in association with the use of major tranquilizers.

§Benzodiazepines have been reported to decrease libido, but in some patients the diminution of anxiety caused by those drugs enhances sexual function.

cavernosography and radioactive xenon penography. These procedures require expert interpretation and are used only for patients who are candidates for vascular reconstructive procedures.

INHIBITED FEMALE ORGASM (ANORGASMIA)

Inhibited female orgasm is defined as the recurrent and persistent inhibition of the female orgasm, as manifested by the absence of orgasm after a normal sexual excitement phase that the clinician judges to be adequate in focus, intensity, and duration. It refers to the inability of the woman to achieve orgasm by masturbation or coitus. Women who can achieve orgasm with one of these methods are not necessarily categorized as anorgasmic, although some degree of sexual inhibition may be postulated (Table 8).

Research on the physiology of the female sexual response has demonstrated that orgasms caused by clitoral stimulation and those caused by vaginal stimulation are physiologically identical. Freud's theory that women must give up clitoral sensitivity for vaginal sensitivity in order to achieve sexual maturity is now considered misleading; but, some women say that they gain a special sense of satisfaction from an orgasm precipitated by coitus. Some workers attribute that to the psychological feeling of closeness engendered by the act of coitus, but others maintain that the coital orgasm is a physiologically different experience. Many women achieve orgasm during coitus by a combination of manual clitoral stimulation and penile vaginal stimulation. Some women who are able to experience orgasm during noncoital clitoral stimulation but who are not able to experience orgasm during coitus in the absence of manual clitoral stimulation may warrant a diagnosis of anorgasmia. However, more and more evidence is forthcoming that this exclusively clitoral orgasm is a normal behavioral variation.

Primary nonorgasmic dysfunction exists when the woman has never experienced orgasm by any kind of stimulation. Secondary orgasmic dysfunction exists if the woman has previously experienced at least one orgasm regardless of the circumstances or

Table 8
Diagnostic Criteria for Inhibited Female Orgasm

A. Persistent or recurrent delay in, or absence of, orgasm in a female following a normal sexual excitement phase during sexual activity that the clinician judges to be adequate in focus, intensity, and duration. Some females are able to experience orgasm during noncoital clitoral stimulation, but are unable to experience it during coitus in the absence of manual clitoral stimulation. In most of these females, this represents a normal variation of the female sexual response and does not justify the diagnosis of Inhibited Female Orgasm. However, in some of these females, this does represent a psychological inhibition that justifies the diagnosis. This difficult judgment is assisted by a thorough sexual evaluation, which may even require a trial of treatment.

B. Occurrence not exclusively during the course of another Axis I disorder (other than a Sexual Dysfunction), such as Major Depression.

Table from DSM-III-R *Diagnostic and Statistical Manual of Mental Disorders,* ed 3, revised. (Current Classification of Mental Disorders, 1987.) Copyright American Psychiatric Association, Washington, D.C., 1987. Used with permission.

means of stimulation, whether by masturbation or during sleep while dreaming. Kinsey found that the proportion of married women over 35 years of age who had never achieved orgasm by any means was only 5 percent. The incidence of orgasm increases with age. According to Kinsey, the first orgasm occurs during adolescence in about 50 percent of women; the rest usually experience orgasm as they get older. Primary anorgasmia is more common among unmarried women than among married women. Increased orgasmic potential in women over 35 has been explained on the basis of less psychological inhibition, greater sexual experience, or both.

Secondary orgasmic dysfunction is a common complaint in clinical populations. One clinical treatment facility described nonorgasmic women as about four times more common in its practice than patients with all other sexual disorders. In another study, 46 percent of the women complained of difficulty in reaching orgasm, and 15 percent described inability to have orgasm. The true prevalence of problems in maintaining excitement is not known, but inhibition of excitement and orgastic problems often occur together. Overall prevalence of inhibited female orgasm from all causes is given as 30 percent in DSM-III-R.

Numerous psychological factors are associated with inhibited female orgasm. They include fears of impregnation, rejection by the sex partner, or damage to the vagina; hostility toward men; and feelings of guilt regarding sexual impulses. For some women, orgasm is equated with loss of control or with aggressive, destructive, or violent behavior; their fear of these impulses may be expressed through inhibition of excitement or orgasm. Cultural expectations and societal restrictions on women are also relevant. Nonorgasmic women may be otherwise symptom free or may experience frustration in a variety of ways, including such pelvic complaints as lower abdominal pain, itching, and vaginal discharge, as well as increased tension, irritability, and fatigue.

INHIBITED MALE ORGASM

In inhibited male orgasm, also called retarded ejaculation, the man achieves ejaculation during coitus with great difficulty, if at all. A man suffers from primary retarded ejaculation if he has never been able to ejaculate during coitus. The disorder is diagnosed as secondary if it develops after previous normal functioning (Table 9).

Some workers suggest that a differentiation should be made between orgasm and ejaculation. Certainly, inhibited orgasm must be differentiated from retrograde ejaculation, in which ejaculation occurs but the seminal fluid passes backward into the bladder. The latter condition always has an organic cause. Retrograde ejaculation can develop after genitourinary surgery and is also associated with medications that have anticholinergic side effects, such as the phenothiazines. Some men ejaculate but complain of a decreased or absent subjective sense of pleasure during the orgasmic experience (orgasmic anhedonia).

The incidence of inhibited male orgasm is much lower than that of premature ejaculation or impotence. Masters and Johnson reported only 3.8 percent in one group of 447 sex dysfunction cases. A general prevalence of 5 percent has been reported.

Table 9
Diagnostic Criteria for Inhibited Male Orgasm

A. Persistent or recurrent delay in, or absence of, orgasm in a male following a normal sexual excitement phase during sexual activity that the clinician, taking into account the person's age, judges to be adequate in focus, intensity, and duration. This failure to achieve orgasm is usually restricted to an inability to reach orgasm in the vagina, with orgasm possible with other types of stimulation, such as masturbation.

B. Occurrence not exclusively during the course of another Axis I disorder (other than a Sexual Dysfunction), such as Major Depression.

Table from DSM-III-R *Diagnostic and Statistical Manual of Mental Disorders*, ed 3, revised. (Current Classification of Mental Disorders, 1987.) Copyright American Psychiatric Association, Washington, D.C., 1987. Used with permission.

Inhibited male orgasm may have physiologic causes and can occur after surgery of the genitourinary tract, such as prostatectomy. It may also be associated with Parkinson's disease and other neurologic disorders involving the lumbar or sacral sections of the spinal cord. The antihypertensive drug guanethidine monosulfate, methyldopa, and the phenothiazines have been implicated in retarded ejaculation.

Primary inhibited male orgasm is indicative of more severe psychopathology. The man often comes from a rigid, puritanical background; he perceives sex as sinful and the genitals as dirty; and he may have conscious or unconscious incest wishes and guilt. There are usually difficulties with closeness that extend beyond the area of sexual relations.

In an ongoing relationship, secondary ejaculatory inhibition frequently reflects interpersonal difficulties. The disorder may be the man's way of coping with real or fantasized changes in the relationship. These changes may include plans for pregnancy about which the man is ambivalent, the loss of sexual attraction to the partner, or demands by the partner for greater commitment as expressed by sexual performance. In some men, the inability to ejaculate reflects unexpressed hostility toward the woman. This problem is more common among men with obsessive-compulsive disorders than among others.

PREMATURE EJACULATION

In premature ejaculation, the man recurrently achieves orgasm and ejaculation before he wishes to. There is no definite time frame within which to define the dysfunction. The diagnosis is made when the man regularly ejaculates before or immediately after entering the vagina. The clinician needs to consider factors that affect duration of the excitement phase, such as age, novelty of the sex partner, and the frequency and duration of coitus (Table 10). Masters and Johnson conceptualize the disorder in terms of the couple and consider a man a premature ejaculator if he cannot control ejaculation for a sufficient length of time during intravaginal containment to satisfy his partner in at least one half of their episodes of coitus. This definition assumes that the female partner is capable of an orgastic response. Like the other dysfunctions, this disturbance is not caused exclusively by organic factors nor is it symptomatic of any other clinical psychiatric syndrome. There is an absence of data on female premature orgasm; no separate category of premature orgasm for women is included in DSM-III-R. The authors have seen a case of multiple spontaneous orgasms occurring in a woman without sexual stimulation that was caused by an epileptogenic focus in the temporal lobe.

Premature ejaculation is more common today among college-educated men than among men with less education and is thought to be related to their concern for partner satisfaction; however, the true incidence of this disorder has not been determined. About 35 to 40 percent of men treated for sexual disorders have premature ejaculation as the chief complaint. Difficulty in ejaculatory control may be associated with anxiety regarding the sex act or with unconscious fears about the vagina. It may also result from negative cultural conditioning. The man who has most of his early sexual contacts with prostitutes who demand that the sex act proceed quickly or in situations in which discovery would be

Table 10
Diagnostic Criteria for Premature Ejaculation

Persistent or recurrent ejaculation with minimal sexual stimulation or before, upon, or shortly after penetration and before the person wishes it. The clinician must take into account factors that affect duration of the excitement phase, such as age, novelty of the sexual partner or situation, and frequency of sexual activity.

Table from DSM-III-R *Diagnostic and Statistical Manual of Mental Disorders,* ed 3, revised. (Current Classification of Mental Disorders, 1987.) Copyright American Psychiatric Association, Washington, D.C., 1987. Used with permission.

embarrassing (e.g., in the back seat of a car or in the parental home) may become conditioned to achieve orgasm rapidly. In ongoing relationships, the partner has been found to have great influence on the premature ejaculator. A stressful marriage exacerbates the disorder. The developmental background and psychodynamics found in this disorder and in impotence are similar.

SEXUAL PAIN DISORDERS: DYSPAREUNIA

Dyspareunia refers to recurrent and persistent pain occurring before, during, or after intercourse in either the man or the woman. Much more common in women, it is related to and often coincides with vaginismus. Repeated episodes of vaginismus may lead to dyspareunia and vice versa, but in either case, somatic causes must be ruled out. Dyspareunia should not be diagnosed when an organic basis for the pain is found, or when, in a woman, it is not caused exclusively by vaginismus or by a lack of lubrication (Table 11). The true incidence of dyspareunia is unknown, but it has been estimated that 30 percent of surgical procedures on the female genital area result in temporary dyspareunia. Additionally, of women with this complaint who are seen in sex therapy clinics, 30 to 40 percent have pelvic pathology.

Organic abnormalities leading to dyspareunia and vaginismus include irritated or infected hymenal remnants, episiotomy scars, Bartholin's gland infection, various forms of vaginitis and cervicitis, endometriosis, and other pelvic disorders. The postmenopausal woman may develop dyspareunia resulting from thinning of the vaginal mucosa and reduced lubrication. In the majority of cases, however, dynamic factors are usually considered causative. Painful coitus may result from tension and anxiety about the sex act that cause the woman to involuntarily contract her vaginal muscles. The pain is real and makes intercourse unpleasant or unbearable. The anticipation of further pain may cause

Table 11
Diagnostic Criteria for Dyspareunia

A. Recurrent or persistent genital pain in either a male or a female before, during, or after sexual intercourse.

B. The disturbance is not caused exclusively by lack of lubrication or by vaginismus.

Table from DSM-III-R *Diagnostic and Statistical Manual of Mental Disorders,* ed 3, revised. (Current Classification of Mental Disorders, 1987.) Copyright American Psychiatric Association, Washington, D.C., 1987. Used with permission.

the woman to avoid coitus altogether. If the partner proceeds with intercourse regardless of the woman's state of readiness, the condition is aggravated. Dyspareunia can also occur in men, but it is uncommon and is usually associated with an organic condition, such as Peyronie's disease, which consists of sclerotic plaques on the penis that cause penile curvature.

SEXUAL PAIN DISORDER: VAGINISMUS

Vaginismus is an involuntary muscle constriction of the outer one third of the vagina that prevents penile insertion and intercourse. This response may occur during gynecological examination when involuntary vaginal constriction prevents introduction of the speculum into the vagina. The diagnosis is not made if the dysfunction is caused exclusively by organic factors or if it is symptomatic of another Axis I psychiatric syndrome (Table 12). Vaginismus is less prevalent than anorgasmia. It most often afflicts highly educated women and those in the higher socioeconomic groups. The woman suffering from vaginismus may consciously wish to have coitus, but she unconsciously prevents the penis from entering her body. A sexual trauma such as rape may result in vaginismus. Women with psychosexual conflicts may perceive the penis as a weapon. In some women, pain or the anticipation of pain at the first coital experience causes vaginismus. A strict religious upbringing that associates sex with sin is frequently noted in these cases. For others, there are problems in the dyadic relationship; if the woman feels emotionally abused by her partner, she may protest in this nonverbal fashion.

SEXUAL DYSFUNCTION NOT OTHERWISE SPECIFIED

This category is for psychosexual dysfunctions that cannot be classified under the categories described above. Examples include persons who experience the physiologic components of sexual excitement and orgasm but report no erotic sensation or even anesthesia (orgasmic anhedonia). Women with conditions analogous to premature ejaculation in the man would be classified here. The orgastic female who desires but has not experienced multiple orgasms can be classified under this heading as well. Also, disorders of excessive rather than inhibited dysfunction, such as compulsive masturbation, might be diagnosed under atypical

Table 12
Diagnostic Criteria for Vaginismus

A. Recurrent or persistent involuntary spasm of the musculature of the outer third of the vagina that interferes with coitus.

B. The disturbance is not caused exclusively by a physical disorder, and is not due to another Axis I disorder.

Table from DSM-III-R *Diagnostic and Statistical Manual of Mental Disorders,* ed 3, revised. (Current Classification of Mental Disorders, 1987.) Copyright American Psychiatric Association, Washington, D.C., 1987. Used with permission.

dysfunctions, as would genital pain occurring during masturbation. Other unspecified disorders are found in persons who have one or more sexual fantasies about which they feel guilty or otherwise dysphoric. However, the range of common sexual fantasies is broad.

Postcoital Headache

This phenomenon is characterized by headache immediately following coitus, which may last for several hours. It is usually described as throbbing in nature and is localized in the occipital or frontal area. The cause is unknown. There may be vascular, muscle contraction (tension), or psychogenic etiologies. Coitus may precipitate migraine or cluster headaches in predisposed persons.

Orgasmic Anhedonia

This refers to a condition in which there is no physical sensation of orgasm even though the physiologic component (e.g., ejaculation) remains intact. Organic causes such as sacral or cephalic lesions that interfere with afferent pathways from the genitalia to the cortex must be ruled out. Psychic causes usually relate to extreme guilt about experiencing sexual pleasure. These feelings produce a type of dissociative response that isolates the affective component of the orgasmic experience from consciousness.

Masturbatory Pain

In some cases, persons may experience pain during masturbation. Organic causes should always be ruled out. A small vaginal tear or early Peyronie's disease may produce a painful sensation. This condition should be differentiated from compulsive masturbation. People may masturbate to the extent that they do physical damage to their genitals and eventually experience pain during subsequent masturbatory acts. Such cases constitute a separate sexual disorder and should be so classified.

Certain masturbatory practices have resulted in what has been called autoerotic asphyxiation. This practice involves masturbating while hanging oneself by the neck to heighten erotic sensations and the intensity of orgasm through the mechanism of mild hypoxia. Although the individual releases himself from the noose after orgasm, an estimated 500 to 1,000 persons per year accidentally kill themselves by hanging. Most who indulge in this practice are male; transvestism is often associated with the habit, and the majority of deaths occur among adolescents. Such masochistic practices are usually associated with severe mental disorders such as schizophrenia and major mood disorders.

OTHER SEXUAL DISORDERS

There are many sexual disorders that are not classifiable in any of the previous categories of sexual disorders (e.g., paraphilia or sexual dysfunction). They are either rare, poorly documented, not easily classified, or not specifically described in DSM-III-R (Table 13).

Postcoital Dysphoria

This condition is not currently listed in DSM-III-R. It occurs during the resolution phase when the person normally experiences a sense of general well-being and muscular and psychological relaxa-

Table 13
Diagnostic Criteria for Sexual Disorder Not Otherwise Specified

Sexual disorders that are not classifiable in any of the previous categories. In rare instances, this category may be used concurrently with one of the specific diagnoses when both are necessary to explain or describe the clinical disturbance.

Examples:

(1) Marked feelings of inadequacy concerning body habitus, size and shape of sex organs, sexual performance, or other traits related to self-imposed standards of masculinity or femininity

(2) Distress about a pattern of repeated sexual conquests or other forms of nonparaphilic sexual addiction, involving a succession of people who exist only as things to be used

(3) Persistent and marked distress about one's sexual orientation

Table from DSM-III-R *Diagnostic and Statistical Manual of Mental Disorders,* ed 3, revised. (Current Classification of Mental Disorders, 1987.) Copyright American Psychiatric Association, Washington, D.C., 1987. Used with permission.

tion. In some persons, however, a postcoital dysphoria occurs. After an otherwise satisfactory sexual experience, they become depressed, tense, anxious, irritable, and show psychomotor agitation. They often want to get away from their partner and may become verbally or even physically abusive. The incidence of the disorder is unknown, but it is more common in men. The causes are several and relate to the attitude of the person toward sex in general, and toward the partner in particular. It may occur in adulterous sex or with prostitutes. More recently, the fear of AIDS may cause some persons to experience this phenomenon postcoitally. Treatment requires insight-oriented psychotherapy to help the patient understand the unconscious antecedents to his behavior and attitudes.

Couple Problems

At times, a complaint must be viewed in terms of the spousal unit or the couple rather than as an individual dysfunction. An example is a couple, one of whom prefers morning sex while the other functions more readily at night; another example is a couple with unequal frequencies of desire.

The Unconsummated Marriage

The couple involved in an unconsummated marriage have never had coitus and are typically uninformed and inhibited about sexuality. Their feelings of guilt, shame, or inadequacy are only increased by their problem, and they are conflicted by a need to seek help and by a need to conceal their difficulty. Couples present with the problem after having been married several months or several years. Masters and Johnson reported an unconsummated marriage of 17 years' duration.

Frequently, the couple do not seek help directly, but the woman may reveal the problem to her gynecologist on a visit ostensibly concerned with vague vaginal or somatic complaints. On examining her, the gynecologist may find an intact hymen. In some cases, the wife may have undergone a hymenectomy to resolve the problem; but, this surgical procedure is another stress and often serves to increase the feelings of inadequacy in the couple. The wife may feel put upon, abused, or mutilated, and the husband's concern about his manliness may increase. The hymenectomy usually aggravates the situation without solving the basic problem. The physician's inquiry, if he is comfortable in dealing with sexual problems, may be the first opening to frank discussion of the couple's distress. Often, the pretext of the medical visit is a discussion of contraceptive methods or—even more ironic—a request for an infertility work-up. Once presented, the complaint can often be successfully treated. The duration of the problem does not significantly affect the prognosis or the outcome of the case.

The causes are varied: lack of sex education, sexual prohibitions overly stressed by parents or society, neurotic problems of an oedipal nature, immaturity in both partners, overdependence on primary families, and problems in sexual identification. Religious orthodoxy, with severe control of sexual and social development or the equation of sexuality with sin or uncleanliness, has also been cited as a dominant cause. Many women involved in unconsummated marriages have distorted concepts about their vaginas. There can be a fear of having no opening, a fear of being too small or too soft, or a confusion of the vagina with the rectum, leading to feelings of being unclean. The man may share in these distortions of the vagina and, in addition, perceive it as dangerous to himself. Similarly, both partners may share distortions about the man's penis, perceiving it as a weapon, as too large, or as too small. Many of these patients can be helped by simple education about genital anatomy and physiology, by suggestions for self exploration, and by correct information from a physician. The problem of the unconsummated marriage is best treated by seeing both members of the couple. Dual-sex therapy (discussed below) involving a male-female cotherapist team has been markedly effective. However, other forms of conjoint therapy, marital counseling, traditional psychotherapy on a one-to-one basis, and counseling from a sensitive family physician, gynecologist, or urologist are all helpful.

Body Image Problems

Persons who are ashamed of their bodies and who experience feelings of inadequacy related to self-imposed standards of masculinity or femininity may develop a sexual disorder. They may insist on sex only during total darkness, not allow certain body parts to be seen or touched, or seek unnecessary operative procedures to deal with their imagined inadequacies. Dysmorphophobia should be ruled out.

Don Juanism

Some men appear to be hypersexual as manifested by their need to have many sexual encounters or conquests. Their sexual activities, however, are used to mask deep feelings of inferiority. Some have unconscious homosexual impulses, which they deny by compulsive sexual contact with women. After having sex, most Don Juans are no longer interested in the woman. The condition is sometimes referred to as "satyriasis."

Nymphomania

This is a descriptive term that signifies excessive or pathological desire for coitus in a woman. There have been few scientific studies of the condition. Those who have been studied usually have one or more sexual disorders, usually anorgasmia. There is often an intense fear over loss of love. The woman attempts to satisfy dependency rather than to gratify the sexual impulse through her actions.

SEXUAL ORIENTATION DISTRESS

Persistent and marked distress about one's sexual orientation is listed as an example of a sexual disorder in DSM-III-R. Previously known in DSM-III as ego-dystonic homosexuality, it was defined as a desire to acquire or increase heterosexual arousal so that a heterosexual relationship could be initiated. The person with the disorder explicitly states that homosexual arousal and behavior is unwanted and a source of distress, hence the term "ego-dystonic." The category was eliminated for several reasons. As stated in DSM-III-R:

> It suggested to some that homosexuality was itself considered a disorder. In the United States, almost all individuals who are homosexual first go through a phase in which their homosexuality is ego-dystonic. Furthermore, the diagnosis of ego-dystonic homosexuality has rarely been used clinically, and there have been only a few articles in the scientific literature that use the concept. Finally, the treatment programs that attempt to help bisexual men become heterosexual have not used this diagnosis. In DSM-III-R, an example of sexual disorder not otherwise specified are cases that in DSM-III would have met the criteria for ego-dystonic homosexuality.

In view of the above, the clinician needs to recognize that persons with an exclusive or predominant preference for same-sex sex partners are not considered to have a mental disorder on the basis of their sexual orientation alone. According to DSM-III-R such persons constitute a substantial portion of the adult and adolescent population. Kinsey reported that 4 percent of adult men were exclusively homosexual throughout their lives and that another 13 percent were predominantly homosexual for at least 3 years between the ages of 16 and 55. More than one in three men had experienced a sexual interaction leading to orgasm with another male during the postpubertal years. For women, the reported rates were approximately half those for men.

Overview of Homosexuality

Etiology

Psychological. The causes of homosexual behavior are enigmatic. Freud viewed homosexuality as an arrest of psychosexual development. Castration fears for the male and fears of maternal engulfment in the preoedipal phase of psychosexual development are mentioned. According to psychodynamic theory, early-life situations that can result in male homosexual behavior include a strong fixation on the mother, lack of effective fathering, inhibition of masculine development by the mother, fixation or regression at the narcissistic stage of development, and losing competition with brothers and sisters. Freud's views on female homosexuality included a lack of resolution of penis envy in association with unresolved oedipal conflicts.

Homosexual females, as compared with heterosexual females have been reported to have fathers who were close and intimate, the converse of that found for male homosexuals. However, the descriptions given of the mothers of female homosexuals were not different from the descriptions given of the mothers of the heterosexuals.

Biological. Based on recent studies, there is strong evidence that genetic and biological components may contribute to homosexual orientation. There are reports that homosexual men exhibit lower levels of circulatory androgen than heterosexual men; but these reports have not been replicated sufficiently. There have also been reports of atypical estrogen feedback patterns among homosexual males. Such males show abnormal rebound increases in luteinizing hormone (LH) levels following estrogen injections. Prenatal hormones appear to play a role in the organization of the central nervous system. The effective presence of androgens in prenatal life is purported to contribute to a sexual orientation toward females, and a deficiency of prenatal androgens (or a tissue insensitivity to them) may lead to a sexual orientation toward males. Preadolescent girls exposed to large amounts of androgens before birth are unusually aggressive and unfeminine, and boys exposed to female hormones in utero are less athletic, less assertive, and less aggressive than other males.

Genetic studies demonstrate a higher incidence of homosexual concordance among monozygotic twins than among dizygotic twins, which suggests a hidden genetic predisposition; but chromosome studies have been unable to differentiate homosexuals from heterosexuals. Male homosexuals also show a familial distribution; homosexual men have more siblings who are also homosexual than heterosexual men.

Sexual Behavioral Patterns. The behavioral features of male and female homosexuals are as varied as those of male and female heterosexuals. Sexual practices engaged in by homosexuals are the same as for heterosexuals, with the obvious limitations imposed by anatomical differences.

Varying ongoing relationship patterns exist among homosexuals, as they do among heterosexuals. Some homosexual dyads live in a common household in either a monogamous or a primary relationship for decades, and other homosexual persons typically have only fleeting sexual contacts. Although more stable male-male relationships exist than were previously thought, it appears that male-male relationships are less stable and more fleeting than are female-female relationships. Many fleeting male relationships are initiated in gay baths and bars, with a smaller number initiated in public restrooms and parks. Comparable female institutions are practically nonexistent. The amount of male homosexual promiscuity has diminished since the onset of acquired immune deficiency syndrome (AIDS) and its rapid spread in the homosexual community through sexual contact. Increased condom use is recommended to decrease the transmission of AIDS.

Homosexual males are subjected to civil and social discrimination and do not have the legal social support system of marriage or the biological capacity for childbearing that bonds some otherwise incompatible heterosexual couples together. Female-female couples, on the other hand, experience less social stigmatization and appear to have more enduring monogamous or primary relationships.

Psychopathology. The range of psychopathology that may be found among distressed homosexuals parallels that found among heterosexuals. Distress about one's sexual orientation is characterized by a dissatisfaction with homosexual arousal patterns, a desire to increase heterosexual arousal, and strong negative feelings about being homosexual.

Occasional statements to the effect that life would be easier if the person were not homosexual do not constitute the syndrome of sexual orientation distress. Also, distress resulting only from conflict between the homosexual and the societal value structure is not classifiable as a disorder. If the distress is sufficiently severe to warrant a diagnosis, an adjustment disorder or a depressive disorder is to be considered. Some homosexuals suffering from a major depressive disorder may experience guilt and self-hatred that becomes directed toward their sexual orientation; then the desire for sexual reorientation is only a symptom of the depressive disorder.

Course and Treatment. Some homosexuals, particularly males, report being aware of same-sex romantic attractions before puberty. According to Kinsey's data, about half of all prepubertal males have some genital experience with a same-sex partner. However, this experience is often of an exploratory nature and typically lacks a strong affective component. Most male homosexuals recall the onset of romantic and erotic attractions to same-sex partners during early adolescence. For females, the age of initial romantic feelings toward same-sex partners may also be pre-adolescent. However, the clear recognition of a same-sex partner preference typically occurs in middle to late adolescence or not until young adulthood. More homosexual women than homosexual men appear to have heterosexual experiences during their primary homosexual careers. In one study, 56 percent of a lesbian sample had heterosexual intercourse before their first genital homosexual experience, compared with 19 percent of a male homosexual sample who had heterosexual intercourse first. Nearly 40 percent of the lesbians had had heterosexual intercourse during the year preceding the survey.

Treatment of sexual orientation distress is controversial. It has been reported that, with a minimum of 350 hours of psychoanalytic therapy, approximately one third of about 100 bisexual or homosexually oriented males achieved a heterosexual reorientation at a five-year follow-up; but, this study has been challenged. Behavior therapy and avoidance conditioning techniques have also been used, but a basic problem with behavioral techniques is that, while the behavior may be changed in the laboratory setting, it may not be changed outside of the laboratory, in real life. Prognostic factors weighing in favor of heterosexual reorientation for men include under age 35 years, some experience of heterosexual arousal, and high motivation for reorientation.

An alternative style of intervention is directed at enabling the person with sexual orientation distress to live more comfortably as a homosexual without shame, guilt, anxiety, or depression. Gay counseling centers are engaged with patients in such treatment programs. At present, outcome studies of such centers have not been reported in detail. As for the treatment of women with sexual orientation distress, there are few data, and those are primarily single case studies with variable outcomes.

TREATMENT OF SEXUAL DISORDERS

Prior to 1970, the most common treatment of psychosexual dysfunction was individual psychotherapy. Classic psychodynamic theory considers sexual inadequacy to have its roots in early developmental conflicts, and the sexual disorder is treated as part of a more pervasive emotional disturbance. Treatment focuses on the exploration of unconscious conflicts, motivation, fantasy, and various interpersonal difficulties. One of the assumptions of therapy is that the removal of the conflicts will allow the sexual impulse to become structurally acceptable to the patient's ego and thereby find appropriate means of satisfaction in the environment. Unfortunately, the symptoms of sexual dysfunction frequently become secondarily autonomous and continue to persist even when other problems evolving from the patient's pathology have been resolved. The addition of behavioral techniques is often necessary to cure the sexual problem.

Four treatment modalities, dual-sex therapy, hypnotherapy, behavior therapy, and group therapy, will be discussed, as well as analytically oriented sex therapy, which integrates the tenets of psychoanalysis with behavioral techniques.

Dual-Sex Therapy

The theoretical basis of the dual-sex therapy approach is the concept of the marital unit or dyad as the object of therapy; the major advance in the diagnosis and treatment of sexual disorders in this century. The methodology was originated and developed by William Masters and Virginia Johnson. In dual-sex therapy, there is no acceptance of the idea of a sick half of a patient couple. Both are involved in a relationship in which there is sexual distress, and both, therefore, must participate in the therapy program.

The sexual problem often reflects other areas of disharmony or misunderstanding in the marriage. The marital relationship as a whole is treated, with emphasis on sexual functioning as a part of that relationship. Psychological and physiologic aspects of sexual functioning are discussed and an educative attitude is used. Suggestions are made for specific sexual activity, and those suggestions are followed in the privacy of the couple's home. The keystone of the program is the roundtable session in which a male and female therapy team clarifies, discusses, and works through the problems with the couple. These four-way sessions require active participation on the part of the patients. The aim of the therapy is to establish or re-establish communication within the marital unit. Sex is emphasized as a natural function that flourishes in the appropriate domestic climate, and improved communication is encouraged toward that end.

Treatment is short term and is behaviorally oriented. The therapists attempt to reflect the situation as they see it, rather than interpret underlying dynamics. An undistorted picture of the relationship presented by the psychiatrist often corrects the myopic, narrow view held by each marriage partner. The new perspective can interrupt the couple's vicious cycle of relating, and improved, more effective communication can be encouraged.

Specific exercises are prescribed for the couple to help them with their particular problem. Sexual inadequacy often involves lack of information, misinformation, and performance fear. Therefore, the couples are specifically prohibited from any sexual play other than that prescribed by the therapists. Beginning exercises usually focus on heightening sensory awareness to touch, sight, sound, and smell. Initially, intercourse is interdicted, and couples learn to give and receive bodily pleasure without the pressure of performance. They are simultaneously learning how to communicate nonverbally in a mutually satisfactory way and learning that sexual foreplay is as important as intercourse and orgasm.

During these *sensate focus* exercises, the couple receive much reinforcement, to reduce their anxiety. They are urged to use fantasies to distract them from obsessive concerns about performance (spectatoring). The needs of both the dysfunctional and the nondysfunctional partner are considered. If either partner becomes sexually excited by the exercises, the other is encouraged to bring him or her to orgasm by manual or oral means. Open communica-

tion between the partners is urged, and the expression of mutual needs is encouraged. Resistances, such as claims of fatigue or not enough time to complete the exercises, are common and must be dealt with by the therapist. Genital stimulation is eventually added to general body stimulation. The couple are instructed sequentially to try various positions for intercourse, without necessarily completing the act, and to use varieties of stimulating techniques before they are instructed to proceed with intercourse.

Roundtable sessions follow each new exercise period, and problems and satisfactions, both sexual and in other areas of the couple's lives, are discussed. Specific instructions and the introduction of new exercises geared to the individual couple's progress are reviewed in each session. Gradually, the couple gain confidence and learn or relearn to communicate, verbally and sexually. Dual-sex therapy is most effective when the sexual dysfunction exists apart from other psychopathology.

Specific Techniques and Exercises. Different techniques are used to treat the various dysfunctions. In cases of vaginismus the woman is advised to dilate her vaginal opening with her fingers or with dilators.

In cases of premature ejaculation, an exercise known as the *squeeze technique* is used to raise the threshold of penile excitability. In that exercise, the man or woman stimulates the erect penis until the earliest sensations of impending ejaculation are felt. At that point, the woman forcefully squeezes the coronal ridge of the glans, the erection is diminished, and ejaculation is inhibited. The exercise program eventually raises the threshold of the sensation of ejaculatory inevitability and allows the man to become more aware of his sexual sensations and confident about his sexual performance. A variant of the exercise is the stop-start technique developed by J. H. Semans in which the woman stops all stimulation of the penis when the man first senses an impending ejaculation. No squeeze is used. Research has shown that the presence or absence of circumcision has no bearing on a man's ejaculatory control; the glans is equally sensitive in either state.

A man with inhibited desire or inhibited excitement is sometimes told to masturbate to demonstrate that full erection and ejaculation are possible. In cases of primary anorgasmia, the woman is directed to masturbate, sometimes using a vibrator. The shaft of the clitoris is the masturbatory site most preferred by women, and orgasm depends on adequate clitoral stimulation. An area on the anterior wall of the vagina has been identified in some women as a site of sexual excitation known as the G-spot; however, reports of an ejaculatory phenomenon at orgasm in woman have not been satisfactorily demonstrated. Men masturbate by stroking the shaft and glans of the penis.

Retarded ejaculation is managed by extravaginal ejaculation initially and gradual vaginal entry after the stimulation to the point of near ejaculation.

Hypnotherapy

Hypnotherapists focus specifically on the anxiety-producing symptom, that is, the particular sexual dysfunction. The successful use of hypnosis enables the patient to gain control over the symptom that has been lowering self-esteem and disrupting psychological homeostasis. The cooperation of the patient is first obtained and encouraged during a series of nonhypnotic sessions with the therapist. These discussions permit the development of a secure doctor-patient relationship, a sense of physical and psychological comfort on the part of the patient, and the establishment of mutually desired treatment goals. During this time, the therapist assesses the patient's capacity for the trance experience. The nonhypnotic sessions also permit the clinician to take a careful psychiatric history and do a mental status examination before beginning hypnotherapy. The focus of treatment is on symptom removal and attitude alteration. The patient is instructed in developing alternative means of dealing with the anxiety-provoking situation, the sexual encounter.

Patients are also taught relaxation techniques to use on themselves before sexual relations. With those methods to alleviate anxiety, the physiologic responses to sexual stimulation can more readily result in pleasurable excitation and discharge. Psychological impediments to vaginal lubrication, erection, and orgasm are removed, and normal sexual functioning ensues. Hypnosis may be added to a basic individual psychotherapy program to accelerate the impact of psychotherapeutic intervention.

Behavior Therapy

Behavior therapists assume that sexual dysfunction is learned maladaptive behavior. Behavioral approaches were initially designed for the treatment of phobias. In cases of sexual dysfunction, the therapist sees the patient as being fearful of sexual interaction. Using traditional techniques, the therapist sets up a hierarchy of anxiety-provoking situations for the patient, ranging from the least threatening to the most threatening situation. Mild anxiety may be experienced at the thought of kissing, and massive anxiety may be felt when imagining penile penetration. The behavior therapist enables the patient to master the anxiety through a standard program of systematic desensitization. The program is designed to inhibit the learned anxious response by encouraging behaviors antithetical to anxiety. The patient first deals with the least anxiety-producing situation in fantasy and progresses by steps to the most anxiety-producing situation. Medication, hypnosis, or special training in deep muscle relaxation is sometimes used to help with the initial mastery of anxiety.

Assertiveness training is helpful is teaching the patient to express sexual needs openly and without fear. Exercises in assertiveness are given in conjunction with sex therapy; the patient is encouraged both to make sexual requests and to refuse to comply with requests perceived as unreasonable. Sexual exercises may be prescribed for the patient to perform at home, and a hierarchy may be established, starting with those activities that have proved most pleasurable and successful in the past.

One treatment variation involves the participation of the patient's sexual partner in the desensitization program. The partner, rather than the therapist, presents items of increasing stimulation value to the patient. In such situations, a cooperative partner is necessary to help the patient carry gains made during treatment sessions to sexual activity at home.

Group Therapy

Methods of group therapy have been used to examine both intrapsychic and interpersonal problems in patients with sexual disorders. The therapy group provides a strong support system for a patient who feels ashamed, anxious, or guilty about a particular sexual problem. It is a useful forum in which to counteract sexual myths, correct misconceptions, and provide accurate information regarding sexual anatomy, physiology, and varieties of behavior.

Groups for the treatment of sexual disorders can be organized in several ways. Members may all share the same problem, such as premature ejaculation; members may all be of the same sex with different sexual problems; or groups may be composed of both men and women who are experiencing different sexual problems. Group therapy may be an adjunct to other forms of therapy or the prime mode of treatment. Groups organized to cure a particular dysfunction are usually behavioral in approach.

Groups composed of sexually dysfunctional married couples have also been effective. The group provides the opportunity to gather accurate information, provides consensual validation of individual preferences, and enhances self-esteem and self-acceptance. Techniques such as role playing and psychodrama may be used in treatment. Such groups are not indicated for couples when one partner is uncooperative, when a patient is suffering from a severe depression or psychosis, when there is a strong repugnance for explicit sexual audiovisual material, or when there is a strong fear of groups.

Analytically Oriented Sex Therapy

One of the most effective treatment modalities is the use of sex therapy integrated with psychodynamic and psychoanalytically oriented psychotherapy. The sex therapy is conducted over a longer than usual time period, and the extended schedule of treatment allows for the learning or relearning of sexual satisfaction under the realities of the patients' day-to-day lives. The addition of psychodynamic conceptualizations to the behavioral techniques used to treat sexual dysfunctions allows for the treatment of patients with sex disorders associated with other psychopathology.

The themes and dynamics that emerge in patients in analytically oriented sex therapy are the same as those seen in psychoanalytic therapy, such as relevant dreams, fear of punishment, aggressive feelings, difficulty with trusting the partner, fear of intimacy, oedipal feelings, and fear of genital mutilation.

The combined approach of analytically oriented sex therapy is used by the general psychiatrist, who carefully judges the optimal timing of sex therapy and the ability of patients to tolerate the directive approach that focuses on their sexual difficulties.

Biological Treatment Methods

Biological forms of treatment have limited application, but more attention is being given to this approach. Intravenous methohexital sodium (Brevital) has been used in desensitization therapy. Antianxiety agents may have application in very tense patients, although these drugs can also interfere with sexual response. Sometimes the side effects of such drugs as thioridazine and the tricyclic antidepressants are used to prolong the sexual response in conditions such as premature ejaculation. The use of tricyclics has also been advocated in the treatment of patients who are phobic about sex.

Pharmacologic approaches also involve treating any underlying psychiatric disorder that may be contributing to the sexual dysfunction. For example, patients whose sexual functioning is impaired as a result of depression will usually show improved performance as their depression responds to antidepressant medication.

Specific medications to deal with the dysfunction are not generally successful. Testosterone, which affects libido, will be of benefit to those patients who have a demonstrated low testosterone level. In women, however, testosterone leads to masculinization, such as deep voice, enlarged clitoris, and hirsutism, not all of which are reversable upon discontinuing the medication. Testosterone is contraindicated when fertility needs to be maintained. There are no known aphrodisiacs. Such substances as powdered rhinoceros horn used in Asia for their alleged stimulant effects are of benefit only through the power of suggestion in a particular culture.

Surgical treatment is even more rarely advocated, but improved penile prosthetic devices are available for men with inadequate erectile response who are resistant to other treatment methods or who have deficiencies of organic origin. Placement of a penile prosthesis in a male who has lost the ability to ejaculate or have an orgasm due to organic causes will not enable him to recover those functions. Men with prosthetic devices have generally reported satisfaction with their subsequent sexual functioning. Their wives, however, report much less satisfaction than do the men. Presurgical counseling is strongly recommended so that the couple have a realistic expectation of what the prosthesis can do for their sex lives. Some physicians are attempting revasculariztion of the penis as a direct approach to treating erectile dysfunction due to vascular disorders. In patients with corporal shunts which allow normally entrapped blood to leak from the corporal spaces leading to inadequate erections (steal phenomenon), such surgical procedures may be indicated. There are limited reports of prolonged success with this technique. Endarterectomy can be of benefit if aortoiliac occlusive disease is responsible for erectile dysfunction.

Surgical approaches to female dysfunctions include hymenectomy in the case of dyspareunia in an unconsummated marriage, vaginoplasty in multiparous women who complain of reduced vaginal sensations, or release of clitoral adhesions in women with inhibited excitement. Such surgical treatments have not been carefully studied and should be considered with great caution. Injections of papaverine into the corporal bodies of the penis produce erections for several hours; however, repeated use may cause vascular damage, and this treatment cannot be recommended on a long-term basis.

Results of Treatment

The reported effectiveness of various treatment methods for problems of sexual dysfunction varies from study to study. Demonstrating the effectiveness of traditional outpatient psychotherapy is just as difficult when therapy is oriented to sexual problems as it is in general. In some cases, the patient improves in all areas except the sexual area. Unfortunately, the more severe the psychopathology associated with a problem of long duration, the more adverse the outcome is likely to be.

The more difficult treatment cases involve couples with severe marital discord. Cases with problems of fear of intimacy, excessive dependency, or excessive hostility are also complex. Other challenges are posed by patients with lack of desire, impulse disorders, unresolved homosexual conflicts, or fetishistic defenses. Patients phobic of sex also present treatment difficulties.

When behavioral approaches are used, empirical criteria that are supposed to predict outcome are more easily isolated. Using these criteria, for instance, it appears that couples who regularly practice assigned exercises have a much greater likelihood of successful outcome than do more resistant couples or couples whose interaction involves sadomasochistic or depressive features or mechanisms of blame and projection. Flexibility of attitude is also a positive prognostic factor. Overall, younger couples tend to

complete sex therapy more often than do older couples. Those couples whose interactional difficulties center on their sex problems, such as inhibition, frustration, fear of failure, or fear of performance, are also likely to respond well to therapy.

Masters and Johnson have reported high positive results for their dual-sex therapy approach. They have studied the failure rates of their patients; failure is defined as the failure to initiate reversal of the basic symptom of the presenting dysfunction. They compared initial failure rates with 5-year follow-up findings for the same couples. Although some have criticized their definition of the percentage of presumed successes, other studies have confirmed the effectiveness of their approach. A single therapist, however, seems to be nearly as effective as a dual-sex therapy team.

In general, methods that have proved effective singly or in combination include training in behavioral-sexual skills, systematic desensitization, directive marital counseling, traditional psychodynamic approaches, and group therapy. Although treating a couple for sexual dysfunctions is the mode preferred by most workers, treatment of individuals has also been successful.

References

Dawkins S, Taylor R: Non-consummåtion of marriage. Lancet *2:*1029, 1961.
Frank E: Frequency of sexual dysfunction in "normal" couples. N Engl J Med *299:*111, 1978.
Freud S: Three essays on the theory of sexuality. In S Freud: *The Complete Psychological Works of Sigmund Freud,* vol 7, p125. Hogarth Press, London, 1953.
Fordney D S: Dyspareunia and vaginismus. Clin Obstet Gynecol *21:*205, 1978.
Furlow W L, editor: Male sexual dysfunction. Urol Clin North Am *8:*1, 1981.
Herman J, Lo Piccolo J: Clinical outcome of sex therapy. Arch Gen Psychiatry *40:*443, 1983.
Person E, Ovesy L: Homosexual cross-dressers. J Am Acad Psychoanal *12:*167, 1984.
Marmor J, editor: *Homosexual Behavior.* Basic Books, New York, 1980.
Masters W H, Johnson V E: *Human Sexual Inadequacy.* Little Brown and Co., Boston, 1970.
Sadock B J, Kaplan H I, Freedman A M, editors: *The Sexual Experience.* Williams & Wilkins, Baltimore, 1976.
Semans J H: Premature ejaculation: A new approach. South Med J *49:*353, 1956.

21.3 _____
Special Areas of Interest

RAPE

The problem of rape is most appropriately discussed under the heading of aggression. Rape is an act of violence and humiliation that happens to be expressed through sexual means. Rape is used to express power or anger. There are rarely rapes in which sex is the dominant issue; sexuality is usually used in the service of nonsexual needs.

A legal definition of rape in the United States is: "The perpetration of an act of sexual intercourse with a female, not one's wife, against her will and consent, whether her will is overcome by force or fear resulting from the threat of force or by drugs or intoxicants; or when because of mental deficiency she is incapable of exercising rational judgment, or when she is below an arbitrary age of consent."

The crime of rape requires slight penile penetration of the victim's outer vulva. Full erection and ejaculation are not necessary. Forced acts of fellatio and anal penetration, although they frequently accompany rape, are legally considered sodomy.

Studies of convicted rapists suggest that the crime is committed to relieve pent-up aggressive energy against persons of whom the rapist is in some awe. Although these awesome persons are usually men, the retaliatory violence is directed toward a woman. This finding dovetails with feminist theory, which proposes that the woman serves as an object for the displacement of aggression that the rapist cannot express directly toward other men. The woman is considered the property or the vulnerable possession of men.

Rape often occurs as an accompaniment to another crime. The rapist always threatens his victim with fists, a gun, or a knife and frequently harms her in nonsexual ways, as well as in sexual ways. The victim may be beaten, wounded, and sometimes killed.

Statistics show that 61 percent of rapists are under 25 years of age, 51 percent are white and tend to rape white victims, 47 percent are black and tend to rape black victims, and the remaining 2 percent come from all other races. Alcohol is involved in 34 percent of all forcible rapes. A composite characterization of the archetypical rapist drawn from police statistics figures portrays a single, 19-year-old man from the lower socioeconomic classes with a police record of acquisitive offenses.

Rape is a highly underreported crime. It is estimated that only one out of four to one out of ten rapes is reported. If the lower estimated figure is used, the reported incidence of 60,000 rapes reported in 1986 increases to over 200,000 rapes a year. The underreporting is attributed to feelings of shame on the part of the victim.

Victims of rape can be of any age. Cases have been reported in which the victims were 15 months old and 82 years old. The greatest danger exists for women aged 10 to 29. Rape most commonly occurs in a woman's own neighborhood, frequently inside her own home. Most rapes are premeditated. About half are committed by strangers, and half by men known, to varying degrees, by the victims; 7 percent of all rapes are perpetrated by close relatives of the victim.

The woman being raped is frequently in a life-threatening situation. During the rape, she experiences shock and fright approaching panic. Her prime motivation is to stay alive. In most cases, rapists choose victims slightly smaller than themselves. The rapist may urinate or defecate on his victim, ejaculate into her face and hair, force anal intercourse, and insert foreign objects into her vagina and rectum.

After the rape, the woman may experience shame, humiliation, confusion, fear, and rage. The type of reaction and duration of the reaction are variable, but women report effects lasting for a year or longer. Many women experience the symptoms of post-traumatic stress disorder.

Some women are able to resume sexual relations with men, particularly if they have always felt sexually adequate. Others become phobic of sexual interaction or develop such symptoms as vaginismus. Few women emerge from the assault completely unscathed. The manifestations and the degree of damage depend on the violence of the attack itself, the vulnerability of the woman, and the support systems available to her immediately after the attack.

The victim fares best when she receives immediate support and is able to ventilate her fear and rage to loving family members and to sympathetic physicians and law enforcement officials. She is helped when she knows that she has socially acceptable means of recourse at her disposal, such as the arrest and conviction of the rapist. Therapy is usually supportive in approach, unless there is a severe underlying disorder. It focuses on restoring the victim's sense of adequacy and control over her life, and relieving the feelings of helplessness, dependency, and obsession with the assault that frequently follow rape. Group therapy with homogeneous groups composed of rape victims is a particularly effective form of treatment.

The rape victim experiences a physical and psychological trauma when she is assaulted. Until recently, she also faced frequent skepticism from those to whom she reported the crime (if she had sufficient ego strength to do so) or accusations of having provoked or desired the assault. In reality, the National Commission on the Causes and Prevention of Violence found discernible victim precipitation of rape in only 4.4 percent of cases. This statistic is lower than in any other crime of violence. The education of police officers and the assignment of policewomen to deal with rape victims have helped increase the reporting of the crime. Rape crisis centers and telephone hot lines are available for immediate aid and information for victims. Volunteer groups work in emergency rooms in hospitals and with physician education programs to assist the treatment of victims.

Legally, women no longer have to prove that they actively struggled against the rapist when they appear in court. Testimony regarding the prior sexual history of the victim has recently been declared inadmissible as evidence in a number of states. Also, penalties for first-time rapists have been reduced, making juries more likely to consider a conviction. In some states wives can now prosecute husbands for rape.

Male Rape

In some states, the definition of rape is being changed to substitute the word "person" for "female." In most states, male rape is legally defined as sodomy. Homosexual rape is much more frequent among men than among women, and it occurs primarily in closed institutions, such as prisons and maximum-security hospitals. The dynamics are identical to those involved in heterosexual rape. The crime enables the rapist to discharge aggression and to aggrandize himself. The victim is usually smaller than the rapist and may be handsome in a feminine way. He is always perceived as passive and unmanly (weaker) and is used as an object.

Homosexual-rape victims often feel, as do raped women, that they have been ruined. In addition, some fear they will become homosexual because of the attack.

Statutory Rape

Intercourse is unlawful between a male over 16 years of age and a female under the age of consent, which varies from 14 to 21 years depending on the jurisdiction. Thus, a man of 18 and a girl of 15 may have consensual intercourse, yet the man may be held for statutory rape. This type of rape may vary dramatically from the crimes described above in being nonassaultive and in being a sexual act, not a violent act. Nor is it a deviant act, unless the age discrepancy is sufficient for the man to be defined as a pedophile—that is, when the girl is less than 13 years old. Charges of statutory rape are rarely pressed by the consenting girl; they are brought by her parents.

SPOUSE ABUSE

Spouse abuse is estimated to occur in from 3 million to 6 million families in the United States. This aspect of domestic violence has been recognized as a severe problem, largely as a result of recent cultural emphasis on civil rights and the work of feminist groups. However, the problem itself is one of long standing.

The major problem in spouse abuse is wife abuse, although some beatings of husbands are reported. In these cases, the husbands complain of fear of ridicule if they expose the problem, fear of charges of counterassault, and inability to leave the situation because of financial difficulties. Husband abuse has also been reported when a frail elderly man is married to a much younger woman.

Wife beating occurs in families of every racial and religious background and in all socioeconomic strata. It is most frequent in families with problems of drug abuse, particularly when there is alcoholism.

Behavioral, cultural, intrapsychic, and interpersonal factors all contribute to the development of the problem. Abusive men are likely to have come from violent homes where they witnessed wife beating or were abused themselves as children. The act itself is reinforcing; once a man has beaten his wife, he is likely to do so again. Abusive husbands tend to be immature, dependent, and nonassertive, and to suffer from strong feelings of inadequacy.

Their aggression is bullying behavior, designed to humiliate their wives to build up their own low self-esteem. The abuse is most likely to occur when the man feels threatened or frustrated at home, at work, or with peers. Impatient and impulsive, abusive husbands physically displace aggression provoked by others onto their wives. The dynamics include identification with an aggressor (father, boss), testing behavior (Will she stay with me no matter how I treat her?), distorted desires to express manhood, and dehumanization of the woman. As in rape, aggression is "permissible" when the woman is perceived as property.

Recently, hot lines, emergency shelters for women, and other organizations (e.g., Respond) have been developed to aid battered wives and to educate the public. A Presidential Commission was established to investigate spouse abuse. A major problem for abused women has been where to find a place to go when they leave home, frequently in fear of their lives. Battering is often severe, involving broken limbs, broken ribs, internal bleeding, and brain damage. When an abused wife tries to leave her husband, he often becomes doubly intimidating and threatening, "I'll get you." If the woman has small children to care for, her problem is compounded.

Some men feel remorse and guilt after an episode of violent behavior, and become particulary loving. This behavior gives the wife hope, and she remains until the next cycle of violence, which inevitably occurs.

Change is initiated only when the man is convinced that the woman will not tolerate the situation, and when she begins to exert control over his behavior. She can do so by leaving for a prolonged period, with therapy for the man as a condition of return. Family therapy is effective in treating the problem. With relatively less impulsive men, external controls, such as calling the neighbors or the police, may be sufficient to stop the behavior.

INCEST

Incest is defined as the occurrence of sexual relations between close blood relatives. A broader definition describes incest as intercourse between participants who are related to one another by some formal or informal bond of kinship, which is culturally regarded as a bar to sex relations. For example, sexual relations between stepparents and stepchildren or among stepsiblings are usually considered incestuous, even though no blood relationship exists.

The strongest and most universal taboo exists against mother-son incest. It occurs much less frequently than any other form of incest. Such behavior is usually indicative of more severe psychopathology among the participants than is father-daughter or sibling incest.

Sociologists have underlined the role of incest prohibitions as socialization factors. Biological factors also support the taboo. Groups that inbreed risk the unmasking of lethal or detrimental recessive genes, and the progeny of inbreeding groups are generally less fit than other progeny. Anthropologists have observed that the particular form of the incest taboo is culturally determined. In *Totem and Taboo*, Freud developed the concept of primal horde, in which the younger men collectively murdered the group's patriarch, who had kept all the women of the tribe to himself. The incest taboo arose both out of guilt after the murder and to prevent a repetition of the act and further rivalry after the murder and subsequent disintegration of the horde.

Accurate figures on the incidence of incest are difficult to obtain because of the general shame and embarrassment of the entire family is involved. Females are victims more often than males. About 15 million women in the United States have been the object of incestuous attention and one third of sexually abused persons have been molested before the age of 9.

Incestuous behavior is reported much more frequently among families of low socioeconomic status than among other families. This difference may be due to greater contact with reporting officials—such as welfare workers, public health personnel, and law enforcement agents—and is not a true reflection of higher incidence in that demographic group. Incest is more easily hidden by economically stable families than by the poor.

Social, cultural, physiologic, and psychological factors all contribute to the breakdown of the incest taboo. Incestuous behavior has been associated with alcoholism, overcrowding, increased physical proximity, and rural isolation that prevents adequate extrafamilial contacts. Some communities may be more tolerant of incestuous behavior than society in general. Major mental illnesses and intellectual deficiencies have been described in some cases of clinical incest. Some family therapists view incest as a defense designed to maintain a dysfunctional family unit. The older and stronger participant in incestuous behavior is usually male. Thus, incest may be viewed as a form of child abuse or as a variant of rape.

Sibling incest is reported to be more common than either father-daughter incest or mother-son incest. Many cases of sibling incest are denied by parents, or involve nearly normal interaction if the activity is prepubertal sexual play and exploration.

The daughter in father-daughter incest has frequently had a close relationship with her father throughout her childhood and is at first pleased when he approaches her sexually. The onset of incestuous behavior usually occurs when the daughter is 10 years old. As the behavior continues, however, the abused daughter becomes more bewildered, confused, and frightened. As she nears adolescence, she undergoes physiological changes that add to her confusion. She never knows whether her father will be parental or sexual. Her mother may be alternately caring and competitive; she often refuses to believe her daughter's reports or to confront her husband with her suspicions. The daughter's relationships with her siblings are also affected as they sense her special position with her father and treat her as an outsider. The father, fearful that his daughter may expose their relationship and often jealously possessive of her, interferes with the development of her normal peer relationships.

The physician must be aware of the possibility of intrafamilial sexual abuse as the cause of a wide variety of emotional and physical symptoms, including abdominal pain, genital irritations, separation anxiety, phobias, nightmares, and school problems. When incest is suspected, it is essential to interview the abused child apart from the rest of the family.

Homosexual Incest

In father-son incest, two cultural sanctions are violated: the taboo against incestuous behavior and that against homosexual behavior.

The family in which such behavior occurs is usually highly disturbed, with a violent, alcoholic, or psychopathic father, a dependent mother who is unable to protect her children, and an absence of the usual family roles and individual identities. Father-son and mother-daughter incest are rarely reported. The son is frequently the eldest child, and, if he has a sister, she is sexually abused by the father as well. The father does not necessarily have any other history of homosexual behavior. The sons in this situation may experience homicidal or suicidal ideation, and may first present to a psychiatrist with self-destructive behavior.

Treatment

The first step in the treatment of incestuous behavior is its disclosure. Once a breakthrough of the denial and collusion or fear by the family members has been achieved, incest is less likely to recur. When the participants suffer from severe psychopathology, treatment must be directed toward the underlying illness. Family therapy is useful to re-establish the group as a functioning unit and to develop healthier role definitions for each member. While the participants are learning to develop internal restraints and more appropriate methods of gratifying their needs, the external control provided by therapy helps prevent further incestuous behavior.

INFERTILITY

It is not one factor or one mate but a combination of several factors in each that contribute to infertility in 80 percent of all cases. A couple is considered infertile if they have had coitus without contraception for a period of 1 year and pregnancy has not occurred. In the United States, 12 percent of all marriages are estimated to be involuntarily childless. Various clinics report that 20 to 50 percent of couples presently facing infertility can be helped.

Until recently, the onus for the failure to conceive was on the woman, and feelings of guilt, depression, and inadequacy frequently accompanied her perception of being barren. Current practice encourages simultaneous investigation of factors preventing conception in both the man and the woman. However, it is still frequently the woman who first presents for an infertility work-up.

A thorough sexual history of the couple—including such factors as frequency of contact, erectile or ejaculatory dysfunction, and coital position—must be obtained. Frequently, conception is less likely simply because the woman rises to void, wash, or even douche immediately after coitus. Preference for coitus with the woman in the superior position is also not conducive to conception because of the lessened retention of semen.

A psychiatric evaluation of the couple may be advisable. Marital disharmony or emotional conflicts around intimacy, sexual relations, or parenting roles can directly affect endocrine function and such physiologic processes as erection, ejaculation, and ovulation.

The stress of infertility itself in a couple who want children can lead to emotional disturbance. When a pre-existing conflict gives rise to problems of identity, self-esteem, and neurotic guilt, the disturbance may be severe. It may manifest itself through regression; extreme dependency on the physician, the mate, or a parent; diffuse anger; impulsive behavior; or depression. The problem is further complicated if hormone therapy is being used to treat the infertility because the therapy may temporarily increase depression in some patients.

People who have difficulty conceiving experience shock, disbelief, and a general sense of helplessness, and they develop an understandable preoccupation with the problem. Involvement in the infertility work-up, and the development of expertise about infertility, can be a constructive defense against feelings of inadequacy and the humiliating, sometimes painful aspects of the work-up itself. Worry about attractiveness and sexual desirability is common. Partners may feel ugly or impotent, and episodes of sexual dysfunction and loss of desire are reported. These problems are aggravated if a couple is scheduling their sexual relations according to temperature charts.

In addition, they are dealing with a narcissistic blow to their sense of femininity or masculinity. An infertile partner may fear abandonment or feel that the spouse is remaining in the relationship resentfully. Single people who are aware of their own infertility may shy away from relationships for fear of being rejected once their "defect" is known. Infertile people may have particular difficulty in their adult relationships with their own parents. The identification and the equality that come from sharing the experience of parenthood must be replaced by internal reserves and other generative aspects of their lives.

Professional intervention may be necessary to help infertile couples ventilate their feelings and go through the process of mourning their lost biological functions and the children they cannot have. Couples who remain infertile must cope with an actual loss. Couples who decide not to pursue parenthood may develop a renewed sense of love, dedication, and identity as a pair. Others may need help in exploring the options of husband or donor insemination, laboratory implantation, and adoption.

STERILIZATION

Sterilization is a procedure that prevents a man or a woman from producing offspring. In a woman, the procedure is usually salpingectomy or ligation of the fallopian tubes. It is a hospital procedure with low morbidity and low mortality. A man is usually sterilized by vasectomy, ligation of the vas deferens. It is a simpler procedure than a salpingectomy and is performed in the physician's office.

A small proportion of patients who elect sterilization may suffer a neurotic poststerilization syndrome. It may manifest itself through hypochondriasis, pain, loss of libido, sexual unresponsiveness, depression, and concerns about masculinity or femininity.

When it occurs, a premorbid psychopathologic state can generally be found.

Involuntary sterilization procedures have been performed to prevent the reproduction of traits considered genetically undesirable. There have been statutes allowing for the sterilization of hereditary criminals, sex offenders, syphilitics, the mentally retarded, and epileptics. Some of these statutes have been declared unconstitutional. In recent years, human rights and civil liberties groups have been challenging the legality and ethical standing of such sterilization procedures with increasing vigor.

References

Becker J V, Skinner L J, Abel G G, Treacy E C: Incidence and types of sexual dysfunctions in rape and incest victims. J Sex Marital Ther 8:65, 1982.

Brownmiller S: *Against Our Will: Men, Women and Rape.* Simon & Schuster, New York, 1975.

Burgess A W, Holmstrom L L: Rape trauma syndrome. Am J Psychiatry *131*:981, 1974.

Ellenberg J J, Koren Z: Infertility and depression. Int J Fertil 27:219, 1982.

Freud S: *Totem and Taboo.* W W Norton, New York, 1950.

Henderson D J: Incest. In *The Sexual Experience,* B J Sadock, H I Kaplan, A M Freedman, editors, p415. Williams and Wilkins, Baltimore, 1976.

Herman J L, Gartrell N, Olarte S, Feldstein M, Cocalio R: Psychiatrist-patient sexual contact: Results of a national survey. II: Psychiatrist's attitudes. Am J Psychiatry *144*:164, 1987.

Herman J, Hirschman L: Families at risk for father-daughter incest. Am J Psychiatry *138*:967, 1981.

Hilberman E: "Wife-beater's wife" reconsidered. Am J Psychiatry *137*:11, 1980.

Johnson R L, Shrier D: Past sexual victimization by females of male patients in an adolescent medicine clinic population. Am J Psychiatry *144*:650, 1987.

Sarrel P M, Masters W H: Sexual molestation of men by women. Arch Sex Behav *11*:117, 1982.

Stewart B D, Hughes C, Frank E, Andersen B, Kendall K, West D: The aftermath of rape. Profiles of immediate and delayed treatment seekers. J Nervous Mental Dis *175*:90, 1987.

Vessey M, Higgins G, Lawless M, McPherson K, Yeates D: Tubal sterilization: Findings in a large prospective study. Br J Obstet Gynecol *90*:203, 1983.

22

Normal Sleep and Sleep Disorders

22.1

Normal Sleep

Sleep can be defined as a regular, recurrent, easily reversible state of the organism that is characterized by relative quiescence and by a great increase in the threshold of response to external stimuli relative to the waking state. Complaints of sleep disturbance are among the most common of all symptoms. Close monitoring of sleep is an important part of clinical practice since sleep disturbance is an early symptom of impending mental illness. Recent advances in sleep research have demonstrated that some mental disorders are associated with characteristic changes in sleep physiology. These changes can provide insights into the underlying pathophysiology of mental disorders as well as determine diagnoses in complex clinical presentations.

NORMAL SLEEP PATTERNS

As a person falls asleep, his brain waves go through certain characteristic changes, classified as stages 1, 2, 3, and 4 (Figure 1). The waking EEG is characterized by α-waves of 8 to 12 cycles a second and low-voltage activity of mixed frequency. As the person falls asleep, α-activity begins to disappear. Stage 1, considered the lightest stage of sleep, is characterized by low-voltage, regular activity at 3 to 7 cycles per second. After a few seconds or minutes, this stage gives way to stage 2, a pattern showing frequent spindle-shaped tracings at 12 to 14 cycles per second (sleep spindles) and slow, triphasic waves known as K-complexes. Soon thereafter, δ waves—high-voltage activity at 0.5 to 2.5 cycles per second—make their appearance and occupy less than 50 percent of the tracing (stage 3). Eventually, in stage 4, δ-waves occupy more than 50 percent of the record. It is common practice to describe stages 3 and 4 as delta sleep or slow-wave sleep (SWS) because of their characteristic appearance on the EEG record.

POLYSOMNOGRAM REM FINDINGS

NREM sleep is composed of stages 1 through 4. As compared to wakefulness, most physiological functions are markedly reduced during NREM sleep. REM sleep is a qualitatively different kind of sleep characterized by a highly active brain, and physiological activity levels similar to wakefulness. About 90 minutes after sleep onset, NREM yields to be the first REM episode of the night. This "REM latency" of 90 minutes is a consistent finding in normal adults. A shortening of REM latency frequently occurs with disorders, such as depression or narcolepsy. The EEG records the rapid conjugate eye movements that are the identifying feature of this sleep state (there are no or few rapid eye movements in NREM sleep); the EEG pattern consists of low voltage, random fast activity with sawtooth waves; the electromyograph (EMG) shows marked reduction in muscle tone.

In normal persons, NREM sleep is a peaceful state relative to waking. Pulse rate is typically slowed, 5 or 10 beats per minute below the level of restful waking, and is very regular. Respiration behaves in the same way. Blood pressure also tends to be low, with few minute-to-minute variations. Resting muscle potential of body musculature is lower in REM sleep than in waking. Episodic, involuntary body movement is present in NREM sleep. There are few rapid eye movements, if any, and seldom any penile erections. Blood flow through most tissues, including cerebral blood flow, is also slightly reduced.

The deepest portions of NREM sleep—stages 3 and 4—are sometimes associated with unusual arousal characteristics. When someone is aroused a half hour to 1 hour after sleep onset—usually in SWS—he is disoriented and his thinking is disorganized. Brief arousals from SWS are also associated with amnesia for events that occur during the arousal. In certain persons, the disorganization during arousal from stage 3 or stage 4 results in specific problems, including enuresis, somnambulism, and stage 4 nightmares or night terrors.

Polygraphic measures during REM sleep show irregular patterns, sometimes close to aroused waking patterns. Indeed, if one was not aware of the behavioral state of the person and one happened to be recording a variety of physiologic measures (but not muscle tone) during REM periods, one would undoubtedly conclude that the person or animal was in an active waking state. It is because of this observation that REM sleep has also been termed "paradoxical sleep." Pulse, respiration, and blood pressure in humans are all high during REM sleep—much higher than during

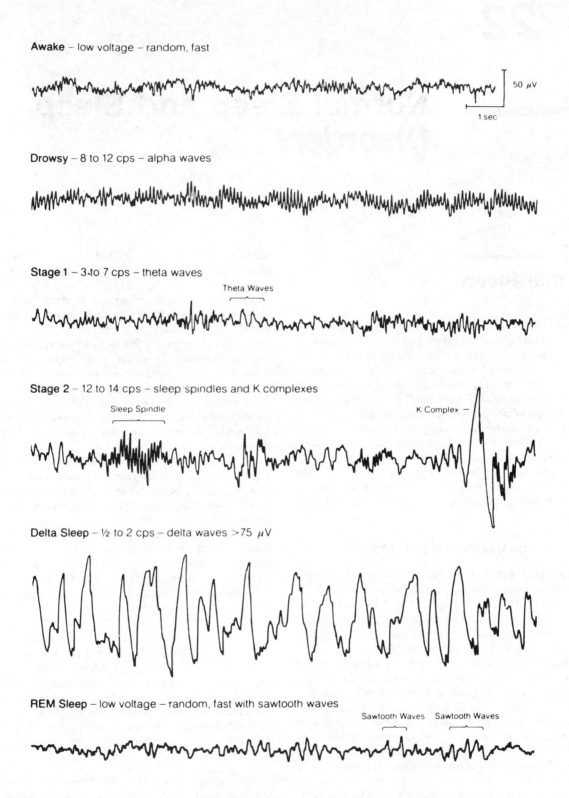

Awake – low voltage – random, fast

50 μV

1 sec

Drowsy – 8 to 12 cps – alpha waves

Stage 1 – 3 to 7 cps – theta waves

Theta Waves

Stage 2 – 12 to 14 cps – sleep spindles and K complexes

Sleep Spindle

K Complex –

Delta Sleep – ½ to 2 cps – delta waves >75 μV

REM Sleep – low voltage – random, fast with sawtooth waves

Sawtooth Waves   Sawtooth Waves

Figure 1.   Human Sleep Stages. Figure from Houri P: *The Sleep Disorders,* p 7. Current Concepts, Upjohn, Michigan, 1982.

NREM sleep and quite often higher than during waking. Even more striking than the level or rate is the variability from minute to minute. Brain oxygen use increases during REM sleep. The ventilatory response to increased levels of CO_2 is depressed during REM sleep, so that there is no increase in tidal volume as PCO_2 increases. Thermoregulation is altered during REM sleep. In contrast to the homeothermic condition of temperature regulation that is present during wakefulness or NREM sleep, a poikilothermic condition (a state in which animal temperature varies with the changes in the temperature of the surrounding medium) is present during REM sleep. Poikilothermia, which is characteristic of reptiles, results in a failure to respond to changes in ambient temperature with shivering or sweating, whichever is appropriate to maintaining body temperature. Almost every REM period is accompanied by a partial or full penile erection. This finding has proven to be of significant clinical value in evaluating the cause of impotence. The nocturnal penile tumescence study is one of the most commonly requested sleep laboratory tests. Another physiologic change that occurs during REM sleep is the near total paralysis of skeletal (postural) muscles. Because of this motor inhibition, body movement is absent during REM sleep. Probably the most distinctive feature of REM sleep is dreaming. Persons awakened during REM sleep frequently (60 to 90 percent of the time) report that they had been dreaming.

The cyclical nature of sleep is quite regular and reliable; a REM period covers about every 90 to 100 minutes during the night (Figure 2). The first REM period tends to be the shortest, usually lasting less than 10 minutes; the later REM periods may last 15 to 40 minutes each. Most REM time occurs in the last third of the night, whereas most stage 4 sleep occurs in the first third of the night.

NREM sleep can be neatly organized according to depth, as measured by arousal threshold and by EEG activity: stage 1 is the lightest stage, and stage 4 is the deepest stage. REM sleep, however-er, does not fit into that continuum. The arousal threshold for REM sleep is similar to that for stage 2 sleep.

Sleep patterns change over the lifespan. In the neonatal period, REM sleep represents more than 50 percent of total sleep time. In addition, newborns pass from wakefulness directly to REM sleep. By 4 months of age, the sleep pattern shifts so that the total percentage of REM drops to less than 40 percent and entry into sleep occurs with an initial period of NREM sleep. By young adulthood, the distribution of sleep stages is as follows:

NREM (75 percent)
    Stage 1: 5 percent
    Stage 2: 45 percent
    Stage 3: 12 percent
    Stage 4: 13 percent
REM (25 percent)

This distribution remains relatively constant into old age, although a reduction occurs in both SWS and REM sleep.

SLEEP REGULATION

The prevailing view at present is that there is not a simple sleep control center but a small number of interconnecting systems or centers that are chiefly located in the brain stem and that mutually activate and inhibit one another. Many studies support the role of serotonin in sleep regulation. Prevention of serotonin synthesis or destruction of the dorsal raphe nucleus of the brain stem which contains nearly all the brain's serotonergic cell bodies, reduces sleep for a considerable time. Synthesis and release of serotonin by serotonergic neurons is influenced by availability of amino acid precursors of that neurotransmitter, such as

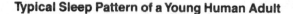

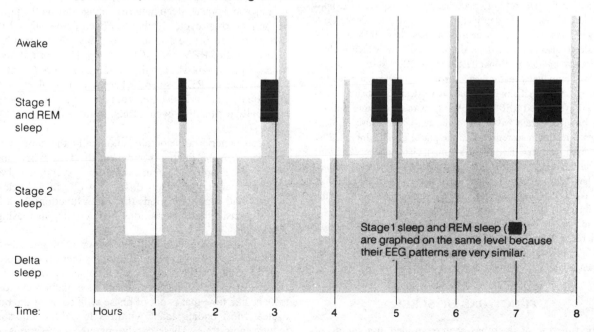

Figure 2. Typical Sleep Pattern of a Young Human Adult. Figure from Houri P: *The Sleep Disorders,* p 8. Current Concepts, Upjohn, Michigan, 1982.

L-tryptophan. Ingestion of large amounts of L-tryptophan (1 to 15 g) have been shown to reduce sleep latency and nocturnal awakenings. Conversely, L-tryptophan deficiency is associated with less time spent in REM sleep. Thus, enhancement of serotonergic neurotransmission may be beneficial in the treatment of sleep disturbances.

In newborns, the addition of L-tryptophan to formula hastens the onset of both REM and NREM sleep. By comparison, feeding valine, which competes with L-tryptophan for entry into the brain, prolongs onset of both sleep states.

Norepinephrine-containing neurons with cell bodies located in the locus ceruleus play an important role in controlling normal sleep patterns. Drugs and manipulations that increase firing of these noradrenergic neurons produce a marked reduction in REM sleep ("REM off" neurons) and an increase in wakefulness. Electrical stimulation of the locus ceruleus in humans with chronically implanted electrodes (for control of spasticity) profoundly disrupts all sleep parameters.

Brain acetylcholine is also involved in sleep, particularly in the production of REM sleep. In animal studies, injection of cholinergic-muscarinic agonists into pontine reticular formation neurons ("REM on" neurons) results in a shift from wakefulness to REM sleep. Disturbances in central cholinergic activity are associated with the sleep changes observed in major depression. As compared to healthy subjects and non-depressed psychiatric controls, depressed patients have marked disruption of REM sleep patterns. These include: shortened REM latency (60 minutes or less); greater percentage of REM; and shift in REM distribution from the last half to the first half of the night. Administration of a muscarinic agonist, such as arecoline, to depressed patients during the first or second NREM periods results in a rapid onset of REM sleep. It is postulated that depression is associated with an underlying supersensitivity to acetylcholine.

Another intriguing observation suggests a link between acetylcholine and depression. Drugs that reduce REM sleep, such as antidepressants, produce beneficial effects in depression. Indeed, about half of the patients with major depression experience temporary improvement when deprived or restricted from sleep. Conversely, reserpine, which is one of the few drugs that increases REM sleep, also produces depression. Narcolepsy, which is characterized by pathological manifestations of REM sleep, is aggravated by compounds that enhance or mimic cholinergic activity.

Patients with Alzheimer's disease have sleep disturbances characterized by reduced REM and SWS. Loss of cholinergic neurons in the basal forebrain has been implicated as the cause of these changes. Melatonin secretion from the pineal gland is inhibited by bright light, so that the lowest serum melatonin concentrations occur during the day. The suprachiasmatic nucleus of the hypothalamus has been identified as the anatomical site of a "circadian pacemaker" that regulates melatonin secretion as well as the entrainment of the brain to a 24-hour sleep-wake cycle.

Evidence shows that dopamine has an alerting effect. Drugs that increase brain dopamine tend to produce arousal and wakefulness. In contrast, dopamine blockers, such as pimozide and the phenothiazines, tend to increase sleep time.

FUNCTIONS OF SLEEP

The function of sleep has been examined in a variety of ways; most investigators conclude that sleep serves a restorative, homeostatic function.

Sleep Deprivation

Prolonged periods of sleep deprivation sometimes lead to ego disorganization, hallucinations, and delusions. Depriving persons of REM sleep by awakening them at the beginning of REM cycles produces an increase in the number of REM periods and in the amount of REM sleep (rebound increase) when the person is allowed to sleep without interruption. REM-deprived patients tend to be irritable and lethargic.

Sleep Requirements

Some persons are normally short sleepers who require less than 6 hours each night and function adequately. Long sleepers are those who sleep more than 9 hours each night in order to function adequately. Long sleepers have more REM periods and more rapid eye movements within each period (known as REM density) than do short sleepers. These movements are sometimes considered a measure of intensity of REM sleep and are related to the vividness of dreaming. Short sleepers are generally efficient, ambitious, socially adept and content. Long sleepers tend to be mildly depressed, anxious, and socially withdrawn. Increased sleep needs occur with physical work, exercise, illness, pregnancy, general mental stress, or increased mental activity. REM periods increase after strong psychological stimuli (e.g., difficult learning situations, stress) and after the use of chemicals or drugs that decrease brain catecholamines.

SLEEP-WAKE RHYTHM

Sleep is influenced by biological rhythms. Within a 24-hour period, adults sleep once, sometimes twice. This rhythm is not present at birth, but develops over the first 2 years of life.

In some women, sleep patterns change during the phases of the menstrual cycle. It also has been demonstrated that naps, taken at different times of the day, differ greatly in their content of REM and NREM sleep. In a normal nighttime sleeper, a nap taken in the morning or at noon contains a great deal of REM sleep, whereas a nap taken in the afternoon or the early evening contains much less. There is apparently a circadian cycle affecting the tendency to have REM sleep.

Sleep patterns are not physiologically the same when one sleeps in the daytime or during the time when one's body is accustomed to being awake; the psychological and behavioral effects of sleep differ as well. In a world of industry and communications that often functions on a 24-hour day basis, these interactions are becoming increasingly significant.

Even in persons who do not work at night, the interference between the various rhythms can produce problems. The best known example is jet lag in which, after flying east-to-west, one tries to convince one's body to go to sleep at a time that is out of phase with some of the body cycles. Most bodies adapt within a few days, but some require more time. These conditions are more serious and apparently involve long-term cycle disruption and interference.

References

Dement W C: *Some Must Watch While Some Must Sleep*. W H Freeman, New York, 1974.

Dubé S, Kumar N, Ehedgui E: Cholinergic REM induction response: Separation of anxiety and depression. Bio/Psychiatry 20:408, 1985.

Karacan I, editor: *Psychophysiological Aspects of Sleep: Proceedings of the Third International Congress of Sleep Research*. Noyes Medical Publications, Park Ridge, NJ, 1981.

Karacan I, Moore C A: Physiology and Neurochemistry of Sleep. In *Annual Review*, A J Frances, R E Hales, editors, vol 4. American Psychiatric Press, Washington, DC, 1985.

Lugaresi E, Medori R, Montagna P: Fatal familial insomnia and dysautonomia with selective degeneration of thalamic nuclei. N Engl J Med 315:997, 1986.

Mellinger G D: Insomnia and its treatment. Arch Gen Psychiatry 42:225, 1985.

Merica H, Gaillard J M: Internal structure of sleep cycles in a healthy population. Sleep, 9:502, 1986.

Moore-Ede M E, Sulzman F M, Fuller C A: *The Clocks That Time Us: Physiology of the Circadian Timing System*. Harvard Press, Cambridge, MA, 1982.

Morrison A R: A window on the sleeping brain. Sci American 248:94, 1983.

22.2 ———
Sleep Disorders

Sleep disorders are major psychiatric disorders that affect many persons. For instance, in the course of a year, up to 30 percent of the population suffer from insomnia and seek help for it. In many sleep disorders, a careful diagnostic workup reveals a specific cause of the insomnia and a specific treatment aimed at the cause may be used.

In DSM-III-R, the nosology of sleep disorders is derived in part from that of the Association of Sleep Disorder Centers (ASDC). There are two major DSM-III-R categories of sleep disorders: the dyssomnias and the parasomnias. The dyssomnias are insomnia, difficulty in falling asleep; hypersomnia, excessive amounts of sleep or complaints about excessive daytime somnolence; and sleep-wake schedule disorders. The parasomnias are a heterogeneous group of episodic nocturnal events that occur during sleep or at the threshold between wakefulness and sleep.

In this section, the current DSM-III-R classification is used, but the reader should be aware of the more detailed ASDC groupings, which many sleep experts favor (Table 1).

DYSSOMNIAS

Insomnia Disorder

Insomnia is a disorder of initiating or of maintaining sleep (DIMS). It may be transient or persistent. In the latter case, according to DSM-III-R, the disturbance occurs at least three times a week for at least 1 month and results in significant daytime fatigue or impaired social or occupational functioning (Table 2). A causal classification of insomnia is presented in Table 3.

A brief period of insomnia most often is associated with anxiety, either as a sequela to an anxious experience or in anticipation of an anxiety-provoking experience (e.g., an examination or an impending job interview). In some persons, transient insomnia of this kind may be related to grief reaction, reaction to loss, or almost any life change. This condition is not likely to be serious, although it should be kept in mind that a psychotic episode or a severe depression may sometimes begin with an acute insomnia. Specific treatment for this condition is usually not required. In cases where treatment with hypnotic medication may be indicated, the physician and patient should both be clear that the treatment is of short duration and that some symptoms, including brief recurrence of the insomnia, may be expected when medication is discontinued.

Persistent insomnia is a fairly common type; it is a category that is not well understood. It refers to a group of conditions in which the problem is most often difficulty falling asleep rather than remaining asleep, and involves two sometimes separable but often intertwined problems: somatized tension and anxiety, and a conditioned associative response. The patients often have no clear complaint other than insomnia. They may not experience anxiety per se but discharge it through physiologic channels. They may complain chiefly of apprehensive feelings or ruminative thoughts that appear to keep them from falling asleep. Usually, these are not patients who experience specific fears or dreads as they fall asleep. Sometimes, but not always, a patient describes how the condition is exacerbated at times of stress at work or at home and remits during vacations.

Treatment of this condition is among the most difficult problems in sleep disorders. In pure cases where the conditioned component is prominent, a deconditioning technique may be useful. The patients are asked to use the bed for sleeping and for nothing else; if they are not asleep after 5 minutes in bed, they are instructed to simply get up and do something else. Sometimes actually changing to another bed or to another room is useful. In some cases where the somatized tension or muscle tension is prominent, relaxation tapes, transcendental meditation, or practicing the relaxation response and biofeedback are occasionally helpful. Psychotherapy has not been very useful in the treatment of this sort of insomnia.

Insomnia Related to Another Mental Disorder (Nonorganic)

Insomnia that is clearly related to the psychological and behavioral symptoms of the clinically well known psychiatric disorders are classified here (Table 4). This category consists of a heterogeneous group of conditions. In these cases, the sleep problem is usually, but not always, difficulty in falling asleep, and is secondary to anxiety that is part of any of the various psychiatric illnesses and conditions listed. Nonorganic insomnia is more common in females than in males. In clear-cut cases where the anxiety has psychological roots, psychiatric treatment of the cause of the anxiety (e.g., individual psychotherapy, group psychotherapy, and family therapy) often relieves the insomnia.

The insomnia associated with depression is well known to psychiatrists. Most common in severe unipolar depression, it involves relatively normal sleep onset, but repeated awakenings during the second half of the night and premature morning awakening, usually with a very uncomfortable mood in the morning.

Table 1
Outline of Diagnostic Classification of Sleep and Arousal Disorders*

(A.) DIMS: Disorders of Initiating and Maintaining Sleep (Insomnias)
1. Psychophysiological
    a. Transient and Situational
    b. Persistent
2. *associated with*
Psychiatric Disorders
    a. Symptom and Personality Disorders
    b. Affective Disorders
    c. Other Functional Psychoses
3. *associated with*
Use of Drugs and Alcohol
    a. Tolerance to or Withdrawal from CNS Depressants
    b. Sustained Use of CNS Stimulants
    c. Sustained Use of or Withdrawal from Other Drugs
    d. Chronic Alcoholism
4. *associated with*
Sleep-induced Respiratory Impairment
    a. Sleep Apnea DIMS Syndrome
    b. Alveolar Hypoventilation DIMS Syndrome
5. *associated with*
Sleep-related (Nocturnal) Myoclonus and "Restless Legs"
    a. Sleep-related (Nocturnal) Myoclonus DIMS Syndrome
    b. "Restless Legs" DIMS Syndrome
6. *associated with*
Other Medical, Toxic, and Environmental Conditions
7. Childhood-Onset DIMS
8. *associated with*
Other DIMS Conditions
    a. Repeated REM Sleep Interruptions
    b. Atypical Polysomnographic Features
    c. Not Otherwise Specified†
9. No DIMS Abnormality
    a. Short Sleeper
    b. Subjective DIMS Complaint without Objective Findings
    c. Not Otherwise Specified†

(B.) DOES: Disorders of Excessive Somnolence
1. Psychophysiological
    a. Transient and Situational
    b. Persistent
2. *associated with*
Psychiatric Disorders
    a. Affective Disorders
    b. Other Functional Disorders
3. *associated with*
Use of Drugs and Alcohol
    a. Tolerance to or Withdrawal from CNS Stimulants
    b. Sustained Use of CNS Depressants
4. *associated with*
Sleep-induced Respiratory Impairment
    a. Sleep Apnea DOES Syndrome
    b. Alveolar Hypoventilation DOES Syndrome
5. *associated with*
Sleep-related (Nocturnal) Myoclonus and "Restless Legs"

a. Sleep-related (Nocturnal) Myoclonus DOES Syndrome
    b. "Restless Legs" DOES Syndrome
6. Narcolepsy
7. Idiopathic CNS Hypersomnolence
8. *associated with*
Other Medical, Toxic, and Environmental Conditions
9. *associated with*
Other DOES Conditions
    a. Intermittent DOES (Periodic) Syndromes
        i. Kleine-Levin Syndrome
        ii. Menstrual-associated Syndrome
    b. Insufficient Sleep
    c. Sleep Drunkenness
    d. Not Otherwise Specified†
10. No DOES Abnormality
    a. Long Sleeper
    b. Subjective DOES Complaint without Objective Findings
    c. Not Otherwise Specified†

(C.) Disorders of the Sleep-Wake Schedule
1. Transient
    a. Rapid Time Zone Change ("Jet Lag") Syndrome
    b. "Work Shift" Change in Conventional Sleep-Wake Schedule
2. Persistent
    a. Frequently Changing Sleep-Wake Schedule
    b. Delayed Sleep Phase Syndrome
    c. Advanced Sleep Phase Syndrome
    d. Non-24-Hour Sleep-Wake Syndrome
    e. Irregular Sleep-Wake Pattern
    f. Not Otherwise Specified†

(D.) Dysfunctions Associated with Sleep, Sleep Stages, or Partial Arousals (Parasomnias)
1. Sleepwalking (Somnambulism)
2. Sleep Terror (Pavor Nocturnus, Incubus)
3. Sleep-related Enuresis
4. Other Dysfunctions
    a. Dream Anxiety Attacks (Nightmares)
    b. Sleep-related Epileptic Seizures
    c. Sleep-related Bruxism
    d. Sleep-related Headbanging (Jactatio Capitis Nocturnus)
    e. Familial Sleep Paralysis
    f. Impaired Sleep-related Penile Tumescence
    g. Sleep-related Painful Erections
    h. Sleep-related Cluster Headaches and Chronic Paroxysmal Hemicrania
    i. Sleep-related Abnormal Swallowing Syndrome
    j. Sleep-related Asthma
    k. Sleep-related Cardiovascular Symptoms
    l. Sleep-related Gastroesophageal Reflux
    m. Sleep-related Hemolysis (Paroxysmal Nocturnal Hemoglobinuria)
    n. Asymptomatic Polysomnographic Finding
    o. Not Otherwise Specified†

*From the Association of Sleep Disorders Centers: Diagnostic classification of sleep and arousal disorders. Sleep **2**: 17, 1979, by permission.
†This entry is intended to leave place in the classification for both undiagnosed ("don't know") conditions and additional (as yet undocumented) conditions that may be described in the future. Table from Hartman E L: Sleep disorders. In *Comprehensive Textbook of Psychiatry*, ed 4, H I Kaplan, B J Sadock, editors, p 1249. Williams & Wilkins, Baltimore, 1985.

Table 2
Diagnostic Criteria for Insomnia Disorders

A. The predominant complaint is of difficulty in initiating or maintaining sleep, or of nonrestorative sleep (sleep that is apparently adequate in amount, but leaves the person feeling unrested).

B. The disturbance in A occurs at least three times a week for at least 1 month and is sufficiently severe to result in either a complaint of significant daytime fatigue or the observation by others of some symptom that is attributable to the sleep disturbance (e.g., irritability or impaired daytime functioning).

C. Occurrence not exclusively during the course of Sleep-Wake Schedule Disorder or a Parasomnia.

Table from DSM-III-R *Diagnostic and Statistical Manual of Mental Disorders,* ed 3, revised. (Current Classification of Mental Disorders, 1987.) Copyright American Psychiatric Association, Washington, D.C., 1987. Used with permission.

(Morning is the worst time of day for these patients.) Polysomnography shows reduced stages 3 and 4 sleep, often a short REM latency, and a long first REM period.

Bipolar depression as well as less severe depression may involve some of the sleep maintenance insomnia described above, but it is also frequently associated with hypersomnia. Depression secondary to other illness often causes sleep maintenance insomnia; the patient awakens during the night but does not display reduced REM latency.

Manic and hypomanic patients appear to be extreme cases of short sleepers. They sometimes appear to have difficulty falling asleep, but most often do not complain of any sleep problem. They awaken refreshed after 2 to 4 hours of sleep and appear to have a true reduction in need for sleep during the course of the manic episode.

Treatment involves treatment of the underlying mania and depression, rather than of the sleep problem. If possible, these patients should not be given sleeping medication in addition to their antidepressants. An antidepressant, such as amitriptyline, given at bedtime often produces an improvement in sleep even before the remainder of the depression is improved.

Insomnia Related to a Known Organic Factor

The essential feature of this classification is that insomnia is due to a known physical condition or to medication or drugs (Table 5).

Physical Condition. Almost any medical condition associated with pain and discomfort (e.g., arthritis, angina) can produce insomnia. A variety of CNS conditions are associated with insomnia even when pain and discomfort are not specifically present. These include neoplasms, vascular lesions, infections and degenerative and traumatic conditions. Likewise, a variety of other conditions, especially endocrine and metabolic diseases, frequently involve some sleep disturbance.

Awareness of the possibility of such conditions and obtaining a good medical history usually lead to a correct diagnosis; the treatment, whenever possible, will be treatment of the underlying medical condition.

Medication. Insomnia is associated with tolerance to or withdrawal from CNS depressants. With sustained use of such agents—usually undertaken to treat insomnia arising from a different source—tolerance increases and the depressants lose their sleep-inducing effects; then, patients often increase the dose. Upon

Table 3
Causes of Insomnia

Symptom	Insomnias Secondary to Medical Conditions	Insomnias Secondary to Psychiatric or Environmental Conditions
Difficulty in falling asleep	Any painful or uncomfortable condition CNS lesions Conditions listed below, at times	Anxiety, common Anxiety, chronic neurotic Anxiety, prepsychotic Tension anxiety, muscular Environmental changes Conditioned (habit) insomnia Sleep-Wake Schedule Disorders
Difficulty in remaining asleep	Sleep apnea syndromes Nocturnal myoclonus and restless legs syndrome Dietary factors (probably) Episodic events (parasomnias) Direct drug effects (including alcohol) Drug withdrawal effects (including alcohol) Drug interactions Endocrine or metabolic diseases Infectious, neoplastic, or other diseases Painful or uncomfortable conditions Brain stem or hypothalamic lesions or diseases Aging	Depression, especially primary depression Environmental changes Sleep-Wake Schedule Disorders Dream interruption insomnia

Table from Hartman E L: Sleep disorders. In *Comprehensive Textbook of Psychiatry,* ed 4, H I Kaplan, B J Sadock, editors, p 1248. Williams & Wilkins, Baltimore, 1985.

Table 4
Diagnostic Criteria for Insomnia Related to Another Mental Disorder (Nonorganic)

Insomnia Disorder, as defined by criteria A, B, and C in Table 2, that is related to another Axis I or Axis II mental disorder, such as Major Depression, Generalized Anxiety Disorder, Adjustment Disorder with Anxious Mood, or Obsessive Compulsive Personality Disorder. This category is not used if the Insomnia Disorder is related to an Axis I disorder involving a known organic factor, such as a Psychoactive Substance Use Disorder (e.g., Amphetamine Dependence).

Table from DSM-III-R *Diagnostic and Statistical Manual of Mental Disorders,* ed 3, revised. (Current Classification of Mental Disorders, 1987.) Copyright American Psychiatric Association, Washington, D.C., 1987. Used with permission.

Table 5
Diagnostic Criteria for Insomnia Related to a Known Organic Factor

Insomnia Disorder, as defined by criteria A, B, and C in Table 2 that is related to a known organic factor, such as a physical disorder (e.g., sleep apnea, arthritis), a Psychoactive Substance Use Disorder (e.g., Amphetamine Dependence), or a medication (e.g., prolonged use of decongestants).

The known organic factor should be listed on Axis III (if a physical disorder or use of a medication that does not meet the criteria for a Psychoactive Substance Use Disorder) or Axis I (if a Psychoactive Substance Use Disorder).

Table from DSM-III-R *Diagnostic and Statistical Manual of Mental Disorders,* ed 3, revised. (Current Classification of Mental Disorders, 1987.) Copyright American Psychiatric Association, Washington, D.C., 1987. Used with permission.

sudden discontinuation of the drug, severe sleeplessness supervenes, often accompanied by the general features of a drug withdrawal syndrome.

Chronic use (over 30 days) of a hypnotic agent is well tolerated by some patients, while others begin to complain of sleep disturbance, most often multiple brief awakenings during the night. Recordings show disruption of sleep architecture, reduced stages 3 and 4 REM sleep, increases of stages 1 and 2, and fragmentation of sleep throughout the night.

It is important to be aware of CNS stimulants as a possible cause for insomnia and to remember that various medications for weight reduction, beverages containing caffeine (including Coca-Cola), and occasionally adrenergic drugs taken by asthmatics may all produce this sort of insomnia.

For reasons that are not always clear, a wide variety of drugs occasionally produce sleep problems as a side effect. These drugs include antimetabolites and other cancer chemotherapeutic agents, thyroid preparations, anticonvulsant agents, monoamine oxidase (MAO) inhibitors, adrenocorticotropic hormone–like (ACTH) drugs, oral contraceptives, α-methyl dopa, β-blocking drugs, and others.

Another group of agents do not produce sleep disturbance while they are being used, but may upon withdrawal. Almost any drug with sedating or tranquilizing agents can have this effect, including at times the benzodiazepines, the phenothiazines, the sedating tricyclics, and various street drugs, including marijuana and the opiates.

Alcohol is a CNS depressant and produces the serious problems discussed above under CNS depressants, both during administration—perhaps related to the development of tolerance—and after withdrawal. The insomnia following long-term alcohol consumption is sometimes extremely severe and lasts for weeks or longer. It is inadvisable to give a patient who has just recovered from an addiction another potentially addicting medication; thus, sleeping medication, if possible, should be avoided at such times.

Primary Insomnia

This is a new category in DSM-III-R used to describe an insomnia disorder not due to any of the causes mentioned above (e.g., psychiatric illness, medical illness, or drug use). The term "primary" indicates that the insomnia occurs independent of any known physical or mental condition (Table 6). Some persons who complain of insomnia may be malingerers; others who have a hypochondriacal condition may choose sleep as the problem on which to concentrate. Aging persons complain because they do not sleep as much as they used to, although they actually have absolutely normal sleep for their age. There are so-called variable sleepers, who have not yet become accustomed to their need for less sleep. They are distinguished from short sleepers who have no complaints, although they may on occasion want to sleep longer. In general, patients with this disorder are preoccupied with getting enough sleep, which may be a lifelong pattern.

Repeated REM Sleep Interruptions. REM–interruption insomnia, originally called dream-interruption insomnia, is quite rare. It has been related to psychological difficulties and periods of nightmares or other disturbing dreams. In these cases, it may actually represent a sort of conditioned avoidance response in which the patient's CNS senses the beginnings of a dream period (REM period), associates it with the oncoming unpleasant dream or nightmare, and produces an immediate arousal response.

Atypical Polysomnographic Features. Atypical polysomnographic features is a condition in which sleep is frequently interrupted and nonrestorative, and the sleep stage structure is marked by abnormal physiologic features.

The diagnosis can be made on the basis of sleep recordings, preferably multiple sleep recordings. Most commonly, the patient describes quality of sleep as poor, light, or unrestful.

Table 6
Diagnostic Criteria for Primary Insomnia

Insomnia Disorder, as defined by criteria A, B, and C in Table 2, that apparently is not maintained by any other mental disorder or any known organic factor, such as a physical disorder, a Psychoactive Substance Use Disorder, or a medication.

Table from DSM-III-R *Diagnostic and Statistical Manual of Mental Disorders,* ed 3, revised. (Current Classification of Mental Disorders, 1987.) Copyright American Psychiatric Association, Washington, D.C., 1987. Used with permission.

Hypersomnia Disorder

Hypersomnia consists of two groups of symptoms: complaints about excessive amounts of sleep and complaints about excessive daytime sleepiness (somnolence). In some situations, both groups of symptoms may be present. The DSM-III-R diagnostic criteria for hypersomnia disorder are presented in Table 7. This condition is also known as disorders of excessive somnolence (DOES). The term "somnolence" should be reserved for patients who complain of sleepiness and have a clear demonstrable tendency to fall asleep suddenly in the waking state, who have sleep attacks, and who cannot remain awake; it should not be used for persons who are simply physically tired or weary. The distinction, however, is not always absolutely clear. The complaints constituting hypersomnolence are much less frequent than are the complaints of insomnia, but they are by no means rare complaints if the clinician is alert to them. It has been estimated that there are more than 100,000 narcoleptics in the United States, and narcolepsy is just one well known condition clearly producing hypersomnolence. If one includes drug-related and alcohol-related conditions, it turns out that hypersomnolence is quite a common symptom.

Table 8 presents a causal classification of hypersomnolence. As with the symptom of insomnia, there are borderline conditions, situations that are hard to classify, and idiopathic cases.

According to a recent survey, the most common conditions responsible for hypersomnolence severe enough to be evaluated by all-night recordings at a sleep disorders center were sleep apnea and narcolepsy. It is worth keeping in mind that sleep requirements vary. Many people, long sleepers, require 9 to 10 hours of sleep a night, but like short sleepers, they do not have any problem.

Transient and situational hypersomnia consists of a disruption of the normal sleep-wake pattern marked by excessive difficulty remaining awake and a tendency to remain in bed for unusually long periods or to return to bed frequently during the day to nap. This change is experienced suddenly in response to an identifiable recent life change, conflict, or loss. It is much less common than insomnia. It is seldom marked by definite sleep attacks or unavoidable sleep, but rather by tiredness or falling asleep sooner than usual and by difficulty in arising in the morning.

Hypersomnia Related to Another Mental Disorder (Nonorganic)

Hypersomnia associated with a mental disorder is found in a variety of conditions including both mood and other depressive (cyclothymic, dysthymic) syndromes. Excessive daytime sleepiness may be reported in the initial stages of many mild depressive disorders and characteristically in the depressed phase of bipolar disorder. It is sometimes associated for a few weeks with uncomplicated grief. *Other mental disorders* such as personality disorders, dissociative and somatoform disorders, fugue, and amnesia, can produce hypersomnia (Table 9).

Hypersomnia Related to a Known Organic Factor

The essential feature is hypersomnia caused by a physical condition, medication, or substance abuse and make up 85 percent of all sleep disorders (Table 10).

Medications. Somnolence related to tolerance or withdrawal from a CNS stimulant is very common in persons withdrawing from amphetamines, cocaine, caffeine, and related drugs. It may be associated with quite severe depression, which occasionally reaches suicidal proportions.

The sustained use of CNS depressants such as alcohol can cause somnolence. Heavy alcohol use in the evening produces sleepiness and difficulty in arising the next day. This reaction may present a diagnostic problem if the patient does not admit to alcohol abuse.

Respiratory Disorders. There are two disorders of the respiratory system that can produce hypersomnia: the sleep apnea syndrome and the alveolar hypoventilation syndrome.

Sleep apnea and related breathing disorders during sleep are major recognized illnesses. For a number of reasons, breathing during sleep is more fragile and more easily compromised than during waking. Thus, many persons—elderly persons and obese persons, even those who do not have clinical symptoms—are likely to have apneic periods and, in general, more respiratory problems in sleep than during waking.

Sleep apnea refers to cessation of air flow at the nose or mouth. By convention, an apneic period is one that lasts 10 seconds or more. Sleep apnea can be of several distinct types. In pure central sleep apnea, both air flow and respiratory effort (abdomen and chest) cease during the apneic episodes and begin again during arousals. In pure obstructive sleep apnea, air flow ceases, but respiratory effort increases during apneic periods, indicating an obstruction in the airway and increasing efforts by the abdominal and thoracic muscles to force air past the obstruction. Again, the episode ceases with an arousal. The mixed types involve elements of both obstructive and central sleep apnea.

Usually, sleep apnea is considered pathological if there are at least five apneic episodes per hour or 30 apneic episodes during the night. In severe cases of obstructive sleep apnea, there may be as many as 300 apneic episodes, each followed by an arousal, so that almost no normal scorable sleep occurs, even though the patients have been in bed and often assume that they have been sleeping for the entire night.

Sleep apnea can be a dangerous condition. It is thought to account for a certain number of unexplained deaths and "crib

Table 7
Diagnostic Criteria for Hypersomnia Disorders

A. The predominant complaint is either (1) or (2):
  (1) excessive daytime sleepiness or sleep attacks not accounted for by an inadequate amount of sleep
  (2) prolonged transition to the fully awake state on awakening (sleep drunkenness)

B. The disturbance in A occurs nearly every day for at least 1 month, or episodically for longer periods of time, and is sufficiently severe to result in impaired occupational functioning or impairment in usual social activities or relationships with others.

C. Occurrence not exclusively during the course of Sleep-Wake Schedule Disorder.

Table from DSM-III-R *Diagnostic and Statistical Manual of Mental Disorders*, ed 3, revised. (Current Classification of Mental Disorders, 1987.) Copyright American Psychiatric Association, Washington, D.C., 1987. Used with permission.

Table 8
Causes of Hypersomnolence

Symptom	Chiefly Medical	Chiefly Psychiatric or Environmental
Excessive sleep (hypersomnia)	Kleine-Levin syndrome Menstrual-associated somnolence Metabolic or toxic conditions Encephalitic conditions Alcohol and other depressant medications Withdrawal from stimulants	Depression (some) Avoidance reactions
Excessive daytime sleepiness	Narcolepsy and narcolepsy-like syndromes Sleep apneas Hypoventilation syndrome Hyperthyroidism and other metabolic and toxic conditions Alcohol and other depressant medications Withdrawal from stimulants Sleep deprivation or insufficient sleep Any condition producing serious insomnia	Depression (some) Avoidance reactions Sleep-Wake Schedule Disorders

Table from Hartman E L: Sleep disorders. In *Comprehensive Textbook of Psychiatry*, ed 4, H I Kaplan, B J Sadock, editors, p 1248. Williams & Wilkins, Baltimore, 1985

Table 9
Diagnostic Criteria for Hypersomnia Related to Another Mental Disorder (Nonorganic)

Hypersomnia, as defined by criteria A, B, and C in Table 7, that is related to another Axis I or II mental disorder, such as Major Depression or Dysthymia.

Table from DSM-III-R *Diagnostic and Statistical Manual of Mental Disorders,* ed 3, revised. (Current Classification of Mental Disorders, 1987.) Copyright American Psychiatric Association, Washington, D.C., 1987. Used with permission.

deaths" of children and infants. It is probably also responsible for a large number of pulmonary and cardiovascular deaths in adults and in the elderly. Episodes of sleep apnea can produce cardiovascular changes, including arrhythmias, and transient alterations in blood pressure for each apneic episode. Longstanding sleep apnea is associated with an increase in pulmonary blood pressure and eventually an increase in systemic blood pressure as well. It is likely that these cardiovascular changes of sleep apnea account for a considerable number of cases in which the diagnosis is essential hypertension.

The prevalence of sleep apnea in the population has not been established, but increasing numbers of cases are discovered as growing awareness of its existence develops. In a recent survey among patients with disorders of excessive somnolence (DOES) that were serious enough to bring them to be evaluated polygraphically at a sleep disorders center, 42 percent were found to be suffering from one of the variants of sleep apnea.

Clinically, one can suspect sleep apnea and sometimes make a tentative diagnosis even without polysomnographic recordings. The most characteristic picture is that of middle-aged or older males who report tiredness and inability to stay awake in the daytime, sometimes associated with depression, mood changes, and daytime sleep attacks. They may or may not complain of anything unusual during sleep. If a history is obtained from a spouse or bed partner, however, it will include reports of loud, intermittent snoring, at times accompanied by gasping. Sometimes,

observers will actually recall apneic periods when patients appeared to be trying to breathe but were unable to do so. Such patients almost certainly have obstructive sleep apnea. With central or mixed apnea, the complaints will be of repeated awakenings during the night, with no difficulty in falling asleep, associated with morning headaches, mood changes, and so on. At onset, there may be no complaints at all by patients, although bed partners or roommates report heavy snoring and very restless sleep. Obese patients with this disorder are referred to as having *Pickwickian syndrome*.

Patients suspected of having sleep apnea should undergo careful laboratory recordings. A number of recording techniques have been developed, which will be discussed here only briefly. The usual all-night sleep recordings, including electroencephalogram (EEG), electromyogram (EMG), electrocardiogram (EKG), and respiratory tracings of various kinds are useful. Recording air flow, as well as respiratory effort, is usually necessary to make a diagnosis. The question of severity of apneic episodes often bears investigation using oximetry to determine oxygen saturation continuously during the night. Twenty-four-hour EKG monitoring is sometimes useful to monitor cardiac changes.

Making an accurate diagnosis of sleep apnea and its severity can be important and sometimes lifesaving for the patient. Treatments for various forms of sleep apnea are available, including medications to stimulate the respiratory centers, a mechanical tongue-retaining device, and surgical procedures for severe obstructive apnea, including tracheotomy and pharyngoplasty. Occasionally, use of oxygen during the night can be helpful, and at times, respiratory assistance by mechanical devices is necessary. Also, when sleep apnea is established or suspected, it is very important to avoid the use of depressant medication, including alcohol, because it can considerably exacerbate the condition and may then become life threatening.

The alveolar hypoventilation syndrome consists of several conditions marked by impaired ventilation, in which the respiratory abnormality appears or greatly worsens only during sleep and in which significant apneic pauses are not present. The ventilatory dysfunction is characterized by inadequate tidal volume or respira-

Table 10
Diagnostic Criteria for Hypersomnia Related to a Known Organic Factor

Hypersomnia Disorder, as defined by criteria A, B, and C in Table 7, that is related to a known organic factor, such as a physical disorder (e.g., sleep apnea), a Psychoactive Substance Use Disorder (e.g., Cannabis Dependence), or a medication (e.g., prolonged use of sedatives or antihypertensives).

The known organic factor should be listed on Axis III (if a physical disorder or use of a medication that does not meet the criteria for a Psychoactive Substance Use Disorder) or Axis I (if a Psychoactive Substance Use Disorder).

Table from DSM-III-R *Diagnostic and Statistical Manual of Mental Disorders,* ed 3, revised. (Current Classification of Mental Disorders, 1987.) Copyright American Psychiatric Association, Washington, D.C., 1987. Used with permission.

tory rate during sleep. Death may occur during sleep (Ondine's curse). Both of these syndromes can also cause insomnia; however, hypersomnolence is more common.

Narcolepsy. Narcolepsy is a syndrome consisting of excessive daytime sleepiness and abnormal manifestations of REM sleep. The latter includes the presence of frequent sleep-onset REM periods, which may be subjectively appreciated as hypnagogic hallucinations, and dissociated REM sleep inhibitory processes cataplexy and sleep paralysis. The appearance of REM sleep within 10 minutes of sleep onset is considered evidence for narcolepsy.

Narcolepsy is not as rare as was once thought. It is estimated to occur at a rate of at least four cases per 10,000 and shows some familial incidence. Twenty-five percent of hypersomnia due to organic conditions is caused by narcolepsy. Narcolepsy is neither a type of epilepsy nor a psychogenic disturbance. It is a minor CNS abnormality of the sleep mechanisms—specifically, REM-inhibiting mechanisms—and it has been demonstrated and studied in dogs as well as in humans.

The most common symptom is sleep attacks: The patient cannot avoid falling asleep. Often associated with this problem (close to 50 percent of long-standing cases) is cataplexy—a sudden loss of muscle tension, such as jaw drop, head drop, weakness of the knees, or paralysis of all skeletal muscles with collapse. The patient often remains awake during brief cataplectic episodes; the longer ones usually merge with sleep and show the EEG of REM sleep. The rarer symptoms include hypnagogic hallucinations: vivid perceptual experiences, either auditory or visual, occurring at sleep onset or on awakening. The patient is often momentarily frightened, but within a minute or two, returns to an entirely normal frame of mind and is quite aware that "nothing was actually there."

Another less common symptom is sleep paralysis, most often occurring upon awakening in the morning, during which the patient is apparently awake and conscious but unable to move a muscle. If this symptom persists for more than a few seconds, as it often does in narcoleptics, it can become extremely uncomfortable. (Note that isolated brief episodes of sleep paralysis occur in many nonnarcoleptic persons). Another rare symptom is blackout, sometimes associated with automatic behavior. Persons find that they have driven to unknown towns miles away and have no idea how they arrived there. Narcoleptics report falling asleep quickly at night, but often report a number of brief awakenings during the night.

Narcolepsy can occur at any age, but it most frequently begins in adolescence or young adulthood, in most instances before the age of 30. The disorder either progresses very slowly or reaches a plateau that is maintained throughout life. Although the condition is not progressive, narcolepsy can be dangerous because it can lead to automobile and industrial accidents.

In cases where the diagnosis is not absolutely clear clinically, a nighttime polysomnographic recording reveals a characteristic sleep-onset REM period or a REM period very shortly after sleep onset. A daytime multiple sleep latency test (several recorded naps at 2-hour intervals) shows very rapid sleep onset and usually one or more REM periods almost at sleep onset.

Occasionally, a regimen of forced naps at a regular time of day can help, and in some cases, it can almost cure the patient without medication. When medication is required, stimulants (e.g., amphetamine or methylphenidate) are most useful, sometimes combined with antidepressants (e.g., protriptyline (Vivactil)) when cataplexy is prominent. Treatment should be conducted very cautiously, avoiding excessive medication, because the medications used have many associated problems.

Idiopathic CNS Hypersomnolence (Non–REM Narcolepsy) Idiopathic CNS hypersomnolence is characterized by recurrent daytime sleepiness, but "sleep attacks" do not occur because the sleepiness is not as irresistible as in narcolepsy. Naps are lengthy, not refreshing, and preceded by long periods of drowsiness. If actual sleep is resisted, automatic behaviors occur due to "microsleeps." There is a familial and an isolated type of this condition. This is not a well understood condition, although it may be almost as common as narcolepsy. According to one group, it may be related to abnormal dopamine metabolism.

Other Conditions Producing Hypersomnolence or Disorders of Excessive Somnolence

Kleine-Levin Syndrome. Kleine-Levin syndrome is a relatively rare condition consisting of recurrent periods of exceedingly prolonged sleep (from which the patient may be aroused) with intervening periods of normal sleep and alert waking. During the hypersomnic episodes, wakeful periods are usually marked by withdrawal from social contacts and a return to bed at the first opportunity; however, the patient may also display apathy, irritability, confusion, voracious eating, loss of sexual inhibitions, delusions and hallucinations, frank disorientation, memory impairment, incoherent speech, excitation or depression, and truculence. Unexplained fevers have occurred in a few patients.

This condition is characterized by recurrent periods of hypersomnia, usually associated with hyperphagia. The hypersomnia is characterized by prolonged sleep from which the patient may usually be aroused. Apathy, irritability, and even confusion may be present during wakefulness; the patient withdraws from social contacts and returns to bed as soon as possible in most cases.

Kleine-Levin syndrome is probably relatively uncommon, although its exact prevalence is undetermined. Almost 100 cases with features suggesting the diagnosis have been reported. In most cases, several periods of hypersomnia, each lasting for one or several weeks, are experienced by the patient in a year. With few exceptions, the first attack occurs between the ages of 10 and 21 years. Rare instances of onset in the fourth and fifth decade of life have been reported. The disorder appears almost invariably self-limited, enduring remission occurring spontaneously before age 40 in early-onset cases. In one instance, narcolepsy was reported to develop as a sequel to periodic hypersomnia. No residual abnormalities have been noted in other cases.

Menstrual-Associated Syndrome. This category is reserved for women who experience intermittent, marked hypersomnolence at or shortly before the onset of their menses. The entity may resemble Kleine-Levin syndrome in other respects, at times involving similar behavioral patterns and voracious eating, but it has not been studied as extensively as Kleine-Levin syndrome. Prolonged polygraphic recording has not been performed in the majority of cases reported in the literature, but nonspecific EEG abnormalities similar to the ones associated with Kleine-Levin syndrome have been documented in several instances. Sleep patterns sometimes include normal proportions of individual stages, but diminished amounts of REM sleep have been described. Endocrine factors are probably involved, but specific abnormalities in laboratory endocrine measures have not been reported. Increased cerebrospinal fluid turnover of 5-hydroxytryptamine was identified in one instance. A relationship between cyclic increases in progesterone levels and the onset of hypersomnolence has been postulated but not established.

Somnolence Associated with Insufficient Sleep. Insufficient sleep is defined as an earnest complaint of DOES and associated waking symptoms by a person who persistently fails to obtain sufficient daily sleep needed to support alert wakefulness. The individual is voluntarily, but often unwittingly, chronically sleep deprived.

This diagnosis can usually be made on the basis of a careful history, including a sleep log. Some persons, especially students and shift workers, who want to maintain an active daytime life as well as perform their nighttime jobs may seriously deprive themselves of sleep, producing somnolence during waking hours.

Sleep Drunkenness. Sleep drunkenness is an abnormal form of awakening in which the lack of a clear sensorium in the transition from sleep to full wakefulness is prolonged and exaggerated. A confusion state develops that often leads to individual or social inconvenience and sometimes to criminal acts. Essential to the diagnosis is the absence of sleep deprivation. It is a rare condition, and there may be a familial tendency. Before making this diagnosis, it is important to examine sleep carefully and to rule out such conditions as apnea, myoclonus, narcolepsy, and an excessive use of drugs and alcohol.

Primary Hypersomnia

This condition is diagnosed when no other cause for excessive somnolence can be found. Some persons are long sleepers who, like short sleepers, show a normal variation. The sleep, although long, is normal in architecture and physiology. Sleep efficiency and sleep-wake schedule are normal. This pattern is without complaints about quality of sleep, daytime sleepiness, or difficulties with awake mood, motivation, and performance.

Long sleep may be a lifetime pattern, and it appears to have a familial incidence. There are many persons, as discussed, who are variable sleepers and who may become long sleepers at certain times of their lives.

Some persons have a subjective complaint of feeling sleepy without objective findings. They do not have a tendency to fall asleep more often than normal or have any objective signs. One should try to rule out more clear-cut causes of excessive somnolence (Table 11).

Table 11
Diagnostic Criteria for Primary Hypersomnia

Hypersomnia, as defined by criteria A, B, and C in Table 7, that is apparently not maintained by any other mental disorder or any known organic factor, such as a physical disorder, a Psychoactive Substance Use Disorder, or a medication.

Table from DSM-III-R *Diagnostic and Statistical Manual of Mental Disorders,* ed 3, revised. (Current Classification of Mental Disorders, 1987.) Copyright American Psychiatric Association, Washington, D.C., 1987. Used with permission.

Sleep-Wake Schedule Disorder

This is a group of sleep disorders that has only recently been studied in detail. Classification is still tentative, although DSM-III-R has three types listed: (1) frequently changing, (2) advanced or delayed, and (3) disorganized (Table 12). The common symptom is that patients cannot sleep when they wish to sleep, although they are able to sleep at other times. Correspondingly, they cannot be fully awake when they want to be fully awake, but they are able to be awake at other times. In this sense, these sleep disorders do not produce precisely insomnia or somnolence. In practice, the initial complaint is often either insomnia or somnolence only, and the above inabilities are elicited only on careful questioning.

The conditions listed below as disorders of the sleep-wake schedule can all be considered as misalignments between sleep and wake behaviors.

Frequently Changing Sleep-Wake Schedule. This condition, increasingly prevalent in recent years, occurs in persons who frequently fly east to west such as flight crews and frequent overseas travelers; in persons who repeatedly and rapidly change their work schedule; and occasionally with self-imposed chaotic sleep schedules. The most frequent symptoms found are a period of mixed insomnia and somnolence; however, many other symptoms and somatic problems, including peptic ulcer, may be associated with this pattern after some time. Some adolescents and young adults appear to withstand changes of this kind remarkably well with few symptoms; however, older persons and persons with sensitivity to change are clearly affected.

Jet lag syndrome usually disappears spontaneously in 2 to 7 days, depending on the length of the east-to-west trip and individual sensitivity, and no specific treatment is required. Some people find they can prevent the symptoms by altering their mealtimes and sleep times in an appropriate direction before traveling. Others find that what appear to be symptoms of jet lag (tiredness and so on) are actually associated with sleep deprivation and that simply obtaining enough sleep will help.

Symptoms of work shift change are generally worst the first few days after shifting to a new schedule, but in some persons, the disrupted sleep-wake patterns persist for a long time. Many persons never adapt completely to unusual shift schedules because they maintain the altered pattern only 5 days a week, returning to the prevailing pattern of the rest of the population on days off and on vacations.

Shift work schedules are an extremely important area that has not received sufficient study considering that a large proportion of the population now works unusual shifts and, sometimes, in chang-

Table 12
Diagnostic Criteria for Sleep-Wake Schedule Disorder

Mismatch between the normal sleep-wake schedule for a person's environment and his or her circadian sleep-wake pattern, resulting in a complaint of either insomnia (criteria A and B of Insomnia Disorder) in Table 2 or hypersomnia (criteria A and B of Hypersomnia Disorder) in Table 7.

Specify Type:

Advanced or Delayed Type: Sleep-Wake Schedule Disorder with onset and offset of sleep considerably advanced or delayed (if sleep-wake schedule is not interfered with by medication or environmental demands) in relation to what the person desires (usually the conventional societal sleep-wake schedule).

Disorganized Type: Sleep-Wake Schedule Disorder apparently due to disorganized and variable sleep and waking times, resulting in absence of a daily major sleep period.

Frequently Changing Type: Sleep-Wake Schedule Disorder apparently due to frequently changing sleep and waking times, such as recurrent changes in work shifts or time zones.

Table from DSM-III-R *Diagnostic and Statistical Manual of Mental Disorders*, ed 3, revised. (Current Classification of Mental Disorders, 1987.) Copyright American Psychiatric Association, Washington, D.C., 1987. Used with permission.

ing shift schedules. People's sensitivities to shifting schedules vary widely and there are a fair number of persons whose bodies simply do not adapt to shift work and who, therefore, should not be assigned to it. Temperamentally, some people are "owls" who like to stay up at night and sleep during the day and other are "larks" who rise early and retire early.

A particular problem occurs in the training of physicians who are often required to work 36 to 48 hours without sleeping. That condition is dangerous to doctors and their patients. It behooves medical educators to develop more shifts for doctors in training.

Advanced or Delayed Type Sleep-Wake Schedule

Delayed sleep phase syndrome. Delayed sleep phase syndrome is marked by sleep-onsets and wake times that are intractably later than desired; actual sleep times at virtually the same daily clock hour; no reported difficulty in maintaining sleep once begun; and inability to advance the sleep phase by enforcing conventional sleep and wake times. The syndrome often presents with the major complaint of difficulty in falling asleep at a desired conventional time and may appear to be similar to a sleep-onset DIMS. Daytime DOES symptoms commence secondary to sleep loss.

Advanced sleep phase syndrome. Advanced sleep phase is characterized by sleep-onsets and wake times that are intractably earlier than desired; actual sleep times at virtually the same daily clock hour; no reported difficulty in maintaining sleep once begun; and inability to delay the sleep phase by enforcing conventional sleep and wake times. Unlike delayed sleep phase, this condition does not interfere with the work or school day. The major presenting complaint is the inability to stay awake in the evening and to sleep in the morning until desired conventional times.

Disorganized type. Irregular sleep-wake pattern is defined as disorganized and variable sleep and waking behavior that disrupts the regular sleep-wake pattern. This condition is associated with frequent daytime naps at irregular times and excessive bed rest. Sleep at night is not of adequate length, and the condition may

present as a DIMS, although total amount of sleep over 24 hours is normal for age.

PARASOMNIAS

Dyssomnias Not Otherwise Specified

According to DSM-III-R, these are insomnias, hypersomnias, or sleep-wake schedule disturbances that cannot be classified in the above categories.

Included here are a group of clinical conditions that are not basically disorders of sleeping and waking, but are unusual or undesirable phenomena that appear suddenly during sleep or that occur at the threshold between waking and sleeping.

Sleepwalking Disorder

Sleepwalking, also known as somnambulism, consists of a sequence of complex behaviors that are initiated in the first third of the night during deep NREM (stages 3 and 4) sleep, and frequently, although not always, progress—without full consciousness or later memory of the episode—to leaving bed and walking about (Table 13).

The patient sits up and sometimes performs perseverative motor acts, such as walking, dressing, going to the bathroom, talking, screaming, and even driving. The behavior occasionally terminates in an awakening with several minutes of confusion; more frequently, the individual returns to sleep and has no recollection of the sleepwalking event. Polysomnography usually shows an arousal from stage 4 sleep, including high-amplitude slow waves preceding muscle activation, and then an arousal pattern. An artificially induced arousal from stage 4 sleep can sometimes produce the condition. For instance, in children, especially children with a history of sleepwalking, an attack can sometimes be provoked by standing the children

Table 13
Diagnostic Criteria for Sleepwalking Disorder

A. Repeated episodes of arising from bed during sleep and walking about, usually occurring during the first third of the major sleep period.

B. While sleepwalking, the person has a blank, staring face, is relatively unresponsive to the efforts of others to influence the sleepwalking or to communicate with him or her, and can be awakened only with great difficulty.

C. On awakening (either from the sleepwalking episode or the next morning), the person has amnesia for the episode.

D. Within several minutes after awakening from the sleepwalking episode, there is no impairment of mental activity or behavior (although there may initially be a short period of confusion or disorientation).

E. It cannot be established that an organic factor initiated and maintained the disturbance (e.g., epilepsy).

Table from DSM-III-R *Diagnostic and Statistical Manual of Mental Disorders*, ed 3, revised. (Current Classification of Mental Disorders, 1987.) Copyright American Psychiatric Association, Washington, D.C., 1987. Used with permission.

on their feet and thus producing a partial arousal during stage 4 sleep.

Sleepwalking usually begins between ages 6 and 12, but is still seen in adolescents and young adults. The disorder is more common in males than in females, and about 15 percent of children have an occasional episode. It tends to run in families. A minor neurologic abnormality probably underlies this condition; the episodes should not be considered purely psychogenic, although there is no question that stressful periods are associated with an increase in sleepwalking in affected individuals. Extreme tiredness or prior sleep deprivation exacerbates attacks. This is occasionally a dangerous condition owing to the possibility of accidental injury.

Sleeptalking (Somniloquy)

Sleeptalking is quite common in children and adults. It has been studied extensively in the sleep laboratory and is found to occur in all stages of sleep. The talking usually involves a few words that are difficult to distinguish. Longer episodes of talking involve the sleeper's life and concerns, but the sleeptalker does not relate his dreams during sleep, nor does he often reveal deep secrets. Episodes of sleeptalking sometimes accompany night terrors and somnambulism. Sleeptalking alone requires no treatment.

Sleep Terror Disorder (Pavor Nocturnus, Incubus)

A sleep terror is an arousal in the first third of the night during deep NREM (stage 3 and 4) sleep. It is almost invariably inaugurated by a piercing scream or cry and accompanied by behavioral manifestations of intense anxiety bordering on panic (Table 14).

Typically, patients sit up in bed with a frightened expression, scream loudly, and sometimes awaken immediately with a sense of intense terror. Sometimes patients remain awake in a disoriented state. More often, patients fall asleep, and as with sleepwalking, they forget the episodes. Not infrequently, a night-terror episode, after the original scream, develops into a sleepwalking episode. Polygraphic recordings of night terrors are somewhat like those of sleepwalking. In fact, the two conditions appear to be closely related. Night terrors, as isolated episodes, are especially frequent in children. About 1 to 4 percent have the disorder, which is more common in males than in females and tends to run in families. It is possible that night terrors represent a minor neurologic abnormality, perhaps in the temporal lobe or underlying structures, because in those cases where night terrors begin in adolescence and young adulthood they turn out to be the first symptom of temporal lobe epilepsy. In a typical case of night terrors, however, no signs of temporal lobe epilepsy or other seizure disorders are seen either clinically or on EEG recordings.

Night terrors are closely related to sleepwalking and are occasionally related to enuresis, but are quite different from nightmares. Night terrors are associated with simply awakening in terror. There is generally no dream recall, but occasionally there may be recall of a single frightening image.

Specific treatment for night terror or sleepwalking episodes is seldom required. Investigation of stressful family situations may be important, and individual or family therapy can sometimes be useful. In the rare cases where medication is required, diazepam (Valium) in small doses at bedtime improves the condition and sometimes completely eliminates attacks.

Table 14
Diagnostic Criteria for Sleep Terror Disorder

A. A predominant disturbance of recurrent episodes of abrupt awakening (lasting 1 to 10 minutes) from sleep, usually occurring during the first third of the major sleep period and beginning with a panicky scream.

B. Intense anxiety and signs of autonomic arousal during each episode, such as tachycardia, rapid breathing, and sweating, but no detailed dream is recalled.

C. Relative unresponsiveness to efforts of others to comfort the person during the episode and, almost invariably, at least several minutes of confusion, disorientation, and perseverative motor movements (e.g., picking at pillow).

D. It cannot be established that an organic factor initiated and maintained the disturbance (e.g., brain tumor).

Table from DSM-III-R *Diagnostic and Statistical Manual of Mental Disorders,* ed 3, revised. (Current Classification of Mental Disorders, 1987.) Copyright American Psychiatric Association, Washington, D.C., 1987. Used with permission.

Dream Anxiety Disorder

A dream anxiety disorder or nightmare is a long, frightening dream from which one awakens frightened (Table 15). As with other dreams, nightmares almost always occur during REM sleep. They usually occur after a long REM period late in the night. Some persons have frequent nightmares as a lifelong condition; others, experience them predominantly at times of stress and illness. According to Vaillant, persons with frequent nightmares as a lifelong condition appear to have a certain vulnerability to schizophrenia, but they are also artistic, creative persons. About 5 percent of the general population report dream anxiety disorders at some time in their lives.

Parasomnia Not Otherwise Specified

Sleep-Related Epileptic Seizures. The relationship of sleep and epilepsy is complex. Almost every form of epilepsy either improves or becomes worse at various times in the sleep cycle. When seizures occur almost exclusively during sleep, the condition is called "sleep epilepsy."

Sleep-Related Bruxism. Bruxism, or tooth grinding, occurs throughout the night, most prominently in stage 2 sleep. According to dentists, 5 to 10 percent of the population suffer from bruxism severe enough to produce noticeable damage to the teeth. The condition often goes unnoticed by the sleeper, except for an occasional feeling of jaw ache in the morning; however, bed partners and roommates are consistently awakened by the sound.

Sleep-Related (Nocturnal) Myoclonus Syndrome. Sleep-related (nocturnal) myoclonus syndrome consists of highly stereotyped abrupt contractions of certain leg muscles during sleep. It is also known as restless legs syndrome because an individual feels deep sensations of creeping inside the calves whenever sitting or lying down. These dysesthesias are rarely painful, but agonizingly relentless, and cause an almost irresistible urge to move the legs, thus interfering with sleep. The diagnosis is made by polygraphic recordings with surface electrodes placed over the tibialis muscles and, occasionally, on other muscles as well.

Table 15
Diagnostic Criteria for Dream Anxiety Disorder

A. Repeated awakenings from the major sleep period or naps with detailed recall of extended and extremely frightening dreams, usually involving threats to survival, security, or self-esteem. The awakenings generally occur during the second half of the sleep period.

B. On awakening from the frightening dreams, the person rapidly becomes oriented and alert (in contrast to the confusion and disorientation seen in Sleep Terror Disorder and some forms of epilepsy).

C. The dream experience or the sleep disturbance resulting from the awakenings causes significant distress.

D. It cannot be established that an organic factor initiated and maintained the disturbance (e.g., certain medications).

Table from DSM-III-R *Diagnostic and Statistical Manual of Mental Disorders*, ed 3, revised. (Current Classification of Mental Disorders, 1987.) Copyright American Psychiatric Association, Washington, D.C., 1987. Used with permission.

There is no established treatment. Very careful medical and drug histories are indicated, because sometimes changing a patient's current medication schedule can be helpful. Because metabolic and perhaps electrolyte changes may be involved, changes of diet could also make a difference, particularly if foods high in L-tryptophan are added. When pharmacotherapy is required, the benzodiazepine clonazepam (Clonopin), is the only drug that has showed some clear positive results; but the effects have been variable, and it cannot be considered a firmly established treatment. Restless legs syndrome may be helped by regular moderate exercise.

Sleep-Related Head Banging (Jactatio Capitis Nocturnus) Sleep-related head banging is the term for a sleep behavior consisting chiefly of rhythmic to-and-fro head rocking, less commonly of total body rocking, occurring just before or during sleep. Usually, it is observed in the immediate presleep period and is sustained into light sleep. It uncommonly persists into or occurs in deep NREM sleep.

Familial Sleep Paralysis. Familial sleep paralysis is characterized by a sudden inability to execute voluntary movements either just at the onset of sleep or on awakening during the night or in the morning.

Sleep-Related Cluster Headaches and Chronic Paroxysmal Hemicrania. Sleep-related cluster headaches are agonizingly severe, unilateral headaches that appear often during sleep and are marked by an on-off pattern of attacks. Chronic paroxysmal hemicrania is a similar unilateral headache that occurs every day with more frequent but short-lived onsets that are without a preponderant sleep distribution. Both types of vascular headache are examples of sleep-exacerbated conditions and appear in

association with REM sleep periods, paroxysmal hemicrania being virtually "REM sleep locked."

Sleep-Related Abnormal Swallowing Syndrome. Abnormal swallowing syndrome is a condition during sleep in which inadequate swallowing results in aspiration of saliva, coughing, and choking. It is intermittently associated with brief arousals or awakenings.

Sleep-Related Asthma. Asthma appears to be exacerbated by sleep in some persons and may result in significant sleep disturbances.

Sleep-Related Cardiovascular Symptoms. Sleep-related cardiovascular symptoms derive from disorders of cardiac rhythm, myocardial incompetence, coronary artery insufficiency, and blood pressure variability, which may be induced or exacerbated by sleep-altered or sleep-stage-modified cardiovascular physiology.

Sleep-Related Gastroesophageal Reflux. Sleep-related gastroesophageal reflux is a disorder in which the patient awakens from sleep either with burning, substernal pain, a feeling of general pain or tightness in the chest, or a sour taste in the mouth. Coughing, choking, and vague respiratory discomfort may also occur repeatedly.

Sleep-Related Hemolysis (Paroxysmal Nocturnal Hemoglobinuria). Paroxysmal nocturnal hemoglobinuria is a rare, acquired, chronic hemolytic anemia in which intravascular hemolysis results in hemoglobinemia and hemoglobinuria. The hemolysis and consequent hemoglobinuria are accelerated during sleep, coloring the morning urine a brownish red. Hemolysis is linked to the sleep period even if the latter is acutely shifted.

References

Association of Sleep Disorders Center: Diagnostic classification of sleep and arousal disorders. Sleep 2:1, 1979.

Dement W C: The effect of dream deprivation. Science 131:1705, 1960.

Emslie G J, Roffwarg H P, Rush A J, Weinberg W A, Parkin-Feigenbaum L: Sleep EEG findings in depressed children and adolescents. Am J Psychiatry 144:668, 1987.

Goetz R R, Puig-Antich J, Nyan N, Rabinovich M, Ambrosini P J, Belson B, Kraeviec V: Electroencephalographic sleep of adolescents with major depression and normal controls. Arch Gen Psychiatry 44:61, 1987.

Guilleminault C: *Sleeping and Waking Disorders: Indications and Techniques.* Addison-Wesley, Menlo Park, CA, 1982.

Hartmann E, Russ D, Oldfield M, Sivan I, Cooper S: Who has nightmares? Arch Gen Psychiatry 44:49, 1987.

Hauri P J: A cluster analysis of insomnia. Sleep 6:326, 1983.

Hefez A, Metz L, Lavie R: Long-term effects of extreme situational stress on sleep and dreaming. Am J Psychiatry 144:344, 1987.

Kales A, Soldatos C, Daldwell A B: Somnambulism. Arch Gen Psychiatry 37:1406, 1980.

Karacan I, editor: *Psychophysiological Aspects of Sleep.* Noyes Medical Publications, Park Ridge, NJ, 1981.

Vogel G W, Vogel F, McAbee R S: Improvement of depression by REM-sleep deprivation. Arch Gen Psychiatry 37:253, 1980.

Weitzman E D: Sleep and its disorders. Annu Rev Neurosci 4:381, 1981.

Williams R L, Karacan I: *Sleep Disorders, Diagnosis and Treatment.* John Wiley and Sons, New York, 1978.

Williams R L, Karacan I, Moore C, editors: *Sleep Disorders and Treatment,* ed 2. John Wiley and Sons, New York, 1987.

23 Factitious Disorders

INTRODUCTION

Factitious disorders are characterized by physical or psychological symptoms that are intentionally produced or feigned. The physical or mental illness is simulated with the sole objective of assuming the role of a patient. Many of these persons make hospitalization itself a primary objective and often a way of life. There is a compulsive quality to these disorders, and the behaviors thus are considered voluntary in that they are deliberate and purposeful, not that they can be controlled.

EPIDEMIOLOGY

The prevalence of factitious disorders is unknown, although some believe that they are more common than acknowledged. They appear to occur more frequently in men and among hospital or health care workers. One study reported a 9 percent rate of factitious illness among patients admitted to a hospital; another study found factitious fever in 3 percent of patients. A data bank of persons who feign illness is being established to alert hospitals about these patients, many of whom travel from place to place seeking admission under different names or simulating different illnesses.

ETIOLOGY

Frequently such patients have a personal history of early deprivation or of serious illness or disability from which they recovered but which provided a series of care-givers (e.g., doctors, nurses, hospital workers) whom they found loving and caring. In contrast, these patients' families of origin usually contains a rejecting mother or an absent father. The usual history reveals that the patient perceives one or both parents as rejecting figures who are unable to form close relationships. The facsimile of genuine illness therefore is used to re-create the desired positive parent–child bond. The disorder is a form of a repetition compulsion—repeating the basic conflict of needing and seeking acceptance and love while expecting that they will not be forthcoming. Hence, the patient transforms the physician and staff into rejecting parents.

Patients who seek out painful procedures, such as surgical operations or invasive diagnostic tests, may have a masochistic personality makeup in which pain serves as punishment for past sins, imagined or real. It has been suggested that some patients attempt to master the past and early trauma of serious medical illness or hospitalization by assuming the role of the patient and reliving the painful and frightening experience over and over again through multiple hospitalizations.

Patients who feign psychiatric illness may have had a relative who was hospitalized with the illness they are simulating. By identifying with that person, these patients hope to reunite with him or her in a magical way.

Many of these patients have a poor identity formation and disturbed self-image, characteristic of the borderline personality. Some are "as if" personalities who have assumed the identify of those around them. If the patient is a health professional, he or she will often be unable to differentiate himself or herself from the patients with whom he or she comes in contact.

The cooperation or encouragement of persons other than the patient in simulating a factitious illness represents a rare variant of the disorder, suggesting another possible causative factor. Although the majority of such patients act alone, in some instances, friends or relatives participate in fabricating the illness.

Significant defense mechanisms are repression, identification, identification with the aggressor, regression and symbolization.

DIAGNOSIS AND CLINICAL FEATURES

Factitious Disorder with Physical Symptoms

Factitious disorder with physical symptoms has been designated by a variety of labels, the most well known being Münchausen's syndrome, named after the German Baron von Münchausen, who lived in the 18th century and wrote many travel and adventure stories. The disorder has also been called hospital addiction, poly-surgical addiction, and professional patient syndrome, among other names.

The essential feature of patients with this disorder is their ability to present physical symptoms so well that they are able to gain admission to and stay in a hospital (Table 1). To support their history, these patients may feign symptoms suggestive of a disorder that may involve any organ system. They are familiar with the diagnoses of most disorders that usually require hospital admission or medication and can give excellent histories capable of deceiving even the most experienced clinician. Clinical presentations are myriad and include hematoma, hemoptysis, abdominal pain, fever, hypoglycemia, "lupus-like" syndromes, nausea, vomiting, dizziness, and seizures. Urine is contaminated with blood or feces; anticoagulants are taken to simulate bleeding disorders; insulin is used to produce hypoglycemia; and so on. Such patients often insist on surgery, claiming adhesions from previous surgical procedures. These people may acquire a "gridiron abdomen" from multiple procedures. Complaints of pain, especially that simulating renal colic, are common, with the patients' wanting narcotics. In about half the reported cases, the patients demand treatment with specific medications, usually analgesics. Once in the hospital, they continue to be demanding and difficult. As each test is returned with a negative result, they may accuse the doctor of incompetence, threaten litigation, and become generally abusive. Some may sign out abruptly shortly before they believe they are going to be confronted with their factitious behavior. They will then go to another hospital in the same or another city and begin the cycle again. According to DSM-III-R, specific predisposing factors are true physical disorders during childhood leading to extensive medical treatment; a grudge against the medical professions; employment as a medical paraprofessional; and an important relationship with a physician in the past.

Factitious Disorder with Psychological Symptoms

Some patients present with psychiatric symptomatology that is judged to be feigned. This determination can be extremely difficult and is often made only after a prolonged investigation (Table 2). Feigned symptomatology often includes depression, hallucinations, dissociative and conversion symptoms, and bizarre behavior. Because there is no response to routine therapeutic measures, patients with this disorder may receive large doses of psychoactive drugs and may undergo electroconvulsive therapy.

Factitious psychological symptoms resemble the phenomenon of pseudomalingering, conceptualized as satisfying the need to maintain an intact self-image, which would be marred by admitting psychological problems that are beyond the person's capacity to master through conscious effort. In that case, deception is a transient ego-supporting device.

Recent findings suggest that factitious psychotic symptoms are more common than was previously suspected. The presence of simulated psychosis as a feature of other disorders, such as affective disorders, indicates a poor overall prognosis.

Psychotic inpatients found to have definite factitious illness with psychological symptoms—that is, exclusively simulated psychotic symptoms—generally have a concurrent diagnosis of borderline personality disorder. In these cases, the outcome appears to be worse than that of manic or schizoaffective disorder.

Patients may present as being depressed, offering as the reason a false history of the recent death of a significant friend or relative.

Table 1
Diagnostic Criteria for Factitious Disorder with Physical Symptoms

A. Intentional production or feigning of physical (but not psychological) symptoms.
B. A psychological need to assume the sick role, as evidenced by the absence of external incentives for the behavior, such as economic gain, better care, or physical well-being.
C. Occurrence not exclusively during the course of another Axis I disorder, such as Schizophrenia.

Table from *DSM-III-R Diagnostic and Statistical Manual of Mental Disorders,* ed 3, revised. (Current Classification of Mental Disorders, 1987.) Copyright American Psychiatric Association, Washington, D.C., 1987. Used with permission.

Table 2
Diagnostic Criteria for Factitious Disorder with Psychological Symptoms

A. Intentional production or feigning of psychological (but not physical) symptoms.
B. A psychological need to assume the sick role, as evidenced by the absence of external incentives for the behavior, such as economic gain, better care, or physical well-being.
C. Occurrence not exclusively during the course of another Axis I disorder, such as Schizophrenia.

Table from *DSM-III-R Diagnostic and Statistical Manual of Mental Disorders,* ed 3, revised. (Current Classification of Mental Disorders, 1987.) Copyright American Psychiatric Association, Washington, D.C., 1987. Used with permission.

Elements of the history that should suggest factitious bereavement include a violent or bloody death, a death under dramatic circumstances, and the dead person's being a child or young adult. Others may present with both recent and remote memory loss or with both auditory and visual hallucinations.

Other symptoms, which also appear in the physical type, include pseudologia fantastica, and impostorship. In pseudologia fantastica, limited factual material is mixed with extensive and colorful fantasies. The listener's interest pleases the patient and thus reinforces the symptom. This distortion of truth is not limited, however, to the history of an illness's symptoms; such patients often give false and conflicting accounts about other areas of their lives (e.g., claiming the death of a parent so as to play on the sympathy of others). Impostorship is commonly related to lying in these cases. Many patients assume the identity of a prestigious person. Men, for example, report being war heroes, attributing their surgical scars to wounds received during battle or other dramatic and dangerous exploits. Similarly, they may represent themselves as having ties with an accomplished or renowned figure.

Factitious Disorder Not Otherwise Specified

Factitious disorder not otherwise specified, is a combination of the characteristics described for each of the single disorders. Many clinicians believe that the pure form of either the physical or the psychological disorder is less common than the combined form (Table 3).

COURSE AND PROGNOSIS

Factitious illness typically begins in early adult life, although it may appear during childhood or adolescence. The actual onset of this disorder, or of discrete episodes of treatment seeking, may follow a real illness, loss, rejection, or abandonment. Usually, there is a hospitalization in childhood or early adolescence for a genuine physical illness of the patient or a close relative. Thereafter, a long pattern of successive hospitalizations unfolds, which is insidious in its beginning. If this is the case, the onset will actually have been earlier than generally reported. As the disorder progresses, the patient will become more knowledgeable about medicine and hospitals.

Table 3
Diagnostic Criteria for Factitious Disorder Not Otherwise Specified

Factitious Disorders that cannot be classified in any of the previous specific categories, e.g., a disorder with both factitious physical and factitious psychological symptoms.

Table from *DSM-III-R Diagnostic and Statistical Manual of Mental Disorders*, ed 3, revised. (Current Classification of Mental Disorders, 1987.) Copyright American Psychiatric Association, Washington, D.C., 1987. Used with permission.

Factitious disorder is extremely incapacitating to the patient, often producing severe trauma or untoward reactions related to treatment. As may seem obvious, a course of chronic hospitalization is incompatible with meaningful vocational work and sustained interpersonal relationships. The prognosis in most cases is poor. A few of these patients occasionally spend time in jail, usually for minor crimes such as burglary, vagrancy, and disorderly conduct. There may also be intermittent psychiatric hospitalization.

Although there are no adequate data about the ultimate outcome for these patients, a few of them probably die as a result of needless medication, instrumentation, or surgery. Given these patients' often expert simulation and the risks that they take, it is possible that some die without this disorder being suspected. Possible features that indicate a favorable prognosis are (1) the presence of a depressive-masochistic character, (2) functioning at a borderline, not a continuously psychotic, level, and (3) the presence of minimal psychopathic antisocial personality attributes. Patients who exhibit a relatively static pattern, as compared with patients who wander, usually have a less severe course of illness.

PSYCHIATRIC EXAMINATION

The psychiatric examination should emphasize securing information from any available friend, relative, or other informant, because interviews with reliable outside sources often reveal the false nature of the patient's illness. Although time-consuming and tedious, it is essential to verify all the facts presented by the patient concerning prior hospitalizations and medical care.

Psychiatric evaluation is requested on a consultation basis in about 50 percent of the cases, usually after the presence of a simulated illness is suspected. The psychiatrist is often asked to confirm the diagnosis of factitious illness. Under these circumstances, it is necessary to avoid pointed or accusatory questioning that may provoke truculence, evasion, or flight from the hospital. There may be a danger of provoking frank psychosis if vigorous confrontation is used, because in some instances, the feigned illness serves an adaptive function and represents a desperate attempt to ward off further disintegration.

DIFFERENTIAL DIAGNOSIS

Any disorder in which physical symptoms are prominent should be considered in the differential diagnosis, and the possibility of authentic or concomitant physical illness must always be explored.

Somatoform Disorders

Factitious disorder is differentiated from somatization disorder (Briquet's syndrome) by the voluntary production of factitious symptoms, the extreme course of multiple hospitalizations, and the patient's seeming willingness to undergo an extraordinary number of mutilating procedures. Patients diagnosed as having a conversion disorder are not usually conversant with medical terminology and hospital routines, and their symptoms have a direct temporal relation or symbolic reference to specific emotional conflicts.

Hypochondriasis differs from factitious illness in that the hypochrondriacal patient does not voluntarily initiate the production of symptoms, and hypochondriasis typically has a later age of onset. As is the case with somatization disorder, patients with hypochondriasis do not usually submit to potentially mutilating procedures.

Personality Disorders

Because of their pathological lying, lack of close relationships with others, hostile and manipulative manner, and associated drug and criminal history, factitious disordered patients are often diagnosed as having an antisocial personality disorder; however, antisocial persons do not usually volunteer for invasive procedures or resort to a way of life marked by chronic hospitalization.

Because of attention seeking and a flair for the dramatic, these patients may be diagnosed as having a histrionic (hysterical) personality disorder. But not all of these patients have this dramatic flair; many are withdrawn and bland.

Consideration of the patient's chaotic life-style, past history of disturbed interpersonal relations, identity crisis, drug abuse, self-damaging acts, and manipulative tactics may lead to the diagnosis of borderline personality disorder.

Schizophrenic Disorders

The diagnosis of schizophrenia is often based on patients' admittedly bizarre life-styles, but these patients do not usually meet the specified criteria of schizophrenia unless they have the fixed delusion that they are actually ill and act on that belief by seeking chronic hospitalization. This practice seems to be the exception, for few patients with a factitious disorder show evidence of a severe thought disorder or bizarre delusions.

These persons usually do not have the eccentricities of dress, thought, or communication that characterize schizotypal personality disorder.

Malingering

Factitious disorder must be distinguished from malingering. Malingerers have an obvious, recognizable environmental goal in producing symptoms. They may seek hospitalization in order to secure financial compensation, evade the police, avoid work, or merely obtain free bed and board for the night; but they always have some apparent end for their behavior. Moreover, they can usually stop producing their symptoms when they are no longer considered profitable or when the stakes rise too high and they risk life and limb.

Drug Abuse

Although patients with a factitious disorder may have a complicating history of drug abuse, they should not be considered merely as drug addicts but, rather, as having coexisting diagnoses.

Ganser's Syndrome

Ganser's syndrome, a controversial condition and most typically associated with prison inmates, is characterized by the use of approximate answers. Such persons respond to simple questions with astonishingly incorrect answers. For example, when asked about the color of a blue car, the person answers "red." Ganser's syndrome may be a variant of malingering, in that the patients avoid punishment or responsibility for their actions. Ganser's syndrome is classified in DSM-III-R as an atypical dissociative disorder and is further discussed in that section.

Psychological Tests

Psychological testing may reveal specific underlying pathology in individual patients. Features that are overrepresented in factitious illness patients include normal or above-average I.Q.; absence of a formal thought disorder; poor sense of identity, including confusion over sexual identity; poor sexual adjustment; poor frustration tolerance; strong dependency needs; and narcissism.

TREATMENT

No specific psychiatric therapy has been effective in treating factitious disorders. It is a clinical paradox that such patients simulate serious illness, seeking and submitting to unnecessary treatment, while denying to themselves and others their true illness. Ultimately, these patients elude meaningful therapy by abruptly leaving the hospital or failing to keep follow-up appointments.

Treatment thus is best focused on management rather than on cure. Perhaps the single most important factor in successful management is a physician's early recognition of the disorder. The physician can then forestall the patient's undergoing a multitude of painful and potentially dangerous diagnostic procedures.

Legal intervention has been obtained in several instances, particularly with children. An obstacle to successful court action is the senselessness of the disorder and the denial of false action by parents, thereby often making conclusive proof unobtainable. In such cases, the child welfare services should be notified and arrangements made for the ongoing monitoring of these children's health.

The personal reactions of physicians and staff members are of great significance in treating and establishing a working alliance with these patients, who invariably evoke feelings of futility, bewilderment, betrayal, hostility, and even contempt. In essence, staff members are forced to abandon a basic element of their relationship with patients: acceptance of the truthfulness of the patient's statements.

Physicians should try not to feel resentment when patients humiliate their diagnostic prowess, and they should avoid any "unmasking ceremony" that sets up these patients as adversaries and precipitates their flight from the hospital.

References

Asher R: Münchausen's syndrome. Lancet *1*:339, 1951.

Cramer B, Gershberg M R, Stern M: Münchausen syndrome: Its relationship to malingering, hysteria, and the physician–patient relationship. Arch Gen Psychiatry *24*:573, 1971.

Eisendrath S J: Factitious illness. Psychosomatics *25*:111, 1984.

Hyler S E, Sussman N: Chronic factitious disorder with physical symptoms (the Münchausen syndrome). Psychiatr Clin North Am *4*:365, 1981.

Ireland P, Sapira J D, Templeton B: Münchausen's syndrome. Am J Med *43*:579, 1967.

Kass F: Masochistic personality. Am J Psychiatry *143*:216, 1986.

Menninger K A: Polysurgery and polysurgical addiction. Psychoanal Q *3*:173, 1934.

Raspe R E: *The Singular Travels, Campaigns, and Adventures of Baron Münchausen.* Cresset Press, London, 1948.

Reich P: Factitious disorders in a teaching hospital. An Intern Med *99*:240, 1983.

Shafer N, Shafer R: Factitious diseases including Münchausen's syndrome. NY State J Med *80*:594, 1980.

24

Impulse Control Disorders Not Elsewhere Classified

INTRODUCTION

According to DSM-III-R, this is a residual diagnostic class for disorders of impulse control that are not classified in other categories, (e.g., psychoactive substance use disorders or paraphilias). Patients with disorders of impulse control are characterized in the following way: (1) They fail to resist an impulse, drive, or temptation to perform some action that is harmful to themselves or others. They may or may not consciously resist the impulse and may or may not plan the act. (2) Before committing the act, they feel an increasing sense of tension or arousal. (3) While committing the act, they feel either pleasure gratification or release. The act is ego-syntonic in that it is consonant with the individual's immediate conscious wish. Immediately after the act, the patients may or may not feel genuine regret, self-reproach, or guilt.

There are five specific categories of this disorder: intermittent explosive disorder, kleptomania, pathological gambling, pyromania, and trichotillomania. There is also a diagnosis of impulse control disorder not otherwise specified for disorders of impulse control that do not meet the criteria for any of the specific disorders.

ETIOLOGY

The causes of impulse disorders are unknown. It is believed that psychodynamic, biological, and psychosocial factors interact to cause these disorders. In all categories of impulse disorders, an act is committed that is injurious to the person committing it and, possibly, to others. The disorders of impulse control share a similar source of tension—that is, the libidinal and aggressive instinctual drives—and a similar episodic lapse in the ego's defense against them. Freud conceptualized the impulse disorders in terms of the pleasure principle and the reality principle.

An impulse is a disposition to act so as to decrease the heightened tension caused by the welling up of instinctual drives or by the diminished ego defenses against them. An impulse often has the qualities of hastiness, lack of deliberation, and impetuosity.

Usually there is a compromise in the drive gratification that includes punishment. For example, the kleptomaniac or pyromaniac is caught; the aggressive person is arrested or beaten up; and the pathological gambler is disgraced or gets into legal trouble because of bad debts. It is as if the patient is free to act on the impulse because his or her superego will have its eventual moment in court, often literally. With the explosive breakthrough of murderous impulses, one can often see the aggressor's suicidal impulse. As demonstrated in repeated episodic impulses, the knowledge of past guilt and pain can often reinforce the behavior. In fact, in some cases the need for punishment is antecedent to the impulse.

The psychodynamics of persons designated as having impulse disorders are varied even when the symptoms are similar. Fenichel believed that impulsive actions defend against danger, including depression, and produce a distorted, sexual or aggressive satisfaction. Such actions are directed less toward achieving a goal than toward getting rid of tension; that is, the acquisition of pleasure is less significant than is the discontinuance of pain. Several therapists have stressed the patients' fixation at the oral stage of development. These patients attempt to master anxiety, guilt, depression, and other painful affects by means of action, but such actions aimed at obtaining relief seldom succeed even temporarily.

Many current writers have focused on a possible organic involvement in the impulse disorders, especially regarding those patients presenting with overtly violent behavior. Experiments have shown that specific brain regions such as the limbic system are associated with impulsive and violent activity and that others are associated with the inhibition of such behaviors. Certain hormones, especially testosterone, have been associated with violent and aggressive behavior. Some reports have described a relationship between temporal lobe epilepsy and certain violent behaviors, an association of aggressive behavior with patients with histories of head trauma, increased numbers of emergency room visits, and other potential organic antecedents. It has been suggested that there is a higher incidence of mixed cerebral dominance in some violent populations. Recent work has suggested the continuance of impulse disorder symptoms into adulthood in persons who were classified as suffering from childhood minimal brain dysfunction syndrome. Lifelong or acquired mental deficiency, epilepsy, and even reversible brain syndromes have long been implicated in lapses of impulse control.

The capacity to undermine ego defenses by means of temporary organic states produced by alcohol and other drugs is well known. Stealing and setting fires "for the fun of it," gambling, and actual physical fighting are common antisocial acts caused by intoxicants.

In some disorders of impulse control, the ego defenses are overwhelmed without actual nervous system pathology. Fatigue, incessant stimulation, and psychic trauma can lower resistance and temporarily suspend the ego's control.

Some workers have stressed the disorder's psychosocial aspects, such as early life events, as being important. Improper models for identification and parental figures who themselves often have difficulty in controlling impulses have also been implicated. In addition, such parental factors as violence in the home, alcohol abuse, promiscuity, and antisocial tendencies have been thought to be significant.

INTERMITTENT EXPLOSIVE DISORDER

Definition and Diagnosis

According to DSM-III-R, intermittent explosive disorder describes individuals who have discrete episodes of losing control of aggressive impulses resulting in serious assault or the destruction of property. The degree of aggressiveness expressed is grossly out of proportion to any stressors that may have helped elicit the episodes. The symptoms, which the patient may describe as "spells" or "attacks," appear within minutes or hours and, regardless of duration, remit spontaneously and quickly. Each episode usually is followed by genuine regret or self-reproach. Signs of generalized impulsivity or aggressiveness are absent between attacks. The diagnosis of intermittent explosive disorder should not be made if the loss of control can be accounted for by schizophrenia, antisocial or borderline personality disorder, conduct disorder, or intoxication with a psychoactive substance (Table 1).

The term "epileptoid personality" has been used to convey the seizure-like quality of its characteristic outbursts, which are not typical of the patient, and to convey the suspicion of an organic disease process. A number of associated features suggest the possibility of an epileptoid state: There may an aura; postictal-like changes in the sensorium, including partial or spotty amnesia; or hypersensitivity to photic, aural, or auditory stimuli. These persons have a higher incidence of hyperactivity, soft neurological signs, nonspecific EEG findings, and accident proneness.

Epidemiology

Intermittent explosive disorder is apparently very rare and appears to be more common in males than in females. The males are likely to be found in a correctional institution, and the females in a psychiatric facility.

There is evidence that intermittent explosive disorder is more common in first-degree biological relatives of persons with the disorder. A variety of factors could be responsible, however, and a simple genetic explanation seems unlikely.

Etiology

Some investigators suggest that disordered brain physiology, particularly in the limbic system, is involved in most cases of episodic violence. It is generally believed, however, that an unfavorable environment in childhood is the major determinant. Predisposing factors in childhood are thought to include perinatal trauma, infantile seizures, head trauma, encephalitis, and hyperactivity. The patients' childhood environment is often filled with alcoholism, beatings, threats to life, and promiscuity.

Those workers who have concentrated on psychogenesis in the etiology of episodic explosiveness have stressed identification with assaultive parental figures or the symbolism of the target of the violence. Early frustration, oppression, and hostility have been noted as predisposing factors. Situations that are directly or symbolically reminiscent of these early deprivations (e.g., persons who directly or indirectly evoke the image of the frustrating parent) become targets for destructive hostility.

Typical patients have been described as physically large but dependent men, whose sense of masculine identity is poor. A sense of being useless and impotent or of being unable to change the environment often precedes the episode of physical violence.

Clinical Features

The diagnosis of intermittent explosive disorder should be the result of careful history taking that reveals several episodes of loss of control associated with aggressive outbursts; a single discrete episode does not justify the diagnosis. This latter condition was referred to in the past as a "catathymic crisis." The history is typically of a childhood in the midst of alcoholism, violence, and emotional instability. Their work history is poor. The patients report job losses, marital difficulties, and trouble with the law. Most have sought psychiatric help in the past, but to no avail. A high level of anxiety, guilt, and depression is usually present after an episode. Neurological examination sometimes reveals soft neurological signs, such as left-right ambivalence and perceptual reversal. Electroencephalographic studies are frequently normal or show nonspecific changes. Psychological tests for organicity are frequently normal.

Table 1
Diagnostic Criteria for Intermittent Explosive Disorder

A. Several discrete episodes of loss of control of aggressive impulses resulting in serious assaultive acts or destruction of property.

B. The degree of aggressiveness expressed during the episodes is grossly out of proportion to any precipitating psychosocial stressors.

C. There are no signs of generalized impulsiveness or aggressiveness between the episodes.

D. The episodes of loss of control do not occur during the course of a psychotic disorder, Organic Personality Syndrome, Antisocial or Borderline Personality Disorder, Conduct Disorder, or intoxication with a psychoactive substance.

Table from DSM-III-R *Diagnostic and Statistical Manual of Mental Disorders*, ed 3, revised. (Current Classification of Mental Disorders, 1987.) Copyright American Psychiatric Association, Washington, D.C., 1987. Used with permission.

Course and Prognosis

According to DSM-III-R, intermittent explosive disorder may begin at any stage of life but usually begins in the second or third decade. In most cases, the disorder decreases in severity with the onset of middle age. Heightened organic impairment, however, can lead to more frequent and severe episodes.

Differential Diagnosis

The diagnosis of intermittent explosive disorder can be made only after other disorders associated with the occasional loss of control of aggressive impulses have been ruled out. These other disorders include psychotic disorders, organic personality syndrome, antisocial or borderline personality disorder, conduct disorder, or intoxication with a psychoactive substance.

One can differentiate intermittent explosive disorder from the antisocial and borderline personality disorders because in the personality disorders, aggressiveness and impulsivity are part of the patient's character and are present between outbursts. In paranoid or catatonic schizophrenia, there may be violent behavior in response to delusions and hallucinations, and there is gross impairment in reality testing. Hostile manic patients may be impulsively aggressive, but their underlying diagnosis is generally clear from their mental status and clinical presentation. Organic disorders, such as epilepsy, brain tumors, degenerative diseases, or endocrine disorders, must be considered and ruled out, as must acute intoxications with such psychoactive substances as alcohol, barbiturates, hallucinogens, or amphetamines. Conduct disorder is ruled out by a repetitive and resistant pattern of behavior, as opposed to an episodic pattern.

Treatment

Those psychiatrists interested in treating patients with intermittent explosive disorder advocate a combined pharmacological and psychotherapeutic approach with an emphasis on the former. Psychotherapy with violent patients is difficult, dangerous, and often unrewarding, as there may be difficulties with countertransference and limit setting. Group psychotherapy with violent outpatients may be of some help, as may family therapy, particularly when the explosive patient is an adolescent or a young adult.

Anticonvulsants have long been used in treating explosive patients, with mixed results. Phenothiazines and antidepressants have been effective in some cases, but then one must wonder whether schizophrenia or mood disorder is the actual diagnosis. When there is a likelihood of subcortical seizure–like activity, these medications can aggravate the situation. Benzodiazepines have been reported to produce a paradoxical reaction of dyscontrol in some cases. Lithium has been reported to be useful in generally lessening aggressive behavior, and carbamepazine (Tegretol) has also been reported to be helpful.

Operative treatments for intractable violence and aggression have been performed by some neurosurgeons; but there is no evidence that such treatment is effective, and the practice appears to have stopped.

KLEPTOMANIA

Definition and Diagnosis

According to DSM-III-R, the essential feature of kleptomania is a recurrent failure to resist impulses to steal objects not needed for personal use or their monetary value. The objects taken are given away, returned surreptitiously, or kept and hidden (Table 2).

Kleptomaniacs usually have the money to pay for the object they impulsively steal. As in other impulse disorders, kleptomania is characterized by mounting tension before the act followed afterward by gratification and less tension with or without guilt, remorse, or depression. The stealing is not planned and does not involve others. Although the thefts do not occur when immediate arrest is probable, kleptomaniacs do not always consider the chances of their apprehension. Although kleptomaniacs may feel guilt and anxiety after the theft, they do not feel anger or vengeance. Furthermore, when the object stolen is the goal, the diagnosis is not kleptomania, for in kleptomania, the act of stealing itself is the goal.

Epidemiology

Kleptomania is apparently quite rare. According to DSM-III-R, fewer than 5 percent of arrested shoplifters give a history consistent with the disorder, and in some of these cases, the history may have been fabricated to conform to the stereotype of the disorder. The sex ratio is unknown, but shoplifting itself is more common among females, and thus kleptomania-related shoplifting is also probably more common in females.

Etiology

As with other disorders of impulse control, brain disease and mental retardation have sometimes been associated with profitless stealing.

Some psychoanalytic writers have stressed the expression of the aggressive impulses in kleptomania; others have discerned a libidinal aspect. Those who focus on symbolism see meaning in the act itself, the object stolen, and the

Table 2
Diagnostic Criteria for Kleptomania

A. Recurrent failure to resist impulses to steal objects not needed for personal use or their monetary value.

B. Increasing sense of tension immediately before committing the theft.

C. Pleasure or relief at the time of committing the theft.

D. The stealing is not committed to express anger or vengeance.

E. The stealing is not due to Conduct Disorder or Antisocial Personality Disorder.

Table from DSM-III-R *Diagnostic and Statistical Manual of Mental Disorders,* ed 3, revised. (Current Classification of Mental Disorders, 1987.) Copyright American Psychiatric Association, Washington, D.C., 1987. Used with permission.

victim of the theft. Kleptomania is often associated with other psychological disturbances, such as chronic depression, anorexia nervosa, bulimia, and pyromania (in females). The symptoms of kleptomania tend to appear in times of significant stress (e.g., losses, separations, and the ending of important relationships).

Analytic writers have focused on stealing by children and adolescents. Anna Freud pointed out that the first thefts from the mother's purse indicate the degree to which all stealing is rooted in the initial oneness between mother and child. Abraham wrote of the central feeling of being neglected, injured, or unwanted. One theoretician established seven categories of stealing in chronically acting-out children: (1) as a means of restoring the lost mother–child relationship, (2) as an aggressive act, (3) as a defense against fears of being damaged (perhaps a search by females for a penis or a protection against castration anxiety in males), (4) as a means of seeking punishment, (5) as a means of restoring or adding to self-esteem, (6) in connection with and as a reaction to a family secret, and (7) as excitement (lust Angst) and a substitute for a sexual act. One or more of these categories can also apply to adult kleptomania.

Clinical Features

In addition to the essential feature of kleptomania noted in DSM-III-R of a recurrent failure to resist impulses to steal unneeded objects, several associated features are often present. Kleptomaniacs may be distressed about the possibility or actuality of their being apprehended and so manifest signs of depression, anxiety, and guilt. They often have serious problems with interpersonal relationships and often, but not invariably, show signs of personality disturbance.

Course and Prognosis

Kleptomania may begin in childhood, although most children or adolescents who steal do not become kleptomaniacs in adulthood. The course of the disease waxes and wanes but tends to be chronic. The spontaneous recovery rate is unknown. Serious impairment and complications are usually secondary to being caught, particularly when linked to being arrested. Many persons seem never to have consciously considered the possibility of having to face the consequences of their acts, a feature in line with those writers who have described kleptomaniacs as people who feel wronged and therefore entitled to steal. And some persons have bouts of being unable to resist the impulse to steal, followed by free periods that last for weeks or months. The prognosis with treatment can be good, but few patients come for help of their own accord. Often, the disease in no way impairs the person's social or work functioning. In quiescent cases, new bouts of the illness may be precipitated by loss or disappointment.

Differential Diagnosis

Because most kleptomaniacs are referred for examination in connection with legal proceedings after apprehen-

sion, the clinical picture may be clouded by subsequent symptoms of depression and anxiety. The major differentiation is between kleptomania and other forms of stealing. For a diagnosis of kleptomania, the stealing must always follow a failure to resist the impulse and be a solitary act, and the stolen articles must be without immediate usefulness or monetary gain. In ordinary stealing, the act is usually planned, and the objects are stolen for their use or financial value. Malingerers may try to simulate the disorder to avoid prosecution. Stealing that occurs in association with conduct disorder, antisocial personality disorder, and manic episodes is clearly related to the pervasive, overlying disorder. Schizophrenics may steal in response to hallucinations and delusions, and patients with organic mental disorders may be accused of stealing because of their forgetting to pay for the object.

Treatment

Because true kleptomania is rare, reports of treatment tend to be individual case descriptions or a short series of cases. Insight-oriented psychotherapy and psychoanalysis have been successful but depend on the patient's motivation. Persons who feel guilt and shame are perhaps most helped by insight-oriented psychotherapy, because of their increased motivation to change the behavior.

Behavior therapy, including systematic desensitization, aversive conditioning, and a combination of aversive conditioning, altered social contingencies, and marital therapy has been reported to be successful, even when motivation was lacking. These reports cite follow-up studies of up to 2 years.

PATHOLOGICAL GAMBLING

Definition and Diagnosis

As currently defined by DSM-III-R, the essential features of pathological gambling are a chronic and progressive failure to resist impulses to gamble and gambling behavior that compromises, disrupts, or damages personal, family, or vocational pursuits. The gambling preoccupation, urge, and activity increase during periods of stress. Problems that arise as a result of the gambling intensify the gambling behavior. Characteristic problems include extensive indebtedness and consequent default on debts and other financial responsibilities, disrupted family relationships, inattention to work, and financially motivated illegal activities to pay for the gambling (Table 3).

Epidemiology

Estimates place the number of pathological gamblers at 2 to 3 percent of the adult United States population. The disorder is more common in men than in women. Both the fathers of males and the mothers of females with the disorder are more likely to have the disorder than is the population at large. Females with the disorder are more likely than are those not so affected to be married to an alcoholic who is

Table 3
Diagnostic Criteria for Pathological Gambling

Maladaptive gambling behavior, as indicated by at least four of the following:

(1) frequent preoccupation with gambling or with obtaining money to gamble

(2) frequent gambling of larger amounts of money or over a longer period of time than intended

(3) a need to increase the size or frequency of bets to achieve the desired excitement

(4) restlessness or irritability if unable to gamble

(5) repeated loss of money by gambling and returning another day to win back losses ("chasing")

(6) repeated efforts to reduce or stop gambling

(7) frequent gambling when expected to meet social or occupational obligations

(8) sacrifice of some important social, occupational, or recreational activity in order to gamble

(9) continuation of gambling despite inability to pay mounting debts, or despite other significant social, occupational, or legal problems that the person knows to be exacerbated by gambling

Table from DSM-III-R *Diagnostic and Statistical Manual of Mental Disorders,* ed 3, revised. (Current Classification of Mental Disorders, 1987.) Copyright American Psychiatric Association, Washington, D.C., 1987. Used with permission.

usually absent from the home. Alcohol dependence in general is more common among the parents of pathological gamblers than among the overall population.

Etiology

There is some evidence that the following may be predisposing factors for the development of the disorders: loss of parent by death, separation, divorce or desertion before the child is 15 years of age; inappropriate parental discipline (absence, inconsistency, or harshness); exposure to and availability of gambling activities to the adolescent; a family emphasis on material and financial symbols; and a lack of family emphasis on saving, planning, and budgeting.

Clinical Features

In addition to the features described above, pathological gamblers most often appear overconfident, somewhat abrasive, very energetic, and "free spending" when there are obvious signs of personal stress, anxiety, and depression. Commonly these persons have the attitude that money is both the cause of and the solution to all of their problems. As their gambling increases, they are usually forced to lie in order to obtain money and to continue gambling, while hiding the extent of their gambling behavior. They make no serious attempt to budget or save money. When their borrowing resources are strained, they are likely to engage in antisocial behavior in order to obtain money for gambling. Any criminal behavior is typically nonviolent, such as forgery, embezzlement, or fraud. The conscious intent is to return or repay the money.

Complications include alienation from family and acquaintances, loss of one's life accomplishments, suicide attempts, and association with fringe and illegal groups. Arrest for nonviolent crimes may lead to imprisonment.

Course and Prognosis

Pathological gambling usually begins in adolescence in males and late in life for females. Its course waxes and wanes and tends to be chronic. There are three phases in pathological gambling: (1) The winning phase, ending with a big win, equal to approximately a year's salary, which hooks the patient. (2) The progressive-loss stage, in which patients structure their life around gambling. They move from being excellent gamblers to being stupid ones—taking considerable risks, cashing in securities, owing money, missing work, and losing jobs. (3) The desperate stage, with the patients gambling in a frenzy with larger amounts of money, not paying debts, becoming involved with loan sharks, writing bad checks, and possibly embezzling. It may take up to 15 years to reach the third phase, but then within a year or two, the patients are totally deteriorated.

Differential Diagnosis

Social gambling is distinguished from pathological gambling in that the former is associated with gambling with friends, on special occasions, and with predetermined acceptable and tolerable losses.

Gambling that is symptomatic of a manic episode can usually be distinguished from pathological gambling by the history of a marked mood change and loss of judgment preceding the gambling. Manic-like mood changes are common in pathological gambling but always follow winning and are usually followed by depressive episodes because of subsequent losses.

Persons with antisocial personality disorder may have problems with gambling, and DSM-III-R suggests that in cases in which both disorders are present, both should be diagnosed.

Treatment

All investigators who write about pathological gambling indicate that the gamblers seldom come forward voluntarily for treatment. Legal difficulties, family pressures, or other psychiatric complaints are what bring the gamblers into treatment. Gamblers Anonymous (G.A.) was founded in Los Angeles in 1957 and modeled on Alcoholics Anonymous; it is accessible—at least in the larger cities—and is probably the most effective treatment for gambling. It is a method of inspirational group therapy, which involves public confession, peer pressure, and the presence of reformed gamblers available (as are sponsors in A.A.) to help individuals resist the impulse to gamble.

It may be helpful in some cases to hospitalize the patients so as to remove them from their environment and not to work to achieve insight until the patients have been away from gambling for 3 months. At this point, pathological gamblers may become excellent candidates for insight-oriented psychotherapy.

PYROMANIA

Definition and Diagnosis

As defined by DSM-III-R, the essential features of pyromania are deliberate and purposeful fire setting on more than one occasion; tension or affective arousal before setting the fires; and intense pleasure, gratification, or relief when setting the fires or seeing fires burn (Table 4). There is also a general fascination with and interest in every aspect of fires. Although the fire setting results from the failure to resist an impulse, there may be considerable advance preparation in order to start the fire.

According to DSM-III-R, a diagnosis of pyromania should not be made when fires are set to make money, to express sociopolitical ideology, to conceal criminal activity, to express anger or vengeance, to improve one's living circumstances, or to respond to a delusion or hallucination.

Epidemiology

No information is available on the prevalence of pyromania, only that a small percentage of those adults who set fires can be classified as having pyromania. The disorder is found far more often in males than in females, and more people who set fires are likely to be mildly retarded than are those who do not set fires. Some studies have noted an increased incidence of alcohol abuse in people who set fires. Fire setters also tend to have a history of antisocial traits, such as truancy, running away from home, and delinquency. Enuresis has been considered to be a common finding in the history of fire setters, although controlled studies have failed to confirm these findings. Rather, studies have suggested a greater association between cruelty to animals and fire setters, as compared with people who do not set fires.

Table 4
Diagnostic Criteria for Pyromania

A. Deliberate and purposeful fire-setting on more than one occasion.

B. Tension or affective arousal before the act.

C. Fascination with, interest in, curiosity about, or attraction to fire and its situational context or associated characteristics (e.g., paraphernalia, uses, consequences, exposure to fires).

D. Intense pleasure, gratification, or relief when setting fires, or when witnessing or participating in their aftermath.

E. The fire-setting is not done for monetary gain, as an expression of sociopolitical ideology, to conceal criminal activity, to express anger or vengeance, to improve one's living circumstances, or in response to a delusion or hallucination.

Table from DSM-III-R *Diagnostic and Statistical Manual of Mental Disorders*, ed 3, revised. (Current Classification of Mental Disorders, 1987.) Copyright American Psychiatric Association, Washington, D.C., 1987. Used with permission.

Etiology

Freud gave unconscious meaning to fire, seeing it as a symbol of sexuality. The warmth that is radiated by fire evokes the same sensation that accompanies a state of sexual excitation, and the shape and movements of a flame suggest a phallus in activity. Other therapists have associated pyromania with an abnormal craving for power and social prestige. Some pyromaniacs are volunteer fire fighters who set fires to prove themselves brave, to force other fire fighters into action, or to demonstrate their power to extinguish a blaze. The incendiary act is a way to vent accumulated rage over the frustration caused by a sense of social, physical, or sexual inferiority. A number of studies have noted that the fathers of pyromanic patients were absent from the home. Thus one explanation of fire setting is that it represents a wish for the absent father to return home as a rescuer, to put out the fire, and to save the child from a difficult existence.

It has also been found that female fire setters, in addition to being much fewer in number than male fire setters, do not start fires to put fire fighters into action, as men frequently do. Rather, promiscuity without pleasure and petty stealing, often approaching kleptomania, were frequently noted delinquent trends in female fire setters.

Clinical Features

In addition to the essential features described above, DSM-III-R lists the following: Individuals with the disorder often are regular watchers at fires in their neighborhoods, frequently set off false alarms, and show interest in fire-fighting paraphernalia. They may be indifferent to the consequences of the fire for life or property, or they may gain satisfaction from the resulting destruction. Frequently they leave obvious clues. Common associated features include alcohol intoxication, psychosexual dysfunctions, lower-than-average I.Q., chronic personal frustrations, and resentment toward authority figures. In some cases, the fire setter becomes sexually aroused by the fire.

Course and Prognosis

Pyromania usually begins in childhood. When the onset is in adolescence or adulthood, the fire setting tends to be more deliberately destructive. The prognosis for treated children is good, and complete remission is not an unrealistic goal. The prognosis for adults is much more guarded, owing to their frequent use of denial and refusal to take responsibility, as well as their possible concurrent alcoholism and lack of insight.

Differential Diagnosis

In discussing the differential diagnosis of pyromania, DSM-III-R notes that there should be little trouble distinguishing between pyromania and the fascination of many young children with matches, lighters, and fire as part of the normal investigation of their environment. Pyromania must also be separated from incendiary acts of sabotage carried out by dissident political extremists or "paid torches," which are legally termed as arson.

When fire setting occurs in conduct disorders and antisocial personality disorders, it is a deliberate act rather than the failure to resist an impulse. Fires thus may be set for profit, sabotage, or retaliation. In schizophrenia, fires may be set in response to delusions or hallucinations. And in organic mental disorders, fires may be set because of failure to appreciate the consequences of the act.

Treatment

Because of pyromania's position as a symptom rather than a disorder, little has been written on its treatment. The treatment of fire setters has been difficult because of their lack of motivation. Incarceration may be necessary as the only method available to prevent a recurrence. Behavior therapy can then be administered in the institution.

Fire setting in children must be treated with the utmost seriousness. Intensive interventions should be undertaken when possible, but as therapeutic and preventive measures rather than as a punishment.

TRICHOTILLOMANIA

Definition and Diagnosis

According to DSM-III-R, the essential feature of trichotillomania is the recurrent failure to resist impulses to pull out one's own hair. The diagnosis should not be made when hair pulling is associated with a preexisting inflammation of the skin or is in response to a delusion or hallucination (Table 5).

Epidemiology

According to DSM-III-R, trichotillomania is apparently more common in females. There is no information on the familial pattern, but one study of children reported that 5 of 19 subjects had a family history of some form of alopecia. Prevalence data are unavailable, but trichotillomania may be more common than is now believed. It is seen more often in mentally retarded people and may be more common in schizophrenia and borderline personality disorder. It has been reported that mainly oldest or

Table 5
Diagnostic Criteria for Trichotillomania

A. Recurrent failure to resist impulses to pull out one's own hair, resulting in noticeable hair loss.

B. Increasing sense of tension immediately before pulling out the hair.

C. Gratification or a sense of relief when pulling out the hair.

D. No association with a preexisting inflammation of the skin, and not a response to a delusion or hallucination.

Table from DSM-III-R *Diagnostic and Statistical Manual of Mental Disorders,* ed 3, revised. (Current Classification of Mental Disorders, 1987.) Copyright American Psychiatric Association, Washington, D.C., 1987. Used with permission.

only children present with the disorder. The disorder usually begins in childhood but can occur at any age.

Etiology

DSM-III-R states that although trichotillomania is regarded as "multidetermined," its onset has been linked to stressful situations in more than one quarter of the cases. Disturbances in mother–child relationships, fear of being left alone, and recent object loss are often cited as critical factors contributing to the condition. Psychoactive substance abuse may encourage the development of this disorder. Depressive dynamics are often cited as predisposing factors. Some see self-stimulation as the primary goal of hair pulling.

Clinical Features

According to DSM-III-R, before engaging in the behavior, trichotillomaniacs experience an increasing sense of tension and achieve a sense of release or gratification from pulling out their hair. All areas of the body may be affected. The most common site is the scalp. Other areas involved are the eyebrows, eyelashes, and beard; less commonly, the trunk, armpits, and pubic area. Such a hair loss is often characterized by short, broken strands appearing together with long, normal hairs in the affected areas. No abnormalities of the skin on the scalp are present.

Trichophagy, or mouthing of the hair, may follow the hair plucking. Hair pulling is not reported to be painful, although pruritus and tingling in the involved areas may be present.

There are characteristic histopathologic changes in the hair follicle, known as trichomalacia, which are demonstrated by biopsy and which help distinguish trichotillomania from other causes of alopecia. Patients usually deny the behavior and often try to hide the resultant alopecia. Head banging, nail biting, scratching, gnawing, excoriation, and other acts of self-mutilation may be present.

Course and Prognosis

Trichotillomania is generally a disorder of childhood, but onsets have been reported much later in adulthood. Some believe that an adult onset is strongly associated with the presence of a psychotic disorder. According to DSM-III-R, the course of the disorder is not well known. In some cases it has been known to persist for more than two decades. Of people presenting for treatment, approximately one third report a duration of 1 year or less. Frequent exacerbations and remissions are common.

Differential Diagnosis

According to DSM-III-R, stroking and playing with one's hair are common and normal activities. In obsessive-compulsive disorders, the behavior has particular meaning and is designed to prevent or produce some future event or situation. Patients with factitious disorder with physical symptoms actively seek medical attention and the "patient" role and deliberately simulate illness toward these ends. Patients with stereotype or habit disorder have stereotypical and rhythmic movements, and they usually do not seem distressed by their behavior. This condition may be difficult to distinguish from alopecia areata.

Treatment

There appears to be no consensus on the best treatment modality for trichotillomania. Treatment usually involves psychiatrists and dermatologists in a joint endeavor. Psychopharmacologic methods that have been used to treat psychodermatologic disorders include hydroxyzine hydrochloride, an anxiolytic with both anxiolytic and antihistamine properties; antidepressants; and neuroleptics. Many psychotropic agents have been used to treat dermatologic manifestations, and their use testifies to the wide belief that emotional factors underlie their etiology. When depression is present, antidepressant agents may lead to dermatological improvement. Successful behavioral treatments have been reported (e.g., biofeedback); however, most of these reports have been individual cases or small series of studies, with relatively short follow-up periods. Further controlled study of these techniques is warranted.

Hypnotherapy has been mentioned as a potentially effective modality in the treatment of dermatologic disorders in which psychologic factors are clearly involved. There have been repeated demonstrations of the skin's susceptibility to hypnotic suggestion. Most of this work has been research oriented, with little impact yet on clinical management.

Finally, there are many reports detailing treatment outcomes with individual, group, and family psychotherapy approaches to psychophysiological skin disorders. Generally, supportive and insight-oriented psychotherapies are effective.

References

Custer R L: Profile of the pathological gambler. J Clin Psychiatry 45:35, 1984.

Fenichel O: *The Psychoanalytic Theory of Neurosis.* Norton, New York, 1945.

Frosch J: The relation between acting out and disorders of impulse control. Psychiatry 40:295, 1977.

Geller J L, Bertsch G: Fire-setting behavior in the histories of a state hospital population. Am J Psychiatry 142:465, 1985.

Greenberg H R, Sarner C A. Trichotillomania: Symptom and syndrome. Arch Gen Psychiat 12:482, 1965.

Jenkins S C, Maruta T: Therapeutic use of propanolol for intermittent explosive disorder. Mayo Clin Proc 62:204, 1987.

Lesieur H R: The compulsive gambler's spiral of options and involvement. Psychiatry 42:79, 1979.

Linden R D: Pathological gambling and major affective disorder. J Clin Psychiatry 47:201, 1986.

Monopolis S, Lion J R. Problems in the diagnosis of intermittent explosive disorder. Am J Psychiatry 140:1200, 1983.

Vikkunen M, Nuutila A, Goodwin F K, Linnoila M: Cerebrospinal fluid monoamine metabolite levels in male arsonists. Arch Gen Psychiatry 44:241, 1987.

25

Adjustment Disorders

DEFINITION

According to DSM-III-R, an adjustment disorder is a maladaptive reaction to a clearly identifiable psychosocial stressor, or stressors, that occurs within 3 months after the stressor's onset. It is a pathological response to what a layperson might call personal misfortune; it is not an exacerbation of a psychiatric disorder that meets other criteria. The disorder is expected to remit soon after the stressor ceases or, if the stressor persists, a new level of adaptation is achieved. The response is maladaptive because of an impairment in social or occupational functioning or because of symptoms or behaviors that are beyond the normal, usual, expected response to such a stressor. Hence, the diagnostic category should not be used if the patient meets the criteria for a more specific disorder.

EPIDEMIOLOGY

Adjustment disorders are quite common. In one study, 5 percent of hospital admissions over a 3-year period were diagnosed as adjustment disorders. They are most frequently diagnosed in adolescents but may occur at any age.

ETIOLOGY

Adjustment disorders are precipitated by one or more stressors. The severity of the stressor or stressors is not always predictive of the severity of the adjustment disorder. Personality organization and cultural or group norms and values contribute to the disproportionate responses to stressors. The severity of a stressor is a complex function of degree, quantity, duration, reversibility, environment, and personal context. As an example, the loss of a parent is quite different for a 10-year-old and a 40-year-old.

Stressors may be single, such as a divorce or the loss of a job, or multiple, such as the death of an important person occurring at the same time as one's own physical illness and loss of a job. Stressors may be recurrent, such as seasonal business difficulties, or continuous, such as chronic illness or living in poverty. A discordant intrafamilial relationship may produce adjustment disorders that affect the whole family system. Or the disorder may be limited to the patient, as when he or she is the victim of a crime or has a physical illness. Sometimes adjustment disorders occur in a group or community setting, and the stressor affects several people, as in a natural disaster or in racial, social, or religious persecution. Specific developmental stages—such

as beginning school, leaving home, getting married, becoming a parent, failing to achieve occupational goals, the last child's leaving home, and retiring—are often associated with adjustment disorders.

Several psychoanalytic researchers have discussed the capacity of the same stress to produce a range of responses in different normal human beings. Throughout his life, Freud remained interested in why the stresses of ordinary life produced illness in some and not in others, why an illness took a particular form, and why some experiences and not others predisposed a person to psychopathology. He gave considerable weight to constitutional factors and viewed them as interacting with a person's life experiences to produce fixation.

Psychoanalytic research has emphasized the role of the mother and the rearing environment in a person's later capacity to respond to stress. Particularly important was Winnicott's concept of the "good-enough mother," a person who adapts to the infant's needs and provides enough support to enable the growing child to tolerate the frustrations in life.

A concurrent personality disorder or organic impairment may make a person more vulnerable to an adjustment experience. Vulnerability is also associated with the loss of a parent during infancy.

DIAGNOSIS

Although by definition an adjustment disorder follows a stressor, the symptoms do not necessarily begin immediately, nor do they always subside as soon as the stressor ceases. If the stressor continues, the disorder may be lifelong. The disorder may occur at any age. Its symptoms vary considerably, with depressive, anxious, and mixed features the most common in adults.

Physical symptoms are most common in children and the elderly but may occur in any age group. Manifestations may also include assaultive behavior and reckless driving, excessive drinking, defaulting on legal responsibilities, and withdrawal. See Table 1 for the DSM-III-R diagnostic criteria for adjustment disorder.

SUBTYPES OF ADJUSTMENT DISORDERS

Adjustment Disorder with Depressed Mood

In adjustment disorder with depressed mood, the predominant manifestations are depressed mood, tearfulness, and hopelessness.

Table 1
Diagnostic Criteria for Adjustment Disorder

A. A reaction to an identifiable psychosocial stressor (or multiple stressors) that occurs within 3 months of onset of the stressor(s).

B. The maladaptive nature of the reaction is indicated by either of the following:
   (1) impairment in occupational (including school) functioning or in usual social activities or relationships with others
   (2) symptoms that are in excess of a normal and expectable reaction to the stressor(s)

C. The disturbance is not merely one instance of a pattern of overreaction to stress or an exacerbation of one of the mental disorders previously described.

D. The maladaptive reaction has persisted for no longer than 6 months.

E. The disturbance does not meet the criteria for any specific mental disorder and does not represent Uncomplicated Bereavement.

Table from DSM-III-R *Diagnostic and Statistical Manual of Mental Disorders,* ed 3, revised. (Current Classification of Mental Disorders, 1987.) Copyright American Psychiatric Association, Washington, D.C., 1987. Used with permission.

This subtype must be distinguished from a major depressive disorder or uncomplicated bereavement.

Adjustment Disorder with Anxious Mood

Symptoms of anxiety such as palpitations, jitteriness, and agitation are present in adjustment disorder with anxious mood, which must be differentiated from anxiety disorders.

Adjustment Disorder with Mixed Emotional Features

Adjustment disorder with mixed emotional features applies when the predominant symptoms involve combinations of anxiety and depression or other emotions. This subtype must be differentiated from depressive and anxiety disorders.

Adjustment Disorder with Disturbance of Conduct

In adjustment disorder with disturbance of conduct, the predominant manifestation involves conduct in which the rights of others are violated or age-appropriate societal norms and rules are disregarded. Examples of behavior in this category are truancy, vandalism, reckless driving, and fighting. This category must be separated from conduct disorders.

Adjustment Disorder with Work or Academic Inhibition

Adjustment disorder with work or academic inhibition is applicable to an inhibition of work or academic functioning in a person who has previously functioned adequately in this area. Frequently, there is anxiety and depression, and so the condition must be differentiated from depressive disorder and phobic disorder.

The clinical features of adjustment disorder with work or academic functioning is presented in Table 2. The following case is an example of adjustment disorder:

A 19-year-old male college sophomore was referred to a West Coast mental health service because of difficulties completing school assignments. He apparently is able to complete a first paragraph that is well written and of high quality, but is unable to go further, and consequently is now in danger of flunking two or three of his courses. He has also had difficulty getting to class because he oversleeps. He states that the difficulty began about two years ago and created problems for him during his freshman year, but he somehow managed to get his papers done and to pass his courses.

The patient attended a private secondary school and did well there until his senior year, when he began to have academic difficulties after his mother had a recurrence of cancer and died. He has no conflict about being in college at this time and very much wants to be able to overcome his difficulty and continue his education toward an eventual career in law.

Discussion

This disturbance in academic functioning is clinically significant because of its persistence and potentially damaging effect on the patient's career. Therefore, it is classified as an adjustment disorder with academic inhibition.

Most cases of work (or academic) inhibition are chronic manifestations of a personality disorder, usually compulsive personality disorder. But in this case, the disturbance apparently marked a sudden change in functioning in response to a psychosocial stressor, and there is no information to support a diagnosis of a personality disorder.

DSM-III-R Diagnosis:
Axis I: Adjustment Disorder with Academic Inhibition

[Adapted with permission from *DSM-III Case Book*. American Psychiatric Association, Washington, D.C., 1981.]

Adjustment Disorder with Withdrawal

Adjustment disorder with withdrawal is used for cases of social withdrawal without significant depressed or anxious mood.

Adjustment Disorder with Physical Complaints

Adjustment disorder with physical complaints is manifested in symptoms such as headache, backache, fatigue, or other bodily complaints.

Adjustment Disorder Not Otherwise Specified

Adjustment disorder not otherwise specified is a residual category for atypical maladaptive reactions to stress. Examples include inappropriate responses to the diagnosis of physical illness, such as massive denial and severe noncompliance with treatment.

DIFFERENTIAL DIAGNOSIS

Adjustment disorders must be differentiated from conditions not attributable to a mental disorder. According to DSM-III-R, conditions not attributable to a mental disorder do not have impairment in social or occupational functioning, symptoms, or other behaviors beyond the normal and expectable reaction to the stressor. Because there are no absolute criteria to aid in distinguishing between an adjust-

Table 2
Clinical Features of Adjustment Disorder with Work or Academic Inhibition

Essential Features	Associated Features
Severe stress interfering significantly with any of the following academic or work tasks and manifested by:	Anxiety and depression
Anxiety related to examinations or other tests	Sleep disturbances
Inability to write papers, prepare reports, or perform in studio arts activities	Compulsive behavior
Difficulty in concentrating on studies or work	Disorganization of daily routine
Avoidance of studying or work that does not seem to be under conscious control	Eating disturbances
Distress not present when the person is not thinking about the academic or work task	Abuse of drugs, alcohol, or tobacco
Adequate intellectual and academic work skills present	Loneliness
Adequate previous academic or work functioning	
Intended academic or work effort, even if secondarily extinguished by above symptoms	

*Based on American Psychiatric Association: *Diagnostic and Statistical Manual of Mental Disorders,* ed 3, American Psychiatric Association, Washington, D.C., 1980.

ment disorder and a condition not attributable to a mental disorder, a clinical judgment is necessary.

Although uncomplicated bereavement often includes temporarily impaired social and occupational functioning, a person's dysfunctioning remains within the expectable bounds of a reaction to the loss of a loved one and thus is not considered an adjustment disorder.

Other disorders from which an adjustment disorder must be differentiated include major depressive disorder, chronic depressive disorder, brief reactive psychosis, generalized anxiety disorder, somatization disorder, various substance use disorders, conduct disorders, specific academic or work inhibition, identity disorder, and post-traumatic stress disorder. These diagnoses should be given precedence in all cases that meet their criteria, even in the presence of a stressor or group of stressors that might have served as a precipitant. However, some patients meet the criteria for both an adjustment disorder and a personality disorder.

In a post-traumatic stress disorder, the symptoms develop after a psychologically traumatizing event or events outside the range of normal human experience. That is, the stressors producing such a syndrome are expected to do so in the average human being. They may be experienced alone, such as rape or assault, or in groups, such as military combat. A variety of mass catastrophes—such as floods, airplane crashes, atomic bombings, and death camps—have also been identified as stressors. The stressor always contains a psychological component and frequently a concomitant physical component that directly damages the nervous system. Clinicians believe that the disorder is more severe and lasts longer when the stressor is of human origin (e.g., rape) than when it is not (e.g., floods).

PROGNOSIS

The overall prognosis of adjustment disorders is generally favorable with appropriate treatment. Most patients return to their previous level of functioning within 3 months. Adolescents usually require a longer time to recover than do

adults. Some persons (particularly adolescents) diagnosed as having an adjustment disorder later develop mood disorders or psychoactive substance abuse disorders.

TREATMENT

Psychotherapy remains the treatment of choice for adjustment disorders. Group therapy for patients who have undergone similar stresses can be particularly useful—for example, a group of retired persons or renal dialysis patients. Individual psychotherapy offers the opportunity to explore the meaning of the stressor to the patient, so that earlier traumas can be worked through. On occasion, after successful therapy, patients emerge from an adjustment disorder stronger than in the premorbid period, although no pathology was evident during that period.

The psychiatrist treating an adjustment disorder must be particularly mindful of problems of secondary gain. The illness role may be rewarding to some normal persons who have had little experience with its capacity to free one from responsibility. Thus the therapist's attention, empathy, and understanding—which are necessary for success—can become rewarding in their own right, thereby reinforcing the symptoms. Such considerations must be weighed before intensive psychotherapy is begun. When a secondary gain has already been established, therapy is more difficult.

Occasionally, antianxiety agents are useful in treating the anxiety often found in adjustment disorders; less frequently, tricyclic antidepressants are effective with the depression. Indeed, when psychiatrists think of instituting a course of antidepressive medication, they should reconsider the diagnosis and contemplate a depressive disorder. Few, if any, adjustment disorders can be adequately treated by medication alone.

Patients whose adjustment disorder includes a conduct disturbance may have difficulties with the law, authorities, or school. It is not advisable for psychiatrists to attempt to rescue such patients from the consequences of their actions. Too often, such kindness only reinforces socially unacceptable means of tension reduction and hinders the acquisition of insight and subsequent emotional growth.

Because a stressor can be clearly delineated in adjustment disorders, it is often believed that psychotherapy is not indicated and that the disorder will remit spontaneously. But such thinking fails to consider that many persons exposed to the same stressor do not develop similar symptoms and that it is a pathological response. Psychotherapy can help the person better adapt to the stressor if it is not reversible or time limited and can serve as a preventive intervention if the stressor does remit.

References

Andreasen N, Hoenk P: The predictive value of adjustment disorders: A follow-up study. Am J Psychiatry *139*:584, 1982.

Andreasen N, Wasek P: Adjustment disorders in adolescents and adults. Arch Gen Psychiatry *37*:1166, 1980.

Elliot C, Eisdorfer C: *Stress and Human Health*. Springer, New York, 1982.

Garmezy N, Rutter M: *Stress, Coping, and Development in Children*. McGraw–Hill, New York, 1983.

Holmes J, Raphe R: The social readjustment rating scale. J Psychosom Res *11*:213, 1967.

Horowitz M J: *Stress Response Syndromes*. Jason Aronson, New York, 1976.

Klerman G L, Weissman M M: Affective response to stressful life events. Program of the NIMH Conference on Prevention of Stress-Related Psychiatric Disorders. University of California, San Francisco, December 1981.

Lewis D: *Vulnerability to Delinquency*. Spectrum Publications, New York, 1981.

Popkin M K, MacKenzie T B, Collies A L: Psychiatric consultation to geriatric medically ill patients in University Hospital. Arch Gen Psychiatry *41*:703, 1984.

Winnicott D W: Translational objects and transitional phenomena. Int J Psychoanal *34*:89, 1953.

26

Psychological Factors Affecting Physical Condition (Psychosomatic Disorders)

INTRODUCTION

The diagnostic criteria in DSM-III and DSM-III-R for psychological factors affecting physical condition (i.e., psychosomatic disorders) are that psychologically meaningful environmental stimuli are significantly—albeit partially—and temporally related to the initiation or exacerbation of a physical disorder. Such a condition has either a demonstrable organic pathology, such as rheumatoid arthritis, or a known pathophysiological process, such as migraine headache. Many believe that the deletion in DSM-III of the nosological term psychophysiological (a synonym for psychosomatic) de-emphasized the interaction of mind (psyche) and body (soma), a concept that emphasizes a unitary or holistic approach to medicine, in that all disease is influenced by psychological factors. The DSM-III-R diagnostic criteria for psychological factors affecting physical condition are presented in Table 1.

Specifically excluded from the DSM-III-R classification are (1) classical psychiatric disorders presenting with physical symptomatology as part of the disorder (e.g., conversion disorder in which a physical symptom is produced by psychological conflict); (2) somatization disorder, in which there are physical symptoms not based on organic pathology; (3) hypochondriasis, in which there is an exaggerated or imagined concern with one's health; (4) physical complaints that are frequently associated with psychological disorders (e.g., dysthymic disorder, which usually has such somatic accompaniments as muscle weakness and exhaustion); and (5) physical complaints associated with habit disorders (e.g., coughing associated with tobacco dependence).

HISTORY AND CURRENT CONCEPTS

Exactly where and how do psyche and soma interact? Representatives from both psychiatry and medicine have agreed for more than 100 years that in some disorders, emotional and somatic activities overlap. These disorders were first called psychosomatic by Heinroth in 1818, when he used the term in regard to insomnia. The word was later popularized by Jacobi, a German psychiatrist. The psy-

chosomatic disorders grew to include ulcerative colitis, peptic ulcer, migraine headaches, bronchial asthma, and rheumatoid arthritis, among others.

The treatment of psychosomatic disorders by psychological methods has not produced enough satisfactory results to recommend psychological treatment as the only treatment. As a result, investigators have questioned the validity of the concept of psychophysiological medicine. Some have suggested that it is too diffuse a term; others say that it is too narrow. Most agree that chronic, severe, and perceived stress may play an etiological role in the development of certain somatic diseases. The character of the stress, the general underlying psychophysiological factors, the nature of the emotional conflicts (whether they are specific or nonspecific), and the way they operate to produce disease are controversial.

General Types of Stress Leading to Psychosomatic Disorders

A stressful or a traumatic life situation is one that generates challenges to which the organism cannot competently respond. Holmes and Rahe devised a social readjustment rating scale that lists 43 life events associated with varying amounts of disruption and stress in the average person's life

Table 1
Diagnostic Criteria for Psychological Factors Affecting Physical Condition

A. Psychologically meaningful environmental stimuli are temporally related to the initiation or exacerbation of a specific physical condition or disorder (recorded on Axis III).

B. The physical condition involves either demonstrable organic pathology (e.g., rheumatoid arthritis) or a known pathophysiologic process (e.g., migraine headache).

C. The condition does not meet the criteria for a Somatoform Disorder.

Table from DSM-III-R *Diagnostic and Statistical Manual of Mental Disorders,* ed 3, revised. (Current Classification of Mental Disorders, 1987.) Copyright American Psychiatric Association, Washington, D.C., 1987. Used with permission.

(e.g., death of a spouse, 100 units; divorce, 73 units; marital separation, 65 units; and death of a close family member, 63 units).

The scale was constructed by asking hundreds of individuals of different backgrounds to rank the relative amount of adjustment necessitated by changing life events. Holmes and Rahe found that an accumulation of over 200 or more life-change units in a single year increased the incidence of psychosomatic disorders. More recent studies have demonstrated that individuals who face these general stresses optimistically rather than pessimistically are less apt to develop a psychosomatic disorder and, if they do, to recover from it more easily.

In addition to general stresses, such as a divorce or the death of a spouse, various therapists have suggested that specific personalities and conflicts are associated with different psychosomatic diseases. Others have held that nonspecific generalized anxiety from any type of conflict may lead to a number of different diseases.

Specific Versus Nonspecific Stress in Psychosomatic Etiology

Specific stress may be defined as a specific personality or unconscious conflict causing a homeostatic dysequilibrium that contributes to the development of a psychosomatic disorder.

Specific personality types were first postulated by Flanders Dunbar, who spoke of the coronary personality (a hard-driving, aggressive individual) who suffers a myocardial occlusion. More recently, Friedman and Rosenman suggested that a type A personality (similar to the coronary personality) is a predisposition to coronary disease. Rather than emphasizing the conscious personality, Franz Alexander hypothesized specific typical unconscious conflicts associated with various disorders (e.g., unconscious dependency conflict predisposed to peptic ulcer). Both the specific personality type and unconscious conflicts fall under the rubric of specific etiological theories of psychosomatic diseases.

On the other hand, chronic nonspecific stress, with the intervening variable of anxiety, is suggested as having physiological correlates that in genetically predisposed individuals may result in a psychosomatic disorder. Alexithymic individuals are particularly vulnerable. These are individuals who have a poor fantasy life and are not conscious of their emotional conflicts, so that psychosomatic disorders may be an outlet for accumulated tension. Nonspecific theories are supported by experimental evidence that under chronic stress, animals develop psychosomatic disorders (e.g., peptic ulcer) and that animals are unlikely to have the specific personality or unconscious psychological conflicts of humans.

Intervening Physiologic Variables between Stress and Psychosomatic Disorders

The mediator between stress and disease may be hormonal, for example, Selye's general adaptation syndrome, in which cortisol is the intervenor. Others have suggested changes in the functioning of the anterior pituitary-hypothalamic-adrenal axis. Alexander pointed to the auto-nomic nervous system (e.g., the parasympathetic nervous system in peptic ulcer and the sympathetic nervous system in hypertension) as the mechanism linking chronic stress and psychosomatic disorder. A description of various classical psychosomatic disorders follows, including a brief discussion of relevant psychosomatic factors.

CARDIOVASCULAR SYSTEM

Coronary Artery Disease

Coronary artery disease causes myocardial ischemia and is characterized by episodic subcordial pain, discomfort, or pressure; it is usually precipitated by exertion or stress.

Personality Type. Flanders Dunbar first described the personality of coronary disease patients as aggressive-compulsive personalities with a tendency to work long hours and to seize authority. Later, Friedman and Rosenman defined type A and type B personalities, type A being more strongly associated with the development of coronary heart disease. Type A personalities are action-oriented individuals who struggle to achieve poorly defined goals by means of competitive hostility. Type B personalities are the opposite—they are relaxed and less aggressive and tend to strive less vigorously to achieve their goals. Type A personalities have increased amounts of low-density lipoprotein, serum cholesterol, triglycerides, and 17-hydroxycorticosteroids, and they tend to develop coronary heart disease.

Treatment. When coronary occlusion occurs, various medications for the patient's cardiac status are used. To alleviate the psychic distress associated with the disease, psychotropics (e.g., diazepam) are indicated. Pain is treated with analgesics (e.g., morphine). Medical management should be supportive and reassuring, with some psychological emphasis on the alleviation of psychic stress, compulsivity, and tension.

Essential Hypertension

Hypertension is a disease characterized by a blood pressure of 160/95 Hg or greater. Twenty percent of the adult population in the United States is hypertensive.

Personality Type. Hypertensives appear to be outwardly congenial, compliant, and compulsive, and although their anger is not expressed openly, they have much inhibited rage. There appears to be a familial genetic predisposition to hypertension; that is, when chronic stress occurs in a genetically predisposed compulsive personality who has repressed and suppressed rage, hypertension may result.

Treatment. Supportive psychotherapy and behavioral techniques (e.g., biofeedback, meditation, and relaxation therapy) have been reported to be useful in treating hypertension. Medically, there must be good compliance in taking antihypertensive medication.

Congestive Heart Failure

Congestive heart failure is a disorder in which the heart fails to move the blood forward normally, causing congestion in the lungs and systemic circulation and decreased tissue blood flow with diminished cardiac output. Psychological factors, such as nonspecific emotional stress or conflict, are frequently significant in the initiation or exacerbation of this disorder. Thus, supportive psychotherapy is important to its treatment.

Vasomotor (Vasodepressor) Syncope

Vasomotor (vasodepressor) syncope is characterized by a sudden loss of consciousness (fainting) caused by a vasovagal attack. Sympathetic autonomic activity is inhibited, and parasympathetic vagal nerve activity is augmented, resulting in decreased cardiac output, decreased vascular peripheral resistance, vasodilation, and bradycardia. According to Franz Alexander, acute fear or fright inhibits the impulse to fight or flee, thereby pooling the blood in the lower extremities, from the vasodilation of the blood vessels in the extremities. This reaction results in decreased ventricular filling and a drop in the blood supply to the brain, and consequent brain hypoxia and loss of consciousness.

Treatment. Because these patients normally put themselves, or fall, into a prone position, the decreased cardiac output is corrected. Raising their legs also helps correct the physiological imbalance. Psychotherapy should be used to determine the cause of the fright or trauma associated with syncope. When syncope is related to orthostatic hypotension, the patient should be advised to shift slowly from a sitting to a standing position.

Cardiac Arryhthmias

Life-threatening arryhthmias, such as ventricular tachycardia and ventricular fibrillation, sometimes occur in conjunction with an emotional upset. Also associated with emotional trauma are sinus tachycardia, ST and T-wave changes, ventricular ectopy, increased plasma catecholamines, and free fatty-acid concentrations. Emotional stress is nonspecific, as is the personality description associated with these disorders.

Treatment. Psychotherapy and β-blocking drugs such as propranolol help protect against these emotionally induced arryhthmias.

Psychogenic Cardiac Nondisease

A different problem is presented by patients who are free of heart disease and yet complain of symptoms suggestive of cardiac disease. They often exhibit a morbid concern about their heart and an exaggerated fear of heart disease. Their fear may range from an anxious concern, manifested by a severe phobia or hypochondriasis, to a delusional conviction about cardiac disease. Many of those patients suffer from an ill-defined syndrome often referred to as neurocirculatory asthenia.

Neurocirculatory asthenia was first described by DaCosta in 1871 and was named irritable heart by him. It has some 20 synonyms, including effort syndrome, DaCosta's syndrome, cardiac neurosis, vasoregulatory asthenia, hyperkinetic heart syndrome, and hyperdynamic-adrenergic circulatory state. Psychiatrists tend to view it as a clinical variant of anxiety disorder, although it does not appear in the official DSM-III-R nomenclature.

Diagnosis. The diagnostic criteria for neurocirculatory asthenia are (1) respiratory complaints, such as sighing respiration, inability to take a deep breath, smothering and choking, or dyspnea; (2) palpitations, chest pain, or discomfort; (3) nervousness, dizziness, faintness, or discomfort in crowds; (4) undue fatigue or limitation of activities; and (5) excessive sweating, insomnia, and irritability. The symptoms usually start in adolescence or the early 20s but may begin in middle age. Such symptoms are twice as common in women as in men and tend to be chronic, with recurrent acute exacerbations.

Treatment. The management of neurocirculatory asthenia may be difficult, and the prognosis is guarded if the condition is chronic. Phobic elements are prominent, and patients often derive primary or secondary gains from this disability. Psychotherapy aimed at uncovering psychodynamic factors—often relating to hostility, unacceptable sexual impulses, dependence, guilt, and death anxiety—may be effective in some cases, but most patients with the condition tend to shun psychiatric help. Other behavioral techniques may be useful. Physical training programs aimed at correcting faulty breathing habits and gradually increasing the patient's effort tolerance may be helpful, especially if the programs are combined with group psychotherapy. Psychopharmacologic treatment focuses on the predominant symptomatology. The use of propranolol may interrupt the vicious cycle of cardiac symptoms and have a positive reinforcement feedback effect on anxiety, which aggravates the symptoms. Antianxiety agents (e.g., diazepam) can be used for major anxiety symptoms. If fatigue, lassitude, and weakness are the major complaints, the judicious use of amphetamines or methylphenidate may be helpful.

RESPIRATORY SYSTEM

Bronchial Asthma

Bronchial asthma is a chronic recurrent obstructive disease of the bronchial airways, which tend to respond to various stimuli by bronchial constriction, edema, and excessive secretion. Genetic factors, allergic factors, infections, and acute and chronic stress all combine to produce the disease. The rate and depth of a healthy person's breathing may be changed voluntarily and may correlate with different emotional states; in asthma, such changes are aggravated and prolonged.

Psychological Factors. Although asthmatics are characterized as having excessive dependency needs, no specific personality type has been identified. Alexander pointed to psychodynamic conflictual factors, as he found in many asthmatics a strong unconscious wish for protection and for envelopment by their mother or surrogate mother. These mother figures tend to be overprotective and oversolicitous, perfectionistic, dominating, and helpful. When protection is sought but is not received, an asthmatic attack occurs.

Treatment. Some asthmatic children improve by being separated from their mother (so-called parentectomy). All standard psychotherapies are used: individual, group, behavioral, and hypnotic. Asthmatics should be treated jointly by internists, allergists, and psychiatrists.

Hay Fever

Strong psychological factors combine with allergic elements to produce hay fever. One factor may dominate over the other, and they may alternate in importance.

Treatment. Psychiatric, medical, and allergic factors must be considered in treating hay fever.

Hyperventilation Syndrome

Normal persons can voluntarily change the rate, depth, and regularity of their breathing, which can also be correlated with different emotional states. Hyperventilative patients breathe rapidly and deeply for several minutes, feel lightheaded, and then faint because of cerebral vasoconstriction and a respiratory alkalosis. Other symptoms, such as paresthesias and carpopedal spasm, may be present. Specific medical differentials for the syndrome are epilepsy, hysteria, vasovagal or hypoglycemic attacks, myocardial attacks, bronchial asthma, acute porphyria, Meniere's disease, and pheochromocytoma. Psychiatric differentials include anxiety attacks, panic attacks, schizophrenia, borderline or histrionic personality disorders, and phobic or obsessive complaints.

Treatment. Instruction or retraining regarding particular symptoms and how they are evoked by hyperventilation should be provided so that patients may consciously avoid precipitating symptoms. Breathing into a paper bag can abort the attack.

GASTROINTESTINAL SYSTEM

Peptic Ulcer

Peptic ulcer is a circumscribed ulceration of the mucous membrane of the stomach or duodenum, penetrating to the muscularis mucosa and occurring in areas exposed to gastric acid and pepsin.

Psychosomatic Psychophysiological Etiologic Theories
Specific theory. Franz Alexander hypothesized that chronic frustration of intense dependency needs results in a characteristic unconscious conflict. This unconscious conflict pertains to intense dependent oral-receptive longings to be cared for and loved, which causes a chronic regressive unconscious hunger and anger. This reaction is manifested physiologically by persistent vagal hyperactivity leading to gastric acid hypersecretion, which is particularly ominous in a genetically predisposed hypersecretor of acid. With the aformentioned equation, ulcer formation may result. Genetic factors as well as preexisting organ damage or disease (e.g., gastritis) is etiologically important. Such gastritis may result from excessive caffeine, nicotine, or alcohol.
Nonspecific theories. Stress and anxiety caused by varied nonspecific conflicts may produce gastric hyperacidity and hypersecretion of pepsin, resulting in an ulcer. Because various traumatic occurrences in animals (e.g., electric shock in dogs), may produce ulcers, such experimental data support a nonspecific approach. Peptic ulcers have been diagnosed in all personality types.

Treatment. Psychotherapy is directed toward the patient's dependency conflicts. Biofeedback and relaxation therapy may be useful. Medical treatment with cimetidine (Tagamet) or ranitidine (Zantac) antacid medications and dietary control (e.g., no alcohol) are indicated in ulcer management.

Ulcerative Colitis

Ulcerative colitis is a chronic inflammatory ulcerative disease of the colon and is usually associated with a bloody diarrhea. Familial incidence and genetic factors are significant. Related diseases include regional ileitis and irritable bowel syndrome.

Personality Type. Most studies show a predominance of compulsive personality traits. Such patients are neat, orderly, clean, punctual, hyperintellectual, timid, and inhibited in expressing their anger.
Specific Theory. Alexander described a typical specific conflictual constellation in ulcerative colitis. The key issue is an inability to fulfill an obligation (usually of accomplishment) to a key dependency figure. Essentially frustrated dependency stimulates oral aggressive feelings, producing guilt and anxiety and resulting in restitution through the "gifting" of diarrhea. In regard to colitis, George Engel described a pathological mother–child relationship, resulting in feelings of "hopelessness–helplessness" and a "giving up–given up complex."
Nonspecific Theory. Nonspecific stress of many types may produce ulcerative colitis.
Treatment. Supportive psychotherapy is indicated during the acute phase of ulcerative colitis, with more interpretative psychotherapy during the more chronic quiescent periods. Medical treatment consists of nonspecific supportive medical measures, such as anticholinergics and antidiarrheal agents. Prednisone therapy is useful in severe cases. Bismuth-containing medications (e.g., Pepto-Bismol) are very useful in managing diarrhea.

OBESITY

Definition

Obesity is a condition characterized by the excessive accumulation of fat (when the body weight exceeds by 20 percent the standard weight listed in the usual height–weight tables).

Psychosomatic Considerations

There is a familial genetic predisposition to obesity as well as early developmental factors seen in childhood obesity. The latter suggests that obese children increase their fat-cell number (hyperplastic obesity), which predisposes them to adult obesity. When obesity occurs first in adult life, it usually is hypertrophic obesity (an increase in fat-cell size) rather than an increase in the number of fat cells. Obesity also tends to limit physical activity, which further aggravates this condition. Psychological factors are important to hyperphagic obesity (overeating). Among the psychodynamics suggested are oral fixation, oral regression, and overvaluation of food. Bulimia—usually associated with binge eating—may be present. In addition, there is often a past history of body-image disparagement and poor early conditioning to food intake.

Treatment

Obesity must be controlled through dietary limitation and the reduction of calorie intake. Emotional support and behavior modification are helpful for the anxiety and depression associated with overeating and dieting. Gastric reduction surgery and similar techniques are of limited value.

ANOREXIA NERVOSA

Anorexia nervosa is characterized by behavior directed toward losing weight, peculiar patterns of handling food, weight loss, intense fear of gaining weight, disturbance of body image, and, in women, amenorrhea. It is one of the few psychiatric illnesses that may have a course unremitting until death. Anorexia nervosa is discussed in Section 38.3.

MUSCULOSKELETAL

Rheumatoid Arthritis

Rheumatoid arthritis is a disease characterized by chronic musculoskeletal pain caused by inflammatory disease of the joints. This disorder has significant hereditary, allergic, immunological, and psychological etiological factors. It has been suggested that psychological stress predisposes patients to rheumatoid arthritis, as well as to other autoimmune diseases. The arthritic feels restrained, tied down, and confined. Because many of these people have had a past history of being very active physically (e.g., dancers), they often have repressed rage about the inhibition of their muscle function, which aggravates their stiffness and immobility.

Treatment. Treatment should include psychotherapy, which is usually supportive during the acute attack and interpretative during the chronic phase. Rest and exercise should be structured, and patients should be encouraged not to become bed bound and to return to their former activities. The rest and exercise program should be coordinated with the medical treatment for pain and inflammation of the joints.

Low Back Pain

Low back pain is felt in the lower lumbar, lumbosacral, and sacroiliac region. It is often accompanied by sciatica, with pain radiating down one or both buttocks or following the distribution of the sciatic nerve. Although low back pain may be caused by a ruptured intervertebral disc, a fracture of the back, congenital defects of the lower spine, or a ligamentous muscle strain, many are psychosomatic in origin. Some reports indicate that 95 percent of cases are psychological in origin.

The examining physician should be particularly alert to a patient who gives a history of minor back trauma followed by severe disabling pain. Very often the low back patient will report that the pain was initiated at a time of psychological trauma or stress. In addition, the patient's reaction to the pain is disproportionately emotional, with excessive anxiety and depression. Furthermore, the distribution of the pain rarely follows a normal neuroanatomic distribution (e.g., of sciatica).

Treatment. Treatment should be conservative. Aspirin—up to a total of 4 g daily is a useful analgesic. Diazepam (Valium), 5 to 10 mg every 4 to 6 hours, acts as both a muscle relaxant and an anxiolytic. A careful exercise and physical therapy regimen, supportive psychotherapy regarding the precipitating emotional trauma, relaxation therapy, or biofeedback are helpful. Patients should be encouraged to return to their usual activities as soon as possible. Surgical intervention is rarely indicated.

HEADACHES

Introduction

Headaches are the most common neurological symptom and one of the most common of all medical complaints. Every year about 80 percent of the population is estimated to suffer from at least one headache, and 10 to 20 percent of the population presents to a physician with headache as their primary complaint. Headaches also are a major cause of absenteeism from work or avoidance of other social or personal activities.

The majority of headaches are not associated with significant organic disease. Many individuals are susceptible to headaches at times of emotional stress. Moreover, many psychiatric disorders, including anxiety and depressive disorders, frequently present with headaches as a prominent symptom. Headache patients are often referred to psychiatrists by primary-care physicians and neurologists after extensive biomedical work-ups, which often include a CT scan of the head. The overwhelming majority of such work-ups for common headache complaints are negative, and such results may be frustrating for both patient and physician. The psychologically unsophisticated physician may attempt to reassure such patients by telling them that there is no disease. But this may often have the opposite effect, increasing the patients' anxiety and even escalating into a disagreement about whether the pain is real or imagined.

Psychological stresses usually exacerbate headaches, whether their primary underlying cause is physical or psychological. Psychosomatic headaches are sometimes differentiated from psychogenic (e.g., anxiety, depression, hypochondriacal, delusional) headaches. For example, headaches may be a conversion symptom of inpatients with hysterical or other types of personality traits. In these patients, the headache symbolizes unconscious psychological conflicts, and the symptoms are mediated through the voluntary sensorimotor nervous system. In contrast, psychosomatic headaches are defined as autonomic responses to conscious or unconscious conflicts and are not symbolic in nature. This distinction is important for psychiatrists to make so as to reach the proper diagnosis which then allows the most specific treatment to be recommended.

Migraine (Vascular) Headaches

Migraine (vascular) headaches are a paroxysmal disorder characterized by recurrent headaches, with or without related visual and gastrointestinal disturbances. They are probably caused by a functional disturbance in the cranial circulation.

Personality Types. Two thirds of patients developing migraine headaches have a family history of similar disorders. Obsessional personalities who are overly controlled and perfectionistic, suppress anger, and are genetically predisposed to migraines may develop such a headache under severe nonspecific emotional conflict or stress.

Treatment. Migraines are best treated during the prodromal period with ergotamine tartrate and analgesics. The prophylactic administration of propranalol (Inderal) or phenytoin (Dilantin) is useful if the headaches are frequent. Psychotherapy to diminish the effect of conflict and stress, and certain behavioral techniques (e.g., biofeedback) have been reported as useful.

Tension (Muscle Contraction) Headaches

Emotional stress is often associated with the prolonged contraction of head and neck muscles, which over several hours may constrict the blood vessels and result in ischemia. A dull, aching pain often begins suboccipitally and may spread over the head, sometimes feeling like a tightening band. The scalp may be tender to the touch, and in contrast with a migraine, the headache is usually bilateral and not associated with prodromata, nausea, and vomiting. The onset is often toward the end of the workday or in early evening, possibly after the individual has been removed from stressful job pressures, has tried to relax, and has focused more on somatic sensations. But if family or personal pressures are equal to or greater than those at work, the headaches may be worse later in the evening, on weekends, or during vacations.

Tension headaches may occur to some degree in about 80 percent of the population during periods of emotional stress. Anxiety and depression frequently are associated with these headaches. Tense, high-strung, competitive, type A personality individuals are especially prone to this disorder. They may be treated in the acute stage with anti-anxiety agents, muscle relaxants, and massage or heat application to the head and neck. If an underlying depression is present, antidepressants may be prescribed. However, psychotherapy is usually the treatment of choice for patients chronically afflicted by tension headaches. Learning to avoid or better cope with tension is the most effective long-term management approach. Electromyogram feedback from the frontalis or temporalis muscles may help some tension-headache patients. Relaxation associated with the practice periods, meditation, or other changes in a pressured life-style may provide symptomatic relief for some patients.

ENDOCRINE SYSTEM

Hyperthyroidism

Hyperthyroidism (thyrotoxicosis) is a syndrome characterized by biochemical and psychological changes that occur as a result of a chronic endogenous or exogenous excess of thyroid hormone.

Psychosomatic Considerations. In a genetically predisposed individual, stress is often associated with the onset of hyperthyroidism. According to psychoanalytic theory, during their childhood, hyperthyroid patients have an unusual attachment and dependence on a parent, usually the mother, and so they find intolerable any threat to their mother's approval. As children, such patients often had inadequate support, because of economic stress, divorce, death, or multiple siblings. This persistent threat to security in early life leads to premature and unsuccessful attempts to identify with an adult object. It also causes early stress and over-utilization of the endocrine system, and further frustration of childhood dependency cravings. Because of this failure, the patients continuously strive toward premature self-sufficiency and tend to dominate others with smothering attention and affection. They need to build defenses against a repetition of the unbearable feelings of rejection and isolation that occurred in childhood. Should these mechanisms break down, requiring a premature stimulation of the body's psychophysiological defense in a genetically predisposed patient, thyrotoxicosis may result.

Treatment. Antithyroid medication, tranquilizers, and supportive psychotherapy are useful. Crisis intervention may be helpful at the acute onset of the disease.

Diabetes Mellitus

Diabetes mellitus is a disorder of metabolism and the vascular system manifested by a disturbance of the body's handling of glucose, lipid, and protein.

Psychosomatic Etiology. Heredity and family history are extremely important in regard to the onset of diabetes. An acute onset is often associated with emotional stress, which disturbs the homeostatic balance in a predisposed patient. Psychological factors that seem significant are those provoking feelings of frustration, loneliness, and dejection. Diabetic patients usually must maintain some sort of dietary control of their diabetes. Thus when they are depressed and dejected, they often overeat or overdrink self-destructively, causing their diabetes to get out of control. This is especially common in juvenile diabetics. In addition, terms such as oral, dependent, seeking maternal attention, and excessive passivity have been applied to diabetics.

Treatment. Supportive psychotherapy is necessary in order to achieve cooperation in the medical management of this complex disease. Therapy should encourage diabetics to lead as normal a life as possible, with the recognition that they have a chronic but manageable disease.

Disorders Associated with Female Endocrine Functions

Premenstrual Syndrome. The premenstrual syndrome (PMS) is characterized by cyclical subjective changes in mood and general sense of physical and psychological well-being correlated with the menstrual cycle. The symptoms usually begin soon after ovulation, increase gradually, and reach a maximum of intensity about 5 days before the menstrual period. Psychological, social, and biological factors have been implicated in the syndrome's pathogenesis. In particular, changes in estrogen, progesterone, androgen, and prolactin levels have been hypothesized to be important to the etiology. Recently, it has been proposed that excessive exposure to and subsequent abrupt withdrawal of endogenous opiate peptides, which fluctuate under the influence of gonadal steroids, may contribute to PMS. An increase in prostaglandins secreted by the uterine musculature have been implicated in the pain

Table 2
Diagnostic Criteria for Late Luteal Phase Dysphoric Disorder

A. In most menstrual cycles during the past year, symptoms in B occurred during the last week of the luteal phase and remitted within a few days after onset of the follicular phase. In menstruating females, these phases correspond to the week before, and a few days after, the onset of menses. (In nonmenstruating females who have had a hysterectomy, the timing of luteal and follicular phases may require measurement of circulating reproductive hormones.)

B. At least five of the following symptoms have been present for most of the time during each symptomatic late luteal phase, at least one of the symptoms being either (1), (2), (3), or (4):

  (1) marked affective lability, e.g., feeling suddenly sad, tearful, irritable, or angry

  (2) persistent and marked anger or irritability

  (3) marked anxiety, tension, feelings of being "keyed up," or "on edge"

  (4) markedly depressed mood, feelings of hopelessness, or self-deprecating thoughts

  (5) decreased interest in usual activities, e.g., work, friends, hobbies

  (6) easy fatigability or marked lack of energy

  (7) subjective sense of difficulty in concentrating

  (8) marked change in appetite, overeating, or specific food cravings

  (9) hypersomnia or insomnia

  (10) other physical symptoms, such as breast tenderness or swelling, headaches, joint or muscle pain, a sensation of "bloating," weight gain

C. The disturbance seriously interferes with work or with usual social activities or relationships with others.

D. The disturbance is not merely an exacerbation of the symptoms of another disorder, such as Major Depression, Panic Disorder, Dysthymia, or a Personality Disorder (although it may be superimposed on any of these disorders).

E. Criteria A, B, C, and D are confirmed by prospective daily self-ratings during at least two symptomatic cycles. (The diagnosis may be made provisionally prior to this confirmation.)

Table from DSM-III-R *Diagnostic and Statistical Manual of Mental Disorders,* ed 3, revised. (Current Classification of Mental Disorders, 1987.) Copyright American Psychiatric Association, Washington, D.C., 1987. Used with permission.

associated with the syndrome. PMS occurs in woman past the menarche and after hysterectomy, providing that the ovaries remain intact. Seventy to 90 percent of all women of childbearing age report at least some symptoms.

Late Luteal Phase Dysphoric Disorder. A new and controversial diagnostic category called Late Luteal Phase Dysphoric Disorder (LLPDD) was suggested to be added to the DSM-III-R. The signs and symptoms of LLPDD are more severe and create more distress than those of PMS, and they are more likely to occur in women over 30. LLPDD is considered to be controversial in that many clinicians do not feel that the menstrual cycle should be associated with a diagnosable mental disorder. Also, there are no data regarding LLPDD's prevalance, predisposing factors, course, or specific treatment. The DSM-III-R cautiously states that the category has a high potential for misapplication and misinterpretation and encourages its further study. Because of this controversy over LLPDD, this classification has been placed in an appendix to DSM-III-R and *not* in DSM-III-R proper.

According to DSM-III-R, LLPDD is characterized by a pattern of significant emotional and behavioral symptoms that are sufficiently severe to cause a marked impairment in social or occupational functioning. The symptoms occur during the last week of the luteal phase of the menstrual cycle (hence the term late luteal) and remit within a few days after the onset of the follicular phase. Among the most commonly experienced symptoms that DSM-III-R lists are affective lability (e.g., sudden episodes of tearfulness, sadness, or irritability; anger and tension); feelings of depression, which may be accompanied by suicidal ideation; decreased energy and greater fatigue; loss of appetite or craving for certain foods such as carbohydrates; sleep disturbances; and physical complaints such as joint or muscle pain, weight gain, headaches, breast tenderness, and a feeling of being bloated. Similar symptoms are seen in PMS, but to a much lesser degree. (DSM-III-R's diagnostic criteria for LLPDD is listed in Table 2). The differential diagnosis of this disorder is listed in DSM-III-R as follows: dysmenorrhea, depressive disorder, and panic disorder. According to the DSM-III-R; dysmenorrhea (painful menses) is characterized by symptoms that occur with the menses, whereas in LLPDD, the onset of the symptoms is premenstrual. The diagnosis of LLPDD should not be made if the symptoms preceding the menses are limited to pain and physical discomfort. Other disorders that are symptomatically similar to LLPDD, such as depressive disorders and panic disorder, do not remit regularly with the onset of menses.

Because of the controversy about LLPDD, this classification was placed in an appendix to DSM-III-R, and is limited by the statement that the syndrome requires further study.

Treatment. The symptoms of PMS or LLPDD are treated symptomatically. Water retention—which accounts for the bloated feeling—weight gain, and edema may be relieved by antidiuretic medication and salt restriction. Pain, such as headaches and, particularly dysmennorhea, respond to analgesics. Acetaminophen is preferable to aspirin because it does not interfere with clotting mechanisms. Mental manifestations (e.g., fatigue, lassitude, and general malaise) respond to small doses of amphetamine, which also appear to act synergistically with analgesics such as aspirin for the better relief of associated pain. Antiprostaglandins help some women whose dysmennorhea is the result of uterine prostaglandin release; however, in order for the medication to be effective, it should be started before the onset of pain. Other drugs, including progesterone, lithium, antidepressants, and antianxiety agents, have been tried with uncertain success. It is helpful to many women to be made aware that premenstrual symptoms represent a recurring syndrome that can be anticipated. Psychotherapy may be helpful in individual cases. In very rare cases, psychotic symptoms have been described that occur exclusively in the latter part of the luteal phase of the menstrual cycle and that respond to antipsychotic medication.

Menopausal Distress. Menopause is a natural physiological event. It is usually dated as having occurred after an absence of menstrual periods for 1 year. Usually the menses taper off during a 2- to 5-year span, most often between the ages of 48 and 55; the median age is 51.4 years. Menopause also occurs immediately after the surgical removal of the ovaries. The term "involutional period" refers to advancing age, and "climacteric" refers to involution of the ovaries.

Clinical description. Many psychological symptoms have been attributed to the menopause, including anxiety, fatigue, tension, emotional lability, irritability, depression, dizziness, and insomnia. There is no general agreement on the relative contribution of those complaints or of the physiological changes to the psychological and social meanings of menopause and this developmental era in a woman's life.

Physical signs and symptoms include night sweats, flushes, and hot flashes. A hot flash is a sudden perception of heat within or on the body that may be accompanied by sweating or color change. The cause of the hot flash is unknown; it may be linked to pulsatile LH secretion. Estrogen-dependent functions are sequentially lost, and there may be atrophic changes in mucosal surfaces, accompanied by vaginitis, pruritus, dypareunia, and stenosis. There are changes in calcium and lipid metabolism, probably as secondary effects of the lower levels of estrogen, and these may be associated with a number of medical problems occurring in the postmenopausal era, such as osteoporosis and coronary atherosclerosis. The physical changes may begin as much as 4 to 8 years before the last menstrual period. During this time, women may have irregular menstrual periods with variations in the menstrual intervals and the quality of the menstrual flow.

Hormonal changes and their relation to clinical manifestations. Blood levels of ovarian hormones decline gradually during the climacteric period, usually over a period of several years. For many years, decreasing estrogen levels were thought to be of primary importance in relation to the clinical manifestations of menopause. Both estrogen and progesterone bind directly to brain tissue and were considered to act directly on brain function. More recently, however, it has been thought that other hormones, such as androgens and LH, are also involved. The effects of estrogen on mood may be indirectly moderated through its influence on androgen production. In any case, the significance of hormonal changes is evidenced by the severe physical and psychological symptoms that follow abrupt (surgical) depletion of ovarian hormones. One difficulty in those studies that have attempted to assess the relationships of changing hormonal levels in normal females is that the date of the last menstrual period is often difficult to establish, as is the menarche, for they merely mark a point on a curve of changing hormonal function. That is, the presence or absence of menstrual bleeding is not an exact measure of hormonal status.

The degree of symptomatology at the menopause seems to be related to the rate of hormone withdrawal; the amount of hormone depletion; a woman's constitutional ability to withstand the overall aging process, including her overall health and level of activity; and the psychological meaning of aging for her.

Psychological and psychosocial factors. Clinically significant psychiatric difficulties may develop during the life cycle's involutional phase. Women who have previously experienced psychological difficulties, such as low self-esteem and low life satisfaction, are likely to be vulnerable to difficulties during menopause. A woman's response to menopause has been noted to parallel her response to other crucial developmental events in her life, such as puberty and pregnancy. Attempts to link the severity of menopausal distress with the premenstrual tension syndrome have been inconclusive.

Women who have invested heavily in childbearing and childrearing activities are most likely to suffer distress during the postmenopausal years. Concerns about aging, loss of childbearing capacity, and changes in appearance all may be focused on the social and symbolic significance attached to the physical changes of the menopause.

Although in the past it was assumed that the incidence of mental illness and depression would increase during the menopause, epidemiological evidence casts some doubt on this assumption as an all-inclusive and complete explanation. Epidemiological studies of mental illness showed no increase in symptoms of mental illness or in depression during the menopausal years, and studies of psychological complaints found no greater frequency in menopausal women than in younger women.

Treatment. Treatment programs must be individualized. Postclimacteric women may be asymptomatic for estrogen deprivation or may manifest estrogen excess (dysfunctional uterine bleeding).

The use of estrogen replacement treatment is still controversial. For women with signs of estrogen depletion, recent studies have been more encouraging in regard to the use of long-term combined estrogen and progesterone replacement therapy, both in estrogen depletion syndrome and to prevent osteoporesis. Topical estrogen cream used to treat mucosal atrophy is readily absorbed systemically. The increased risk of cancer, particularly endometrial cancer, has been implicated in the use of exogenous estrogen, but the addition of a progestational agent to the replacement estrogen regime is thought to reduce this increased risk.

Exercise, diet, and symptomatic treatment all are helpful in reducing physical discomfort. Psychological distress should be evaluated and treated primarily by appropriate psychotherapeutic and sociotherapeutic measures. Psychotherapy should include an exploration of the life stage and the meaning of aging and reproduction to the patient. The patient should be encouraged to accept the menopause as a natural life event and to develop new activities, interests, and gratifications. Psychotherapy should also attend to family dynamics and enlist family and other social support systems when necessary.

Idiopathic Amenorrhea. The cessation of normal menstrual cycles in nonpregnant, premenopausal women with no demonstrable structural abnormalities in their brain, pituitary, or ovaries is termed idiopathic amenorrhea.

The diagnosis is made first by exclusion and then, if possible, by identifying the primary psychogenic cause. Amenorrhea may occur as one feature of complex clinical psychiatric syndromes, such as anorexia nervosa and pseudocyesis. Other conditions associated with amenorrhea include massive obesity, diseases of the pituitary and hypothalamus, and, in some cases, excessive amounts of running or jogging. Drugs such as reserpine and chlorpromazine can block ovulation and so delay the menses. Drug-induced amenorrhea is almost always accompanied by galactorrhea and elevated levels of prolactin.

The patterns of hormone defect that result in psychogenic amenorrhea are not well understood. Disturbed menstrual function with delayed or precipitate menses is a well-known response by healthy women to stress. The stress can be as minor as going away to college or as catastrophic as being put into a concentration camp.

In most women, mentrual cycling returns without medical intervention, sometimes even in continuing stressful conditions. Psychotherapy should be undertaken for psychological reasons, not just in response to the symptom of amenorrhea and also to determine its cause. However, if the amenorrhea has been protracted and refractory, psychotherapy may be helpful in restoring regular menses.

CHRONIC PAIN

Definition

Persistent pain is the most frequent complaint of patients, yet it is one of the most difficult symptoms to treat because of differing etiologies and individual responses to pain.

Pain is affected by a myriad of subjective, unmeasurable factors, including level of attention, emotional state, personality, and past experiences. Pain may simultaneously serve as a symptom and as a defense against psychological stress. Psychological factors may cause a person to become somatically preoccupied and magnify even normal sensations to chronic pain. Patients may be excessively responsive to pain for personal, social, or financial secondary gain. Chronic pain may be a way of justifying failure of establishing relationships with others. Cultural, ethnic, or religious affiliations may influence the degree and manner in which individuals express pain and the way in which their families react to the symptoms. Therefore, in evaluating and treating persistent pain, the physician should realize that pain is not a simple stimulus–response phenomenon. Rather, the perception of a reaction to pain is multifactorial, combining many biopsychosocial variables.

Pain Threshold and Perception Peripheral sensations are transmitted via the pain pathways (e.g., lateral spinothalamic tract, posterior thalamus of the diencephalon) to cortical somatosensory regions of the central nervous system for conscious perception. The parietal cortex both localizes pain and perceives intensity. However, psychogenic pain may be entirely of central origin. More complex reactions to pain involve other areas of the cortex responsible for memory, and conscious and unconscious elements of an individual's personality.

The threshold for perception of pain is the same for most people but may be decreased by about 40 percent by biofeedback, a positive emotional state, relaxation exercises, physical therapy or other physical activity, meditation, guided imagery, suggestion, hypnosis, placebos, or analgesics. The beneficial response to placebos is sometimes falsely thought to differentiate organic from functional etiologies. In fact, about one-third of normal persons, or those with organic causes of pain, have at least a transient positive response to a placebo.

Variations in the effectiveness and responsiveness of persons' endorphin or other neurotransmitter systems may modulate pain perception and tolerance. A gate-control theory has been proposed, which suggests that large peripheral afferent nerve fibers modulate sensory input by inhibiting hypothetical sensory transmitting neurons (gateway cells) in the substantia gelatinosa of the spinal cord. Relief of pain by transcutaneous or dorsal column electrical stimulators may result from this system's activation.

Classification

DSM-III-R classifies chronic pain patients under somatoform disorders (see Chapter 19). If patients have multiple recurrent pains of at least several years' duration that began before age 30, they are considered to have a somatization disorder. If the patients' pain suggests a physical illness but may be attributed to psychological factors alone, their diagnosis is conversion disorder or somatoform pain disorder (if pain is the only symptom). Patients with somatization, depressive or schizophrenic disorders complain of various aches and pains but pain is not the major complaint. In conversion disorders, the distribution and referral of pain are inconsistent.

Treatment

Patients are often undermedicated with analgesia because of a lack of knowledge of the pharmacology of analgesics, an unrealistic fear of causing addiction (even in terminal patients), and the ethical judgment that only bad physicians prescribe large doses of narcotics. In this regard, it is critical to separate patients with chronic benign pain (who tend to do much better with psychotherapy and psychotropic drugs) from those with chronic pain due to cancer or other chronic medical disorders. The former often respond to the combination of an antidepressant and a phenothiazine. The latter usually respond better to analgesics or nerve blocks. Many cancer patients may be kept relatively active, alert, and comfortable with the judicious use of morphine, avoiding costly and incompletely effective surgical procedures, such as peripheral nerve section, cordotomy, or stereotaxic thalamic ablations.

A behavior modification, deconditioning program may also be useful. Analgesia should be prescribed at regular intervals, rather than only as needed. Otherwise, patients must suffer before receiving relief, which only increases their anxiety and sensitivity to pain. Standing orders dissociate experiencing pain from receiving medical medication. The deconditioning of needed care from experiencing increased pain should also extend to patients' interpersonal relationships. Patients should receive as much or more attention for displaying active and healthy behavior as they receive for passive, dependent, pain-related behaviors. Their spouses, bosses, friends, physicians, health care, or social agencies should not reinforce chronic pain and penalize patients (including threatening to discontinue disability payments) if the patients begin to relinquish their sick role. Patients should be assured of regular and supportive appointments that are not contingent on pain. Hospitalization should be avoided, if possible, to prevent further regression.

Pain clinics with a multispecialty staff evaluate and treat patients with complex pain disorders. These clinics include the early involvement of psychiatrists, rather than only after the real causes of pain have been ruled out and the patient and physicians are frustrated. The patients are managed without addictive drugs although many patients commence treatment already addicted. Exploratory or neurodestructive surgery are not encouraged, especially if the patient has a hysterical personality or a history of multiple surgical procedures. Pain clinics also recognize that most chronic pain patients experience a vicious cycle of biological and psychosocial factors, so that the most effective treatment involves a systems approach that addresses each biopsychosocial component relevant to the patient.

IMMUNE DISORDERS

Introduction

There is considerable evidence of a relationship among psychosocial factors, immune function, and health and illness. It seems that psychosocial processes, including a range of the person's life experiences and state and trait characteristics, influence the central nervous system, thereby encouraging the suppression of immune activity.

Immune Response. Immunological responses *in vivo* can be divided into two types—immediate hypersensitivity and delayed hypersensitivity. An immediate response is exemplified by the wheal-and-flare reaction that takes place 10 to 15 minutes after an extract of pollen is injected into the skin of a person with hay fever. An example of delayed response is the erythema and induration elicited 24 to 48 hours after the injection of tuberculin into the skin of a patient with tuberculosis.

Immediate and delayed hypersensitivity responses may be further distinguished by the ability to produce these responses in immunologically naive recipients. The immediate wheal-and-flare response can be transferred to an apparently healthy person by the serum of a hypersensitive person. In contrast, delayed hypersensitivity may be transferred by cells (lymphocytes) but not by serum. As a result, delayed hypersensitivity is referred to as "cell-mediated immunity," and immediate hypersensitivity is referred to as "humoral immunity," as it is mediated by antibodies in the serum.

Mediation of Psychosocial Influences on the Immune Function. The endocrine system is highly responsive to both life experiences and the psychological state, and it has a significant, although complicated, effect on immune responses. The most widely studied hormones are those of the pituitary-adrenocortical system. A wide variety of stressors associated with the elicitation of emotional changes within the organism induce the classical stress response characterized by the rapid release of adrenocorticotrophic hormone (ACTH), followed by the release of corticosteroids. Corticosteroids have been found to alter various immune functions and usually suppress but occasionally may enhance the immune response.

Infectious Diseases

Clinical studies have reported that psychological variables influence the rate of recovery from infectious mononucleosis and influenza, and the susceptibility to rhinovirus-induced common cold symptoms and tularemia. Recurrent herpes simplex and herpes genitalis lesions have been shown to occur most frequently in patients with clinical depression or who experience unusual stress. Stressful life events and a poor psychological state have been found to decrease resistance to tuberculosis and to influence the course of the illness. Social supports have also been shown to play a role in recovery from tuberculosis. Life experiences that induce anger have been noted to alter the intestine's bacterial composition. College students who respond to upsetting events with maladaptive aggression or affective changes were found to have a higher incidence of subsequent upper respiratory infections. It should be noted that in these studies the primary immune response was cell mediated. In AIDS, transmitted by the HIV virus, psychiatric symptoms are common and there are many who feel that the progress of the disease is influenced by the person's psychological state. See Chapter 12 for further discussion of the psychiatric aspects of AIDS.

Allergic Disorders

Considerable clinical evidence suggests that psychological factors are related to the precipitation of many allergic disorders. Bronchial asthma is a prime example of a pathological process involving immediate hypersensitivity that is associated with psychosocial processes. Emotional reactions to life experience, personality patterns, and conditioning have been reported to contribute to the onset and course of asthma.

Organ Transplantation

Psychosocial factors seem to play a role in organ transplantation. A number of clinical studies have reported that stressful life events, anxiety, and depression precede some cases of graft rejection. Psychosocial effects on the immune system may contribute to the mechanisms involved in such rejections.

Autoimmune Diseases

A prime function of the immune system is to distinguish between self and nonself and to reject foreign antigens (nonself). Occasionally, for reasons that are unclear at the present time, a cell-mediated or humoral immune response develops against a person's own cells. This reaction results in a variety of pathological effects that are known clinically as autoimmune diseases. Disorders in which an autoimmune component has been implicated include Graves' disease, Hashimoto's disease, rheumatoid arthritis, ulcerative colitis, regional ileitis, systemic lupus erythematosus, psoriasis, myasthenia gravis, and pernicious anemia.

Cancer

There is now a large literature on the relationship between psychosocial factors and cancer. It has been reported that stressful life experiences, particularly experiences of separation and loss, frequently precede the clinical onset of various neoplasms, including cancer of the cervix, leukemia, and lymphoma.

In contrast, several studies have found no association between life experience and the onset of breast cancer. In one of these studies, however, there was a relationship between life events and benign breast disease. A similar observation was reported in an investigation of benign prostatic hypertrophy, in which a relatively high rate of life change was found to precede the onset of benign prostatic hypertrophy, in contrast with a lower rate of life change before the onset of bladder cancer.

Numerous studies have attempted to relate personality traits and susceptibility to cancer. Patients with lung cancer have been reported to be less able to discharge emotions than are patients without cancer. A 30-year prospective study of medical students who developed cancer showed that they tended not to express their emotions readily. Other studies reported that cancer patients used excessively the defenses of denial and repression.

The growing information on the immunological aspects of cancer raises the possibility that psychosocial influences are important to the mediation of immunological mechanisms in the susceptibility and course of neoplastic disease.

Immunity and Psychiatric Disorders

Although a number of investigators have found evidence suggesting altered immunity and autoimmunity in patients with schizophrenia, the specific findings have been difficult to replicate. Whether the immune abnormalities are involved in the pathogenesis of some or all types of schizophrenia or whether such abnormalities are related to a wide range of factors, including chronic institutionalization and neuroleptic agents, remains to be determined.

Immune phenomena in psychiatric disorders other than schizophrenia have been less extensively studied. Work indicates that psychiatric patients manifest increased IgM and IgA levels. These findings indicate the need for further study. The notion that patients with depression have an increased incidence of autoimmune antibodies has sparked some controversy. In some studies, the frequency of antinuclear antibodies, commonly found in patients with autoimmune disorders, such as systemic lupus erythematosus, has been reported as increased in patients with depression.

SKIN DISORDERS

Definition

Psychosomatic skin disorders include a great variety of abnormal skin sensations. Emotional factors are important as regards skin manifestation aggravation, and responses of skin disease.

Generalized Pruritus

It has been shown that itch, tickle, and pain are all conveyed by the same afferent fibers and are differentiated only by the frequency of electrical impulse.

The itching dermatoses include scabies, pediculosis, bites of insects, urticaria, atopic dermatitis, contact dermatitis, lichen rubor planus, and miliaria. Internal disorders that frequently cause itching are diabetes mellitus, nephritis, diseases of the liver, gout, diseases of the thyroid gland, food allergies, Hodgkin's disease, leukemia, and cancer. Itching can also occur during pregnancy and senility.

The term "generalized psychogenic pruritus" denotes that no organic cause for the itching exists or, at least, no longer exists, and that on psychiatric examination, emotional conflicts have been established that convincingly account for its occurrence.

The emotions that most frequently lead to generalized psychogenic pruritus are repressed anger and repressed anxiety. Whenever persons consciously or preconsciously experience anger or anxiety, they scratch themselves, often violently. An inordinate need for affection is a common characteristic of these patients. Frustrations of this need elicit aggressiveness that is inhibited. The rubbing of the skin provides a substitute gratification of the frustrated need, and the scratching represents aggression turned against the self.

Localized Pruritus

Pruritus Ani. The investigation of this disorder commonly yields a history of local irritation (e.g., thread worms, irritant discharge, fungal infection) or general systemic factors (e.g., nutritional deficiencies, drug intoxication). However, after running a conventional course, pruritus ani often fails to respond to therapeutic measures and acquires a life of its own, apparently perpetuated by scratching and superimposed inflammation. It is a distressing complaint that often interferes with work and social activity. Careful investigation of large numbers of these patients has revealed that personality deviations often precede this condition, and that emotional disturbances often precipitate and maintain it.

Pruritus Vulvae. As in pruritus ani, specific physical causes, either localized or generalized, may be demonstrable in pruritus vulvae, and the presence of glaring psychopathology in no way lessens the need for adequate medical investigation. In some patients, pleasure derived from rubbing and scratching is quite conscious—they realize that it is a symbolic form of masturbation—but more often than not the pleasure element is repressed. Most of the patients studied gave a long history of sexual frustration, which was frequently intensified at the time of the onset of pruritus.

Hyperhidrosis

States of fear, rage, and tension can induce an increase of sweat secretion. It has been demonstrated that perspiration in the human has two distinct forms: thermal and emotional. Emotional sweating appears primarily on the palms, soles, and axillae; thermal sweating is most evident on the forehead, neck, trunk, and dorsum of hand and forearm. The sensitivity of the emotional sweating response serves as the basis for the measurement of sweat by the galvanic skin response (an important tool of psychosomatic research), biofeedback, and the polygraph (lie detector test).

Under conditions of prolonged emotional stress, excessive sweating (hyperhidrosis) may lead to secondary skin changes, rashes, blisters, and infections; therefore, it may underlie a number of other dermatological conditions that are not primarily related to emotions. Basically, hyperhidrosis may be viewed as an anxiety phenomenon mediated by the autonomic nervous system; it must be differentiated from drug-induced states of hyperhidrosis.

CONSULTATION–LIAISON PSYCHIATRY

Definition

In consultation–liaison (C–L) psychiatry, the psychiatrist serves as a consultant to a medical colleague (either another psychiatrist or, more commonly, a nonpsychiatric physician) or another mental health professional (psychologist, social worker, or psychiatric nurse). In addition, the C–L psychiatrist consults in regard to patients in medical or surgical settings and provides follow-up psychiatric treatment as needed. In general, C–L psychiatry is associated with all of the diagnostic, therapeutic, research, and teaching services that the psychiatrist performs in the general hospital and serves as a bridge between psychiatry and other specialties.

Diagnosis

Knowledge of psychiatric diagnosis is essential to the liaison psychiatrist. Both dementia and delirium frequently complicate organic medical illness, especially among hospital patients. Psychoses and neuroses often complicate the treatment of medical illness. And deviant illness behavior, such as suicide, is a common problem in organically ill patients. The C–L psychiatrist must be aware of the many medical illnesses that can present with psychiatric symptoms. (A list of such medical problems is presented in Table 3.) The tools that the consulting psychiatrist has for diagnosis are the interview and serial clinical observations. The purposes of the diagnosis are to identify psychiatric disorders and psychological responses to the physical illness, to identify the patient's personality features, and to identify the patient's characteristic coping techniques in order to recommend the therapeutic intervention that is most appropriate to the patient's needs.

Patient Management

The liaison psychiatrist's principal contribution to medical management is a comprehensive analysis of the patient's response to illness, psychological and social resources, coping style, and psychiatric illness, if any.

This assessment is the basis of the plan for patient

Table 3
Medical Problems That Present with Psychiatric Symptoms

Disease	Sex and Age Prevalence	Common Medical Symptoms	Psychiatric Symptoms and Complaints	Impaired Performance and Behavior	Diagnostic Problems
Acquired Immune deficiency syndrome (AIDS)	Males>Females; IV drug abusers, homosexuals, female sex partners of bisexual men	Lymphademopathy, fatigue, opportunistic infections, Kaposi's sarcoma	Depression, anxiety, disorientation	Dementia with global impairment	Seropositive HIV virus is diagnostic when clinical signs are present
Hyperthyroidism (thyrotoxicosis)	Females 3 : 1, 20 to 50	Tremor, sweating, loss of weight and strength, heat intolerance	Anxiety, depression	Occasional hyperactive or grandiose behavior	Long lead time; rapid onset resembles anxiety attack
Hypothyroidism (myxedema)	Females 5 : 1, 30 to 60	Puffy face, dry skin, cold intolerance	Lethargy anxiety with irritability, thought disorder, somatic delusions, hallucinations	Myxedema madness, delusional, paranoid, belligerent behavior	Madness may mimic schizophrenia; mental status is clear, even during most disturbed behavior
Hyperparathyroidism	Females 3 : 1, 40 to 60	Weakness, anorexia, fractures, calculi, peptic ulcers			Anorexia and fatigue of slow-growing adenoma resemble involutional depression
Hypoparathyroidism	Females, 40 to 60	Hyperreflexia, spasms, tetany	Either state may cause anxiety, hyperactivity, and irritability or depression, apathy, and withdrawal	Either state may proceed to a toxic psychosis: confusion, disorientation, and clouded sensorium	None; rare condition except after surgery
Hyperadrenalism (Cushing's disease)	Adults, both sexes	Weight gain, fat alteration, easy fatigability	Varied; depression, anxiety, thought disorder with somatic delusions	Rarely produces aberrant behavior	Bizarre somatic delusions caused by bodily changes resemble schizophrenia
Adrenal cortical insufficiency (Addison's disease)	Adults, both sexes	Weight loss, hypotension, skin pigmentation	Depression— negativism, apathy; thought disorder— suspiciousness	Toxic psychosis with confusion and agitation	Long lead time; weight loss, apathy, despondency resemble involutional depression

Table 3 *continued*
Medical Problems That Present with Psychiatric Symptoms

Disease	Sex and Age Prevalence	Common Medical Symptoms	Psychiatric Symptoms and Complaints	Impaired Performance and Behavior	Diagnostic Problems
Porphyria—acute intermittent type	Females, 20 to 40	Abdominal crises, paresthesias, weakness	Anxiety—sudden onset, severe; mood swings	Extremes of excitement or withdrawal; emotional or angry outbursts	Patients often have truly neurotic lifestyles; crises resemble conversion reactions or anxiety attacks
Pernicious anemia (Addisonian anemia)	Females, 40 to 60	Weight loss, weakness, glossitis, extremity neuritis	Depression—feelings of guilt and worthlessness	Eventual brain damage with confusion and memory loss	Long lead time, sometimes many months; easily mistaken for involutional depression; normal early blood studies may give false reassurance
Hepatolenticular degeneration (Wilson's disease)	Males 2:1, adolescence	Liver and extrapyramidal symptoms	Mood swings—sudden and changeable; anger—explosive	Eventual brain damage with memory and I.Q. loss; combativeness	In late teens, may resemble adolescent storm, incorrigibility, or schizophrenia
Hypoglycemia (islet cell adenoma)	Adults, both sexes	Tremor, sweating, hunger, fatigue, dizziness	Anxiety—fear and dread, depression with fatigue	Agitation, confusion; eventual brain damage	Can mimic anxiety attack or acute alcoholism; bizarre behavior may draw attention away from somatic symptoms
Intracranial tumors	Adults, both sexes	None early; headache, vomiting, papilledema later	Varied; depression, anxiety, personality changes	Loss of memory, judgment, self-criticism; clouding of consciousness	Tumor location may not determine early symptoms
Pancreatic carcinoma	Males 3:1, 50 to 70	Weight loss, abdominal pain, weakness, jaundice	Depression, sense of imminent doom but without severe guilt	Loss of drive and motivation	Long lead time; exact age and symptoms of involutional depression
Pheochromocytoma	Adults, both sexes	Headache, sweating during elevated blood pressure	Anxiety, panic, fear, apprehension, trembling	Inability to function during an attack	Classic symptoms of anxiety attack, intermittently normal blood pressures may discourage further studies
Multiple sclerosis	Females, 20 to 40	Motor and sensory losses, scanning speech, nystagmus	Varied; personality changes, mood swings, depression; bland euphoria uncommon	Inappropriate behavior due to personality changes	Long lead time; early neurological symptoms mimic hysteria or conversion disorders
Systemic lupus erythematosus	Females 8:1, 20 to 40	Multiple symptoms of cardiovascular, genitourinary, gastrointestinal, other systems	Varied; thought disorder, depression, confusion	Toxic psychosis unrelated to steroid treatment	Long lead time, perhaps many years; psychiatric picture variable over time; thought disorder resembles schizophrenia, steroid psychosis

Adapted from table prepared by Maurice J. Martin, M.D.

management. In discussing that plan, the consultation–liaison psychiatrist makes known his or her assessment of the patient to nonpsychiatric health professionals. The psychiatrist's recommendations should be clear, concrete guidelines for action. The consultation–liaison psychiatrist may recommend a specific therapy, may suggest areas for further medical inquiry, may inform doctors and nurses of their role in the patient's psychosocial care, may recommend a transfer to a psychiatric facility for long-term psychiatric treatment, or may suggest or undertake brief psychotherapy on the medical ward.

The range of problems with which the C–L psychiatrist must deal is very broad. Studies show that up to 65 percent of medical inpatients have psychiatric disorders, the most common symptoms being anxiety, depression, and disorientation. Management problems account for 50 percent of the consultation requests made of psychiatrists. (Table 4 covers the most common C–L problems with which the psychiatrist must deal.)

Special Settings

Intensive Care Units (ICUs). The central psychological aspect of ICUs is that their patients are suffering life-threatening illnesses to which the psychological responses are predictable and which, if untreated, could threaten life or recovery. Coronary and medical ICU staffs see reactions to acute unexpected illnesses. At first there is fear and anxiety, followed by the psychological behaviors associated with denial, such as acting out, signing out, hostility, and excessive dependency. Staff working in burn units encounter patients going through the problems of acute unexpected illness and, later, depression, grief, and disassociation related to pain and disfigurement. Staff in surgical ICUs see patients recovering from major surgery with the expected disorientation of delirium, depression, and adjustment reactions to surgery.

Treatment of the psychological problems in the ICU requires close attention to diagnostic possibilities and de-

Table 4
Common Consultation-Liaison Problems

Reason for Consultation	Comments
Suicide attempt or threat	High-risk factors are males over 45, no social support, alcoholism, previous attempt, incapacitating medical illness with pain, and suicidal ideation. If risk is present, transfer to psychiatric unit or start 24-hour nursing care.
Depression	Suicidal risks must be assessed in every depressed patient (see above); presence of cognitive defects in depression may cause diagnostic dilemma with dementia (pseudodementia); check for history of substance abuse or depressant drugs (e.g., reserpine, propranolol); use antidepressants cautiously in cardiac patients because of conduction side effects, orthostatic hypotension.
Agitation	Often related to organic mental disorder, withdrawal from drugs, (e.g., opioids, alcohol, sedative-hypnotics); haloperidol most useful drug for excessive agitation; use physical restraints with great caution; examine for command hallucinations or paranoid ideation to which patient is responding in agitated manner; rule out toxic reaction to medication (e.g., cortisol paranoia, anticholinergic delirium).
Hallucinations	Most common cause in hospital is delirium tremens; onset 3 to 4 days after hospitalization. In intensive care units, check for sensory isolation; rule out brief reactive psychosis, schizophrenia, organic brain disorder. Treat with antipsychotic medication.
Sleep disorder	Common cause is pain; early morning awakening associated with depression; difficulty falling asleep associated with anxiety. Use antianxiety or antidepressant agent depending on cause. These drugs have no analgesic effect, so prescribe adequate painkillers. Rule out early drug withdrawal reaction.
No organic basis for symptoms	Rule out conversion disorder, somatization disorder, factitious disorder or malingering; glove and stocking anesthesia with autonomic nervous system symptoms seen in conversion; multiple body complaints seen in somatization; wish to be hospitalized seen in factitious disorder; obvious secondary gain in malingering (e.g., compensation case).
Disorientation	Delirium versus dementia; review metabolic status, neurologic findings, drug history. Prescribe small dose of antipsychotics for major agitation; benzodiazepines may worsen condition and cause sundowner syndrome (ataxia, confusion); modify environment so patient does not experience sensory deprivation.
Noncompliance or refusal to consent to procedure	Explore relationship of patient and treating doctor; negative transference is most common cause of noncompliance; fears of medication or procedure require education and reassurance. Refusal to give consent is issue of judgment; if impaired, patient can be declared incompetent, but only by judge; organic mental disorder is main cause of impaired judgment in hospitalized patients.

tails of the environment, as well as careful team communication. Clinicians clearly are helped by familiarity with the patient's premorbid character, because the reactions to disease and illness are influenced by prior conditioning. The most common initial reactions to acute medical disasters include shock, fear, and anxiety. These reactions in many patients will respond to the manner of the care team coupled with succinct, authoritative, and consistent reassurance. When these are insufficient, benzodiazepines—preferably the shorter-acting forms—should be considered and used cautiously. When fear leads to panic or psychotic loss of control, fast-acting major tranquilizers (e.g., haloperidol) should be used.

Denial and associated behaviors of acting out, hostility, dependency, and demanding behavior must be dealt with individually, based on knowledge of the patient and the reasons for these reactions. Several general points are pertinent. Direct communication with the patient, which allows but does not force a discussion of feelings, often eliminates disruptive behaviors without dealing with them directly. Allowing patients as much mastery as they want and can handle is more reassuring than anything else is. Permitting a person to make small choices restores some sense of control over the self and the future and calms patients far beyond the meaning of the specific choices. They feel a symbolic sense of progress. For example, allowing patients to control pain medications, the lighting level, or where they sit reassures and relaxes them. Whether the disruptive behavior is hostility, dependency, or panic, allowing some to be shown while setting limits on their extremes reassures patients. Thus, the independent patient can be allowed to move around, but not too far; the dependent patient can be allowed a limited number of interactions, such as use of the call button; and the hostile patient can be permitted some disagreement and ventilation but be limited in disruptive acts.

All ICUs deal mainly with anxiety, depression, and delirium. ICUs also impose extraordinarily high stress, both on the staff and on the patients, related to the intensity of the problems. Patients and staff alike frequently observe cardiac arrests, deaths, and medical disasters, which leave all autonomically aroused and psychologically defensive. ICU nurses and their patients experience particularly high levels of anxiety, depression, turnover, and burnout.

Attention is often given, especially in the nursing literature, to the problem of stress in the ICU staff. Much less attention is given to the house staff, especially on the surgical services. All persons in ICUs need to be able to deal directly with their feelings about the extraordinary experiences they are having and the difficult emotional and physical circumstances they are experiencing. Regular support groups in which these persons are able to discuss how they are feeling are important to the ICU staff and the house staff. Such groups are needed to protect the staff from the otherwise predictable psychiatric morbidity that some will experience and also to protect their patients from the loss of concentration, decreased energy, and psychomotor-retarded communications that some staff will otherwise come to exhibit.

Hemodialysis Units. Hemodialysis units represent a paradigm of complex modern medical treatment settings.

Patients are coping with lifelong, debilitating, and limiting disease; they are totally dependent on a multiplex group of care providers for access to a machine controlling their well-being. Dialysis is scheduled 3 times per week and takes 4 to 6 hours, thereby disrupting their previous living routine.

In this context, such patients' major struggle is with the disease. Invariably, however, they also have to come to terms with a level of dependency on others, a dependency they probably have not experienced since childhood. Predictably, patients entering dialysis struggle for their independence; regress to childhood states; show denial by acting out against doctor's orders or by breaking their diet or missing sessions; show anger directed against staff; bargain and plead or become infantilized and obsequious; but most often are accepting and courageous. The determinants of the patients' responses to entering dialysis include personality styles and their prior experience with this or another chronic illness. Patients who have had time to react and adapt to their chronic renal failure face less new psychological work of adaptation than do those to whom renal failure and machine dependency are new. Although little has been written about social factors, the effect of cultural factors in reaction to dialysis and the management of the dialysis unit are important. Units that are run with a firm hand, are consistent in dealing with patients, have clear contingencies for behavioral failures, and have adequate psychological support for staff tend to do the best. Complications of dialysis treatment can include psychiatric problems, such as depression, and suicide is not rare. Sexual problems can be neurogenic, psychogenic, or related to gonadal dysfunction and testicular atrophy.

Dialysis dementia is a rare condition that consists of loss of memory, disorientation, dystonias, and seizures. It occurs in patients that have been on dialysis for many years. The cause is unknown.

The psychological treatment of dialysis patients falls into two areas. First, careful preparation before dialysis, including the work of adaptation to chronic illness, is important, especially in dealing with denial and unrealistic expectations. All predialysis patients should have a psychosocial evaluation. Second, once in dialysis, periodic specific inquiry about adaptation, which does not encourage dependence or the sick role, may be helpful. The staff should be sensitive to the likelihood of depression and sexual problems. Group sessions function well for support, and patient self-help groups serve to restore a useful social network, self-esteem, and self-mastery. When needed, tricyclic antidepressants or phenothiazines can be used for dialysis patients. Psychiatric care is best if brief and problem oriented.

The use of home dialysis units has been of great help. The patients are better able to integrate the treatment into their daily lives and feel more autonomous and less dependent on others for their care.

Surgical Patients. Some surgeons believe that patients who expect to die during surgery will do so. This belief now seems less superstitious than it did earlier. Kimball and others have studied the premorbid psychological adjustment of patients headed for surgery and have shown that those who show evident depression or anxiety, despite denying it, have a higher risk for morbidity and mortality than do those who, given similar depression or anxiety, are able to express it. Even better is to have a positive attitude toward impending surgery. The factors that contribute to an improved outcome for surgery are informed consent, the education of patients so that they know what to expect concerning what they will feel, where they will be (e.g., it is useful to show patients the recovery room), what loss of function to expect, what tubes and gadgets will be in place, and how to cope with the anticipated pain. In cases in which the patients will not be able to talk or see, it is extremely helpful to explain before the surgery what they can do to compensate for these losses. If postoperative states such as confusion, delirium, or pain can be predicted, they should be discussed with the patients in advance to avoid their experiencing them as unwarranted or as a sign of danger. The presence of constructive family support members is helpful both before and after the surgery. Table 5 lists various surgical conditions with which the C–L psychiatrist must deal.

Psychotherapy of Patients with Medical Illness

The type of therapy selected depends on the patients' short-term and long-term needs, their illness, their coping responses, and the intervention's setting. However, usually the liaison psychiatrist provides therapy on a time-limited basis, using crisis intervention modalities. Patients requiring long-term therapy are referred to other psychotherapists. The techniques most commonly used by liaison psychiatrists are of the brief short-term dynamic type. The techniques are largely supportive, focusing on identifying appropriate strategies for resolving reality-based problems and mobilizing social support. In the majority of cases that the liaison psychiatrist sees, no psychotherapy is undertaken, and the patient is counseled by other members of the health care team, who follow the psychiatrist's management recommendations. Some patients may benefit from a behavioral therapy technique or from hypnosis.

Patients with chronic medical disorders can benefit from long-term psychoanalytically oriented psychotherapy in a

Table 5
Transplantation and Surgical Problems

Organ	Biological Factor	Psychological Factor
Kidney	50 to 90% success rate. May not be done if patient over age 55. Increasing use of cadaver kidneys rather than those from living donors.	Living donors must be emotionally stable; parents are best donors, siblings may be ambivalent; donors are subject to depression. Patients who panic before surgery may have poor prognosis; altered body image with fear of organ rejection is common. Group therapy for patients is helpful.
Bone Marrow	Used in aplastic anemias and immune system disease.	Patients are usually very ill and must deal with death and dying; compliance important. Commonly done in children who present problems of prolonged dependency; siblings are often donors who may be angry or ambivalent about procedure.
Heart	End-stage coronary artery disease and cardiomyopathy.	Donor is legally dead; relatives of deceased may refuse permission or be ambivalent. No fall-back position if organ rejected; kidney rejection can go on hemodialysis. Some patients seek transplant hoping to die. Postcardiotomy delirium in 25 percent of patients.
Breast	Radical mastectomy versus lumpectomy.	Reconstruction of breast at time of surgery leads to better postoperative adaptation; veteran patients used to counsel new patients; lumpectomy patients more open about surgery and sex than are mastectomy patients; group support helpful.
Uterus	Hysterectomy performed on 10% of women over 20.	Fear of loss of sexual attractiveness with sexual dysfunction may occur in small percentage of women; loss of childbearing capacity upsetting.
Brain	Anatomic location of lesion determines behavioral change.	Environmental dependency syndrome in frontal lobe tumors characterized by inability to show initiative; memory disturbances involved in periventricular surgery; hallucinations in parieto-occipital area.
Prostate	Cancer surgery has more negative psychobiological effects and is more technically difficult than is surgery for benign hypertrophy.	Sexual dysfunction common except in transurethral prostatectomy (TUP). Perineal prostatectomy produces absence of emission, ejaculation, and erection; penile implant may be of use.
Colon and Rectum	Colostomy and ostomy is common outcome, especially for cancer.	One-third of patients with colostomy feel worse about themselves than before bowel surgery; shame and self-consciousness about stoma can be alleviated by self-help groups that deal with those issues.
Limbs	Amputation performed for massive injury, diabetes, or cancer.	Phantom limb phenomenon occurs in 98% of cases; experience may last for years; sometimes sensation may be painful, and neuroma at stump should be ruled out; no known cause or treatment, may stop spontaneously.

variety of ways: It provides an ongoing relationship with a trusted physician with whom the patient can discuss emotional reactions to the effects of the illness. Defense mechanisms that may develop in response to chronic illness can be examined. For example, denial is a useful defense, but if excessive, the patient may forget appointments for follow-up visits or may not take the prescribed medication. Studies have shown that patients who have chronic pain associated with physical illness benefit from psychotherapy and behavior therapy, by requiring less analgesic medication, being more mobile, and making greater attempts to maintain their premorbid life-style than do those chronic medical patients who do not receive therapy.

References

Ader R, editor: *Psychoneuroimmunology*. Academic Press, New York, 1981.

Alexander F: *Psychosomatic Medicine*. W W Norton, New York, 1950.

Bauer M, Droba M, Whybrow P C: Disorders of thyroid and parathyroid. In *Handbook of Clinical Psychoneuroendocrinology*, C B Nemeroff, P T Loosen, editors. Guillard Press, New York, 1987.

Blackwell B, Galbraith J R, Dahl D S: Chronic pain management. Hosp Community Psychiatry *35*:999, 1984.

Cecil Textbook of Medicine, ed 17, J B Wyngaarden, L H Smith Jr. editors, W B Saunders, Philadelphia, 1985.

Green R L, McAllister T W, Bernal J L: A study of crying in medically and surgically hospitalized patients. Am J Psychiatry *144*:442, 1987.

Hackett T P, Rosenbaum J F: Emotion, psychiatric disorders, and the heart. In *A Textbook of Cardiovascular Medicine*, E Braunwald, editor, p 1826. W B Saunders, Philadelphia, 1984.

Linder A E: *Emotional Factors in Gastrointestinal Illness*. Excerpta Medica, Amsterdam, 1973.

Lipowski Z J: Consultation–liaison psychiatry: The first half century. Gen Hosp Psychiatry *8*:305, 1986.

Lipowski Z J: *Psychosomatic Medicine and Liaison Psychiatry: Selected Papers*. Plenum, New York, 1985.

Maciewicz R, Martin J B: Pain: Pathophysiology and management. In *Harrison's Principles of Internal Medicine*, ed 11, E Braunnold, K J Isselbacher, R G Petersdorf, J D Wilson, J B Martin, A S Fauci, editors, McGraw–Hill, New York, 1987.

Popkin M K, Callies A L: Psychiatric consultation to inpatients with "early-onset" type I diabetes mellitus in a university hospital. Arch Gen Psych *44*:169, 1987.

Wallen J, Pincus H A, Goldman H H, Marcus S E: Psychiatric consultations in short-term general hospitals. Arch Gen Psych *44*:163, 1987.

Weiner H: *The Psychobiology of Human Disease* Elsevier/North Holland, New York, 1977.

27 Personality Disorders

INTRODUCTION

Patients with personality disorders are commonly encountered in psychiatric practice, and they are among the most difficult to treat. According to DSM-III-R, such patients show deeply ingrained, inflexible, and maladaptive patterns of relating to and perceiving both the environment and themselves.

Personality disorders are recognizable by adolescence or earlier and continue throughout most of adult life. Those with personality disorders uniformly have trouble working and loving. If clinicians are able to penetrate the protective armor of the personality disorder, they often will find anxiety and depression. Patients with these disorders consistently fail to see themselves as others see them, and they lack empathy with other people. As a result, their behavior consistently annoys others. Thus, characteristic of personality disorders is the tendency to create a vicious circle in which already precarious interpersonal relationships are made worse by the person's mode of adaptation. In general, it is not easy to understand people with personality disorders. In contrast, neurotics are aware of their problems. In technical terminology, neurotics' symptoms are autoplastic (i.e., the process of adapting by changing the self), and their symptoms are experienced as ego-dystonic (i.e., unacceptable to the self). However, people with a personality disorder are far more likely to refuse psychiatric help and to deny their problems. Their symptoms are alloplastic (i.e., the process of adapting and altering the external environment) and ego-syntonic (i.e., acceptable to the ego); they do not feel anxiety about their maladaptive behavior.

Because persons with a personality disorder do not routinely acknowledge pain from what society perceives as their symptoms, they are often regarded as unmotivated for treatment and impervious to recovery. Such traits are unlikely to engage mental health professionals, many of whom do not like to work with such patients.

CLASSIFICATION

DSM-III-R groups the personality disorders into three clusters. The first cluster (A) includes the paranoid, schizoid, and schizotypal personality disorders. Persons with these disorders often appear odd and eccentric. The second cluster (B) includes the histrionic, narcissistic, antisocial, and borderline personality disorders. Persons with these disorders often appear dramatic, emotional, and erratic. The second cluster, with the possible exception of the borderline, captures Carl Jung's concept of extroversion. The third cluster (C) includes the avoidant, dependent, obsessive-compulsive, and passive-aggressive personality disorders. Persons with these disorders often appear anxious or fearful. The third cluster captures Jung's dimension of introversion.

According to DSM-III-R, many people exhibit traits that are not limited to a single personality disorder, and if a patient meets the criteria for more than one disorder, each one should be diagnosed. Personality disorders are coded on Axis II of DSM-III-R.

ETIOLOGY

Genetic Factors

The best evidence that genetic factors contribute to the genesis of personality disorders comes from the investigations of psychiatric disorders in 15,000 pairs of American twins. Among monozygotic twins, the concordance for personality disorders was several times higher than that among dizygotic twins.

Cluster A illnesses (paranoid, schizoid, and schizotypal) are more common in the biological relatives of schizophrenics. Significantly more relatives with schizotypal personality disorder are found in the family histories of persons with schizophrenia than among control groups. There is less correlation between paranoid and schizoid personality disorders and schizophrenia.

Cluster B illnesses (histrionic, narcissistic, antisocial, and borderline) demonstrate a genetic predisposition for antisocial personality disorder, which is also associated with alcoholism. Depression is more common in the family background of borderline patients. There is also a strong association between histrionic personality disorder and somatization disorder (Briquet's syndrome), in that patients with each disorder show an overlap of symptoms.

Borderline patients have more relatives with mood disorders than do control groups, and borderline personality disorder and mood disorder often coexist.

Cluster C disorders (obsessive-compulsive, passive-aggressive, dependent and avoidant) may also have a genetic base. Obsessive-compulsive traits are more common in monozygotic than in dizygotic twins, and obsessive-compulsive personalities show some signs associated with depression (e.g., shortened REM latency period, abnormal dexamethasone suppression test). The avoidant personality is often associated with a high anxiety level.

Temperamental Factors

Temperamental factors have been identified in childhood that may be associated with personality disorders in adulthood. For example, children who are temperamentally fearful may develop avoidant personalities.

Central nervous dysfunction in childhood associated with soft neurological signs is more common in antisocial and borderline personalities. Children with minimal brain damage are at risk for developing personality disorders, particularly the antisocial types.

Biochemical Studies

Hormones. Persons who show impulsive traits often also show increased levels of testosterone, 17-estradiol, and estrone. In nonhuman primates, androgens increase the likelihood of aggression and sexual behavior; however, the role of testosterone in human aggression is not clear. The dexamethasone suppression test (DST) is abnormal in some borderline patients with depressive symptoms.

Platelet Monoamine Oxidase. Low platelet MAO has been associated with activity and sociability in monkeys. Low platelet MAO college students report spending more time in social activities than do high platelet MAO students.

Smooth Pursuit Eye Movements (SPEM). Smooth pursuit eye movements are abnormal in persons with the traits of introversion, low self-esteem, and withdrawal and in schizotypal personality disorder. Movements are saccadic (i.e., jerky). These findings have no clinical application, but they do indicate the role of inheritance.

Neurotransmitters. Endorphins have an effect similar to that of exogenous morphine, including analgesia and suppression of arousal. High endogenous endorphins might be associated with a phlegmatic passive individual. Studies of personality traits and the dopaminergic and serotonergic systems indicate an arousal-activating function for these neurotransmitters. Levels of 5-hydroxyindoleacetic acid (5-HIAA), a metabolite of serotonin, is low in persons who attempt suicide and in patients who are impulsive and aggressive.

Psychoanalytic Theory

Freud believed that personality traits resulted from a fixation at one of the psychosocial stages of development and from the interplay between impulses and persons in the environment (known as object choices). He used the term "character" to describe the organization of the personality and identified several character types: (1) oral characters who are passive and dependent and who take in food or other substances excessively; (2) anal characters who are precise, parsimonious, punctual (the three "Ps" of the anal triad), and stubborn; (3) obsessional characters who are rigid and dominated by a harsh superego; and (4) narcissistic characters who are aggressive and self-serving.

Wilhelm Reich used the term "character armor" to describe defensive mechanisms that protect people from internal impulses and that must be analyzed if psychotherapy is to be successful. Carl Jung used the term "introvert" to describe solitary introspective types and "extrovert" to describe outgoing sensation-seeking types. Erik Erikson believed that the inability to establish basic trust led to para-

noid disorders and the failure to become autonomous led to dependent characters.

In its effort to avoid inference and to remain based on objective data, DSM-III-R ignores the psychodynamic domain of the classification of personality disorders. Reliable diagnosis depends on what the psychiatrist can observe with certainty; however, the successful management of patients who insist that nothing is the matter must be based on what the clinician can infer. Therapeutically, the psychiatrist cannot afford to miss the covert dependence concealed behind the insistent independence of the paranoid character, nor can the psychiatrist afford to ignore the unexpressed fearfulness that manifests itself as bland affect in the schizoid character.

Defense Mechanisms. To help patients with personality disorders, the psychiatrist needs to appreciate their underlying defenses. Defenses are unconscious mental processes that the ego uses to resolve conflicts among the four lodestars of the inner life—instinct (wish or need), reality, important people, and conscience. When defenses are most effective, especially in personality disorders, they can abolish anxiety and depression. Thus, a major reason that patients with personality disorders are so reluctant to alter their behavior is that to abandon a defense is to increase conscious anxiety and depression.

In addition, defenses are dynamic and reversible. Although defenses are labeled pathological, just as pus and fever are so labeled, defenses serve health, just as pus and fever do.

Although patients with personality disorders may be characterized by their most dominant or most rigid mechanism, each patient uses several defenses. Thus, the management of the defense mechanisms used by patients with personality disorders is discussed here as a general topic, rather than under the specific disorders. Many of the formulations presented here in the language of psychoanalytic psychiatry can be translated into principles consistent with cognitive and behavioral approaches.

The defenses of patients with personality disorders have been part of the warp and woof of their life histories and of their personality identities. However, maladaptive their defenses may be, they represent homeostatic solutions to inner problems. Neurotics may value insight and see interpretation of their defenses as helpful. In contrast, patients with personality disorders meet interpretation of their defenses with anger. Breaching their defenses evokes enormous anxiety and depression, and carelessly threatening such patients' defenses ruptures therapist-patient relationships. Thus, attempts to breach such defenses should be either mitigated by such strong social supports as AA or replaced by such alternative defenses as helping a Hell's Angel use reaction formation and become a motorcycle policeman.

Fantasy. Many persons, especially eccentric, lonely, frightened persons who are often labeled schizoid, make extensive use of the defense of fantasy. They seek solace and satisfaction within themselves by creating an imaginary life, especially imaginary friends, within their minds. Often, such persons seem strikingly aloof. One needs to understand the unsociability of such persons as resting on a fear of intimacy, rather than to criticize them or feel rebuffed by their rejection. The therapist should maintain a quiet, reassuring, and considerable interest in them without insisting on reciprocal response. Recognition of their fear of closeness and respect for their eccentric ways are useful.

Dissociation. The second defense, dissociation or neurotic denial, consists of a Pollyanna-like replacement of unpleasant affects with pleasant ones. Frequent users of dissociation are often seen as dramatizing and as emotionally shallow; they may be labeled histrionic personalities. Their behavior is reminiscent of the stunts of anxious adolescents who, to erase anxiety, carelessly expose themselves to exciting dangers. Accepting such patients as exuberant and seductive is to miss their anxiety; but confronting them with their vulnerabilities and defects is to make them still more defensive. Because they seek appreciation of their attractiveness and courage, the therapist should not be too reserved. At the same time, while remaining calm and firm, the therapist should realize that these patients are often inadvertent liars. Patients who use dissociation benefit from having a chance to ventilate their own anxieties; in the process they may "remember" what they "forgot." Often dissociation and denial are best dealt with by the therapist using displacement. Thus, the clinician may talk with patients about the same affective issue but in a context of a less threatening circumstance. Empathizing with the denied affect of such patients without directly confronting them with the facts may allow the patients to raise the original topic themselves.

Isolation. A third, very different defense is isolation. It is characteristic of the orderly, controlled person, often labeled a compulsive personality, who, unlike the histrionic personality, remembers the truth in fine detail but without affect. In a crisis, there may be an intensification of self-restraint, overformal social behavior, and obstinacy. The patient's quest for control may be annoying or boring to the clinician. Often, such patients respond well to precise, systematic, and rational explanations. They value efficiency, cleanliness, and punctuality as much as they do the clinician's affective responsiveness. Whenever possible, clinicians should allow such patients to control their own care, rather than engage in a battle of wills.

Projection. A fourth defense commonly met with in the personality disorders is projection, in which the patients attribute their own unacknowledged feelings to others. Excessive fault finding and sensitivity to criticism may seem to be prejudiced, hypervigilant injustice collecting, but should not be met by defensiveness and argument. Instead, even minor mistakes on the part of the examiner and the possibility of future difficulties should be frankly acknowledged. Strict honesty, concern for the patient's rights, and maintaining the same formal, concerned distance as with a patient using fantasy are helpful. Confrontation guarantees a lasting enemy and an early termination of the interview. The therapist, however, need not agree with the patient's injustice collecting, but should ask if they can agree to disagree.

The technique of counterprojection is especially helpful. In that technique the clinician acknowledges and gives paranoid patients full credit for their feelings and for their perceptions. Further, the clinician neither disputes the patient's complaints nor reinforces them, but acknowledges that the world the paranoid describes can be imagined. The interviewer can then talk about the real motives and feelings, even though they are misattributed to someone else, and begin to cement an alliance with the patient.

Hypochondriasis. A fifth mechanism commonly seen in patients with personality disorders—especially those with a borderline, dependent, or passive-aggressive diagnosis—is hypochondriasis. In contrast to the usual supposition, a patient does not make hypochondriacal complaints for simple secondary gain. A moment's reflection reveals that a hypochondriac's complaints can rarely be relieved. The initial response of clinicians to that state of affairs is guilt, followed by anger and rejection. In other words, hypochondriasis disguises reproach. Often the hypochondriac's complaint that others do not provide help conceals bereavement, loneliness, or unacceptable aggressive impulses. The first step is

self-reproach followed by unrelievable complaints of pain, somatic illness, and neurasthenia or by the repetition of insoluble life dilemmas. The mechanism of hypochondriasis permits covert punishment of others with the patient's own pain and discomfort. By concealing the real unmet wishes for dependency, the hypochondriacal complaints allow the patient to feel perpetually justified in an angry reproach of others.

Splitting. A sixth mechanism commonly seen in patients with personality disorders, especially in those with borderline personalities, is splitting. In splitting, instead of synthesizing and assimilating less-than-perfect past care-givers and instead of responding to important people in the current environment as they are, the patient divides ambivalently regarded people, both past and present, into good people and bad people. For example, in an inpatient setting some staff members are idealized, and others are uniformly disparaged. The effect of that defensive behavior on a hospital ward can be highly disruptive; it ultimately provokes the staff to turn against the patient. Splitting is best mastered if the staff members anticipate the process, discuss it at staff meetings, and gently confront the patient with the fact that no one is all good or all bad.

Passive aggression. A seventh mechanism, commonly seen in patients with borderline and passive-aggressive personality disorders, is turning anger against the self. In military psychiatry and DSM-III-R, such behavior is called passive-aggressive; in psychoanalytic terminology it is most often described as masochism. It includes failure, procrastinations, silly or provocative behavior, and self-demeaning clowning, as well as more frankly self-destructive behavior. The hostility in such behavior is never entirely concealed; indeed, the mechanism, as in the case of wrist cutting, engenders such anger in others that they feel themselves have been assaulted and view the patient as a sadist, not a masochist.

Passive aggression is best dealt with by trying to get the patients to ventilate their anger. It is seldom wise to respond to provocatively suicidal patients as though they were simply depressed or to isolate them in a seclusion room or state hospital for their angry gestures. The pleasure and the relief of anxiety that some patients obtain from repeatedly cutting themselves should be accepted as matter of factly as masturbatory behavior. Rather than treating such behavior as perverse, staff members should say gently, "I wonder if there's some other way you could make yourself feel better. Can you put what you are feeling into words?"

Sometimes long-suffering, self-sacrificing patients are able to cooperate in a medical regimen out of a readiness to add to the burden that they carry, rather than for the benefits that might accrue to themselves. Recovery may be usefully presented to the patient as a special additional task. In every interaction with self-defeating patients, it is important to avoid humiliating comments about foolish, inexplicable behavior. If stubborn passive-aggressive patients are reluctant to help themselves, it is sometimes useful to take time out. Leaving the room or postponing the next appointment breaks the pattern of struggle and underscores the point that passive-aggressive struggles result in less attention, rather than more attention. After a short time-out, the interviewer, too, is able to continue the relationship in a less angry and covertly sadistic manner.

Acting out. An eighth defense common to personality disorders is acting out. The mechanism represents the direct expression through action of an unconscious wish or conflict to avoid being conscious of either the idea or the affect that accompanies it. Tantrums, apparently motiveless assaults, child abuse, and pleasureless promiscuity are common examples. Because the behavior occurs outside of reflective awareness, acting out often appears to the observer to be unaccompanied by guilt. In responding to such behavior, the clinician should forcibly remember the maxim, "nothing human is alien to me." As in conversion hysteria, anxiety and pain exist behind *la belle indifférence,* but unlike conversion hysteria, acting out must be controlled as rapidly as possible. Prolonged acting out is frightening to patient and staff alike. Once acting out is not possible, the conflict behind the defense may be accessible. Faced with acting out, either aggressive or sexual, in an interview situation, the clinician must recognize (1) that the patient has lost control; (2) that anything the interviewer says will probably be misheard; and (3) that getting the patient's attention is of paramount importance. Depending on the circumstances, the clinician's response can be, "How can I help you if you keep screaming?" Or, if the interviewer feels that the patient's loss of control is escalating, "If you continue screaming, I'll leave." Or if the interviewer feels genuinely frightened of the patient, simply leaving and asking for help, including the police. Invariably, acting out begets fear in the observer, and nobody working with psychiatric patients should bear fear alone.

Other stereotyped behaviors. Narcissism, dependency, and no-win relationships are repetitive behaviors that also threaten the patient's quest for help. Unlike the eight mechanisms of defense cited above, these three behaviors offer little of homeostatic value.

NARCISSISM. When threatened, many patients with personality disorders see themselves as powerful and all important. To the observer, that behavior may be labeled vanity, grandiosity, entitlement, or narcissism. It may lead patients to be unusually critical of the therapist. Some patients suggest that the therapist pay for the privilege of caring for them. In response, the therapist may become defensive, contemptuous, or rejecting. Nobody likes being belittled. The mere fact that the therapist is telling patients that they are sick and potentially helpless is likely to increase such patients' superior responses. Clinical progress is facilitated if, instead of belittling patients or defending themselves, the clinicians acknowledge that patients are persons in their own right, offer them consultation with an expert if that seems appropriate, and matter of factly reassure them of the competence of the treatment team or approach.

DEPENDENCY. A second stereotyped behavior in personality disorders is dependency, however vehemently denied. Dependency is often manifested first by a sense of entitlement and then by resentment when unreasonable wants are not met. Pessimism, self-doubt, and immaturity are common, and they lead to a dependent, demanding relationship that the staff are likely to mock behind the patient's back. Usually, the resentment and the needy behavior of the dependent patient are analogous to that of a person who justly calls in a bad debt. The problem, however, lies in the fact that it is a bad debt, and thus repayment is impossible. When the patient reexperiences the old resentment outside of the original relationship in which the bad debt was incurred, the demanding behavior and entitlement seem highly inappropriate. Because personality disorders are frustrating to begin with, unreasonable wants are met by withdrawal on the part of the physician, and a vicious cycle is begun.

The contagion of an overly dependent patient may evoke dependency needs in the clinician, who must realize this. Obviously, to meet a patient's every wish for boundless interest and abundant care does not help a dependent patient, neither does it help if the clinician feels overwhelmed and withdraws in fear. In general, dependent patients are best managed by observing three rules.

First, for self-protection the clinician must set realistic limits. F example, one may say, "Today I can see you for only 15 minutes, but I'll be able to see you for 30 minutes tomorrow at 11:00." Second, the clinician should never present limits as if they were an expression of impatience and punitiveness. They should never seem to be a withdrawal of interest or consideration; nothing should be taken away from patients without something else being given. Third, at the same time the limits are set, care-givers should convey their readiness to care for the patient as completely as is reasonable. Rather than telling a demanding patient that barbiturates are not allowed for sleep because they are addicting, a care-giver should tell the patient that 50 mg of diphenhydramine is allowed, which is "better" than barbiturates because it is nonaddicting. The solution is not to remind dependent patients that they cannot have what they want, but to focus on trying to give them what they need.

NO-WIN RELATIONSHIPS. The third stereotyped behavior that creates therapeutic problems for patients with personality disorders may be summed up by the no-win learning paradigm. A no-win situation is one in which two people take positions that neither will modify. Without compromise or changes in behavior, both parties must lose what they otherwise could gain if they reached a fair agreement. If two confidence men ensnare each other in their respective resentments and entitlements, if both have larceny in their hearts, then both will be cheated. The person with a personality disorder frequently seeks out relationships that offer a promise of something for nothing. In choosing people from whom the patient feels entitled to take, there is the risk of recreating past cheats and defeating interactions. Consequently, those with personality disorders seem perennially entangled in troublesome relationships in which there is neither satisfaction nor escape.

Sociocultural Factors

Certain personality disorders may arise from poor parental fit, that is, a poor match between temperament and child-rearing practices. For example, an anxious child reared by an equally anxious mother is more vulnerable to a personality disorder than would be the same child raised by a tranquil mother. Stella Chess and Alexander Thomas referred to this as "goodness of fit." Cultures that encourage aggression may unwittingly reinforce and thereby contribute to paranoid or antisocial personality disorders. The physical environment may also play a role. For example, an active young child may appear hyperactive if kept in a small, closed apartment but may appear normal in a larger, middle-class house with a fenced-in yard.

INDIVIDUAL PERSONALITY DISORDERS

Paranoid Personality Disorder

Definition. Paranoid personalities are characterized by long-standing suspiciousness and mistrust of people in general. They refuse responsibility for their own feelings and assign responsibility to others. This category includes many of life's least lovable character types—the bigot, the injustice collector, the pathologically jealous spouse, and the litigious crank.

Epidemiology. The prevalence of this disorder is not known. Persons with paranoid personality disorder rarely seek treatment themselves; when referred to treatment by a spouse or an employer, they can often pull themselves together and not appear distressed. Relatives of schizophrenic patients show a higher incidence of paranoid personalities than do controls. The disorder is more common in men than in women, and it does not appear to have a familial pattern. There is no higher incidence among homosexuals, as was once thought, but it is believed to be more common among minority groups, immigrants, and the deaf.

Clinical Features. According to DSM-III-R, the essential feature of this disorder is a pervasive and unwarranted tendency—beginning by early adulthood and present in a variety of contexts—to interpret other people's actions as deliberately demeaning or threatening. Almost invariably they expect to be exploited or harmed by others in some way. Frequently persons with this disorder will question, without justification, the loyalty or trustworthiness of friends or associates. Often such persons are pathologically jealous, questioning without justification the fidelity of their spouse or sexual partner.

These patients externalize their own emotions and use the defense of projection in that they attribute to others impulses and thoughts that they are unable to accept in themselves. Ideas of reference and logically defended illusions are common.

Paranoid patients are affectively restricted and appear unemotional. They pride themselves on being rational and objective, but such is not the case. Such patients lack warmth and are impressed with and pay close attention to power and rank, expressing disdain for those who are seen as weak, sickly, impaired, or defective in some way. In social situations, persons with paranoid personality disorder may appear businesslike and efficient, but they often generate fear or conflict in others.

Diagnosis. On psychiatric examination, paranoid characters may appear quite formal and baffled at having been required to seek psychiatric help. Muscular tension, inability to relax, and a need to scan the environment for clues may be evident. Their affect is often humorless and serious. Although some of the premises of their arguments may be false, their speech is goal directed and logical. Their thought content shows evidence of projection, prejudice, and occasional ideas of reference. The DSM-III-R diagnostic criteria are listed in Table 1.

Course and Prognosis. There are no adequate and systematic long-term studies of the paranoid personality. In some, the paranoid personality disorder is lifelong. In others, it is a harbinger of schizophrenia. In still others, as they mature or as stress diminishes, paranoid traits give way to reaction formation, appropriate concern with morality, and altruistic concerns. In general, however, these patients have lifelong problems working and living with others. Occupational and marital problems are common.

Differential Diagnosis. Paranoid personality disorder can usually be differentiated from the delusional disorders because fixed delusions are absent in paranoid personality disorder. It can be differentiated from paranoid schizophrenia because hallucinations and formal thought disorder are absent in the personality disorders. Paranoid personality disorder can be distinguished from borderline personality disorder because the paranoid patient is rarely as capable as the borderline patient is of overinvolved, if tumultuous, relations with others. Paranoid patients lack the antisocial character's long history of antisocial behavior. Schizoid personalities are withdrawn and aloof and do not have paranoid ideation.

Treatment. Psychotherapy is the treatment of choice. Therapists should be straightforward in all their dealings with the

Table 1
Diagnostic Criteria for Paranoid Personality Disorder

A. A pervasive and unwarranted tendency, beginning by early adulthood and present in a variety of contexts, to interpret the actions of people as deliberately demeaning or threatening, as indicated by at least *four* of the following:
(1) expects, without sufficient basis, to be exploited or harmed by others
(2) questions, without justification, the loyalty or trustworthiness of friends or associates
(3) reads hidden demeaning or threatening meanings into benign remarks or events, e.g., suspects that a neighbor put out trash early to annoy him
(4) bears grudges or is unforgiving of insults or slights
(5) is reluctant to confide in others because of unwarranted fear that the information will be used against him or her
(6) is easily slighted and quick to react with anger or to counterattack
(7) questions, without justification, fidelity of spouse or sexual partner

B. Occurrence not exclusively during the course of Schizophrenia or a Delusional Disorder.

Table from DSM-III-R *Diagnostic and Statistical Manual of Mental Disorders,* ed 3, revised. (Current Classification of Mental Disorders, 1987.) Copyright American Psychiatric Association, Washington, D.C., 1987. Used with permission.

patient. If a therapist is accused of some inconsistency or fault, such as lateness for an appointment, honesty and an apology are better than a defensive explanation. Therapists must remember that trust and toleration of intimacy are troubled areas for these patients. Individual psychotherapy thus requires a professional and not overly warm style from the therapist. Paranoid patients do not do well in group psychotherapy, nor are they likely to tolerate the intrusiveness of the behavior therapies. Too zealous a use of interpretation—especially interpretation concerning deep feelings of dependency, sexual concerns, and wishes for intimacy—significantly increases the patient's mistrust.

At times, paranoid patients' behavior becomes so threatening that it is important to control it or set limits on it. Delusional accusations must be dealt with realistically but gently and without humiliating the patient. It is profoundly frightening for paranoid patients to feel that those trying to help them are weak and helpless; therefore, therapists should never threaten to take over control unless they are both willing and able to do so.

Pharmacotherapy is useful in dealing with agitation or anxiety. In most cases, an antianxiety agent such as diazepam is sufficient. But it may be necessary to use an antipsychotic such as thioridazine or haloperidol, in small doses and for brief periods of time, to manage severe agitation or quasidelusional thinking.

Schizoid Personality Disorder

Definition. Schizoid personality disorder is diagnosed in patients who display a lifelong pattern of social withdrawal. Their discomfort with human interaction, their introversion, and their bland, constricted affect are noteworthy. Schizoid personalities are often seen by others as eccentric, isolated, or lonely.

Epidemiology. The prevalence of schizoid personality is not clearly established. Schizoid disorders may affect 7.5 percent of the general population. The sex ratio of the disorder is unknown, although some studies report a two-to-one, male-to-female ratio. Persons with the disorder tend to gravitate toward solitary jobs that involve little or no contact with others. Many prefer night work to day work so that they do not have to deal with as many people.

Clinical Features. Schizoid personalities give an impression of being cold and aloof and display a remote reserve and a lack of involvement with everyday events and the concerns of others. They appear quiet, distant, seclusive, and unsociable. They may pursue their own lives with remarkably little need or longing for emotional ties with others. They are the last to catch on to changes in popular fashion.

The life histories of such persons reflect solitary interests and success at noncompetitive, lonely jobs that others find difficult to tolerate. Their sexual life may exist exclusively in fantasy, and they may postpone mature sexuality indefinitely. Men may not marry because they are unable to achieve intimacy; women may passively agree to marry an aggressive man who wishes to do so. Usually, schizoid persons reveal a lifelong inability to express anger directly. Schizoid personalities are able to invest enormous affective energy in nonhuman interests such as mathematics and astronomy, and they may be very attached to animals. They are often engrossed in dietary and health fads, philosophical movements, and social improvement schemes, especially those that require no personal involvement.

Although schizoid personalities appear self-absorbed and engaged in excessive daydreaming, they show no loss of capacity to recognize reality. Because aggressive acts are rarely included in their repertoire of usual responses, most threats, real or imagined, are dealt with by fantasied omnipotence or resignation. Others experience schizoid personalities as aloof; yet at times, such persons are able to conceive, develop, and give to the world genuinely original, creative ideas.

Diagnosis. On initial psychiatric examination, patients may appear ill at ease. They rarely tolerate eye contact. The interviewer may surmise that such patients are eager for the interview to end. Their affect may be constricted, aloof, or inappropriately serious. But underneath the aloofness, the sensitive clinician may recognize fear. These patients find it difficult to act lightheartedly: their efforts at humor may seem adolescent and off the mark. The patients' speech is goal directed, but they are likely to give short answers to questions and avoid spontaneous conversation. Occasionally, they may use an unusual figure of speech, such as an odd metaphor. Their mental content may reveal a sense of unwarranted intimacy with people they do not know well or whom they have not seen for a long time. They may be fascinated with an overvaluation of inanimate objects or metaphysical constructs. The patients' sensorium is intact; their memory functions well; and their proverb interpretations are abstract. The DSM-III-R diagnostic criteria are listed in Table 2.

Course and Prognosis. The onset of schizoid personality disorder usually begins in early childhood. Like all personality disorders, a schizoid personality disorder is long lasting but not necessarily lifelong. The proportion of patients who go on to develop schizophrenia is unknown.

Differential Diagnosis. In contrast with patients with schizophrenia or schizotypal personality disorder, patients with schizoid personality disorder do not have schizophrenic relatives, and they may have very successful, if isolated, work histories. Schizophrenic patients also differ by exhibiting thought disorder or

Table 2
Diagnostic Criteria for Schizoid Personality Disorder

A. A pervasive pattern of indifference to social relationships and a restricted range of emotional experience and expression, beginning by early adulthood and present in a variety of contexts, as indicated by at least *four* of the following:

(1) neither desires nor enjoys close relationships, including being part of a family
(2) almost always chooses solitary activities
(3) rarely, if ever, claims or appears to experience strong emotions, such as anger and joy
(4) indicates little if any desire to have sexual experiences with another person (age being taken into account)
(5) is indifferent to the praise and criticism of others
(6) has no close friends or confidants (or only one) other than first-degree relatives
(7) displays constricted affect, e.g., is aloof, cold, rarely reciprocates gestures or facial expressions, such as smiles or nods

B. Occurrence not exclusively during the course of Schizophrenia or a Delusional Disorder.

Table from DSM-III-R *Diagnostic and Statistical Manual of Mental Disorders,* ed 3, revised. (Current Classification of Mental Disorders, 1987.) Copyright American Psychiatric Association, Washington, D.C., 1987. Used with permission.

delusional thinking. Although they share many traits with the schizoid, paranoid personalities exhibit more social engagement, a history of aggressive verbal behavior, and a greater tendency to project their feelings onto others. If just as emotionally constricted, the compulsive and avoidant personalities experience loneliness as dysphoric, possess a richer history of past object relations, and do not engage as much in autistic reverie. Theoretically, the chief distinction between the schizotypal personality and the schizoid personality is that the schizotypal shows a greater similarity to the schizophrenic patient in the oddities, of perceptions, thoughts, behaviors, and communications. Avoidant personalities are isolated but strongly wish to participate in activities, which is absent in schizoid persons.

Treatment. The treatment of schizoid personalities is similar to that of paranoid personalities. However, schizoid patients' tendencies toward introspection are consistent with the psychotherapist's expectations, and schizoid patients may become devoted, if distant, patients. As trust develops, schizoid patients may, with great trepidation, reveal a plethora of fantasies, imaginary friends, and fears of unbearable dependency—even of merging with the therapist.

In group therapy settings, schizoid patients may be silent for long periods of time; nonetheless, they do become involved. These patients should be protected against aggressive attack by group members in regard to their proclivity for silence. With time, the group members become important to the patients and may provide the only social contact in their otherwise isolated existence.

Schizotypal Personality Disorder

Definition. Persons with schizotypal personality disorder are strikingly odd or strange, even to laypersons. Magical thinking, peculiar ideas, ideas of reference, illusions, and derealization are part of their everyday world.

Epidemiology. The epidemiology, prevalence, and sex ratio of schizotypal personality disorders are unknown. There is an increased association of cases among the biological relatives of chronic schizophrenic patients than among controls and a higher incidence among monozygotic than among dizygotic twins (33 percent versus 4 percent in one study).

Clinical Features. In schizotypal personality disorder, thinking and communicating are disturbed. Like schizophrenic patients, persons with schizotypal personalities may not know their own feelings; yet they are exquisitely sensitive to detecting the feelings of others, especially negative affects, like anger. They may be superstitious or claim clairvoyance. Their inner world may be filled with vivid imaginary relationships and childlike fears and fantasies. They may believe that they have special powers of thought and insight. Although frank thought disorder is absent, their speech may often require interpretation. They may admit that they have perceptual illusions or macropsia or that people appear to them as wooden and alike.

The speech of schizotypal personalities may be odd or peculiar and have meaning only to them. They show poor interpersonal relationships and may act inappropriately. As a result, they are isolated and have few if any friends. According to DSM-III-R, these patients may show features of borderline personality disorder, and indeed, both diagnoses can be made. Under stress, schizotypal personalities may decompensate and have psychiatric symptoms, but they are usually of brief duration. In severe cases, anhedonia and severe depression may occur.

Diagnosis. Schizotypal personalities are diagnosed on the basis of their peculiarities of thinking, behavior, and appearance. History taking may be difficult because of the patients' unusual way of communicating. The DSM-III-R diagnostic criteria for schizotypal personality are outlined in Table 3.

Course and Prognosis. A long-term study by Thomas McGlashan reported that 10 percent of persons with schizotypal personality disorder eventually committed suicide. In retrospective studies, many patients suffering from schizophrenia were actually schizotypal personalities, and the current clinical thinking suggests the schizotype to be the premorbid personality of the schizophrenic patient. Many of these patients, however, maintain a stable schizotypal personality throughout their lives and marry and work despite their oddities.

Differential Diagnosis. Theoretically, those with schizotypal personality disorder can be distinguished from schizoid and avoidant personalities by the presence of oddities in their behavior, thinking, perception, and communication and perhaps by a clear family history of schizophrenia. Schizotypal personalities may be distinguished from schizophrenic patients by their absence of psychosis. If psychotic symptoms do appear, they will be brief and fragmentary in nature. At present, some patients meet the criteria for both schizotypal personality disorder and borderline personality disorder. The paranoid personality is characterized by suspiciousness but lacks the odd behavior of the schizotype.

Treatment. The principles of treatment of schizotypal personality disorder should be no different from those of schizoid personality disorder. However, their odd and peculiar thinking must be handled carefully. Some patients will be involved in cults, strange religious practices, and the occult. Therapists cannot ridicule such activities and must not be judgmental about these beliefs or activities.

Antipsychotic medication may be useful in dealing with ideas of reference, illusions, and other symptoms of the disorder and can be used in conjunction with psychotherapy.

Table 3
Diagnostic Criteria for Schizotypal Personality Disorder

A. A pervasive pattern of deficits in interpersonal relatedness and peculiarities of ideation, appearance, and behavior, beginning by early adulthood and present in a variety of contexts, as indicated by at least *five* of the following:
 (1) ideas of reference (excluding delusions of reference)
 (2) excessive social anxiety, e.g., extreme discomfort in social situations involving unfamiliar people
 (3) odd beliefs or magical thinking, influencing behavior and inconsistent with subcultural norms, e.g., superstitiousness, belief in clairvoyance, telepathy, or "sixth sense," "others can feel my feelings" (in children and adolescents, bizarre fantasies or preoccupations)
 (4) unusual perceptual experiences, e.g., illusions, sensing the presence of a force or person not actually present (e.g., "I felt as if my dead mother were in the room with me")
 (5) odd or eccentric behavior or appearance, e.g., unkempt, unusual mannerisms, talks to self
 (6) no close friends or confidants (or only one) other than first-degree relatives
 (7) odd speech (without loosening of associations or incoherence), e.g., speech that is impoverished, digressive, vague, or inappropriately abstract
 (8) inappropriate or constricted affect, e.g., silly, aloof, rarely reciprocates gestures or facial expressions, such as smiles or nods
 (9) suspiciousness or paranoid ideation

B. Occurrence not exclusively during the course of Schizophrenia or a Pervasive Developmental Disorder.

Table from DSM-III-R *Diagnostic and Statistical Manual of Mental Disorders,* ed 3, revised. (Current Classification of Mental Disorders, 1987.) Copyright American Psychiatric Association, Washington, D.C., 1987. Used with permission.

Histrionic Personality Disorder

Definition. Histrionic personality disorder is characterized by colorful, dramatic, extroverted behavior in excitable, emotional persons. Accompanying their flamboyant presentation, however, is often an inability to maintain deep, long-lasting attachments. This is also known as hysterical personality.

Epidemiology. The exact prevalence of histrionic personality disorder is unknown. It is diagnosed more frequently in women than in men. Some studies have found an association with somatization disorder and alcoholism.

Clinical Features. Patients with histrionic personality disorder show a high degree of attention-seeking behavior. They tend to exaggerate their thoughts and feelings, making everything sound more important than it really is. They will display temper tantrums, tears, and accusations if they are not the center of attention or are not receiving praise or approval.

Seductive behavior is common in both sexes. Sexual fantasies about persons with whom they are involved are common, but they are inconsistent about verbalizing these fantasies and may be coy or flirtatious rather than sexually aggressive. In fact, histrionic patients may have a psychosexual dysfunction: the women may be anorgasmic, and the men may be impotent. They may act on their sexual impulses to reassure themselves that they are attractive to the other sex. Their need for reassurance is endless. Their relationships tend to be superficial, however, and these persons can be vain, self-absorbed, and fickle. Their strong dependency needs makes them overly trusting and gullible.

The major defenses of histrionic personalities are repression and dissociation. Accordingly, such patients are unaware of their true feelings and are unable to explain their motivations. Under stress, reality testing becomes easily impaired.

Diagnosis. In their interview, histrionic patients are generally cooperative and eager to give a detailed history. Gestures and dramatic punctuation in their conversation are common. They may make frequent slips of the tongue, and their language is colorful. Affective display is common, but when pressed to acknowledge certain feelings (e.g., anger, sadness, and sexual wishes), they may respond with surprise, indignation, or denial. The results of the cognitive examination are usually normal, although a lack of perserverance may be shown on arithmetic or concentration tasks, and their forgetfulness of affect-laden material may be astonishing. The DSM-III-R diagnostic criteria are listed in Table 4.

Course and Prognosis. With age, patients with histrionic personalities tend to show fewer symptoms, but because they lack the same energy they had when younger, that difference may be more apparent than real. These patients are sensation seekers and may get into trouble with the law, abuse drugs, and act promiscuously.

Differential Diagnosis. The distinction between histrionic personality and borderline personality is difficult. In the latter, suicide attempts, greater identity diffusion, and brief psychotic episodes are more likely. Although DSM-III-R states that both conditions may be diagnosed in the same patient, it is preferable that the clinician try to separate the two. Somatization disorder

Table 4
Diagnostic Criteria for Histrionic Personality Disorder

A pervasive pattern of excessive emotionality and attention-seeking, beginning by early adulthood and present in a variety of contexts, as indicated by at least *four* of the following:
  (1) constantly seeks or demands reassurance, approval, or praise
  (2) is inappropriately sexually seductive in appearance or behavior
  (3) is overly concerned with physical attractiveness
  (4) expresses emotion with inappropriate exaggeration, e.g., embraces casual acquaintances with excessive ardor, uncontrollable sobbing on minor sentimental occasions, has temper tantrums
  (5) is uncomfortable in situations in which he or she is not the center of attention
  (6) displays rapidly shifting and shallow expression of emotions
  (7) is self-centered, actions being directed toward obtaining immediate satisfaction; has no tolerance for the frustration of delayed gratification
  (8) has a style of speech that is excessively impressionistic and lacking in detail, e.g., when asked to describe mother, can be no more specific than, "She was a beautiful person."

Table from DSM-III-R *Diagnostic and Statistical Manual of Mental Disorders*, ed 3, revised. (Current Classification of Mental Disorders, 1987.) Copyright American Psychiatric Association, Washington, D.C., 1987. Used with permission.

(Briquet's syndrome) may occur in conjunction with histrionic personality disorder. Patients with brief reactive psychoses and dissociative disorders may warrant a coexisting diagnosis of histrionic personality disorder.

Treatment. Patients with histrionic personality disorder are often unaware of their own real feelings; therefore, clarification of their inner feelings is an important therapeutic process. Psychoanalytically oriented psychotherapy, whether group or individual, is probably the treatment of choice for this personality disorder. Pharmacotherapy can be adjunctive when symptoms are targeted (e.g., antidepressants for depression and somatic complaints, antianxiety agents for anxiety, and antipsychotics for derealization or illusions).

Narcissistic Personality Disorder

Definition. Persons with narcissistic personality disorder are characterized by a heightened sense of self-importance and grandiose feelings that they are unique in some way.

Epidemiology. There are no data on the prevalence, sex ratio, and familial pattern of narcissistic personality disorder. There may be a higher risk in the offspring of parents with this disorder who impart to them an unrealistic sense of omnipotence, grandiosity, beauty, and talent. The number of cases reported is increasing steadily.

Clinical Features. According to DSM-III-R, persons with this disorder have a grandiose sense of self-importance. They consider themselves special people and expect special treatment. They handle criticism poorly and may become enraged that anyone would dare to criticize them, or they may appear to be completely indifferent to it. They want their own way and are frequently ambitious, desiring fame and fortune. Their sense of entitlement is striking. Their relationships are fragile, and they can make others furious because they refuse to obey the conventional rules of behavior. They are unable to show empathy, and they feign sympathy only to achieve their selfish ends. Interpersonal exploitiveness is commonplace. These patients have fragile self-esteem and are prone to depression. Interpersonal difficulties, rejection, loss, and occupational problems are among the stresses that narcissists commonly produce by their behavior stresses they are least able to handle.

Diagnosis. See Table 5 for the DSM-III-R diagnostic features for narcissistic personality disorder.

Course and Prognosis. This disorder is chronic and difficult to treat. These patients must constantly deal with blows to their narcissism resulting from their own behavior or from life experiences. Aging is handled poorly, as these patients value beauty, strength, and youthful attributes, to which they cling inappropriately. They may be more vulnerable, therefore, to mid-life crises than are other groups.

Differential Diagnosis. According to DSM-III-R, borderline, histrionic, and antisocial personality disorders are often present together with narcissistic personality disorder, which means that a differential diagnosis is difficult. Patients with narcissistic personality disorder have less anxiety than do patients with borderline personalities, and their lives tend to be less chaotic. Suicidal attempts are also more likely to be associated with borderlines than with narcissists. Antisocial personalities give a history of impulsive behavior often associated with alcohol or drug abuse that frequently gets them into trouble with the law. And histrionic patients show features of exhibitionism and interpersonal manipulativeness that

Table 5
Diagnostic Criteria for Narcissistic Personality Disorder

A pervasive pattern of grandiosity (in fantasy or behavior), lack of empathy, and hypersensitivity to the evaluation of others, beginning by early adulthood and present in a variety of contexts, as indicated by at least *five* of the following:

(1) reacts to criticism with feelings of rage, shame, or humiliation (even if not expressed)
(2) is interpersonally exploitative: takes advantage of others to achieve his or her own ends
(3) has a grandiose sense of self-importance, e.g., exaggerates achievements and talents, expects to be noticed as "special" without appropriate achievement
(4) believes that his or her problems are unique and can be understood only by other special people
(5) is preoccupied with fantasies of unlimited success, power, brilliance, beauty, or ideal love
(6) has a sense of entitlement: unreasonable expectation of especially favorable treatment, e.g., assumes that he or she does not have to wait in line when others must do so
(7) requires constant attention and admiration, e.g., keeps fishing for compliments
(8) lack of empathy: inability to recognize and experience how others feel, e.g., annoyance and surprise when a friend who is seriously ill cancels a date
(9) is preoccupied with feelings of envy

Table from DSM-III-R *Diagnostic and Statistical Manual of Mental Disorders,* ed 3, revised. (Current Classification of Mental Disorders, 1987.) Copyright American Psychiatric Association, Washington, D.C., 1987. Used with permission.

are similar to those of narcissist patients who have, however, a greater capacity for empathy and genuine warmth.

Treatment. The treatment of narcissistic personality disorder is extremely difficult, as these patients must renounce their narcissism if progress is to be made. Psychiatrists such as Otto Kernberg and Heinz Kohut advocate using psychoanalytic approaches to effect change; however, much research is required to validate the diagnosis and determine the best treatment.

Antisocial Personality Disorder

Definition. Antisocial personality disorder is characterized by continual antisocial or criminal acts, but it is not synonomous with criminality. Rather, it is an inability to conform to social norms that involves many aspects of the patient's adolescent and adult development.

Epidemiology. The prevalence of antisocial personality disorder is 3 percent in men and 1 percent in women. It is most common in poor urban areas and among mobile residents of those areas. Boys with the disorder come from larger families than do girls. The onset of the disorder is before the age of 15. Females usually develop symptoms before puberty, and males, even earlier. In prison populations, the prevalence of antisocial personality may be as high as 75 percent. A familial pattern is present in that it is five times more common among first-degree relatives of males with the disorder than among controls.

Clinical Features. Antisocial personalities often present a normal and even a charming and ingratiating exterior. Their histories reveal, however, many areas of disordered life functioning.

Lying, truancy, running away from home, thefts, fights, drug abuse, and illegal activities are typical experiences that the patients report as beginning in childhood. Often, antisocial personalities impress opposite-sex clinicians with the colorful, seductive aspects of their personalities, but same-sex clinicians may regard them as manipulative and demanding. Antisocial personalities demonstrate a lack of anxiety or depression that may seem grossly incongruous with their situation, and their own explanations of their antisocial behavior make it seem mindless. Suicide threats and somatic preoccupations may be common. Nevertheless, the patients' mental content reveals the complete absence of delusions and other signs of irrational thinking. In fact, they frequently demonstrate a heightened sense of reality testing. They often impress observers as having good verbal intelligence.

Antisocial personalities are highly represented by so-called "con men." They are highly manipulative and are frequently able to talk others into participating in schemes that involve easy ways to make money or to achieve fame or notoriety, which eventually may lead the unwary to financial ruin, social embarrassment, or both. Antisocial personalities do not tell the truth and cannot be trusted to carry out any task or adhere to any conventional standard of morality. Promiscuity, spouse abuse, child abuse, and drunk driving are common events in these patients' lives. A notable finding is a lack of remorse for those actions; that is, these patients appear to lack a conscience.

Diagnosis. As mentioned, these patients may appear composed and credible in the interview. However, beneath the veneer (or, to use Hervey Cleckley's term, the "mask of sanity"), there is tension, hostility, irritability, and rage. Stress interviews, in which patients are vigorously confronted with inconsistencies in their history, may be necessary to reveal the pathology. Even the most experienced clinicians have been fooled by such patients.

A diagnostic work-up should include a thorough neurologic exam. Because these patients often show abnormal EEGs and soft neurologic signs suggestive of minimal brain damage in childhood, these findings can be used to confirm the clinical impression. The DSM-III-R diagnostic criteria are listed in Table 6.

Once an antisocial personality disorder develops, it runs an unremitting course, with the height of antisocial behavior usually occurring in late adolescence. The prognosis is variable. There are reports that symptoms decrease as patients grow older. Many patients develop somatization disorder and have multiple physical complaints. Depression, alcoholism, and substance abuse are common.

Differential Diagnosis. Antisocial personality disorder can be distinguished from illegal behavior in that antisocial personality disorder involves many areas of the person's life. If antisocial behavior is the only manifestation, such patients are diagnosed in the DSM-III-R category called conditions not attributable to a mental disorder. Dorothy Lewis has demonstrated, however, that many of these patients have a neurological or mental disorder that has either been overlooked or not diagnosed. More difficult is the differentiation of antisocial personality disorder from substance abuse disorder. When both substance abuse and antisocial behavior begin in childhood and continue into adult life, both disorders should be diagnosed. When, however, the antisocial behavior is clearly secondary to premorbid alcohol abuse or drug abuse, the diagnosis of antisocial personality disorder is not warranted.

In diagnosing antisocial personality disorder, it is important to adjust for the distorting effects of social class, cultural background, and sex on its manifestations. Furthermore, the diagnosis of antisocial personality disorder is not warranted if mental retardation, schizophrenia, or mania can explain the symptoms.

Treatment.   If antisocial personalities are immobilized, or if they are approached by understanding peers, then—instead of appearing incorrigible, inhuman, unfeeling, guiltless, and unable to learn from experience—they will become only too human. Once antisocial personalities feel that they are among peers, their lack of motivation for change disappears. Perhaps this is why self-help groups have been more useful than jails and psychiatric hospitals have been in alleviating these disorders.

Before treatment can begin, firm limits are essential. The therapist must find some way of dealing with the patient's self-destructive behavior. And to overcome the antisocial personality's fear of intimacy, the therapist must frustrate the patient's wish to run from the tenderness and the honest pain of human encounter. In doing so, the therapist faces the challenge of separating control from punishment and of separating help and confrontation from social isolation and retribution.

Antisocial personalities are made worse by good defense lawyers, as they are not helped by the consequences of their behavior.

Table 6
Diagnostic Criteria for Antisocial Personality Disorder

A. Current age at least 18.

B. Evidence of Conduct Disorder with onset before age 15, as indicated by a history of *three* or more of the following:
   (1) was often truant
   (2) ran away from home overnight at least twice while living in parental or parental surrogate home (or once without returning)
   (3) often initiated physical fights
   (4) used a weapon in more than one fight
   (5) forced someone into sexual activity with him or her
   (6) was physically cruel to animals
   (7) was physically cruel to other people
   (8) deliberately destroyed others' property (other than by fire-setting)
   (9) deliberately engaged in fire-setting
   (10) often lied (other than to avoid physical or sexual abuse)
   (11) has stolen without confrontation of a victim on more than one occasion (including forgery)
   (12) has stolen with confrontation of a victim (e.g., mugging, purse-snatching, extortion, armed robbery)

C. A pattern of irresponsible and antisocial behavior since the age of 15, as indicated by at least *four* of the following:
   (1) is unable to sustain consistent work behavior, as indicated by any of the following (including similar behavior in academic settings if the person is a student):
      (a) significant unemployment for 6 months or more within five years when expected to work and work was available
      (b) repeated absences from work unexplained by illness in self or family
      (c) abandonment of several jobs without realistic plans for others
   (2) fails to conform to social norms with respect to lawful behavior, as indicated by repeatedly performing antisocial acts that are grounds for arrest (whether arrested or not), e.g., destroying property, harassing others, stealing, pursuing an illegal occupation

   (3) is irritable and aggressive, as indicated by repeated physical fights or assaults (not required by one's job or to defend someone or oneself), including spouse- or child-beating
   (4) repeatedly fails to honor financial obligations, as indicated by defaulting on debts or failing to provide child support or support for other dependents on a regular basis
   (5) fails to plan ahead, or is impulsive, as indicated by one or both of the following:
      (a) traveling from place to place without a prearranged job or clear goal for the period of travel or clear idea about when the travel will terminate
      (b) lack of a fixed address for a month or more
   (6) has no regard for the truth, as indicated by repeated lying, use of aliases, or "conning" others for personal profit or pleasure
   (7) is reckless regarding his or her own or others' personal safety, as indicated by driving while intoxicated, or recurrent speeding
   (8) if a parent or guardian, lacks ability to function as a responsible parent, as indicated by one or more of the following:
      (a) malnutrition of child
      (b) child's illness resulting from lack of minimal hygiene
      (c) failure to obtain medical care for a seriously ill child
      (d) child's dependence on neighbors or nonresident relatives for food or shelter
      (e) failure to arrange for a caretaker for young child when parent is away from home
      (f) repeated squandering, on personal items, of money required for household necessities
   (9) has never sustained a totally monogamous relationship for more than one year
   (10) lacks remorse (feels justified in having hurt, mistreated, or stolen from another)

D. Occurrence of antisocial behavior not exclusively during the course of Schizophrenia or Manic Episodes.

Table from DSM-III-R *Diagnostic and Statistical Manual of Mental Disorders,* ed 3, revised. (Current Classification of Mental Disorders, 1987.) Copyright American Psychiatric Association, Washington, D.C., 1987. Used with permission.

Rather, antisocial personalities should be encouraged to find alternative defense mechanisms. As with a young child, the therapist does not tell an antisocial personality to stop doing something but provides the patient with an alternative.

Only group membership or caring for others or both can eventually provide adults with the parenting they never received. Antisocial personalities have been generally neglected during childhood, and the group can provide what they experience as a caring family. Pharmacotherapy is used to deal with incapacitating symptoms such as anxiety, rage, or depression, but because these patients are often substance abusers, drugs must be used judiciously.

Borderline Personality Disorder

Definition.   Borderline patients stand on the border between neurosis and psychosis and are characterized by extraordinarily unstable affect, mood, behavior, object relationships, and self-image. The disorder has also been called ambulatory schizophrenia, "as if" personality (a term coined by Helene Deutsch), pseudoneurotic schizophrenia (described by Paul Hoch and Phillip Politan), psychotic character (described by John Frosch), and emotionally unstable personality.

Epidemiology. No definitive prevalence studies are available, but this disorder is thought to be present in about 1 or 2 percent of the population and is twice as common in women as in men. There is an increased prevalence of unibipolar depression, alcoholism, and substance abuse in first-degree relatives of subjects with borderline personality.

Clinical Features. Borderline patients almost always appear to be in a state of crisis. Mood swings are common. The patients can be argumentative at one moment, depressed at another, or complain of having no feelings at still another time.

There may be short-lived psychotic episodes (so-called micropsychotic episodes) rather than full-blown psychotic breaks, and their psychotic symptoms are almost always circumscribed, fleeting, or in doubt. The behavior of borderline personalities is highly unpredictable; consequently, they rarely achieve up to the level of their abilities. The painful nature of their lives is reflected in repetitive self-destructive acts. Such patients may perform wrist slashing and other self-mutilations in order to elicit help from others, to express anger, or to numb themselves to overwhelming affect.

Because they feel both very dependent and hostile, borderline personalities have tumultuous interpersonal relationships. They can be very dependent on those to whom they are close, and they can express enormous anger at their intimate friends when frustrated. Borderline personalities cannot tolerate being alone, however, and prefer a frantic search for companionship, no matter how unsatisfactory, to sitting by themselves. To assuage loneliness, if only for brief periods of time, they will accept a stranger as a friend or will be promiscuous. They often complain about chronic feelings of emptiness and boredom, the lack of a consistent sense of identity (identity diffusion), and, when pressed, how depressed they feel most of the time, despite the flurry of other affects.

Most therapists agree that borderline patients demonstrate ordinary reasoning abilities on structural tests, such as the Wechsler Adult Intelligence Scale, and demonstrate deviant processes only on unstructured projective tests such as the Rorschach.

Functionally, adult borderline patients distort their present relationships by putting every person into either an all-good or an all-bad category. They see people as either nurturant and attachment figures or hateful and sadistic persons who deprive them of security needs and threaten them with abandonment whenever they feel dependent. As a result of this splitting, the good person is idealized, and the bad person is devalued. Shifts of allegiance from one person or group to another are frequent.

Some clinicians use panphobia, pananxiety, panambivalence and chaotic sexuality to describe the borderline personality's characteristics.

Diagnosis. According to DSM-III-R, the diagnosis of borderline personality can be made by early adulthood when the patient shows at least five of the criteria listed in Table 7.

Biological studies may aid in the diagnosis, as some borderline patients show shortened REM latency and sleep continuity disturbances, an abnormal dexamethasone suppression test, and an abnormal thyrotropin releasing hormone test. But these changes are also seen in some cases of depression.

Course and Prognosis. The disorder is fairly stable in that patients change little over time. Longitudinal studies do not

Table 7
Diagnostic Criteria for Borderline Personality Disorder

A pervasive pattern of instability of mood, interpersonal relationships, and self-image, beginning by early adulthood and present in a variety of contexts, as indicated by at least *five* of the following:

(1) a pattern of unstable and intense interpersonal relationships characterized by alternating between extremes of overidealization and devaluation
(2) impulsiveness in at least two areas that are potentially self-damaging, e.g., spending, sex, substance use, shoplifting, reckless driving, binge eating (Do not include suicidal or self-mutilating behavior covered in [5].)
(3) affective instability: marked shifts from baseline mood to depression, irritability, or anxiety, usually lasting a few hours and only rarely more than a few days
(4) inappropriate, intense anger or lack of control of anger, e.g., frequent displays of temper, constant anger, recurrent physical fights
(5) recurrent suicidal threats, gestures, or behavior, or self-mutilating behavior
(6) marked and persistent identity disturbance manifested by uncertainty about at least two of the following: self-image, sexual orientation, long-term goals or career choice, type of friends desired, preferred values
(7) chronic feelings of emptiness or boredom
(8) frantic efforts to avoid real or imagined abandonment (Do not include suicidal or self-mutilating behavior covered in [5].)

Table from DSM-III-R *Diagnostic and Statistical Manual of Mental Disorders*, ed 3, revised. (Current Classification of Mental Disorders, 1987.) Copyright American Psychiatric Association, Washington, D.C., 1987. Used with permission.

show a progression toward schizophrenia, but there is a high incidence of major depressive episodes in these patients. The diagnosis is usually made before the age of 40, when these patients are attempting to make occupational, marital, or other choices and are unable to deal with these normal stages in the life cycle.

Differential Diagnosis. The differentiation from schizophrenia is made on the basis of there being no prolonged psychotic episodes, thought disorder, or other classic schizophrenic signs. Schizotypes show marked peculiarities of thinking, strange ideation, and recurrent ideas of reference. Paranoid personalities are marked by extreme suspiciousness. Histrionic and antisocial personalities are difficult to distinguish from borderline personalities. In general, the borderline will show chronic feelings of emptiness, impulsivity, self-mutilation, short-lived psychotic episodes, manipulative suicide attempts, and unusually demanding involvement in close relationships.

Treatment. Psychotherapy for borderline personalities is an area of intensive investigation and has been the treatment of choice. More recently, pharmacotherapy has been added to the treatment regimen.

Psychotherapy is difficult for patient and therapist alike. Regression occurs easily in such patients, who act out their impulses and show labile or fixed negative or positive transferences, which are difficult to analyze. Splitting as a mechanism of defense causes the borderline to alternately love or hate the therapist and others in the environment. A reality-oriented approach is more effective than are in-depth unconscious interpretations. Special support systems such as day hospitals, night hospitals, and halfway houses have been useful. Prolonged hospitalization, in conjunction with intensive individual and group therapy, helps patients understand themselves and sets limits on the extent and frequency of acting out during the psychotherapeutic process.

Pharmacotherapy of borderline disorders is useful to deal with specific personality features that interfere with the patients' overall functioning. Antipsychotics have been used to control anger, hostility, and brief psychotic episodes. Antidepressants improve the depressed mood that is common in these patients. The monoamine oxidase inhibitors have been effective in modulating impulsive behavior in some patients. Benzodiazepines, particularly alprazolam (Xanax), help anxiety and depression, but some patients show a disinhibition with this class of drugs. Anticonvulsants such as carbamazepine (Tegretol) may improve global functioning in some patients.

Avoidant Personality Disorder

Definition. Persons with avoidant personalities show an extreme sensitivity to rejection, which may lead to a socially withdrawn life. They are not asocial but are shy and show a great desire for companionship; they need unusually strong guarantees of uncritical acceptance. Such persons are commonly referred to as having an inferiority complex.

Epidemiology. The prevalence of avoidant personality disorder is unknown; as defined, it is common. No information is available on sex ratio or familial pattern. Infants classified as having a timid temperament may be more prone to the disorder than are those high on activity-approach scales.

Clinical Features. Hypersensitivity to rejection by others is the central clinical feature of this disorder. Such persons desire the warmth and security of human companionship but justify their avoidance of forming relationships by their alleged fear of rejection. When talking with someone, they express uncertainty and a lack of self-confidence and may speak in a self-effacing manner. They are afraid to speak up in public or to make requests of others, because they are hypervigilant about rejection. They are apt to misinterpret other people's comments as derogatory or ridiculing. The refusal of any request leads them to withdraw from others and to feel hurt.

In the vocational sphere, avoidant personalities often take a job on the sidelines. They rarely attain much personal advancement or exercise much authority. Instead, at work they may seem simply shy and eager to please.

According to DSM-III-R, these persons are generally unwilling to enter relationships unless they are given an unusually strong guarantee of uncritical acceptance. Consequently, they often have no close friends or confidants. In general, their main personality trait is timidity.

Diagnosis. In the clinical interview, the most striking aspect is the patient's anxiety about talking with the interviewer. These patients' nervous and tense manner appears to wax and wane with their perception of whether or not the interviewer likes them. They seem vulnerable to the interviewer's comments and suggestions and may consider a clarification or an interpretation as a criticism. The DSM-III-R diagnostic criteria for avoidant personality are listed in Table 8.

Table 8
Diagnostic Criteria for Avoidant Personality Disorder

A pervasive pattern of social discomfort, fear of negative evaluation, and timidity, beginning by early adulthood and present in a variety of contexts, as indicated by at least *four* of the following:
  (1) is easily hurt by criticism or disapproval
  (2) has no close friends or confidants (or only one) other than first-degree relatives
  (3) is unwilling to get involved with people unless certain of being liked
  (4) avoids social or occupational activities that involve significant interpersonal contact, e.g., refuses a promotion that will increase social demands
  (5) is reticent in social situations because of a fear of saying something inappropriate or foolish, or of being unable to answer a question
  (6) fears being embarrassed by blushing, crying, or showing signs of anxiety in front of other people
  (7) exaggerates the potential difficulties, physical dangers, or risks involved in doing something ordinary but outside his or her usual routine, e.g., may cancel social plans because she anticipates being exhausted by the effort of getting there

Table from DSM-III-R *Diagnostic and Statistical Manual of Mental Disorders*, ed 3, revised. (Current Classification of Mental Disorders, 1987.) Copyright American Psychiatric Association, Washington, D.C., 1987. Used with permission.

Course and Prognosis. Many avoidant personalities are able to function, providing they are in a protected environment. Some marry, have children, and live their lives surrounded only by family. Should their support system fail, however, they are subject to depression, anxiety, and anger. Phobic avoidance is common, and avoidant personalities may give a history of social phobias or develop such phobias during the course of their illness.

Differential Diagnosis. Avoidant personalities desire social interaction, compared with schizoid persons who want to be alone. Avoidant persons are not as demanding, irritable, or unpredictable as are borderline or histrionic personalities. The avoidant personality and dependent personality are very similar. The dependent personality is presumed to have a greater fear of being abandoned or not loved than does the avoidant personality; however, the clinical picture may be indistinguishable. The term "avoidant personality disorder" originated with DSM-III and requires further study to distinguish it from dependent personality disorder.

Treatment. Psychotherapeutic treatment depends on solidifying an alliance with the therapist. As trust develops, the therapist conveys an accepting attitude toward the patient's fears, especially that of rejection. The therapist eventually encourages the patient to move out into the world to take what are perceived as great risks of humiliation, rejection, or failure. But the therapist should be cautious when giving assignments to exercise new social skills outside therapy, because failure may reinforce the patient's already poor self-esteem. Group therapy may help such patients understand the effect that their sensitivity to rejection has on themselves and others. Assertiveness training is a form of behavior therapy that may teach patients to express their needs more openly and improve their self-esteem.

Dependent Personality Disorder

Definition. Persons with dependent personality disorder subordinate their own needs to those of others, get others to assume responsibility for major areas in their lives, lack self-confidence, and may experience intense discomfort when alone for more than a brief period of time. In DSM-I, this condition was called passive-dependent personality. Freud described an oral-dependent dimension to personality characterized by dependence, pessimism, fear of sexuality, self-doubt, passivity, suggestibility, and lack of perseverance, which is similar to the DSM-III-R categorization of dependent personality disorder.

Epidemiology. This disorder is more common in women than in men. One study diagnosed 2.5 percent of all personality disorders as falling into this category. It is more common in younger children than in older children. Persons with chronic physical illness in childhood may be more prone to the disorder.

Clinical Features. According to DSM-III-R, dependent personality disorder is characterized by a pervasive pattern of dependent and submissive behavior. Persons with the disorder are unable to make decisions without an excessive amount of advice and reassurance from others.

Dependent personalities avoid positions of responsibility and become anxious if asked to assume a leadership role. They prefer to be submissive. When on their own, they find it difficult to persevere at tasks but may find it easy to perform those tasks for someone else.

These persons do not like to be alone. They will seek out others on whom they can depend, and their relationships are thus distorted by their need to be attached to that other person. In *folie à deux* (or shared delusional disorder), one member of the pair is usually suffering from a dependent personality disorder, and the submissive partner takes on the delusional system of the more aggressive, assertive partner on whom he or she is dependent.

Pessimism, self-doubt, passivity, and fears of expressing sexual and aggressive feelings characterize the behavior of the dependent personality. An abusive, unfaithful, or alcoholic spouse may be tolerated for long periods of time in order not to disturb the sense of attachment.

Diagnosis. In the interview, these patients appear to be very compliant. They try to cooperate, welcome specific questions, and look for guidance. The DSM-III-R diagnostic criteria for dependent personality disorder are listed in Table 9.

Course and Prognosis. Little is known about the course of this disorder. There tends to be impaired occupational functioning, as there is an inability to act independently and without close supervision. Social relationships are limited to those on whom such persons can depend, and many suffer physical or mental abuse because they cannot assert themselves. They risk severe depression if they sustain the loss of a person on whom they are dependent. The prognosis with treatment, however, is favorable.

Differential Diagnosis. The traits of dependency are found in many types of psychiatric disorders, which makes the differential diagnosis difficult. Dependency is a prominent factor in histrionic and borderline personalities; however, dependent personalities will usually have a long-standing relationship with one person on whom they are dependent, rather than on a series of persons, and they do not tend to be overtly manipulative. Schizoid and schizotypal personalities tend to be isolated. As mentioned, dependent personalities may be indistinguishable from avoidant personalities.

Dependent behavior may occur in patients with agoraphobia, but there tends to be a much higher level of overt anxiety or even panic in agoraphobic patients.

Treatment. The treatment of dependent personality traits can often be very successful. Insight-oriented therapies enable patients to understand the antecedents of their behavior, and with the support of a therapist, such patients can become more independent, assertive, and self-reliant.

A pitfall in the treatment may occur when the therapist encourages the patient to change the dynamics of a pathological relationships (e.g., that a physically abused wife seek help from the police). At that point, the patient may become too anxious, be unable to cooperate in therapy, and feel torn between complying with the therapist and losing a pathological external relationship. The therapist must show great respect for a dependent patient's feelings of attachment, no matter how pathological those feelings may seem.

Behavior therapy, assertiveness training, family therapy, and group therapy all have been used, with successful outcomes in many cases. Pharmacotherapy has been used to deal with such specific symptoms as anxiety or depression, which are common associated features of this disorder.

Obsessive-Compulsive Personality Disorder

Definition. The obsessive-compulsive personality disorder is characterized by emotional constriction, orderliness, perseverance, stubbornness, and indecisiveness. According to DSM-III-R, the essential feature of this disorder is a pervasive pattern of perfectionism and inflexibility.

Table 9
Diagnostic Criteria for Dependent Personality Disorder

A pervasive pattern of dependent and submissive behavior, beginning by early adulthood and present in a variety of contexts, as indicated by at least *five* of the following:
(1) is unable to make everyday decisions without an excessive amount of advice or reassurance from others
(2) allows others to make most of his or her important decisions, e.g., where to live, what job to take
(3) agrees with people even when he or she believes they are wrong, because of fear of being rejected
(4) has difficulty initiating projects or doing things on his or her own
(5) volunteers to do things that are unpleasant or demeaning in order to get other people to like him or her
(6) feels uncomfortable or helpless when alone, or goes to great lengths to avoid being alone
(7) feels devastated or helpless when close relationships end
(8) is frequently preoccupied with fears of being abandoned
(9) is easily hurt by criticism or disapproval

Table from DSM-III-R *Diagnostic and Statistical Manual of Mental Disorders*, ed 3, revised. (Current Classification of Mental Disorders, 1987.) Copyright American Psychiatric Association, Washington, D.C., 1987. Used with permission.

Epidemiology. The prevalence of the obsessive-compulsive personality disorder is unknown. It is more common in males than in females and is diagnosed most often in oldest children. The disorder also occurs more frequently in first-degree biological relatives of persons with the disorder than in the general population. Patients often have backgrounds characterized by harsh discipline. Freud hypothesized that the disorder is associated with difficulties in the anal stage of psychosexual development, generally around the age of 2. However, in various studies, that theory has not been validated.

Clinical Features. Persons with this disorder are preoccupied with rules, regulations, orderliness, neatness, details, and the achievement of perfection. These traits account for a general constriction of the entire personality. Such persons are formal and serious and often lack a sense of humor. They insist that rules be followed rigidly and are unable to tolerate what they perceive to be infractions. Accordingly, they lack flexibility and are intolerant. They are capable of prolonged work, providing it is routinized and does not require changes to which they cannot adapt.

Obsessive-compulsive persons' interpersonal skills are extremely limited. They alienate people, are unable to compromise, and insist that others submit to their needs. They are, however, eager to please those who they see as more powerful than themselves and carry out their wishes in an authoritarian manner. Because of their fear of making mistakes, they are indecisive and ruminate about making decisions. Although a stable marriage and occupational adequacy are common, obsessive-compulsive persons have few friends.

Anything that threatens to upset the routine of these patients' lives or their perceived stability can precipitate a great deal of anxiety that is otherwise bound up in the rituals that they impose on their lives and try to impose on others.

Diagnosis In the interview, obsessive-compulsive personalities may have a stiff, formal, and rigid demeanor. Their affect is not blunted or flat but can be described as constricted. They lack spontaneity. Their mood is usually serious. Such patients may be anxious about not being in control of the interview. Their answers to questions are unusually detailed. The defense mechanisms they use are rationalization, isolation, intellectualization, reaction formation, and undoing. (See Table 10 for the DSM-III-R diagnostic criteria of obsessive-compulsive personality.)

Course and Prognosis. The course of obsessive-compulsive personality disorder is variable and not predictable. From time to time, obsessions or compulsions may develop in the course of the personality disorder. Some obsessive-compulsive adolescents evolve into warm, open, and loving adults; but in others, these traits can be either the harbinger of schizophrenia or—decades later and exacerbated by the aging process—severe depression and melancholia.

These persons may do well in positions demanding methodical, deductive, or detailed work, but they are vulnerable to unexpected changes, and their personal lives may remain barren. Major depressive disorders, especially those of late onset, are common.

Differential Diagnosis. When recurrent obsessions or compulsions are present, the obsessive-compulsive disorder should be noted on Axis I. Perhaps the most difficult distinction is between the outpatient with some obsessive-compulsive traits and one with obsessive-compulsive personality disorder. The diagnosis of personality disorder is reserved for those patients with a significant impairment in their occupational or social effectiveness. In some cases, schizoid and paranoid disorders coexist with the personality disorder, and if they do, they should be noted.

**Table 10
Diagnostic Criteria for Obsessive-Compulsive Personality Disorder**

A pervasive pattern of perfectionism and inflexibility, beginning by early adulthood and present in a variety of contexts, as indicated by at least *five* of the following:

(1) perfectionism that interferes with task completion, e.g., inability to complete a project because own overly strict standards are not met

(2) preoccupation with details, rules, lists, order, organization, or schedules to the extent that the major point of the activity is lost

(3) unreasonable insistence that others submit to exactly his or her way of doing things, **or** unreasonable reluctance to allow others to do things because of the conviction that they will not do them correctly

(4) excessive devotion to work and productivity to the exclusion of leisure activities and friendships (not accounted for by obvious economic necessity)

(5) indecisiveness: decision making is either avoided, postponed, or protracted, e.g., the person cannot get assignments done on time because of ruminating about priorities (do not include if indecisiveness is due to excessive need for advice or reassurance from others)

(6) overconscientiousness, scrupulousness, and inflexibility about matters of morality, ethics, or values (not accounted for by cultural or religious identification)

(7) restricted expression of affection

(8) lack of generosity in giving time, money, or gifts when no personal gain is likely to result

(9) inability to discard worn-out or worthless objects even when they have no sentimental value

Table from DSM-III-R *Diagnostic and Statistical Manual of Mental Disorders*, ed 3, revised. (Current Classification of Mental Disorders, 1987.) Copyright American Psychiatric Association, Washington, D.C., 1987. Used with permission.

Treatment. Unlike patients with the other personality disorders, obsessive-compulsive personalities often know that they are suffering, and they seek treatment on their own. Free association and nondirective therapy are highly valued by the overtrained, oversocialized obsessive-compulsive personality. However, the treatment of these patients is often long and complex, and countertransference problems are common.

Group and behavioral therapy occasionally offer certain advantages. In both contexts, it is easy to interrupt such patients in the midst of their maladaptive interactions or explanations. Preventing the completion of their habitual behavior raises their anxiety and leaves them susceptible to learning new coping strategies. Patients can also receive direct rewards for change in group therapy, something less often possible in individual psychotherapies.

Clonazepam (Clonopin) is a benzodiazepine with anticonvulsant use that has reduced symptoms in patients with severe obsessive-compulsive disorder. Whether it is of use in the personality disorder is not known.

Passive-Aggressive Personality

Definition. The passive-aggressive personality is characterized by covert obstructionism, procrastination, stubbornness, and inefficiency. Such behavior is a manifestation of underlying aggression, which is expressed passively.

Epidemiology. No data are available about the epidemiology of this disorder. Sex ratio, familial patterns, and prevalence have not been adequately studied.

Clinical Features. Passive-aggressive persons characteristically procrastinate, resist demands for adequate performance, find excuses for delays, and find fault with those on whom they depend; yet they refuse to extricate themselves from the dependent relationship. They usually lack assertiveness and are not direct about their own needs or wishes. They fail to ask needed questions about what is expected of them and may become anxious when forced to succeed or when their usual defense of turning anger against themselves is removed.

In interpersonal relationships, passive-aggressive personalities attempt to manipulate themselves into a position of dependency, but their passive, self-detrimental behavior is often experienced by others as punitive and manipulative. Others must do their errands and carry out their routine responsibilities. Friends and clinicans may become enmeshed in trying to assuage the patient's many claims of unjust treatment. The close relationships of passive-aggressive personalities are rarely tranquil or happy. Because passive-aggressive personalities are bound to their resentment more closely than to their satisfaction, they may never even formulate what they want for themselves in regard to enjoyment.

According to DSM-III-R, people with this disorder lack self-confidence and are typically pessimistic about the future.

Diagnosis. The diagnostic criteria for passive-aggressive personality disorder are presented in Table 11.

Course and Prognosis. In a follow-up study, averaging 11 years, of 100 passive-aggressive inpatients, Small demonstrated that passive-aggressive personality was the primary diagnosis in 54 of them, 18 were also alcoholic, and 30 could be clinically labeled as depressed. Of the 73 former patients located, 58 (79 percent) had persistent psychiatric difficulties, and 9 (12 percent) were considered symptom free. Most seemed irritable, anxious, and depressed; somatic complaints were numerous. Only 32 (44 percent) were employed full time as workers or homemakers. Although neglect of responsibility and suicide attempts were common, only 1 patient had committed suicide in the interim. Although 28 (38 percent) were readmitted to a hospital, only 3 patients were called schizophrenic.

Differential Diagnosis. Passive-aggressive personality disorders need to be differentiated from histrionic and borderline patients; however, the passive-aggressive personality is less flamboyant, dramatic, affective, and openly aggressive than are the histrionic and borderline personalities. Patients with oppositional defiant disorder are similar to passive-aggressive personalities, but that diagnosis is reserved, according to DSM-III-R, to persons under age 18.

Treatment. Passive-aggressive patients who receive supportive psychotherapy have good outcomes. However, psychotherapy for patients with passive-aggressive personality disorder has many pitfalls: to fulfill their demands is often to support their pathology but to refuse their demands is to reject them. The therapy session can thus become a battleground in which the patient expresses feelings of resentment against a therapist on whom he or she wishes to become dependent. In passive-aggressive patients, it is important to treat suicide gestures as one would any covert expression of anger, and not as one would treat object loss in primary depression.

Table 11
Diagnostic Criteria for Passive-Aggressive Personality Disorder

A pervasive pattern of passive resistance to demands for adequate social and occupational performance, beginning by early adulthood and present in a variety of contexts, as indicated by at least *five* of the following:

(1) procrastinates, i.e., puts off things that need to be done so that deadlines are not met
(2) becomes sulky, irritable, or argumentative when asked to do something he or she does not want to do
(3) seems to work deliberately slowly or to do a bad job on tasks that he or she really does not want to do
(4) protests, without justification, that others make unreasonable demands on him or her
(5) avoids obligations by claiming to have "forgotten"
(6) believes that he or she is doing a much better job than others think he or she is doing
(7) resents useful suggestions from others concerning how he or she could be more productive
(8) obstructs the efforts of others by failing to do his or her share of the work
(9) unreasonably criticizes or scorns people in positions of authority

Table from DSM-III-R *Diagnostic and Statistical Manual of Mental Disorders*, ed 3, Revised. (Current Classification of Mental Disorders, 1987.) Copyright American Psychiatric Association, Washington, D.C., 1987. Used with permission.

Antidepressants should be prescribed only when there are clinical indications of depression and the possibility of suicide exists. The therapist must point out the probable consequences of passive-aggressive behaviors as they occur. Such confrontations may be more helpful in changing the patient's behavior than is a correct interpretation.

Personality Disorder Not Otherwise Specified

Personality disorder not otherwise specified includes disorders of personality functioning that cannot be classified as a specific personality disorder. In DSM-III this was called mixed personality disorder, a useful and frequently diagnosed personality disorder. A person may have features of more than one personality disorder that do not meet the full criteria for any one yet cause significant impairment in social or occupational functioning or subjective distress (Table 12).

This category can also be used when the clinician judges that a specific personality disorder is not included in any of the preceding categories or, for that matter, is not part of the official DSM-III-R nomenclature.

Sadomasochistic Personality. Some personality types are characterized by elements of sadism, masochism, or a combination of both. It is listed here because it is of major clinical and historical interest in psychiatry. It is not an official diagnostic category in DSM-III-R or its Appendix, but would be classified as personality disorder not otherwise classified.

Sadism (named after the Marquis de Sade, who wrote about persons who experienced sexual pleasure while inflicting pain on others) is the desire to cause others pain, by being either sexually abusive or physically or psychologically abusive in general. Freud believed that sadists ward off castration anxiety and are

Table 12
Diagnostic Criteria for Personality Disorder Not Otherwise Specified

Disorders of personality functioning that are not classifiable as a specific Personality Disorder. An example is features of more than one specific Personality Disorder that do not meet the full criteria for any one, yet cause significant impairment in social or occupational functioning, or subjective distress. In DSM-III, this was called Mixed Personality Disorder.

This category can also be used when the clinician judges that a specific Personality Disorder not included in this classification is appropriate, such as Impulsive Personality Disorder, Immature Personality Disorder, Self-Defeating Personality Disorder (see p. 444), or Sadistic Personality Disorder (see p. 445). In such instances the clinician should note the specific personality disorder in parentheses, e.g., Personality Disorder NOS (Self-defeating Personality Disorder).

Table from DSM-III-R *Diagnostic and Statistical Manual of Mental Disorders,* **ed 3, revised. (Current Classification of Mental Disorders, 1987.) Copyright American Psychiatric Association, Washington, D.C., 1987. Used with permission.**

able to achieve sexual pleasure only when they able to do to others what they fear will be done to them.

Masochism (named after Leopold Von Sacher–Masoch, a 19th-century Austrian novelist) is the achievement of sexual gratification by inflicting pain upon the self. More generally, the so-called moral masochist seeks humiliation and failure rather than physical pain.

Freud believed that masochists' ability to achieve orgasm is disturbed by anxiety and guilt feelings about sex that are alleviated by their own suffering and punishment.

Clinical observations indicate that elements of both sadistic and masochistic behavior are usually present in the same person. Treatment with insight-oriented psychotherapy, including psychoanalysis, has been effective in some cases. As a result of therapy, the patients become aware of the need for self-punishment secondary to excessive unconscious guilt and also come to recognize their repressed aggressive impulses, which originate in early childhood.

Self-Defeating Personality Disorder. DSM-III-R includes the self-defeating personality disorder in its Appendix for Diagnostic Categories Requiring Further Study. It is not considered an official part of DSM-III-R because it is controversial. In order to receive this diagnosis, an individual must have a pervasive pattern of self-defeating behavior, beginning by early adulthood and present in a variety of contexts. Such individuals may often avoid or undermine pleasurable experiences and be drawn to situations or relationships in which they will suffer.

Persons with this disorder choose persons and situations that lead to disappointment, failure, or mistreatment, even when better options are clearly available to them. They reject the attempts of others to offer help. After positive personal events (e.g., new achievement), these persons respond with depression, guilt, or a behavior that produces pain (e.g., an accident). They also invite rejecting responses from others and then feel hurt, defeated, or humiliated (e.g., they may make fun of their spouse in public, provoking an angry retort, and then feel devastated). In general, they engage in excessive self-sacrifice that is unsolicited and discouraged by others.

Self-defeating personalities do not derive any sexual pleasure from humiliation; those persons who do are classified as having a

Table 13
Diagnostic Criteria for Self-Defeating Personality Disorder

A. A pervasive pattern of self-defeating behavior, beginning by early adulthood and present in a variety of contexts. The person may often avoid or undermine pleasurable experiences, be drawn to situations or relationships in which he or she will suffer, and prevent others from helping him or her, as indicated by at least five of the following:
   (1) chooses people and situations that lead to disappointment, failure, or mistreatment even when better options are clearly available
   (2) rejects or renders ineffective the attempts of others to help him or her
   (3) following positive personal events (e.g., new achievement), responds with depression, guilt, or a behavior that produces pain (e.g., an accident)
   (4) incites angry or rejecting responses from others and then feels hurt, defeated, or humiliated (e.g., makes fun of spouse in public, provoking an angry retort, then feels devastated)
   (5) rejects opportunities for pleasure, or is reluctant to acknowledge enjoying himself or herself (despite having adequate social skills and the capacity for pleasure)
   (6) fails to accomplish tasks crucial to his or her personal objectives despite demonstrated ability to do so, e.g., helps fellow students write papers, but is unable to write his or her own
   (7) is uninterested in or rejects people who consistently treat him or her well, e.g., is unattracted to caring sexual partners
   (8) engages in excessive self-sacrifice that is unsolicited by the intended recipients of the sacrifice
B. The behaviors in A do not occur exclusively in response to, or in anticipation of, being physically, sexually, or psychologically abused.
C. The behaviors in A do not occur only when the person is depressed.

Table from DSM-III-R *Diagnostic and Statistical Manual of Mental Disorders,* **ed 3, revised. (Current Classification of Mental Disorders, 1987.) Copyright American Psychiatric Association, Washington, D.C., 1987. Used with permission.**

paraphilia. See Table 13 for the DSM-III-R diagnostic criteria for self-defeating personality disorder.

As mentioned above, the use of this diagnostic label (self-defeating personality disorder) is controversial, as there is concern that victims of abuse might be "blamed" for being abused when, in fact, they are true victims (i.e., blameless). There is also concern about whether a new diagnosis is necessary or whether the disorder could be subsumed under an existing classification.

J. Christopher Perry and George Vaillant believe that most patients diagnosed as self-defeating will concurrently meet the criteria for dependent or passive-aggressive personality disorders.

Because there are no studies of patients diagnosed by the most recent criteria, it is not possible to comment on the epidemiology of the disorder.

Sadistic Personality Disorder. Sadistic personality disorder is also a controversial addition to DSM-III-R. It is in the

Table 14
Diagnostic Criteria for Sadistic Personality Disorder

A. A pervasive pattern of cruel, demeaning, and aggressive behavior, beginning by early adulthood, as indicated by the repeated occurrence of at least four of the following:

(1) has used physical cruelty or violence for the purpose of establishing dominance in a relationship (not merely to achieve some noninterpersonal goal, such as striking someone in order to rob him or her)

(2) humiliates or demeans people in the presence of others

(3) has treated or disciplined someone under his or her control unusually harshly, e.g., a child, student, prisoner, or patient

(4) is amused by, or takes pleasure in, the psychological or physical suffering of others (including animals)

(5) has lied for the purpose of harming or inflicting pain on others (not merely to achieve some other goal)

(6) gets other people to do what he or she wants by frightening them (through intimidation or even terror)

(7) restricts the autonomy of people with whom he or she has a close relationship, e.g., will not let spouse leave the house accompanied or permit teen-age daughter to attend social functions

(8) is fascinated by violence, weapons, martial arts, injury, or torture

B. The behavior in A has not been directed toward only one person (e.g., spouse, one child) and has not been solely for the purpose of sexual arousal (as in Sexual Sadism).

Table from DSM-III-R *Diagnostic and Statistical Manual of Mental Disorders*, ed 3, revised. (Current Classification of Mental Disorders, 1987.) Copyright American Psychiatric Association, Washington, D.C., 1987. Used with permission.

appendix of DSM-III-R but is not a part of it. Persons with this personality show a pervasive pattern of cruel, demeaning, and aggressive behavior, beginning in early adulthood, that is directed toward others. Physical cruelty or violence is used to inflict pain on others and not to achieve some other goal (e.g., mugging someone in order to steal). Such persons like to humiliate or demean people in front of others and usually have treated or disciplined someone unusually harshly, especially children. In general, sadistic personalities are fascinated by violence, weapons, injury, or torture. To be included in this category, such persons are not supposed to derive sexual arousal from their behavior; if they do, a paraphilia should be diagnosed. See Table 14 for the DSM-III-R diagnostic criteria of sadistic personality disorder.

References

Gardner D, Lucas P B, Cowdry R W: Soft sign neurological abnormalities in borderline personality disorder and normal control subjects. J Nervous and Mental Dis *175*:177, 1987.

Hirschfeld R M A, sec editor: Personality disorders. In *Annual Review*, A J Frances, R E Hales, editors, vol. 5. American Psychiatry Press, Washington, DC, 1985.

Horowitz M: *Stress Response Syndromes*. Jason Aronson, New York, 1976.

Kernberg O: *Severe Personality Disorders: Psychotherapeutic Strategies*. Yale University Press, New Haven, CT, 1984.

Kohut H: *The Analysis of Self*. International University Press, New York, 1971.

Kohut H, Wolff E S: The disorders of the self and their treatment: An outline. Int J Psychoanal *59*:413, 1978.

Lion J R, ed.: *Personality Disorders, Diagnosis and Management*, ed 2, Williams and Wilkins, Baltimore, 1981.

McGlashan, T H: Testing DSM-III symptom criterion for schizotypal and borderline personality disorders. Arch Gen Psych *44*:143, 1987.

Millon T: *Disorders of Personality DSM III—Axis II*. Wiley, New York, 1981.

Perry J C: Depression in borderline personality disorders: Lifetime prevalence of interview and longitudinal course of symptoms. Am J Psychiatry *142*:15, 1982.

Reich J, Noyer, R Jr, Troughton E: Dependent personality disorder associated with phobic avoidance in patients with panic disorder. Am J Psych *144*:323, 1987.

Reich J: Sex distribution of DSM-III personality disorders in psych outpatients. Am J Psych *144*:485, 1987.

Vaillant, G E: *Adaptation to Life*. Little, Brown, Boston, 1977.

Waldinger R J: Intensive psychodynamic therapy with borderline patients: An overview. Am J Psych *144*:267, 1987.

Zuckerman M, Ballenger J C, Post R M: The neurobiology of some dimensions of personality. Int Rev Neurobiology *1*:391, 1984.

28

Conditions Not Attributable to a Mental Disorder

INTRODUCTION

As defined in DSM-III-R, conditions not attributable to a mental disorder have led to contact with the mental health care system, but without sufficient evidence to justify a diagnosis of any of the mental disorders noted previously. In some instances, one of these conditions will be noted because after thorough evaluation, no mental disorder has been found. In other instances, the diagnostic evaluation has not been able to determine adequately the presence or absence of a mental disorder, but there is a need to note the primary reason for contact with the mental health care system.

In some cases a mental disorder may eventually be found, but the focus of attention or treatment is on a condition that is not caused by a mental disorder. For example, a patient with an anxiety disorder may receive treatment for a marital problem that is unrelated to the anxiety disorder itself.

ANTISOCIAL BEHAVIOR

Definition

Antisocial behavior is characterized by activities that are illegal, immoral, or both and that violate the society's legal system. Examples include thievery, racketeering, drug dealing, and prostitution. According to DSM-III-R, the diagnosis should not be made if the behavior is caused by a mental disorder (e.g., conduct disorder, antisocial personality disorder) or a disorder of impulse control (e.g., kleptomania). In children and adolescents this condition is also known as juvenile delinquency.

Epidemiology

Estimates of the prevalence of antisocial behavior range from 5 to 15 percent of the population, depending on the criteria and sampling. Within the prison population, investigators report prevalence figures of between 20 and 80 percent.

Etiology

Antisocial behaviors in childhood and adulthood are characteristic of a variety of persons, ranging from those with no demonstrable psychopathology to those who are severely impaired, suffering from psychosis, organic brain syndromes, and retardation, among other conditions. A comprehensive neuropsychiatric assessment of antisocial persons usually reveals a myriad of potentially treatable psychiatric and neurological impairments that can easily be overshadowed by offensive behaviors and thus be overlooked. But as DSM-III-R cautions, only in the absence of organic, psychotic, neurotic, or intellectual impairment should patients be categorized as displaying antisocial behavior.

Antisocial behavior may be influenced by genetic, environmental, or psychological factors.

Genetic Factors. Data supporting the genetic transmission of antisocial behavior are based on studies that demonstrate a 60 percent concordance rate in monozygotic twins and about a 30 percent concordance rate in dizygotic twins. Adoption studies show a higher rate of antisocial behavior in the biological relatives of adoptees identified with antisocial behavior and a higher incidence of antisocial behavior in the adopted-away offspring of those with antisocial behavior.

There is a high incidence of abnormalities during the prenatal and perinatal periods in children who subsequently develop antisocial behavior. There also is an association between attention-deficit hyperactivity disorder and antisocial behavior.

Environmental Factors. Studies note that in neighborhoods in which low socioeconomic status (SES) families predominate, the sons of unskilled workers are more likely to commit more numerous and more serious criminal offenses than are the sons of middle-class or skilled workers, at least during adolescence and early adulthood. These data are not as clear for females, but the findings are generally similar in studies from many different countries. Areas of family training that have been particularly cited as differing by SES group are the use in middle-SES parents of more love-oriented techniques in discipline, the withdrawal of affection versus physical punishment, negative parental attitudes toward aggressive behavior, and more attempts to curb it, and the verbal ability to communicate the various reasons for the values and proscriptions of behavior.

Delinquent children are more likely to come from broken homes. Indeed, homes broken by divorce or separation seem to produce higher rates of delinquency than do homes disrupted by the death of a parent. Thus, the important factor seems to be family discord and disharmony rather than parental absence.

Psychological Factors. If the parenting experience is poor, children will experience emotional deprivation, which leads to low self-esteem and unconscious anger. They are not given any limits, and their consciences are deficient because they have not internalized parental prohibitions that account for superego formation. Therefore they have so-called superego lacunae, which allow them to commit antisocial acts without guilt. At times, such children's antisocial behavior represents a vicarious source of pleasure and gratification for parents who act out through the children their own forbidden wishes and impulses.

Clinical Features

Persons with antisocial behaviors have difficulties in work, marriage, money matters, and conflicts with various authorities. The adult symptoms of antisocial (also known as sociopathic) behavior are summarized in Table 1.

The childhood behaviors most associated with antisocial behavior are theft, incorrigibility, truancy, running away, associating with undesirable persons, and staying out late at night. The greater the number of symptoms present in childhood is, the greater the probability of adult antisocial behavior will be; however, the presence of greater numbers of symptoms is also indicative of the development of other psychiatric illnesses in adult life.

Diagnosis

The diagnosis of antisocial behavior is one of exclusion. The intertwining of alcoholism and drug dependence in such behavior often makes it difficult to separate out the antisocial behavior, related primarily to drug abuse or alcoholism, from disordered behavior that occurred either before drug or alcohol use or during episodes unrelated to alcoholism or drug abuse.

During the manic phases of bipolar disorder, certain aspects of behavior can be similar to antisocial behavior, such as wanderlust, sexual promiscuity, and financial difficulty. Schizophrenia, especially in childhood, may often manifest itself as antisocial behavior. Adult schizophrenic patients may have episodes of anti-social behavior, but the symptom picture is usually clear, especially with regard to thought disorder, delusions, and hallucinations on the mental status examination.

Neurological conditions may cause antisocial behavior, and so EEGs, CT scans, and a complete neurological examination should be done. Temporal lobe epilepsy is often considered in the differential diagnosis. When a clear-cut diagnosis of temporal lobe epilepsy or encephalitis can be made, that may account for the antisocial behavior.

Conduct disorder, which should be differentiated from antisocial disorder, is discussed in Section 36.1. Antisocial personality disorder is discussed in Chapter 27.

Treatment

In general, antisocial behavior provokes great therapeutic pessimism. That is, it is difficult for therapists to have much hope of changing a pattern of behavior that has been present almost continuously throughout the patient's life. Psychotherapy has not been effective, and there have been no major breakthroughs with biological treatments, including the use of medications.

There is more enthusiasm for the use of therapeutic communities and other forms of group treatment, even though the data provide little basis for enthusiasm. Many delinquents and adult criminals who are incarcerated and in institutional settings have shown some response to group therapy approaches. The history of violence, criminality, and antisocial behavior has shown that they seem to decrease after age 40. Recidivism in criminals, which can reach 90 percent in some studies, also decreases in middle age.

ACADEMIC PROBLEM

Definition

The term academic problem is listed in the DSM-III-R as a condition in which the focus or attention of treatment is an academic problem that is apparently not due to a mental disorder. Examples include failing grades and underachievement in a person with adequate intellectual capacity. In order to make the diagnosis, there must not be another mental disorder that would account for the problem.

Etiology

Academic problems may result from a variety of causes and may arise at any time in life, although they occur most often between the ages of 5 and 21, a span that includes the school years.

During this period, the school setting occupies a major portion of the person's time. School is an important social and educational instrument, being interconnected with the major developmental issues of childhood, adolescence, and young adulthood. Boys and girls must cope with the process of separation, adjustment to new environments, adaptation to social contacts, competition, assertion, intimacy, and a myriad of other issues. There is often a reciprocal relationship between how well these developmental tasks are mastered and the level of school performance.

Achievement-related anxiety represents a significant source of academic problems. In psychoanalytic terms, some students exhibit evidence of inner conflict believed to be connected with the Oedipus complex. Described by Freud as "those wrecked by success," such persons fear the consequences that are imagined to accompany

Table 1
Adult Symptoms of Antisocial Behavior

Life Area	Percentage of Antisocials with Significant Problems in This Area
Work problems	85
Marital problems	81
Financial dependency	79
Arrests	75
Alcohol abuse	72
School problems	71
Impulsiveness	67
Sexual behavior	64
Wild adolescence	62
Vagrancy	60
Belligerency	58
Social isolation	56
Military record (of those serving)	53
Lack of guilt	40
Somatic complaints	31
Use of aliases	29
Pathological lying	16
Drug abuse	15
Suicide attempts	11

*Data from L. Robins: *Deviant Children Grown Up: A Sociological and Psychiatric Study of Sociopathic Personality.* Williams & Wilkins, Baltimore, 1966.

the attainment of success. Behaviorists may interpret the conflict as a learned disposition to fear success. An example might be a woman whose motive to avoid success in school is linked to a fear of social rejection or loss of femininity or both, especially when success necessitates aggression and competition with males.

The loss of parents as substitute teachers and the diminished role of the parents themselves as a primary reference group may also undermine academic efforts. Studies revealed that boredom in school is often the result of identity diffusion. Lacking any real and stable sense of themselves and their goals, students become bored and unable to perform their student role.

The teachers' expectations concerning their students' performance influence that performance. Teachers serve as causal agents whose varying expectations can shape the differential development of students' skills and abilities. Such conditioning early in school, especially if negative, can disturb academic performance. Thus, a teacher's affective response to a child can prompt the appearance of academic problems. Most important is the teacher's humane approach to the student. This applies to all levels of education, including medical school.

Treatment

Although not considered a diagnosable psychiatric disorder, academic problems can best be alleviated by psychological means. Psychotherapeutic techniques can be used successfully for scholastic difficulties, including those related to poor motivation, poor self-concept, and underachievement.

Early efforts at relieving the problem should outweigh all other considerations, as sustained problems in learning and school performance frequently are compounded and precipitate more severe difficulties. Feelings of anger, frustration, shame, loss of self-respect, and helplessness—emotions that most often accompany school failures—emotionally and cognitively damage self-esteem, disabling future performance and clouding expectations for success.

Tutoring is an extremely effective technique in dealing with academic problems and should be considered in all cases. Tutoring is of proven value in preparing for objective multiple-choice examinations, such as the SAT, MCAT, and National Boards. Diminishing anxiety by repetitively taking such examinations or by using relaxation skills are two behavioral techniques of great value.

Academic problems should be differentiated from adjustment disorder with academic or work inhibition, which is characterized by a change from previously adequate academic or work performance after a psychosocial stressor. That disorder is discussed in Chapter 25.

BORDERLINE INTELLECTUAL FUNCTIONING

As described in DSM-III-R, borderline intellectual functioning can be identified when the focus of attention or treatment is based on a deficit in functioning associated with borderline intellectual functioning, defined as an I.Q. in the 71 to 84 range. The problem is often masked when a mental disorder is present, especially the residual type of schizophrenia.

Only about 6 to 7 percent of the population are found to have a borderline I.Q., as determined by the Stanford-Binet test or the Wechsler scales. The premise behind the inclu-

sion of this category is that these persons may experience difficulties in their adaptive capacities, which may ultimately produce impaired social and vocational functioning. Thus, in the absence of specific intrapsychic conflicts, developmental traumas, biochemical abnormalities, or other factors linked to mental disorder, such persons may experience severe emotional distress. Frustration and embarrassment over their difficulties may shape their life choices and lead to circumstances warranting psychiatric intervention.

Once the underlying problem is known to the therapist, psychiatric treatment can be quite useful. Many persons with borderline intellectual functioning are able to function at a superior level in some areas while being markedly deficient in others. By directing such persons to appropriate areas of endeavor, by pointing out socially acceptable behavior, and by teaching them living skills, the therapist can help improve their self-esteem.

MALINGERING

Definition

Malingering is characterized by the voluntary production and presentation of false or grossly exaggerated physical or psychological symptoms. There is always an external motivation, which falls into one of three categories: (1) to avoid difficult or dangerous situations, responsibilities, or punishment; (2) to receive compensation, free hospital room and board, a source of drugs, or haven from the police; and (3) to retaliate when the victim feels guilt or suffers a financial loss, legal penalty, or job loss. The presence of a clearly definable goal is the main factor that differentiates malingering from a factitious illness.

Epidemiology

The incidence of malingering is unknown, but it is not uncommon. It occurs most frequently in settings in which there is a preponderance of men—the military, prisons, factories, and other industrial settings—although it also occurs in women.

Diagnosis

According to DSM-III-R, malingering should be strongly suspected if any combination of the following is noted: (1) medicolegal context of presentation (e.g., the person's being referred by his or her attorney to the physican for examination); (2) marked discrepancy between the person's claimed stress or disability and the objective findings; (3) lack of cooperation during the diagnostic evaluation and in complying with the prescribed treatment regimen; and (4) the presence of antisocial personality disorder.

Many malingerers express mostly subjective, vague, ill-defined symptoms—for example, headache; pains of the neck, lower back, chest, or abdomen; dizziness; vertigo; amnesia; anxiety; and depression—and symptoms often having a family history, in all likelihood not organically based but incredibly difficult to refute. Malingerers may complain bitterly, describing how much the symptoms impair their normal function and how much they are disliked. They may use the very best doctors, who are the most trusted (and perhaps most easily fooled), and promptly and willingly pay all their bills, even if excessive, to impress them with their integrity. To seem credible, malingerers must give the same report of symptoms but tell their physicians as little as possible. But often they complain of misery without objective signs or other symptoms congruent with recognized diseases or syndromes; if they do describe all symptoms, the symptoms are said to come and go. Malingerers are often preoccupied with cash, rather than cure, and have a knowledge of the law and precedents relative to their claims.

Objective tests—such as audiometry, brain stem audiometry, auditory and visually evoked potentials, galvanic skin response, electromyography, and nerve conduction studies—may be helpful in sorting out auditory, labyrinthine, ophthalmological, neurological, and other problems.

Differential Diagnosis

According to DSM-III-R, malingering differs from factitious disorder in that there are external incentives in malingering, whereas in factitious disorder, there is an absence of external incentives. Rather, evidence of an intrapsychic need to maintain the sick role suggests factitious disorder.

Conversion and somatoform disorders do not show intentionality; there are no obvious, external incentives. Moreover, the symptoms in malingering are less likely to be symbolically related to an underlying emotional conflict.

Treatment

A patient suspected of malingering should be thoroughly and objectively evaluated, and the physician should refrain from demonstrating his or her suspicions. If the doctor becomes angry (a common response to malingerers), a confrontation may occur, with two consequences: (1) The doctor–patient relationship is disrupted, and no further positive intervention is possible. (2) The patient will be even more on guard, and proof of deception may become virtually impossible. If the patient is accepted and not discredited, subsequent observation, while hospitalized or an outpatient, may reveal the versatility of the symptoms, which are consistently present only when the patient knows he or she is being observed. Preserving the doctor–patient relationship is often essential to the diagnosis and long-term management of the patient. Careful evaluation usually reveals the relevant issue without the need for a confrontation. It is usually best to use an intensive treatment approach, as though the symptoms were real. The symptoms can then be given up in response to treatment, without the patient's losing face.

MARITAL PROBLEMS

According to DSM-III-R, the category of marital problems can be used when the focus of attention or treatment is a marital problem that is apparently not due to a mental disorder.

One of the evaluations that the clinician must make is whether the presenting complaint is engendered by the marriage or is part of a greater disturbance. The developmental, family, sexual, personal, and occupational history, as well as the marital history, should be enlightening in this regard.

Marriage involves many stressful situations that tax the partners' adaptive capacities. If the partners have different backgrounds and have been raised in different value systems, conflicts are more likely to arise than if they have similar backgrounds. The areas to be explored include sexual relations; attitudes toward contraception, childbearing, and child rearing; handling of money; relations with in-laws; and attitudes toward social life. One possible problem period in a marriage is precipitated by the birth of children, especially the first child, as it is a stressful time for both parents. Economic stresses, moves to new areas, unplanned pregnancies, and abortions may upset a seemingly healthy marriage. Differing attitudes toward religion can also present a problem.

The institution of marriage is influenced by cultural changes. When there are external pressures to remain married for religious, economic, or family reasons, the pair may be willing to seek counseling. A new factor is the fear of AIDS, which for many persons limits their extramarital sexual behavior. It may serve as motivation for improving a relationship, or it may contribute to the distress of the partner whose marital stability was precariously predicated on such behavior. The effects of these fears require further research.

NONCOMPLIANCE WITH MEDICAL TREATMENT

Compliance, also known as adherence, is the degree to which a patient carries out the clinical recommendations of the treating physician. Examples include keeping appointments, entering into and completing a treatment program, taking medications correctly, and following recommended changes in behavior or diet. Compliance behavior depends on the specific clinical situation, the nature of the illness, and the treatment program. In general, approximately one third of patients comply with treatment; one third sometimes comply with certain aspects of treatment; and one third never comply with treatment. An overall figure assessed from a number of studies indicates that 54 percent of patients will comply with treatment at any given time. A study of compliance among hypertensive patients indicates that up to 50 percent of such patients do not follow up at all with treatment, and 50 percent of those who do follow up will leave treatment within 1 year.

In an attempt to understand why such a high percentage of patients fails to comply regularly, a number of variables have been investigated. For example, an increased complexity of regimen, plus an increased number of required behavioral changes, appear to be associated with noncompliance. Psychiatric patients also exhibit a higher degree of noncompliant behavior than do medical patients. However, there is no clear association between compliance and the patient's sex, marital status, race, religion, socioeconomic status, intelligence, or educational level. Compliance is increased by such physician characteristics as enthusiasm, permissiveness, age, experience, time spent talking to the patient, and short waiting room time.

The doctor–patient relationship, or what has been termed the doctor–patient "match," is the most important factor in compliance issues. When the doctor and the patient have different priorities and beliefs, different styles of communication including a different understanding of medical advice, and different medical expectations, the patient's compliance diminishes. Compliance can be increased if the physician can ascertain both the value to the patient of a particular treatment outcome and his or her expectation that a given recommendation will produce that outcome. Compliance can also increase if the patient knows the names and the effects of each drug he or she is taking. A highly significant factor in compliance seems to be the patient's subjective feeling of distress or illness, as opposed to the doctor's often more objective, medical estimate of disease and required therapy. The patient must believe that he or she is ill. Thus, asymptomatic patients such as those with hypertension will be at greater risk for noncompliance. Simply stated, when there are problems in communication, compliance decreases; when there is effective communication, coupled with close patient supervision and the patient's subjective sense of satisfaction that the doctor has met expectations, compliance increases. Studies have shown that noncompliance is associated with doctors who are perceived as rejecting and unfriendly. Noncompliance is also associated with asking a patient for information without giving feedback, and failing to explain a diagnosis or the cause of the presenting symptoms. A doctor who is aware of the patient's belief system, feelings, and habits and who enlists the patient in establishing a treatment regimen will increase compliant behavior.

Strategies suggested to improve compliance include asking patients directly to describe what they themselves believe is wrong with them, what they believe should be done, what they understand about what the doctor believes should be done, and what they believe to be the risks and benefits of following the prescribed treatment. Common errors are patients' not taking medications as often or as long as they are supposed to, as well as not taking the right number of pills or treatments. Patients are generally noncompliant if they have to take more than three types of medications a day or if their medications must be taken more than four times a day. Purely verbal instructions by the doctor or the presentation of treatment prescriptions to the patient in the few hours immediately before being discharged from the hospital is associated with increased error. Elderly people who may have trouble hearing or reading small type may become noncompliant if they cannot hear verbal instructions or read prescription labels. In these instances, it has proved helpful to print the instructions on a piece of paper, ask the patient to read them back, ask if there are any questions, and ask the patient to explain when specifically and in what amounts the medication is to be taken. Sometimes instead of errors, patients will deliberately change the treatment regimen, such as not showing up for appointments or taking medications differently than recommended. In these instances, in which there may be competing pressures from family or work, or lack of understanding about the details of the doctor's advice, the doctor will need to negotiate a compromise with the patient, or what has been termed a "patient contract." In this case, the doctor and patient together will specify what they can expect from each other. Implicit in this approach is the idea that the contract can be renegotiated, and the patient can be assured that suggestions can be made by either the doctor or the patient to improve compliance.

OCCUPATIONAL PROBLEMS

According to DSM-III-R, the category of occupational problems is used when the focus of attention or treatment is an occupational problem that is apparently not due to a

mental disorder. Examples are job dissatisfaction and uncertainties about career choices.

An occupational history is part of the total psychiatric interview. On occasion, dissatisfaction with work is the presenting complaint. Because some work situations can be stressful and unpleasant in themselves, because there is evidence that mental effort under such conditions can produce emotional problems, and because economic necessity may force people to accept work essentially distasteful to them, it is possible for someone with this complaint to be otherwise psychiatrically normal.

Maladaption at work may arise from psychodynamic conflicts, which can be reflected in the patient's inability to accept the authority of competent superiors or, conversely, in an over-dependency on authority figures to fulfill infantile needs. People with unresolved conflicts over their competitive and aggressive impulses may have great difficulty in the work area. They may suffer from a pathological envy of others' success or fear success for themselves. These conflicts are also manifest in other areas of life as well, and so the maladaptation is not limited to occupation.

Job-related stress is most likely to develop when work objectives are not clear, when workers are pressured by conflicting demands, when they have too much or too little to do, and when they are responsible for the professional development of others and have little control over decisions that affect them.

Special problems to be considered are the adjustments of those about to face retirement, the dissatisfaction of the housewife, and the minority group member blocked from position or advancement because of sex, race, religion, or ethnic background.

PARENT–CHILD PROBLEMS

According to DSM-III-R, parent–child problems can apply to either a parent or a child when they are apparently not due to a mental disorder of the person being evaluated.

Difficulties can arise in a variety of situations that stress the usual parent–child interaction beyond the adaptations necessary for individual development. For instance, in a family in which the parents are divorced, parent–child problems may arise in the relationship with either the custodial or the noncustodial parent. The remarriage of a divorced or widowed parent can also lead to a parent–child problem. The resentment of a stepparent and the favoring of a natural child are usual in the initial phases of adjustment of a new family.

Other situations that may cause a parent–child problem are the development of a fatal, crippling, or chronic illness in either the parent or the child, such as leukemia, epilepsy, sickle-cell anemia, spinal cord injury, or the birth of a child with congenital defects (e.g., cerebral palsy, blindness, deafness). Although these situations are not rare, they challenge the emotional resources of the people involved. The parents and the child have to face present and potential loss and adjust their day-to-day lives physically, economically, and emotionally. These situations can try the healthiest families and produce parent–child problems, not just with the affected child, but with the unaffected siblings as well. These siblings may be resented, preferred, or neglected because the ill child requires so much time and attention.

OTHER SPECIFIED FAMILY CIRCUMSTANCES

According to DSM-III-R, other specified family circumstances can be used when the focus of attention or treatment is apparently not due to a mental disorder and is not a parent–child or a marital problem.

For instance, a particular stress may arise in dual-career families. The mothers in these families—defined as families in which both spouses have careers, rather than jobs—are found to be particularly vulnerable to guilt and anxiety regarding their maternal role. These women usually accept middle-class or upper-middle-class values that emphasize the importance of the child's individual development and psychological health. The middle-class family system is particularly demanding of the wife and mother who has significant time commitments outside the home.

Another stressful family situation may develop when adults must care for aging parents. Adults often assume this responsibility while they are still caring for their own children. Such an adaptation involves the adjustment to a reversal of roles, recognition of the aging and potential loss of the parent, and coping with the evidence of one's own mortality.

Other circumstances that overlap the categories of marital problems and parent–child problems include families with steprelations, adoptive families, families with special children, and families whose members have significantly differing values, in which there are immigrant parents and native born children or in which family members belong to different religious groups.

OTHER INTERPERSONAL PROBLEMS

The category of other interpersonal problems can be used when the focus of attention or treatment is an interpersonal problem (other than marital or parent–child) that is apparently not due to a mental disorder.

Problems causing sufficient strain to bring a person into contact with the mental health care system may arise in relations with romantic partners, co-workers, neighbors, teachers, students, friends, and social groups. The stress-inducing circumstances, coping mechanisms, and symptoms that have brought someone to seek consultation or treatment must be individually evaluated.

PHASE OF LIFE PROBLEMS OR OTHER LIFE CIRCUMSTANCE PROBLEMS

According to DSM-III-R, phase of life problems or other life circumstance problems can be used when the focus of attention or treatment is due to problems related to stresses in the life cycle.

External events are most likely to overwhelm a person's adaptive capacities if they are unexpected, if they are numerous—that is, a number of stresses occurring within a short time—if the strain is chronic and unremitting, or if one loss actually heralds a myriad of concomitant adjustments that strain a person's recuperative powers.

The strains most likely to produce anxiety and depression relate to major life cycle changes: marriage, occupation, and parenthood. Those events affect both men and women, but women, the poor,

and minority groups seemed particularly vulnerable to adverse reactions. Again, the change creates significant strain when it is unexpected and when it involves not only adjustment to a loss (spouse or job) but also the need to adjust to a new status that entails further hardships and problems.

In general, people have demonstrated their ability to adjust to life changes if they have mature defense mechanisms, such as altruism, humor, and a capacity for sublimation. Flexibility, reliability, strong family ties, regular employment, adequate income, job satisfaction, a pattern of regular recreation and social participation, realistic goals, and a history of adequate performance—in short, a full and satisfying life—create resilience to deal with life changes.

There is some suggestion that periods of cultural transition, with changing mores and fluidity of role definition, increase the individual's vulnerability to life strain. Extreme cultural transition can create a condition of severe distress. This problem, also called culture shock, occurs when a person is suddenly thrust into an alien culture or has divided loyalties to two different cultures. On a less extreme basis, culture shock occurs when young men enter the army, when people change jobs, when families move or undergo a significant change in income, when children have their first day in school, and when black ghetto children are bused to white middle-class schools.

Persons undergoing culture shock experience a variety of emotions—isolation, anxiety, and depression—often accompanied by a sense of loss close to mourning. The degree of adjustment that such persons can make to their new environment depends on their underlying personality structure and strengths. For a further discussion of these issues, see Chapter 25 on Adjustment Disorders.

UNCOMPLICATED BEREAVEMENT

Immediately or within a few months after the loss of a loved one, a normal period of bereavement or grief begins. Feelings of sadness, preoccupation with thoughts about the deceased, tearfulness, irritability, insomnia, and difficulties in concentrating and carrying out one's daily activities are some of the signs and symptoms. A grief reaction is limited to a varying period of time based on one's cultural group (usually no longer than 6 months). Normal grief, however, may lead to a full depressive syndrome, which requires treatment.

References

Bash I Y, Alpert M: The determination of malingering. Ann NY Acad Sci 347:86, 1980.
Gittleman R, Feinbold I: Children with reading disorders. I. Efficacy of reading remediation. J Child Psychol Psychiatry 24:167, 1983.
Gorman W F: Defining malingering. J Forensic Sci 27:401, 1982.
Grant I, Yager J, Sweetwood H, Olshen R: Life events and symptoms. Arch Gen Psychiatry 39:598, 1982.
Holmes T: Life situations, emotions, and disease. J Acad Psychosom Med 19:747, 1978.
Karabenick S A: Fear of success, achievement and affiliation dispositions and the performance of men and women under individual and competitive conditions. J Pers 45:117, 1977.
Lewis D O, editor: Vulnerabilities to Delinquency. Spectrum Publications, New York, 1981.
Lieberman M, Pearlin L: Life stresses. Am J Community Psychol 6:1, 1978.
Pincus J H, Tucker G J: Behavioral Neurology, ed 3, Oxford University Press, New York, 1985.
Vaillant G: Adaptation to Life. Little, Brown, Boston, 1977.

29

Psychiatric Emergencies

29.1

Suicide

INTRODUCTION

Suicidal patients are probably the most frequent cause of psychiatric emergencies and are difficult to identify with certainty. They are often unmanageable in an outpatient setting, resistant to hospitalization, and subject to recurrent crises in management. A thorough knowledge of the demographics of suicidal patients will help the clinician recognize potential victims.

EPIDEMIOLOGY

Incidence and Prevalence

In 1985, about 28,500 deaths were attributed to suicide in the United States. This figure represents successful suicides; the number of attempted suicides is estimated to exceed that number by eight to ten times. Lost in the reporting are the intentional misclassification of cause of death, accidents of undetermined cause, and the so-called chronic suicides—for example, alcoholism, drug abuse, and consciously poor adherence to medical regimens for diabetes, obesity, and hypertension.

Between 1970 and 1980, there were over 230,000 suicides in the United States—about 1 every 20 minutes. The total suicide rate has remained fairly constant over the years. The rate in 1970 was 11.6 suicide deaths per 100,000; in 1980, it was 11.9 deaths per 100,000; and in 1985, it was 12.5 per 100,000 persons. In 1977, suicide was at a peak of 13.3 per 100,000. Since then, there has been a slight decline. Currently, suicide is ranked as the eighth overall cause of death in this country, after heart disease, cancer, stroke, accidents, pneumonia, diabetes mellitus, and cirrhosis.

Suicide rates in the United States are at the midpoint of national rates reported to the United Nations by industrialized countries. Internationally, suicide rates range from highs of more than 25 per 100,000 people in Scandanavia, Switzerland, West Germany, Austria, the Eastern European countries (the suicide belt), and Japan to fewer than 10 per 100,000 in Spain, Italy, Ireland, Egypt, and the Netherlands.

A state-by-state analysis of suicides from 1979 to 1981 among those aged 15 to 44 revealed that New Jersey had the nation's lowest suicide rates for both sexes. Nevada and New Mexico had the highest rates for men, and Nevada and Wyoming, the highest rates for women. Women in Nevada killed themselves at a higher frequency than did men in New Jersey.

Sex. Men commit suicide more than three times as often as do women, a rate that is stable over all ages. Women, on the other hand, are four times as likely to attempt suicide as are men.

Methods. The higher rate of successful suicide for men is related to the methods they use. Men use firearms, hanging, or jumping from high places. Women are more likely to take an overdose of drugs or a poison, but they are beginning to use firearms more often. The use of guns has decreased as a method of suicide in those states with gun control laws.

Age. The significance of the mid-life crisis is underscored by suicide rates. Among men, suicides peak and continue to rise after age 45; among women, the greatest number of completed suicides occurs after age 55. Rates of 40 per 100,000 population are found in men age 65 and older. The elderly attempt suicide less often than do younger people but are successful more often. The elderly account for 25 percent of the suicides, although they make up only 10 percent of the total population. The rate for those 75 or older is more than three times the rate of that among the young.

The suicide rate is rising most rapidly in young people. For males 15 to 24 years old, there was a 40 percent increase between 1970 and 1980, and it is still rising. The suicide rate for females in the same age group showed only a slight increase. Among males 25 to 34 years old, the suicide rate increased almost 30 percent. Suicide is the third leading cause of death in the 15- to 24-year-old group after accidents and homicides. Attempted suicides in this age group number between 1 and 2 million annually. The majority of suicides now occur among those aged 15 to 44.

Race. The rate of suicide among whites is nearly twice that among nonwhites, but these figures are being questioned, as the suicide rate among blacks is increasing. Among ghetto youth and certain native American and Alaskan Indian groups, suicide rates have greatly exceeded the national rate. Suicide among immigrants is higher than in the native-born population. Two out of every three suicides are white males.

Religion. Historically, suicide rates among Catholic populations have been lower than rates among Protestants and Jews. It may be that a religion's degree of orthodoxy and integration is a more accurate measure of risk in this category than is simple institutional religious affiliation.

Marital Status. Marriage reinforced by children seems to lessen significantly the risk of suicide. Among married persons, the rate is 11 per 100,000. Single, never-married persons register an overall rate of nearly double the rate of married persons. However, previously married persons show sharply higher rates than do never-married persons: 24 per 100,000 among the widowed; 40 per 100,000 among divorced persons, with divorced men registering 69 suicides per 100,000, as compared with 18 per 100,000 for divorced women. Suicide is more common in persons who have a history of suicide (attempted or real) in the family and who are socially isolated. So-called anniversary suicides are suicides by persons who take their lives on the same day as did a member of their family.

Occupation. Among occupational rankings with respect to risk for suicide, professionals, and particularly physicians, have traditionally been considered to stand out. Among physicians, psychiatrists are considered to be at greatest risk, followed by ophthalmologists and anesthesiologists, but the trend is toward an equalization among all specialties. Special at-risk populations are musicians, dentists, law enforcement officers, lawyers, and insurance agents. Suicide is higher among unemployed persons than among employed persons. During economic recessions, depressions, and times of high unemployment, the suicide rate increases. During times of high employment and during war, the rate decreases. The suicide rate is also high among prisoners, especially those who have no visitors.

Climate. No seasonal correlation with suicide has been found. There is a slight increase in the spring and fall, but contrary to popular belief, there is no increase in suicide during December or holiday periods.

Physical Health. The relationship of physical health and illness to suicide is significant. Prior medical care appears to be a positively correlated risk indicator of suicide. 32 percent of suicides have had medical attention within 6 months of death. Seventy percent of victims have suffered one or more active—and, for the most part, chronic illnesses at the time of death. Among the suicide attempts studied, more than one third of the persons were actively ill at the time of the attempt, and more than 90 percent of the attempts were influenced by the illness. A particular group at risk are patients on renal dialysis. Factors associated with illness and contributing to both suicides and attempts are loss of mobility among persons to whom physical activity is occupationally or recreationally important; disfigurement, particularly among women; and chronic, intractable pain. In addition to the direct effects of illness, it has been noted that the secondary effects of illness—for example, disruption of relationships and loss of occupational status—are prognostic factors.

Certain drugs can produce depression, which may lead to suicide in some cases. Among these are reserpine, corticosteroids, antihypertensives (e.g., propranolol), and some anticancer agents.

Mental Health. Highly significant factors in suicide also include alcoholism, other drug abuse, depression, schizophrenia, and other mental illnesses.

Almost 95 percent of patients who commit or attempt suicide have a diagnosed mental illness. Depressive disorders account for 80 percent of that figure; schizophrenia for 10 percent; and dementia or delirium for 5 percent. Patients who suffer from delusional depression are at the highest risk for suicide. The risk of suicide in patients with depressive disorder is about 15 percent. Twenty-five percent of all suicides who have a history of impulsive behavior or violent acts are also at high risk for suicide. Previous psychiatric hospitalization for any reason increases the risk of suicide.

Suicide Attempts. There are eight times more suicide attempts than successful suicides, and about 70 percent of these attempts are made by women. Most are made by depressed young adults. About 1 percent of persons who attempt suicide eventually kill themselves, but 30 percent make subsequent attempts. The risk of a patient's making a second suicide attempt is highest within 3 months of the first attempt.

The suicide attempt often represents a kind of psychological drama. The communication of the suicidal intent is often an integral part of the method employed. Such communication can be coercive, can be a cry for help, or can involve a gamble with death in which another person is empowered to decide whether the potential suicide will live or die. Disorganized or multiple suicide methods or those carried out in a chaotic manner and lasting several days are usually chosen by disorganized, schizoid, or schizotypal patients.

THEORIES OF SUICIDE

Sociological Factors

Durkheim. The first major contribution to the study of suicide was made at the end of the last century by the French sociologist Émile Durkheim. In an attempt to explain the statistical patterns, Durkheim divided suicides into three social categories: egoistic, altruistic, and anomic. Egoistic suicide applies to those who are not strongly integrated into any social group. The lack of family integration can be used to explain why the unmarried are more vulnerable to suicide than are the married and why couples with children are the best protected group of all. Rural communities have more social integration than do urban areas, and thus less suicide. Protestantism is a less-cohesive religion than Catholicism is, and so Protestants have a higher suicide rate than do Catholics.

Altruistic suicide describes the group whose proneness to suicide stems from their excessive integration into a group. That is, Durkheim had in mind the kind of suicide that some people expect of certain classes in Japanese society.

Anomic suicide applies to those persons whose integration with society is disturbed, thereby depriving them of the customary norms of behavior. Anomie can explain why the greatest incidence of suicide is among the divorced, as compared with the married, and why those whose economic situation has changed drastically are more vulnerable. Anomie also refers to social unstability with a breakdown of society's standards and values.

Psychological Factors

Freud. The first important psychological insight into suicide came from Freud. He described only one patient who actually made a suicide attempt, but he did see many depressed patients. In his 1917 paper, *Mourning and Melancholia,* Freud stated that the self-hatred seen in depression originated in anger toward a love object, anger that such persons turned back on themselves. Freud regarded suicide as the ultimate form of this phenomenon and doubted that there would be a suicide without the earlier repressed desire to kill someone else.

Menninger. Building on Freud's concepts, Karl Menninger in *Man Against Himself* conceived of suicide as a retroflexed murder, inverted homicide as a result of the patient's anger toward another person, which is either turned inward or used as an excuse for punishment. He also described a self-directed death instinct (Freud's concept of *thanatos*).

The relationship between suicide and depression can be best understood by the need for atonement that can underlie both. Depressed persons may attempt suicide just as they appear to be recovering from their depression. And a suicide attempt can cause a long-standing depression to disappear, especially if it fulfills the patient's need for punishment. That is, one form of atonement appears to substitute for another. Of equal relevance, many suicide patients use a preoccupation with suicide as a way of fighting off intolerable depression and a sense of hopelessness. In fact, hopelessness was found, in a study by Aaron Beck, to be one of the most accurate indicators of long-term suicidal risks.

Persons who have survived suicide attempts have provided important clues to the psychodynamics of suicide. Edwin Schneidman and Neal Farberow (two eminent suicidologists) divided suicides into four groups: (1) patients who conceive of suicide as a means to a better life; (2) patients who commit suicide as a result of psychosis with associated delusions or hallucinations; (3) patients who commit suicide out of revenge against a loved person; and (4) patients who are old, infirm, or both, for whom suicide is a release.

Other Theories. Suicide may also represent a need to atone for a real or imagined crime. Some patients who kill themselves hope for a reunion with a loved one who has died. Others hope to punish or to make those whom they leave behind feel guilty.

Physiological Factors

Genetics. A genetic factor in suicide has been suggested. In one study of 51 monozygotic twin pairs, there were nine cases of suicide, and no dizygotic twins were concordant for suicide. A longitudinal study of an Amish community found 26 suicides committed in just four families, all of whom exhibited heavy genetic loading for unipolar, bipolar, and other mood disorders. Whether the genetic loading in those families was for suicide or for

mood disorders associated with suicide remains to be determined.

Neurochemistry. A serotonin deficiency, measured as a decrease in the metabolism 5-hydroxyindole acetic acid (5-HIAA), was found in a subgroup of depressed patients who attempted suicide. Those patients who attempted suicide by violent means (e.g., guns, jumping) had a lower 5-HIAA level in the cerebrospinal fluid than did those depressed patients who were not suicidal or who attempted suicide in a less violent manner (e.g., drug overdose). A few studies have demonstrated ventricular enlargement and abnormal EEGs in some suicidal patients.

Blood samples analyzed for platelet monoamine oxidase, from a group of normal volunteers, revealed that those persons with the lowest level of this enzyme in their platelets had eight times the prevalence of suicide in their families, compared with persons with high levels of the enzyme. There is strong evidence for an alteration of platelet MAO activity in depressive disorders.

PREDICTION

It remains the clinician's task to assess an individual patient's risk of suicide, on the basis of a careful clinical examination. The most predictive items associated with high suicide risk are listed in Table 1. Among the high-risk characteristics are age over 45, male sex, alcoholism (the suicide rate is 50 times higher in alcoholics), violent behavior, prior suicidal behavior, and previous psychiatric hospitalization.

In a survey of 3,800 attempted suicides, Tuckman and Youngman divided categories of suicide risk into high risk–related and low risk–related factors (Table 2).

Table 1
Factors Associated with Suicide Risk

Variable in Rank Order	Content of Item
1	Age (45 and older)
2	Alcoholism
3	Irritation, rage, violence
4	Prior suicidal behavior
5	Sex (male)
6	Unwilling to accept help
7	Longer duration of current episode of depression
8	Prior inpatient psychiatric treatment
9	Recent loss or separation
10	Depression
11	Loss of physical health
12	Unemployed/retired
13	Single, widowed, divorced

Modified from Litman R E, Faberow N L, Wold C I, and Brown T R: Prediction models of suicidal behaviors. In *The Prediction of Suicide,* H Beck, L P Resnik, D J Lettieri, editors, p. 141. Charles Press, Bowie, MD 1974.

The clinician should always ask about suicide ideation as part of every mental status exam, especially if the patient is depressed. The patient should be asked directly, are you or have you ever been suicidal? Do you want to die? Eight out of ten persons who eventually kill themselves give warnings of their intent. Fifty percent say openly that they want to die. If the patient admits to a plan of action, that is a particularly dangerous sign. Also, if a patient who has been threatening suicide becomes quiet and less agitated, that may be an ominous sign. The clinician should be especially concerned with the factors listed in Table 3.

CHILD AND ADOLESCENT SUICIDE

The number of children under 15 who kill themselves each year increased from fewer than 40 in 1950 to 300 in 1985. However, suicide in children under the age of 12 is an exceedingly rare event. Suicidal thoughts (e.g., a child's talking about wanting to harm himself or herself) or suicidal threats (e.g., a child's stating that he or she wants to jump in front of a car) are more common than is successful suicide. In the United States, about 12,000 children are hospitalized each year because of suicidal threats or behavior. According to one study of a group of randomly selected normal children, about 13 percent had occasional ideas of suicide.

Among adolescents (aged 15 to 24), suicide is the third leading cause of death, and there are about 6,000 adolescent suicides each year. Boys commit suicide three times more often than girls do, but girls attempt suicide three times more often than boys do.

Among children and adolescents who attempt or complete suicide, there is a high incidence of parental physical abuse or neglect. Suicide is higher in single-parent homes as

Table 2
Suicide Rate Per 1000 Population Among 3800 Attempted Suicides, By High- and Low-Risk Categories of Risk-Related Factors

Factor	High-risk category	Suicide rate	Low-risk category	Suicide rate
Age	45 years of age and older	24.0	Under 45 years of age	9.4
Sex	Male	19.9	Female	9.2
Race	White	14.3	Nonwhite	8.7
Marital status	Separated, divorced, widowed	12.5	Single, married	8.0
Living arrangements	Alone	48.4	With others	10.1
Employment status[1]	Unemployed, retired	16.8	Employed[2]	14.3
Physical health	Poor (acute or chronic condition in the 6-month period preceding the attempt)	14.0	Good[2]	12.4
Mental condition	Nervous or mental disorder, mood or behavioral symptoms, including alcoholism	19.1	Presumably normal, including brief situational reactions[2]	7.2
Medical care (within 6 months)	Yes	16.4	No[2]	10.8
Method	Hanging, firearms, jumping, drowning	28.4	Cutting or piercing, gas or carbon monoxide, poison, combination of other methods	12.0
Season	Warm months (April–September)	14.2	Cold months (October–March)	10.9
Time of day	6:00 A.M.–5:59 P.M.	15.1	6:00 P.M–5:59 A.M.	10.5
Where attempt was made	Own or someone else's home	14.3	Other type of premises, out-of-doors	11.9
Time interval between attempt and discovery	Almost immediately, reported by person making attempt	10.9	Later	7.2
Intent to kill (self-report)	No[2]	14.5	Yes	8.5
Suicide note	Yes	16.7	No[2]	12.3
Previous attempt or threat	Yes	25.2	No[2]	11.0

[1]Does not include housewives and students.
[2]Includes cases for which information on this factor was not given in the police report.
Table by Tuckman J, Youngman W F: A scale for assessing suicide risk of attempted suicides. J Clin Psychol 24:17, 1968.

Table 3
History, Signs, and Symptoms of Suicidal Risk

1. Previous attempt or fantasized suicide
2. Anxiety, depression, exhaustion
3. Availability of means of suicide
4. Concern for effect of suicide on family members
5. Verbalized suicidal ideation
6. Preparation of a will, resignation following agitated depression
7. Proximal life crisis such as mourning or impending surgery
8. Family history of suicide

a result of separation or divorce. Sixty percent of adolescent suicides live with only one parent, and the suicide risk is higher when one or more family members have a chronic illness.

According to most studies, depressive illnesses are associated with suicidal behavior in children and adolescents. Feelings of abandonment, desires to be reunited with lost loved ones, and feelings of despair and hopelessness are common. All children evaluated psychiatrically should be asked about suicidal ideas. Major risk factors for suicide include depression, a preoccupation with death and dying, and suicidal tendencies in the child's family. A child who has lost a parent by any means before the age of 13 has a higher risk for affective disorders and suicide.

Clusters of suicides among adolescents who know one another and go to the same school have been reported. Suicidal behavior may precipitate other such attempts within a peer group via identification—so-called copy-cat suicides. A 1986 study by David Shaffer indicated that there was an increase in adolescent suicide after television programs were shown whose main theme was the suicide of a teenager. In general, however, many other factors are involved, including a necessary substrate of psychopathology.

The tendency of disturbed young persons to imitate highly publicized suicides has been called the "Werther syndrome" after the protagonist in Goethe's novel *The Sorrows of Young Werther*. The novel, in which the hero kills himself, was banned in some European countries after its publication nearly 200 years ago because of a rash of suicides by young men who had read it, some, when they killed themselves, having dressed like Werther or having left the book open to the passage describing his death.

MANAGEMENT

Whether to hospitalize the patient with suicidal ideation is the most important clinical decision to be made. Not all such patients require hospitalization; some may be managed on an outpatient basis. But the absence of a strong social support system, a history of impulsive behavior, or a suicidal plan of action are indications for hospitalization. To determine whether outpatient treatment is feasible, a straightforward clinical approach is best. Ask the patient considered suicidal whether he or she will agree to call

when reaching a point beyond which he or she is uncertain of controlling suicidal impulses. If the patient can make such an agreement, he or she will be reaffirming the belief that he or she has sufficient strength to control such impulses and seek help.

In return for the patient's commitment, the clinician should be available to the patient 24 hours a day. If a patient who is considered seriously suicidal cannot make this commitment, immediate and emergency hospitalization is indicated, and both the patient and the patient's family should be so advised. If, however, the patient is to be managed on an outpatient basis, it is often useful for the therapist to note the patient's home and work phone numbers for emergency reference; occasionally, a patient hangs up unexpectedly during a late night call or gives only a name to the answering service. If the patient refuses hospitalization, the family must take the responsibility to be with the patient 24 hours a day.

According to Edwin Schneidman, there are several practical preventive measures for dealing with a suicidal person: (1) reduce the psychological pain by modifying the patient's stressful environment, by enlisting the aid of a spouse, employer, or friend; (2) build realistic support by recognizing that the patient may have a legitimate complaint; and (3) offer alternatives to suicide.

Many psychiatrists believe that any patient who has made a suicidal attempt, regardless of its lethality, should be hospitalized. Although most of these patients will voluntarily enter the hospital, a danger to self is one of the few clear-cut indications currently acceptable in all states for involuntary hospitalization.

In the hospital, the patient can receive antidepressant or antipsychotic medications as indicated; individual, group, and family therapy are available; and the patient receives the hospital's social support and sense of security. Other therapeutic measures depend on the patient's underlying diagnosis. For example, if alcoholism is an associated problem, treatment must be directed toward alleviating that condition.

Although patients classified as acutely suicidal may have favorable prognoses, chronically suicidal patients are difficult to treat, and they exhaust the caretakers. Constant observation by special nurses, seclusion, and restraints will not prevent a determined suicide. Electroconvulsive therapy (ECT) may be necessary for some severely depressed patients, who may require several treatment courses.

Patients recovering from a suicidal depression are at particular risk. As the depression lifts, patients become more energized and are thus able to put their suicidal plans into action. Sometimes, depressed patients, with or without treatment, suddenly appear to be at peace with themselves, because they have reached a secret decision to commit suicide. The clinician should be especially suspicious of such a dramatic clinical change, which may portend a suicidal attempt.

Finally, a patient may commit suicide even when in the hospital. According to one survey, approximately 1 percent of suicides occurred in patients who were being treated in general medical-surgical or psychiatric hospitals; however, the annual suicide rate in psychiatric hospitals is only 0.003 percent.

LEGAL AND ETHICAL CONSIDERATIONS

Liability issues stemming from suicides in psychiatric hospitals frequently involve questions about the rate of deterioration of psychiatric status, the presence during hospitalization of clinical signs indicating risk, and the psychiatrist's and the staff's awareness of and response to these clinical signs.

In about half the cases in which suicide occurs while the patient is on a psychiatric unit, a lawsuit results. What the courts require is not that suicide never occur but that the patient be periodically evaluated for suicidal risk, that a treatment plan with a high level of security be formulated, and that the staff follow this treatment plan.

At present, suicide and attempted suicide are variously viewed as a felony and a misdemeanor; in some states, the acts are considered not crimes but unlawful under common law and statutes. The role of an aider and abettor in suicide adds another dimension to the legal morass; some court decisions have held that although neither suicide nor attempted suicide is punishable, anyone who assists in the act may be punished.

COMMUNITY ORGANIZATIONS

Community organizations seem to have fewer problems than do individual therapists with the ethics and legalities of helping suicidal people. Prevention centers, crisis listening posts, and so-called suicide telephone hot lines are a clear attempt to intervene and diminish the isolation, withdrawal, and loneliness of the suicidal patient. Outreach programs enable highly motivated laypersons to respond to cries for help in a variety of ways. But it would be wrong to believe that such responses do more than just diminish an acute crisis; highly suicidal people place fewer than 10 percent of such calls, and most of these calls are made by distressed young women. No accurate statistical data are available on whether the national rate of suicide has decreased as a result of these programs; however, there are instances in which suicidal persons with high-risk characteristics have been hospitalized as a result of these efforts.

References

Barraclough B, Bunch J, Nelson B, Sainsbury P: A hundred cases of suicide: Clinical aspects. Br J Psychiatry *125*:355, 1974.
Beck A T: Hopelessness and eventual suicide. Am J Psychiatry *142*:559, 1985.
Braverman E R, Pfeiffer C C: Suicide and biochemistry. Biol Psychiatry *20*:123, 1985.
Farberow N L, Shneidman E, editors: *The Cry for Help*. McGraw-Hill, New York, 1961.
Fawcett J, Scheftner W, Clark D, Hedeker D, Gibbons R, Coryell W: Clinical predictors of suicide in patients with major affective disorders: A controlled prospective study. Am J Psych *144*:35, 1987.
Fishbain D A, Fletcher J R, Aldrich T E, Davis J H: Relationship between Russian roulette deaths and risk-taking behavior: A controlled study. Am J Psych *144*:563, 1987.
Hawton K, Catalan J, editors: *Attempted Suicide*. Oxford University Press, New York, 1975.
Hollnger P C, Offer D, Ostrov E: Suicide and homicide in the United States: An epidemiologic study of violent death, population changes, and the potential for prediction. Am J Psych *144*:215, 1987.
Murphy G E, Robins E: Social factors in suicide. JAMA *199*:303, 1967.
Perlin S, editor: *A Handbook for the Study of Suicide*. Oxford University Press, New York, 1975.
Roy A, editor: *Suicide*. Williams & Wilkins, Baltimore, 1986.
Shaffer J W, Perlin S, Schmidt C W Jr, Stevens J A: The prediction of suicide in schizophrenia. J Nerv Ment Dis *150*:349, 1974.
Shneidman E: *Definition of Suicide*. Wiley, New York, 1985.

29.2 _____
Other Psychiatric Emergencies

DEFINITION

A psychiatric emergency is a disturbance in thoughts, feelings, or actions for which immediate treatment is necessary. Most often, the patients themselves express this need. However, a state of psychiatric emergency may be declared by family members, teachers, or the public. This section discusses common conditions for which patients come or are brought to the psychiatric emergency room or admitting office.

EPIDEMIOLOGY

Psychiatric emergency rooms are used equally by men and women and more by single persons than married persons. About 20 percent of patients are suicidal, and about 10 percent are violent. The most common diagnoses are mood disorder, schizophrenia, and alcoholism. About 40 percent of all patients seen in psychiatric emergency rooms require hospitalization. Most visits occur during the night hours, but there is no utilization difference based on day of the week or month of the year. Contrary to popular belief, studies have not demonstrated a higher utilization of psychiatric emergency rooms during a full moon or during the Christmas holiday.

DOCTOR–PATIENT RELATIONSHIP

Emergency room physicians must be aware of their own feelings and attitudes that may adversely affect their relationship with their patients and thus impair their clinical judgment. For example, physicians may respond with condemnatory attitudes toward patients whose psychiatric emergency has been precipitated by alcohol or drug abuse or whose chronic mental illness has led to social deterioration and a lack of personal cleanliness. Many acutely disturbed patients are irritable, demanding, hostile, and provocative. Physicians may react with understandably negative feelings, but such feelings should alert them to be especially careful in their examination of the patient. If a patient causes the doctor excessive anxiety, the doctor should try to understand the cause. Frequently, it stems from a fear of the patient's becoming violent. In those instances, it is appropriate for the doctor to see the patient with an attendant or guard nearby should the patient become assaultive. About 25 percent of all mental health workers report being assaulted some time in their career. A significant number of physicians and psychiatrists have been murdered in the performance of their duties.

PSYCHIATRIC INTERVIEW

The emergency room interview is similar to the standard psychiatric interview and mental status except for the time limitation imposed by the other patients waiting to be seen. In general, the psychiatrist focuses on the presenting complaint and the reasons that the patient with a chronic condition has come to the emergency room at this time. The time constraint requires that the clinician structure the interview, particularly with patients who suffer from chronic emotional disturbances and so may respond with long rambling accounts of their illness. If friends, relatives, or the police accompany the patient, a supplemental history should be obtained from them. That is especially necessary if the patient is negativistic, uncooperative, or otherwise unable to give a coherent history.

The greatest potential error of emergency room psychiatry is overlooking a physical illness as the cause of the emotional illness. Head trauma, drug abuse (including alcohol), stroke, metabolic abnormalities, and medication all may cause abnormal behavior, and a concise medical history concentrating on those areas should be taken. Studies have demonstrated that 5 to 30 percent of patients in psychiatric emergency rooms have medical disorders that account for all or most of their symptoms.

Sometimes the contact to the emergency room is by telephone. In such cases, the psychiatrist should obtain the number from which the call is made, as well as the exact address. These items are important in case the call is interrupted, and they allow the psychiatrist to direct help, depending on the circumstances. If the patient is alone, the police should be alerted. If possible, an assistant should call the police on another line while the psychiatrist keeps the patient engaged until help arrives. The patient should not be told to drive alone to the hospital. Rather, an emergency medical team should be dispatched to bring the patient to the hospital.

PSYCHOLOGICAL EMERGENCY STATES

Suicide

Suicidal depression is the single most important category in emergency psychiatry, and the evaluation of suicidal risk is a major task for the clinician.

One must be alert to the danger signs of suicidal depression, namely, suicidal ideas, early-morning insomnia and agitation, a loss of all appetites and interests, feelings of hopeless despair, an inability to express one's thoughts or feelings, and progressive social withdrawal. The appearance of delusions, such as having committed an unpardonable sin or of hallucinations telling the patient to harm himself or herself, is a particularly ominous sign. Hospitalization is indicated if a patient is actively suicidal and if many risk factors (e.g., previous attempt, plan, command hallucinations) are present. Many clinicians believe that every patient should be hospitalized for observation after a suicidal attempt. (See Section 29.1 for a more complete discussion of the management of the suicidal patient.)

Violence and Assaultive Behavior

Violence and assaultive behavior is very difficult to predict. However, the fear with which some people regard all psychiatric patients is completely out of proportion to the rather small group representing an authentic danger to others. The best predictors of potential violent behavior are (1) excessive alcohol intake, (2) a history of violent acts with arrests or criminal activity, and (3) a history of childhood abuse. Although violent patients can arouse a realistic fear in the psychiatrist, they can also touch off irrational fears that impair clinical judgment and that may lead to the premature and excessive use of sedation or physical restraint. Violent patients are usually frightened by their own hostile impulses and desperately seek help to prevent loss of control. Nevertheless, restraints should be applied if there is a reasonable risk of violence.

Management

Patients in the grip of a violent episode pay no attention to the rational intercessions of others and probably do not even hear them. When armed, they are particularly dangerous and capable of murder. Such patients should be disarmed by trained law enforcement personnel without harming the patients, if at all possible. If unarmed, such patients should be approached with sufficient help and with overwhelming strength so that there is, in effect, no contest. In the emergency room, armed police should always remove bullets from their weapons. There have been numerous instances of disturbed patients' grabbing a loaded gun and randomly killing others.

Violent struggling patients are most effectively subdued with an appropriate sedative or antipsychotic. Diazepam (Valium) 5 to 10 mg, or lorazepam (Ativan) 2 to 4 mg, may be given slowly intravenously (IV) over 2 minutes. It is most important to give IV medication with great care so that respiratory arrest does not occur. Patients who require intramuscular (IM) medication can be sedated with haloperidol, 5 to 10 mg IM, or with chlorpromazine, 25 mg IM. If the furor is due to alcohol or is part of a postseizure psychomotor disturbance, the sleep produced by a relatively small amount of IV medication may go on for hours. On awakening, such patients are often entirely alert and rational and typically have a complete amnesia for the violent episode.

If the furor is part of an ongoing psychotic process and returns as soon as the IV medication wears off, continuous medication may be given. It is sometimes better to use small intramuscular or oral doses at one-half- to one-hour intervals—for example, haloperidol, 2 to 5 mg, or diazepam, 10 mg—until the patient is controlled, than to use larger doses initially and end up with an overmedicated patient. As the patient's disturbed behavior is brought under control, successively smaller and less frequent doses should be used. During the preliminary treatment, the patient's blood pressure and other vital signs should be carefully monitored. The use of medication is contraindicated in acutely agitated patients who have suffered head injury, because medication can confuse the clinical picture. In general, intramuscular haloperidol is one of the most useful emergency treatments for violent psychotic patients. ECT has also been used in emergencies to control psychotic violence. The administration of one or several ECT treatments within several hours usually ends an episode of psychotic violence.

Violent psychotic patients are sometimes placed in mechanical restraints. The danger of that procedure should be noted. Not only does it create a vicious cycle by intensifying the patient's psychotic terror, but if prolonged, mechanical restraints can cause hyperthermia, and in some instances of catatonic excitement, they can cause death. Mechanical restraints should also be used with due regard to local laws—that is, with permission from the proper authorities and with careful monitoring of the patient's physical condition.

Adjustment disorders in all age groups may result in tantrum-like outbursts of rage. These outbursts are seen particularly in marital quarrels. Police are often summoned by neighbors distressed by the sounds of a violent altercation. Such family quarrels should be approached with great caution, because they may be complicated by the use of alcohol and the presence of dangerous weapons. The warring couple frequently turns their combined fury on the unwary outsider. Wounded self-esteem is a big issue. Therefore, patronizing or contemptuous attitudes must be avoided, and an effort must be made to communicate an attitude of respect and an authentic peacemaking concern.

In family violence, the special vulnerability of selected close relatives should be noted. A wife or a husband may have a curious masochistic attachment to the spouse and provoke violence by taunting and otherwise undermining the partner's self-esteem. Such relationships often end in the murder of the provoking partner and sometimes in the suicide of the other partner, the dynamics behind most so-called suicide pacts.

As in the case of suicidal patients, violent patients require hospitalization and usually accept the offer of inpatient care with a sense of relief.

Amnesia

Patients are occasionally brought to emergency rooms with an expression of bewilderment on their faces. Despite negative findings on physical and laboratory examinations, such patients describe a total amnesia for the events of the preceding several hours or days. Often, the patients claim to have forgotten all personal identification data. In military settings, these patients may be enlisted men wandering in the streets, found by military police. These patients usually suffer from a dissociative disorder or fugue state.

Such patients should be hospitalized, and the life circumstances preceding the fugue state should be scrutinized. The history usually will reveal that the patient has taken

flight from an unbearable life situation. The traumatic situation often involves a personal interaction filled with rage, threats to self-esteem, and the danger of losing impulse control. Such patients can often be hypnotized, and in their induced trance state, they may be able to reconstruct the missing details in their personal history, including their feelings. An amytal interview can be conducted, which also will aid in restoring memory.

Amnesia from trauma (e.g., head injury) or secondary to an organic lesion (e.g., epilepsy or tumor) must always be ruled out.

Panic

Panic reactions without psychotic content can occur alone or as part of agoraphobia. These episodes may present clinically as a fear of an impending fatal heart attack. They may be associated with localized inframammary chest pain and sensations of a lump in the throat (globus hystericus). Typically, there is a history of anxiety and depression during the preceding months, based on an increasingly stressful life circumstance related to difficulties at work, at school, or in the home. Some patients with mitral valve prolapse have associated panic attacks.

Treatment of the acute episode is by simple reassurance because the attack remits in about 30 minutes. Alprazolam (Xanax) and propranolol (Inderal) are also useful in managing panic. Proper long-term treatment depends on a careful diagnostic evaluation. Tricyclic antidepressants and monoamine oxidase inhibitors have been used successfully in agoraphobia.

Homosexual Panic. Homosexual panic refers to a disorder of adult life characterized by massive anxiety, delusions, and hallucinations that accuse the patient, in derisive and contemptuous terms, of a variety of homosexual practices. The panic typically occurs in heterosexual males who have difficulty dealing with homosexual impulses or ideas. The breakdown may occur in a setting of enforced intimacy, such as a college dormitory or a military barracks. There may be a history of alcohol or drug use preceding the acute episode.

If anxiety is predominant, a benzodiazepine will ameliorate the condition. An antipsychotic agent will be necessary if the patient is having delusions or hallucinations. If possible, a physician of the opposite sex to the patient is preferable if extensive interviewing is necessary. Touching the patient or performing a physical exam may be misinterpreted as a homosexual advance and precipitate violence.

Post-Traumatic Stress Disorder

Post-traumatic stress disorder designates the acute anxiety symptoms that start after a near escape from death in combat, an accident, or a natural catastrophe. Usually, the patient retains self-control during the actual period of danger. But some persons have a panic reaction at the time, characterized by terror and ineffective efforts at flight, that may precipitate panic reactions in others. Such panic stricken patients are extraordinarily suggestible and easily hypnotized, and so they usually follow firm instructions concerning their appropriate behavior. Treatment should encourage an immediate return to their previous assignments and responsibilities. Most of all, prolonged diagnostic and therapeutic inpatient procedures should be avoided, as these encourage regression and chronic invalidism.

Mania

Manic excitement occurs in the manic phase of a bipolar disorder. In the emergency room, it is usually possible to quiet such patients long enough for them to accept medications and hospitalization, if necessary. Haloperidol, 2 to 20 mg, is used to quiet agitation, and the patient is admitted. After the patient is hospitalized, the psychiatrist should start lithium carbonate by mouth in sufficient quantity to achieve therapeutic blood levels, as determined by laboratory testing.

Mania may be induced by antidepressant medication in bipolar patients, and so a careful history to determine the cause of the mania should always be taken.

Paranoid Schizophrenia

Paranoid schizophrenics occasionally display psychotic excitement, in which they may barricade themselves against imagined enemies or declare themselves the principal figure in some grandiose plot—political, religious, or otherwise. They may harm themselves or others when in an agitated state. It may be possible to establish contact with them and persuade them to accept medication and hospitalization. Sometimes these patients will have to be physically subdued and given medication intramuscularly (haloperidol, 2 to 10 mg). Hospitalization is almost always indicated. Paranoid agitation may also be caused by chronic cocaine and amphetamine use and PCP toxicity.

Catatonic Schizophrenia

A subtype of schizophrenic patients may present a psychiatric emergency in the stage of catatonic stupor. Such patients are becoming rare. They are usually mute and display automatic obedience. Waxy flexibility (catalepsy) is present. Their symptoms respond rapidly to antipsychotic medication, but such patients should be admitted to the hospital for further evaluation. At times catatonic stupor spontaneously and suddenly develops into catatonic excitement, during which the patient is agitated, hyperactive, and assaultive. If not controlled, patients have been known to exhaust themselves and die. Hospital admission and antipsychotic medication such as haloperidol usually resolve the condition. ECT has also been used to interrupt the excitement phase.

A rare condition of psychotic withdrawal consists of the patient's being brought into the emergency room completely immobile—in a rigid state, not speaking, sometimes keeping their eyes tightly closed, and not responding to questions or commands. This is a variant of catatonic schizophrenia, and such patients may be dangerous because they may suddenly erupt into an excited assaultive state. They should be admitted to the psychiatric unit and given antipsychotic medication as soon as possible. The condition should be differentiated from akinetic mutism caused by lesions of the diencephalon. Such patients are immobile and mute and cannot voluntarily respond. They are not negativistic, however, and their eyes may follow persons around the room as they try to make contact. The possibility of organic brain disease as a cause of catatonic stupor or excitement should be excluded by careful physical and laboratory examinations.

Insomnia

Insomnia may occur as a relatively benign symptom in relation to a period of unusual personal stress. But it may mark the onset of a more severe depressive reaction, in which case it is associated with early-morning agitation and other signs and symptoms of depression. There may be a fear of falling asleep because of frightening dreams as part of a traumatic neurosis after a battle, accident, or other personal catastrophe. The differential diagnosis depends on a careful history. However, the accumulating fatigue of successive sleepless nights can complicate the clinical picture, whatever the diagnosis. Sleep disorders and their management are discussed in Chapter 22. In general, hypnotics are not indicated except for brief periods of time. Sedatives of the benzodiazepine class, such as triazolam (Halcion) 0.25 to 0.5 mg at bedtime for up to 10 days, can be used. Any underlying mental disorder should be treated.

Anorexia Nervosa and Bulimia Nervosa

The key symptom of anorexia nervosa is an obsessional preoccupation with the desire to be thin. It usually occurs in females. The victim of the condition may become physically fragile and cachectic. It may be combined with bulimia nervosa in which the patient tries to lose weight by means of self-induced vomiting or purges with laxatives or enemas. The compulsive avoidance of food may reduce the patient to such an extreme degree of inanition that death occurs. Patients may be seen in the emergency room in a state of starvation, dehydration, and electrolyte imbalance. For this reason, hospitalization and forced feeding may become necessary.

Headache

Patients who come to the emergency room with complaints of headache require careful study to rule out organic disease. Psychiatric diagnoses commonly associated with headache include somatization disorder, hypochondriasis, and depression. Narcotic analgesics should be avoided at all costs because of the risk of dependency. Patients with factitious disorder will feign somatic symptoms (including headache) to gain admittance.

Dysmenorrhea

A patient who presents herself at a psychiatric emergency room with a complaint of dysmennorhea is usually suffering from an associated depression. Suicidal ideation should be considered. In DSM-III-R a new controversial diagnostic category called late luteal phase dysphoric disorder (LLPDD) (in Chapter 26) describes the patient who may be seriously depressed, hostile, and agitated around the time of the menses. There may be suicidal attempts or brief reactive psychoses. If a suicidal depression is diagnosed and if there have been suicidal attempts in the past, suicidal precautions, especially hospitalization, are indicated.

Hyperventilation

Anxious patients may sometimes pant in terror. After a few seconds of overbreathing, a state of alkalosis sets in, caused by excess carbon dioxide output. Consciousness is reduced, with giddiness, a tingling feeling in the extremities, carpopedal spasm, faintness, and blurring of vision. These symptoms further terrify the already panic-stricken patient. Overbreathing tends to continue automatically and uncontrollably. There are electroencephalogram and electrocardiogram changes during the attack, reflecting the metabolic derangement.

The classic remedy is to have the patient breathe into a paper bag, which restores the blood bicarbonate level by the inhalation of CO_2. More effective is a behavior modification approach, in which the patient is encouraged to hyperventilate in the doctor's office in the presence of a friend or relative. However, lasting results depend on further reinforcement where the attacks usually occur, outside the doctor's office. The patient's understanding of the mechanisms of the symptom (i.e., hyperventilation) lays the best foundation for effective therapy.

Grief and Bereavement

Symptoms of normal grief and bereavement include guilt feelings, irritability, insomnia, and somatic complaints. The patient who comes to the emergency room should be encouraged to ventilate those feelings and be reassured that they are normal. Antidepressants block the grief process and so are contraindicated. A mild tranquilizer for insomnia, such as triazolam (Halcion) 0.25 mg or flurazepam (Dalmane) 15 mg, given at bedtime for 3 or 4 days, may be useful. Grief needs to be differentiated from depression, which is characterized by feelings of hopelessness, vegetative signs, and suicidal ideation, and which requires more vigorous treatment.

ORGANIC EMERGENCY STATES

Delirium and Dementia

Delirium and dementia are organic brain disorders characterized by global cognitive impairment, altered emotionality and impulsivity, and disturbances in alertness and wakefulness. The causes are multifactorial, and the emergency room psychiatrist's first task after ensuring that the patient is medically stable is to determine the cause of the disorganized brain function. An agitated, restless, fearful, or belligerent delirious patient needs to be sedated to prevent complications and accidents. Haloperidol (Haldol) in doses of from 2 to 10 mg IM may be given and repeated hourly if the patient continues to be agitated. Benzodiazepines are used for their sedative effect and their anticonvulsant properties (diazepam 5 to 10 mg PO or IM, lorazepam 2 to 4 mg). It is important, however, that treatment of both conditions be directed primarily to the cause. Admission to the hospital is usual for both delirium and dementia. Glucose (for hypoglycemia), thiamine (for Wernicke's encephalopathy) and Narcan (for opioid overdose) can be given to this type of patient to rule out and definitively treat the acute delirium. Organic mental disorders (their causes and treatment) are more fully covered in Chapter 11.

Alcoholism

Alcoholics are probably the most mistreated group of patients in the emergency room. They are often dirty, malodorous, and are either belligerent or unresponsive. They often engender negative feelings in the emergency room staff, who respond by not giving them the attention they require. A careful medical examination is important because the alcohol may disguise behavioral abnormalities caused by schizophrenia, hypoglycemia, or subdural hemorrhage. The analgesic effect of alcohol may obscure the presence of broken bones and other serious injuries.

The physician should be alert to the problem of mixed addiction, the alcoholic who is also on barbiturates and other tranquilizers. In addition, antidepressants, phenothiazines, and related psychotropic agents potentiate the effects of alcohol. Thus, a careful drug and medication history is important. A regimen for barbiturate withdrawal may be the primary treatment indicated.

When the possibility of a major physical disease requiring inpatient care has been eliminated, the treatment of the acute alcoholic in the emergency room is aimed at making the patient ambulatory as swiftly as possible.

Acute Intoxication. Acute intoxication, also known as simple drunkenness, is characterized by an unsteady gait, slurred speech, poor attention, and labile affect. Blood alcohol levels vary between 100 to 200 mg per dl. No specific treatment is necessary because most persons fall asleep and awaken in 3 to 4 hours without sequelae. There may be memory defects (blackouts) for the period while drunk. Pathological intoxication is treated with haloperidol. Mixed intoxication syndromes, with more than one substance should always be considered.

Alcohol Withdrawal. When the obvious signs of intoxication have subsided, it is necessary to watch for withdrawal symptoms, coarse tremors, hyperreflexia, a tendency to startle in response to minor stimuli, and nausea. Pulse rate and blood pressure tend to be elevated at this time.

The severity of the withdrawal syndrome depends on the chronicity and the severity of the preceding alcoholic state. When there is doubt, the patient should be hospitalized. A benzodiazepine is administered by mouth and repeated in 1 to 6 hours, depending on the patient's condition. There is no need for parenteral medication if the patient is cooperative. When the patient has been stable for 24 to 36 hours, the medication should be gradually discontinued by reducing the dose over several days. If withdrawal symptoms do not appear but are expected, a benzodiazepine should be administered every 6 hours for 24 hours. If the symptoms have not occurred after 24 hours, the medication should be gradually discontinued over several days.

Alcohol Withdrawal Delirium. Alcohol withdrawal delirium, also known as delirium tremens, has a mortality rate of 5 to 20 percent if not treated. It is a medical emergency because of the possibility of cardiac or circulatory collapse. Treatment involves inpatient care with the maintenance of good hydration, nutrition, and electrolyte balance, particularly magnesium and potassium. Delirium is managed with sedatives, such as diazepam 10 to 20 mg orally or IM every 1 to 4 hours, which is also of value in preventing withdrawal seizures. Delirium tremens should be differentiated from alcoholic hallucinosis in which there are auditory hallucinations in a clear sensorium. Those hallucinations respond to antipsychotic medication.

Wernicke's Encephalopathy. Wernicke's encephalopathy, seen in chronic alcoholics, is characterized by dementia, ophthalmoplegia, and ataxia. Thiamine (100 mg daily) reverses the disorder after several months.

Drug Abuse Emergencies

Opioids. Overdosed heroin patients are pale and cyanotic. They have pinpoint pupils and are areflexic. They may not be breathing at all or may take three or four shallow gasping breaths a minute. Vital signs should be noted—that is, level of consciousness, deep tendon reflexes, pupil size and reactivity, blood pressure, pulse rate, and respiration. An open airway should be maintained.

Blood should be drawn for a study of drug levels, and the patient given intravenous naloxone hydrochloride (Narcan), 0.4 mg in a 1-ml dose. Naloxone is a narcotic antagonist that reverses the opiate effects, including respiratory depression, within 2 minutes of the injection. If the desired degree of counteraction and respiratory improvement is not obtained, the dose may be repeated after 2 or 3 minutes. Failure to obtain significant improvement after two or three such doses suggests that the condition may be due partly or completely to other disease processes or to nonnarcotic sedative drugs. Patients who respond to naloxone should be carefully observed, lest they lapse into coma again.

If the overdose is due to methadone, breathing should be monitored for 24 hours because the toxicity may last that long and the naloxone action is quite brief. It may be necessary in a methadone overdose to provide naloxone in the form of a continuous intravenous drip overnight, 2.0 mg of naloxone in 500 mg of 0.45 normal saline, injected at a rate of 0.4 mg every 30 minutes.

The family or friends who bring the patient to the emergency room must remain available to provide pertinent information, such as the patient's drug preferences and customary doses. If a sample of the patient's drug is available, it should be forwarded for laboratory assay. A urine analysis should be done as soon as a specimen can be obtained. It is important to consider the possibility of a physical condition that may mimic a drug reaction, such as diabetes or a postseizure state. See Section 13.4 for a further discussion of the opioids.

Sedative-Hypnotic Withdrawal. The use of barbiturates, nonbarbiturates, and the so-called minor tranquilizers is widespread. The first symptoms of withdrawal may start about 8 hours after the last pill has been taken and may consist of anxiety, confusion, and ataxia. In time, gross tremors appear, with headache, nausea, and vomiting. Seizures, including status epilepticus, may occur sometime after the first 12 hours of withdrawal; they are a serious complication, as head injuries may be incurred. Whenever seizures occur in a previously nonepileptic adult, withdrawal should be considered in the differential diagnosis.

As the withdrawal continues, a psychotic state erupts, characterized by hallucinations, panic, and disorientation. Nystagmus is almost invariably present. During the delirium, the patient may leap to his or her death in an attempt to escape from the frightening psychotic experience.

The simplest way to institute the withdrawal procedure is to ask the patient directly about the usual daily drug intake, divide that reported figure in half, and administer it to the patient in four doses every 6 hours. In a case of mixed addiction, the withdrawal procedure is most simply accomplished with a barbiturate, because there is a cross-tolerance of all antianxiety agents and similar substances. Patients should be closely observed and the dose decreased if they become drowsy and increased if withdrawal signs appear. From then on, the dose is reduced every other day in small steps, for 7 to 10 days, enabling the patient to reach a dose of one pill a day. This dosage is continued for 2 days; then all further sedation is terminated.

If it is not possible to learn from the patient what his or her customary daily dose is, it has been suggested that the patient receive by mouth a 200-mg test dose of pentobarbital sodium and be observed 1 hour later. If the patient is clearly drowsy or asleep, it may be concluded that his or her intake is minimal, equivalent to 200 mg a day; if there is nystagmus, ataxia, and drooping eyelids without verbal responsiveness, that suggests moderate abuse in the range of 500 mg a day; if the patient is able to speak but is dysarthric, that suggests heavy use in the 600- to 700-mg daily dose range; and if the patient shows minimal effects, it may be concluded that there is extremely heavy use in the range of 900 mg or more per day. The withdrawal schedule can then be planned accordingly.

Amphetamine and Cocaine. Patients brought to the emergency room may be agitated, psychotic, or delirious as a result of cocaine or amphetamine intoxication. These drugs produce dilated pupils that are reactive to light, elevated blood pressure and temperature, dry mouth, tachycardia and cardiac arrhythmias, and hyperactive tendon reflexes. The patients are often paranoid, subject to tactile hallucinations, irritable, and capable of violent aggressive behavior. Delusions and hallucinations from cocaine are usually more transitory than are those from amphetamine. Treatment is to reduce autonomic hyperactivity with diazepam (5 to 10 mg orally or IM) and to prescribe antipsychotic medication (haloperidol, 2 to 10 mg) for delusions and hallucinations.

Hallucinogens. Hallucinogens include LSD, phencyclidine (PCP), psilocybin, and mescaline. New substances appear sporadically. These drugs produce dilated pupils that react to light, elevated blood pressure, hyperactive reflexes, fever, tachycardia, sweating, and nystagmus. Psychotic reactions are associated with perceptual distortions and hallucinations. Panic may occur, with impulsive flight and suicide. Occasionally, there may be impulsive acts of violence.

Next to alcohol, phencyclidine (PCP, angel dust, hog) has become the most common cause of psychotic drug-related emergency hospital admissions. The presence of dissociative phenomena, nystagmus (horizontal, vertical, rotary), muscular rigidity, and elevated blood pressure in a patient who is agitated, psychotic, or comatose and whose respirations are not depressed strongly suggests PCP intoxication. Treatment of the condition with phenothiazine tranquilizers is contraindicated. The so-called talking-down process does not help, as such patients are out of contact with reality. The following steps are recommended: (1) sensory isolations with the patient in a quiet room on a floor pad; (2) gastric lavage to recover the drug; (3) diazepam to reduce anxiety; (4) an acidifying diuretic program consisting of ammonium chloride and furosemide (Lasix), which will enhance PCP excretion; and (5) treatment of hypertension with propranolol (Inderal). Restraints should not be used because of the danger of hyperthermia.

Central Anticholinergic Syndrome (CAS). Atropine, scopolamine, belladonna, and the antihistamines are the active ingredients in over-the-counter—that is, nonprescription—sleeping pills and in antiparkinsonian medications, including L-dopa. As a result of overdose or drug sensitivity, these so-called anticholinergic substances may produce an acute psychotic reaction. This syndrome may also be caused by antidepressant and antipsychotic medication. Apart from the psychotic symptoms that may be confused with schizophrenia, the patient shows fixed dilated pupils, a flushed skin, blurred vision, fever, delirium, and urinary retention.

Based on these telltale signs, a physician may administer physostigmine, 4.0 mg IM, for diagnostic purposes and swift symptomatic relief. In anticholinergic psychotic states, improvement after a single injection lasts for about 2 to 3 hours. In any event, the psychotic reaction usually subsides within 3 days. Perhaps the most important aspect of this psychotic category is that the use of phenothiazines is contraindicated; patients are intolerant of these tranquilizers, because of their anticholinergic effects, tending to react with more delirium and sometimes with dangerous hypotension. When in doubt, one should avoid the phenothiazines and, instead, use chlordiazepoxide (Lithium), diazepam (Valium), or phenobarbital. Physostigmine is generally avoided if the CAS is due to tricyclics because most of the dosage is from the cardiotoxic effects.

MAOIs. A hypertensive crisis can occur in patients being treated for depression with a monoamine oxidase inhibitor (MAOI) if they have eaten food with a high tyramine content (strong cheese, smoked or pickled fish, spiced meats, red wines, chicken liver, yeast extract, excessive amounts of coffee) or if they have taken sympathomimetic drugs, particularly by injection. The hypertensive crisis is characterized by a severe occipital headache that may radiate frontally, palpitations, neck stiffness and soreness, nausea, vomiting, sweating, photophobia, constricting chest pain, and dilated pupils. Intracranial bleeding, sometimes fatal, has been associated with hypertensive crisis.

If a hypertensive crisis occurs, the MAOI should be discontinued at once, and therapy should be instituted to reduce blood pressure. Chlorpromazine, a 50-mg tablet, may be carried by the patient and taken orally if a severe headache occurs after a dietary infraction. If the crisis is severe and the patient is brought to a hospital emergency room, 5 mg of phentolamine should be administered intravenously, slowly, to avoid producing an excessive hypotensive effect.

There is a toxic interaction between MAOIs and meperidine hydrochloride (Demerol), which can be fatal. When patients combine these two drugs, they become agitated, disoriented, cyanotic, hyperthermic, hypertensive, and tachycardic. Should this occur, chlorpromazine has been used as an effective treatment. There have been no clinical reports of the same severe toxic interactions with other narcotics. Should narcotics be needed for a patient on a MAOI, meperidine must be avoided. A careful history of MAOI use should be taken in the emergency room before giving narcotics.

Exhaustion and Hyperthermia

Since first reported in 1832, a syndrome known as lethal (or fatal, mortal, or pernicious) catatonia, delirious state, hypertoxic schizophrenia, or exhaustion syndrome is characterized by extreme excitement or catatonic stupor or both, with an elevated temperature (as high as 108°F). Such a hyperthermia can quickly progress to death. The violent, hyperagitated state can progress to an exhaustion death in 1.5 to 14 days unless effective treatment is given. Electroconvulsive therapy is recommended. The cause of this state is unknown. Because patients are invariably treated with chemotherapy, drugs have been falsely implicated without evidence of a causal connection. The fact that the syndrome occurred before 1952 makes it likely that it is not caused by drug treatment but, rather, by a viral or unknown cause.

Hypothermia

Persons may be brought to the emergency room suffering from hypothermia. This condition often overlooked and misdiagnosed as mental illness because confusion, lethargy, and combativeness are early signs.

The diagnosis is made on the basis of low body temperature (94°F or 34.4°C) and shivering. Patients with a very low body temperature (under 92°F or 33.3°C) may not feel cold; a paradoxical feeling of warmth occurs that causes some persons to undress (paradoxical undressing).

Treatment in the emergency room consists of administering intravenous fluids and rewarming, by total body immersion in a warm tub of water from 90° to 106°F (32.2° to 41.1°C) or by warming blankets. Cardiac status must be carefully monitored because ventricular fibrillation occurs with low body temperature. Alcohol should be avoided because it leads to further heat loss as a result of peripheral vasodilating effects.

AUTHOR'S NOTE: For the sake of brevity and to avoid repetition and reduplication, not all psychiatric emergencies are covered in this section (e.g., neuroleptic malignant syndrome, akathesia, tardive dyskinesia, among others). The reader is referred to the index to find the area of the text that covers these and other emergencies in a more thorough manner.

References

Bellak L, Siegel H: *The Handbook of Intensive, Brief, and Emergency Psychiatry*. CRS, Larchmont, New York, 1983.

Hanke N: *Handbook of Emergency Psychiatry*. Health, Boston, 1984.

McNiel D E, Binder R L: Predictive validity of judgments of dangerousness in emergency civil commitment. Am J Psych *144*:197, 1987.

Rund D A, Hutzler J C: *Emergency Psychiatry,* Mosby, St. Louis, 1983.

Slaby A E: Crisis-oriented therapy. In *Emergency Psychiatry at the Crossroads: New Directions for Mental Health Services,* F R Lipton, S M Goldfinger, editors, p 21, Jossey–Bass, San Francisco, 1985.

Slaby A E: Emergency psychiatry in the general hospital: Staffing, training, and leadership issues. Gen Hosp Psych *3*:306, 1981.

Slaby A E: Emergency psychiatry: An update. H & C Psych *32*:687, 1981.

Slaby A E, Glicksman A S: *Adapting to Life-threatening Illness*. Praeger, New York, 1985.

Slaby A E, Lieb J, Tancredi L: *Handbook of Psychiatric Emergencies,* ed 3. Medical Examination Publishing, New York, 1985.

Weissman A: *Coping Capacity: On the Nature of Being Mortal*. Human Sciences Press, New York, 1984.

30

Psychotherapies

30.1

Psychoanalysis and Psychoanalytic Psychotherapy

INTRODUCTION

Psychoanalysis and psychoanalytic psychotherapy apply the principles of psychoanalysis to understanding and modifying human behavior. The two forms of treatment are similar in that both examine psychodynamics, which studies the ideas, impulses, emotions, and defense mechanisms that explain how the mind works and adapts. Psychoanalysis attempts to rely primarily on interpretation as its technical modality and concentrates on the transference (the relationship between the psychiatrist and the patient). Psychoanalytic psychotherapy also uses interpretation but concentrates less on the transference and more on real-life events. In addition, psychoanalytic psychotherapy emphasizes current interpersonal activities, whereas psychoanalysis tries to reconstruct the patient's past life. There is, however, a continuum between the two treatment modalities, so that it may be difficult to decide whether a particular method is psychoanalysis or psychoanalytic psychotherapy.

PSYCHOANALYSIS

Background of Psychoanalysis

Psychoanalysis began with the treatment of patients by hypnosis. In 1881, Anna O, a neurotic young woman who suffered from multiple visual and motor disturbances, as well as alterations of consciousness, was treated by the Viennese internist Josef Breuer. He observed that the patient's symptoms disappeared when she expressed them verbally while hypnotized. Freud used the technique with Breuer, and they reported their findings in 1895 in *Studies on Hysteria*. They explained hysteria as the result of a traumatic experience, which was usually sexual in nature and associated with a large quantity of affect, that was barred from consciousness and that expressed itself in a disguised form through various symptoms. Freud eventually gave up placing his patients in a hypnotic trance; instead, he urged them to recline on a couch and concentrate with their eyes closed on past memories related to their symp-

toms. This concentration method eventually became the technique of free association. Freud instructed his patients to say whatever came into their minds, without censoring any of their thoughts. This method is still used today and is one of the hallmarks of psychoanalysis through which thoughts and feelings that are kept in the unconscious are brought into consciousness.

In the *Interpretation of Dreams*, Freud described the topographical model of the mind as consisting of a conscious, preconscious, and unconscious. The conscious mind was conceptualized as awareness; the preconscious, as thoughts and feelings that are easily available to consciousness; and the unconscious, as thoughts and feelings that cannot be made conscious without overcoming strong resistances. The unconscious contains nonverbal forms of thought function and gives rise to dreams, parapraxes (slips of the tongue), and psychological symptoms. Psychoanalysis emphasizes the conflict between unconscious drives and moral judgments that patients might make about their impulses. That conflict accounts for the phenomenon of repression, which is regarded as pathological. Free association allows repressed memories to be recovered and thereby contributes to cure.

In 1923, Freud described his structural theory of the mind in *The Ego and the Id*. He saw the ego as a group of functions accessible to consciousness that mediate among the demands of the id, the superego, and the environment. He viewed anxiety as the ego's reaction to the threatened breakthrough of forbidden impulses.

Modern advances in psychoanalysis have focused on the increased understanding of the ego's functions (ego psychology), the role of early relationships (object relations), and the relationship between the analyst and the patient.

Goal of Psychoanalysis

The chief requirement of psychoanalysis is the gradual integration of the previously repressed material into the total structure of the personality. It is a slow process, which requires the analyst to maintain a balance between the interpretation of unconscious material and the patient's ability to deal with increased awareness. If the work proceeds too rapidly, there is a danger that the patient will experience the analysis as a new trauma. The work of analysis initially is preparing the patient to deal with the material that has been uncovered, which produces anxiety. The patient is taught to be aware of innermost thoughts and feelings and to recognize that there are natural resistances to the mind's willingness or ability to deal directly with noxious psychic material. The patient and analyst seldom follow a straight path to insight. Instead, the process of analysis is more like putting together the pieces of an immense and complicated jigsaw puzzle.

Analytic Setting

The usual analytic setting is for the patient to lie on a couch or sofa and the analyst to sit behind, partially or totally outside the patient's field of vision. The couch helps the analyst produce the controlled regression that favors the emergence of repressed material. The patient's reclining position in the presence of an attentive analyst also re-creates symbolically the early parent–child situation, which varies from patient to patient. This position also helps the patient focus more on inner thoughts, feelings, and fantasies, which can then become the focus of free associations. Moreover, the use of the couch introduces an element of sensory deprivation because the patient's visual stimuli are limited and the analyst's verbalizations are relatively few. That state promotes regression. There has been some disagreement, however, about the use of the couch as always characteristic of psychoanalysis. Fenichel stated that whether or not the patient lies down or sits and whether or not certain rituals of procedure are used do not matter. The best condition is that most appropriate to the analytic task.

Role of the Analyst

For the most part, the analyst's activity is limited to timely interpretation of the patient's associations. Ideally, the analyst—who has undergone a personal psychoanalysis as part of his or her training—is able to maintain an attitude of benevolent objectivity toward the patient, trying not to impose his or her own personality or system of values. Nevertheless, it is not possible or desirable for the analyst to be a so-called blank screen, *tabula rasa,* or analyst incognito. A real relationship underlies the analytic setting, and the handling of this real relationship may make the difference between success and failure in treatment.

Duration of Treatment. The patient and psychoanalyst must be prepared to persevere in this process for an indefinite period. Psychoanalysis takes time—between 2 and 5 years, sometimes even longer. Sessions are usually held four or more times a week for 45 to 50 minutes each. Some analyses are conducted with less frequency and with the sessions varying from 20 to 30 minutes. The French psychoanalyst Jacques Lacan introduced sessions of variable length (3 to 45 minutes) which he believed to be equally effective.

Treatment Methodology

Fundamental Rule of Psychoanalysis. The fundamental rule is that the patient agrees to be completely honest with the analyst. All ideas, impulses, thoughts, and feelings are to be verbalized. This principle implies that all action based on impulse be avoided without adequate prior discussion with the analyst.

Free Association. Free association refers to the patient's saying everything that comes to mind without any censoring, regardless of whether they believe the thought to be unacceptable, unimportant, or embarrassing. Associations are directed by three kinds of unconscious forces: the pathogenic conflicts of the neurosis, the wish to get well, and the wish to please the analyst. The interplay among these factors become very complex. For example, a thought or impulse that is unacceptable to the patient and that is a part of his or her neurosis may conflict with the patient's wish to please the analyst, who, the patient assumes, also finds the impulse unacceptable. But if the patient follows the fundamental rule, he or she will overcome that resistance.

Free-floating Attention. The analyst's counterpart to the patient's free association is a special way of listening called "free-floating attention." The analyst allows the patient's associations to stimulate his or her own associations and is thereby able to discern a theme in the patient's free associations that he or she may reflect back to the patient then or at some later time. The analyst's careful attention to his or her own subjective experiences is an indispensable part of analysis.

Rule of Abstinence. The rule of abstinence refers to the patient's being able to delay gratifying any instinctual wishes so as to talk about them in treatment. The tension thus engendered produces relevant associations that the analyst uses to increase the patient's awareness. The rule does not refer to sexual abstinence but, rather, to not allowing the treatment setting to gratify the patient's infantile longing for love and affection. That is, the analyst cannot play the role of the indulgent parent if the work of analysis is to proceed.

Analytic Process

Transference. A major criterion by which psychoanalysis can be differentiated in principle from other forms of psychotherapy is the management of the transference. Indeed, psychoanalysis has been defined as the analysis of transference to emphasize that point.

Transference was first described by Freud and refers to the patient's feelings and behavior toward the analyst that are based on infantile wishes the patient has toward parents or parental figures. These feelings are unconscious but are revealed in the transference neurosis in which the patient struggles to gratify his or her unconscious infantile wishes through the analyst. The transference may be positive, in which the analyst is seen as a person of exceptional worth, ability, and character, or it may be negative, in which he or she is despised and seen as not having any redeeming qualities. Both situations reflect the patient's need to repeat unresolved childhood conflicts.

One criterion by which psychoanalysis can be differentiated in principle from other forms of psychotherapy, including psychoanalytic psychotherapy, is the management of transference. In general psychiatry, the term transference has come to be used as a loose designation for all aspects of the patient's feelings and behavior toward the physician. It includes rational and adaptive aspects, as well as those irrational distortions that arise from unconscious strivings. When it is used in this encompassing sense, it may be more appropriate to refer to transference as a relationship. In contrast, transference in psychoanalysis is conceived of as an endopsychic phenomenon that occurs entirely within the mind.

Narcissistic transference. Freud found that some patients were unable to form a transference neurosis because they were fixated at a narcissistic stage of development and could not attach themselves to another person. Heinz Kohut elaborated on that concept and described the narcissistic transference that occurs in borderline and narcissistic personality disorders. Such patients have extremely labile feelings for the analyst that vacillate between extremes of love and hate, called "splitting."

Interpretation. In psychoanalysis, the analyst provides the patient with interpretations about psychological events that were neither previously understood by nor meaningful to the patient. The transference constitutes a major frame of reference for interpretation. A complete psychoanalytic interpretation includes meaningful statements of current conflicts and the historical factors that influenced them. However, complete interpretations of this kind constitute a relatively small part of the analysis. Most interpretations are more limited in scope and deal with matters of immediate concern.

Interpretations must be well timed. The analyst may have a formulation in mind, but the patient may not be prepared to deal with it directly because of a variety of factors, such as anxiety level, negative transference, and external life stress. The analyst may decide to wait until the patient can fully understand the interpretation. The proper timing of interpretations requires great clinical skill.

Dream interpretation. In his classic work *Interpretation of Dreams,* Freud referred to the dream as the "royal road to the unconscious." The manifest content of a dream is what the dreamer reports. The latent content represents the unconscious meaning of the dream after the condensations, substitutions, and symbols are analyzed. The dream arises from what Freud referred to as the "day's residue" (i.e., the events of the preceding day that stimulated the patient's unconscious mind). Dreams may serve as a wish-fulfillment mechanism as well as a way of mastering anxiety about a life event.

Freud outlined several technical procedures to use in dream interpretation: (1) have the patient associate to elements of the dream in the order in which they occurred; (2) have the patient associate to a particular dream element that he (or she) or the therapist chooses; (3) disregard the content of the dream, and ask the patient what events of the previous day could be associated with the dream (the day's residue); and (4) avoid giving any instructions and leave it to the dreamer to begin. The analyst uses the patient's associations to find a clue to the workings of the unconscious mind.

Countertransference. Just as the term transference is used to encompass the patient's total range of feelings for and against the analyst, countertransference refers to a broad spectrum of the analyst's reactions to the patient. Countertransference has unconscious components based on conflicts of which the analyst is not aware. Ideally, the analyst ought to be aware of countertransference issues, which may interfere with his or her ability to remain detached and objective. The analyst should remove such impediments by either further analysis or self-analysis. For

whatever reasons, however, there are some patients or groups of patients with whom a particular analyst does not work well, and the experienced clinician, recognizing this fact, will refer such patients to a colleague.

Therapeutic Alliance. In addition to transferential and countertransferential issues, there is a real relationship between the analyst and the patient that represents two adults entering into a joint venture, referred to as the "therapeutic or working alliance." Both commit themselves to exploring the patient's problems, establishing mutual trust, and to cooperating with each other to achieve a realistic goal of cure or the amelioration of symptoms.

Resistance. Freud believed that unconscious ideas or impulses were repressed and prevented from reaching awareness because they were unacceptable to consciousness for some reason. He referred to that phenomenon as resistance, which had to be overcome if the analysis was to proceed. Resistance may sometimes be a conscious process manifested by withholding relevant information. Other examples of resistance are remaining silent for a long time, being late or missing appointments, and paying bills late or not at all. The signs of resistance are legion, and almost any feature of the analytic situation can be used to represent resistance. Freud once said that any treatment can be considered psychoanalysis that works by undoing resistance and interpreting transferences.

Indications for Psychoanalytic Treatment

The primary indications for psychoanalysis are longstanding psychological conflicts that have produced a symptom or disorder. The connection between the conflict and the symptom may be direct or indirect. Psychoanalysis is considered effective in treating anxiety disorders (especially phobias and obsessive-compulsive disorders), mild depressions (dysthymia), some personality disorders, impulse disorders, paraphilias, and other sexual disorders. More important than diagnosis, however, is the patient's ability to form an analytic pact and to maintain a commitment to a progressively deepening analytic process that brings about internal change through increasing self-awareness. Freud believed that the patient also had to be able to form a transference neurosis, without which analysis was not possible. That excluded most psychotic patients because of the difficulty they have in forming the affective and realistic bonds that are essential to the transference neurosis. The ego of a patient in analysis must be able to tolerate the frustrations of his or her impulses without responding with some serious form of acting out or by shifting from one pathological pattern to another. That would exclude most drug-dependent patients, who are regarded as unsuitable because their egos are unable to tolerate the frustrations of primitive impulses.

Contraindications for Psychoanalytic Treatment

The various contraindications to psychoanalysis are relative, but each must be considered before embarking on a course of treatment:

1. Age. Adults over 40 may lack sufficient flexibility for major personality changes, although some analyses of

older patients report favorable results. The ideal candidates are generally young adults. Children are unable to follow the rule of free association, but with modifications of technique (e.g., play therapy), they have been successfully analyzed.

2. Intelligence. Patients must be intelligent enough to be able to understand the procedure and to cooperate in the process.

3. Life circumstances. If the patient's life situation cannot be modified, analysis may only make it worse. For example, it can be hazardous to create goals for patients who are unable to fulfill them because of external limitations.

4. Time constraints. Unless the patient has time to participate and to wait for change, another type of therapy should be considered. This constraint applies especially to emergency symptoms or to those that the patient can no longer tolerate, including those that are dangerous (e.g., strong suicidal impulses).

5. Nature of the relationship. The analysis of friends, relatives, or acquaintances generally should be avoided because it may distort the transference and the analyst's objectivity.

Finally, some patients work better with some analysts than others. Sometimes this determination can be made after a single consultation, but often a trial analysis of several sessions may be necessary. This time may also allow the patient to see whether he or she wishes to continue. Experience has shown that it does not matter whether the analyst is a man or woman, although some patients may initially prefer to see one or the other, a preference that is eventually understood as the analysis proceeds.

Dynamics of Therapeutic Results

The process of cure or improvement involves the release of repression safely and effectively. The structural apparatus of the mind—id, ego and superego—are modified. The ego has little to fear from repressed impulses, as it is finally in a position to accept or renounce them.

Frequently toward the end of an analysis, a patient will recall some positive memories about the parent figure that he or she has consistently maligned. It seems possible that by erecting defensive processes to repress the memory of some childhood experiences, the ego shrinks away from both negative and positive memories. The analysis then may be able to rescue from repression the nontraumatic memories as well as the traumatic ones. Such a process may help develop stronger ego functioning.

The impulses themselves change. Once freed from repression, their infantile forms are modified. Analysis helps reduce the intensity of the conflicts and helps find more acceptable ways of handling impulses that cannot be reduced. Instead of a more acceptable method of channeling unmodified infantile strivings, the drives' primary process quality itself is lessened, and they become better adapted to reality. The goal of analysis with respect to these drives is to transfer them from the transference to progressive neutralization. The ultimate goal is the elimination of symptoms, thereby increasing the patient's capacity for work, enjoyment and self-understanding.

PSYCHOANALYTIC PSYCHOTHERAPY

Definition

Psychoanalytic therapy is psychotherapy based on psychoanalytic formulations that has been modified conceptually and technically. Unlike psychoanalysis, which has as its ultimate concern the uncovering and subsequent working through of infantile conflicts as they may arise in the transference neurosis, psychoanalytic therapy takes as its focus the current conflicts and current dynamic patterns—that is, the analysis of the patient's problems with other persons and with himself or herself. Also unlike psychoanalysis, which has as its technique the use of free association and the analysis of the transference neurosis, psychoanalytic therapy is characterized by interviewing and discussion techniques that use free association much less frequently. And again unlike analysis, the work on transference in psychoanalytic therapy is usually limited to a discussion of the patient's reactions to the psychiatrist and others. The reaction to the psychiatrist is not interpreted to as great a degree as it is in psychoanalysis. Nevertheless, transference attitudes and responses to the therapist may arise from time to time and can be used productively. For example, spontaneous transferences in the therapeutic situation may give valuable clues to the patient's behavior in extratherapeutic situations and, at times, to his or her childhood. These transferences may tell the therapist the probable focus for the patient at any given time, inside or outside the treatment relationship.

Treatment Techniques

One way in which psychoanalytic therapy differs from classical analysis is that the former does not usually use a couch. The stimulation of temporary regressive patterns of feeling and thinking, which is valuable to psychoanalysis, is much less necessary in psychoanalytic therapy, with its greater focus on current dynamic patterns. In psychoanalytic therapy, the patient and therapist are usually in full view of each other, which may make the therapist seem more real and less a composite of projected fantasies. This type of therapy is much more flexible, and it may be used in conjunction with psychotropic medication, more often than in psychoanalysis.

Psychoanalytic psychotherapy can range from a single supportive interview, centering on a current but pressing problem, to many years of treatment with one or two interviews a week of varying length sessions. In contrast with psychoanalysis, a list of disorders treated by psychoanalytic psychotherapy would cover a major portion of the field of psychopathology.

Types of Psychoanalytic Psychotherapy

Insight-Oriented Psychotherapy. Insight is the patient's understanding of his or her psychological functioning and personality. It is important to specify the area or level of understanding or experience into which the patient is to achieve insight. The psychiatrist's emphasis in insight-oriented therapy (also called expressive therapy and intensive psychoanalytic psychotherapy) is on the value to the patient of gaining a number of new insights into the current dynamics of his or her feelings, responses, behavior, and especially current relations with other persons. To a lesser extent, the emphasis is on the value of developing some insight into the patient's responses to the therapist and responses in childhood.

Insight therapy is the treatment of choice for a patient who has fairly adequate ego strength but who, for one reason or another, should not or cannot undergo psychoanalysis.

The therapy's effectiveness does not depend solely on the insights developed or used. The patient's therapeutic response is also based on such factors as the ventilation of feelings in a nonjudgmental but limit-setting atmosphere, identification with the therapist, and other relationship factors. A therapeutic relationship does not, however, require an indiscriminate acceptance of all that a patient says and does. Rather, the therapist represents long-term as well as short-term values, for the reality principle as well as the pleasure principle. At times, the therapist must intervene on the side of a relatively weak ego by giving unmistakable evidence that the patient could try to achieve a better adjustment or by setting realistic limits to the patient's maladaptive behavior. In so doing, the therapist tries to be guided by his or her dynamic assessment of the situation and not by his or her countertransference responses.

Inevitably, the therapist's attitudes and responses to the patient are different from those of important figures in the patient's childhood. At times, the therapist discusses these differences. Patients may come to see that they have generalized their parents' attitudes as being universal and have generalized their own responses so that they have become automatic responses to all parental or older figures.

Insight psychotherapy is frequently complicated by spontaneous strong transferences to the therapist that at times threaten to disrupt the treatment. The insight therapist may decide to deal for a limited time with transference material essentially as it is in psychoanalysis, that is, the significance of the transference as it relates to the patient's contemporary life and problems, with only limited reference to his or her childhood.

Supportive Psychotherapy

Supportive psychotherapy (also called relationship or superficial psychotherapy) offers support by an authority figure during a period of illness, turmoil, or temporary decompensation. It has the goal of restoring or strengthening the defenses and integrating capacities that have been impaired. It provides a period of acceptance and dependence for a patient who is acutely in need of help in dealing with guilt, shame, and anxiety and in meeting the frustration or the external pressures that have been too great to handle.

Supportive therapy uses such measures as warm, friendly, strong leadership, gratification of dependency needs if that can be done without evoking undue shame, support in the development of legitimate independence, help in the development of hobbies and pleasurable but nondestructive sublimations, adequate rest and diversion, the removal of excessive external strain if that is a productive step, hospitalization when it is indicated, medication that may alleviate symptoms, and guidance and advice in current issues. It uses those techniques that help the patient feel more secure, accepted, protected, encouraged, and safe and less anxious and alone.

One of the greatest dangers lies in the possibility of fostering too great a regression and too strong a dependency. From the beginning, the psychiatrist must plan to wean the patient. But some patients require supportive therapy indefinitely, often with just the goal of maintaining a marginal adjustment outside the hospital.

The verbalization of unexpressed strong emotions may bring considerable relief. The goal of such talking out is not primarily to gain insight into the unconscious dynamic patterns that may be intensifying current responses. Rather, the reduction of inner tension and anxiety may result from the expression of emotion and its subsequent discussion and may lead to a greater insight into and objectivity in evaluating a current problem. The relationship between the therapist and the patient gives the therapist an opportunity to display behavior different from the destructive or unproductive behavior of the patient's parents. At times, such experiences seem to neutralize or reverse some of the effects of the parents' mistakes. If the patient had overly authoritarian parents, the therapist's friendly, flexible, nonjudgmental, nonauthoritarian—but at times firm and limit-setting—attitude means that the patient has an opportunity to adjust to, be led by, and identify with a new type of parent figure. Franz Alexander called this process a corrective emotional experience.

This treatment is suitable for a variety of psychogenic illnesses. For example, it may be useful when a patient is very resistive to an expressive psychotherapy or is considered too emotionally disturbed for such a procedure. Supportive therapy may be chosen when the diagnostic assessment indicates that a gradual maturing process based on the elaboration of new foci for identification is the most promising path toward improvement.

For a summary of the points made in this section the reader is referred to Table 1 for a comparison and description of different types of therapies.

Table 1
Psychoanalysis and Psychoanalytic Psychotherapy

Features	Psychoanalysis	Psychoanalytic Psychotherapy	
		Insight-oriented (Expressive)	Supportive (Relationship)
Basic Theory	Psychoanalytic Psychology	Psychoanalytic Psychology	Psychoanalytic Psychology
Frequency and duration	4 to 5 times weekly, 2 to 5+ years. Sessions usually about 50 minutes. New modifications: shorter sessions	1 to 3 times weekly, few sessions to several years. Sessions usually from 20 minutes to 50 minutes	Daily sessions to once every few months, one session to a lifelong process. Sessions may be brief, ranging from a few minutes to an hour
Activity of patient and therapist	Freely hovering attention by the analyst, free association by the patient. Interpretation of transference and resistance. Analyst assumes neutral role	Freely hovering attention by the therapist but with more focusing than in analysis. Less emphasis on free association, more on discussion by the patient. Analyst is more active	Expressive techniques generally avoided except for some cathartic effects. Therapist actively intervenes, advises, fosters discussion, selects focus. Therapist participates as a real person around current issues
Interpretive emphasis	Focus on resistance and transference to the analyst	Greater emphasis on interpersonal events and external events, less on transferences to the analyst than in analysis, but transference interpretation often effective. Transferences to persons other than the therapist often effectively interpreted	Interpretations of transferences by therapist generally avoided unless significantly interfering with the therapeutic relationship. Strong focus on external events. Clarification of interpersonal events
Transference	Transference neurosis fostered on foundation of the therapeutic alliance. Minimal reality orientation to external events	Transference neurosis discouraged; therapeutic alliance fostered. Considerably more reality oriented	Transference neurosis discouraged. Real relationship and therapeutic alliance emphasized. Almost totally reality oriented
Regression	Fostered in the form of the transference neurosis	Generally discouraged except as necessary to gain access to fantasy material and other derivatives of the unconscious	Regression generally discouraged
Adjuncts	Couch. The use of psychotropic drugs is controversial; some psychoanalysts will not use drugs, others will. Will not see family members or do group psychotherapy	Couch less used. Mostly face-to-face therapy. Psychotropic drugs used as needed. May do combined group and individual therapy	Always face-to-face therapy. Couch contraindicated. Group methods, family therapy, or family contacts on a planned basis. Other therapists and agencies may be involved. Psychotropic drugs used frequently and as needed
Confidentiality	Absolute. May be compromised by third-party payers	Absolute. May be compromised by third-party payers	Absolute. May be compromised by third-party payers
Prerequisites	Relatively mature personality, favorable life situation, motivation for long undertaking, capacity to tolerate frustration, capacity for stable therapeutic alliance, psychological mindedness	Relatively mature personality, capacity for therapeutic alliance, some capacity to tolerate frustration, adequate motivation, and some degree of psychological mindedness	Some capacity for therapeutic alliance, personality capable of growth, reality situation not too unfavorable Personality organization may range from psychotic to mature

Table 1 *continued*

Features	Psychoanalysis	Psychoanalytic Psychotherapy	
		Insight-oriented (Expressive)	Supportive (Relationship)
Basic Theory	Psychoanalytic Psychology	Psychoanalytic Psychology	Psychoanalytic Psychology
Diagnostic indications	Neuroses, personality disorders, paraphilias, sexual disorders	Neuroses, personality disorders (especially borderline and narcissistic), paraphilias, sexual disorders, latent schizophrenia, cyclothymia, psychosomatic disorders	Psychoses, adjustment disorders, Impulse disorders, Psychophysiologic conditions, psychosomatic disorders
Goals	Reorganization of character structure, with diminution of pathological defenses, integration or ultimate rejection of warded-off strivings and ideation. Understanding rather than symptom relief the objective, but symptom relief usually results. Correction of developmental lags in otherwise relatively mature personalities	Resolution of selected conflicts and limited removal of pathological defenses. Understanding the primary goal, usually with secondary relief of symptoms	Growth of the relatively immature personality through catalytic relationship with therapist counteracts the neurotogenic effects of prior significant relationships Restoration of prior equilibrium, reduction of anxiety and fear in new situations. Help in tolerating unalterable situations

References

Alexander F, French T M: *Psychoanalytic Therapy*. Ronald Press, New York, 1956.

Blum H P, editor: *Psychoanalytic Explorations of Technique: Discourse on the Theory of Therapy*. International Universities Press, New York, 1980.

Brenner C: *Psychoanalytic Technique and Psychic Conflict*. International Universities Press, New York, 1976.

Fenichel O: *The Psychoanalytic Theory of Neurosis*. W W Norton, New York, 1945.

Freud S: *The Standard Edition of the Complete Psychological Works of Sigmund Freud*, 24 vols. Hogarth Press, London, 1953–1974.

Hartmann H: *Ego Psychology and the Problem of Adaptation*. International Universities Press, New York, 1959.

Jones E: *The Life and Work of Sigmund Freud*, 3 vols. Basic Books, New York, 1953–1957.

Karasu T B: Psychotherapies: An overview. Am J Psychiatry *134*:851–873, 1977.

Kohut H H: *The Analysis of the Self*. International Universities Press, New York, 1984.

Perry S, Cooper A M, Michels R: The psychodynamic formulation: Its purpose, structure, and clinical application. Am J Psych *144*:543, 1987.

Sullivan H S: *Interpersonal Theory of Psychiatry*. Norton, New York, 1953.

Wylie H W Jr, Wylie M L: An effect of pharmacotherapy on the psychoanalytic process: Case report of a modified analysis. Am J Psych *144*:489, 1987.

30.2 _____

Brief Dynamic Psychotherapy and Crisis Intervention

INTRODUCTION

Brief dynamic psychotherapy has assumed greater importance for several reasons. Long-term treatment extending over several years has become too expensive for many patients; third-party payers have pressed the psychiatric profession to develop brief psychotherapies; and this type of therapy has been proved effective for a wide range of psychiatric disorders.

Most of the basic characteristics of brief dynamic psychotherapy were identified by Franz Alexander and Thomas French in 1946. They described a therapeutic experience that puts the patient at ease, manipulates the transference, and uses trial interpretations in a flexible manner. The emphasis is aimed at developing a corrective emotional experience capable of repairing traumatic events of the past and convincing the patient that new ways of thinking, feeling, and behaving are possible.

At about the same time, Eric Lindemann established a consultation service at the Massachusetts General Hospital for persons experiencing a crisis. New treatment methods were developed to deal with those situations and were eventually applied to persons who were not in crisis but who were experiencing emotional distress from a variety of sources.

PRINCIPLES OF SHORT-TERM DYNAMIC PSYCHOTHERAPY

Selection Criteria

The most valuable predictor for a successful outcome is the patients' motivation for treatment. In addition, patients must be able to deal with psychological concepts, to respond to interpretation, and to concentrate on and resolve the conflict around the central issue or focus that underlies their basic problem. Patients must also be able to develop a therapeutic alliance and work with the therapist toward achieving emotional health.

TYPES OF BRIEF DYNAMIC PSYCHOTHERAPY

Brief Psychotherapy (Tavistock–Malan)

Brief psychotherapy was originally developed by the Michael Balint team at the Tavistock Clinic in London in the 1950s. Daniel Malan, a member of that team, reported the results of the therapy in his three outstanding books. Malan's selection criteria for treatment are eliminating absolute contraindications; rejecting patients for whom certain dangers seem inevitable; clearly assessing the patient's psychopathology; and determining the patient's capacity to consider his or her problems in emotional terms and face disturbing material, respond to interpretations, and endure the stress of the treatment. Malan found that high motivation invariably correlated with successful outcome.

Contraindications to treatment are serious suicidal attempts, drug addiction, chronic alcoholism, incapacitating chronic obsessional symptoms, incapacitating chronic phobic symptoms, and gross destructive or self-destructive acting out.

Requirements and Techniques. Malan emphasizes using the following routine: make the transference early and interpret it. Interpret also the negative transference. Link the transference to the patient's relation to his or her parents. Both patient and therapist must be willing to become deeply involved and to bear the ensuing tension. Successful dynamic interaction predominates. A circumscribed focus is formulated, and a termination date is set in advance. Grief and anger about termination are worked through.

About 20 sessions is suggested as an average length for this kind of therapy, for an experienced therapist, and about 30 sessions for a trainee. However, Malan does not go beyond 40 interviews.

Time-Limited Psychotherapy (Boston University–Mann)

A psychotherapeutic model of exactly 12 interviews focusing on a specified central issue was developed at Boston University by Mann and his colleagues in the early 1970s. In contrast with Malan's emphasis on clear-cut selection and rejection criteria, Mann has not been as explicit as to who is a good candidate to receive time-limited psychotherapy.

The main points that Mann considers important are a reasonably correct central conflict in the patient and, in young people, maturational crises with many psychological and somatic complaints.

Mann also mentioned a few exceptions, which are similar to Malan's rejection criteria. These exceptions are a serious depression that interferes with the treatment agreement, an acute psychotic state, and a desperate patient who needs, but is incapable of tolerating, object relations.

Requirements and Techniques. The following are Mann's technical requirements: strict limitation to 12 sessions; positive transference predominating early; specification and strict adherence to a central issue involving transference; positive identifications, making separation a maturational event for the patient; absolute prospect of termination, avoiding development of dependence; clarification of present and past experiences and resistances; an active therapist who supports and encourages the patient; and education of the patient through direct information, reeducation, and manipulation.

The conflicts likely to be encountered include independence versus dependence, activity versus passivity, unresolved or delayed grief, and adequate versus inadequate self-esteem.

Short-Term Dynamic Psychotherapy (McGill University–Davanloo)

As conducted by Habib Davanloo at McGill University, short-term dynamic psychotherapy encompasses all the varieties of brief dynamic psychotherapy and crisis intervention. Patients treated in Davanloo's series are classified as those whose psychological conflicts are predominantly oedipal, those whose conflicts are not oedipal, or those whose conflicts have more than one focus.

In addition, Davanloo devised a specific psychotherapeutic technique for patients suffering from severe, long-standing neurotic problems, specifically those suffering from incapacitating obsessive-compulsive and phobic disorders.

Davanloo's criteria emphasize the evaluation of those ego functions that are of primary importance to the psychotherapeutic work: the establishment of a psychotherapeutic focus; the psychodynamic formulation of the patient's psychological problem; the ability to get involved in emotional interaction with the evaluator; the history of a give-and-take relationship with a significant person in the patient's life; the extent to which the patient's emotional life is close to conscious awareness; the patient's ability to experience and tolerate anxiety, guilt, and depression; the patient's motivation for change; the patient's psychological mindedness; and the patient's ability to respond to interpretation and to link the evaluator with people in the present and in the past.

Both Malan and Davanloo emphasize the patient's response to interpretation and considers it both an important selection criterion and a prognostic criterion.

Requirements and Techniques. The highlights of this psychotherapeutic approach are flexibility (the therapist should adapt his or her technique to the patient's needs); control of the patient's regressive tendencies; active intervention, so as not to allow the development of overdependence on the therapist; and intellectual insight plus emotional experiences by the patient in the transference. These emotional experiences become corrective as a result of the interpretation.

Short-Term Anxiety-Provoking Psychotherapy (Harvard University–Sifneos)

Short-term anxiety-provoking psychotherapy, or STAPP, was first developed at the Massachusetts General Hospital by Peter Sifneos, during the 1950s. The following criteria for selection are used: circumscribed chief complaint (this implies an ability to select one out of a variety of problems to which the patient assigns top priority and which he or she wants to resolve in the treatment); one meaningful or give-and-take relationship during early childhood; the ability to interact flexibly with the evaluator and to express feelings appropriately; above-average psychological sophistication (this implies not only an above-average intelligence but also an ability to respond to interpretations); a specific psychodynamic formulation (this usually means a set of psychological conflicts underlying the patient's difficulties and centering on an oedipal focus), a contract between the therapist and the patient to work on the specified focus and the formulation of minimal expectations of outcome; and good-to-excellent motivation for change and not for symptom relief.

Requirements and Techniques. The treatment can be divided into four major phases: patient–therapist encounter, early therapy, height of the treatment, and evidence of change and termination. The therapist uses the following techniques during these four phases:

Patient–therapist encounter. The therapist establishes a working alliance by using the quick rapport and the positive feelings for the therapist that appear at this phase. Judicious use of open-ended and forced-choice questions enables the therapist to outline and concentrate on a therapeutic focus. The therapist specifies the minimum expectations of outcome to be achieved by the therapy.

Early therapy. In transference, feelings for the therapist are clarified as soon as they appear, leading to the establishment of a true therapeutic alliance.

Height of the treatment. This phase emphasizes active concentration on the oedipal conflicts that have been chosen as the therapeutic focus for this kind of therapy; repeated use of anxiety-provoking questions and confrontations; avoidance of pregenital characterological issues, which the patient uses defensively to avoid dealing with the therapist's anxiety-provoking techniques; avoidance at all costs of a transference neurosis; repetitive demonstration to the patient of his or her neurotic ways or maladaptive patterns of behavior; concentration on the anxiety-laden material, even before the defense mechanisms have been clarified; repeated demonstration of parent–transference links by the use of properly timed interpretations based on material given by the patient; establishment of a corrective emotional experience; encouragement and support of the patient, who becomes anxious while struggling to understand his or her conflicts; new learning and problem-solving patterns; and repeated presentation and recapitulation of the patient's psychodynamics until the defense mechanisms used in dealing with oedipal conflicts are understood.

Evidence of change and termination of psychotherapy. This phase emphasizes the tangible demonstration of change in the patient's behavior outside the therapy, evidence that more adaptive patterns of behavior are being used, and initiation of talk about terminating the treatment.

OUTCOME

The techniques that all of these kinds of brief dynamic psychotherapy share far outdistance their differences. They include the therapeutic alliance or dynamic interaction between the therapist and the patient, the use of transference, the active interpretation of a therapeutic focus or central issue, the repetitive links between parental and transference issues, and the early termination of the therapy.

More than in any other form of psychotherapy, the outcomes of these brief dynamic treatments have been investigated extensively. Contrary to prevailing ideas that the therapeutic factors in psychotherapy are nonspecific, controlled studies and other assessment methods (e.g., interviews with unbiased evaluators, patients' self-evaluations) point to the importance of the specific techniques

used. Malan summarized the results in five major generalizations: (1) The capacity for genuine recovery in certain patients is far greater than was thought. (2) A certain type of patient receiving brief psychotherapy can benefit greatly from a practical working through of his or her nuclear conflict in the transference. (3) Such patients can be recognized in advance through a process of dynamic interaction, because they are responsive and motivated and able to face disturbing feelings to live independently of therapy; and a circumscribed focus can be formulated for them. (4) The more radical the technique is in terms of transference, depth of interpretation, and the link to childhood, the more radical the therapeutic effects will be. (5) For some disturbed patients, a carefully chosen partial focus can be therapeutically effective.

In regard to this last generalization, Davanloo's successful psychotherapeutic technique in treating chronic incapacitating obsessive-compulsive patients with multiple phobias clearly points to the possible psychotherapeutic results of a judicious use of these techniques. It also points out that the limits of short-term dynamic psychotherapy have not been reached.

SHORT-TERM INTERPERSONAL PSYCHOTHERAPY

A specific type of short-term psychotherapy called interpersonal psychotherapy (IPT), described by Myrna Weissman and Gerald Klerman, is used to treat depression. Therapy consists of 45- to 50-minute sessions held weekly over a 3- to 4-month period. It is called IPT because interpersonal behavior is emphasized as a cause of depression and as a method of cure. Patients are taught to evaluate realistically their interactions with others and to become aware of how they isolate themselves, which contributes to or aggravates the depression about which they complain. The therapist offers direct advice, aids the patient in making decisions, and helps clarify areas of conflict. Little or no attention is given to the transference. The therapist attempts to be consistently supportive, empathic, and flexible. Studies of IPT have shown that in selected cases of depression, it compares favorably with drug therapy with antidepressant agents.

CRISIS THEORY

A crisis is a response to hazardous events and is experienced as a painful state. Consequently, it tends to mobilize powerful reactions to help the person alleviate the discomfort and return to the state of emotional equilibrium that existed before its onset. If this takes place, the crisis can be overcome, but in addition, the person learns how to use adaptive reactions. Furthermore, it is possible that by resolving the crisis, the patient may be in a better state of mind, superior to that before the onset of the psychological difficulties. If, on the other hand, the patient uses maladaptive reactions, the painful state will intensify, the crisis will deepen, and a regressive deterioration will take place, producing psychiatric symptoms. These symptoms, in turn, may crystallize into a neurotic pattern of behavior that restricts the patient's ability to function freely. At times, however, the situation cannot be stabilized; new maladaptive reactions are introduced; and the consequences can be of catastrophic proportions, leading at times to death by suicide.

It is in this sense that psychological crises are painful and may be viewed as turning points for better or for worse.

A crisis is self-limited and can last anywhere from a few hours to about 6 weeks. The crisis as such is characterized by an initial phase, in which anxiety and tension rise. This phase is followed by a phase in which problem-solving mechanisms are set in motion. These mechanisms may be successful, depending on whether they are adaptive or maladaptive.

Conservation of energy is another feature of a person in a state of crisis. All the available resources at one's disposal are used for only one purpose, namely, the resolution of the crisis and the diminution of its pain. Such a successful resolution has important mental health implications. The person who has been able to use resources efficiently, either alone or with the help of another person, not only has learned how to deal with the crisis by becoming acquainted with the ways in which to go about resolving it, but has also discovered ways to anticipate future trouble and to avoid its recurrence. In this way, the crisis resolution has also become a preventive intervention.

Patients during a period of turmoil are receptive to minimal help and obtain meaningful results. All sorts of services, therefore, have been devised for such purposes. Some are open ended; others limit the time available or the number of sessions.

Crisis theory helps one understand healthy normal people, as well as to develop therapeutic tools aimed at preventing future psychological difficulties.

Crisis Intervention

Crisis intervention is offered to persons who are incapacitated or severely disturbed by a crisis.

Criteria for Selection. The criteria used to select patients are a history of a specific hazardous situation of recent origin that produced the anxiety, a precipitating event that intensified this anxiety, clear-cut evidence that the patient is in a state of psychological crisis as previously defined, high motivation to overcome the crisis, a potential for making a psychological adjustment equal or superior to the one that existed before the development of the crisis, and a certain degree of psychological sophistication—an ability to recognize psychological reasons for the present predicament.

Requirements and Techniques. Crisis intervention deals with persons in the midst of a crisis and rapidity is of the essence. Therapy is a joint understanding of the psychodynamics involved and an awareness of how they are responsible for the crisis. The participants work together, aiming at resolving the crisis. In addition, the patient, as well as the therapist, actively participates in the treatment.

Techniques include reassurance, suggestion, environmental manipulation, and psychotropic medications and may even be combined with brief hospitalization as part of the treatment plan. All these therapeutic maneuvers are aimed at decreasing the patient's anxiety. The length of crisis intervention varies from one or two sessions to several interviews over a period of 1 or 2 months. The technical requirements for crisis intervention involve rapidly

establishing rapport with the patient, aimed at creating a therapeutic alliance; reviewing the steps that have led to the crisis; understanding the maladaptive reactions that the patient is using to deal with the crisis; focusing only on the crisis; learning to use different and more adaptive ways to deal with crises; avoiding the development of symptoms; using the predominating positive transference feelings for the therapist so as to transform the work into a learning experience; teaching the patient how to avoid hazardous situations that are likely to produce future crises; and ending the intervention as soon as evidence indicates that the crisis has been resolved and that the patient clearly understands all the steps that led to its development and its resolution.

Outcome. The most striking result of crisis therapy pertains to the patient's ability to become better equipped to avoid or, if necessary, to deal with future hazards. In addition, on the basis of some patients' objective observations, this therapeutic experience has enabled them to attain a level of emotional functioning that is superior to that before the onset of the crisis. In this sense, therefore, one may view crisis intervention as being not only therapeutic but also preventive.

References

Bellack L, Siegel H: *Handbook of Intensive, Brief, and Emergency Psychiatry.* CRS, Larchmont, NY, 1983.

Binder J, Strupp H, Schacht: Counter-transference in time-limited dynamic psychotherapy. Contemp Psychoanal *19*:605, 1983.

Davanloo H, editor: *Short-term Dynamic Psychotherapy.* Jason Aronson, New York, 1980.

Horowitz M: *Personality Styles and Brief Psychotherapy.* Basic Books, New York, 1984.

Hirschowitz R: Crisis theory: A formulation. Psychiatr Ann *3*:33, 1973.

Malan D H: *The Frontier of Brief Psychotherapy.* Plenum, New York, 1976.

Marmor J: Short-term dynamic psychotherapy. Am J Psychiatry *2*:149, 1979.

Rogawski A S: Current status of brief psychotherapy. Bull Menninger Clin *46*:331, 1982.

Schram P C, Burti, L: Crisis intervention techniques designed to prevent hospitalization. Bull Menninger Clin *50*:194, 1986.

Sifneos P E: *Short-term Dynamic Psychotherapy Evaluation and Technique.* Plenum, New York, 1979.

30.3 _____

Group Psychotherapy, Combined Individual and Group Psychotherapy, and Psychodrama

GROUP PSYCHOTHERAPY

Definition

Group psychotherapy is a treatment in which carefully selected emotionally ill persons are placed into a group, guided by a trained therapist, to help one another effect personality change. By using a variety of technical maneuvers and theoretical constructs, the leader uses the group members' interactions to make that change.

Classification

At the present time, there are many approaches to the group method of treatment. Many clinicians work within a psychoanalytic frame of reference. Other therapy techniques include transactional group therapy, which was devised by Eric Berne and emphasizes the "here-and-now" interactions among group members; behavioral group therapy, which relies on conditioning techniques based on learning theory; gestalt group therapy, which was created from the theories of Frederick Perls and enables patients to get in touch with their feelings and express themselves openly and honestly; and client-centered group psychotherapy, which was developed by Carl Rogers and is based on the nonjudgmental expression of feelings among group members. Table 1 outlines the major group therapy approaches.

Patient Selection

To determine a patient's suitability for group psychotherapy, the therapist needs a great deal of information, which is gathered in

Table 1
Comparison of Different Types of Group Psychotherapy

Parameters	Supportive Group Therapy	Analytically Oriented Group Therapy	Psychoanalysis of Groups	Transactional Group Therapy	Behavioral Group Therapy
Frequency	Once a week	1 to 3 times a week	1 to 5 times a week	1 to 3 times a week	1 to 3 times a week
Duration	Up to 6 months	1 to 3+ years	1 to 3+ years	1 to 3 years	Up to 6 months
Primary indications	Psychotic and neurotic disorders	Neurotic disorders, borderline states, personality disorders	Neurotic disorders, personality disorders	Neurotic and psychotic disorders	Phobias, passivity, sexual problems
Individual screening interview	Usually	Always	Always	Usually	Usually
Communication content	Primarily environmental factors	Present and past life situations, in tragroup and extragroup relationships	Primarily past life experiences, intragroup relationships	Primarily intragroup relationships; rarely, past history, here and now stressed	Specific symptoms without focus on causality
Transference	Positive transference encouraged to promote improved functioning	Positive and negative transference evoked and analyzed	Transference neurosis evoked and analyzed	Positive relationships fostered, negative feelings analyzed	Positive relationships fostered, no examination of transference
Dreams	Not analyzed	Analyzed frequently	Always analyzed and encouraged	Analyzed rarely	Not used
Dependency	Intragroup dependency encouraged; members rely on leader to great extent	Intragroup dependency encouraged, dependency on leader variable	Intragroup dependency not encouraged, dependency on leader variable	Intragroup dependency encouraged, dependency on leader not encouraged	Intragroup dependency not encouraged; reliance on leader is high
Therapist activity	Strengthen existing defenses, active, give advice	Challenge defenses, active, give advice or personal response	Challenge defenses, passive, give no advice or personal response	Challenge defenses, active, give personal response, rather than advice	Create new defenses, active and directive
Interpretation	No interpretation of unconscious conflict	Interpretation of unconscious conflict	Interpretation of unconscious conflict extensive	Interpretation of current behavioral patterns in the here and now	Not used
Major group processes	Universalization, reality testing	Cohesion; transference, reality testing	Transference, ventilation, catharsis, reality testing	Abreaction, reality testing	Cohesion, reinforcement, conditioning
Socialization outside of group	Encouraged	Generally discouraged	Discouraged	Variable	Discouraged
Goals	Better adaptation to environment	Moderate reconstruction of personality dynamics	Extensive reconstruction of personality dynamics	Alteration of behavior through mechanism of conscious control	Relief of specific psychiatric symptoms

a screening interview. The psychiatrist should take a careful psychiatric history and perform a mental status examination to obtain certain dynamic, behavioral, and diagnostic factors.

Authority Anxiety. Those patients whose primary problem is their relationship to authority and who are extremely anxious in the presence of authority figures may or may not do well in group therapy. However, they often do better in a group setting than in a dyadic (one-to-one) setting because they are more comfortable in a group. Patients with a great deal of authority anxiety may be blocked, anxious, resistant, and unwilling to verbalize thoughts and feelings in an individual setting, generally for fear of censure or disapproval from the therapist. Thus, they may welcome the suggestion of group psychotherapy so as to avoid the scrutiny of the dyadic situation. Conversely, if the patient reacts negatively to the suggestion of group psychotherapy or is openly resistant to the idea, the therapist should consider the possibility of a high degree of peer anxiety.

Peer Anxiety. Patients, such as schizoid personalities, who have destructive relationships with their peer group or who have been extremely isolated from peer group contact generally react negatively or more anxiously when placed in a group setting. If such patients can work through their anxiety, however, group therapy can be very beneficial.

Diagnosis. The diagnosis of patients' disorders is important to determining the best therapeutic approach and to evaluating their motivation for treatment, capacity for change, and their personality structures' strengths and weaknesses.

There are few contraindications to group therapy. Antisocial patients generally do poorly because they cannot adhere to group standards. Depressed patients do better after they have established a trusting relationship with the therapist. Manic patients are disruptive, but once under pharmacologic control, they do well in the group setting. Patients who are delusional and who may incorporate the group into their delusional system should be excluded, as should patients who pose a physical threat to other members because of uncontrollable aggressive outbursts.

Preparation

Patients who are prepared by the therapist for a group experience tend to continue in treatment longer and report less initial anxiety than do those who are not so prepared. This preparation consists of the therapist's explaining, before the first session, the procedure in as much detail as possible and answering any questions the patient may have.

Structural Organization

Size. Group therapy has been successful with as few as 3 members and as many as 15, but most therapists consider 8 to 10 members the optimal size. With fewer members, there may not be enough interaction, unless they are especially verbal. But with a larger group, the interaction may be too great for the members or the therapist to follow.

Frequency of Sessions. Most group psychotherapists conduct group sessions once weekly. It is important to maintain continuity in sessions. When alternate sessions are used, the group meets twice a week, once with and once without the therapist.

Length of Sessions. In general, group sessions last anywhere from 1 to 2 hours, with the average length being 1½ hours. However, the time limit set should be constant.

Time-extended therapy (marathon group therapy) is a method in which the group meets continuously for 12 to 72 hours. Enforced interactional proximity and, during the longer time-extended sessions, sleep deprivation, break down certain ego defenses, release affective processes, and promote more open communication. However, time-extended groups may be dangerous for patients with weak ego structures, such as schizophrenic or borderline patients. Marathon groups were most popular in the 1970s but are much less often used today.

Homogenous versus Heterogeneous Groups. In general, most therapists believe that the group should be as heterogeneous as possible, to ensure maximum interaction. Thus, the group should be composed of members from different diagnostic categories and with varied behavioral patterns; from all races, social levels, and educational backgrounds; and of varying ages and both sexes.

In general, patients between ages 20 and 65 can be effectively included in the same group. Age differences aid in the development of parent–child and brother–sister models. Moreover, patients have the opportunity to relive and rectify interpersonal difficulties that may have appeared insurmountable.

Both children and adolescents are best treated in groups composed mostly of patients of their own age group. Some adolescent patients are quite capable of assimilating the material of the adult group, regardless of content, but they should not be deprived of a constructive peer experience that they might otherwise not have.

Mechanisms of Group Psychotherapy

Group Formation. Each patient approaches the group differently, and in this sense, the group is a microcosm. Patients use typical adaptive abilities, defense mechanisms, and ways of relating, which are ultimately reflected back to them by the group, thus allowing them to become introspective about their personality functioning. But a process inherent in group formation requires that the patients suspend their previous ways of coping. In entering the group, they allow their executive ego functions—reality testing, adaptation to and mastery of the environment, and perception—to be assumed to some degree by the collective assessment provided by the total membership, including the leader.

Therapeutic Factors. The following group processes account for therapeutic change.

Reality testing. The group setting serves as a reality-testing forum for each member to verbalize his or her thoughts and feelings toward the others, which are examined by the leader and the membership.

Transference. The feelings evoked among members of the group and between the members and the therapist are transferential when they are irrational and not consonant with reality.

Stimulation of transference. As patients observe one another's interactions, feelings that may have been repressed or suppressed can emerge. In general, negative feelings are expressed sooner in the group setting than in the one-to-one situation. A group patient may be reassured as he or she observes the therapist's nonpunitive reaction to another patient's anger and so be willing to express similar feelings of which he or she may not have been aware.

Multiple transferences. A variety of group members—each with his or her own genetic, dynamic, and behavioral patterns—may stand for the people significant in a particular patient's past or current life situation. Group members may take the roles of wife, mother, father, sibling, or employer. The patient can then work through actual or fantasized conflicts with the surrogate figures to a successful resolution. Role-playing techniques use this concept extensively.

Collective transference. A member's pathological personification of the group as a single transferential figure, generally the mother or father, is a phenomenon unique to group therapy. Or the member may see the therapist as one figure and the group as a whole as another. The collective transference may be either positive or negative in feeling. The therapist should encourage the patient to respond to members as individuals and to differentiate them in order to work through his or her particular distortion.

Transference neurosis. When a patient's transferential attachment to the therapist or, in group therapy, to another patient becomes excessively strong, a transference neurosis is said to exist. A strong negative transference by a patient toward the therapist may require an individual psychotherapy session to resolve the distortion. The therapist should not allow one or several patients to attack him or her in a group but should insist that the negative transference be discussed in individual sessions.

Identification. In individual therapy, many patients attempt to learn new modes of adaptation by taking on qualities of the therapist. In the group setting, a variety of other models are available, and patients identify with certain qualities of those other members, a process that may occur consciously, by simple imitation, or unconsciously, outside awareness. Whether identification constructively influences personality growth depends on whom the patient chooses for a model. Most important, the leader must be a suitable model.

Universalization. In the group, patients recognize that they are not alone in having an emotional problem and that others may be struggling with the same or similar problems. It is generally agreed that the process of universalization is one of the most important in group psychotherapy. The simple sharing of experiences, regardless of whether they are labeled as pathological, is an important human need.

Cohesion. All groups, not only psychotherapy groups, are marked by some amount of cohesion. Members feel a "we-ness," a sense of belonging. They value the group, which engenders loyalty and friendliness among them. They are willing to work together and to take responsibility for one another in achieving their common goals. They are also willing to endure a certain degree of frustration in order to maintain the group's integrity. A cohesive psychotherapy group is one in which members are accepting and supportive and have meaningful relationships with one another. Indeed, cohesion is the single most important factor in group therapy. The more cohesion the group has, the more likely it will have a successful outcome, for the patient will then be more receptive to the mechanisms that group therapy has to offer.

Group pressure. All group members are susceptible to group pressures to alter their behavior, thinking, or feeling; how susceptible they are depends on how attracted they are to the other members of the group and how much they value their group membership.

Much of the effectiveness of the behavioral approach to group psychotherapy rests on the observation that a patient is motivated by the reinforcement of the members' and the therapist's approval to embark on a new behavioral pattern.

Intellectualization. Intellectualization implies a cognitive awareness of oneself, others, and the various life experiences—both good and bad—that account for current functioning. Feed-

back, in which each member confronts the others with his or her immediate responses to events as they occur, serves as a learning device. All of the members are helped thereby to evaluate their own and the other members' defense mechanisms and ways of coping. Confrontation groups rely extensively on the feedback mechanism.

Interpretation, a derivative of intellectualization, also gives patients a cognitive framework within which they can better understand themselves, whether this interpretation comes from the therapist or from the other group members.

Intellectualization does not necessarily lead to change; experiential factors must be added if effective learning is to take place. The concept of the corrective emotional experience, first formulated by Franz Alexander, combines both these factors, the intellectual and the experiential, into a functional theoretical framework.

Ventilation and catharsis. Each group develops its own mix of ventilatory and cathartic processes, the mix depending on the group's composition, the style of leadership, and the theoretical framework. Some group therapists adhere to a style of leadership that encourages emotional release almost exclusively; others, equally rigid in their position, actively suppress the expression of strong affect. It is important that the leader be flexible so as to meet the needs of a particular group and so be able to determine which member will benefit from a greater emphasis on one of these processes. However, both processes should operate within any group.

Abreaction. Abreaction brings about an awareness, often for the first time, of degrees of emotion previously blocked from consciousness. It is often a highly therapeutic experience, even though it may produce an unavoidable sense of distress in all group members as the process unfolds.

Techniques geared to release strong emotion must be well timed and used only when the patient is well integrated into a group capable of providing as much support as is necessary to allow the patient to pass through the abreacted experience. When the experience is not well timed, a serious risk is involved, one that may result in psychological decompensation.

Role of the Therapist

Although opinions differ regarding how active or passive the therapist should be, it is generally agreed that the therapist's role is primarily a facilitative one. Ideally, the group members themselves are the primary source of cure and change.

The climate produced by the therapist's personality is a potent agent of change. The therapist is more than an expert applying techniques but is exerting a personal influence that taps variables such as empathy, warmth, and respect.

Inpatient Group Psychotherapy

Group therapy is also an important part of the hospitalized patient's therapeutic experience. Groups may be organized on a ward in a variety of ways: An entire inpatient unit can meet with all staff members (e.g., psychiatrists, psychologists, nurses) which is known as a community meeting; a group can consist of 15 to 20 patients and staff, which is called a team meeting; and a regular or small group composed of 8 to 10 patients may meet with one or two therapists, as in traditional group therapy. Although the goals of each type of group vary, they all have a common purpose: (1) to increase the patients' awareness of themselves through their interactions with the other group members, who provide feedback about their behavior; (2) to provide patients with improved interpersonal and social skills; (3) to help the members adapt to the inpatient setting; and (4) to improve communication between the patients and the staff. In addition, there is a type of group meeting composed only of the inpatient hospital staff that is used to improve communication among the staff members and to provide mutual support and encouragement in their day-to-day work with the patients. The community meeting and the team group are more helpful in dealing with patient management problems than they are for providing insight-oriented therapy, which is more the province of the small group therapy meeting.

Inpatient versus Outpatient Groups. Although the therapeutic factors that account for change in the small inpatient group are similar to those in the outpatient setting, there are qualitative differences. For example, the relatively high turnover of patients in the inpatient group complicates the process of cohesion. But the fact that all the members of the group are together in the hospital aids this cohesion, as do efforts by the therapist to foster this process, emphasizing other similarities. Sharing of information, universalization, and catharsis are the main therapeutic factors at work in inpatient groups. Although insight is more likely to occur in outpatient groups because of their long-term nature, it is possible within the confines of a single group session for some patients to obtain a new understanding of their psychological makeup. A unique quality of the inpatient group is the contact that patients have outside the regularly scheduled group meetings, which is extensive, as they live together on the same ward. If they verbalize their thoughts and feelings about such contacts in the therapy sessions, this will encourage interpersonal learning. In addition, conflicts between patients or between patients and staff can be anticipated and resolved.

Group Composition. Two key factors of the inpatient group are the heterogenity of its members and the rapid turnover of patients, which is common to all short-term therapies. Outside the hospital, however, the therapist has a larger caseload from which to select patients for group therapy. On the ward, the therapist has a limited number of patients from which to draw and is restricted further to those patients who are both willing to participate in and suitable for a small group experience. In certain settings, group participation may be mandatory (e.g., substance abuse and alcoholism units). But this is not usually true for a general psychiatry unit, and in fact, most group experiences are better when the patients themselves choose to enter them.

More sessions are preferable to fewer sessions. During a patient's hospital stay, groups may meet daily, allowing for interactional continuity and the carryover of themes from one session to the next. A new member of the group can quickly be brought up to date, either by the therapist in an orientation meeting or by one of the members. It is not uncommon for a newly admitted patient to have learned many details about the small group program from another patient before actually attending the first session. The less frequently the group sessions are held, the greater will be the need for the therapist to structure the group, and be active. In any case, that is a requirement for the therapist who practices short-term therapy either inside or outside the hospital.

Self-Help Groups

Self-help groups are composed of persons who want to cope with a specific problem or life crisis. Usually organized with a particular task in mind, such groups do not attempt to explore individual psychodynamics in great depth or to change personality functioning significantly. But self-help groups have improved the emotional health and well-being of many people.

A distinguishing characteristic of the self-help group is its homogeneity. The members suffer from the same disorders, and they share their experiences—good and bad, successful and unsuccessful—with one another. By so doing, they educate one another, provide mutual support, and alleviate the sense of alienation that is usually felt by the person drawn to this type of group.

Self-help groups emphasize cohesion, which is exceptionally strong in these groups. Because of the group members' similar problems and symptoms, a strong emotional bond and the group's own characteristics develop, to which magical qualities of healing may be attributed. Examples of self-help groups are Alcoholics Anonymous (A.A.), Gamblers Anonymous (G.A.), and Overeaters Anonymous (O.A.).

The self-help group movement is in its ascendency. The groups meet their members' needs by providing acceptance, mutual support, and help in overcoming maladaptive patterns of behavior or states of feeling with which traditional mental health and medical professionals have not been generally successful. Self-help groups and therapy groups have begun to converge: The self-help groups have enabled their members to give up a pattern of unwanted behavior; the therapy groups also help their members understand why and how they got to be the way they were or are.

COMBINED INDIVIDUAL AND GROUP PSYCHOTHERAPY

In combined individual and group psychotherapy, patients are seen individually by the therapist and also take part in group sessions. The therapist for the group and individual sessions is usually the same.

Groups can vary in size, from 3 to 15 members, but the best size is 8 to 10. It is important that patients attend all group sessions. Attendance at individual sessions is also important, and the failure to attend either group or individual sessions should be examined as part of the therapeutic process.

Combined therapy is a particular treatment modality. It is not a system by which individual therapy is augmented by an occasional group session, nor does it mean that a participant in group therapy meets alone with the therapist from time to time. Rather, it is an ongoing plan in which the group experience interacts meaningfully with the individual sessions and in which there is reciprocal feedback that helps form an integrated therapeutic experience. Although the one-to-one, doctor–patient relationship enables a deep examination of the transference reaction for some patients, it may not provide the corrective emotional experiences necessary for therapeutic change for others. The group gives patients a variety of persons to whom they can develop transferential reactions. In the microcosm of the group, patients can relive and work through familial and other important influences.

Techniques

Various techniques based on different theoretical frameworks have been used in the combined therapy format. Some clinicians increase the frequency of the individual sessions to encourage the emergence of the transference neurosis. In the behavioral model, individual sessions are regularly scheduled but tend to be less frequent. Depending on the therapist's orientation, during the individual sessions, the patient may use a couch or a chair. Techniques such as alternate meetings may be used in the group setting. Harold Kaplan and Benjamin Sadock developed a combined therapy approach called structured interactional group psychotherapy, in which a different member is the focus at each weekly group session.

Results

Most workers in the field believe that combined therapy has the advantages of both the dyadic setting and the group setting, without sacrificing the qualities of either. Generally, the dropout rate in combined therapy is lower than that of group therapy alone. In many cases, combined therapy appears to bring problems to the surface and to resolve them more quickly than may be possible with either method alone.

PSYCHODRAMA

Psychodrama is a method of group psychotherapy originated by Jacob Moreno, in which personality makeup, interpersonal relationships, conflicts, and emotional problems are explored by means of special dramatic methods. The therapeutic dramatization of emotional problems includes (1) the protagonist or patient, the person who acts out problems with the help of (2) auxiliary egos, persons who enact different aspects of the patient, and (3) the director, psychodramatist, or therapist, the person who guides those in the drama toward the acquisition of insight.

Roles

Director. The director is the leader or therapist and so must be active and participating. He or she encourages the members of the group to be spontaneous and so has a catalytic function. The director must be available to meet the group's needs and not superimpose his or her values on it. Of all the group psychotherapies, psychodrama requires of the therapist the most participation and ability to lead.

Protagonist. The protagonist is the patient in conflict. The patient chooses the situation to portray in the dramatic scene, or the therapist may choose it if the patient so desires.

Auxiliary Ego. The auxiliary egos are other group members who represent something or someone in the protagonist's experience. The auxiliary egos help account for the great range of therapeutic effects available in psychodrama.

Group. The members of the psychodrama and the audience make up the group. Some are participants, and others are observers, but all benefit from the experience to the extent that they can identify with the ongoing events. The concept of spontaneity in psychodrama refers to the ability of each member of the group, especially the protagonist, to experience the thoughts and feelings of the moment and to communicate emotion as authentically as possible.

Techniques

The psychodrama may focus on any special area of functioning (e.g., a dream, a family, or community situation), a symbolic role, an unconscious attitude, or an imagined future situation. Such symptoms as delusions or hallucinations can also be acted out. Techniques to advance the therapeutic progress, productivity, and creativity include the soliloquy (a recital of overt and hidden thoughts and feelings), role reversal (the exchange of the patient's role for the role of a significant person), the double (an auxiliary ego acting as the patient), the multiple double (several egos acting as the patient did on different occasions), and the mirror technique (an ego imitating the patient and speaking for him or her). Other modifying techniques include the use of hypnosis or psychoactive drugs to modify the acting behavior in various ways.

References

American Psychiatric Association: *Task Force Report on Encounter Groups and Psychiatry.* American Psychiatric Association, Washington, DC, 1970.

Bloch S, Crouch E: *Therapeutic Factors in Group Psychotherapy.* Oxford University Press, New York, 1985.

Cartright D, Zander A, editors: *Group Dynamics and Research Theory.* Harper & Row, New York, 1960.

Freud S: *Group Psychology and Analysis of the Ego.* Hogarth Press, London, 1962.

Grotjohn M, Freedman C T H, editors: *Handbook of Group Therapy.* Van Nostrand–Reinhold, New York, 1983.

Kaplan H I, Sadock B J, editors: *Comprehensive Group Psychotherapy.* ed 2. Williams & Williams, Baltimore, 1983.

Lieberman M A: Effects of large group awareness training on participants' psychiatric status. Am J Psych *144*:460, 1987.

Moreno J L: *Psychodrama.* Beacon House, Beacon, NY, 1947.

Olsen P A, Barth P A: New uses of psychodrama. J Operational Psychiatry *14*:95, 1983.

Roback H B, Smith M: Patient attention in dynamically oriented treatment groups. Am J Psych *144*:426, 1987.

Wolf A, Schwartz M: *Psychoanalysis in Groups.* Grune & Stratton, New York, 1962.

Yalom I: *The Theory and Practice of Group Psychotherapy,* ed 2. Basic Books, New York, 1975.

30.4 _____

Family Therapy and Marital Therapy

FAMILY THERAPY

General Considerations

Despite differences in specific models, what is unique to family therapy is its family orientation. All the members of the family are interrelated, and so one part of the family cannot be isolated from the rest. A family's structure and organization therefore must be viewed as a unit and are important to determining the behavior of the individual family members. Modern-day family therapy originated from the pioneering work of Nathan Ackerman.

Initial Consultation

Family therapy is well-enough known that families with a high level of conflict may request it specifically. When the initial complaint is about an individual, however, pretreatment work may be necessary. Typical fears underlying resistance to a family approach are fear (1) by parents that they will be blamed for their child's difficulties, (2) that the entire family will be pronounced "sick," (3) that a spouse will object, and (4) that open discussion of one child's misbehavior will have a negative influence on younger siblings. Refusal by an adolescent or young adult patient to participate in family therapy is frequently a disguised collusion with the fears of one or both parents.

Interview Technique

The special quality of the family interview proceeds from two important facts: (1) The family comes to treatment with its history and dynamics firmly in place. To the family therapist, it is this established nature of the group, more than the symptoms, that constitutes the clinical problem; (2) Family members usually live together and, at some level, depend on one another for physical and emotional well-being. Whatever transpires in the therapy session is known to all. Central principles of technique derive from these facts. For example, the catharsis of anger by one family member toward another must be carefully channeled by the therapist. This is because the person who is the object of the anger is present and will react to the attack, either in the interview or at home, running the danger of escalation toward violence, fractured relationships, or withdrawal from therapy. Free association is likewise not appropriate because it would encourage one person to dominate the session. In short, the family interview must always be controlled and directed by the therapist.

Frequency and Length of Treatment

Unless an emergency arises, sessions are usually held no more than once a week. Each session, however, may require 1½ or 2 hours. Long sessions can include an intermission to give the therapist time to organize the material and plan a response. A flexible schedule is necessary when geography or personal circumstances make it physically difficult for the family to get together. The length of treatment depends not only on the nature of the problem but also on the therapeutic model. Therapists who use problem-solving models exclusively may accomplish their goals in a few sessions; therapist using growth-oriented models, however, may work with a family for years, with sessions at long intervals.

Models of Intervention

Psychodynamic-Experiential Models. Psychodynamic-experiential models emphasize individual maturation in the context of the family system, free from unconscious patterns of anxiety and projection rooted in the past. Therapists seek to establish an intimate bond with each family member, alternating between their exchanges with the members and the members' exchanges with one another. Clarity of communication and honestly admitted feelings are given high priority; toward this end, family members may be encouraged to change their seats, to touch one another, and to make direct eye contact. Their use of metaphor, body language, and parapraxes help reveal the unconscious pattern of family relationships. The therapist may also use *family sculpting,* in which family members physically arrange one another in tableaus depicting their personal view of relationships, past or present. The therapist both interprets the sculpture and modifies it in a way to suggest new relationships. In addition, the therapist's subjective responses to the family are given great importance. At appropriate moments, they are expressed to the family to form yet another feedback loop of self-observation and change.

Bowen Model. Bowen calls his model simply "family systems," but in the field it has rightfully been given the name of its originator. Its hallmark is personal differentiation from the family of origin, the ability to be one's true self in the face of familial or other pressures that threaten the loss of love or social position. The problem family is assessed on two levels: (1) the degree of their enmeshment versus the degree of their ability to differentiate and (2) the analysis of emotional triangles in the presenting problem. An emotional triangle is defined as a three-party subsystem (of which there can be many within a family), arranged so that the closeness of two members tends to exclude a third. The closeness may be expressed as either love or repetitive conflict. In either case, emotional cross-currents are activated when the excluded third party attempts to join with one of the others or when one of the involved parties shifts in the direction of the excluded one. The role of the therapist is, first, to stablize or shift the "hot" triangle—the one that relates to the presenting symptoms—and, second, to work with the most psychologically available family members, individually if necessary, on achieving enough personal differentiation so that the hot triangle does not recur. In order to stay neutral in their triangles, the therapist minimizes emotional contact with family members. Bowen originated the *genogram,* which is a historical survey of the family going back several generations.

Structural Model. In a structural model, the family is viewed as a single interrelated system assessed along the following lines: (1) significant alliances and splits among family members, (2) hierarchy of power (i.e., the parents "in charge" of the children), (3) the clarity and firmness of boundaries between the generations, and (4) the family's tolerance of one another. The structure model uses concurrent individual and family therapy.

General Systems Model. Based on general systems theory, the general systems model holds that the family is a system and that every action in the family produces a reaction in one or more of its members. Every member is presumed to play a role (e.g., spokesperson, persecutor, victim, rescuer, symptom bearer, nuturer), which is relatively stable; however, the member who fills each role may change. Some families try to scapegoat one member by blaming him or her for the family's problems (indicated patient). If the indicated patient improves, another scapegoated family member may be found. The family is defined as having external boundaries and internal rules. The system model overlaps with some of the others models presented, particularly the Bowen and structural models.

An overview of family therapy models, techniques, and goals is given in Table 1.

Recent Modifications

Family Group Therapy. Family group therapy combines several families into a single group. Mutual problems are shared, and families compare their interactions with those of the other families in the group. Parents of disturbed children may also be gathered together to share their situations.

Social Network Therapy. Social network therapy gathers together the social community or network of a disturbed individual, all of whom meet in group sessions with the patient. The

Table 1
Major Models of Family Therapy: Normality, Dysfunction, and Therapeutic Goals

Model of Family Therapy	View of Normal Family Functioning	View of Dysfunction/Symptoms	Goals of Therapy

Structural
Minuchin
Montalvo
Aponte
	1. Boundaries clear and firm.
	2. Hierarchy with strong parental subsystem.
	3. Flexibility of system for
	  a. Autonomy and interdependence.
	  b. Individual growth and system maintenance.
	  c. Continuity, and adaptive restructuring in response to changing internal (developmental) and external (environmental) demands.
		Symptoms result from current family structural imbalance:
		a. Malfunctioning hierarchical arrangement, boundaries.
		b. Maladaptive reaction to changing requirements (developmental, environmental).
			Reorganize family structure:
			a. Shift members' relative positions to disrupt malfunctioning pattern and strengthen parental hierarchy.
			b. Create clear, flexible boundaries.
			c. Mobilize more adaptive alternative patterns.

Strategic
Haley
Milan team
Palo Alto group
	1. Flexibility.
	2. Large behavioral repertoire for
	  a. Problem resolution.
	  b. Life-cycle passage.
	3. Clear rules governing hierarchy (Haley).
		Multiple origins of problems; symptoms maintained by family's
		a. Unsuccessful problem-solving attempts.
		b. Inability to adjust to life-cycle transitions (Haley).
		c. Malfunctioning hierarchy: triangle or coalition across hierarchy (Haley).
		Symptom is a communicative act embedded in interaction pattern.
			Resolve presenting problem only; specific behaviorally defined objectives.
			Interrupt rigid feedback cycle: change symptom-maintaining sequence to new outcome.
			Define clearer hierarchy (Haley).

Behavioral-social exchange Liberman Patterson Alexander	1. Maladaptive behavior is not reinforced. 2. Adaptive behavior is rewarded. 3. Exchange of benefits outweighs costs. 4. Long-term reciprocity.	Maladaptive, symptomatic behavior reinforced by a. Family attention and reward. b. Deficient reward exchanges (e.g., coercive). c. Communication deficit.	Concrete, observable behavioral goals: change contingencies of social reinforcement (interpersonal consequences of behavior). a. Rewards for adaptive behavior. b. No rewards for maladaptive behavior.

Table 1 *continued*
Major Models of Family Therapy: Normality, Dysfunction, and Therapeutic Goals

Model of Family Therapy	View of Normal Family Functioning	View of Dysfunction/Symptoms	Goals of Therapy

Psychodynamic
Ackerman
Boszormenyi-
  Nagy
Framo
Lidz
Meissner
Paul
Stierlin
	1. Parental personalities and re-
	  lationships well differentiated.
	2. Relationship perceptions
	  based on current realities,
	  not projections from past.
	Boszormenyi-Nagy: Relational
	equitability.
	Lidz: Family task requisities:
	a. Parental coalition.
	b. Generation boundaries.
	c. Sex-linked parental roles.
		Symptoms due to family projec-
		tion process stemming from un-
		resolved conflicts and losses in
		family of origin.
			1. Insight and resolution of
			  family of origin conflict and
			  losses.
			2. ↓Family projection processes.
			3. Relationship reconstruction
			  and reunion.
			4. Individual and family growth.

Family systems
  therapy
Bowen
	Differentiation of self.
	Intellectual/emotional balance.
		Functioning impaired by rela-
		tionships with family of origin:
		a. Poor differentiation.
		b. Anxiety (reactivity).
		c. Family projection process.
		d. Triangulation.
			1. Differentiation.
			2. ↑Cognitive functioning.
			3. ↓Emotional reactivity.
			4. Modification of relationships
			  in family system:
			  a. Detriangulation.
			  b. Repair cut-offs.

Experiential
Satir
Whitaker
	Satir:
	1. Self-worth: high.
	2. Communication: clear,
	  specific, honest.
	3. Family rules: flexible, human,
	  appropriate.
	4. Linkage to society: open,
	  hopeful.
	Whitaker: Multiple aspects of
	family structure and shared ex-
	perience.
		Symptoms are nonverbal mes-
		sages in reaction to current
		communication dysfunction in
		system.
			1. Direct, clear communication.
			2. Individual and family growth
			  through immediate shared
			  experience.

Table from Walsh F: Conceptualizations of normal family functioning. In *Normal Family Processes,* F Walsh, editor. Guilford Press, New York, 1982. Copyright of Guilford Press, and reprinted by permission.

network includes those persons with whom the patient comes into contact in daily life, not only his or her immediate family, but also relatives, friends, tradespeople, teachers, and co-workers.

Goals

The goals of treatment are as follows: (1) to resolve or reduce pathogenic conflict and anxiety within the matrix of interpersonal relationships, (2) to enhance the perception and fulfillment by family members of one another's emotional needs, (3) to promote more appropriate role relations between the sexes and between the generations, (4) to strengthen the capacity of individual members and the family as a whole to cope with destructive forces inside and outside the surrounding environment, and (5) to influence family identity and values so that members are oriented toward health and growth.

A final goal is to integrate the family into the larger systems in the society, which include not only the extended family but also society as represented by such systems as schools, medical facilities, and social, recreational, and welfare agencies, so that the family is not isolated.

MARITAL THERAPY

Introduction

Marital therapy is a form of psychotherapy designed to modify psychologically the interaction of two people who are in conflict with each other over one or a variety of parameters—social, emotional, sexual, economic. In marital therapy, a trained person establishes a therapeutic contract with the patient-couple and, through definite types of communication, attempts to alleviate the disturbance, to reverse or change maladaptive patterns of behavior, and to encourage personality growth and development.

Marriage counseling may be considered more limited in scope than is marital therapy in that only a particular familial conflict is discussed. Marriage counseling also may be primarily task oriented, geared to solving a specific problem such as child rearing. Marriage therapy emphasizes restructuring the interaction between the couple, sometimes exploring the psychodynamics of each partner. Both therapy and counseling stress helping the marital partners cope more effectively with their problems. Most important is the definition of appropriate and realistic goals, which may involve extensive reconstruction of the union, problem-solving approaches, or a combination of both.

Types of Therapy

Individual Therapy. In individual therapy, the marital partners may be seen by different therapists, who may not necessarily communicate with each other. Indeed, they may not even know each other. The goal of the treatment is to strengthen each partner's adaptive capacities. At times, only one of the partners is in treatment; in such cases, a visit by the spouse who is not in treatment with the therapist may be helpful. The visiting partner may give the therapist data about the patient that may otherwise be overlooked; overt or covert anxiety in the visiting partner as a result of change in the patient can be identified and dealt with; irrational beliefs about treatment events can be corrected; and conscious or unconscious attempts by the partner to sabotage the patient's treatment can be examined.

Individual Marital Therapy. In individual marital therapy, each of the marriage partners is in therapy. When the same therapist conducts the treatment, it is called concurrent therapy; when the partners are seen by different therapists, it is called collaborative therapy.

Conjoint Therapy. Conjoint therapy is the treatment of partners in joint sessions conducted by either one or two therapists; it is the treatment method most frequently used in marital therapy. Co-therapy with therapists of both sexes prevents a particular patient from feeling ganged up on when confronted by two members of the opposite sex.

Four-Way Session. In a four-way session, each partner is seen by a different therapist, with regular joint sessions in which all four persons participate. A variation of the four-way session is the round-table interview, developed by William Masters and Virginia Johnson for the rapid treatment of sexually dysfunctional couples. Two patients and two opposite-sex therapists meet regularly. (See Section 21.2b for a discussion of dual sex therapy.)

Group Psychotherapy. Therapy for married couples placed in a group allows a variety of group dynamics to affect the couples. The group usually consists of three to four couples and one or two therapists. The couples identify with one another and recognize that others have similar problems; each gains support and empathy from fellow group members of the same or opposite sex; they explore sexual attitudes and have an opportunity to gain new information from their peer group; and each receives specific feedback about his or her behavior, either negative or positive, that may have more meaning and be better assimilated coming from a neutral nonspouse member.

When only one partner is in a therapy group, the spouse may occasionally visit the group, so as to allow the members to test reality more effectively. At times, a group may be so organized that only one married couple is part of the larger group.

Combined Therapy. Combined therapy refers to any or all of the preceding techniques used concurrently or in combination. Thus, a particular patient-couple may begin treatment with one or both partners in individual psychotherapy, continue to conjoint therapy with the partner, and terminate therapy after a course of treatment in a married couples group. The rationale for combined therapy is that no single approach to marital problems has been demonstrated as superior to another. A familiarity with a variety of approaches thus allows the therapist a degree of flexibility that will provide maximum benefit for the couple in distress.

Indications

Regardless of the specific therapeutic technique used, certain indications for initiating marital therapy have been agreed on: (1) when individual therapy has failed to resolve the marital difficulties, (2) when the onset of distress in one or both partners is clearly related to marital events, and (3) when marital therapy is requested by a couple in conflict. Problems in communication between partners are a prime indication for marital therapy. In such instances, one spouse may be intimidated by the other, may become anxious when attempting to tell the other about thoughts or feelings, or may project unconscious expectations onto the other. The therapy is geared toward enabling each of the partners to see the other realistically.

Conflicts in one or several areas, such as the partners' sexual life, also are indications for treatment. Similarly, difficulty in establishing satisfactory social, economic, parental, or emotional roles is an indication for help. The clinician should evaluate all aspects of the marital relationship before attempting to treat only one problem, as it may be a symptom of a more pervasive marital disorder.

Contraindications

Contraindications for marital therapy include patients with severe forms of psychosis, particularly patients with paranoid elements and those in whom the marriage's homeostatic mechanism is a protection against psychosis; one or both of the partners really wants to divorce; or one spouse refuses to participate because of anxiety or fear.

Goals

Nathan Ackerman defined the aims of marital therapy as follows: The goals of therapy for marital disorders are to alleviate emotional distress and disability and to promote the levels of well-being of both partners together and each as an individual. In a general way, the therapist moves toward these goals by strengthening the shared resources for problem solving; by encouraging the substitution of more adequate controls and defenses for pathogenic ones; by enhancing both the immunity against the disintegrative effects of emotional upset and the complementarity of the relationship; and promoting the growth of the relationship and each partner.

Part of the therapeutic task is to persuade each partner in the marriage to take responsibility in understanding the psychodynamic makeup of his or her personality. Accountability for the effects of behavior on one's own life, the life of the spouse, and the lives of others in the environment is emphasized, which often results in a deeper understanding of the problems that created the marital discord and in a working through of individual psychotherapy.

Marital therapy does not ensure the maintenance of any marriage. Indeed, in certain instances, it may show the partners that they are in a nonviable union that should be dissolved.

References

Berkowitz D: An overview of the psychodynamics of couples—Bridging concepts. In *Marriage and Divorce—A Contemporary Perspective*, C C Nadelson, D C Polonsky, editors. Guilford Press, New York, 1984.

Berman E, Lief H I, Williams A: A model of marital interactions. In *The Handbook of Marriage and Marital Therapy*, G P Sholevar, editor, p 3. SP Medical and Scientific Books, New York, 1981.

Bowen M: *Family Therapy in Clinical Practice*. Jason Aronson, New York, 1978.

Dicks H V: Concepts of marital diagnosis of therapy as developed at the Tavistock family psychiatric Clinic, London, England. In *Marriage Counseling in Medical Practice*, E M Nas, L Jessner, D W Abse, editors. University of North Carolina Press, Chapel Hill, 1964.

Green R J, Framo J L, editors: *Family Therapy: Major Contributions*. International Universities Press, New York, 1981.

Meissner W W: The conceptualization of marriage and family dynamics from a psychoanalytic perspective. In *Marriage and Marital Therapy*, Paolino T, McCrady B, editors, p. 35. Brunner/Mazel, New York, 1987.

Minuchin S: *Families and Family Therapy*. Harvard University Press, Cambridge, MA, 1974.

Nadelson C C, Polonsky D C, Mathews M A: Marriage as a developmental process. In *Marriage and Divorce—A Contemporary Perspective*, C C Nadelson, D C Polonsky, editors. Guilford Press, New York, 1984.

Rogers C R: A theory of therapy, personality, and interpersonal relationships as developed in the client-centered framework. In *Psychology: A Study of a Science, vol 3, Formulations of the Person and Their Social Context*, S Koch, editor, p 184. McGraw–Hill, New York, 1959.

Sonne J C: Transference considerations in marriage and marital therapy. In *The Handbook of Marriage and Marital Therapy*, G P Sholevar, editor, p 103. SP Medical and Scientific Books, New York, 1981.

30.5 _____
Behavioral Medicine and Biofeedback

INTRODUCTION

Behavioral medicine is the application of principles of behavior therapy to the prevention, diagnosis, treatment, and rehabilitation of medical disorders. It is unusual in that it focuses on physical disorders rather than mental disorders, and it applies to such areas as stress prevention and reduction, adult patient management and compliance, pediatric management, pain control, and psychiatric disorders associated with medical problems. Behavioral medicine also helps prevent disease through the reduction of health risk factors and the modification of life-style. For example, many of the risk factors in coronary artery disease have components that can be influenced by behavior. Such factors include hypercholesterolemia, which can be reduced by a low-fat diet; hypertension, which can be reduced by a low-salt diet and exercise; and obesity, which can also be corrected by diet and exercise. Although medication can be used to correct these conditions, it is preferable to attend to the behavioral factors that contribute to and maintain these risk factors.

The major areas within behavioral medicine are the so-called disorders of self-control, such as obesity, cigarette smoking, and psychoactive substance use disorders, including alcoholism. The clinician attempts to help the patient better control self-destructive behavior by such methods that enable the patient to become aware of behavioral patterns and the factors that reinforce these patterns and so develop new patterns that are constructive and health promoting.

The term "behavioral medicine" was introduced by Bick in 1973 in *Biofeedback: Behavioral Medicine*. Since then, the field has developed a perspective broader than biofeedback, although feedback remains an important concept. Feedback is fundamental to biological adaptation, feedback not only from the environment but also from the body itself. Homeostasis is maintained and neurohumoral behavior is regulated also through feedback loops or servomechanism systems. Biofeedback is a special type of feedback that refers to information provided externally to a person about normally subthreshold biological or physiological processes.

In addition to biofeedback, relaxation training, behavior therapy, and hypnosis are important treatment modalities in behavioral medicine, as described in Sections 30.6 and 30.7.

BIOFEEDBACK THEORY

Neal Miller demonstrated the medical potential of biofeedback by showing that the normally involuntary autonomic nervous system (ANS) could be operantly conditioned using appropriate feedback. By means of instruments, the patient is given information about the status of certain involuntary biological functions such as skin temperature and electrical conductivity, muscle tension, blood pressure, heart rate, and brain wave activity. The patient is then taught to regulate one or more of these biological states, which affects a symptom. For example, the ability to raise the temperature of one's hands may be used to reduce the frequency of migraine headaches, palpitations, or angina pectoris. A presumptive mechanism would be a lowering of sympathetic activation and a voluntary self-regulation of arterial smooth muscle vasoconstrictive tendencies in predisposed persons.

BIOFEEDBACK METHODS

The type of feedback instrument used depends on the patient and the specific problem. The most effective instruments are the electromyograph (EMG), which measures the electrical potentials of muscle fibers; the electroencephalograph (EEG), which measures alpha waves that occur in relaxed states; the galvanic skin response gauge (GSR), which shows decreased skin conductivity during a relaxed state; and the thermister, which measures skin temperature which drops during tension owing to peripheral vasoconstriction. The patient is attached to one of the measuring instruments, which measures a physiologic function and translates the impulse into an audible or visual signal that the patient uses to gauge his or her responses. For example, in treating bruxism, an EMG is attached to the masseter muscle. The EMG emits a high tone when the muscle is contracted and a low tone when at rest. The patient can learn to alter the tone to indicate relaxation. He or she receives feedback about the masseter muscle; the tone reinforces the learning; and the condition ameliorates, all of these events interacting synergistically.

BIOFEEDBACK APPLICATIONS

Neuromuscular Rehabilitation

Mechanical devices or an EMG measurement of muscle activity displayed to a patient increases the effectiveness of traditional therapies, as documented by relatively long clinical histories in peripheral nerve–muscle damage, spasmodic torticollis, selected cases of tardive dyskinesia, cerebral palsy, and upper motor neuron hemiplegias.

Fecal Incontinence and Enuresis

The timing sequence of internal and external anal sphincters has been measured using triple lumen rectal catheters providing feedback to incontinent patients in order for them to reestablish normal bowel habits in a relatively small number of biofeedback sessions. An actual precursor of biofeedback dating to 1938 was the sounding of a buzzer for sleeping enuretic children at the first sign of moisture (the pad and bell).

Raynaud's Syndrome

Cold hands and cold feet are frequent concomitants of anxiety and also occur in Raynaud's syndrome, caused by vasospasm of arterial smooth muscle. A number of studies report that thermal feedback from the hand, an inexpensive and benign procedure compared with surgical sympathectomy, is effective in about 70 percent of cases of Raynaud's syndrome.

Migraine Headaches

The most common biofeedback strategy with classic or common vascular headaches has been thermal biofeedback from a digit accompanied by autogenic self-suggestive phrases encouraging hand warming and head cooling. The mechanism is thought to help prevent excessive cerebral artery vasoconstriction, often accompanied by an ischemic prodromal symptom, such as scintillating scotomata, followed by rebound engorgement of arteries and stretching of vessel wall pain receptors.

Tension Headaches

Muscle contraction headaches are most frequently treated with two fairly large active electrodes spaced on the forehead to provide visual or auditory information about levels of muscle tension. This frontal electrode placement is sensitive to EMG activity regarding the frontalis and occipital muscles which the patient learns to relax.

Cardiac Arrhythmias

Specific biofeedback of the electrocardiogram has permitted patients to lower the frequency of premature ventricular contractions.

Idiopathic Hypertension and Orthostatic Hypotension

A variety of specific (direct) and nonspecific biofeedback procedures, including blood pressure feedback, galvanic skin response, and foot hand thermal feedback combined with relaxation procedures, have been used to teach patients to increase or decrease their blood pressure. Some follow-up data indicate that these changes may persist for at least 2 years and often permit the reduction or elimination of antihypertensive medications.

Myofacial and Temporomandibular Joint (TMJ) Pain

Increased levels of EMG activity over the powerful muscles associated with bilateral temporomandibular joints have been decreased using biofeedback in patients diagnosed as being jaw clenchers or demonstrating bruxism.

Grand Mal Epilepsy

A number of electroencephalographic biofeedback procedures have been used experimentally to suppress seizure activity prophylactically in patients not responsive to anticonvulsant medication. The procedures permit patients to enhance the sensorimotor brain wave rhythm or to normalize brain activity as computed in real-time power spectrum displays.

Hyperactivity

EEG biofeedback procedures have been used on children with attention deficit hyperactivity disorder, to train them to reduce their motor restlessness. Biofeedback of this disorder is still experimental.

Asthma

Both frontal EMG and airway resistance biofeedback have been reported as producing relaxation from the panic associated with asthma, as well as improving air flow rate.

As can be seen from this overview, a wide variety of biofeedback modalities have been used to treat numerous conditions. Many less specific clinical applications, such as treating insomnia, dysmenorrhea, and speech problems; improving athletic performance; treating volitional disorders, achieving altered states of consciousness; managing stress; and using biofeedback as an adjunct to psychotherapy for anxiety associated with somatoform disorders, use a model in which frontalis muscle EMG biofeedback is combined with thermal biofeedback along with verbal instructions in progressive relaxation.

RELAXATION TRAINING

Relaxation produces physiological effects that are opposite to those of anxiety (i.e., slow heart rate, increased peripheral blood flow, and neuromuscular stability). A variety of relaxation methods have been developed, although some, such as yoga and Zen, have been known for centuries. Jacobson developed a method in which various parts of the body are alternately tensed and relaxed. Another method is hypnosis (see Section 30.7). Autogenic methods include phrases that a person repeats (or that are on tape) that instill a sense of muscular and mental relaxation. Type A personalities, as described by Friedman and Rosenman, are hard-driving, ambitious, time-conscious persons who are prone to coronary artery disease. Such persons can benefit from autogenic training that teaches them to relax.

Mental imagery is another relaxation method in which the patient is instructed to imagine himself or herself in a place associated with pleasant relaxed memories. Such images allow the patients to enter a relaxed state or experience, or as Benson termed it, the relaxation response.

References

Basmajian J V, editor: *Biofeedback: Principles and Practice for Clinicians.* Williams & Wilkins, Baltimore, 1983.
Butler F: *Biofeedback: A Survey of the Literature.* Plenum, New York, 1978.
Gaarder K R, Montgomery S: *Clinical Biofeedback: A Procedural Manual for Behavioral Medicine.* Williams & Wilkins, Baltimore, 1981.
Olton D S, Noonberg A R: *Biofeedback: Clinical Applications in Behavioral Medicine.* Prentice–Hall, Englewood Cliffs, NJ, 1980.
Orne M T, editor: *Task Force Report no. 19: Biofeedback.* American Psychiatric Association, Washington, DC, 1980.
Peper E, Ancoli S, Quinn M, editors: *Mind/Body Integration: Essential Readings in Biofeedback.* Plenum, New York, 1979.
Pomerleau O F, Brady J P, editors: *Behavioral Medicine: Theory and Practice.* Williams & Wilkins, Baltimore, 1979.
Runck B: *Biofeedback—Issues and Treatment Assessment.* National Institute of Mental Health (DDHS Pub. no. ADM 80-1032), Rockville, MD, 1980.
Stroebel C F, editor: Biofeedback and behavioral medicine and biofeedback in clinical practice. Psychiatr Ann *11,* 1981.

30.6 _____
Behavior Therapy

INTRODUCTION

The use of behavior therapy to treat mental disorders is relatively new, having come to the fore within the last decade, and is of increasing importance. It is based on the principles of learning theory and uses classical and operant conditioning techniques. Behavior therapy is directed at specific problems and works best when those problems are clearly delineated and the desired goals are clearly defined.

HISTORY

As early as the 1920s, scattered reports began to appear on the application of learning principles to the treatment of behavioral disorders. These reports, however, had little effect on the mainstream of psychiatry or clinical psychology. It was not until the 1960s that behavior therapy emerged as a systematic and comprehensive approach to psychiatric (behavioral) disorders. It is curious that these latter developments arose quite independently of one another and on three different continents. Joseph Wolpe and his colleagues in Johannesburg, South Africa, used largely Pavlovian techniques to produce and eliminate experimental neuroses in cats. It is from this research that Wolpe developed systematic desensitization, the prototype of many current behavioral procedures for the treatment of maladaptive anxiety that is produced by identifiable stimuli in the environment. At about the same time, a group at the Institute of Psychiatry of the University of London, particularly H. J. Eysenck and M. B. Shapiro, stressed the importance of an empirical, experimental approach to the understanding and treatment of the individual patient, using own-control, single-case experimental paradigms, as well as modern learning theory. The third origin of behavior therapy was work inspired by

the research of Harvard psychologist, B. F. Skinner. Skinner's students began to apply his operant-conditioning technology, which was developed in animal-conditioning laboratories, to human subjects in clinical settings.

SYSTEMATIC DESENSITIZATION

Systematic desensitization was developed by Joseph Wolpe and is based on the behavioral principle of counterconditioning, which states that a person can overcome maladaptive anxiety elicited by a situation or object by approaching the feared situations gradually and in a psychophysiological state that inhibits anxiety.

In systematic desensitization, the patient attains a state of complete relaxation and then is exposed to the stimulus that elicits the anxiety response. The negative reaction of anxiety is then inhibited by the relaxed state, a process called *reciprocal inhibition*.

Rather than use actual situations or objects that elicit fear, the patient and the therapist prepare a graded list or hierarchy of anxiety-provoking scenes associated with the patient's fears. Finally the learned relaxation state and the anxiety-provoking scenes are systematically paired in the treatment. Thus, systematic desensitization consists of three steps: relaxation training, hierarchy construction, and the desensitization of the stimulus.

Relaxation Training

Most methods of achieving relaxation are based on a method called progressive relaxation. The patient relaxes major muscle groups in a fixed order, beginning with the small muscle groups of the feet and working cephalad, or vice versa. Some clinicians use hypnosis to facilitate relaxation or use tape-recorded procedures to allow the patient to practice relaxation on his or her own.

Hierarchy Construction

When constructing the hierarchy, the clinican determines all the conditions that elicit anxiety and then has the patient create a list or hierarchy of 10 to 12 scenes in order of increasing anxiety. For example, the acrophobic hierarchy may begin with the patient's imagining standing near a window on the second floor and end with being on the roof of a 20-story building, leaning on a guard rail and looking straight down.

Desensitization of the Stimulus

The desensitization is done systematically by having the patient proceed through the list from the least anxiety-provoking scene to the most anxiety-provoking one, while in a deeply relaxed state. The rate at which the patient progresses through the list is determined by his or her responses to the stimuli. When the patient can vividly imagine the most anxiety-provoking scene of the hierarchy with equanimity, he or she will experience little anxiety in the corresponding real-life situation.

Adjunctive Use of Drugs

Various drugs have been used to hasten desensitization. The widest experience is with the ultrarapidly acting barbiturate sodium methohexital (Brevital), which is given intravenously in subanesthetic doses. Usually, up to 60 mg of the drug are given in divided doses in a session. Intravenous diazepam (Valium) may also be used. If the procedural details are carefully followed, almost all patients will find the procedure pleasant, with few unpleasant side effects. The advantages of pharmacological desensitization are that preliminary training in relaxation can be shortened; almost all patients are able to become adequately relaxed; and the treatment itself seems to proceed more rapidly.

Indications of Densitization

This technique works best when there is a clearly identifiable anxiety-provoking stimulus. Phobias, obsessions, compulsions, and certain sexual disorders have been successfully treated with this use of drugs.

FLOODING

Flooding is based on the premise that escaping from an anxiety-provoking experience reinforces the anxiety, through conditioning. Thus by not allowing the person to escape, anxiety can be extinguished, and the conditioned avoidance behavior can be prevented.

The technique is to encourage the patient to imagine or actually to confront the feared situation. No relaxation exercises are used, as in systematic desensitization. The patient experiences fear, which gradually subsides after a period of time. The success of the procedure depends on the patient's remaining in the fear-generating situation until he or she is calm and feeling a sense of mastery. Prematurely withdrawing from the situation or prematurely terminating the fantasized scene is equivalent to an escape, and then both the conditioned anxiety and the avoidance behavior will be reinforced, opposite to what was intended. A variant of flooding is called *implosion*, in which the imagined or real event is made worse than it actually is (e.g., a patient with a fear of snakes imagines not only seeing one but also seeing it crawling on his or her body), in order to desensitize the person.

Many patients refuse flooding because of the psychological discomfort involved. It also is contraindicated in patients for whom intense anxiety would be hazardous (e.g., patients with heart disease or fragile psychological adaptation). These techniques work best with specific phobias.

GRADED EXPOSURE

Graded exposure is similar to flooding except that the phobic object or situation is approached through a series of small steps. Unlike systematic desensitization, however, relaxation training is not involved, and the treatment is usually carried out in a real-life context.

PARTICIPANT MODELING

Participant modeling refers to having the patient learn by imitation. The patient learns a new behavior by observation alone, without performing the behavior and without direct external reinforcement. Just as irrational fears may be acquired by learning, they can be unlearned by observing a fearless model confront the feared object. The technique has been useful with phobic children who are placed with other children of their own age and sex who approach the feared object or situation. With adults, a therapist may describe the feared activity in a calm manner with which the patient can identify, or the therapist may act out with the patient the process of mastering the feared activity. Sometimes a hierarchy of activities may be established, with the least anxiety-provoking activity being dealt with first. The participant-modeling technique has been used successfully with agoraphobia by having a therapist accompany the patient into the feared situation. A variant of this procedure is called *behavior rehearsal*, in which real-life problems are acted out under the therapist's observation or direction. The technique is useful for more complex behavioral patterns, such as job interviews and shyness.

ASSERTIVENESS AND SOCIAL SKILLS TRAINING

To be assertive requires that persons have confidence in their judgment and sufficient self-esteem to express their opinions. Assertiveness and social skills training teaches people how to respond appropriately in social situations, to express their opinions in acceptable ways, and to achieve their goals. A variety of techniques, including role modeling, desensitization, and positive reinforcement (reward of desired behavior), are used to increase assertiveness. Social skills training deals with assertiveness but also attends to a variety of real-life tasks, such as food shopping, looking for work, interacting with other people, and overcoming shyness.

AVERSION THERAPY

When a noxious stimulus (punishment) is presented immediately after a specific behavioral response, the response is eventually inhibited and extinguished. There are many types of noxious stimuli: electric shocks, substances that induce vomiting, corporeal punishment, social disapproval, and other punishing stimuli. The negative stimulus is paired with the behavior, which is thereby suppressed. The unwanted behavior usually disappears after a series of such sequences. Aversion therapy has been used for alcoholism, paraphilias, and other behaviors with impulsive or compulsive qualities.

POSITIVE REINFORCEMENT

If a behavioral response is followed by a generally rewarding event—for example, food, avoidance of pain, or praise—it tends to be strengthened and to occur more frequently. That principle has been applied in a variety of situations. On inpatient hospital wards, mental patients have been rewarded for performing a desired behavior with tokens that they may use to purchase luxury items or certain privileges. The process has been successful in altering behavior and is known as a *token economy*. Some workers have suggested that psychotherapy is effective, in part because patients want to please the therapist and so change their behavior in order to receive the therapist's praise. Freud stated that in treating phobias, the patient needs to be encouraged to face the phobia at some point based upon the positive relationship between the doctor and patient.

SPECIFIC DISORDERS

Agoraphobia

Graded exposure and flooding can reduce the fear of being in crowded places. About 60 percent of patients so treated are improved. In some cases, the spouse can serve as the therapist while accompanying the patient into the fear situation; however, there cannot be a secondary gain in which the patient attempts to keep the spouse nearby, by displaying symptoms.

Other Phobias

Systematic desensitization has been effective in treating simple phobias, such as fears of heights, animals, and fear of flying. Social skills training has also been used for shyness and fear of other people.

Schizophrenic Disorders

The token economy procedure, in which tokens are awarded for desirable behavior and can be used to buy ward privileges, has been useful in treating inpatient schizophrenic patients. Social skills training teaches schizophrenic patients how to interact with others in a socially acceptable way so that negative feedback is eliminated. In addition, the aggressive behavior of some schizophrenic patients can be diminished through these methods.

Sexual Dysfunctions

Dual sex therapy, developed by William Masters and Virginia Johnson, is a behavioral therapy technique used for various sexual dysfunctions, especially impotence, anorgasmia, and premature ejaculation. It uses relaxation, desensitization, and graded exposure as the primary techniques. (See Section 21.2b for a further discussion of these therapies.)

Alcoholism

Aversion therapy in which the alcoholic is made to vomit (by adding an emetic to the alcohol) every time a drink is ingested is effective in treating alcoholism. Disulfiram therapy (Antabuse) can be given to alcoholics when they are alcohol free. Such patients are warned of the severe physiological consequences of drinking (e.g., nausea, vomiting, hypotension, collapse) with Antabuse in the system.

Paraphilias

Electric shocks can be applied at the time of a paraphilic impulse, and eventually the impulse will subside. Shocks can be administered by either the therapist or the patient. The results are satisfactory but must be reinforced at regular intervals.

RESULTS OF BEHAVIOR THERAPY

Behavior therapy has been successful in a variety of disorders and can be easily taught. It requires less time than other therapies do, such as psychoanalysis and psychoanalytic therapy, and is less expensive to administer. A limitation of the method is that it is useful for circumscribed symptoms rather than for global areas of dysfunction (e.g., personality disorders). As with other forms of treatment, a careful evaluation of the patient's problems, motivation, and psychological strengths should be ascertained before instituting any of the behavior therapy approaches described.

References

Ayllon T, Azrin N H: *The Token Economy: A Motivational System for Therapy and Rehabilitation.* Appleton–Century–Crofts, New York, 1968.
Brady J P: Psychiatry as the behaviorist views it. In *Psychiatry: Areas of Promise and Advancement,* J P Brady, J Mendels, M T Orne, W Rieger, editors. Spectrum Publications, New York, 1977.
Brady J P: Social skills training for psychiatric patients: Concepts, methods, and clinical results. Am J Psychiatry *141*:333, 1984.
Kazdin A E: *History of Behavior Modification.* University Park Press, Baltimore, 1978.
Liberman R P: Behavioral modification of schizophrenia: A review. Schizophr Bull 6:37, 1972.
Paul G L, Lentz R J: *Psychosocial Treatment of Chronic Mental Patients.* Harvard University Press, Cambridge, MA, 1977.
Pomerleau O F, Brady J P, editors: *Behavioral Medicine: Theory and Practice.* Williams & Wilkins, Baltimore, 1979.
Stuart R B, editor: *Behavioral Self-Management: Strategies, Techniques and Outcomes.* Brunner/Mazel, New York, 1977.
Wolpe, J: Misrepresentation and underemployment of behavior therapy. Comp. Psychiatry *27*:192, 1986.
Wolpe J: *The Practice of Behavior Therapy,* ed 2, Pergamon Press, New York, 1973.

30.7 _____
Hypnosis

DEFINITION

Hypnosis is a complex mental phenomenon that has been defined as a state of heightened focal concentration and receptivity to the suggestions of another person. It has also been called an altered state of consciousness, a dissociated state, and a stage of repression. However, there is no known psychophysiologic basis for hypnosis as there is for sleep, in which there are characteristic EEG changes. Martin Orne defines hypnosis as that state or condition in which an individual is able to respond to appropriate suggestions by experiencing alterations of perception, memory, or mood. The essential feature of hypnosis is the subjective experiential change.

HISTORY

Modern hypnosis originated with the Austrian physician Anton Mesmer (1734–1815), who believed the phenomenon to be the result of animal magnetism or an invisible fluid that passed between the subject and the hypnotist, and was known as Mesmerism. The term hypnosis originated in the 1840s with a Scottish physician, James Braid (1795–1860), who believed the subject to be in a particular state of sleep (*hypnos* is the Greek word for sleep). In the late 19th century, the French neurologist Jean Charcot (1825–1893) thought hypnotism to be a special physiological state, and his contemporary Hippolyte Bernheim (1840–1919) believed it to be a psychological state of heightened suggestibility.

Freud, who studied with Charcot, used hypnosis early in his career to help patients recover repressed memories. He noted that patients would relive traumatic events while under hypnosis, a process known as abreaction. Freud later replaced hypnosis with the technique of free association.

Today, hypnosis is a method that is used as a form of therapy (hypnotherapy), a method of investigation to recover lost memories, and a research tool.

HYPNOTIC CAPACITY AND INDUCTION

Hypnotizability is a person's ability to be hypnotized and to respond to suggestion. Herbert Spiegel described an eye-roll sign for hypnotizability, which is the ability to roll one's eyes upward while they are closed. Easily hypnotizable persons have this ability. Other signs are the ability to use visual imagery and a willingness to participate in the procedure.

Induction techniques vary but share the quality of having the patient concentrate his or her attention on an image, an idea, or a part of the body. Persons can also be taught self-hypnosis (also called autogenic training) in which they learn to relax.

HYPNOTHERAPY

The patient in a hypnotic trance can recall memories that are not available to consciousness in the nonhypnotic state. Such memories can be used in therapy to corroborate psychoanalytic hypotheses regarding the patient's dynamics or to enable the patient to use such memories as a catalyst for new associations. It is possible with some patients to induce age regression, during which they reexperience events that occurred at an earlier time in life. Whether or not the patient is experiencing the events as they actually occurred is controversial; however, the material elicited can be used to further the therapy. Patients in a trance state may describe an event with an intensity similar to that when it occurred (abreaction) and experience a sense of relief as a result. It plays a role in the treatment of amnesia and fugue, although the clinician should be aware that it may be hazardous to bring the repressed memory into consciousness so quickly, as the patient may be overwhelmed by anxiety.

ROLE IN BEHAVIORAL MEDICINE

Hypnosis has been used, with varying degrees of success, to control substance use disorders, alcoholism, smoking, and obesity. It has been used to induce anesthesia, and major surgery has been performed with no anesthetic except hypnosis. It has also been used to manage chronic pain conditions. A variety of other conditions respond positively to hypnosis: asthma, warts, pruritis, aphonia, and a great variety of other conversion symptoms.

Relaxation can be achieved easily with hypnosis, so that patients may deal with phobic situations by controlling their anxiety. It also has been used to induce relaxation in systematic desensitization.

TRANCE STATE

Persons under hypnosis are said to be in a trance state, which may be light, medium, or heavy (deep). In the light trance, there are changes in motor activity such that the patients' muscles can feel relaxed, the hands can levitate, and paraesthesia can be induced. A medium trance is characterized by diminished pain sensation and partial or complete amnesia. A deep trance is associated with induced visual or auditory experiences, age regression, and deep anesthesia. Time distortion occurs at all trance levels but is most profound in the deep trance.

Posthypnotic suggestion is characterized by the patient's being instructed to perform a simple act or to experience a particular sensation after awakening from the trance state. It may be used to give a bad taste to cigarettes or a particular food, thus aiding in the treatment of obesity or nicotine dependence. Posthypnotic suggestions are associated with deep trance states.

CONTRAINDICATIONS

Hypnotized patients are in a state of atypical dependency on the therapist, and so strong transference may develop, characterized by a positive attachment that must be respected and interpreted. In other instances, a negative transference may erupt in patients who are fragile or who have difficulty testing reality. Patients who have difficulty with basic trust, such as paranoid patients, or who have problems giving up control, such as obsessive-compulsive patients, are not good candidates for hypnosis. A secure ethical value system is important to all therapy and particularly to hypnosis in which patients (especially those in a deep trance) are extremely suggestible and malleable. There is controversy about whether patients will perform acts during a trance state that they otherwise find repugnant or that run contrary to their moral code.

References

Barber T X: Hypnosuggestive procedures in the treatment of clinical pain: Implications for theories of hypnosis and suggestive therapy. In *Handbook of Clinical Health Psychology*, T Millon, editor, p. 521, Plenum Press, New York, 1982.
Braun B G: The uses of hypnosis in psychiatry. Psych Ann *16*:75, 1986.

Crasilneck H, Hall J: *Clinical Hypnosis: Principles and Applications,* ed 2. Grune & Stratton, Orlando, FL, 1985.

Erickson M H: *Advanced Techniques of Hypnosis and Therapy: Selected Papers of Milton H. Erickson, M.D.* J Haley, editor. Grune & Stratton, New York, 1976.

Kroger W: *Clinical and Experimental Hypnosis,* ed 2. Lippincott, Philadelphia, 1977.

Orne M, Dinges D: Hypnosis. In *Textbook of Pain,* P Wall, R Melzack, editors, p 806. Churchill Livingston, London, 1984.

Spiegel H, Speigel D: *Trance and Treatment: Clinical Uses of Hypnosis.* Basic Books, New York, 1978.

Wain H J: *Clinical Hypnosis in Medicine.* Symposia Specialists, Chicago, 1980.

Wester W C II, Smith A H, editors: *Clinical Hypnosis: A Multidisciplinary Approach.* Lippincott, Philadelphia, 1984.

30.8 _____
Cognitive Therapy

INTRODUCTION

Normal reactions are mediated by cognitive processes that enable persons to perceive reality accurately. In psychopathology, this ability is impaired, and errors in cognition are made. Aaron Beck used the term 'schemas' to describe stable cognitive patterns through which one interprets experiences. Cognitive errors produce negative schemas that persist despite contradictory evidence. Thus, depressogenic schemas may involve viewing experience as black or white, without shades of gray, as categorical imperatives that allow no options or as expectations that people are either all good or all bad.

GENERAL CONSIDERATIONS

Cognitive therapy developed by Aaron Beck is a short-term structured therapy that uses active collaboration between the patient and the therapist to achieve the therapeutic goals. It is oriented toward current problems and their resolution. Therapy is usually conducted on an individual basis, although group methods are also used. Therapy may also be used in conjunction with drugs.

Cognitive therapy has been applied mainly to depression (with or without suicidal ideation); however, it is also used with other conditions such as panic attacks, obsessive-compulsive disorders, paranoid disorders, and somatoform disorders. The treatment of depression can serve as a paradigm of the cognitive approach.

COGNITIVE THEORY OF DEPRESSION

The cognitive theory of depression holds that cognitive dysfunctions are the core of depression and that affective and physical changes and other associated features of depression are consequences of the cognitive dysfunctions. For example, apathy and low energy are results of a person's expectation of failure in all areas. Similarly, paralysis of will stems from a person's pessimism and feelings of hopelessness.

The cognitive triad of depression consists of (1) a negative self-percept that sees oneself as defective, inadequately deprived, worthless, and undesirable; (2) a tendency to experience the world as a negative, demanding, and self-defeating place and to expect failure and punishment; and (3) the expectation of continued hardship, suffering, deprivation, and failure.

The goal of therapy is to alleviate depression and to prevent its recurrence, by helping the patient (1) to identify and test negative cognitions, (2) to develop alternative and more flexible schemas, and (3) to rehearse both new cognitive and new behavioral responses. The goal is also to change the way a person thinks and, subsequently, to alleviate the depressive syndrome.

STRATEGIES AND TECHNIQUES

Overall, therapy is relatively short, lasting about 5 to 7 weeks, twice a week. If there is no response in that time, the diagnosis should be reevaluated. Maintenance therapy can be carried out over a period of years.

As with other psychotherapies, the therapists' attributes are important to successful therapy. The therapists must be able to exude warmth, understand the life experience of each patient, and be truly genuine and honest with themselves, as well as with their patients. Therapists must be able to relate skillfully and interactively with their patients.

Cognitive therapy sets the agenda at the beginning of each session, assigns homework to be performed between sessions, and teaches new skills. The therapist and the patient actively collaborate. Cognitive therapy has three components: didactic aspects, cognitive techniques, and behavioral techniques.

Didactic Aspects

The didactic aspects include explaining to the patient the cognitive triad, schemas, and faulty logic. The therapist must discuss with the patient that they will formulate hypotheses together and test them over the course of the treatment. Cognitive therapy requires a full explanation of the relationship between depression and thinking, affect, and behavior, as well as the rationale for all aspects of the treatment. This explanation contrasts with the more psychoanalytically oriented therapies, which require very little explanation.

Cognitive Techniques

The cognitive approach includes four processes: (1) eliciting automatic thoughts, (2) testing automatic thoughts, (3) identifying maladaptive underlying assumptions, and (4) testing the validity of maladaptive assumptions.

Eliciting Automatic Thoughts. Automatic thoughts are cognitions that intervene between external events and the individual's emotional reaction to the event. An example of an automatic thought is the belief that "everyone is going to laugh at me when they see how badly I bowl"—a thought that occurs to someone who has been asked to go bowling and responds negatively. Another example is a person's thought that "she doesn't like me" if someone passes that person in the hall without saying hello.

Testing Automatic Thoughts.   Acting as a teacher, the therapist helps the patient test the validity of automatic thoughts. The goal is to encourage patients to reject inaccurate or exaggerated automatic thoughts after careful examination.

Patients often blame themselves for things that go wrong that may well have been outside their control. The therapist reviews with the patient the entire situation and helps reattribute more accurately the blame or cause of the unpleasant events. Generating alternative explanations for events is another way of undermining inaccurate and distorted automatic thoughts.

Identifying Maladaptive Assumptions.   As the patient and therapist continue to identify automatic thoughts, patterns usually become apparent, representing rules or maladaptive general assumptions that guide the patient's life. Samples of such rules are "In order to be happy, I must be perfect," or "If anyone doesn't like me, I'm not lovable." Such rules inevitably lead to disappointments and failure and then to depression.

Testing the Validity of Maladaptive Assumptions. Similar to the testing of the validity of automatic thoughts is the testing of the accuracy of maladaptive assumptions. One particularly effective test is for the therapist to ask the patient to defend the validity of an assumption. For example, if a patient stated that he should always work up to his potential, the therapist might ask, "Why is that so important to you?"

Behavioral Techniques

Behavioral techniques go hand in hand with cognitive techniques: Behavioral techniques are used to test and change maladaptive or inaccurate cognitions. The overall purpose of such techniques is to help the patients understand the inaccuracy of their cognitive assumptions and learn new strategies and ways of dealing with issues.

Among the behavioral techniques used in therapy are scheduling activities, mastery and pleasure, graded task assignments, cognitive rehearsal, self-reliance training, role playing, and diversion techniques.

Among the first things done in therapy is to schedule activities on an hourly basis. A record of these activities is kept and reviewed with the therapist.

In addition to scheduling activities, patients are asked to rate the amount of mastery and pleasure of their activities. Patients are often surprised at how much more mastery and pleasure they get out of activities than they had otherwise believed.

In order to simplify the situation and allow for miniaccomplishments, tasks are often broken down into subtasks, as in graded task assignments, to demonstrate to patients that they can succeed.

Cognitive rehearsal has the patient imagine the various steps in meeting and mastering a challenge and rehearse the various aspects of it.

Patients, especially inpatients, are encouraged to become more self-reliant by doing such simple things as making their own beds, doing their own shopping, or preparing their own meals rather than relying on other people. This is known as self-reliance training.

Role playing is a particularly powerful and useful technique to elicit automatic thoughts and to learn new behaviors.

Diversion techniques are useful in helping patients get through particularly difficult times and include physical activity, social contact, work, play, or visual imagery.

IMAGERY

Imagery is a phenomenon that affects behavior, as first discussed by Paul Schilder in his book *The Image and Appearance of the Human Body,* in which he described images as having physiologic components. According to Shilder, visualizing oneself running activates subliminally the same muscles used in running, which can be measured with electromyography. This phenomenon is used in sports training, in which athletes visualize every conceivable event in a performance and develop a muscle memory for the activity. It can also be used to master anxiety or to deal with feared situations, by combining behavioral and cognitive theories.

Impulsive or obsessive behavior has been treated with thought stoppage. For instance, patients imagine a stop sign, a police officer nearby, or another image that evokes inhibition at the same time that they recognize an impulse or obsession that is alien to the ego. Similarly, obesity can be treated by having patients visualize themselves as thin, athletic, trim, and well muscled and then training them to evoke that image whenever they have an urge to eat. Such imagery can be enhanced with hypnosis or autogenic training. A technique called guided imagery is used in psychotherapy whereby patients are encouraged to develop fantasies that can be interpreted as wish fulfillments or attempts to master disturbing affects or impulses.

EFFICACY

Cognitive therapy can be used alone or in conjunction with antidepressant medication for severe depression. Studies have clearly demonstrated that cognitive therapy is effective and in some cases is superior or equal to medication alone. It is one of the most useful psychotherapeutic interventions currently available for depression and shows promise in the treatment of other disorders.

References

Bandura A: *Social Learning Theory.* Prentice–Hall, Englewood Cliffs, NJ, 1977.

Beck A T, Emery G: *Anxiety Disorders and Phobias: A Cognitive Perspective.* Basic Books, New York, 1985.

Beck A T: *Cognitive Therapy and the Emotional Disorders.* International Universities Press, New York, 1976.

Beck A T: *Depression: Causes and Treatment.* University of Pennsylvania Press, Philadelphia, 1972.

Beck A T, Rush A J: Cognitive approaches to depression and suicide. In *Cognitive Defects in the Development of Mental Illness,* G Serban, editor, p. 235. Brunner/Mazel, New York, 1978.

Beck A T, Rush A J, Shaw B F, Emery G: *Cognitive Therapy of Depression.* Guilford Press, New York, 1979.

Ellis A: *Reason and Emotion in Psychotherapy.* Lyle Stuart, 1962.

Kelly G: *The Psychology of Personal Constructs.* Norton, New York, 1955.

Rush A J. Cognitive therapy in combination with antidepressant medication. In *Combining Psychotherapy and Drug Therapy in Clinical Practice,* B D Beitman, G L Klerman, editors, p 121. Spectrum Publications, New York, 1984.

31

Biological Therapies

31.1

General Principles of Psychopharmacology

HISTORY

Organic therapies such as electroconvulsive therapy (pioneered by Ugo Cerletti and Lucio Bini), insulin coma therapy (developed by Manfred Sakel), and psychosurgery (introduced by Egas Moniz) all began in the first third of the 20th century and heralded the biological revolution in psychiatry (Table 1). In 1917, Julius von Wagner-Jauregg introduced malaria toxin to treat syphilis and is the only psychiatrist to have won a Nobel prize.

In the second half of the 20th century, chemotherapy as a treatment for mental illness became a major field of research and practice. Almost immediately after the introduction of chlorpromazine (Thorazine) in the early 1950s, psychotherapeutic drugs became a mainstay of psychiatric treatment, particularly for the more seriously mentally ill patients.

In 1949, the Australian psychiatrist John Cade described the treatment of manic excitement with lithium, which is widely accepted as a pivotal moment in the history of psychopharmacology. While conducting animal experiments, Cade had somewhat incidentally noted that lithium carbonate made the animals lethargic, thus prompting him to administer this drug to several agitated psychiatric patients.

In 1950, Charpentier synthesized chlorpromazine (an aliphatic phenothiazine antipsychotic) in an attempt to develop an antihistaminergic drug that would serve as an adjuvant in anesthesia. Laborit reported the ability of this drug to induce an "artificial hibernation." Reports by Paraire and Sigwald (1951), Delay and Deniker (1952), and Lehmann and Hanrahan (1954) described the effectiveness of chlorpromazine in treating severe agitation and psychosis. Chlorpromazine was quickly introduced into American psychiatry, and many similarly effective drugs have since been synthesized, including haloperidol (a butyrophenone antipsychotic) in 1958 by Janssen.

Imipramine (a tricyclic antidepressant) is structurally related to the phenothiazine antipsychotics. While carrying out clinical research on chlorpromazine-like drugs, Thomas Kuhn found that although imipramine was not very effective in reducing agitation, it did seem to reduce depression in some patients. The introduction of monoamine oxidase inhibitors (MAOIs) to treat depression evolved from the observation that the antituberculous agent iproniazid had mood-elevating effects in some patients. Nathan Kline (1958) was one of the first investigators to report the efficacy of MAOI treatment in depressed psychiatric patients.

By 1960, with the introduction of chloridazepoxide (a benzodi-

azepine antianxiety agent synthesized by Sternbach at the Roche laboratories in the late 1950s), the psychiatric armamentarium of drugs included antipsychotics (e.g., chlorpromazine and haloperidol), tricyclic (e.g., imipramine) and MAOI (e.g., iproniazid) antidepressants, an antimanic agent (lithium), and antianxiety agents (e.g., the benzodiazepines in addition to the older drugs, such as the barbiturates). The following 25 years have been devoted primarily to clinical studies demonstrating the efficacy of these drugs and to the development of related compounds in each category. The efficacy of each of these classes of drugs for treating relatively specific psychiatric syndromes and for elucidating their pharmacodynamic effects provided the impetus to develop the various neurotransmitter hypotheses of mental disorders (e.g., the dopamine hypothesis of schizophrenia, the monoamine hypothesis of mood disorders).

Table 1
Some Historical Events in Psychopharmacology, 1845–1960

1845—Hashish intoxication proposed as a model of insanity (Moreau)

1869—Chloral hydrate introduced as a treatment for melancholia and mania

1875—Cocaine proposed as a treatment in psychiatry (Freud)

1882—Paraldehyde introduced

1892—Research with morphine, alcohol, ether, and paraldehyde in normal individuals (Kraepelin)

1903—Barbiturates introduced

1917—Psychosis of syphilis treated with malaria fever therapy (Julius von Warner Jauregg)

1922—Barbiturate-induced coma (Jacob Klaesi)

1927—Insulin shock for schizophrenia (Manfred Sakel)

1931—*Rauwolfia serpentina* (reserpine) introduced (Sen and Bose) (confirmed as a treatment for schizophrenia in 1953 by Nathan Kline)

1934—Pentylenetetrazol-induced convulsions (Laszlo von Meduna)

1936—Frontal lobotomies (Egas Moniz)

1938—Electroconvulsive therapy (Ugo Cerletti and Lucino Bini)

1940—Dilantin introduced as anticonvulsant (Tracy Putnam)

1943—Lysergic acid diethylamide (LSD) synthesized (Albert Hofmann)

1949—Lithium introduced

1952—Chlorpromazine introduced

1955–1958—Tricyclic antidepressants and monoamine oxidase inhibitors introduced

1960—Chlordiazepoxide introduced

Since 1960, the major addition to the psychotherapeutic drugs has been the anticonvulsants, particularly carbamazepine and valproic acid, which are effective in treating some patients with bipolar disorder. Buspirone, a nonbenzodiazepine anxiolytic, was introduced for clinical use in America in 1986. A number of atypical antidepressant drugs have been marketed, although several have been removed from clinical use because of their dangerous adverse effects. It is expected, however, that the burgeoning knowledge of basic neuroscience and neuropharmacology will lead to the development of new psychotherapeutic drugs during the next decade.

CLASSIFICATION OF DRUGS

This textbook uses the traditional division of psychotherapeutic drugs into antipsychotics, antidepressants, antimanics, and anxiolytics and hypnotics. Although these divisions make valid historical sense, there are at least four reasons that this system may impede the understanding of current clinical practice. First, a drug in one class may also alleviate the characteristic symptoms for another class. For instance, lithium treats both the mania and the psychosis of a bipolar patient. Second, drugs of one class are, in fact, used to treat patients with symptoms associated with other classes. For example, antidepressants may reduce depression in some patients with schizophrenia. Third, drugs from all the classes are used to treat other clinical disorders, such as eating disorders, panic disorders, and impulse disorders. Finally, drugs such as clonidine, propranolol, and verapamil may be effective in a variety of clinical situations and do not fit easily into the current classification of drugs. Indeed, it is perhaps more useful for a clinician to be able to describe the pharmacotherapeutic approach to a specific disorder than it is to be able to list all of the drugs in a certain class.

PHARMACOKINETICS AND PHARMACODYNAMICS

Pharmacokinetic interactions describe how the body handles a drug; pharmacodynamic interactions describe the effects of a drug on the body. In a parallel fashion, pharmacokinetic drug interactions refer to the drugs' plasma concentrations, and the pharmacodynamic drug interactions refer to the drugs' receptor activities.

Pharmacokinetics

The principal divisions of pharmacokinetics are drug absorption, distribution, metabolism, and excretion.

Absorption. A psychotherapeutic drug first must reach the blood on its way to the brain, unless it is directly administered into the cerebrospinal fluid or the brain. Orally administered drugs must dissolve in the fluid of the gastrointestinal (GI) tract before the body can absorb them. Drug tablets can be designed to disintegrate either quickly or slowly, the absorption depending on the drug's concentration and lipid solubility and the GI tract's local pH, motility, and surface area. Depending on the drug's pK_a and the GI tract's pH, the drug may be present in an ionized form that limits its lipid solubility. If the pharmacokinetic absorption factors are favorable, the drug may reach therapeutic blood concentrations more quickly if it is administered intramuscularly. If a drug is coupled with an appropriate carrier molecule, intramuscular administration can sustain the drug's release over a long period of time. Some antipsychotic drugs are available in such depot forms that allow the drug to be administered only once every 1 to 4 weeks. Even though intravenous administration is the quickest route to achieve therapeutic blood levels, it also carries the highest risk of sudden and life-threatening adverse effects.

Distribution. Drugs can be freely dissolved in the blood plasma, bound to dissolved plasma proteins (primarily albumin) and dissolved within the blood cells. But if a drug is bound too tightly to plasma proteins, it may have to be metabolized and excreted before it can leave the bloodstream, thus greatly reducing the amount of active drug reaching the brain. The lithium ion is an example of a water-soluble drug that is not bound to plasma proteins. The distribution of a drug to the brain is determined by the blood–brain barrier, the brain's regional blood flow, and the drug's affinity with its receptors in the brain. Both high blood flow and affinity favor the distribution of the drug to the brain. Drugs may also reach the brain after passively diffusing into the cerebrospinal fluid from the bloodstream. The volume of distribution is a measure of the apparent space in the body available to contain the drug. The volume of distribution can also vary with the patient's age, sex, and disease state.

Metabolism and Excretion. Metabolism is somewhat synonymous with the term "biotransformation." The four major metabolic routes for drugs are oxidation, reduction, hydrolysis, and conjugation. Although the usual result of metabolism is to produce inactive metabolites that are more readily excreted than is the parent compound, there are many examples of active metabolites produced from psychoactive drugs. The liver is the principal site of metabolism, and bile, feces, and urine are the major routes of excretion. Psychoactive drugs are also excreted in sweat, saliva, tears, and milk; therefore, mothers who are taking psychotherapeutic drugs should not nurse their children. Disease states or coadministered drugs that affect the ability of the liver or kidneys to metabolize and eliminate drugs can both raise and lower the blood concentrations of a psychoactive drug.

Four important concepts regarding metabolism and excretion are time of peak plasma level, half-life, first pass effect, and clearance. The time between the administration of a drug and the appearance of peak concentrations of the drug in plasma varies primarily according to the route of administration and absorption. A drug's half-life is defined as the amount of time it takes for one half a drug's peak plasma level to be metabolized and excreted from the body. A general guideline is that if a drug is administered repeatedly in doses separated by time intervals shorter than its half-life, the drug will reach 97 percent of its steady-state plasma concentrations in a time equal to five times its half-life. The first pass effect refers to the extensive initial metabolism of some drugs within the portal circulation or liver, thereby reducing the amount of unmetabolized drug that will reach the systemic circulation. Clearance is a measure of the amount of drug excreted per unit of time. If some disease process or other drug interferes with the clearance of a psychoactive drug, then the drug may reach toxic levels.

Pharmacodynamics

The major pharmacodynamic considerations include receptor mechanism; the dose response curve, the therapeutic index; and the development of tolerance, dependence, and withdrawal phenomena. The receptor for a drug can be defined generally as the cellular component that binds to the drug and initiates the drug's pharmacodynamic effects. A drug can be an agonist for its receptor, thereby stimulating a physiologic effect; conversely, a drug can be an antagonist for the receptor, most often by blocking the receptor so that an endogenous agonist cannot affect the receptor. The receptor site for most psychotherapeutic drugs is also a receptor site for an endogenous neurotransmitter. For example, the primary receptor site for chlorpromazine is the dopamine receptor. However, for other psychotherapeutic drugs, this may not be the case. The receptor for lithium may be the enzyme inositol-1-phosphatase, and the receptor for verapamil (a calcium channel inhibitor) is presumably the calcium channel.

The dose response curve plots the drug concentration against the effects of the drug (Figure 1). The potency of a drug refers to the relative dose required to achieve a certain effect. Haloperidol, for example, is more potent than is chlorpromazine because generally only 5 mg of haloperidol is required to achieve the same therapeutic effect as does 100 mg of chlorpromazine. Both haloperidol and chlorpromazine, however, are equal in their maximal efficacies, that is, the maximum clinical response achievable by the administration of a drug.

The side effects of most drugs are often a direct result of their primary pharmacodynamic effects and are better conceptualized as adverse effects. The therapeutic index is a relative measure of a drug's toxicity or safety. It is defined as the ratio of the median toxic dose (TD_{50}) to the median effective dose (ED_{50}). The TD_{50} is the dose at which 50 percent of individuals experience toxic effects, and the ED_{50} is the dose at which 50 percent of individuals have a therapeutic effect. Haloperidol, for example, has a very high therapeutic index, as evidenced by the wide range of doses in which it is prescribed. Conversely, lithium salts have a very low therapeutic index, thereby requiring careful

Examples of Dose-Response Curves

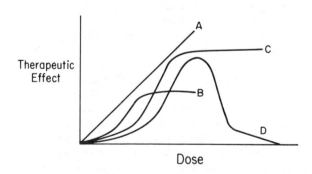

Figure 1. This dose-response curve plots the therapeutic effect as a function of increasing dose, often calculated as the log of the dose. Drug A has a linear dose response; Drugs B and C have sigmoidal curves; and drug D has a curvilinear dose response curve. Although smaller doses of drug B are more potent than are equal doses of drug C, drug C has a higher maximum efficacy than does drug B. Drug D has a "therapeutic window," such that both low and high doses are less effective than are mid-range doses.

monitoring of serum lithium levels when prescribing this drug. There can be both inter- and intraindividual variation in the response to a specific drug. An individual patient may be hyporeactive, normally reactive, or hyperreactive to a particular drug. For example, some patients with schizophrenia require 1 mg a day of haloperidol, others require a more typical 10 mg a day, and still others require 100 mg a day to achieve a therapeutic response. Idiosyncratic drug responses occur when a person experiences a particularly unusual effect from the drug. For example, some patients become quite agitated when given benzodiazepines (e.g., Valium).

A person may become less responsive to a particular drug as it is administered over time, which is referred to as tolerance. The development of tolerance is associated with the appearance of physical dependence, which may be defined as the necessity to continue administering the drug in order to prevent the appearance of withdrawal symptoms.

CLINICAL GUIDELINES

The practice of clinical psychopharmacology requires skill as both a diagnostician and a psychotherapist, knowledge of the available drugs, and the ability to plan a pharmacotherapeutic regimen. The selection and initiation of drug treatment should be based on the patient's past history, current clinical state, and the treatment plan. The psychiatrist should know the purpose or goal of a drug trial, the length of time that the drug needs to be administered in order to assess its efficacy, the approach to be taken to reduce any adverse effects that may occur, alternative drug strategies should the current one fail, and whether long-term maintenance of the patient on the drug is indicated. In almost all cases, the psychiatrist should explain the treatment plan to the patient and often to his or her family and other care-givers. The patient's reaction to and ideas about a proposed drug trial should be considered. However, if the psychiatrist feels that accommodating the patient's wishes would hinder treatment, then this should be explained to the patient. This method contrasts with the psychotherapeutic approach which usually discourages the psychiatrist from telling the patient what he or she thinks the patient should do.

Choice of Drug

The first two steps in selecting a drug treatment, the diagnosis and identification of target symptoms, should be carried out when the patient has been in a drug-free state for 1 to 2 weeks. The drug-free state should include the absence of medications for sleep (e.g., hypnotics), as the quality of sleep can be both an important diagnostic guide and a target symptom. If a patient is hospitalized, however, insurance guidelines may make a drug-free period difficult or even impossible to obtain. Psychiatrists often evaluate symptomatic patients who are already on one or more psychoactive medications, and so it is usually necessary to wean the patient from current medications and then to make an assessment. An exception to this practice occurs when a patient presents to the psychiatrist on a suboptimal regimen of an otherwise appropriate drug. In such cases, the psychiatrist may decide to continue the drug at a higher dose in order to complete a full therapeutic trial.

In the United States, it is a common practice to diagnose a patient according to DSM-III-R and then to base the pharmacologic treatment on recommendations for that disorder. This approach contrasts with the former simplicity of psychopharmacology, in which antidepressants were used for depression, lithium for mania, and antipsychotics for schizophrenia. Although this classification of drug indications is not completely incorrect, it does not adequately represent the complexity and flexibility of current clinical practice.

From among the drugs appropriate to a particular diagnosis, the specific drug should be selected according to the patient's past history of drug response (compliance, therapeutic response, and adverse effects), the patient's family history of drug response, the profile of adverse effects for that drug with regard to a particular patient, and the psychiatrist's usual practice. If a drug has previously been effective in treating a patient or a family member, it should be used again unless there is some specific reason not to use the drug. A past history of adverse effects from a specific drug is a strong indicator that the patient would not be compliant with that drug regimen. It is unfortunate that patients and their families are often quite ignorant of what drugs have been used before, in what doses, and for how long. This finding may reflect the tendency of psychiatrists not to explain drug trials to their patients, and should encourage psychiatrists to give their patients written records of drug trials for their personal medical records. A caveat to obtaining a past history of drug response from patients is that because of their mental disorder, they may inaccurately report the effects of a previous drug trial. If possible, therefore, the patients' medical records should be obtained to confirm their reports. Most psychotherapeutic drugs of a single class have been demonstrated to be equally efficacious; however, these drugs do differ in their adverse effects on individuals. A drug thus should be selected that minimally exacerbates any preexisting medical problems that a patient may have.

Combination Drugs. Some combination drugs (Table 2) may actually increase the patient's compliance by simplifying the drug regimen. A problem with combination drugs, however, is that the clinician has less flexibility in adjusting the dose of one of the components. That is, the use of combination drugs may cause two drugs to be administered when only one continues to be effective.

Nonapproved Dosages and Uses. It is common clinical practice for drugs to be used for indications that are not approved, and in higher doses than approved, by the Food and Drug Administration (FDA). The FDA's view is that it is generally appropriate for clinicians to prescribe within the guidelines of community norms. Psychiatrists should explain this practice to their patients and should document the details of this discussion in a written record. If clinicians are in doubt about a drug treatment plan, they should consult with a colleague or suggest that the patient obtain a second opinion. The DEA has classified drugs according to abuse potential (Table 3), and clinicians are advised to be more cautious when prescribing Class II drugs than when prescribing less controlled substances.

Therapeutic Trials. A drug's therapeutic trial should last for a previously determined length of time. Because behavioral symptoms are more difficult to assess than are other physiologic symptoms (e.g., hypertension), it is particularly important for specific target symptoms to be identified at the initiation of a drug trial. The psychiatrist and the patient can then assess these target symptoms over the course of the drug trial to help determine whether the drug has been effective. There are a number of objective rating scales (e.g., BPRS, SADS) available to assess a patient's progress over the course of a drug trial. If a drug has not been effective in reducing target symptoms within the specified length of time and if other reasons for the lack of response can be eliminated, the drug should be tapered and stopped. The brain is not a group of on-and-off neurochemical switches; rather, it is an interactive network of neurons in a complex homeostasis. Thus the abrupt discontinuation of virtually any psychoactive drug is likely to disrupt further the brain's functioning. Another common clinical mistake is the routine addition of medications without the discontinuation of a prior drug. Although this practice is indicated in specific circumstances (e.g., lithium potentiation of an unsuccessful trial of antidepressants), it often results in increased noncompliance and adverse effects, as well as the clinician's not knowing whether it was the second drug alone or the combination of drugs that resulted in a therapeutic success.

Therapeutic Failures. The failure of a specific drug trial should prompt the clinician to consider a number of possibilities. First, was the original diagnosis correct? This reconsideration should include the possibility of an undiagnosed organic mental disorder, including illicit drug abuse. Second, are the observed remaining symptoms actually the drug's adverse effects and not related to the original disease? Antipsychotic drugs, for example, can produce both akinesia, which resembles psychotic withdrawal, or akathisia and neuroleptic malignant syndrome, which resemble increased psychotic agitation. Third, was the drug administered in sufficient dosage for an appropriate period of time? Patients can have vastly different drug absorption and metabolic rates for the same drug, and plasma drug levels should be obtained to assess this variable. Fourth, was there a pharmacokinetic or pharmacodynamic interaction with another drug the patient was taking that reduced the efficacy of the psychotherapeutic drug? Fifth, did the patient actually take the drug as directed? Drug noncompliance is a very common clinical problem. Reasons for drug noncompliance are complicated drug regimens (more than one drug in more than one daily dose), adverse side effects (especially if unnoticed by the clinician), and poor patient education about the drug treatment plan.

Patient Education

As stated previously, patients should know their diagnosis, the target symptoms that the drug is supposed to reduce, the length of time they will be on the drug, both expected and unexpected adverse effects, and the treatment plan to be followed if the current drug is unsuccessful. Although some psychiatric disorders interfere with patients' ability to comprehend this information, the psychiatrist should relay as much of this information as possible. The clear presentation of this material is often less frightening than are patients' fantasies about drug treatment. It is important to tell patients how long it will take for them to receive benefits from the drug trial. This factor is perhaps most critical when patients have a mood disorder and may not observe therapeutic effects for 3 to 4 weeks.

Table 2
Combination Drugs Used in Psychiatry

Ingredients	Preparation	Manufacturer	Amount of Each Ingredient	Recommended Dosage*	Indications	D.E.A.† Control
Perphenazine and amitriptyline	Triavil	Merck, Sharp & Dohme	Tablet—2:25, 4:25, 4:50, 2:10, 4:10	Initial therapy Tablet of 2:25 or 4:25 q.i.d.	Depression and associated anxiety	0
	Etrafon	Schering		Maintenance therapy Tablet 2:25 or 4:25 b.i.d. or q.i.d.		
Meprobamate and benactyzine	Deprol	Wallace	Tablet—400:1	Initial therapy One tablet q.i.d. Maintenance therapy Initial dosage may be increased to six tablets a day then gradually reduced to the lowest levels that provide relief	Depression and associated anxiety	IV
Meprobamate and trihexethyl chloride	Milpath	Wallace	Tablet—400:25, 200:25	Tablet of 400:25 at mealtimes and two tablets at bedtime	Peptic ulcer and irritable bowel syndrome	0
	Pathibamate	Lederle		One tablet t.i.d. at mealtime, and two tablets at bedtime		
Secobarbital and amobarbital	Tuinal	Lilly	Capsule—25:25, 50:50, 100:100	50 to 200 mg. at bedtime or 1 hour preoperatively	Insomnia; preoperative sedation	II
Dextroamphetamine and amphetamine	Biphetamine‡	Pennwalt	Sustained release capsule—6.25:6.25	1 capsule in the morning	Exogenous obesity	II
Chlordiazepoxide and clinidium bromide	Librax	Roche	Capsule—5:2.5	One or two capsules t.i.d. or q.i.d. before meals and at bedtime	Peptic ulcer, gastritis, duodenitis, irritable bowel syndrome, spastic colitis, and mild ulcerative colitis	0
Chlordiazepoxide and amitriptyline	Limbitrol	Roche	Tablet—5:12.5, 10:25	Tablet of 5:12.5 t.i.d. or q.i.d. Table of 10:25 t.i.d. or q.i.d. initially, then may increase to six tablets daily as required	Depression and associated anxiety	IV

*t.i.d., q.i.d., and b.i.d.
†D.E.A., Drug Enforcement Administration.
‡The United States Food and Drug Administration recommends the use of amphetamine for weight reduction. However, various states (California, New York) allow these medications for short term use as an appetite suppressant and in depression for a 2- to 3-day trial to gauge the effectiveness of certain tricyclics. The authors, based upon their clinical experience, recommend a broader use of amphetamines in selected cases of depression, although such use is controversial.

Table 3
Characteristics of Drugs at Each Drug Enforcement Administration (D.E.A.) Control Level

D.E.A. Control Level (Schedule)	Characteristics of Drug at Each Control Level	Examples of Drugs at Each Control Level
I	High abuse potential No accepted use in medical treatment in the United States at the present time and therefore not for prescription use	LSD, heroin, marijuana, peyote, mescaline, psilocybin, tetrahydrocannabinols, nicocodeine, nicomorphine, and others
II	High abuse potential Severe physical dependence liability Severe psychological dependence liability	Amphetamine, opium, morphine, codeine, hydromorphine, phenmetrazine, cocaine, amobarbital, secobarbital, pentobarbital, methylphenidate, and others
III	Abuse potential less than levels I and II Moderate or low physical dependence liability High psychological liability	Glutethimide, methyprylon, PCP, nalorphine, sulfonmethane, benzphetamine, phendimetrazine, clortermine, mazindol, chlorphentermine, compounds containing codeine, morphine, opium, hydrocodone, dihydrocodeine and others
IV	Low abuse potential Limited physical dependence liability Limited psychological dependence liability	Barbital, phenobarbital, benzodiazepines, chloral hydrate, ethchlorvynol, ethinamate, meprobamate, paraldehyde, and others
V	Lowest abuse potential of all controlled substances	Narcotic preparations containing limited amounts of nonnarcotic active medicinal ingredients

Adverse Effects. Patients will generally have less trouble with adverse effects if they have previously been told to expect them. It is not unreasonable to explain the appearance of adverse effects as evidence that the drug is working. But clinicians should distinguish between probable or expected adverse effects and rare or unexpected adverse effects.

An extreme adverse effect of drug treatment is an attempt by a patient to kill himself by overdosing on a psychotherapeutic drug. One psychodynamic theory of such behavior is that such patients may be angry at their therapists for not having been able to help them. Whatever the motivation, psychiatrists should be aware of this risk and attempt to prescribe the safest possible drugs. It is good practice to write nonrefillable prescriptions for small quantities of drugs when suicide is a consideration. In extreme cases, attempts should be made to verify that patients are actually taking the medication and not hoarding the pills for a later overdose attempt. It is a common clinical observation that patients may attempt suicide just as they are beginning to get better. Clinicians, therefore, should continue to be careful about prescribing large quantities of medication until the patient is almost completely recovered. Another consideration for psychiatrists is the possibility of accidental overdose, particularly by children in the household. Patients should also be advised to keep psychotherapeutic medications in a safe place.

Patients' Attitudes Toward Drugs. Some patients' ambivalent attitudes toward drugs often reflect the confusion about drug treatment that exists in the field of psychiatry. Patients often feel that taking a psychotherapeutic drug means that they are really sick or not in control of their lives or that they may become addicted to the drug and have to take it forever. A simplified approach to these concerns is to describe the psychiatric disorder partially as a brain disease analogous to diabetes as a disease of the pancreas. It is often helpful to draw pictures of neurons to demonstrate how the drug is working in the brain. Psychiatrists should explain the difference between drugs of abuse that affect the normal brain, and psychiatric drugs that are used to treat emotional disorders. They should point out to patients that antipsychotics, antidepressants, and antimanic drugs are not addictive in the way that heroin is addictive, for example. The psychiatrist's clear and honest explanation of how long the patient should take the drug will help the patient adjust to the idea of chronic maintenance medication if that, in fact, is the treatment plan. In some cases, it is appropriate for the psychiatrist to give the patient increasing responsibility for adjusting the medications as the treatment progresses. This can often help the patient feel less controlled by the drug.

Informed Consent. Informed consent is a legal term indicating that the patient has agreed to the suggested drug trial after having been advised of both the potential benefits and the risks of the treatment. Some states require patients to sign a document stating that they have given informed consent, and some clinicians have adopted this practice in states that do not require a form. Clearly, the capacity of a psychiatric patient to understand this information is often difficult to assess. This problem represents an ethical dilemma that can best be met by psychiatrists attempting to meet the letter and spirit of the law to the best of their abilities. When in doubt about a patient's ability to make such a decision, the patient's family, friends, caretakers, or legal counsel should be consulted.

Special Considerations

Children. Special care must be given when administering psychotherapeutic drugs to children. Although the small volume of distribution in children suggests the use of lower doses than in adults, children's higher rate of metabolism suggests that higher ratios of milligrams of drug to kilograms of body weight should be used. In practice, it is best to begin with a small dose and to increase the dose until clinical effects are observed. The clinician, however, should not hesitate to use adult doses in children if the dose is effective and there are no side effects.

Geriatric Patients. The two major concerns when treating geriatric patients with psychotherapeutic drugs are that elderly persons may be more susceptible to adverse side effects (particularly adverse cardiac effects) and may metabolize drugs more slowly, thus requiring lower doses of medication. Another concern is that geriatric patients are often taking other medications, thereby requiring psychiatrists to consider carefully possible drug interactions. In practice, psychiatrists should begin treating geriatric patients with a small dose, usually approximately one half the usual dose. The dose should be raised in small amounts more slowly than in middle-aged adults until either a clinical benefit is achieved or unacceptable adverse effects appear. Although many geriatric patients do require a small dose of medication, many others require the usual adult dosage.

Pregnant and Nursing Women. The basic rule is to avoid administering any drug to a woman who is pregnant (particularly during the first trimester) or who is nursing a child. This rule, however, occasionally needs to be broken when the mother's psychiatric disorder is too severe. If psychotherapeutic medications need to be administered during a pregnancy, then the possibility of a therapeutic abortion should be discussed. The two most teratogenic drugs in the psychopharmacopeia are lithium and anticonvulsants. Lithium administration during pregnancy is associated with a higher incidence of birth abnormalities, including Ebstein's malformation, a serious abnormality in cardiac development. Other psychoactive drugs (antidepressants, antipsychotics, and anxiolytics), although less clearly associated with birth defects, should also be avoided during pregnancy if at all possible. The most common clinical situation occurs when a pregnant woman becomes psychotic. If a decision is made not to terminate the pregnancy, it would seem preferable to administer antipsychotics rather than lithium.

The administration of psychotherapeutic drugs at or near delivery may cause the baby to be overly sedated at delivery, requiring a respirator, or to be physically dependent on the drug, requiring detoxification and treatment of a withdrawal syndrome. Virtually all psychotropic drugs are secreted in the milk of a nursing mother; therefore, mothers on these agents should be advised not to nurse their children.

Medically Ill Patients. Considerations in administering psychotropic drugs to medically ill patients include a possible increased sensitivity to side effects, either increased or decreased metabolism and excretion of the drug, and interactions with other medications. As with children and geriatric patients, the most reasonable clinical practice is to begin with a small dose, increase it slowly, and watch for both clinical and adverse effects. The application of plasma drug levels may be a particularly helpful clinical test in these patients.

PSYCHOPHARMACOLOGY AND PSYCHOTHERAPY

The goal of both clinical psychopharmacology and psychotherapy is to help the patients. If either modality impedes the attainment of that goal, then psychiatrists must try to remedy the situation. The integration of the nondirected approach of some psychotherapies and the doctor-directed approach of psychopharmacology requires the talents of a sophisticated clinician. Two unfortunate clinical mistakes are the avoidance of a time-limited drug trial, in order to maintain the purity of some types of psychotherapeutic

relationships, and the psychiatrist's ambivalence about a drug trial, contributing to a therapeutic failure or the patient's noncompliance.

CONTINUING EDUCATION

The practice of psychopharmacology is continually changing, and so psychiatrists must keep abreast of developments in the field and be able to evaluate research reports about the efficacy of new agents. Whenever a psychiatrist does try a new drug, he or she should review all the available current literature on the agent and possibly consult colleagues.

References

Baldessarini R J: *Chemotherapy in Psychiatry: Principles and Practice.* Harvard University Press, Cambridge, MA, 1985.
Bassuk E L, Schooner S C, Gelenberg A J: *The Practitioner's Guide to Psychoactive Drugs,* ed 2. Plenum, New York, 1983.
Costa E, Greengard P, editors: *Advances in Biochemical Psychopharmacology,* vol. 1. Raven Press, New York, 1987.
Gilman A G, Goodman L S, Rall T W, Morad F: *Goodman and Gilman's: The Pharmacological Basis of Therapeutics,* ed 7. Macmillan, New York, 1985.
Gold M S, Lydiard R B, Carman J S: *Advances in Psychopharmacology: Predicting and Improving Treatment Response.* CRC Press, Boca Raton, FL, 1984.
Klein D F, Gilleman R, Quitkin F, Rifkin A: *Diagnosis and Drug Treatment of Psychiatric Disorders: Adults and Children,* ed 2. Williams & Wilkins, Baltimore, 1980.
Lake C R, editor: *Clinical Psychopharmacology,* vols. 1, 2. Psychiatr Clin of North Am 7:3, 7:4. Saunders, Philadelphia, 1984.
Lipton M, DiMascio A, Killam K F: *Psychopharmacology: A Generation of Progress.* Raven Press, New York, 1978.
Meltzer H Y: *Psychopharmacology: The Third Generation of Progress,* Raven Press, New York, 1987.
Schatzberg A F, Cole J O: *Manual of Clinical Psychopharmacology.* American Psychiatric Press, Washington, DC, 1986.

31.2 _____
Drugs Used to Treat Psychosis

INTRODUCTION

Drugs used to treat psychosis are variously referred to as antipsychotics, neuroleptics, and major tranquilizers. The term "antipsychotic" is used in this chapter because it most accurately describes the major therapeutic effect of these drugs. The term "neuroleptic" refers more to the neurologic or motor effects of these drugs. The term "major tranquilizer" inaccurately implies that the primary effect of these drugs is merely to sedate patients and also confounds these drugs with the so-called minor tranquilizers, such as the benzodiazepines. A common mistake is to use the term "phenothiazine" as synonymous with the term "antipsychotic," since the phenothiazine antipsychotics are only one subclass of antipsychotic drugs.

The major use of antipsychotics is to treat schizophrenia, although these drugs are also used to treat agitation and psychosis associated with other psychiatric and organic disorders. Antipsychotics have little or no abuse potential and thus are not classified as controlled substances. Although antipsychotics do not permanently cure schizophrenia, they greatly benefit many patients in a way that no treatment ever did before their introduction. The clinical use of antipsychotics has reduced the population of inpatients in psychiatric hospitals from over 500,000 in 1950 to approximately 100,000 in 1985. This decline in the inpatient population, often referred to as deinstitutionalization, is largely attributed to the introduction of antipsychotic drugs. Nonetheless, although antipsychotics have allowed many patients to remain out of the hospital and to function in the community, these same drugs are also partly responsible for the problem of the homeless mentally ill. The antipsychotics have made these patients just barely well enough not to require hospitalization; yet the deinstitutionalization plan did not adequately provide for the outpatient treatment of these still impaired individuals.

CLASSIFICATION

There are nine classes of drugs that can be grouped together as antipsychotic drugs (Figure 1).

Phenothiazines

All the phenothiazines have the same three-ring phenothiazine nucleus but differ in the side chains joined to the nitrogen atom of the middle ring. The phenothiazines are subtyped according to the aliphatic (e.g., chlorpromazine), piperazine (e.g., fluphenazine), or piperidine (e.g., thioridazine) nature of the side chain.

Thioxanthenes

The thioxanthene three-ring nucleus differs from the phenothiazine nucleus by the substitution of a carbon atom for the nitrogen atom in the middle ring. The two available thioxanthenes have either an aliphatic (chlorprothixene) or a piperazine (thiothixene) side chain.

Dibenzoxazepines

The dibenzoxazepines are based on another modification of the three-ring phenothiazine nucleus. The only dibenzoxazepine available in the United States is loxapine, which has a piperazine side chain.

Dihydroindoles

The only dihydroindole available in the United States, molindone, has somewhat unusual properties, such as not inducing weight gain and perhaps being less epileptogenic than the phenothiazines are.

Butyrophenones

Only two butyrophenones are available in the United States—haloperidol and droperidol. The former is perhaps the most widely used antipsychotic, and the latter is used as an adjuvant in anesthesia. Some research groups, however, have been using droperidol (Inapsine) as an intravenous (IV) antipsychotic drug in emergency settings. Spiroperidol is a butyrophenone compound widely used in research studies to label dopamine receptors.

Diphenylbutylpiperidines

Diphenylbutylpiperidines are somewhat similar structurally to the butyrophenones. Only one diphenylbutylpiperidine, pimozide

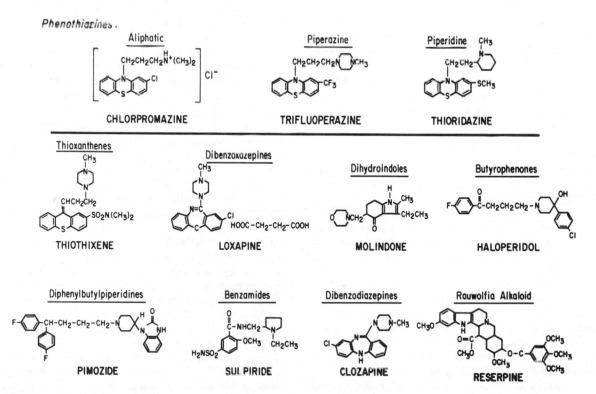

Figure 1. Molecular structure of representative antipsychotics.

(Orep), is available in the United States and is approved only for treating Tourette's syndrome. In Europe, however, pimozide has been shown to be an effective antipsychotic agent. Pimozide and thioridazine (a piperidine phenothiazine) are the most potent calcium channel inhibitors among the antipsychotics. A controversial clinical and research observation about pimozide is that it may be more effective in reducing the deficit symptoms of schizophrenia than are the other antipsychotics.

Benzamides

No benzamide derivatives are available in the United States; however, there is considerable evidence that sulpiride is an effective antipsychotic associated with significantly fewer neurological side effects than are the other antipsychotics.

Dibenzodiazepines

Clozapine is not currently available for clinical use in the United States because it has been associated with agranulocytosis. Clozapine, however, is of research interest because it lacks the neurological side effects associated with most other antipsychotics. This unique characteristic may prompt the FDA to approve clozapine for clinical use. Clozapine should not be confused with clonazepam, a benzodiazepine.

CLINICAL EFFICACY

Antipsychotics are superior to placebos in the treatment of acute and chronic schizophrenia, as well as in the control of other agitated and psychotic behavior. Approximately 70 percent of patients improve significantly with antipsychotic treatment. The onset of sedation is rapid, often within 1 hour after intramuscular (IM) administration of these drugs. Antipsychotic activity has a slower onset, but most therapeutic gain occurs in the first 6 weeks of therapy. Patients may continue to improve, however, for up to 6 months. Antipsychotics are most effective against the positive symptoms of psychosis, such as agitation and hallucinations. Although the negative symptoms are less affected by antipsychotic treatment, with continued treatment, many patients become less socially withdrawn.

PHARMACOKINETICS

Although the pharmacokinetic details for the different antipsychotics vary widely (e.g., half-lives ranging from 10 to 20 hours), the most important clinical generalization is that all the antipsychotics currently available in the United States can be given in one daily dose once the patient is in a stable condition and has adjusted to any adverse effects. Most antipsychotics are incompletely absorbed following oral administration. In addition, most have high binding to plasma proteins, volumes of distribution, and lipid solubilities. Antipsychotic drugs are metabolized in the liver and reach steady-state plasma levels in 5 to 10 days. There is some evidence that after a few weeks of administration, chlorpromazine, thiothixene, and thioridazine induce metabolic enzymes, thereby decreasing the plasma concentrations. Chlorpromazine is notorious among psychopharmacologists for having over 150 metabolites, some of which are active. The nonaliphatic phenothiazines and the butyrophenones have very few metabolites, but the activity of these metabolites is still controversial. The potential presence of active metabolites complicates the interpretation of plasma drug levels that report the presence of only the parent compound.

PHARMACODYNAMICS

The potency of antipsychotic drugs to reduce psychotic symptoms is most closely correlated with the affinity of these drugs with the dopamine type-2 (D_2) receptor. The mechanism of therapeutic action for antipsychotic drugs is thought to be as D_2 receptor antagonists, preventing the binding of endogenous dopamine to this subtype of dopaminergic receptor. The mesolimbic, and possibly the mesocortical dopaminergic, pathways are likely to be the site of action for the antipsychotic effects. There are three caveats to this hypothesis. First, although the antipsychotics' dopamine receptor blocking effect occurs immediately, the full antipsychotic effects may take weeks to develop. This observation suggests that some more slowly developing homeostatic change in the brain is the actual mechanism of action for the antipsychotic effects of these drugs. Second, an individual patient may respond to one antipsychotic but not another. This variation in an individual's response is not explained by a D_2 receptor blocking model, thereby suggesting that other neurotransmitter systems may be involved in therapeutic effects of these drugs. Third, although the correlation of dopamine blocking effects with the antipsychotics' clinical potency has led to the dopamine hypothesis of schizophrenia, it is also true that these drugs will reduce psychotic symptoms regardless of the patient's diagnosis. The therapeutic effects of dopamine receptor blockade, therefore, are not unique to the pathophysiology of schizophrenia.

Most of the neurological and endocrinological adverse effects of antipsychotics can also be explained by the blockade of dopamine receptors. Various antipsychotics, however, also block noradrenergic, cholinergic, and histaminergic receptors, thus accounting for the variation in adverse effects profiles seen among these drugs (Table 1).

Although the potency of the antipsychotics varies widely (Table 2), all available antipsychotics are equally efficacious in the treatment of schizophrenia. No subtype of schizophrenia or subset of symptoms has been demonstrated conclusively to be more effectively treated by any single class of antipsychotics (with the controversial exception of pimozide for negative symptoms). The therapeutic index for antipsychotics is very favorable and has contributed to the unfortunate practice of routinely using high doses of these drugs. More recent investigations of the dose response curve for antipsychotics indicate that the equivalent of 5 to 10 mg of haloperidol is usually efficacious for either the acute or the chronic treatment of schizophrenia. Antipsychotics, particularly haloperidol, may have a bell-shaped dose response curve. Overly high doses of antipsychotics may lead to neurological side effects such as akinesia or akathisia that are difficult to distinguish from an exacerbation of psychosis. Moreover, excessively high doses of some antipsychotics become less effective in reducing psychotic symptoms. Haloperidol, in particular, may have such a therapeutic window (plasma levels of 8 to 18 mg per ml).

Although patients can develop a tolerance to most of the adverse effects caused by antipsychotics, patients do not develop a tolerance to the antipsychotic effect. It is wise, nevertheless, to taper the dose of neuroleptics when the drugs are being discontinued, as there may be rebound effects from the other neurotransmitter systems that the drug blocked. Cholinergic rebound, for example, can produce a flu-like syndrome in patients. It is also theoretically possible that abruptly withdrawing antipsychotics could exacerbate psychotic symptoms.

INDICATIONS

Idiopathic Psychosis

Idiopathic psychoses include schizophrenia, schizophreniform disorder, schizoaffective disorder, delusional disorder, brief reactive psychosis, mania, and psychotic depression. Antipsychotics are effective in both the acute and chronic management of these conditions; that is, antipsychotics both reduce acute symptoms and prevent future exacerbations. Antipsychotics are often used in combination with antimanic drugs to treat mania and in combination with antidepressants to treat psychotic depressions. Because of the potential adverse effects of repeatedly administering antipsychotics, maintenance treatment with these drugs is indicated primarily for schizophrenia and some cases of schizoaffective disorder.

Secondary Psychosis

Secondary psychoses are associated with an identified organic etiology, such as a brain tumor or drug intoxication. The higher potency antipsychotics are usually safer to use in such patients because of their lower cardiogenic and epileptogenic potential. Antipsychotic drugs should not be used to treat drug intoxications or withdrawals when there is an increased risk of seizures. The drug of choice in such cases is usually a benzodiazepine. Psychosis secondary to amphetamine intoxication, however, is an indication for neuroleptic treatment if a pharmacological treatment is required.

Severe Agitation or Violent Behavior

The administration of antipsychotics will calm most severely agitated or violent individuals, although the use of a sedative drug (e.g., benzodiazepines or barbiturates) might be preferable in some cases. The agitation associated with delirium and dementia, most common in elderly patients, is an indication for antipsychotics. Small doses of high-potency drugs (e.g., 0.5 to 1 mg a day of haloperidol) are usually the best choice. The repeated administration of antipsychotics to control disruptive behavior in mentally retarded children is a controversial indication.

Movement Disorders

Both the psychosis and the movement disorder of Huntington's disease are often treated with antipsychotics. These drugs are also used to treat the motor and vocal tics of Tourette's syndrome.

Other Psychiatric Indications

The use of thioridazine to treat depression with marked anxiety or agitation has been approved by the FDA. Some clinicians use small doses of antipsychotics (0.5 mg of haloperidol or 25 mg of chlorpromazine 2 to 3 times a day) to treat severe anxiety. In addition, some investigators have reported using antipsychotics to control the behavioral turmoil in patients with borderline personality disorder. But because of the possible long-term adverse effects

Table 1

Affinity* of Certain Antipsychotic Agents for Several Neurotransmitter Receptors[†]

Antipsychotic agent: generic name (trade name)	Receptor						
	Dopamine D_2	Histamine		Adrenergic			Muscarinic
		H_1	H_2	α_1	α_2		
Chlorpromazine (Thorazine)	5.3	11	0.033	38	0.13		14
Chlorprothixene (Taractan)	13	...	...	...	...		...
Fluphenazine (Permitil, Prolixin)	125	4.8	...	22	0.064		0.053
Haloperidol (Haldol)	25	0.053	0.0034	16	0.026		0.0042
Loxapine (Loxitane)	1.4	20	...	3.6	0.042		0.22
Mesoridazine (Serentil)	5.3	55	...	50	0.062		1.4
Molindone (Moban)	0.83	0.00081	0.00142	0.040	0.16		0.00026
Perphenazine (Trilafon)	71	12	...	10	0.20		0.067
Prochlorperazine (Compazine)	14	5.3	...	4.2	0.059		0.18
Thioridazine (Mellaril)	3.8	6.2	...	20	0.12		5.6
cis-Thiothixene (Navane)	222	17	0.0213	9.1	0.50		0.034
Trifluoperazine (Stelazine)	38	1.6	...	4.2	0.038		0.15

*$10^{-7} \times 1/K_d$, in which K_d is the equilibrium dissociation constant in molarity. All receptors were from human brain except the histamine H_2 receptor, which was from guinea pig brain.
[†]A higher numerical value indicates greater binding and greater antagonism of a given receptor.
Table from Black J L, Richelson E, Richardson J W: Antipsychotic agents—A clinical update. Mayo Clin Proc 60:777–789, 1985. Used with permission.

of antipsychotics, they should be used in these other psychiatric conditions only after more conventional drugs have been tried.

CLINICAL GUIDELINES

Antipsychotic drugs are remarkably safe, and if necessary, a clinician can administer these drugs without conducting a physical or laboratory examination of the patient. The major contraindications to antipsychotics are (1) a history of a serious allergic response; (2) the possibility that the patient may have ingested a drug that will interact with the antipsychotic to induce CNS depression (e.g., alcohol, opioids, barbiturates, benzodiazepines) or anticholinergic delirium (e.g., scopolamine, possibly phencyclidine); (3) the presence of a severe cardiac abnormality; (4) a high risk of seizures from organic or idiopathic causes; and (5) the presence of narrow-angle glaucoma if an anticholinegic antipsychotic is to be used. In the usual assessment, however, it is best to obtain a CBC with white blood cell indices, liver function tests, and an EKG, especially in women over 40 and men over 30.

Choice of Drug

The general guidelines for choosing a particular psychotherapeutic drug should be followed (Section 32.1).

If no other rationale prevails, the choice should be based on adverse effect profiles, as described below, and the psychiatrist's preference. Although high-potency neuroleptics are associated with more neurological adverse effects, current clinical practice greatly favors their use because of the higher incidence of other adverse effects (e.g., cardiac, hypotensive, epileptogenic, sexual, and allergic) with the low-potency drugs. There is a myth in psychiatry that hyperexcitable patients respond best to chlorpromazine because it is more sedating, whereas withdrawn patients respond best to high-potency antipsychotics such as fluphenazine. This belief has never been proved true; furthermore, if sedation is a desired goal, then either the antipsychotic can be given in divided doses or a sedative drug (e.g., a benzodiazepine) can also be administered.

A clinical observation that is supported by some research is that an unpleasant experience by the patient to the first dose of an antipsychotic correlates highly with future poor response and noncompliance. Such experiences include a subjective negative feeling, oversedation, and acute dystonia. If a patient reports such a reaction, the clinician may be well advised to switch to a different antipsychotic.

Failure of a Drug Trial. In the acute state, virtually all patients will respond eventually to repeated doses of an antipsychotic (every 1 to 2 hours with IM administration or every 2 to 3 hours with per oral (PO) administration), sometimes with a ben-

Table 2
Antipsychotic Drugs, Trade Names, and Potencies

Generic	Trade	Potency* mg of drug equivalent to 100 mg chlorpromazine
Phenothiazines		
Aliphatic		
Chlorpromazine	Thorazine & Generic	100
Triflupromazine	Vesprin	25–50
Piperazime		
Prochlorperazine	Compazine	15
Perphenazine	Trilafon	10
Trifluoperazine	Stelazine	3–5
Fluphenazine	Prolixin & Permitil	1.5–3
Acetophenazine	Tindal	25
Butaperazine	Repoise	10
Carphenazine	Proketazine	25
Piperidine		
Thioridazine	Mellaril	100
Mesoridazine	Serentil	50
Piperacetazine	Quide	10
Thioxanthenes		
Chlorprothixene	Taractan	50
Thiothixene	Navane	2–5
Dibenzoxazepine		
Loxapine	Loxitane	10–15
Dihydroindole		
Molindone	Moban & Lidone	6–10
Butyrophenone		
Haloperidol	Haldol	2–5

*Recommended adult doses are 200 to 400 mg/day of chlorpromazine or an equivalent amount of another drug.

zodiazepine. The failure of a patient to respond in the acute situation should cause the clinician to seriously consider the possibility of an organic lesion.

A major reason for a failed drug trial is insufficient length of the trial. It is generally a mistake to increase the dose or change antipsychotic medications in the first 2 weeks of treatment. If a patient is improving on the current regimen at the end of this time, then continued treatment with the same regimen will likely result in steady clinical improvement. If, however, a patient has truly shown little or no improvement in 2 weeks, then the possible reasons for a drug failure, including noncompliance, should be considered (See Section 31.1). In a truly noncompliant patient, the use of liquid preparations or depot forms of fluphenazine or haloperidol may be indicated. Because of the great individual diversity in the metabolism of these drugs, it is reasonable to obtain plasma levels if this laboratory capability is available. The therapeutic plasma range for haloperidol is 8 to 18 mg per ml; the therapeutic range for the other antipsychotics is less certain and can best be obtained from the testing facility.

Having eliminated other possible reasons for an antipsychotic's therapeutic failure, it is reasonable to try a second antipsychotic with a structure different from that of the first one. Additional strategies include adding or removing co-administered anticholinergic drugs; supplementing the antipsychotic with lithium, carbamazepine, or a benzodiazepine; and so-called megadose therapy. Megadose therapy refers to the use of very high doses of antipsychotics (in the range of 100 to 200 mg a day of haloperidol). If this strategy is used, a specified time (approximately 1 month) should be set for the drug trial. If no improvement is seen, then the high doses should be discontinued. Electroconvulsive therapy may be an alternative if no satisfactory pharmacological treatment can be found.

Combinations of Antipsychotics. It has not been experimentally demonstrated that combining two antipsychotics produces a treatment superior to comparable amounts of a single antipsychotic alone; however, it also has not been demonstrated that this practice is harmful. The only reasonable indication for this practice would be the use of a nonsedating, high-potency antipsychotic during the day and a sedating, low-potency antipsychotic at bedtime. This drug regimen would rarely be indicated, as the single bedtime dose should almost always result in antipsychotic activity throughout the following day.

Dosage and Schedule

Various patients may respond to widely different doses of antipsychotics; therefore, there is no set dose for any given antipsychotic drug. It is reasonable clinical practice to start each patient at a low dose and increase it as necessary. It is important to remember that the maximal effects of a particular dosage may not be evident for 4 to 6 weeks.

Acute Treatment. The equivalent of 5 mg of haloperidol is a reasonable dose for an adult patient in an acute state. A geriatric patient might benefit from as little as 1 mg of haloperidol. The administration of more than 50 mg of chlorpromazine in one injection, however, may result in serious hypotension. The administration of the antipsychotic IM will result in peak plasma levels in approximately 30 minutes, versus 90 minutes with the oral route. The patient should be observed for 1 hour, at which time most clinicians administer a second dose of the antipsychotic.

Rapid neuroleptization is the practice of administering hourly IM doses of antipsychotic medications until the desired clinical

effect is achieved. Several research studies have shown, however, that merely waiting several more hours following one dose of antipsychotics will result in the same clinical improvement as seen with repeated doses of antipsychotics. The clinician must be very careful to prevent patients from becoming violent while they are psychotic. Psychiatrists can do this by temporarily using physical restraints until such patients can control their behavior.

Because the administration of very high doses of high-potency antipsychotics is not associated with a higher incidence of adverse effects, the practice of giving very large cumulative antipsychotic doses in the emergency setting has become quite common. Physicians, therefore, may be pressured by their staff to use repeated administrations of antipsychotics. But hypotension can be a very serious complication resulting from the repeated administration of low-potency antipsychotics.

Clinicians usually attempt to achieve sedation, in addition to the reduction of psychosis, with repeated administrations of antipsychotics. It may be reasonable, therefore, to use a sedative agent, rather than an antipsychotic, following one or two doses of the antipsychotic. Possible sedatives include lorazepam (2 mg IM) or amobarbital (50 to 250 mg IM).

Early Treatment. The equivalent of 10 to 20 mg of haloperidol or 400 mg of chlorpromazine per day is adequate treatment for most patients with schizophrenia. Some research suggests that 5 mg of haloperidol or 200 mg of chlorpromazine may in fact be just as effective. It is wise to use divided doses when initiating the therapy. This practice reduces the incidence and severity of adverse effects and may also help sedate the patient. The sedative effects of antipsychotics last only a few hours, in contrast to the antipsychotic effects which last for 1 to 3 days. After approximately 1 week of treatment, it is usually helpful to give the entire dose of antipsychotic at bedtime. This practice usually helps the patient sleep and reduces the incidence of adverse effects. In older patients treated with low-potency antipsychotics, however, this practice may increase the risk of their falling if they get out of the bed during the night.

It is common clinical practice to order medications to be given as needed, or PRN. Although this practice may be reasonable during the first few days that a patient is hospitalized, it has been shown that the time on antipsychotic drugs rather than an increase in dosage is what produces therapeutic improvement. Again, clinicians may feel pressured by their staff to write PRN antipsychotic orders. The orders for PRN medications should include the specific symptoms, how often they should be given, and how many PRNs can be given each day. Clinicians may choose to use small doses for the PRNs (e.g., 2 mg of haloperidol) or may use a benzodiazepine (e.g., 2 mg lorazepam IM).

Maintenance Treatment. A patient with schizophrenia should be continued on an effective dosage of antipsychotics for at least 6 months following improvement. For a patient who has had only one or two psychotic episodes and has been in a stable clinical state for 6 months, it is reasonable to attempt to reduce the dosage by 50 percent gradually over 3 to 6 months. After another 6 months in a stable clinical state, another 50 percent dosage reduction may be indicated. There is some research data that suggest that many patients with schizophrenia can be maintained on the equivalent of 5 mg of haloperidol per day. It is wise for the clinician to know enough about the patient's life to try to predict upcoming stressors, during which times the patient's antipsychotic dosage should perhaps be increased.

Patients who have had three or more exacerbations of schizophrenic symptoms should probably be continued on antipsychotics indefinitely, although attempts to reduce the dosage may be warranted every 4 to 5 years if the patient has been clinically stable. Although antipsychotic drugs may be quite effective, patients may report that they actually prefer being off of the drugs because they feel better without them. It is true that normal individuals who have taken antipsychotic drugs report a sense of dysphoria. The clinician must thus discuss maintenance medication with the patients and take into account the patients' wishes, the severity of their illness, and the quality of their support systems.

Alternative Maintenance Regimens. Alternative maintenance regimens have been designed to reduce both the risk of long-term adverse effects and any unpleasantness associated with taking antipsychotic medications. "Intermittent medication" refers to the use of antipsychotics only when patients require them. This arrangement requires that the patients or their care providers be both willing and able to watch carefully for early signs of clinical exacerbations. At the earliest signs of such problems, antipsychotic medications should be reinstituted for a reasonable period, usually 1 to 3 months.

"Drug holidays" are regular 2- to 7-day periods during which the patient is not given antipsychotic medications. There is currently no evidence that drug holidays reduce the risk of long-term adverse effects from antipsychotics, and it is possible that drug holidays increase the incidence of noncompliance.

Long-acting Depot Antipsychotics. Because some patients with schizophrenia will not reliably comply with oral antipsychotic regimens, it may be reasonable to treat them with long-acting depot preparations of antipsychotics. These preparations are usually administered IM once every 1 to 4 weeks by a clinician. The clinician, therefore, will immediately know if a patient has missed a dose of medication. Depot antipsychotics may be associated with more adverse effects, including tardive dyskinesia. Although this concern is controversial, clinicians should probably refrain from using depot forms unless the patient is unable to comply with oral medications.

Two depot preparations (a decanoate and an enanthate) of fluphenazine (Prolixin) and a decanoate preparation of haloperidol (Haldol) are available in the United States. These preparations of the antipsychotics are injected IM into an area of large muscle tissue, from where they are absorbed slowly into the blood. Decanoate preparations can be given less frequently than are enanthate preparations because they are absorbed more slowly. Although it is not absolutely necessary to stabilize a patient on the PO preparation of the specific drug before initiating the depot form, it is good practice to give at least one PO dose of the drug to assess the possibility of any untoward adverse effect, such as an allergic reaction.

It is very difficult to predict the correct dosage or time interval for depot preparations. It is reasonable to begin with 12.5 mg (0.5 cc) of either fluphenazine preparation or 25 mg (0.5 cc) of haloperidol decanoate. If symptoms emerge in the next 2 to 4 weeks, the patient can be treated temporarily with additional oral medications or with additional small depot injections. After 3 to 4 weeks, the depot injection can be increased to include the supplemental doses given during this initial period.

A good reason to initiate depot treatment with low doses is that the absorption of these preparations may be faster at the onset of treatment, resulting in frightening episodes of dystonia that will eventually discourage compliance with the medication. Some clinicians actually keep patients drug free for 3 to 7 days before initiating depot treatment and give very small doses of the depot preparations (3.125 mg fluphenazine or 6.25 mg haloperidol) every

few days to avoid these initial problems. Because the major indication for depot medication is poor compliance with oral forms, it may be wise to go slowly with what is just about the last method of achieving compliance.

Prevention and Treatment of Some Neurological Adverse Effects

A variety of drugs (Table 3) may be used to prevent and treat neurological adverse effects caused by antipsychotics. Most acute dystonias and parkinson-like symptoms are effectively treated by these drugs, and akathisia may also respond in some cases. All but two of the available drugs act through their anticholinergic effects; amantadine (a dopaminergic agonist) and ethopropazine (a phenothiazine derivative) presumably act through dopaminergic systems.

It is not known whether prophylatic treatment with these drugs is warranted when starting a patient on antipsychotic treatment. The proponents of prophylactic treatment argue that the increased likelihood of avoiding adverse neurological effects is more humane to the patient and increases the possibility of future compliance. The opponents of this practice argue that the increased likelihood of anticholinergic adverse effects from these drugs offsets any possible gain. A reasonable compromise is to use these drugs in patients under age 45 who are more at risk of developing neurological adverse effects and not to use these drugs prophylactically in patients over 45 who are at increased risk for anticholinergic toxicity. If a patient does develop dystonias, parkinson-like symptoms, or akathisia, then a trial of these drugs is warranted.

Once a patient has been started on these drugs, he or she should be treated for 4 to 6 weeks. At that point, there should be an attempt to taper and stop the medication over 1 month. Many patients will have become tolerant to the neurological adverse effects and will no longer require the drug. Some patients will experience the return of neurological symptoms and will have to be restarted on these drugs. And some patients will state that they feel less anxious or depressed while on these medications, so it may be reasonable to restart them even in the absence of neurological symptoms.

Most clinicians will use one of the anticholinergic drugs, including diphenhydramine, to provide prophylaxis or treatment for neurological adverse effects. Of these drugs, diphenhydramine is the most sedating; biperiden is neutral; and trihexyphenidyl may be slightly stimulating. In fact, trihexyphenidyl, benztropine, and diphenhydramine can be abused, as some patients report obtaining a euphoria from these drugs. Amantadine and ethopropazine are most often used when one of the anticholinergic drugs does not work. Although amantadine does not exacerbate the psychosis of schizophrenia, some patients may become tolerant of its antiparkinsonian effects. Amantadine is also a sedating drug in some patients.

ADVERSE EFFECTS

Nonneurological Adverse Effects

One generalization about the adverse effects from antipsychotics is that low-potency drugs cause more nonneurological adverse effects and that high-potency drugs cause more neurological adverse effects.

Sedation. Sedation is primarily a result of the blockade of histamine type-1 receptors. Chlorpromazine is the most sedating antipsychotic; thioridazine, chlorprothixene, and loxapine are also

Table 3
Drugs Used to Treat Neurological Adverse Effects from Antipsychotics

Generic	Trade	Usual Adult Dose, mg/day	Usual Adult Single Dose (mg)
Biperiden	Akineton	2–6	2
Procyclidine	Kemadrin	10–20	2–5
Trihexyphenidyl	Artane & Other Brands	4–15	2–3
Benztropine	Cogentin	1–6	1–2
Diphenhydramine	Benadryl	50–300	10–50
Orphenadrine	Disipal & Norflex	50–150	50
Amantadine	Symmetral	100–300	100
Ethopropazine	Parsidol	100–400	50–100

very sedating; and the high-potency antipsychotics are much less sedating. Patients should be warned about driving or operating machinery when first treated with antipsychotics. Giving the entire antipsychotic dosage at bedtime will usually eliminate any problems from sedation, and tolerance to this adverse effect often develops.

Orthostatic (Postural) Hypotension. Orthostatic (postural) hypotension is mediated by adrenergic blockade and is most common with chlorpromazine and thioridazine. It occurs most frequently during the first few days of treatment, and patients readily develop a tolerance to it. It is most apt to occur when high doses of intramuscular, low-potency antipsychotics are given. The chief dangers of this adverse effect are that the patients may faint, fall, and injure themselves, although such occurrences are uncommon. When using IM low-potency antipsychotics, it is prudent to measure the patients' blood pressure (lying and standing) before and after the first dose and during the first few days of treatment. When appropriate, patients should be warned of the adverse effects and given the usual instructions: "Rise from bed gradually, sit at first with your legs dangling, wait for a minute, and sit or lie down if you feel faint." Support hose may help with this symptom. If low-potency antipsychotics are used by patients with cardiac problems, then the dose should be increased very slowly.

If hypotension does occur in patients receiving these medications, the symptom can usually be managed by having the patients lie down with their feet higher than their head. On rare occasions, volume expansion or vasopressor agents, such as norepinephrine, may be indicated. Because hypotension is produced by α-adrenergic blockade, these drugs also block the α-adrenergic stimulating properties of epinephrine, leaving the β-adrenergic stimulating effects untouched. Therefore, administering epinephrine to these patients results in a paradoxical worsening of hypotension and so is contraindicated in cases of antipsychotic-induced hypotension. Pure α-adrenergic pressors such as metaraminol or norepinephrine (levarterenol) are the drugs of choice in the treatment of this disorder.

Peripheral Anticholinergic Effects. Peripheral anticholinergic effects are quite common and consist of dry mouth and nose, blurred vision, constipation, urinary retention, mydriasis, and mydriasis. Some patients also have nausea and vomiting. Chlorpromazine, thioridazine, mesoridazine, and trifluoperazine are potent anticholinergics. Anticholinergic effects can be particularly severe if a low-potency antipsychotic is used with a tricyclic antidepressant and an anticholinergic drug; such a practice is seldom warranted.

Dry mouth can be quite a troubling symptom for patients. They should be advised to rinse out their mouth frequently with water and not to chew gum or candy containing sugar, as this can result in fungal infections of the mouth or an increased incidence of dental caries. Constipation should be treated with the usual laxative preparations, but this condition can progress to paralytic ileus. Pilocarpine may be used in such situations, although the relief is only transitory. A decrease in the antipsychotic or a change to another drug would be warranted in such cases.

Central Anticholinergic Effects. The symptoms of central anticholinergic activity include severe agitation; disorientation to time, person, or place; hallucinations; seizures; high fever; and dilated pupils. Stupor and coma may ensue. The treatment consists of discontinuing the causal agent, close medical supervision, and physostigmine (2 mg by slow IV infusion, repeated within 1 hour as necessary). Too much physostigmine is dangerous, and symptoms of physostigmine toxicity include hypersalivation and sweating. Atropine sulfate (0.5 mg) can reverse these effects.

Endocrine Effects. Blockade of the dopamine receptors in the tuberoinfundibular tract results in increased secretion of prolactin, which can result in breast enlargement, galactorrhea, impotence in males, and amenorrhea in females. Both sexes may report decreased libido, and females may have a false pregnancy test while on some antipsychotics. Thioridazine is particularly associated with decreased libido and retrograde ejaculation in male patients. Psychiatrists may not find out about the disturbing sexual adverse effects of an antipsychotic if they do not ask about them specifically. Another adverse effect of antipsychotics is the inappropriate secretion of antidiuretic hormone. Some patients' glucose tolerance tests shift in a diabetic direction because of antipsychotic administration.

Skin Effects. Allergic dermatitis and photosensitivity occur in a small percentage of patients, most commonly those on low-potency drugs, particularly chlorpromazine. A variety of skin eruptions—urticarial, maculopapular, petechial, and edematous eruptions—have been reported. These eruptions occur early in treatment, generally in the first few weeks, and remit spontaneously. A photosensitivity reaction that resembles a severe sunburn also occurs in some patients on chlorpromazine. Patients should be warned of this adverse effect, should spend no more than 30 to 60 minutes in the sun, and should use sun screens. Chlorpromazine is also associated with some cases of blue-gray discoloration of the skin over areas exposed to sunlight. The skin changes often begin with a tan or golden brown color and progress to such colors as slate gray, metallic blue, or purple.

Ophthalmologic Effects. Thioridazine is associated with irreversible pigmentation of the retina when given in doses over

800 mg a day. This pigmentation is quite similar to that seen in retinitis pigmentosa, and it can progress even after the thioridazine is stopped and can result in blindness.

Chlorpromazine may induce whitish-brown granular deposits concentrated in the anterior lens and posterior cornea, visible only by slit-lens examination. They progress to opaque white and yellow-brown granules, often stellate in shape. Occasionally, the conjunctiva is discolored by a brown pigment. Retinal damage is not seen in these patients, and their vision is almost never impaired. The majority of patients who show the deposits are those who have ingested 1 to 3 kg of chlorpromazine throughout their life.

Cardiac Effects. Low-potency antipsychotics are more cardiotoxic than are high-potency drugs. Chlorpromazine causes prolongation of the Q-T and P-R intervals, blunting of T waves, and depression of the S-T segment. Thioridazine, in particular, has marked effects on the T wave, and these unique cardiac effects may be why overdoses of the piperazine phenothiazines are the most lethal among the antipsychotics.

Sudden Death. The cardiac effects of antipsychotics have been hypothesized to be related to sudden death in patients treated with these drugs. Careful evaluation of the literature, however, suggests that it is premature to attribute these sudden deaths to the antipsychotic drugs. Supporting this view is the observation that the introduction of antipsychotics had no effect on the incidence of sudden death in schizophrenic patients. In addition, both low- and high-potency drugs were involved in the cases. Furthermore, many reports were of patients with other medical problems, treated with other drugs.

Weight Gain. A very common adverse effect of treatment with antipsychotics is weight gain, which can be quite significant in some cases. Molindone and, perhaps, loxapine are not associated with this symptom and may be indicated in patients for whom weight gain is a serious health hazard or a reason for noncompliance.

Hematologic Effects. A leukopenia with a white blood count (WBC) around 3,500 is a common but not serious problem. A life-threatening hematologic problem is agranulocytosis, occurring most often with chlorpromazine and thioridazine but seen with almost all antipsychotics. It occurs most frequently during the first 3 months and with an incidence of 1 per 500,000. Routine complete blood counts (CBCs) are not indicated; however, if a patient reports a sore throat and fever, a CBC should be done immediately to check for this possibility. If the blood indices are low, the antipsychotic should be stopped, and the patient should be transferred to a medical facility. The mortality rate for this complication may be as high as 30 percent. Thrombocytopenic or nonthrombocytopenic purpura, hemolytic anemias, and pancytopenia may also occur rarely in patients treated with antipsychotics.

Jaundice. In the early days of chlorpromazine treatment, jaundice was not unusual, occurring in about 1 out of every 100 patients treated. More recently, for unexplained reasons, the incidence of chlorpromazine-induced jaundice has dropped considerably. Although accurate data are lacking, the incidence is probably in the range of 1 out of every 1,000 patients treated.

The jaundice occurs most often in the first 5 weeks of treatment and is generally preceded by a flu-like syndrome. It is generally wise to discontinue chlorpromazine if patients develop jaundice, although the value of this practice has never been proved. Indeed, patients have been maintained on chlorpromazine throughout the illness, without adverse effects. Chlorpromazine-associated jaundice has also recurred in patients as long as 10 years later.

Jaundice has also been reported to occur with promazine, thioridazine, mepazine, and prochlorperazine and very rarely with fluphenazine and trifluoperazine. No convincing evidence indicates that haloperidol or many of the other nonphenothiazine antipsychotics can produce jaundice. The majority of the cases reported in the literature are still associated with the use of chlorpromazine.

Overdoses of Antipsychotics. With the exception of overdoses from thioridazine and mesoridazine, the outcome of antipsychotic overdoses is favorable, unless the patient has also ingested other CNS depressants, such as alcohol or benzodiazepines. The symptoms of overdose include drowsiness, which may progress to delirium, coma, dystonias, and seizures. The pupils are mydriatic; deep tendon reflexes are decreased; tachycardia and hypotension are present; and the EEG shows diffuse slowing and low voltage. The piperazine phenothiazines can lead to heart block and ventricular fibrillation, resulting in death.

The treatment should include gastric lavage and activated charcoal followed by catharsis. Convulsions can be treated with IV diazepam or diphenylhydantoin. Hypotension should be treated with either norepinephrine or dopamine, and not epinephrine.

Neurological Adverse Effects

Epileptogenic Effects. Antipsychotic administration is associated with a slowing and an increased synchronization of the EEG. This effect may be the mechanism by which some antipsychotics decrease the seizure threshold. Chlorpromazine, loxapine, and other low-potency antipsychotics are thought to be more epileptogenic than are high-potency drugs, especially molindone. The risk of inducing a seizure by antipsychotic administration warrants consideration in patients who already have a seizure disorder or an organic brain lesion.

Dystonias. Approximately 10 percent of patients will experience dystonias as an adverse effect of antipsychotics, usually in the first few hours or days of treatment. Dystonic movements result from a slow, sustained muscular contraction or spasm that can result in an involuntary movement. Dystonias can involve the neck (spasmodic torticollis or retrocollis), jaw (forced opening resulting in a dislocation, or also trismus), tongue (protrusions, twisting), or entire body (opisthotonos). Involvement of the eyes can result in an oculogyric crisis, characterized by their upward lateral movement. (Unlike other dystonias, an oculogyric crisis may occur later in treatment as well.) Other dystonias include blepharospasm and glossopharyngeal dystonias, resulting in dysarthria, dysphagia, and even cyanosis. Children may be particularly likely to evidence opisthotonos, scoliosis, lordosis, and writhing movements. Dystonias can be painful and quite frightening and often result in later noncompliance.

Dystonias are most common in younger males but can occur at any age in either sex. Although they are most common with IM doses of high-potency antipsychotics, dystonias can occur with any antipsychotic but are rare with thioridazine. The mechanism of action is thought to be the dopaminergic hyperactivity in the basal ganglia that occurs when the CNS levels of the antipsychotic begin to fall. Dystonias can fluctuate spontaneously, responding to reassurance and resulting in the clinician's false impression that the movement is hysterical. The differential diagnosis should include seizures and tardive dyskinesia. Prophylaxis with anticholinergics usually prevents the development of dystonias. Treatment with IM anticholinergics or IV or IM diphenhydramine (50 mg) will almost always relieve the symptoms. Diazepam (10 mg IV), amobarbital, caffeine sodium benzoate, and hypnosis have also been reported to be effective. Although tolerance to this adverse effect usually develops, it is sometimes prudent to change the antipsychotic if the patient is particularly concerned about the reaction's recurrence.

Parkinsonian Effects. Parkinsonian adverse effects occur in approximately 15 percent of patients, usually within 5 to 90 days of the treatment's initiation. Symptoms include muscle stiffness, cogwheel rigidity, shuffling gait, stooped posture, and drooling. The pill-rolling tremor of idiopathic parkinsonism is rare, but a regular, coarse tremor similar to essential tremor may be present. Rabbit syndrome is a focal, perioral tremor that resembles the other parkinsonian effects of antipsychotics but can occur late in treatment. The mask-like facies, bradykinesia, and akinesia of this parkinsonian syndrome are often misdiagnosed as being part of the negative symptom picture of schizophrenia and are therefore not treated.

Women are affected about twice as often as men are, and the syndrome can occur at all ages, although more frequently after age 40. All antipsychotics can cause the symptoms, especially high-potency drugs with low anticholinergic activity. Chlorpromazine and thioridazine are less likely to be involved. The blockade of dopaminergic transmission in the nigrostriatal tract is the cause of drug-induced parkinsonism. Because not all patients develop this syndrome, those who do seem not to be able to compensate for the presence of antipsychotic blockade in the nigrostrital tract. The differential diagnosis should also include other causes of idiopathic parkinsonism, other organic causes of parkinsonism, and depression. The syndrome can be treated with anticholinergic agents, amantadine, or ethopropazine. Although amantadine may have fewer side effects, it may be less effective at reducing muscular rigidity. Levodopa does not work in these cases, and it may exacerbate the psychosis. Anticholinergics should be withdrawn after 4 to 6 weeks to assess whether the patient has developed a tolerance to the parkinsonian effects; approximately 50 percent of patients will need continued treatment. Even after antipsychotics are withdrawn, parkinsonian symptoms may last for up to 2 weeks, and even up to 3 months in elderly patients. In such patients, it is reasonable to continue the anticholinergic drug after stopping the antipsychotic.

Akathisia. Akathisia is a subjective feeling of muscular discomfort that can cause the patient to be agitated, pace relentlessly, stand and sit continually, and feel quite dysphoric. The symptoms are primarily motor and cannot be controlled by the patient's will. Akathisia can appear at any time during treatment. It is probably underdiagnosed because the symptoms are mistakenly attributed to psychosis, agitation, or lack of cooperation. The mechanism underlying akathisia is poorly understood, although it presumably involves dopamine receptor blockade. The antipsychotic dose and treatment with anticholinergics and amantadine should be reduced, although this latter approach is often not effective. Propranolol (30 to 120 mg a day) and benzodiazepines have been shown to be effective in several research studies. In some cases of akathisia, no treatment seems to be effective.

Tardive Dyskinesia. Tardive dyskinesia is a delayed effect of antipsychotics, rarely occurring until after 6 months of treatment. The syndrome consists of abnormal, involuntary, irregular, choreoathetoid movements of muscles of the head, limbs, and trunk. The severity of these movements ranges from minimal—often missed by patients and their families—to grossly incapacitating. Perioral movements are the most common and include darting, twisting, and protruding movements of the tongue, chewing and

lateral jaw movements, lip puckering, and facial grimacing. Finger movements and hand clenching are also quite common. Torticollis, retrocollis, trunk twisting, and pelvic thrusting are seen in more severe cases. Respiratory dyskinesias have also been reported. Dyskinesias are exacerbated by stress and disappear during sleep. Other tardive or late-occurring syndromes may include tardive dystonias, tardive parkinsonism, and tardive behavioral syndromes, although the last of these is quite controversial.

All of the neuroleptics have been associated with causing tardive dyskinesia, although there is some evidence that thioridazine is less likely to be involved. The longer that patients are on antipsychotics, the more likely they are to develop tardive dyskinesia. Women are more affected than are men, and patients over 50 years of age, patients with brain damage, and patients with mood disorders also seem to be at a higher risk. The incidence increases by approximately 3 to 4 percent per year after 4 to 5 years of treatment. Approximately 50 to 60 percent of chronically institutionalized patients have the syndrome. It is an interesting observation that 1 to 5 percent of schizophrenic patients had similar abnormal movements before the introduction of antipsychotics in 1955. Tardive dyskinesia is hypothesized to be caused by dopaminergic receptor supersensitivity in the basal ganglia resulting from chronic blockade of dopamine receptors by antipsychotics. This hypothesis, however, has not been proved.

The three basic approaches to tardive dyskinesia are prevention, diagnosis, and management. Prevention is best achieved by using antipsychotic medications only when clearly indicated and in the lowest effective doses. Patients on antipsychotics should be checked regularly for the appearance of abnormal movements, preferably by using a standardized rating scale (Table 4). When abnormal movements are detected, a differential diagnosis should be considered (Table 5).

Once a diagnosis of tardive dyskinesia is made, it becomes imperative to complete regular objective ratings of the movement disorder. Although tardive dyskinesia often emerges while the patient is taking a steady dosage of medication, it is even more likely to emerge when the dosage is reduced. Some investigators have called the latter dyskinesias "withdrawal" dyskinesias. Once tardive dyskinesia is recognized, consideration should be given to reducing or stopping the antipsychotic if at all possible. Between 5 and 40 percent of all tardive dyskinesias will eventually remit, and between 50 and 90 percent of mild cases will remit. It is not thought at this time that tardive dyskinesia is a progressive condition.

There is no single effective treatment for tardive dyskinesia. If the movement disorder is severe, an attempt should be made to decrease or stop the antipsychotic. Lithium, carbamazepine, or benzodiazepines may be effective in reducing both the psychotic symptoms and the movement disorder. Various studies have reported that cholinergic agonists and antagonists, dopaminergic agonists, and GABAergic drugs (e.g., sodium valproate) are useful.

Neuroleptic Malignant Syndrome. Neuroleptic malignant syndrome (NMS) is a life-threatening complication of antipsychotic treatment, with a variable time of onset during treatment. Symptoms include muscular rigidity and dystonia, akinesia, mutism, obtundation, and agitation. Autonomic symptoms include hyperpyrexia (up to 107°F), sweating, and increased pulse and blood pressure. Laboratory findings include increased WBC, blood creatinine phosphokinase, liver enzymes, and myoglobin in plasma resulting in renal shutdown. The symptoms usually evolve over 24 to 72 hours, and the untreated syndrome lasts 10 to 14 days. The diagnosis is often missed in the early stages, and the withdrawal or

Table 4
AIMS* Examination Procedure

Patient Identification	Date

Rated by

Either before or after completing the examination procedure, observe the patient unobtrusively at rest (e.g., in waiting room).

The chair to be used in this examination should be a hard, firm one without arms.

After observing the patient, he may be rated on a scale of 0 (none), 1 (minimal), 2 (mild), 3 (moderate) and 4 (severe) according to the severity of symptoms.

Ask the patient whether there is anything in his/her mouth (i.e., gum, candy, etc) and if there is to remove it.

Ask patient about the *current* condition of his/her teeth. Ask patient if he/she wears dentures. Do teeth or dentures bother patient *now?*

Ask patient whether he/she notices any movement in mouth, face, hands or feet. If yes, ask to describe and to what extent they *currently* bother patient or interfere with his/her activities.

0	1	2	3	4	Have patient sit in chair with hands on knees, legs slightly apart and feet flat on floor. (Look at entire body for movements while in this position.)
0	1	2	3	4	Ask patient to sit with hands hanging unsupported. If male, between legs, if female and wearing a dress, hanging over knees. (Observe hands and other body areas.)
0	1	2	3	4	Ask patient to open mouth. (Observe tongue at rest within mouth.) Do this twice.
0	1	2	3	4	Ask patient to protrude tongue. (Observe abnormalities of tongue movement.) Do this twice.
0	1	2	3	4	Ask the patient to tap thumb, with each finger, as rapidly as possible for 10–15 seconds; separately with right hand, then with left hand. (Observe facial and leg movements.)
0	1	2	3	4	Flex and extend patient's left and right arms. (One at a time)
0	1	2	3	4	Ask patient to stand up. (Observe in profile. Observe all body areas again, hips included.)
0	1	2	3	4	†Ask patient to extend both arms outstretched in front with palms down. (Observe trunk, legs and mouth.)
0	1	2	3	4	†Have patient walk a few paces, turn and walk back to chair. (Observe hands and gait.) Do this twice.

*Abnormal Involuntary Movement Scale †Activated movements

agitation may be mistakenly considered as increased psychosis. Males are affected more frequently than are females, and the mortality rate is between 15 to 25 percent. The pathophysiology of NMS is unknown, although it may be related to hyperthermic crises that were seen in psychotic patients before the advent of antipsychotic drugs.

The treatment is the immediate discontinuation of antipsychotic drugs, medical support to cool the patient, and the monitoring of vital signs and renal output. Dantrolene, a skeletal muscle relaxant (200 mg a day) may reduce the muscle spasms, and bromocriptine (5 mg every 4 hours, up to 60 mg a day) has also been reported to be of some benefit in treating this syndrome.

DRUG INTERACTIONS

Antacids

Antacids and cimetidine, administered in intervals of 1 to 2 hours of antipsychotic administration reduce the absorption of antipsychotic drugs.

Anticholinergics

Anticholinergics may decrease the absorption of antipsychotics. The additive anticholinergic activity of antipsychotics, anticholinergics, and tricyclic antidepressants may result in anticholinergic toxicity.

Anticonvulsants

Phenothiazines, especially thioridazine, may decrease the metabolism of diphenylhydantoin, resulting in toxic levels of the latter. Barbiturates may increase the metabolism of antipsychotics, and antipsychotics may lower the seizure threshold.

Antidepressants

Tricyclic antidepressants and antipsychotics may decrease each other's metabolism, resulting in increased plasma concentrations of both. The anticholinergic, sedative, and hypotensive effects of these drugs may also be additive.

Antihypertensives

Antipsychotics may inhibit the uptake of guanethidine into the synapse and may also inhibit the hypotensive effects of clonidine and α-methyldopa. Conversely, antipsychotics may have an additive effect on some hypotensives. Antipsychotics have a variable effect on clonidine.

CNS Depressants

Antipsychotics potentiate the CNS depressant effects of sedatives, antihistamines, opiates, and alcohol, particularly in patients with an impaired respiratory status.

Other Drugs

Cigarette smoking may decrease the plasma levels of antipsychotic drugs. Epinephrine has a paradoxical hypotensive effect in patients on antipsychotics. The co-administration of lithium and antipsychotics may result in symptoms similar to those of lithium intoxication or neuroleptic malignant syndrome. There is no reason to believe that these two syndromes are more common with co-administration than when these agents are administered alone and that the interaction is no more common with one antipsychotic than another. Propranolol co-administration with antipsychotics increases the blood concentrations of both. Antipsychotics decrease the blood concentration of warfarin, resulting in decreased bleeding time.

OTHER DRUGS USED TO TREAT PSYCHOSIS

As previously mentioned, reserpine and clozapine have been used to treat psychosis, especially schizophrenia. Reserpine is a less potent and perhaps less effective drug than the other antipsychotics. It has a slow onset of activity (up to 2 months) and is associated with depression and even suicide. Clozapine is an interesting drug because it does not cause the usual neurological adverse effects; however, it is not currently available because of the increased incidence of agranulocytosis associated with its use.

Lithium

Lithium may be effective in further reducing psychotic symptoms in up to 50 percent of patients with schizophrenia. Lithium may also be a reasonable drug to use if patients are unable, for some reason, to take antipsychotics.

Carbamazepine

Carbamazepine may be used alone or in combination with lithium. It has not been shown to be effective in treating the psychosis of schizophrenia; however, there is evidence that it may reduce the episodic violence associated with some cases of schizophrenia.

Propranolol

Propranolol in doses ranging from 600 to 2,000 mg a day is a controversial treatment for schizophrenia. However, some patients are helped by this drug when they are either not able to take antipsychotics or nonresponsive to antipsychotics.

Table 5
Differential Diagnosis for Tardive Dyskinesia-like Movements

Common—Schizophrenic mannerisms and stereotypies
  Dental problems (e.g., ill-fitting dentures)
  Meige's syndrome and other senile dyskinesias

Drug induced—Antidepressants
  Antihistamines
  Antimalarials
  Antipsychotics
  Diphenylhydantoin
  Heavy metals
  Levodopa
  Sympathomimetics

CNS—Anoxia induced
Hepatic failure
Huntington's disease
Parathyroid hypoactivity
Postencephalitic
Pregnancy (chorea gravidarum)
Renal failure
Sydenham's chorea
Systemic lupus erythematosus
Thyroid hyperactivity
Torsion dystonia
Tumors
Wilson's disease

Benzodiazepines

There is increasing interest in the possibility of co-administering alprazolam with antipsychotics in patients who do not respond to the antipsychotic alone. There are also reports of schizophrenic patients' responding to high doses of diazepam alone.

References

Adler L A, Angrist B, Perelow E, Reitano J, Rotrosen J: Clonidine in neuroleptic induced akathisia. Am J Psych 144:235, 1987.
Black J L, Richelson E, Richardson J W: Antipsychotic agents: A clinical update. Mayo Clin Proc 60:777, 1985.
Cole J O, Gardos G: Alternatives to neuroleptic drug therapy. McLean Hosp J 10:112, 1985.
Delva N, Letemendia F: Lithium treatment in schizophrenic and schizoaffective disorders. Brit J Psychiatry 141:387, 1982.
Jeste D V Wyatt R J: Understanding and Treating Tardive Dyskinesia. Guilford Press, New York, 1982.
Kane J M, editor: Developing rational maintenance therapy for schizophrenia. J Clin Psychopharm 6:1, 1986.
Lipinski J F, Zubenko G, Cohen B M: Propranolol in the treatment of neuroleptic-induced akathisia. Am J Psychiatry 141:412, 1984.
Pearlman C A: Neuroleptic malignant syndrome: A review of the literature. J Clin Psychopharm 6:257, 1986.
Picker D, Wolkowitz O M, Doran A R, Labarca R, Roy A, Breier A, Narorj P K: Clinical and biochemical effects of verapamil administration to schizophrenic patients. Arch Gen Psych 44:113, 1987.
Prosser E S, Csernonsky J G, Kaplan J, Thiemann S, Becker T J, Hollister L E: Depression, parkinsonian symptoms, and negative neuroleptics. J Ner and Men Dis 175:100, 1987.
Richelson E: Neuroleptic affinities for human brain receptors and their use in predicting adverse effects. J Clin Psychiatry 45:331, 1984.
Van Putten T: Why do schizophrenic patients refuse to take their drugs? Arch Gen Psychiatry 31:67, 1978.

31.3 ——————
Drugs Used to Treat Depression

INTRODUCTION

The drugs referred to as antidepressants include the heterocyclic antidepressants (HCAs), monoamine oxidase inhibitors (MAOIs), several atypical antidepressants, and the sympathomimetics (e.g., amphetamine).

The heterocyclic group contains both tricyclic and tetracyclic drugs. The tricyclic antidepressants and the MAOIs are considered the classic antidepressant drugs; however, they all have a 2- to 3-week onset of action and are associated with various unpleasant adverse effects. Although the development of new antidepressants has been directed toward finding quicker-acting drugs with fewer adverse effects, this search has yet to be particularly successful.

The principal indication for antidepressants is a major depressive episode. The first symptoms to improve are usually poor sleep and appetite. Then agitation, anxiety, depression, and hopelessness are reduced. Other target symptoms include low energy, poor concentration, helplessness, and decreased libido. The use of these drugs as antidepressants approximately doubles the chance that a depressed patient will recover within 1 month. More recent indications for antidepressant medications (e.g., eating disorders, anxiety) make somewhat confusing the grouping of these drugs under a single label of antidepressants.

The antidepressant drugs do not markedly influence the brain of a mentally healthy human but, rather, correct an abnormal condition. The HCAs and MAOIs are antidepressants for depressed individuals but have relatively little or no effect as general euphoriants or stimulants in most mentally healthy persons. In contrast, sympathomimetic antidepressants are euphoriants in such persons.

HETEROCYCLIC ANTIDEPRESSANTS

Classification

All the tricyclic compounds have a three-ring nucleus (Figure 1). Imipramine, amitriptyline, trimipramine, and doxepin are tertiary amines because there are two methyl groups on the nitrogen atom of the side chain. Desipramine, nortriptyline, and protriptyline are secondary amines because there is only one methyl group in this position. Amoxapine, a dibenzoxazepine, is a derivative of the antipsychotic loxapine and has a cyclic side chain off the three-ring nucleus. Maprotiline is a tetracyclic with the same side chain as desipramine; its fourth ring actually bridges the center ring of the standard tricyclic nucleus. Mianserin is a tetracyclic drug whose side chain has been cyclicized to form the fourth ring; mianserin is not currently available for clinical use.

Pharmacokinetics

Absorption from oral administration of most HCAs is incomplete, and there is a significant metabolism from the first pass

effect. Imipramine pamoate is a depot form of the drug for IM administration; indications for the use of this preparation are limited. Protein binding is usually over 75 percent; the lipid solubility is quite high; and the volume of distribution ranges from 10 to 30 L per kg for tertiary amines to 20 to 60 L per kg for secondary amines. The tertiary amines are demethylated to form the related secondary amines. The ratio of methylated to demethylated forms varies widely from individual to individual. The tricyclic nucleus is oxidized in the liver, conjugated with glucuronic acid, and excreted. The 7-hydroxymetabolite of amoxapine has potent dopamine blocking activity, thus causing the antipsychotic-like neurological and endocrinological adverse effects that are seen with this drug. The half-lives vary from 10 to 70 hours, although nortriptyline, maprotiline, and particularly proptriptyline can have longer half-lives. The long half-lives allow for all of these compounds to be given once daily and means that 5 to 7 days are needed to reach steady-state plasma levels.

Pharmacodynamics

The acute effects of HCAs are to reduce the re-uptake of norepinephrine and serotonin and to block muscarinic acetylcholine and histamine receptors. The different HCAs vary in their pharmacodynamic effects (see Table 1). It should be noted that amoxapine and maprotiline have the least anticholinergic activity and that doxepin has the most antihistaminergic activity. The reuptake blockade of norepinephrine and serotonin by the HCAs, and the monoamine oxidase inhibition by the MAOIs, led to the development of the monoamine hypothesis of mood disorders. Chronic administration of HCAs results in a decrease in the number of β-adrenergic receptors and, perhaps, a similar decrease in the number of serotonin type-2 receptors. It is this downregulation of receptors after repeated administration that most closely correlates with the time that clinical effects appear in patients. This downregulation of β-adrenergic receptors occurs whether the initial

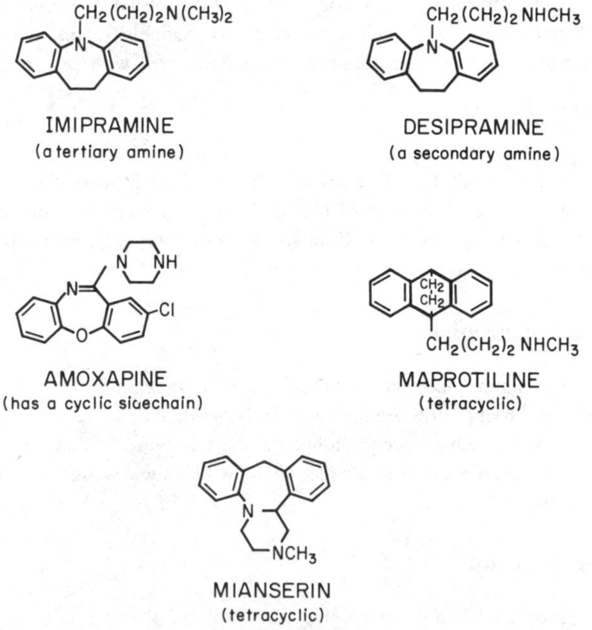

Figure 1. Molecular structures of selected HCAs.

Table 1
Neurotransmitter Effects of HCAs

	Reuptake Blockade		Receptor Blockade		
	NE	5HT	muscarinic ACh	H₁	H₂
Imipramine	+	+	+ +	±	±
Desipramine	+ + +	±	±	−	−
Trimipramine	±	±	+ +	+ +	?
Amitriptyline	±	+ +	+ + +	+ +	+ +
Nortriptyline	+ +	±	+	±	±
Protriptyline	+ + +	±	+	+ + +	−
Amoxapine	+ +	±	+	±	?
Doxepin	+	±	+ +	+ + +	+
Maprotiline	+ + +	−	+	±	?

Table 2
Clinical Information for the HCAs

Generic Names	Trade Names	Usual Adult Dose Range mg/day	Therapeutic Plasma Levels* mg/ml
Imipramine	Tofranil Other Brands Generic	150–300†	150–300
Desipramine	Norpramine Pertofrane	150–300†	150–300
Trimipramine	Surmontil	150–300†	?
Amitriptyline	Elavil, Other Brands Generic	150–300†	100–250†
Nortriptyline	Pamelor, Aventyl	50–150	50–150 (maximum)
Protriptyline	Vivactil	15–60	75–250
Amoxapine	Asendin	150–400	?
Doxepin	Adapin, Sinequan	150–300†	100–250
Maprotiline	Ludiomil	150–225	150–300

*Exact range may vary among laboratories.
†Includes parent compound and desmethyl metabolite.

effect is blocking noradrenergic or serotonin receptors. Research with animals has demonstrated, however, that intact noradrenergic and serotonergic systems are required for the downregulation to occur.

Plasma Levels

Research has defined the dose response curves for HCAs. Clinical determinations of HCA plasma levels should be conducted 8 to 12 hours after the last dose, after 5 to 7 days on the same dosage of medication. Because of variation in absorption and metabolism, there is a 30- to 50-fold difference in the plasma levels of humans given the same dose of an HCA. The therapeutic ranges for HCA plasma levels have been determined (Table 2). Nortriptyline is unique in its association with a therapeutic window; that is, plasma levels over 150 mg per ml may reduce the efficacy. It is important that clinicians follow the directions for collection from the testing laboratory and have confidence in the assay procedures used.

The use of HCA plasma levels in clinical practice is still an evolving skill. HCA plasma levels may be useful in confirming compliance, assessing reasons for drug failures, and documenting effective plasma levels for future treatment. Clinicians should al-

ways treat the patient, and never the plasma level. Some patients may have perfectly adequate clinical responses on seemingly subtherapeutic plasma levels, and other patients may have a response only at supratherapeutic plasma levels without experiencing adverse effects. The latter situation, however, should alert clinicians to monitor carefully the patient's condition (e.g., EKG).

Indications

Major Depressive Episode. A major depressive episode in both unipolar and bipolar patients is the major indication for using HCAs. Symptoms of melancholia and prior episodes of depression increase the likelihood of a therapeutic response.

Secondary Depression. Depressions associated with organic syndromes may respond to HCAs. These include depressions following cerebrovascular accidents and CNS trauma, as well as the depressive symptoms seen in some dementias and movement disorders (e.g., Parkinson's disease). Depression associated with AIDS may also respond to these drugs.

Agoraphobia with Panic Attacks. Imipramine has been the HCA most studied for agoraphobia with panic attacks, although other HCAs may also be effective. Early reports suggested that small dosages of imipramine (50 mg a day) were often effective;

however, more recent studies indicate that the usual antidepressant dosages are usually required.

Generalized Anxiety. The use of doxepin for the treatment of anxiety is approved by the FDA. There are some research data showing that imipramine may also be useful, and many clinicians use a combination drug containing chlordiazepoxide and amitriptyline (Limbitrol) for mixed anxiety and depressive disorders.

Obsessive-Compulsive Disorder. Obsessive-compulsive disorder is classified under the anxiety disorders in DSM-III-R and appears to respond somewhat specifically to clomipramine. Clomipramine is not available in the United States but is available in Canada. It is possible to obtain this drug for a particular patient through a special arrangement with the FDA and the drug company. It does not appear that any of the other HCAs are nearly as effective as clomipramine.

Eating Disorders. Both anorexia nervosa and bulimia have been successfully treated with imipramine and desipramine, although other HCAs may also be effective.

Pain. Chronic pain syndromes, including headaches (e.g., migraines), are often treated with HCAs.

Other Syndromes. Childhood enuresis is often treated with imipramine. Peptic ulcer disease, a psychosomatic condition, can be treated with doxepin, which has marked antihistaminergic effects. Other indications for HCAs are narcolepsy and nightmares.

Clinical Guidelines

Choice of Drug. The specific choice of which HCA or other antidepressant to use should be based on the general guidelines outlined in Section 31.1. All available HCAs are equally effective in the treatment of groups of depressed patients. Because of its antidopaminergic effects, some clinicians recommend using amoxapine in psychotic depressions. The side effect profiles for the HCAs differ. The choice of a specific HCA for an indication other than depression should be based on a knowledge of that clinical syndrome, and a review of the recent literature.

Initiation of Treatment. A routine physical and laboratory examination of a patient to be started on HCAs should be conducted. The routine laboratory tests include a complete blood count (CBC) with differential, a white blood cell count (WBC), and serum electrolytes (SMA=G) with liver function tests (SMA=12). An EKG probably should be obtained for all patients, but especially women over 40 and men over 30. The initial dose should be small and should be raised gradually. The clinician can raise the dosage for inpatients more quickly than for outpatients because of their closer clinical supervision.

It should be explained to patients that although sleep and appetite may improve in 1 to 2 weeks, HCAs usually take 3 to 4 weeks to have antidepressant effects, and a complete trial should last 6 weeks. It may be important to explain to some patients what the drug treatment plan will entail if there is no clinical response at that time.

Dosage (Table 2). Imipramine, amitriptyline, doxepin, desipramine, and trimipramine can be started at 75 mg a day. Divided doses at first will reduce the severity of the side effects, although most of the dose should be given at night to help induce sleep if a sedating HCA (e.g., amitriptyline) is used. Eventually the entire dose can be given at bedtime. Protriptyline and less-sedating HCAs should be given not less than 2 to 3 hours before a patient goes to sleep. For outpatients, the dose can be raised to 150 mg a day the second week, 225 mg a day the third week, and 300 mg a day the fourth week. A very common clinical mistake is to stop increasing the dose at less than 250 mg a day in the absence of clinical improvement. This can result in a further delay in obtaining a therapeutic response, disenchantment with the treatment, and even premature discontinuation of the drug. The clinician should routinely assess the patient's baseline pulse and postural hypotension while the dose is being raised.

Other HCAs have different guidelines for dosage. Nortriptyline should be started at 50 mg at day and be raised to 150 mg a day over 3 or 4 weeks. Amoxapine should be started at 150 mg a day and be raised to 400 mg a day. Protriptyline should be started at 15 mg a day and be raised to 60 mg a day. Maprotiline has been associated with an increased incidence of seizures if the dose is raised too quickly or is maintained at too high a level. Maprotiline should be started at 75 mg a day and be maintained at that level for 2 weeks. The dose can be increased over 4 weeks to 225 mg a day but should be kept at that level for only 6 weeks and then reduced to 175 to 200 mg a day.

Failure of Drug Trial. If an HCA has been used for 4 weeks at maximal doses without a therapeutic effect, the clinician should obtain a plasma level and adjust the dose accordingly. If plasma levels are adequate, then supplementation with lithium or L-triiodothyronine (T_3, Cytomel) should be considered.

Lithium. Lithium (900 to 1200 mg a day, serum level between 0.6 to 0.8 mEq per liter) can be added to the HCA dose for 7 to 14 days. This approach converts a significant number of HCA-nonresponders into responders. The mechanism of action is not known, although it has been hypothesized that the lithium potentiates the serotonergic neuronal system. Some data indicate that the pretreatment with HCAs is necessary for this effect and that starting the treatment with both drugs is not as effective.

L-triiodothyronine. The addition of 25 to 50 μg a day of T_3 to the HCA regimen for 7 to 14 days also may convert HCA-nonresponders into responders. The adverse effects from T_3 are minor but may include a headache and feeling warm. The mechanism of action for T_3 augmentation is not known, although the modulation of β-adrenergic receptors and the presence of undetectable thyroid axis abnormalities have been suggested. If T_3 augmentation is successful, the T_3 should be continued for 2 months and then tapered at the rate of 12.5 μg a day every 3 to 7 days.

Maintenance. HCAs should be continued at maximal dose for 3 to 4 months following a successful therapeutic recovery. At that point, it may be reasonable to reduce the dose to three-fourths the maximal dose for 1 month, then one-half the maximal dose for another month. At this time, if no symptoms are present, the HCA can be tapered by 25 mg (5 mg for protriptyline) every 2 to 3 days. This slow tapering process is indicated for most psychotherapeutic drugs, and in the case of most HCAs, it avoids a cholinergic-rebound syndrome consisting of nausea, upset stomach, sweating, headache, neck pain, and vomiting. The appearance of this syndrome can be treated by reinstituting a small dose of the antidepressant and tapering more slowly. There are also several case reports of rebound mania or hypomania following the abrupt discontinuation of HCAs. If a patient has been treated with HCA and lithium augmentation, it would seem reasonable to taper and stop the lithium first and then the HCA. Clinical studies supporting this approach are lacking, however, and the guidelines may change as more physicians report their experience with this drug combination.

Both HCAs and lithium are useful in preventing the recurrence of depressive episodes. The decision to use a prophylactic treatment is based on the severity and nature of the disorder in a particular patient. Some data suggest that the chronic use of antidepressants may induce a rapid cycling bipolar disorder. Lithium prophylaxis, therefore, may be an alternative treatment in a patient who has frequent, episodic, and serious depressive episodes.

Several investigators have suggested that neuroendocrine tests may be a guide for deciding when to maintain a patient on HCAs and other antidepressants. Specifically, the normalization of a previously abnormal dexamethasone suppression test or a thyroid-releasing hormone stimulation test may indicate that a patient can be safely discontinued from drug treatment. This use of neuroendocrine monitoring is still being investigated.

Drug Combinations

In addition to the combination of HCAs with lithium, T_3, and benzodiazepines mentioned above, HCAs are also used with antipsychotics, MAOIs, and electroconvulsive therapy. A combination of HCAs and antipsychotics is the treatment of choice for psychotic depression, although some clinicians recommend using amoxapine as a single agent. The neuroleptic should be tapered and discontinued as early as possible once the HCA has been clinically effective at reducing the depression. HCAs are sometimes used as adjuvants to ECT and as a therapy after ECT to prolong the clinical improvement.

The combination of an HCA and an MAOI is sometimes used in patients who have not been responsive to several other pharmacologic treatments. This is not a treatment of first or second choice because of the high incidence of adverse effects. It is best to initiate treatment with these two drugs simultaneously at very low doses of each and to raise the dosage very slowly. Imipramine or trimipramine and an MAOI should not be used in combination because of the particularly high incidence of toxic effects, including restlessness, dizziness, tremulousness, muscle twitching, sweating, convulsions, hyperpyrexia, and sometimes death.

If a patient has been on an HCA, the dose of the HCA should be quartered for 5 to 7 days, and then the MAOI can slowly be added to the regimen. If the patient has been on a MAOI, the drug should be stopped for 2 weeks, and both drugs started together at that point. The reason for this latter strategy is that MAOIs irreversibly inhibit monoamine oxidase, and it takes approximately 2 weeks for normal MAO activity levels to be achieved.

Adverse Effects

Psychiatric. A major adverse effect of all HCAs is the possibility of inducing a manic episode in both bipolar patients and patients without a previous history of bipolar disorder. The clinician should watch carefully for this effect in bipolar patients, especially if HCA-induced mania has been a problem in the past. It is prudent to use very low doses of HCAs in such patients.

Anticholinergic. Patients should be warned that anticholinergic effects are quite common but that they may develop a tolerance to them with continued treatment. Amitriptyline, imipramine, trimipramine, and doxepin are the most anticholinergic; amoxapine, nortriptyline, and maprotiline are less anticholinergic;

and desipramine may be the least anticholinergic HCA. HCAs differ in their ability to cause dry mouth, constipation, blurred vision, and urinary retention. Sugarless gum or candy, or fluoride lozenges can alleviate the dry mouth. Bethanechol (urecholine), 25 to 50 mg three times a day (t.i.d.) or four times a day (q.i.d.) may reduce urinary hesitancy and may be helpful for impotence when taken 30 minutes before sex. Narrow-angle glaucoma can also be aggravated by anticholinergic drugs, and the precipitation of glaucoma requires emergency treatment with a miotic agent. HCAs can be used in patients with glaucoma providing that pilocarpine eye drops are administered concurrently. More severe anticholinergic effects can lead to a CNS anticholinergic syndrome with confusion and delirium, especially if HCAs are administered with antipsychotics and anticholinergics. Some clinicians have used IM or IV physostigmine as a diagnostic tool to confirm the presence of anticholinergic delirium.

Sedation. Sedation is a common effect of antidepressants and may be welcomed if sleeplessness has been a problem. The sedative effect of HCAs is a result of serotonergic, cholinergic, and histaminergic (H_1) activity. Amitriptyline, trimipramine, doxepin, and trazodone are the most sedating; imipramine, amoxapine, nortriptyline, and maprotiline have some sedating effects; and desipramine and protriptyline are the least sedating.

Autonomic. The most common autonomic effect, partly due to α_1-adrenergic blockade, is orthostatic hypotension, which can result in falls and injuries in affected patients. Nortriptyline may be the HCA least likely to cause this problem, and some patients respond to fludrocortisone (Florinef) 0.025 to 0.05 mg twice a day. Other possible autonomic effects are profuse sweating, palpitations, and increased blood pressure.

Cardiac Effects. When administered in their usual therapeutic doses, the HCAs may cause tachycardia, flattened T-waves, prolonged Q-T intervals, and depressed S-T segments in the electrocardiogram. Imipramine has been shown to have a quinidine-like effect at therapeutic plasma levels and, indeed, may reduce the number of premature ventricular contractions. Because these drugs prolong conduction time, their use in patients with preexisting conduction defects is contraindicated. In patients with a cardiac history, HCAs should be initiated at low doses, with gradual increases in dose and careful monitoring of cardiac functions. At high plasma levels, as seen in overdoses, the drugs become arrhythmogenic.

Neurological. In addition to the sedation induced by HCAs and the possibility of anticholinergic-induced delirium, two HCAs—desipramine and protriptyline—are associated with psychomotor stimulation. Myoclonic twitches and tremors of the tongue and upper extremities are fairly common. Rarer effects include speech blockage, paresthesias, peroneal palsies, and ataxia.

Amoxapine is unique in causing parkinsonian-like symptoms, akathisia, and even dyskinesias because of the dopaminergic blocking activity of one of its metabolites. Maprotiline may cause seizures when the dose is increased too quickly or is kept at high levels for too long. Amoxapine may also be a bit more epileptogenic than are the other HCAs. All HCAs, however, may induce seizures in patients who have epilepsy or organic brain lesions. Although HCAs can still be used in such patients, the initial doses should be lower and be raised more slowly.

Allergic. Exanthematous skin rashes are seen in 4 to 5 percent of patients treated with maprotiline. Jaundice is very rare. Agranulocytosis, leukocytosis, leukopenia, and eosinophilia are rare complications of HCA treatment. However, a patient who develops a sore throat or fever during the first few months of HCA treatment should have a CBC done immediately.

Other Adverse Effects. Weight gain, primarily an effect of blockade of histamine type-2 receptors, is quite common. If this is a major problem, then changing to trazodone, an atypical antidepressant, may help. Impotence, an occasional problem, is perhaps most often associated with amoxapine because of its blockade of dopamine receptors in the tuberoinfundibular tract. Amoxapine can also cause hyperprolactinemia, galactorrhea, anorgasmia, and ejaculatory disturbances. Other HCAs have also been associated with gynecomastia and amenorrhea. Inappropriate secretion of antidiuretic hormone has also been reported with HCAs.

Overdose Attempts. Overdose attempts with HCAs are very serious and can often be fatal. Prescriptions for HCAs should be nonrefillable and for no longer than a week at a time. Amoxapine may be more likely than the other HCAs to result in death when taken in an overdose attempt.

Symptoms of overdose include agitation, delirium, convulsions, hyperactive deep tendon reflexes, bowel and bladder paralysis, dysregulations of blood pressure and temperature, and mydriasis. The patient then progresses to coma and may develop respiratory depression. Cardiac arrhythmias may not respond to treatment. Because of the long half-lives of HCAs, these patients are at risk of developing cardiac arrhythmias for 3 to 4 days after the overdose attempt, and so they should be monitored carefully in an intensive medical setting.

Drug-Drug Interactions

Antihypertensives. HCAs block the neuronal re-uptake of guanethidine, which is required for antihypertensive activity. The antihypertensive effects of propranolol and clonidine may also be blocked by HCAs. Co-administration of HCAs with alpha methyldopa may cause behavioral agitation.

Antipsychotics. The plasma levels of both HCAs and antipsychotics are increased by their co-administration. Antipsychotics also add to the anticholinergic and sedative effects of the HCAs.

CNS Depressants. Opioids, alcohol, anxiolytics, hypnotics, and over-the-counter cold medications have additive effects by causing CNS depression when co-administered with HCAs.

Oral Contraceptives. Birth control pills may decrease HCA plasma levels through the induction of hepatic enzymes.

Other Pharmacokinetic Interactions. HCA plasma levels may also be increased by acetazolamide, acetylsalicylic acid, thiazide diuretics, and sodium bicarbonate. Decreased HCA plasma levels may be caused by ascorbic acid, ammonium chloride, barbiturates, cigarette smoking, chloral hydrate, lithium, and primidone.

MONOAMINE OXIDASE INHIBITORS

Although controversial, the monoamine oxidase inhibitors (MAOIs) are probably as effective as the HCAs are in treating depression. When first introduced into clinical practice, there was a lack of awareness of the risk of developing tyramine-induced hypertensive crises, thus leading to fatalities and the temporary withdrawal of these drugs from the marketplace. It is now appreciated that these drugs are as safe as are HCAs, providing that reasonable dietary precautions are followed. Some clinicians believe that

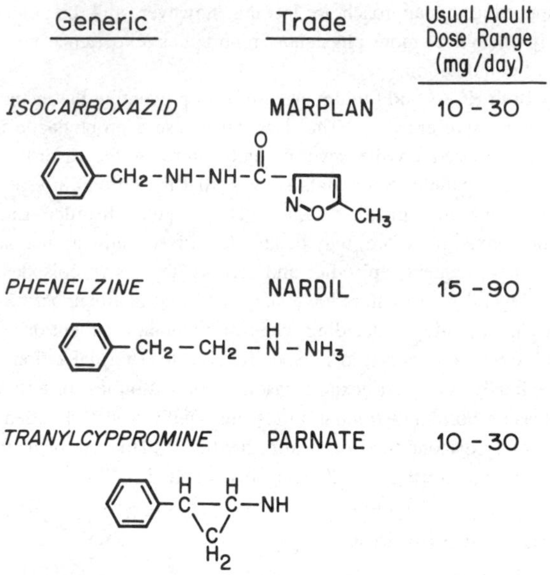

Figure 2. Monoamine oxidase inhibitors.

MAOIs are underused as effective antidepressant treatment.

Classification

There are three MAOIs available in the United States (Figure 2). Phenelzine and isocarboxazid are derivatives of hydrazine (-CNN is the hydrazine moiety), and tranylcypromine is a derivative of amphetamine. Clorgyline is a specific inhibitor of MAO-A (enzyme subtype more specific for norepinephrine and serotonin). Clorgyline may be particularly effective in treating depression in rapid cycling bipolar patients, but it is not available for clinical use in the United States. Deprenyl is a specific inhibitor of MAO-B (enzyme subtype more specific for dopamine) but is not available in the United States and does not appear to be an effective antidepressant.

Pharmacokinetics

MAOIs are readily absorbed when administered orally. The hydrazine MAOIs are metabolized by acetylation. About one-half of North American and European persons, and even a higher proportion of Asians, are slow acetylators, which may explain why when given these drugs, some patients have more adverse effects than do others.

Pharmacodynamics

MAOIs irreversibly inhibit monoamine oxidase, reaching maximum inhibition 5 to 10 days on the medication. Antidepressant effects, however, take 3 to 6 weeks to develop. The measurement of MAO activity in platelets can be used as an indicator of MAO inhibition. Platelet MAO activity needs to be reduced 80 percent to achieve a therapeutic response. Because platelet MAO is of the B-type, this measurement cannot be used if the effects of clorgyline are being studied. Because the MAO inhibition by MAOIs is irreversible, it takes approximately 2 weeks after their discontinuation before the body has synthesized enough new MAO to restore its baseline concentrations.

Indications

The indications for MAOIs are quite similar to those for HCAs. MAOIs may be particularly effective in agoraphobia with panic attacks, post-traumatic stress syndromes, eating disorders, and pain syndromes. Some investigators have reported that MAOIs may actually be preferable to HCAs in the treatment of atypical depression, characterized by hypersomnia, hyperphagia, anxiety, and the absence of vegetative symptoms. These depressions are often less severe, and the patients present with less functional impairment. A trial of MAOIs may be indicated in any depressed patient if a trial of an HCA has been unsuccessful.

Clinical Guidelines

There is no definitive rationale for choosing one MAOI over another, except that tranylcypromine may be the most activating of the drugs. Phenelzine should be started with a test dose of 15 mg on the first day. On an outpatient basis, the dose can be increased to 45 mg a day during the first week and increased by 15 mg a day each week thereafter, until 90 mg a day is reached by the end of the fourth week. Tranylcypromine and isocarboxazid should begin with a test dose of 10 mg and may be increased to 30 mg a day by the end of the first week. Upper limits of 50 mg for isocarboxazid and 40 mg for tranylcypromine have been suggested by some researchers. If an MAOI trial is not successful after 6 weeks, then lithium or T_3 augmentation, as decribed for HCAs, is warranted. The guidelines for maintenance treatment with MAOIs are similar to those for HCAs. Combined treatment with MAOIs and HCAs is described in the previous section on HCAs.

Adverse Effects

Adverse effects from MAOI administration are quite similar to those for HCAs. The most frequent adverse effects are orthostatic hypotension, weight gain, edema, sexual dysfunction, and insomnia. The orthostatic hypotension, if severe, may respond to treatment with fludrocortisone (Florinef), a mineralocorticoid, 0.1–0.2 mg a day; support stockings; corsets; hydration; and increased salt intake. Weight gain, edema, and sexual dysfunction are often not responsive to any treatment and may warrant switching from a hydrazine to a nonhydrazine MAOI, or vice versa. When switching from one MAOI to another, it is prudent to taper and stop the first one for 10 to 14 days before beginning the second one. Insomnia and behavioral activation can be treated by dividing the dose, not giving medication after dinner, and using a benzodiazepine hypnotic if necessary. Insomnia may paradoxically be accompanied by sedation during the day. Myoclonus, muscle pains, and parathesias are also occasionally seen in patients treated with MAOIs. Occasionally patients complain of feeling drunk or confused, perhaps indicating that the dose should be reduced and then increased more gradually. There are uncommon reports of the hydrazine MAOIs being associated with hepatotoxic effects. It may be that MAOIs are less cardiotoxic and less epileptogenic than are HCAs.

Tyramine-induced Hypertensive Crisis. When patients on MAOIs ingest foodstuffs rich in tyramine (Table 3), they may have a hypertensive reaction that can be life threatening

Table 3
Tyramine-Rich Foods to Be Avoided While Taking MAOIs

Very high tyramine content:

Alcohol (particularly beer and wines, especially chianti; a small amount of scotch, gin, vodka, or sherry is permissible.)

Fava or broad beans

Aged cheese (e.g., Camembert, Liederkranz, Edam, and cheddar; cream cheese and cottage cheeses are permitted.)

Beef or chicken liver

Orange pulp

Pickled or smoked fish, poultry, or meats

Soups (packaged)

Yeast vitamin supplements

Meat extracts (e.g., Marmite, Bovril)

Summer (dry) sausage

Moderately high tyramine content (no more than one or two servings per day):

Soy sauce

Sour cream

Bananas (green bananas can be included only if cooked in their skins; ordinary peeled bananas are fine.)

Avocados

Eggplant

Plums

Raisins

Spinach

Tomatoes

Yogurt

(e.g., cerebrovascular accident). Patients should also be warned that bee stings may cause a hypertensive crisis. The mechanism is MAO inhibition in the gastrointestinal (GI) tract, resulting in the increased absorption of tyramine, which then acts as a false neurotransmitter. Increased concentrations of noradrenaline in presynaptic endings is a result of MAO-A inhibition and may be an even more significant mechanism in producing this hypertensive effect.

Patients should be warned about the dangers of ingesting tyramine-rich foods while taking MAOIs, and they should be advised to continue the dietary restrictions for 2 weeks after they stop MAOI treatment in order to allow the body to resynthesize the enzyme. The prodromal symptoms of a hypertensive crisis may include headache, stiff neck, sweating, nausea, and vomiting. If these symptoms occur, a patient should seek immediate medical treatment. Treatment should include administration of α-adrenergic blockers, such as phentolamine. Chlorpromazine may also be used, and some clinicians give their patients several 50 mg tablets of chlorpromazine to use in an emergency. A headache from the hypotensive effects of MAOIs may confuse the patient, however, and taking the chlorpromazine could result in more severe hypotension, fainting, and possibly injury.

Overdose Attempts. In general, intoxication caused by MAOIs is characterized by agitation that progresses to coma with hyperthermia, hypertension, tachypnea, tachycardia, dilated pupils, and hyperactive deep tendon reflexes. Involuntary movements may be present, particularly in the face and jaw.

Table 4
Drugs to Be Avoided During MAOI Treatment

Never Use:

Anesthesia—never spinal anesthesia or locals containing epinephrine (Lidocaine and procaine are safe.)

Antiasthmatic medications

Antihypertensives (α-methyldopa, guanethidine, reserpine, pargyline)

L-dopa, L-tryptophan

Narcotics (especially meperidine [Demerol]; morphine or codeine may be less dangerous.)

Over-the-counter cold, hay fever, or sinus medications, especially those containing dextromethorphan. (Aspirin, acetaminophen, and menthol lozenges are safe.)

Sympathomimetics (amphetamine, cocaine, methylphenidate, dopamine, metaraminol, epinephrine, norepinephrine, isoproterenol)

Use carefully:

Antihistamines

Hydralazine

Propranolol

Terpin hydrate with codeine

There is often an asymptomatic period of 1 to 6 hours after the ingestion of the drugs before the occurrence of toxicity. Acidification of the urine markedly hastens the excretion of MAOIs, and dialysis may be of some use. Phentolamine and chlorpromazine may be useful if hypotension is a problem.

Drug-Drug Interactions

The inhibition of MAO can cause severe and even fatal interactions with various other drugs (Table 4). Patients should be instructed to tell any other physicians who are treating them that they are taking an MAOI.

ATYPICAL ANTIDEPRESSANTS

Atypical antidepressants are also referred to as second-generation antidepressants (Figure 3). Although the available atypical antidepressants have been demonstrated to be clinically effective, it still is wise to use an HCA or MAOI before conducting a trial with one of the second-generation drugs.

Trazodone

Trazodone (Desyrel) is available in the United States and is approved for the treatment of depression. Trazodone is a triazolopyridine derivative and therefore contains the same triazolo ring as does alprazolam, another atypical antidepressant. Some clinicians believe that trazodone is less effective than are HCAs or MAOIs; however, they may not have used trazodone in high enough doses, which are approximately twice that for HCAs. Trazodone inhibits serotonin reuptake and is also an α-adrenergic receptor blocker. It has very low anticholinergic activity and may be the drug of choice if benign prostatic hypertrophy or closed-angle glaucoma is present.

Because trazodone is very sedating, it has been suggested as a good drug to try if patients have severe insomnia. The starting dose should be 50 mg a day and be increased to 150 mg a day by the end of the first week. The dose can then be raised 75 to 100 mg a day every week until a maximal dose of 600 mg a day is reached.

Common side effects include sedation and dry mouth (secondary to α-adrenergic blockade). Acute dizziness, headache, and nausea have also been reported. Trazodone may be relatively less lethal compared with HCAs when taken in overdose attempts. Trazodone is associated with the unusual adverse effect of priapism, and patients should be told to seek immediate medical attention if an erection lasts more than 1 hour. Untreated priapism can result in impotence. Trazodone may also be associated with cardiac arrhythmias in patients with preexisting mitral valve prolapse.

Alprazolam

Alprazolam (Xanax) is a triazolo benzodiazepine that appears to have potent antipanic activity and has been demonstrated to have moderate antidepressant effects in a number of studies. Alprazolam may act by altering the function of G-proteins and adenylate cyclase. The starting dose should be 1 to 1.5 mg a day and be raised 0.5 mg a day every 3 to 4 days. The maximal dose is usually 4 to 5 mg a day, although some investigators and clinicians have used dosages as high as 10 mg a day. It is particularly important to taper,

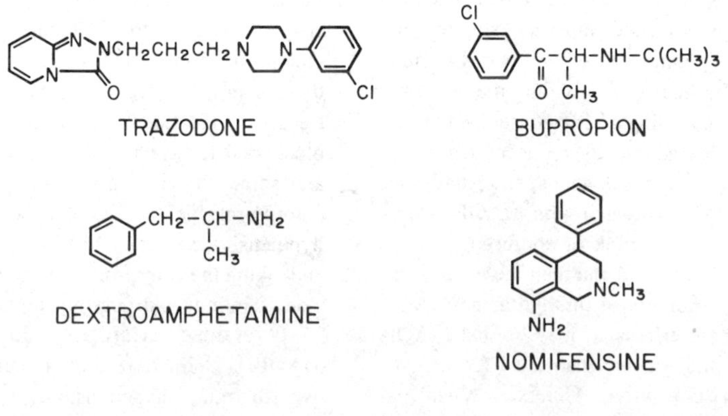

Figure 3. Molecular structures of selected atypizal and sympathomimetic antidepressants.

rather than abruptly stop alprazolam, usually at the rate of 0.5 mg a day every 3 to 4 days. The major adverse effect of alprazolam is sedation.

Buproprion

Buproprion is a unicyclic compound that was introduced in the United States but then withdrawn because of its toxic adverse effects. Its mechanism of action is unclear, but may block dopamine re-uptake. Although it did not improve insomnia very quickly, it was associated with fewer adverse effects, including the absence of orthostatic hypotension, weight gain, or anticholinergic effects.

Nomifensine

Nomifensine is a tetrahydroisoquinoline compound that was introduced in the United States but then withdrawn because of the occurrence of hemolytic anemias and deaths in patients treated with this drug. Nomifensine is a potent re-uptake blocker of norepinephrine and dopamine. Because of its stimulating effects, it seemed particularly appropriate for anergic patients. There were generally few adverse effects, although some patients reported sleep disturbances, tachycardia, and mild hypertension. The drug has a relatively short half-life, requiring dosages 2 to 3 times a day.

Other Atypical Antidepressants

Although not yet available clinically in the United States, a number of atypical antidepressants are in various stages of research and development. Fluoxetine blocks serotonin re-uptake as its primary acute effect. The use of this drug is associated with the usual anticholinergic adverse effects, and therapeutic effects take 2 to 3 weeks to develop. Fluoxetine is not sedating and may even be somewhat activating for patients. This drug is associated with weight loss, in contrast with the weight gain associated with most other antidepressants. The standard dose is 60 to 80 mg a day in divided doses. Zimeldine and citalopram are also potent inhibitors of serotonin re-uptake. Mianserin may act as a blocker of presynaptic α2-adrenergic receptors, and the mechanism of action for iprindole is unknown.

SYMPATHOMIMETICS

Dextroamphetamine (Dexedrine), methylphenidate (Ritalin), and magnesium pemoline (Cylert) are sympathomimetics that may be useful in treating some patients with depression (Figure 3). Dextro-amphetamine and methylphenidate are Class II drugs and require triplicate prescriptions. Fenfluramine is an amphetamine-like drug that primarily affects serotonin and may be useful in treating autism. Generally these drugs are thought to be less effective in treating depression than are the previously discussed drugs, and all three drugs have a high abuse potential. Sympathomimetic drugs work by decreasing the re-uptake and by increasing the release of catecholamines. The use of these drugs may be indicated in treatment-resistant patients, elderly patients, medically ill patients, and in situations in which a quick response is required and ECT is not acceptable. Sympathomimetics are also effective in treating attention-deficit hyperactivity disorder.

Some clinicians try magnesium pemoline first because it has less abuse potential. Pemoline should be started at 37.5 mg twice daily, with the second dose around 2 P.M. The dose can be raised to 75 mg a day over a week, and improvement can be assessed at the end of 2 weeks. Dextroamphetamine can be started at 10 mg a day and raised to 30 mg a day; methylphenidate can be started at 20 mg a day and raised to 60 mg a day.

Adverse effects include increased pulse and blood pressure, decreased appetite and sleep, and sometimes a feeling of being "wired." Some patients develop a tolerance to the antidepressant effects of these drugs. Physical dependence and symptoms of depression on withdrawal can occur with all three of these drugs.

OTHER DRUGS USED TO TREAT DEPRESSION

When administered alone, lithium is successful in treating some patients with depression, including approximately 50 percent of depressed bipolar patients. The onset of action, however, is usually quite slow, and supplementation with HCAs is usually indicated.

Carbamazepine has been demonstrated to be quite similar to lithium in the treatment of bipolar patients. Although there is very little information about the use of carbamazepine to treat depression, a trial of this drug might be indicated in unusual circumstances.

References

Callies A L, Popkin M K: Antidepressant treatment of medical and surgical inpatients by nonpsychiatrc physicians. Arch Gen Psychiatry 44:157, 1987.
Cassem N: Cardiovascular effects of antidepressants. J Clin Psychiatry 43:11, 22, 1982.
Chiarello R J, Cole J O: The use of psychostimulants in general psychiatry: A reconsideration. Arch Gen Psychiatry 44:286, 1987.
Garvey M J, Tolletson G D: Occurrence of myoclonus in patients treated with cyclic antidepressants. Arch Gen Psychiatry 44:269, 1987.
Georgotas A, McCue R E, Friedman E, Cooper T: Prediction of response to nortriptyline and phenelzine by platelet MAO activity. Am J Psychiatry 144:338, 1987.
Jabbari B, Bryan G E, Marsh E E, Gunderson C H: Incidence of seizures with tricyclic antidepressants. Arch Neurology 42:480, 1985.
Maas J W, Koslow S H, Davis J, Katz M, Krazer A, Bowden C L, Berman N, Gibbons R, Stokes P, Landis D M: Catecholamine metabolism and disposition in healthy and depressed subjects. Arch Gen Psychiatry 44:337, 1987.
McDaniel K D: Review: Clinical pharmacology of monoamine oxidase inhibitors. Clin Neuropharmacology 9:207, 1986.
NIMH/NIH Consensus Development Panel: Mood disorders: Pharmacologic prevention of recurrences. Am J Psychiatry 142:469, 1985.
Potter W Z, Murphy D L, Wehr T A: Clorgyline. Arch Gen Psychiatry 39:505, 1982.
Rabkin J, Quitkin F, Harrison W: Adverse Reactions to monoamine oxidase inhibitors. J Clin Psychopharm Part I, 4:270, 1984; II, 4:270, 5:2, 1984, 1985.
Rickels K, Feighner J P, Smith W T: Alprazolam, amitriptyline, doxepin, and placebo in the treatment of depression. Arch Gen Psychiatry 42:143, 1985.
Robertson M, Trimble M: Major tranquilizers used as antidepressants—A review. J Affective Disorders 4:173, 1982.
Roose S P, Glassman A H, Giardina E G V, Walsh B T, Woodring S, Bigger J T: Tricyclic antidepressants in depressed patients with cardiac conduction disease. Arch Gen Psychiatry 44:273, 1987.
Roy A, Everett D, Pickar D, Paul S M: Platelet initiated imipramine binding and serotonin uptake in depressed patients and controls. Arch Gen Psychiatry 4:22, 1987.
White K, Simpson G: Combined MAOI-tricyclic antidepressant treatment. A reevaluation. J Clin Psychopharm 1:264, 1981.

31.4 ————
Drugs Used to Treat Bipolar Disorder

INTRODUCTION

A variety of drugs are now available to treat bipolar disorder (Table 1). Lithium containing salts (e.g., lithium carbonate and citrate) are the major pharmacologic treatments for bipolar disorder. In the last five years, anticonvulsants (carbamazepine and sodium valproate) have also been used to treat this disorder. Levothyroxine is sometimes used to augment the clinical response to these drugs in patients with rapid cycling. Finally, several studies and case reports have reported calcium channel inhibitors (e.g., verapamil), a benzodiazepine anticonvulsant (clonazepam), and an α-2-adrenergic agonist (clonidine) to be effective treatments.

LITHIUM

Classification

Lithium is an element and is the lightest of the alkali metals (group Ia of the periodic table), similar to sodium, potassium, magnesium, and calcium. Lithium is a monovalent ion and is available as a carbonate (Li_2CO_3) for oral use in both rapidly acting and slow-release tablets and capsules. Lithium citrate is available in a liquid form for oral administration.

Pharmacokinetics

Following ingestion, lithium is completely absorbed by the gastrointestinal tract. Serum levels peak in 0.5 to 2 hours, and in 4 to 4.5 hours for the slow-release preparation. Lithium does not bind to plasma proteins and is distributed nonuniformly throughout body water. The half-life of lithium is around 20 hours, and equilibrium is reached after 5 to 7 days of regular intake. Lithium is almost entirely eliminated by the kidneys. Renal clearance of lithium is decreased with renal insufficiency and in the puerperium, and increased during pregnancy. Lithium is excreted in breast milk and in insignificant amounts in feces and sweat.

Pharmacodynamics

The therapeutic mechanism of action for lithium remains uncertain. The most accepted current theory is that lithium works by blocking the enzyme inositol-1-phosphatase within neurons, thus reducing the reformation of phosphatidylinositol from inositoltriphosphate. This inhibition results in decreased cellular responses to neurotransmitters that are linked to the phosphatidyl inositol second messenger system.

Indications

Bipolar Disorder. Lithium has been proved effective in both the acute treatment and prophylaxis of bipolar disorder in approximately 70 to 80 percent of patients. Both manic and depressive episodes often respond to lithium treatment alone. However, because treatment with lithium alone can take a relatively longer time, manic episodes are usually treated with both lithium and an antipsychotic, and depressive episodes are treated with a combination of lithium and an antidepressant. The clinician should be aware of the risk of inducing a manic episode with antidepressant treatment. Most studies have reported that lithium maintenance halves the number of recurrences, and that the recurrences that do occur are less severe. The prophylactic effect of lithium, however, does not develop for several months. A recurrence of symptoms, therefore, before that time should not be taken as an indication that the lithium is not effective. In severe cases of cyclothymia, treatment with lithium may be indicated.

Schizoaffective Disorder. The use of lithium for schizoaffective disorder (manic type) is certainly indicated. If such patients' schizoaffective disorder (depressed type) demonstrates a particularly cyclic nature, a lithium trial may also be warranted.

Major Depression. The major indication for lithium in depression is as an adjuvant treatment to HCAs or MAOIs in order to convert an antidepressant-nonresponder into a responder. Lithium alone may also be an effective treatment for depressed patients who are actually bipolar patients but who have not yet had their first manic episode. Moreover, lithium has been reported to be effective in unipolar depressed patients whose illness has a marked cyclicity.

Schizophrenia. The symptoms of approximately one fifth to one half of schizophrenic patients are further reduced when lithium is added to their antipsychotic drug. Some schizophrenic patients who cannot take antipsychotics may benefit from lithium treatment. Intermittent angry outbursts in schizophrenic patients may also be reduced by lithium.

Impulse Disorders. The impulse disorders include episodic violence and rage. Patients whose episodes are not premeditated and seemingly untriggered may respond to lithium. Episodic angry outbursts in patients with mental retardation may also be reduced with lithium.

Other Disorders. A few studies have reported that the episodic disorder characterizing the premenstrual syndrome, the intermittent behaviors seen in borderline personality disorder, and episodes of binge drinking respond to lithium treatment.

Clinical Guidelines

Lithium is the drug of first choice to treat bipolar disorder unless there is a specific reason not to use lithium or a specific reason to use another drug.

Initial Medical Work-up. Before starting lithium, a routine laboratory and physical examination should be conducted. The laboratory examination should include a serum creatinine level (or a 24-hour urine creatinine if there is any reason to be concerned about renal function), an electrolyte screen, thyroid functions tests (T_4, T_3RU, FT_4I, and TSH), CBC, EKG, and a pregnancy test if there is any risk of the patient's being pregnant.

Dosage. If a patient has previously been treated with lithium and the former dose is known, then it is reasonable to use that dose in the current episode unless there have been changes in the patient's pharmacokinetic parameters for lithium clearance. For most adult patients, it is reasonable to start lithium at 300 mg t.i.d. The starting dose in patients who are elderly or who have renal impairment should be 300 mg once or twice daily. The usual eventual dose range is between 900 and 2,100 mg a day. Serum concentrations of lithium can be obtained after 5 days, and the dose can be adjusted to obtain a serum level between 0.8 and 1.2 mEq

Table 1
Drugs Used to Treat Bipolar Disorder

Class	Generic	Preparation	Trade Name
Lithium salts	Lithium carbonate	Tablets and capsules	Eskalith Lithane Lithotabs
		Sustained release	Eskalith Lithobid
	Lithium citrate	Oral concentrate	Cibalith-S
Anticonvulsants	Carbamazepine	Tablets and capsules	Tegretol
	Valproic acid	Tablets and capsules	Depakene Depokate
	Clorazepam (a benzodiazepine)	Tablets and capsules	Clonopin
Calcium channel inhibitors	Verapamil	Tablets and capsules	Isoptin Calan
α-2-adrenergic agonist	Clonidine	Tablets and capsules	Catapres

per liter during the acute episode. Lithium levels should be obtained 12 hours after the last dose. Lithium levels in patients treated with slow-release preparations are approximately 30 percent higher. The use of divided doses (3 to 4 doses a day) reduces gastric upset and avoids having a single large peak in lithium levels. There is currently a debate over whether multiple smaller daily peaks are less likely to cause adverse effects than is a single large daily peak. Single daily dosing, however, is not considered standard practice at this time. Slow-release lithium preparations can be given two to three times daily and result in lower peak levels of lithium, but this procedure has not yet been demonstrated to be of special value. A therapeutic trial of lithium should last a minimum of 4 to 6 weeks. If there is some response within that time, improvement may continue for another 5 months. If the lithium treatment has been successful, it should be continued for a minimum of 6 to 9 months, then tapered over a month unless the patient is to be maintained on lithium prophylaxis.

Lithium Levels. The patient's lithium level should be monitored weekly for the first month and then biweekly for another 2 months. After 6 months, it may be appropriate to check the patient's lithium level every 2 months. If a patient has been stable on lithium for a year, then lithium levels three to four times a year may be sufficient.

Patient Education. The patient should be advised that changes in the body's water and salt content could affect the amount of lithium excreted, resulting in either increases or decreases in lithium levels. Excessive intake of sodium (e.g., a dramatic dietary change) will lower lithium levels. Conversely, too little sodium (e.g., fad diets) may lead to potentially toxic levels of lithium. Decreases in body fluid (e.g., excessive sweating) can lead to dehydration and lithium intoxication.

Failure of Drug Treatment. If the drug produces no clinical response after 4 weeks at therapeutic levels, then slightly higher serum levels (up to 1.4 mEq per liter) may be tried if there are no severe adverse effects. If after 2 weeks at a higher serum concentration, the drug is still ineffective, then the patient should be tapered off the drug over 1 to 2 weeks. Other drugs should be given therapeutic trials at this point.

Rapid Cycling. One type of treatment failure is the rapid cycling of manic and depressive episodes (more than three or four a year) that are not adequately controlled by lithium treatment. It has been hypothesized that rapid cycling may be a late-appearing adverse effect of HCA administration. Rapid cycling may respond to the addition of levothyroxine (T_4) 0.3 to 0.5 mg a day. The mechanism for this response is not known. The substitution or addition of carbamazepine for lithium may also be effective in reducing the frequency of episodes.

Maintenance. The decision to maintain a patient on lithium prophylaxis is based on the severity of the patient's illness, the risk of adverse effects from lithium, and the quality of the patient's support systems. Maintenance serum levels of lithium can be lower than those needed for acute treatment. Such levels usually are kept between 0.6 and 0.8 mEq per liter, although some researchers have reported successful prophylaxis with serum levels as low as 0.4 mEq per liter. In addition to periodic measurements of lithium levels, serum creatinine and TSH levels should be monitored every 3 to 6 months.

Adverse Effects

The most common adverse effects from lithium treatment are gastric distress, weight gain, tremor, fatigue, and mild cognitive impairment. Gastric distress may include nausea, vomiting, and diarrhea and can often be reduced by further dividing up the dosage, administering the lithium with food, or switching among the various lithium preparations. Weight gain and edema can be impossible to treat other than by encouraging the patient to eat less and to exercise moderately. The tremor affects mostly the fingers and sometimes can be worse at peak levels of the drug. It can be reduced by further dividing the dose. Propranolol (30 to 160 mg a day in divided doses) reduces the tremor significantly in most patients. The fatigue and mild cognitive impairment may decrease with time. Rare neurological adverse effects include symptoms of mild parkinsonism, ataxia, and dysarthria. Leukocytosis is a common and not worrisome effect of lithium treatment.

Renal Effects. The most common adverse renal effect of lithium is polyuria with secondary polydipsia. This symptom is particularly problematic in 20 to 25 percent of treated patients. The polyuria is secondary to the decreased resorption of fluid from the distal tubules of the kidney. When polyuria is a significant problem, the patient's renal function should be carefully evaluated and followed with 24-hour urine collections for creatinine clearance, and with consultation with a nephrologist.

Lithium-induced nephrogenic diabetes insipidus is not responsive to vasopressin treatment and results in urine volumes up to 8L a day and difficulty maintaining adequate lithium levels. This syndrome can be treated with chlorothiazide 500 mg a day, hydrochlorothiazide (50 mg a day), or amiloride (5 to 10 mg a day). The lithium dose should be halved and the diuretic not started for 5 days, because the diuretic is likely to increase the retention of lithium.

The most serious renal adverse effects that were thought to be associated with lithium administration were minimal change glomerulopathy, interstitial nephritis, and renal failure. The original concern about these adverse effects was based on postmortem studies of kidneys from patients who had been treated with lithium. Although it is now generally considered that serious renal disorders are not associated with lithium administration, the clinician should vigorously explore any clinical changes in renal function.

Thyroid Effects. Lithium also affects thyroid function, causing a generally benign and often transient diminution in the concentrations of circulating thyroid hormones. Reports of goiter (5 percent), benign reversible exophthalmos, and hypothyroidism (3 to 4 percent) have also been attributed to lithium. About 50 percent of patients on chronic lithium treatment have an abnormal TRH response, and approximately 30 percent have elevated levels of TSH. If laboratory values of thyroid hormone indicate dysfunction, then thyroid supplementation can be administered safely. TSH levels should be measured and checked periodically. Hyperthyroidism has been reported rarely.

Cardiac Effects. The cardiac effects of lithium, which resemble those of hypokalemia on EKG, are caused by displacement of intracellular potassium by the lithium ion. The most common changes on EKG are T-wave flattening or inversion. They are benign and disappear after the lithium is excreted from the body. Nevertheless, baseline EKG's are essential and should be repeated yearly.

Because lithium depresses the sinus node's pacemaking activity, lithium treatment is strongly contraindicated in patients with sick sinus syndrome. In rare cases, ventricular arrhythmias and congestive heart failure have been associated with lithium therapy.

Dermatologic Effects. Several cutaneous adverse effects, which may be dose dependent, have been associated with lithium treatment. The more prevalent effects include acneiform, follicular, and maculopapular eruptions; pretibial ulcerations; and worsening of psoriasis. Alopecia has also been reported. Many of these conditions respond to changing to another lithium preparation or the usual dermatological measures. Lithium levels should be monitored if tetracycline is used because of several reports of its increasing the retention of lithium. Occasionally, the aggravated psoriasis or acneiform eruptions may force the discontinuation of lithium treatment.

Use in Pregnancy. Lithium should not be administered to pregnant women in the first trimester because of the increased incidence of birth defects, specifically Ebstein's anomaly, which occurs in 3 percent of babies exposed to lithium *in utero*. Adminis-

tration of lithium to the mother during the final months of pregnancy can result in babies who are lithium toxic at birth. The syndrome consists of lethargy, cyanosis, abnormal reflexes, and sometimes hepatomegaly.

Lithium Toxicity. The symptoms of lithium toxicity are severe manifestations of the aforementioned pharmacodynamic organ interactions. These include vomiting, abdominal pain, profuse diarrhea, severe tremor, ataxia, coma, and seizures. Initial neurological signs of mental confusion, hyperreflexia, focal neurological signs, and dysarthria can proceed to coma and death. Cardiac arrhythmias also may occur.

Overdoses. Overdoses of lithium result in symptoms of severe lithium toxicity. Treatment should include lavage with a wide-bore tube because of the drug's clumping in the stomach. Activated charcoal does not help in this condition. Osmotic diuresis, intravenous sodium bicarbonate, and peritoneal or hemodialysis can also be used.

Drug-Drug Interactions

Most diuretics (e.g., thiazides, potassium sparing, and loop) and prostaglandin synthetase inhibitors (e.g., indomethacin) can increase lithium levels to toxic levels. Osmotic diuretics, carbonic anhydrase inhibitors, and xanthines (including caffeine) may reduce lithium levels to below therapeutic levels.

When co-administered, antipsychotics and lithium may result in a synergistic increase in the symptoms of lithium-induced neurological adverse effects. This interaction is not, as initially thought, specifically associated with the co-administration of lithium and haloperidol. The co-administration of lithium with anticonvulsants, including carbamazepine, may also aggravate neurological symptoms. Although it is reasonable practice to stop drug administration if serious symptoms of toxicity are noted, it is usually possible to restart both medications at lower doses without the recurrence of the adverse effects.

ANTICONVULSANTS

The FDA does not currently approve the use of anticonvulsants to treat psychiatric disorders. A therapeutic trial with these drugs may be undertaken if indicated, and the reasons for using the specific drug should be included in the written record. The clinician should be familiar with the most recent literature on the anticonvulsant treatment of bipolar patients before initiating such treatment.

Carbamazepine

Carbamazepine (Figure 1) is approved for use in the United States to treat temporal lobe epilepsy and trigeminal neuralgia. Although experience with carbamazepine in psychiatry is still relatively limited, this drug is a reasonable alternative to the lithium treatment of bipolar patients. Studies have indicated that carbamazepine is effective in both the acute treatment and the maintenance of bipolar patients. Bipolar patients who respond to this drug usually have completely normal EEGs. Other possible psychiatric indications for carbamazepine include borderline personality disorder and atypical depression characterized by feelings of depersonalization and perceptual disturbances.

Pharmacokinetics and Pharmacodynamics. Carbamazepine is absorbed slowly and erratically; peak plasma levels

CARBAMAZEPINE

VALPROIC ACID

VERAPAMIL

CLONIDINE

Figure 1. Molecular structures of carbamazepine, valproic acid, verapamil and clonidine

may be reached 4 to 24 hours after an oral dose. Binding to plasma proteins and volume of distribution are high. The metabolism of this drug is complicated by the presence of an active metabolite and by the induction of hepatic enzymes with continued administration during the first month. The pharmacodynamic effects of carbamazepine are uncertain, but it may act through the GABAergic system or by altering the activity of calcium-calmodulin–dependent protein kinases.

Clinical Guidelines. The pretreatment work-up should include a routine physical and laboratory examination, with special attention to the CBC (with differential) and liver function tests. The initial dose is 200 mg twice daily, increased by 200 mg a day each week, until plasma levels of 6 to 8 mg per liter are achieved. Some reports have suggested plasma levels as high as 12 mg per liter. Most clinicians have reported that these levels are hard to achieve, but they should be strived for if the patient is not clinically responsive at lower levels. The usual daily dose range is 1,200 to 2,000 mg a day in divided doses. It is reasonable to assume—but not yet demonstrated—that a patient who responds in acute situations to carbamazepine can be maintained for a long time at plasma levels lower than those required for acute treatment.

Drug Combinations. If a patient does not respond to lithium or carbamazepine separately, then a combination of the two drugs may be effective. Because of a few cases of synergistic neurotoxicity, the doses should be raised more slowly than when either drug is used alone. The usual therapeutic blood levels of both drugs should be achieved before determining that this drug combination is ineffective.

Adverse Effects. The most frequent adverse effects from carbamazepine are nausea, vomiting, drowsiness, dizziness, ataxia, and blurred vision. These symptoms may be reduced by increasing the dose more slowly. Some tolerance also develops to the neurological adverse effects. Because of the minor risk of hepatotoxicity, liver function tests should be done every 3 to 6 months. Carbamazepine treatment may result in a false positive result on the dexamethasone suppression test.

The most serious adverse effects associated with carbamazepine are aplastic anemia and agranulocytosis. A transient leukopenia or thrombocytopenia may develop in some patients. A persistent leukopenia requires consultation with a hematologist and may force discontinuation of the drug. The incidence of aplastic anemia is approximately 1 in 50,000, and 50 percent of the cases result in death. Despite the seriousness of the problem, monitoring of the CBC every 3 to 6 months after the first 3 months of treatment seems adequate.

Valproic Acid

There are fewer data supporting the use of valproic acid (Figure 1) for bipolar disorder than there are for carbamazepine. Nevertheless, in treatment-resistant patients, a therapeutic trial with this drug may be indicated. Valproic acid is currently approved in the United States only for the treatment of simple and complex partial seizures. The clinician should refer to the most recent psychiatric and pharmacological literature before initiating a trial of this drug.

Clonazepam

Clonazepam is a benzodiazepine anticonvulsant approved for the treatment of akinetic and myoclonic seizures, refractory absence seizures, and the Lennox–Gastaut variant of petit mal seizures. There are a few reports that this anticonvulsant is effective in treating mania in bipolar patients.

OTHER DRUGS

Verapamil and clonidine (Figure 1) may also be useful in treating bipolar disorder; however, this indication should be considered preliminary at this time. The FDA has not approved these drugs for this indication, and clinicians should consult the most recent pharmacologic and psychiatric literature for specific therapeutic guidelines. There is perhaps more evidence supporting the efficacy of verapamil than there is for clonidine.

Verapamil

Verapamil is a calcium channel inhibitor that acts by inhibiting the inward flux of calcium into neurons. There have been four double-blind, placebo-controlled studies and six uncontrolled reports of the efficacy of verapamil in the treatment of mania. Verapamil doses from 320 to 480 mg a day have been used for both acute and maintenance treatment, including some patients who had been incompletely responsive to or who had experienced intolerable adverse effects from lithium. The adverse effects of verapamil have been limited to slightly decreased blood pressure and increased pulse.

References

Bond W S: Psychiatric indications for clonidine: The neuropharmacologic and clinical basis. J Clin Psychopharm 6:81, 1986.

Chouinard G, Young S N, Annable L: Antimanic effects of clonazepam. Biol Psychiatry 18:451, 1983.

Dubovsky S L: Calcium antagonists: A new class of psychiatric drugs? Psychiat Ann 16:724, 1986.

Goodnick P J, Fieve R R, Schlegel A, Baxter N: Predictors of interepisodic symptoms and relapse in affective disorder patients treated with lithium carbonate. Am J Psychiatry 144:367, 1987.

Hart R G, Easton J D: Carbamazepine and hematological monitoring. Ann Neurol 11:309, 1982.

Jefferson J W, Greist J H, Ackerman D L: Lithium Encyclopedia for Clinical Practice, ed 2. American Psychiatric Press, Washington, D.C., 1986.

Kishimoto A, Ogura C, Hazama H: Long-term prophylactic effects of carbamazepine in affective disorder. Br J Psychiatry *143*:327, 1983.

Post R M, Uhde T W: Carbamazepine in bipolar illness. Psychopharm Bull *21*:10, 1985.

Puzynski S, Klosiewicz L: Valproic acid amide in the treatment of affective and schizoaffective disorders. J Affective Disorders *6*:115, 1985.

Ramsey T A, Cox M: Lithium and the kidney. Am J Psychiatry *139*:443, 1982.

Samiy A H, Rosnick P B: Early identification of renal problems in patients receiving chronic lithium treatment. Am J Psychiatry *144*:670, 1987.

Stancer H C, Persad E: Treatment of intractable rapid-cycling manic depressive disorder with levothyroxine. Arch Gen Psychiatry *39*:311, 1981.

Swann A C, Koslow S H, Katz M M, Maas J W, Javaid J, Secunda S K, Robins E: Lithium carbonate treatment of mania. Arch Gen Psychiatry *44*:345, 1987.

31.5 ————
Drugs Used to Treat Anxiety and Insomnia

INTRODUCTION

Some of the drugs used to treat anxiety disorders are referred to as antianxiety agents, anxiolytics, or minor tranquilizers. The term minor tranquilizer is generally regarded as misleading because it confuses this class of drugs with the major tranquilizers, a faulty, but commonly used, term for the antipsychotic drugs. Heterocyclic drugs, monoamine oxidase inhibitors, phenothiazines, and propranolol are also used to treat various anxiety disorders. However, these drugs are not generally classified as antianxiety drugs.

Almost all of the antianxiety drugs are also classified as sedative/hypnotics. A sedative drug reduces daytime activity, tempers excitement, and generally quiets the patient. A hypnotic drug produces drowsiness and facilitates the onset and maintenance of sleep. In general, most of the drugs discussed in this chapter act as hypnotics in high doses, anxiolytics in moderate doses, and sedatives in low doses. In addition to these actions, the benzodiazepines and barbiturates are used as anesthetics in doses above those used for hypnosis, and both of these drugs are also used as anticonvulsants. Benzodiazepines are also clinically used as muscle relaxants.

Buspirone is an important exception to the usual rule that anxiolytic drugs are also sedatives and hypnotics. Buspirone is an azaspirodecanedione that is pharmacologically distinct from the benzodiazepines. In addition to lacking sedative/hypnotic properties, buspirone has a much longer onset of anxiolytic action (1 to 3 weeks) and seems to have less abuse potential or withdrawal symptoms associated with it. Buspirone, however, is a very new drug, and the early enthusiasm may diminish after further clinical experience. Nevertheless, this drug has stimulated much interest in basic neuroscience because it dissociates anxiolytic effects from sedative properties.

Although a number of drug classes are included in this group, only a few of these drugs are currently used in routine clinical psychiatric practice. The benzodiazepines

account for the overwhelming majority of prescriptions for anxiolytic, sedative, and hypnotic drugs. Buspirone may also gain wide acceptance as an anxiolytic. Barbiturates have several specific indications, and chloral hydrate—and perhaps the antihistamines—continue to be used as mild sedative/hypnotics. The remaining drugs in this class are seldom used.

BENZODIAZEPINES

The benzodiazepines have become the usual drug of first choice because they have a higher therapeutic index and significantly less abuse potential than do many of the other drugs in this class.

Classification

The benzodiazepine nucleus consists of a benzene ring fused to the seven-sided diazepine ring. All clinically important benzodiazepines also have a second benzene ring attached to the carbon at position 5 on the diazepine ring (Figure 1). The benzodiazepines can be subclassified as 2-keto, 3-hydroxy, or triazolo benzodiazepines (Table 1). The 2-keto benzodiazepines have a keto group off the carbon atom in position 2 in the diazepine ring. Although chlordiazepoxide has a different substitution (-NHCH$_3$) at this position, it is useful to classify it along with the 2-keto derivatives. The 3-hydroxy benzodiazepines have a hydroxy group on the carbon at position 3 of the diazepine ring. The triazolo benzodiazepines have a triazolo ring fused to the nitrogen at position 1 and to the carbon at position 2 of the diazepine ring.

Pharmacokinetics

With the exception of clorazepate, all of the benzodiazepines are completely absorbed unchanged from the GI tract. Clorazepate

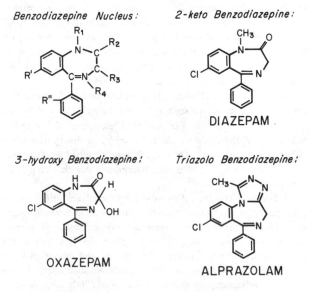

Figure 1. Representative benzodiazepine structures.

Table 1
Classification of Benzodiazepines

2-keto	3-hydroxy	Triazolo
chlordiazepoxide	oxazepam	alprazolam
diazepam	lorazepam	triazolam
prazepam	temazepam	
clorazepate		
halazepam		
flurazepam		

pate is converted to desmethyldiazapam in the GI tract and absorbed in that form. Absorption, attainment of peak levels, and onset of action are quickest for the following drugs in each class: 2-keto—diazepam; 3-hydroxy—lorazepam; triazolo— both alprazolam and triazolam have rapid effects. The rapid onset of effects is important to patients who take a single dose of benzodiazepines to calm an episodic burst of anxiety. The rapid onset of effects for these drugs can be partly attributed to their high lipid solubility, a characteristic that varies 5-fold among the different benzodiazepines. The range of time to peak plasma levels is 1 to 3 hours, although prazepam may take up to 6 hours. There may also be a secondary peak plasma level 6 to 12 hours after enterohepatic recirculation. Although several benzodiazepines are available in parenteral forms for IM administration, only lorazepam has rapid and reliable absorption from this route. The use of IM lorazepam is beginning to replace the use of IV diazepam in psychiatric emergency settings, with the possible exception of the management of PCP intoxication.

The metabolism of benzodiazepines differs for the three subclasses. Chlordiazepoxide is metabolized to diazepam, then to desmethyldiazepam (nordiazepam), then to oxazepam, and finally to the glucuronide. Diazepam, clorazepate, prazepam, and halazepam are metabolized first to desmethyldiazepam and then follow the same route as chlordiazepoxide does. The metabolism of flurazepam follows similar biochemical steps. As a result of the slow metabolism of desmethyldiazepam, all of the 2-keto benzodiazepines have plasma half-lives of 30 to 100 hours and are therefore the longest-acting benzodiazepines. The plasma half-life can be as high as 200 hours in individuals who are genetically slow metabolizers of these compounds. Because it can take up to 2 weeks to reach steady plasma levels of these drugs, patients may develop toxicity after 7 to 10 days of treatment with a dose that may have seemed therapeutic to the clinician. Patients with hepatic disease and elderly patients are particularly likely to become toxic on benzodiazepines if administered in repeated or high doses.

The 3-hydroxy benzodiazepines have short half-lives (10 to 30 hours) because they are directly metabolized by glucuronidation and thus have no active metabolites. The triazolo benzodiazepines are hydroxylated before they undergo glucuronidation. Alprazolam has a half-life of 10 to 15 hours, and triazolam has the shortest half-life (2 to 3 hours) of all the benzodiazepines.

Pharmacodynamics

The benzodiazepines bind to specific receptor sites that are associated with GABA binding sites and chloride channels. Benzodiazepine binding increases the affinity of the GABA receptor for GABA, thereby increasing the flow of chloride ions into the neurons.

Tolerance, Dependence, and Withdrawal. When benzodiazepines are used for short periods of time (1 to 2 weeks) in moderate doses, there is usually no evidence of tolerance, dependence, or withdrawal. The very short acting benzodiazepines (e.g., triazolam) may be a slight exception to this rule, as some patients have reported increased anxiety the day after taking this drug. Some patients also report developing a tolerance to the anxiolytic effects of benzodiazepines and require increased doses to maintain clinical remission. There is also a cross-tolerance among most of the different classes of antianxiety drugs, with the notable exception of buspirone.

The appearance of a withdrawal syndrome from benzodiazepines depends on the length of time a patient has taken the drug, the dose the patient has been on, the rate at which the drug is tapered, and the half-life of the particular compound. The withdrawal syndrome consists of peripheral and subjective symptoms of anxiety. Other symptoms include irritability, tinnitus, hypertension, headache, rebound insomnia, and unpleasant dreams. More serious symptoms may include depression, paranoia, delirium, and seizures. The incidence of this syndrome is controversial; however, some features of this syndrome may occur in as many as 50 percent of the patients treated with these drugs. The development of a severe withdrawal syndrome is seen only in patients who have taken high doses for long periods of time. The appearance of the syndrome may be delayed for 1 to 2 weeks in patients who had been taking 2-keto benzodiazepines with very long half-lives. A number of clinicians have reported that alprazolam seems to be particularly associated with a withdrawal syndrome.

Indications

Anxiety. The major clinical application for these drugs in psychiatry is the treatment of anxiety—both idiopathic generalized anxiety disorder and anxiety associated with specific life events (e.g., adjustment reaction with anxious mood). Most patients should be treated for a specific and relatively brief period. Some patients, however, may actually have a disorder that requires maintenance on these drugs. Alprazolam is the only benzodiazepine that may be effective in the treatment of panic disorders.

Insomnia. Flurazepam, temazepam, and triazolam are the three benzodiazepines approved for use as hypnotics. They differ principally in their half-lives, with flurazepam having the longest and triazolam having the shortest. Flurazepam may be associated with minor cognitive impairment on the day after its administration, and triazolam may be associated with mild rebound anxiety. Temazepam may represent a reasonable compromise between these two adverse effects for the usual adult patient.

Other Psychiatric Indications. Chlordiazepoxide is used to manage the symptoms of alcohol withdrawal. The benzodiazepines (especially IM lorazepam) are used to manage both drug-induced (except amphetamine) and psychotic agitation in the emergency room. Alprazolam is approved for use in patients with mixed symptoms of anxiety and depression. There are a few reports of the use of high doses of benzodiazepines in patients with schizophrenia who had not responded to antipsychotics or who were unable to take more traditional drugs because of adverse effects.

Medical Indications. Benzodiazepines are used as anticonvulsants, muscle relaxants, and adjuvants in anesthesia. Diazepam is also used for its minor analgesic properties.

Clinical Guidelines

The clinical decision to initiate treatment with a benzodiazepine should be a considered and specific one. The patient's diagnosis, the specific target symptoms, and the duration of treatment all should be defined, and this information should be shared with the patient. Treatment for most anxiety conditions lasts for 2 to 6 weeks, followed by 1 to 2 weeks of tapering the drug before it is discontinued. The most common clinical mistake with benzodiazepine treatment is to decide passively to continue treatment indefinitely.

For the treatment of anxiety, it is usual to begin a drug at the low end of its therapeutic range (Table 2) and to increase the dose to achieve a therapeutic response. The use of divided doses prevents the development of adverse effects associated with high peak plasma levels. The improvement produced by benzodiazepines may go beyond a simple antianxiety effect. For example, these drugs may cause the patient to regard various occurrences in a positive light. The drugs may also have a mild disinhibiting action, similar to that observed after modest amounts of alcohol.

Alcohol withdrawal is usually treated with chlordiazepoxide, 50 mg every 6 hours. The use of alprazolam to treat panic attacks or depression often requires doses higher (4 to 10 mg a day) than those for anxiolytic effects. It is important to taper patients very slowly from high doses of alprazolam, in order to avoid withdrawal symptoms.

Plasma levels of benzodiazepines are not available in clinical practice at this time.

Drug Combinations

The most common drug combination is the use of benzodiazepines as a hypnotic in patients who are also being treated with other drugs for schizophrenia or mood disorders. The combination of a benzodiazepine and an antidepressant may be indicated in the treatment of markedly anxious depressed patients. There are several reports that the combined use of alprazolam with antipsychotics may further reduce psychotic symptoms in patients who had not responded adequately to the antipsychotic alone.

Adverse Effects   The most common adverse effect of benzodiazepines is drowsiness, and patients should be advised not to drive or use dangerous machinery while taking these drugs. Some patients also experience dizziness and ataxia. The most serious adverse effects of benzodiazepines occur when other sedative drugs (e.g., alcohol) are taken concurrently. These combinations can result in marked drowsiness, disinhibition, or even respiratory depression. Other relatively common adverse effects include weakness, nausea, vomiting, blurred vision, and epigastric distress. There have been several reports of mild cognitive deficits that could impair job performance in patients who are taking benzodiazepines. A rare, paradoxical increase in aggression has been reported in patients given a benzodiazepine. Allergic reactions to these drugs are also rare, but there are a few reports of maculopapular rashes and generalized itching.

Abuse and Dependence.   Mentally healthy individuals may take single doses of benzodiazepines for recreational purposes. Patients who take prescribed benzodiazepines may develop both a physical and a psychological dependence on these drugs and insist on taking them against the clinician's advice. As previously mentioned, withdrawal syndromes do occur, although much less often than with many other drugs in this class (e.g., barbiturates, carbamates).

Overdoses.   Overdoses with benzodiazepines have a predictably favorable outcome unless other drugs (e.g., alcohol, antipsychotics, antidepressants) have also been ingested. In this case, respiratory depression, coma, seizures, and death are much more likely.

Drug Interactions

Cimetidine, disulfiram, isoniazid, and estrogens increase the plasma levels of 2-keto benzodiazepines. Antacids and food may decrease the absorption of benzodiazepines, and smoking may increase the metabolism of benzodiazepines. The benzodiazepines may increase the plasma levels of phenytoin and digoxin. All benzodiazepines have additive CNS depressant effects with other sedative drugs.

Table 2
Benzodiazepine Trade Names and Dose Ranges

Generic	Trade	Usual Adult Dose Range mg/day	Adult Single Dose Range mg
Alprazolam	Xanax	0.5–6	0.25–1
Chlordiazepoxide*	Librium	15–100	5–25
Clorazepate	Tranxene	7.5–60	3.25–22.5
Diazepam*	Valium	2–60	2–10
Flurazepam[†]	Dalmane	15–30	15–30
Halazepam	Paxipam	60–160	20–40
Lorazepam	Ativan	2–6	0.5–2
Oxazepam	Serax	30–120	10–30
Prazepam	Centrax	20–60	10–20
Temazepam[†]	Restoril	15–30	15–30
Triazolam[†]	Halcion	0.125–0.5	0.125–0.5

*Also available for parenteral administration. Diazepam is available for IV administration in 5 mg/ml syringes. Lorazepam is available for IM administration in 2 and 4 mg/ml syringes.
[†]FDA approved for use as an hypnotic.

BUSPIRONE

Buspirone (Buspar) is the first azaspirodecanedione to be approved by the FDA for the treatment of anxiety in the United States (Figure 2). Additional drugs of this class are likely to be introduced in the next few years. The efficacy of this drug for treating panic disorders is not known. Buspirone does not have the sedative, hypnotic, or anticonvulsant effects of the benzodiazepines, and it is thought to have very low abuse potential. It is possible that drugs of this class will eventually replace the benzodiazepines for the treatment of anxiety. It should be cautioned, however, that buspirone is a recently released drug and that further clinical experience may eventually uncover new problems.

Pharmacokinetics and Pharmacodynamics. Buspirone is well absorbed following oral administration. Its mechanism of action is unclear, but it may act through serotonergic mechanisms. Presynaptic dopamine antagonism and direct binding to the chloride channel have also been suggested as possible mechanisms.

Clinical Guidelines. Buspirone should be started at a dose of 5 mg twice daily and increased to 15 to 60 mg daily in divided doses. The antianxiety effects of buspirone may take 1 to 3 weeks to appear, thereby paralleling the delayed therapeutic effects of antipsychotic and antidepressant medications. Some clinicians suggest that buspirone may be the drug of first choice for the treatment of anxiety in patients who have not received benzodiazepines in the past. Patients who have previously received benzodiazepines often complain that buspirone is not as effective. This response may be due to the absence, with buspirone treatment, of some of the nonanxiolytic effects of benzodiazepines (e.g., muscle relaxation, additional sense of well-being). Although data are currently lacking, it is almost certain that buspirone is not an effective treatment for benzodiazepine withdrawal.

Adverse Effects. The most common adverse effects of buspirone treatment are reported to be headache, nausea, dizziness, and a subjective sense of tension. Buspirone does not seem to impair motor function, but it may be associated with an exacerbation of psychotic symptoms.

BARBITURATES

The clinical use of barbiturates in psychiatry has been essentially eclipsed by the benzodiazepines. This change in clinical practice is based on the higher abuse potential and lower therapeutic index for barbiturates, compared with that for benzodiazepines. There are currently six indications for barbiturate administration. First, amobarbital (50 to 250 mg IM) may be used in emergency settings to control agitation. The use of IM lorazepam or diazepam, however, seems to be replacing this application of amobarbital. Second, amobarbital interviews are sometimes used for diagnostic purposes. Several studies report that other sedative drugs, including the benzodiazepines, may also be effective in this application. Third, there are several reports that barbiturates can activate some catatonic patients, although benzodiazepines may also have this effect. Fourth, barbiturates may be indicated for use in patients who have serious adverse effects from benzodiazepines or buspirone. Fifth, some patients who do not respond adequately to benzodiazepines or buspirone may respond to barbiturates. Sixth, some patients, particularly older persons, who have received barbiturates in the past may insist on taking barbiturates rather than trying a benzodiazepine or buspirone.

Pharmacokinetics and Pharmacodynamics

The barbiturates (Figure 3) are well absorbed after oral administration. The binding of barbiturates to plasma proteins is high, but lipid solubility varies. The individual barbiturates are differentially metabolized by the liver and excreted by the kidney. The half-lives of specific barbiturates range from 1 to 2 hours to 80 to 120 hours. Barbiturates may also induce hepatic enzymes, thereby reducing levels of both the barbiturate and any other concurrently administered drugs metabolized by the liver. The mechanism of action for the barbiturates is thought to involve the GABA receptor/benzodiazepine receptor/chloride ion channel complex.

Clinical Guidelines

The dosages for barbiturates vary (Table 3), and treatment should begin with low doses that are increased to achieve a clinical effect. Barbiturates with half-lives in the 15- to 40-hour range are preferable because longer-acting drugs will build up in the body. The patient should be clearly instructed about the adverse effects and potential for dependence associated with barbiturate treatment.

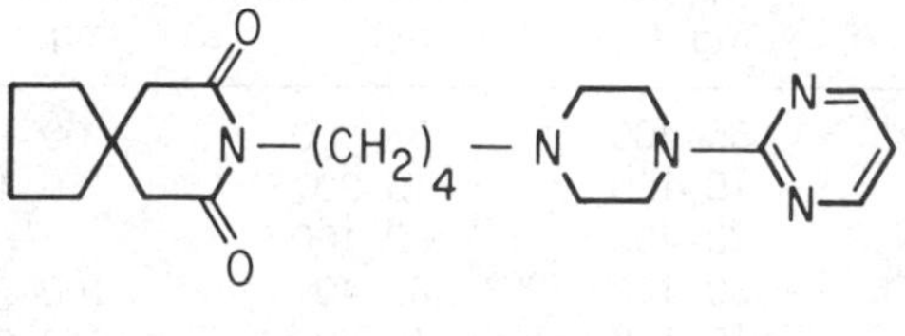

Barbiturate Nucleus

The different barbiturates are synthesized by substituting specific side chains at R_1 and R_2

Figure 2. Molecular structure of buspirone.

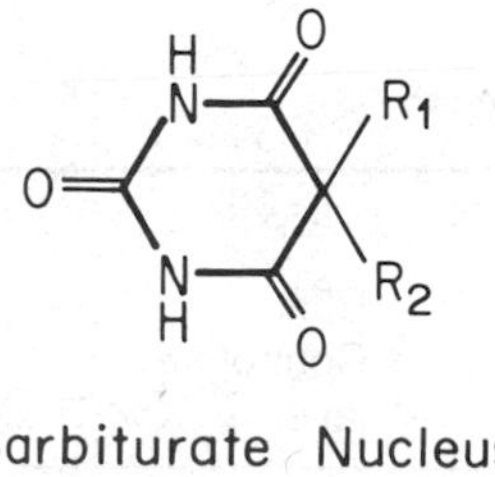

Figure 3. Molecular structure of the barbiturate nucleus.

Adverse Effects

The adverse effects of barbiturates are similar to those for benzodiazepines, including paradoxical dysphoria, hyperactivity, and cognitive disorganization. The barbiturates differ from the benzodiazepines in their high abuse potential, marked development of dependence, and low therapeutic index. The symptoms of barbiturate withdrawal are similar to, but more marked than, those for benzodiazepine withdrawal. Barbiturates are often lethal in overdoses because of respiratory depression, especially if combined with alcohol intake, as is often seen clinically.

Drug-Drug Interactions

Barbiturates interact with many other drugs, and the clinician should consult a reference text for these interactions when prescribing barbiturates. The two most important interactions are the additive effects of other sedatives and the increased metabolism of many cardiac-related drugs and heterocyclic antidepressants.

ALCOHOLS

The alcohols that are used clinically are chloral hydrate (Noctec, other brands, and generic), ethanol, and ethclhorvynol (Placidyl). Although they possess sedative effects, these drugs are used primarily as hypnotics. Chloral hydrate is the most commonly used of these drugs, although some clinicians use ethclhorvynol or even a glass of sherry to treat insomnia.

Chloral hydrate is the oldest hypnotic, having been introduced into medicine in 1869. It is a relatively short acting drug that is useful in treating mild complaints of initial insomnia, but it has less value as a daytime sedative. Chloral hydrate is rapidly converted to an active metabolite trichloroethanol. Trichloroacetic acid is a toxic metabolite of chloral hydrate that can accumulate in the body if this drug is taken repeatedly. The therapeutic dose ranges from 500 to 2000 mg, and the lethal dose is 5 to 10 times that amount. Although physical dependence does occur, it is unusual. Tolerance to the hypnotic effect of chloral hydrate seems to develop quickly. The major adverse effect is occasional severe gastritis or ulceration.

ANTIHISTAMINES

A variety of over-the-counter medicines are marketed for relief from insomnia and for the control of nervousness. These drugs usually contain a sedative antihistamine and hydrobromides. Bromism, a toxic psychotic state, can occur as a side effect. One controlled study of the ingredients in one over-the-counter medicine, Compoz, found the drug to be ineffective when prescribed by physicians as a tranquilizer. Antihistamines have sedative effects in some adults, and one such drug, diphenhydramine (Benadryl, other brands, and generic), is used as a sedative in children and the elderly. Another antihistamine, hydroxyzine (Atarax, other brands, and generic), is also used as an antianxiety agent. The adult dose range of both diphenhydramine and hydroxyzine is 25 to 400 mg a day; 50 mg is the usual hypnotic dose. These agents may be indicated in patients with mild symptoms or in patients who cannot tolerate more traditional drugs.

CARBAMATES

Meprobamate (Miltown, other brands, and generic), ethinamate (Valmid), and carisoprodol (Soma, other brands, and generic) are carbamates that are effective as anxiolytics, sedatives, hypnotics, and muscle relaxants. These drugs have a lower therapeutic index and a higher abuse potential than do benzodiazepines, and their use is indicated only if the previously described drugs are not an option. The carbamates may have even more abuse potential and may be more dependence inducing than are the barbiturates.

The usual dose of meprobamate is 400 mg, three or four times daily. Drowsiness is a common adverse effect, and patients should be warned of the additive effects of sedative drugs. Sudden withdrawal may cause anxiety, restlessness, weakness, delirium, and convulsions. Adverse effects can include urticarial or erythematous rashes, anaphylactoid and other allergic reactions, angioneurotic edema, dermatitis, blood dyscrasias, gastrointestinal upsets, and extraocular muscular paralysis. Fatal overdoses can occur with meprobamate in dosages as low as 12 g (thirty 400 mg tablets) without any other sedatives ingested.

PIPERIDINEDIONES

Glutethimide (Doriden and generic) and methyprylon (Noludar) are piperidinediones that are effective as hypnotics, sedatives, and anxiolytics but are even more subject to abuse and more lethal in overdoses than are the barbiturates and carbamates. Glutethimide has a slow and unpredictable absorption following oral administration. Seizures, shock, and anticholinergic toxicity are more com-

Table 3
Selected Barbiturates

| Generic | DEA Control level | Trade | Half-life hrs | Sedative | | Hypnotic |
				Adult Dose Range mg/day	Adult Single Dose range mg	Dose Range mg
Amobarbital	II	Amytal, Generic	8–42	65–400	65–100	100–200
Butabarbital	III	Butisol	34–42	15–120	15–30	50–100
Mephobarbital	IV	Mebaral	11–67	32–400	32–100	—
Pentobarbital	II	Nembutal, Generic	15–48	30–120	30–40	100–200
Phenobarbital	IV	Luminal, Generic	80–120	15–600	15–60	100–200
Secobarbital	II	Seconal, Generic	15–40	—	—	100–300

mon in glutethimide than barbiturate overdoses. It would be a very rare patient for whom treatment with these drugs would be indicated.

CYCLIC ETHERS

Paraldehyde was introduced in 1882 as a hypnotic. When 5 ml are given intramuscularly, or 5 to 10 ml administered orally, it as an effective, albeit old-fashioned, treatment for alcohol withdrawal symptoms, anxiety, and insomnia. Paraldehyde is mostly metabolized, but its excretion in the unmetabolized form by the lungs limits its usefulness because of its offensive taste and ubiquitous odor.

OTHER DRUGS USED TO TREAT ANXIETY DISORDERS AND INSOMNIA

Heterocyclic and MAOI Antidepressants

Doxepin is approved for the treatment of mixed depression and anxiety syndromes. Antidepressants are also the drug of choice for agoraphobia with and without panic attacks. Clomipramine is the drug of choice for the treatment of obsessive-compulsive disorder.

Noradrenergic Drugs

Propranolol, a β-adrenergic blocker, is useful in treating the peripheral symptoms of anxiety (e.g., palpitations, sweating, tremor) and in reducing the performance anxiety of musicians and others. Propranolol may also be effective in treating generalized anxiety, but not panic disorders. The dose ranges from 10 mg twice daily to 80 to 160 mg a day in divided doses. Adverse effects include lethargy, depression, bradycardia, hypotension, weakness, confusion, GI upset, and bronchospasm. The use of propranolol is contraindicated in patients with asthma, diabetes, sinus bradycardia, congestive heart failure, thyroid disease, conduction defects, or Raynaud's disease. When this drug has been used chronically, it should always be tapered off rather than abruptly discontinued.

Clonidine, an α_2-adrenergic agonist, may also be useful in treating some anxious patients. A dosage of 0.1 mg twice daily up to 0.4 to 0.6 mg a day in divided dosages is the range that has been used in the several reports of this drug. Adverse effects include dry mouth, fatigue, and hypotension. Clonidine should always be tapered rather than abruptly discontinued.

L-tryptophan

L-tryptophan is an amino acid that when taken in a dosage of 1 to 6 g is an effective hypnotic. This amino acid is thought to work by increasing the concentrations of brain serotonin. L-tryptophan is a relatively expensive and not particularly potent hypnotic; a reasonable loading dose of L-tryptophan can be obtained from a large glass of milk.

References

Allgulander C, Borg S, Vikander B: A 4–6 year follow-up of 50 patients with primary dependence on sedative and hypnotic drugs. Am J Psychiatry *141*:1580, 1984.

Fyer A J, Liebowtiz M R, Gorman J M, Camplas R, Levin A, Davies S O, Goetz D, Klein D F: Discontinuation of alprazolam treatment in panic patients. Am J Psych *144*:303, 1987.
Hollister L: A symposium on benzodiazepine hypnotics. J Clin Psychopharm *3*:127, 1983.
Liebowitz M R, Fyer A J, Gorman J M: Alprazolam in the treatment of panic disorders. J Clin Psychopharm *6*:13–20, 1986.
Linnoila M, Erwin C W, Brendle A, Simpson D: Psychomotor effects of diazepam in anxious patients and healthy volunteers. J Clin Psychopharm *3*:88, 1983.
Lydiard R B, Laraia M T, Ballenger J C, Howell E F: Emergence of depressive symptoms in patients receiving alprazolam for panic disorder. Am J Psych *144*:664, 1987.
Martin I L: The benzodiazepines: A critical review. Prog Neuro-Psychopharm and Biol Psychiatry *7*:421, 1983.
Mitler M M, Seidel W F, van den Hoed J: Comparative hypnotic effects of flurazepam, triazolam, and placebo: A long-term simultaneous nighttime and daytime study. J Clin Psychopharm *4*:2, 1984.
Naylor M W, Grahnaus L, Cameron O: Single case study. Myoclonic seizures after abrupt withdrawal from phenelzine and alprazolam. J Ner Men Dis *175*:111, 1987.
Noyes R: Beta-blocking drugs and anxiety. Psychosomatics *23*:155, 1982.

31.6 _____
Electroconvulsive Therapy

INTRODUCTION

Electroconvulsive therapy (ECT) is one of the most effective treatments available in psychiatry; nevertheless, it has become a controversial treatment modality. There may be at least two reasons for this public sentiment. First, ECT requires the use of electricity and the production of convulsive fits, both of which may sound frightening to the layperson. Second, there have been several inaccurate reports of permanent brain damage resulting from ECT. Although these reports have been largely disproved, this specter remains.

The decision to suggest ECT to a patient, as with all treatment recommendations, should be based on both the treatment options and the risk–benefit considerations of ECT. The major alternatives to ECT usually are pharmacotherapy and psychotherapy, both of which have their own risks and benefits. The growing feeling among many psychiatrists is that ECT is underutilized as a safe and effective treatment for depression. Conversely, some psychiatrists and allied health professionals continue to believe strongly that ECT should be a treatment of last resort. In regard to those patients for whom ECT has been an effective treatment in the past, clinicians should not allow their biases to deprive them of this effective treatment.

HISTORY

In April 1938 in Rome, Ugo Cerletti and Lucio Bini administered the first electroconvulsive treatment. Initially the treatment was referred to as electroshock therapy (EST) but later became known as ECT. Although Cerletti and Bini had been doing research on animal models of epilepsy, their work with humans was influenced primarily by the work of Lazlo von Meduna in

Budapest. In 1934, von Meduna had reported the successful treatment of catatonia and other acute schizophrenic symptoms with pharmacologically induced seizures. Von Meduna began by using intramuscular injections of camphor suspended in oil but quickly switched to intravenously administered pentylenetetrazol (Metrazol). Von Meduna had attempted this treatment method based on two observations. First, it had been clinically observed that schizophrenic symptoms often decreased following a seizure. Such seizures were often accidentally or iatrogenically induced in psychiatric patients secondary to withdrawal from medications (e.g., barbiturates). Second, there was the incorrect belief that schizophrenia and epilepsy could not coexist in the same patient. They reasoned, therefore, that the induction of seizures might rid the patient of the schizophrenia. Pentylenetetrazol-induced seizures had been used as an effective treatment for 4 years before the introduction of electrically induced seizures.

The major problems associated with ECT were the patients' discomfort from the procedure and fractures resulting from the seizures' motor activity. These problems were eventually eliminated by the use of general anesthesia and muscle relaxants during the treatments. Interestingly, an American psychiatrist, A. E. Bennett, had helped develop the method of extracting curare from plant material. Bennett had suggested the use of spinal anesthesia during ECT, as well as the use of curare to paralyze the muscles so as to prevent fractures. In 1951, succinylcholine was introduced and became the most widely used muscle relaxant for ECT. In 1957, hexafluorinated diethylether (Indokolon) was introduced as a new pharmacological means of inducing seizures, by administering the compound as a gas. The lack of superiority to ECT, together with the introduction of antidepressant drugs in the 1950s, led to the removal of Indokolon from the market, as well as a decline in the number of patients given ECT.

CLASSIFICATION

Electroconvulsive therapy can be conducted with either bilaterally or unilaterally placed electrodes. Bilateral electrodes, which were introduced first, are applied with one stimulating electrode over both hemispheres of the brain. Unilateral ECT involves both electrodes over the nondominant hemisphere. Although controversial, bilateral ECT may be somewhat more effective than unilateral ECT, especially for more seriously ill patients. However, bilateral ECT is also more closely associated with adverse cognitive effects. In sum, unilateral ECT is probably as effective as bilateral ECT for most depressed patients and is associated with less severe adverse cognitive effects.

Another way of classifying ECT treatments is by the shape of the electric current as projected by an oscilloscope. The two major shapes are the sine wave and the brief pulse. The brief pulse method of stimulus delivery induces a seizure using less energy than is used in the sine wave method. The administration of less electric current is associated with fewer cognitive effects; therefore, the brief pulse method is becoming the method of choice.

Two other variations in ECT treatments are (1) the threshold dosage schedule and (2) the placement of the two electrodes within a hemispheric region. Both variations in treatment are aimed at reducing the cognitive effects associated with the treatment. A threshold dosage schedule adjusts the current for each treatment

session to just above the amount needed to produce the seizure. Because the amount of current needed to induce a seizure increases with the number of treatments, the current setting should be low at the initiation of treatment and increased during the course of treatment. Whether threshold dosage schedules are as effective as constant dosage schedules, and whether they are associated with fewer adverse effects are currently not known and are under investigation. Unfortunately, the placement of the two electrodes within a hemisphere does not seem to be associated with any reduction in cognitive adverse effects.

MECHANISMS OF ACTION

The induction of a bilateral generalized seizure is necessary for both the beneficial and adverse effects of ECT. The two main research approaches to finding the relationship between these seizures and the reduction of psychiatric symptoms have been neurochemical and neurophysiological.

The neurochemical hypotheses suggest that the clinical improvement from a series of ECT treatments results from changes in neurotransmitter function. A series of ECT treatments results in a downregulation of postsynaptic β-adrenergic receptors, the same receptor change observed with chronic antidepressant treatment. ECT is associated with an increase in postsynaptic $5HT_2$ receptors, however, which is opposite to the direction of change seen from some antidepressants. ECT has also been shown to downregulate the number of muscarinic acetylcholine receptors. Some investigators suggest that the balance among noradrenergic, serotonergic, and cholinergic transmission is important, rather than the change in any individual neurotransmitter system. There is some research evidence that ECT may decrease the synthesis and release of GABA, as well as increase endogenous opioid activity.

The neurophysiologic approach to idiopathic epilepsy has demonstrated that brain regions that are metabolically hyperactive during the seizure are actually quite hypoactive immediately after the seizure. This change has been demonstrated by PET scans and cerebral blood flow imaging and is consistent with computed topographic maps of brain electrical activity. An observation that perhaps relates the neurochemical and neurophysiological findings is that ECT acts as an anticonvulsant; that is, repeated treatments with ECT actually raise the individual's seizure threshold.

INDICATIONS

Major Depression

The most common indication for ECT is major depression. Over 80 percent of ECT patients in the United States have this diagnosis. The response rate to ECT for patients with major depression is 80 to 90 percent, at least equal to (and probably greater than) the response rate for antidepressant drugs. ECT treatment yields a quicker therapeutic response and fewer adverse effects than does treatment with antidepressants. ECT is effective for both unipolar and bipolar depressions and in both male and female patients. Delusional or psychotic depression is particularly responsive to ECT, whereas the response of this disorder to antidepressants alone is quite poor. Depressions with features of melancholia (e.g., markedly severe symptoms, psychomotor retardation, early morning awakening, diurnal variation (worse in morning), decreased appetite and weight, and agitation) are the most likely to respond to ECT. Patients with nonsuppression on the dexamethasone suppression test and a blunted response of TSH to TRH infusion are also more likely to respond. Older patients tend to respond to ECT more slowly than do younger patients. It needs to be realized, however, that ECT is a treatment for an episode of depression and does not provide prophylaxis. The question of maintenance ECT treatments to sustain clinical remission has not yet been answered.

Other Indications

Schizophrenia. Approximately 15 to 20 percent of patients receiving ECT are being treated for schizophrenia. Schizophrenic patients with acute, catatonic, or affective symptoms are the most likely to respond. The efficacy of ECT in such patients is approximately equal to that of antipsychotics; however, ECT is effective in only 5 to 10 percent of chronic patients.

Mania. There is increasing evidence from controlled clinical trials that ECT is an effective treatment for acute mania. Because the pharmacological management of mania is so effective and reasonably safe, ECT is utilized only when there is a specific contraindication to the pharmacological approach.

Other Indications and Considerations. In countries outside the United States, ECT has been reported effective in treating delirium tremens and conversion disorder. ECT is probably the safest treatment in certain special circumstances, including pregnancy, the elderly, and in the presence of extreme symptoms requiring immediate relief. ECT can be administered safely during pregnancy. In medically ill and elderly patients, ECT has less cardiotoxicity than do currently available pharmacological treatments.

CLINICAL GUIDELINES

The patients and their families are often fearful and apprehensive of ECT; therefore, its beneficial and adverse effects, as well as alternative treatment approaches, should be explained to them. This informed consent process should be documented in the patient's medical record. The use of involuntary ECT is rare today and should be reserved only for patients for which the treatment is urgent and a legally appointed guardian has agreed to its use. Relevant local, state, and federal laws must always be considered.

Pretreatment Evaluation

Pretreatment evaluation should include a standard physical examination and medical history, blood and urine chemistries, a chest x-ray, and an electrocardiogram. Spine and skull x-rays, CT scan, MRI, or EEG may be indicated in special circumstances.

The patient's ongoing medications should be carefully assessed for possible drug interactions with adjunctive agents used with ECT. Anticholinesterase ophthalmic solutions, monoamine oxidase inhibitors, and lithium may alter succinylcholine metabolism. Hypotensive collapse with reserpine and increased CNS sequelae with lithium have been reported. Sedative-hypnotic drugs and anticonvulsants interfere with the electricity's ability to induce the seizure. The issue of whether to continue a patient's antidepressant or antipsychotic medications during ECT treatment remains unsettled. Most clinicians, however, discontinue antidepressants before administering ECT.

Premedication, Anesthesia, and Muscular Relaxation

Thirty minutes before the actual treatment, an anticholinergic agent (e.g., atropine) is administered to minimize secretions and to create a mild tachycardia which helps prevent treatment-related bradycardia. Some ECT treatment centers have stopped the routine use of anticholinergics as a premedication. Their use is still indicated in patients on β-adrenergic blocking drugs and in patients with ventricular ectopic beats.

The administration of an ECT treatment requires general anesthesia, muscular relaxation or paralysis, and oxygenation. ECT patients are usually given oxygen from the onset of anesthesia to the resumption of adequate spontaneous respiration, except for the brief interval of electrical stimulation.

The depth of anesthesia should be as light as possible, not only to minimize adverse effects, but also to avoid elevating the seizure threshold associated with many anesthetics. In most settings, methohexital (Brevital) or thiopental (Pentothal) are used. The former is probably preferable, as it is associated with fewer incidents of ECT-associated cardiac arrhythmias. A typical dose of methohexital for a medium-sized adult is 60 mg, although the range is from 30 to 160 mg.

Following the onset of anesthetic effect, usually within a minute, the muscle relaxant is injected intravenously. Succinylcholine, an ultra-fast-acting depolarizing blocking agent, has gained virtually universal acceptance for this purpose. The optimal succinylcholine dose provides enough relaxation to stop most, but not all, of the major ictal body movements. A typical starting dose is 60 mg for a medium-sized adult. Because succinylcholine is a depolarizing blocking agent, its action is marked by the presence of muscle fasciculations, which move in a rostrocaudal progression. The disappearance of these movements indicates that maximal relaxation has been achieved. If musculoskeletal or cardiac disease necessitates the use of total relaxation, the addition of curare (3 to 6 mg IV) may be given several minutes before the anesthetic, along with an increased succinylcholine dosage. If necessary, a peripheral nerve stimulator can be used to ascertain the presence of a complete neuromuscular block.

Because of the short half-life of succinylcholine, the duration of apnea following its administration generally is shorter than the delay in regaining consciousness caused by the anesthesia and the postictal state. In cases of inborn or acquired pseudocholinesterase deficiency, or when the metabolism of succinylcholine is disrupted by drug interaction, a prolonged apnea may occur, and the treating physician should always be prepared to manage this problem.

Stimulus Electrode Placement

As mentioned previously, there are two types of electrode placement, bilateral and unilateral. Because unilateral ECT appears to be associated with fewer adverse cognitive effects, some clinicians now routinely start patients on it and switch to bilateral placement if no significant improvement appears after five or six treatments.

Traditional bilateral ECT places electrodes bifrontotemporally, each with its center approximately 1 inch above the midpoint of an imaginary line drawn from the tragus of the ear to the external canthus of the eye. With unilateral ECT, one stimulus electrode is typically placed over the nondominant frontotemporal area. Although several locations for the second stimulus electrode have been proposed, placement on the nondominant centroparietal scalp, just lateral to the midline vertex, appears to provide a configuration associated with a relatively low seizure threshold.

Which cerebral hemisphere is dominant can generally be determined by a simple series of performance tasks (e.g., handedness, footedness, stated preference). Right body responses correlate very highly with left brain dominance. If the responses are mixed or if they clearly indicate left body dominance, clinicians should alternate the polarity of unilateral stimulation during successive treatments. They should also monitor the time that it takes for patients to recover consciousness and to answer simple orientation and naming questions. The side of stimulation associated with less rapid recovery and return of function is considered dominant.

The Electrical Stimulus

ECT machines operate on either a constant current or a constant voltage. Which type of machine is preferable is not clear. The two main types of stimulation are sine wave and brief pulse. The brief pulse method can evoke a seizure with about one-third as much energy as needed with sine wave stimulation. The brief pulse method is now the preferred method in the United States. The precise stimulus settings depend on the machine used and the individual patient's seizure threshold. The resultant seizure should last for 30 to 60 seconds. Seizures of more than 60 seconds sometimes indicate that the stimulus intensity is suprathreshold and can be diminished at a later treatment session. At other times, however, even a small decrease in stimulus intensity can lead to no seizure at all. If no seizure is produced after about 20 seconds, a higher intensity setting should be tried. Waiting too long before restimulation may cause the effects of the anesthetic or muscle relaxant agents to wear off.

The Induced Seizure

A brief muscular contraction, usually strongest in the jaw and facial muscles, is seen concurrently with the flow of stimulus current, regardless of whether a seizure occurs. The first behavioral sign of the seizure is often a plantar extension, which lasts up to 10 to 20 seconds and marks the tonic phase. This phase is then followed by rhythmic (i.e., clonic) contractions that decrease in frequency and finally disappear. The tonic phase is marked by high-frequency, sharp electroencephalographic activity on which may be superimposed an even higher-frequency muscle artifact. During the clonic phase, bursts of polyspike activity occur simultaneously with the muscular contractions but usually persist for at least a few seconds after the clonic movements stop. There is often some postictal transient suppression and occasionally even an apparent absence of background EEG activity. Such suppression is much less likely to occur with unilateral ECT, particularly over the nonstimulated hemisphere.

It is important to have an objective measure that there actually has been a bilateral generalized seizure after the stimulation. The physician should be able to observe either some evidence of tonic-clonic movements or to detect electrophysiological evidence of seizure activity from the EEG or electromyogram (EMG). Seizures with unilateral ECT are asymmetrical, demonstrating higher ictal EEG amplitude over the stimulated hemisphere. Occasionally, unilateral seizures are induced, and for this reason, it is important that at least a single pair of EEG electrodes be placed over the contralateral hemisphere when using unilateral ECT.

Prolonged seizures (seizures lasting more than 5 minutes) or status epilepticus can be terminated either with additional doses of anesthetic agent or with intravenous diazepam. Management of such complications should be accompanied by intubation because the oral airway is insufficient to maintain adequate ventilation over an extended apneic period. In clinical practice, a more common problem is difficulty in generating a seizure. This problem can be resolved using hyperventilation, less anesthesia, a low-intensity stimulus before a high-intensity stimulus, or additional stimulating agents (e.g., caffeine).

Number and Spacing of ECT Treatments

Rather than using a fixed number of treatments, the length of the ECT course should be determined on the basis of clinical response. Patients being treated for depression typically show some signs of improvement after the first few treatments, with maximum responses after 5 to 10 treatments. Depressed patients are usually treated with 2 to 3 treatments per week. Manic and schizophrenic patients may require more frequent treatments (sometimes daily) and more treatments (up to as many as 25).

Maintenance Treatment

An acute course of ECT induces a remission but does not, in itself, prevent relapse. Post-ECT maintenance treatment should always be considered. Generally, this maintenance therapy is pharmacological, as the effectiveness of maintenance ECT has not yet been clarified.

ADVERSE EFFECTS

Contraindications

There are no absolute contraindications to ECT, only situations in which there is increased risk. Patients with intracranial masses and evolving strokes are likely to deteriorate neurologically with ECT because of an ECT-associated transient breakdown of the blood–brain barrier and an increase in intracranial pressure. ECT for such patients should only be done in the presence of measures (e.g., antihypertensives, steroids, and careful monitoring) designed to minimize these potential adverse sequelae. The presence of a recent myocardial infarction increases the risk of further cardiac decompensation with ECT, because of the increased cardiovascular demands associated with the procedure. Severe underlying hypertension can be a concern because ECT markedly increases blood pressure. Bringing the blood pressure into a normal range at the time of each treatment is essential in such cases.

Mortality

The mortality rate with ECT has been variously estimated to be between 1 in 1,000 and 1 in 10,000 patients, roughly the same as the mortality rate associated with brief general anesthesia itself. Death is usually from cardiovascular complications and is more likely to occur in patients whose cardiac status is already compromised.

Central Nervous System Effects

The greatest concern of both professional and lay groups regarding ECT is the potential adverse CNS effects, especially memory function. Although memory impairment during a course of treatment is almost the rule, follow-up data indicate that virtually all patients are back to their cognitive bascline after 6 months. Some patients, however, do complain of persistent memory difficulties. The degree of cognitive impairment during treatment and the time it takes to return to baseline are related in part to the amount of electrical stimulation used during the treatment.

Systemic Effects

Occasional, although usually quite mild, transient cardiac arrhythmias occur during ECT, particularly in patients with existent cardiac disease. These arrhythmias are usually a by-product of the brief postictal bradycardia and therefore often can be prevented by increasing the dosage of anticholinergic premedication. At other times, arrhythmias may be secondary to a tachycardia present during the seizure and may occur as the patient returns to consciousness. The prophylactic administration of propranolol can be useful in such cases. As mentioned earlier, an apneic state may be prolonged if the metabolism of succinylcholine is impaired. Toxic or allergic reactions to the pharmacological agents used in the ECT procedure have rarely been reported.

References

Abrams R, Taylor M A, Volavka J. ECT-induced EEG asymmetry and therapeutic response in melancholia: Relation to treatment electrode placement. Am J Psych 144:327, 1987.
American Psychiatric Association Task Force on ECT: Task Force Report 14: Electroconvulsive Therapy. American Psychiatric Association, Washington, DC, 1978.
Blain J D, Clark S M, editors: Report of the NIMH–NIH consensus development conference on electroconvulsive therapy. Psychopharm Bull 22:445, 1986.
Fink M: Meduna and the origins of convulsive therapy. Am J Psychiatry 141:1034, 1984.
Horne R L, Pettinati H M, Sugerman A A, Varga E: Comparing bilateral to unilateral electroconvulsive therapy in a randomized study with EEG monitoring. Arch Gen Psychiatry 42:1087, 1985.
Hyram V, Palmer L H, Cernik J. ECT: The search for the perfect stimulus. Biol Psychiatry 20:634, 1985.
Kanamatsu T, McGinty J F, Mitchell C L. Dynorphin and enkephalin-like immunoreactivity is altered in limbic-basal ganglia regions of rat brain after repeated electroconvulsive shock. J Neurosci 6:644, 1986.
Lerer B: Studies on the role of brain cholinergic systems on the therapeutic mechanisms and adverse effects of ECT and lithium. Biol Psychiatry 20:20, 1985.
Malitz S, Sackeim H A, editors: Electroconvulsive Therapy: Clinical and Basic Research Issues. Annals of the New York Academy of Sciences 1:462, 1986.
Sackheim H, Decina P, Prohovnik I, Malitz S. Seizure threshold in electroconvulsive therapy. Arch Gen Psych 44:355, 1987.
Squire L R, Zouzounis J A: ECT and memory: Brief pulse versus sinewave. Am J Psychiatry 143:596, 1986.
Thompson J W, Blaine J D. Use of ECT in the United States in 1975 and 1980. Am J Psych 144:557, 1987.
Weiner R D: Does electroconvulsive therapy cause brain damage? Behav Brain Sci 7:1, 1984.

31.7
Other Organic Therapies

PSYCHOSURGERY

Introduction and History

Psychosurgery is surgically modifying the brain in order to reduce the symptoms of severely ill psychiatric patients who have not responded adequately to more traditional treatments. Psychosurgical procedures destroy either specific brain regions (e.g., lobotomies, cingulotomies) or connecting tracts (e.g., tractotomies, leukotomies). Both these techniques and the implantation of stimulating devices are used in the neurosurgical treatment of pain and epilepsy.

In 1935, following the demonstration by Jacobsen and Fulton at Yale University that frontal lobe ablation in a monkey had a calming effect, Moniz and Lima, working in Portugal, severed frontal lobe white matter in 20 psychotic patients and reported a decrease in their tension and psychotic symptoms. In 1936, Freeman and Watts at George Washington University introduced the psychosurgical technique of prefrontal lobotomy to the United States. Although earlier procedures required burr holes or other exposure of the brain, Freeman eventually developed the technique of transorbital leukotomy that involved the introduction and lateral movement of a sharp instrument (actually an ice pick) through the eye socket as a method of sectioning the white matter of the frontal lobes. By the late 1940s, psychosurgery was being performed worldwide, and an estimated 5,000 patients were being operated on each year. In 1949, Egas Moniz won the Nobel Prize for his work in developing psychosurgical techniques. Shortly thereafter, the introduction of anti-psychotic drugs and the increasing public concern about the ethics of psychosurgery led to a near abandonment of these techniques. Although psychosurgical approaches to pain and epilepsy continued to be used, the interest in psychosurgical approaches to psychiatric disorders has only recently been rekindled. This renewed interest is based on several factors, including much improved techniques that allow the neurosurgeon to make more exact stereotactically placed lesions, better preoperative diagnoses, more comprehensive preoperative and postoperative psychological assessments, and more complete follow-up data.

Indications

The major indication for psychosurgery is the presence of a debilitating, chronic psychiatric disorder that has not responded to any other treatment. A reasonable guideline is that the disorder should have been present for 3 years during which a variety of alternative treatment approaches were attempted. Chronic depression and obsessive-compulsive disorder are the two disorders most responsive to psychosurgery. The presence of vegetative symptoms and marked anxiety further increases the likelihood of success. Whether psychosurgery is a reasonable treatment for intractable and extreme aggression is still controversial. Psychosurgery does not appear to be indicated for the treatment of mania or schizophrenia.

Modern Psychosurgical Techniques

Stereotactic neurosurgical equipment now allows the neurosurgeon to place discrete lesions in the brain. Radioactive implants, cyroprobes, electrical coagulation, proton beams, and ultrasonic waves are used to make the actual lesion. The most commonly performed procedure is an anterior cingulotomy, thought to work by disrupting the thalamofrontal tracts. Indeed, it has been suggested that thalamotomy is the most useful psychosurgical procedure to treat depression. This lesion destroys the dorsomedial nucleus of the thalamus. A third procedure is the lesioning of the substantia innominata. Most modern neurosurgeons believe that bilateral lesions are necessary for optimal results.

Therapeutic and Adverse Effects

When patients are carefully selected, between 60 and 90 percent have significant therapeutic improvement with psychosurgery. Fewer than 3 percent become worse. Continued improvement is often noted for 1 to 2 years following surgery, and patients are often more responsive than they were before psychosurgery to traditional pharmacologic and behavioral treatment approaches. Postoperative seizures are present in fewer than 1 percent of patients, and these are easily controlled with diphenylhydantoin. As measured by I.Q. scores, cognitive abilities improve after surgery, probably because of an increased ability to attend to cognitive tasks. Undesired changes in personality have not been noted with the modern limited procedures.

LIGHT THERAPY

Light therapy, also called phototherapy, involves exposing patients to artificial light sources. The major indication for this treatment is seasonal affective disorder (SAD), also known as seasonal mood disorder, a constellation of depressive symptoms that occurs during the fall and winter in some persons.

Mechanism of Action

Human circadian rhythms result from the entrainment of endogenous pacemakers by exogenous *zeitgebers*. The suprachiasmatic nucleus of the hypothalamus is thought to be the major endogenous pacemaker; the light-dark cycle is thought to be the major exogenous *zeitgeber*. Exposure to light at the beginning of night results in a phase delay—that is, rhythms are shifted to a later time—and exposure to light during the second half of the night results in a phase advance—that is, rhythms are shifted to an earlier time. Therefore, the entrainment of the endogenous pacemakers by light is the result of a phase advance at dawn and a phase delay at dusk. Melatonin is secreted by the pineal gland during the night. It is stopped by exposure to light during the night but is not stimulated by exposure to darkness during the day.

It is not known how light therapy works, although there are three hypotheses, and conflicting data for all three. First, the suppression of melatonin secretion may be the effective agent. Second, exposure to light in the morning may produce a phase advance, thus treating a phase-delay syndrome manifested as a seasonal mood disorder. Third, because of conflicting data regarding the most effective exposure times, the mere exposure to more photons (through the skin as well as the eyes) may be the key mechanism.

Indications

The major indication for light therapy at this time is seasonal mood disorder, seen predominantly (80 percent) in women. The mean age of presentation is 40, although this age may decrease with better recognition of the disorder. The symptoms appear during the winter and remit spontaneously in the spring. The most common symptoms include depression, fatigue, hypersomnia, hyperphagia, carbohydrate craving, irritability, and interpersonal difficulties. One third to one half of patients with seasonal mood disorder have not previously sought psychiatric help. The remainder are most often diagnosed as having a mood disorder. Over 50 percent of these patients have a first-degree relative with a mood disorder.

Clinical Guidelines

The treatment requires exposure to bright light (2,500 lux) that is approximately 200 times brighter than usual indoor lighting. The initial experiments exposed patients to the light for 2 to 3 hours before dawn and 2 to 3 hours after dusk every day. The patients were instructed not to look directly into the light but to glance at it only occasionally. Some experimenters have suggested that exposure to light in the morning is both necessary and sufficient for therapeutic effects. Conversely, other investigators have suggested that 2 to 3 hours of light exposure anytime during the day will be effective. Patients usually respond after 2 to 4 days of treatment and relapse in 2 to 4 days after the treatment is stopped. The only adverse effect reported with any frequency is irritability. This adverse effect can usually be managed by reducing the length of time that the patient is exposed to the light.

SLEEP DEPRIVATION AND ALTERATION OF SLEEP SCHEDULES

Another treatment involves depriving a patient of one night's sleep. A variation is to deprive the patient only of REM sleep. The alteration of sleep schedules means either advancing or delaying the time a patient goes to sleep each night. These treatments presumably alter the phase relationships between different circadian rhythms. It is hypothesized that a state in which circadian rhythms are out of phase is itself pathogenic and that by altering the sleep-wake cycle, it is possible to reestablish normal phase relationships.

The major indication for these treatments is depression. A phase advance of the sleep cycle may also be an adjuvant for the pharmacotherapy of depression. The loss of one night's sleep has been demonstrated as an effective therapy; however, the beneficial effects usually last only one day. In contrast, it has been reported that advancing a patient's sleep by 3 to 5 hours for 2 to 4 days can have therapeutic effects that last for one week.

DRUG-ASSISTED INTERVIEWING

Introduction

To make it easier to gather information during a psychiatric interview, some psychiatrists advocate drug-assisted interviewing. The common use of an intravenous injection of sodium amytal led to the popular name of "amytal interview" for this technique. Narcotherapy, or narcoanalysis, consists of a series of drug-assisted psychotherapy sessions. Both sedatives (e.g., barbiturates, benzodiazepines) and stimulants (e.g., methylphenidate) have been used. Narcotherapy was thought to benefit patients by allowing them to experience the catharsis of having a repressed memory or thought brought to conscious awareness. Although narcotherapy is very rarely used in modern psychiatry, there has been renewed interest in it. Some noted psychiatrists have proposed that MDMA ("ecstasy") may be beneficial when used as an agent for drug-assisted psychotherapy.

Indications

Although there is much literature on drug-assisted interviewing, it consists mainly of uncontrolled studies and anecdotal reports, thus making difficult a definitive statement about its indications. Furthermore, several controlled trials have shown that the use of drugs does not guarantee that patients will tell the truth, despite the popular misconception of sodium amytal as a "truth serum." A few studies have shown, in fact, that drug-assisted interviews are no better at eliciting information than are an empathic interviewer, hypnosis, or the administration of a placebo.

The most common reasons for drug-assisted interviews in modern practice are uninformative or mute patients, catatonia, and supposed conversion reactions. Although drug-assisted interviews will often elicit information sooner, there is no evidence that this technique has a positive effect on the therapeutic outcome. Patients may be silent because of excessive anxiety about recounting a traumatic event (e.g., rape, accident), and drug-assisted interviews have been used in such cases. But hypnosis, daytime sedation, an empathic and supportive approach, and time will also help elicit information, without the risks of drug-assisted interviewing.

Mute patients with a psychiatric disorder may have catatonic schizophrenia, a conversion reaction, or be malingering. Barbiturates seem to help in temporarily activating catatonic patients; therefore, catatonic schizophrenia may be a reasonable indication for using a drug-assisted interview. Patients with any type of conversion reaction or malingering may or may not improve during a drug-assisted interview. The commonly held but controversial belief is that a functional disorder will improve during a drug-assisted interview, whereas an organic disorder will not improve or will even worsen. If such patients do improve, there is no indication that this technique facilitated their treatment, and if they do not improve or even worsen, the information gained from the interview will be of very little help in guiding the patients' treatment.

Another indication for drug-assisted interviewing is the differential diagnosis of confusion, based on the assumption that functional confusion will clear during the procedure and that organic confusion will not. False positives occur when a confused patient is withdrawing from alcohol or barbiturates or when a patient has an epileptic disorder. False negatives occur when the interviewer uses too much drug or sometimes when the patient has a conversion disorder or is a malingerer. Another proposed indication for drug-assisted interviewing is to differentiate between schizophrenia and depression. It had been thought that when given sodium amytal, schizophrenic patients would recall more bizarre material, and depressed patients would recall more depressed material. This hypothesis has not been confirmed in controlled studies. Sodium amytal has also been suggested as an adjuvant in supportive therapy. In this procedure, the drug is used to reinforce a therapeutic suggestion (e.g., you will stop smoking). However, hypnosis has been found to be more effective in this regard. Furthermore, muscle relaxation has been found to be more powerful than is sodium amytal as an adjuvant in behavioral therapy.

Clinical Guidelines

A 10 percent solution of sodium amytal is administered at a rate of about 0.5 to 1.0 ml a minute. The rate and the total dose should be adjusted for each patient. The total dose may vary between 0.25 and 0.5 g, although occasionally some patients need up to 1.0 g. The end point is a state of mild sedation, but not sleep. The benzodiazepines (e.g., diazepam) may be just as effective and less dangerous than are the barbiturates.

Barbiturates should not be used in patients with liver, renal, or cardiopulmonary diseases or in patients with porphyria or a history of sedative abuse. Patients may have allergic reactions or respiratory suppression during barbiturate interviews, and the clinician must be prepared for both of these possibilities. Furthermore, the use of what patients may perceive as a truth serum may increase their paranoia and interfere with transference and countertransference.

OTHER ORGANIC TREATMENTS

Placebos

Placebos are substances that have no known pharmacological activity. Although it is usually thought that placebos act through suggestion rather than biological action, this idea is based on an artificial distinction between the mind and the body. Virtually every treatment modality is accompanied by poorly understood factors affecting its outcome (e.g., the taste of a medicine, emotional response to a physician). Indeed, both these poorly understood factors and the effects of placebos might better be called nonspecific therapeutic factors. For example, it has recently been demonstrated that naloxone, an opioid antagonist, can block the analgesic effects of a placebo, thus suggesting that a release of endogenous opioids may explain some placebo effects.

Chronic treatment with placebos should never be undertaken when patients have clearly stated an objection to such treatment. Furthermore, deceptive treatment with placebos seriously undermines the patients' confidence in their physicians. Finally, placebos should never be used when an effective therapy is available, as they can lead to both a dependence on pills and various adverse effects.

Acupuncture and Acupressure

An ancient Chinese treatment, acupuncture is the stimulation of specific points on the body with electrical stimulation or the twisting of a needle. Acupressure is the stimulation of these same points with pressure; however, acupressure was not a legitimate part of traditional Chinese medicine. The stimulation of specific points is associated with the relief of certain symptoms and is identified with particular organs. Many Chinese doctors have reported therapeutic success with these treatments in combination with herbal treatment (given orally, topically, or intradermally) for a variety of disorders, including psychiatric disorders. Several American investigators have reported that acupuncture is an effective treatment for some patients with depression or chemical addictions (e.g., nicotine, caffeine, cocaine, heroin). Although it is difficult to approach these

Eastern treatments with a Western mind, it is also true that history has demonstrated that many folk remedies have a firm biological basis.

Orthomolecular Therapy

Megavitamin therapy is treatment with large doses of niacin, ascorbic acid, pyridoxine, folic acid, vitamin B_{12}, and various minerals. Special diets and hormone treatments are often part of these treatment protocols as well. Uncontrolled reports of successful treatment of schizophrenia with niacin have not been replicated in controlled, collaborative studies. Despite claims to the contrary, megavitamin and diet therapies currently have no clinical use in psychiatry. However, a balanced diet reasonably supplemented with vitamins is a good prescription for all patients and physicians.

Hemodialysis

Because of anecdotal reports of therapeutic success in treating schizophrenia with hemodialysis, a double-blind, placebo-controlled study of this modality was undertaken. This carefully conducted study, as well as other attempts to replicate the initial findings, have been unable to demonstrate any positive effects from hemodialysis for patients with schizophrenia.

HISTORICAL TREATMENTS

A variety of treatments were used before the introduction of effective pharmacologic agents. Although most never underwent controlled therapeutic trials, many clinicians report that the treatments were, in fact, quite effective. But because most of them were associated with unpleasant or dangerous adverse effects, they have been virtually supplanted by pharmacotherapy.

Subcoma Insulin Therapy

Psychiatrists used to inject small doses of insulin to induce mild hypoglycemia and the resultant sedative effects. Because of the possible complications of this treatment, as well as the introduction of sedating drugs, this treatment has been abandoned.

Coma Therapy

Insulin coma therapy was introduced in 1933 by Manfred Sakel following his observation that schizophrenic patients who went into coma appeared to have less severe psychiatric symptoms after the coma. Insulin was thus used to induce a comatose state lasting 15 to 60 minutes. The risk of death and intellectual impairment, as well as the introduction of antipsychotic drugs, led to the abandonment of this treatment in the United States.

Atropine sulfate was first used in 1950 to induce coma in psychiatric patients. These atropine-induced comas lasted for 6 to 8 hours, and the patients took warm and cold showers after awakening. Atropine coma is no longer used in the United States.

Carbon Dioxide Therapy

Carbon dioxide therapy was first used in 1929 and involved having the patient inhale carbon dioxide, resulting in an abreaction with severe motor excitement after removing the breathing mask. This treatment was used principally for neurotic patients, and there was doubt even when it was in use that the treatment was effective. Carbon dioxide therapy is no longer used in the United States.

Electrosleep Therapy

Electrosleep therapy is applying a low level of current through electrodes applied to the patient's head. The patient usually feels a tingling sensation at the sites of electrode placement, but sleep is not necessarily induced. This treatment is applied to a wide variety of disorders, with mixed reports of efficacy, but it is not used in the United States.

Continuous Sleep Treatment

Continuous sleep treatment is a symptomatic method of treatment in which the patient is sedated with any of a variety of drugs in order to induce 20 hours of sleep per day, sometimes for as long as 3 weeks for severely agitated patients. Klaesi introduced the name in 1922 and used barbiturates to obtain a fairly deep narcosis. This treatment is not used in the United States.

References

Brody H: The lie that heals: The ethics of giving placebos. Ann Int Med *97*:112, 1982.

Dysken M W, Chang S S, Casper R C. Barbiturate-facilitated interviewing. Biol Psychiatry *14*:421, 1979.

Lewy A J, Sack R L: Light therapy and psychiatry. Proc Soc Exp Biol Med *183*:11, 1986.

Lewy A J, Sack R L, Miller S. Antidepressant and circadian phase-shifting effects of light. Science *235*:352, 1987.

Pflug B: The effect of sleep deprivation on depressed patients. Acta Psychiatr Scand *53*:148, 1976.

Rosenthal N E, Sack D A, Gillin J C. Seasonal affective disorder: A description of the syndrome and preliminary findings with light therapy. Arch Gen Psych *41*:72, 1984.

Sack D A, Nurnberger J, Rosenthal N E. Potentiation of antidepressant medications by phase advance of the sleep-wake cycle. Am J Psychiatry *142*:606, 1985.

Sweet W H, Obrador S, Martin-Rodriguez J G, editors: *Neurosurgical Treatment in Pain and Epilepsy.* University Park Press, Baltimore, 1975.

Tippin J, Henn F A: Modified leukotomy in the treatment of intractable obsessional neurosis. Am J Psychiatry *139*:1601, 1982.

Wehr T A, Wirz-Justice A, Goodwin F K. Phase advance of the circadian sleep-wake cycle as an antidepressant. Science *206*:710, 1979.

32

Child Psychiatry: Assessment, Examination, and Psychological Testing

INTRODUCTION

The psychiatric assessment of children is aimed at elucidating their mental state and adaptive behavioral pattern in disorder as well as in health, by using a biopsychosocial paradigm. The psychiatrist evaluates the child's emotional and cognitive developmental progress, capacity to deal with feelings, thoughts, and wishes; physical development; and social experiences and competence.

There are currently three groups of methods for the psychiatric assessment of children: (1) clinical interviews (2) structured interviews using rating scales and question naires, and (3) standardized tests.

EXAMINATION OF THE CHILD

Clinical interview and direct observation are the first steps and primary means of examining child patients and include history taking, a mental status examination, and direct behavioral observation.

Parents are usually first interviewed, particularly in the cases of infants and young children, as such children cannot remember and communicate various crucial facts and past experiences essential to evaluation. Adolescents should be given the choice of being seen first or being present during the initial interview with their parents.

Children in early developmental stages often are articulate. But even articulate and cooperative children may be reluctant to talk and may conceal, minimize, or even deny their problems out of fear and guilt. As in most child referral cases, if the children have been coerced, if they are confused, or if they associate the psychiatric examination with a threat of abandonment and rejection by their parents, they are likely to behave as normally as they can, reveal as little as possible, or be uncooperative.

Even under the most favorable circumstances with an articulate child who is eager to talk, there is much necessary information that the child alone cannot provide. Interviews with parents and family may not only supplement further information but also help clarify areas of disagreement on salient points of the presenting problems. Each parent should be seen in a separate interview in order to discern the differences in his or her view of the child's problem.

In general, historical and factual data (e.g., age, sex, race, legal status, birth history information, developmental milestones, and previous illnesses) are best gathered by asking specific questions, whereas data about feelings and relationships are best elicited by an open-ended and indirect approach. Parents frequently recall historical dates incorrectly, although they may offer comparisons of their children (e.g., "David was much slower in getting toilet trained than Susan was.") In order to ensure the accuracy of the historical information, data should be gathered from as many objective sources as possible (e.g., school reports, hospital records, previous test reports) and from various observers (e.g., mother, father, siblings). Under special circumstances of child abuse, neglect, broken home, physical or mental illness, or institutionalization, the information provided by adults other than the child's parents is important to the examination and assessment.

In addition, a comprehensive pediatric and psychiatric history is essential. This history should include a careful description of the presenting problem (as seen by the child and his or her parents), personal and developmental history, illness history, and social history. Tables 1 and 2 are suggested outlines for a complete assessment of the child, including the interview with parents and a history-taking guide.

Interview and Observation

The strategy and the clinician's manner of the interview should be flexible and adjusted to the child's age, his or her developmental stage, and the types of presenting problems. The clinician, however, has to make every effort to provide children with a comfortable emotional and physical setting in which they can easily interact in order to facilitate the children's verbal expressions and the interviewer's observations.

Clinical Interviews with Infants and Younger Children. The parents of infants should be present to share in the observation and to learn. The parents' presence will also allow the examiner to observe the parent–child interactions. An evaluation of the parents' child-rearing skills is particularly important to the assessment of an infant. Information should be gathered about the parents' physical health, self-esteem, competence, flexibility, and ability to provide a safe, nurturing, and appropriately stimulating environment for the child. Particular attention has to be paid to the parents' perception of, and sensitivity to, the infant's needs; the

Table 1
Outline for Interview with Parents*

Child's history:
> Parents' main concerns about the child (chief complaint or presenting problem)
>
> Course of symptoms and current adjustment
>
> Past developmental, medical, social, and psychological history, including peer and school adjustments
>
> Child's relationships with siblings and each parent

Parents' marital history

Parents' personal history:
> Parents' primary family, past and present
>
> School and vocational adjustment
>
> Social and avocational interests and activities
>
> Review of any specific medical or psychological problems suffered by either parent

Other family problems:
> Other children
>
> Previous marriages
>
> In-laws
>
> Neighbors

Parents' opinions about possible causes and a review of their feelings about various treatments that may be proposed

*Based on Simmons J E: *The Psychiatric Examination of Children.* Lea & Febiger, Philadelphia, 1969.

Table 2
History Guide*

		Date:
		Referral:
Name:	Sex:	Date of birth:
Address:		
Father's name:	Mother's name:	
Occupation:	Occupation:	
Siblings:	Sex:	Grade:
	Age:	

Informants:
Presenting problems:
Birth and Infancy:
Parents' ages when child was born:
Length of marriage when child was born:
Planned baby? Problems of conception:
History of pregnancy, labor, and delivery:
Birth weight and neonatal history:
Feeding history:
Daily care of the baby given by:
Developmental Milestones (Ages Of):
Sitting: Standing: Walking:
First word: First phrase or sentence:
Toilet training: Time of initiation, mode of procedure:
Temperament in Infancy:
Temperament at Later Stages:
Health:
Operations:
Childhood disease:
Other illnesses:
Accidents:
School History:
Nursery:
Kindergarten:
First grade:
Present:
Interpersonal Relationships:
Additional Factors of Importance:
Further Development of Behavior Problems:
Impression of Parents:

*Based on Chess S: *An Introduction to Child Psychiatry,* ed 2, Grune & Stratton, New York, 1969.

identification of the infant's temperamental characteristics to determine the "goodness of fit" between parent and child; the parents' ability to respond rapidly to the infant's expressed needs; the quality of play between parent and infant; and the amount of support, encouragement, and assistance ("scaffolding") that the parent can provide for the child. The parents' ability to provide a "stimulus shelter" to prevent the child from being overwhelmed should also be evaluated. Observation of infants under the age of 18 months in spontaneous free play, using such games as peek-a-boo and pat-a-cake, should immediately follow the clinical interview. Children between 18 months and 3 years of age can participate more readily in regular unstructured play interviews. The play items should look reasonably realistic, as children at this age have a limited capacity for abstraction and symbolic play. A more thorough and detailed assessment requires the use of standardized developmental scales and psychological tests.

Clinical Interviews with School-Age Children. Interviews with school-age children usually require a minimum of 45 to 60 minutes for each session. The examination room should be open and spacious enough to allow the physical activity required in the assessment, but not so large as to reduce a reasonably intimate contact between the examiner and the child. Toys and materials should be available to suit children of different ages, sexes, and interests. Only necessary and appropriate play items should be made available, as too great a choice may be overstimulating or distracting and too little may fail to accommodate important fantasies or interests.

The unstructured play sessions help the examiner make further inferences about the child's intrapsychic life, such as wishes, fears, impulses, conflicts, defenses, affects, and capacity to relate to others. At the beginning of the interview, the clinician should ask the child what his or her understanding is of the reason for the visit, and the clinician should tell the child his or her own understanding. Next, the clinician should tell the child what will take place in the interview. The clinician should avoid taking notes during the interview, as it may not only inhibit the child but also interfere with the clinician's ability to observe. Leading questions or any kind of demanding interrogation is unproductive and may inhibit the play and communication. Open-ended questions are better than leading questions or questions that require only a single-word answer.

Clinical Interviews with Adolescents. Interviews with adolescents require an even more open and explicit approach. The clinician may tell the adolescent of his or her parents' having come to see the clinician to discuss their concerns, but the clinician wants to learn directly the adolescent's views of what his or her parents have said or what the problem is. The clinician should show genuine interest, acceptance, and candor and give the adolescent undivided and uninterrupted attention. If the adolescent talks in terms of a third person, the clinician should answer matter-of-factly, in the same third-person way.

Many adolescents are rejecting, even hostile, on the first few visits. The clinician should be patient and not jump to any conclusions. This rejection is often a test of how much the clinician can be trusted, a defense against anxiety, or a transference phenomenon. Silence should not be allowed to continue for too long, however, as it may start a power game to see who can hold out longer. Similarly, it is important not to be rigid about the length of the interview session.

Eventually, the clinician must inquire about such sensitive areas as suicidal thoughts, hallucinations, use of drugs, and sexual experiences. This should be done in a matter-of-fact, straightforward manner.

Limit Setting. At the outset, the clinician must set certain limits so as to avoid amplifying anxiety and guilt feelings, with which the child may have no immediate help. Therefore, destructive or unduly regressive behavior may have to be restrained—directly but compassionately—at the beginning of the interview.

Confidentiality. In child psychiatric practice, the younger the child, the more information will have to be shared between the psychiatrist and the parents as to what the child has said and done. Latency-age and preadolescent children, as well as adolescents, can rightfully expect the therapist to keep confidential some private information (e.g., masturbatory fantasies, sexual and aggressive urges and actions, and oedipal wishes). Absolute confidentiality is unrealistic with young children, but a reasonably trusting relationship can be achieved with them. Whenever possible and appropriate, the child and adolescent should be informed of the extent or limits of confidentiality, particularly in the case of a court-referred or court-remanded psychiatric evaluation.

Countertransference. During clinical interviews with children and adolescents, the clinician should be aware of possible countertransference and transference phenomena. For example, aggressive children often make the clinician defensive; mentally retarded children are often overlooked or inadequately served; and deformed children may initially repel some clinicians.

Mental Status Examination

How and what the child plays, says, and does constitute the raw data for the mental status examination. An outline of the mental status examination is presented in Table 3.

Another useful organizing principle is to keep in mind the major categories of psychopathology that should be covered. A list of such categories is shown in Table 4.

The presenting symptoms and history may indicate important areas for close attention. Clinicians should use their clinical judgment about what they should look for and how fast and in what detail they should proceed, considering, when assessing a response, the age and developmental level of the infant, child, or adolescent.

Physical Appearance. The child's size, stature, head size, physical stigmata, bruising, nutritional state, level of anxiety—manifested by hyperalertness and other behavioral signs—attention span, gait, dress, and conflicts are expressed in attitudes, behavior, dress, and mannerisms.

Separation. Too much ease in separating may indicate superficial relationships associated with frequent separations or maternal deprivation. Difficulty in separating may indicate an ambivalent parent–child relationship.

Manner of Relating. Most children relate to the interviewer cautiously at first. Indiscriminate friendliness and shallow relatedness may indicate deprivation or child abuse. Autistic children appear to "look through" people or may avoid eye contact altogether.

Orientation to Time, Place, and Person. Impairments in time, place, and person indicate organic brain factors, low intelligence, anxiety, or a thought disorder.

Central Nervous System Functions. Soft (nonfocal) neurological signs in such areas as speech, gross or fine motor coordination, right-left discrimination, decreased muscle tone, strabismus, nystagmus, asymmetry of muscle tones or reflexes, laterality, handedness, footedness, tremors, eye tracking, motor overflow, and activity level should be explored.

Reading and Writing. Some children may struggle to read or write and may spell poorly. At the same time, many normal first graders (6-year-olds) reverse letters. Clinicians should look for signs of general reading backwardness, with a broadly retarded reading level (2 to 2.5 years below the predicted level) and specific reading retardation. Children exhibiting reading and writing disorders should be evaluated further by means of standardized tests.

Language and Speech. Children who do not use words by 18 months or phrases by 2.5 to 3 years but who have a history of normal babbling and who understand commands and can use and respond to nonverbal cues are

Table 3
Mental Status Examination

Outline	
1. Physical appearance	11. Fantasies and inferred conflicts
2. Separation	12. Affects
3. Manner of relating	13. Object relations
4. Orientation to time, place, and person	14. Drive behavior
5. Central nervous system functions	15. Defense organization
6. Reading and writing	16. Judgment and insight
7. Speech and language	17. Self-esteem
8. Intelligence	18. Adaptive capacities
9. Memory	10. Positive attributes
10. Quality of thinking and perception	

Table 4
Categories of Psychopathology

Developmental delay
Organic brain dysfunction
Thought disorder
Anxiety and neurotic conflict
Mood disorder
Temperament and personality (character) problems
Psychophysiological disorder
Mental retardation
Reaction to unfavorable environment

probably developing normally. However, delays beyond these ages or disturbances in these and other forms of communication should be evaluated further.

Intelligence. An appropriate idea of the child's intelligence may be assessed by his or her general vocabulary, responsiveness, level of comprehension and curiosity, and drawing ability and may be confirmed by a standardized intelligence test.

Memory. At age 8, normal children can count five digits forward and two or three digits backward; at age 10, they can count six digits forward and four digits backward. Minor difficulties may simply reflect anxiety. But very poor performance on the digit span test may indicate brain damage (particularly left hemisphere damage) or mental retardation.

Thinking Processes and Perception. Three major clinical dimensions in the thinking process should be evaluated: actual thought content, speed of thinking, and ease of flow. A variation in any of these dimensions may be of such a degree and duration as to constitute a thought disorder.

Hallucinations in childhood are almost always pathological and may also be secondary to drug intoxication, seizure disorder, metabolic disorder, infection, immaturity, stress, anxiety, mood disorder, and schizophrenia.

Fantasies and Inferred Conflicts. Fantasies and inferred conflicts can be assessed by direct questioning about the child's dreams, drawings, doodles, or spontaneous play.

Affects. The interviewer should observe affects such as anxiety, depression, apathy, guilt, and anger. Suicidal risk may be part of a major depressive disorder. Whenever suspected, suicidal fantasies, actions, the presence or absence of previous suicidal behavior, motivation, the child's experiences and concept of death, nature of depression, other affects, and the family and environmental situations should be carefully explored. A useful tool for suicide assessment in children is the Corder–Haizlip Child Suicide Checklist.

Object Relations. The interviewer may discuss the child's relations with family, peers, and teachers.

Drive Behavior. Basic drive behavior in sexual and aggressive areas may be explored.

Defense Organization. Defense organization may be studied by assessing the presence or absence of phobias, obsessive-compulsive behavior, denial, and reaction formation.

Judgment and Insight. To assess the child's judgment and insight, the following should be explored: What

the child thinks caused his or her problem; how upset the child appears to be about the problem; what the child thinks might help solve the problem; and how the child thinks the clinician can help.

Self-esteem. The child who has low self-esteem often makes such remarks as "I can't do that" or "I am no good at all."

Adaptive Capacity. The child may be adept at many different kinds of problem-solving activities.

Positive Attributes. Positive attributes include physical health, attractive appearance, normal height and weight, normal vision and hearing, even temperament, normal intelligence, appropriate emotional responses without extreme mood swings, recognition of feelings and fantasies, a good command of language and a capacity to verbalize thoughts and feelings, and good academic and social performance at school.

DIAGNOSIS AND CLASSIFICATION

The DSM-III-R classification of disorders, usually first evident in infancy or childhood, includes all the childhood and adolescent psychiatric disorders. The Committee on Child Psychiatry of the Group for the Advancement of Psychiatry (GAP) proposed a diagnostic classification that divides childhood and adolescent disorders into ten major diagnostic categories (Table 5). It is the first system to include healthy responses as a diagnostic category, pointing up the need to recognize when signs that may cause concern are manifestations of adaptation and do not indicate failure to maintain mental growth. The first six categories, arranged more or less in ascending order of seriousness, deal essentially with the total personality, following as closely as possible the unitary view underlying the system. In contrast, the next three categories reflect end organ or organ system responses, even though the personality of the child with such a disorder is almost always significantly involved.

Anna Freud's system of classification divides the psychiatric disorders of children into two major groups (Table 6). She defined symptoms more narrowly than does the GAP system. For Anna Freud, symptoms were only those manifestations of disorder that result from the failure of an essential step in mental development to take place at

Table 5
Group for the Advancement of Psychiatry Classifications*

1. Healthy responses
2. Reactive disorders
3. Developmental deviations
4. Psychoneurotic disorders
5. Personality disorders
6. Psychotic disorders
7. Psychosomatic disorders
8. Brain syndromes
9. Mental retardation
10. Other disorders

*Based on Group for the Advancement of Psychiatry: *Psychopathological Disorders in Childhood*, Report 62. Group for the Advancement of Psychiatry, New York, 1966.

Table 6
Anna Freud's System of Classification

Symptoms

Symptoms resulting from initial nondifferentiation between somatic and psychological processes: psychosomatics

Symptoms resulting from compromise formation between id and ego: neurotic symptoms

Symptoms resulting from the irruption of id derivatives into the ego: psychotic or delinquent symptoms if complete irruption, borderline symptoms if parital irruption

Symptoms resulting from changes in the libido economy or direction of cathexis: symptoms of some personality disorders and hypochondriasis

Symptoms resulting from changes in the quality or direction of aggression: inhibited or destructive symptoms

Symptoms resulting from undefended regressions: infantile symptoms

Symptoms resulting from organic causes

Other signs of disturbance and other reasons for a child's referral

Fears and anxieties

Delays and failures in development

School failures

Failures in social adaptation

Aches and pains

---

the normal time. She defined symptoms in terms of the specific step that failed and at which the child's development took its pathological turn.

DEVELOPMENTAL AND PSYCHOLOGICAL TESTING

Psychological testing may not be always necessary for an effective examination. However, it is valuable in determining an infant's or child's developmental status, level of intelligence, and revelation of inner states otherwise obscured by defenses or inhibitions in communication. Psychological testing is particularly indicated when there are questions pertaining to learning difficulties, mental retardation, brain damage, a severe disturbance of thinking, or behavioral problems related to the personality disorder.

Intelligence Tests

Infant and Preschool Child Testing. Tests applicable to preschool children are divided into (1) developmental tests designed for infants 18 to 24 months and (2) preschool tests for children aged 24 to 60 months. In the infant tests, the clinician's speech is of little or no use in giving test instructions, although the child's own speech development provides relevant developmental data. Most of the infant tests are controlled observations of the infant's sensorimotor development, especially in the first year, with some additional social and language assessment. On the other hand, preschool children can actively participate in the test, because of their better ability to walk, sit at a table, manipulate test objects, and communicate verbally with the tester.

The Gesell Developmental Schedules cover ages 8 weeks to 3.5 years. Data are obtained by direct observation of the child's responses to standard toys and other controlled stimulus objects and are supplemented by developmental information provided by the mother or primary caretaker. The schedules yield scores indicating the child's level of development in four separate areas: motor, adaptive, language, and personal and social.

A more test-oriented approach is the Cattell Infant Scale for Intelligence, applicable to infants and children aged 2 to 30 months. This scale was developed as a downward extension of the Stanford–Binet Test and also includes some items from the Gesell Schedules.

School-age Testing. Intelligence tests for school-age children measure primarily those abilities essential to academic achievement. They are often more accurately described as tests of scholastic aptitude.

In the United States, the earliest intelligence test was the Stanford–Binet Test, adapted from the original Binet–Simon Scales. The Stanford–Binet Test relies heavily on verbal performance and covers the ages of 2 years to adulthood. It yields both a mental age and an intelligence quotient (I.Q.). Objects, pictures, and drawings are used mostly at the younger ages; and printed, verbal, and numerical materials are used more at the older ages.

Another individual intelligence test, perhaps currently the most widely used test for children aged 6 to 17 years, is the Wechsler Intelligence Scale for Children–Revised (WISC-R). This scale provides verbal and performance subscale scores as well as a full-scale I.Q. score.

Both the Stanford–Binet and the WISC-R require a highly trained tester and are administered individually to each subject. Group tests are designed for mass testing. Most group tests enable a single examiner to test a large group in one session, and they are relatively easy to administer and score. They are mainly for screening purposes and useful when a crude index of intellectual level suffices or when more extensive individual testing is not available.

Long-term Stability of Intelligence. Most children's I.Q.s remain fairly constant throughout the developmental periods. In theory, if all of a child's biological, social, and psychological givens remain stable, his or her I.Q. will also remain the same. However, scores on infant tests are not reliable in predicting the child's intelligence in late childhood or adolescence. Infant tests are valuable only for the early detection of developmental deviations, including mental retardation and other developmental disorders of hereditary or adverse environmental origin. Infant tests rely heavily on sensorimotor functions, which bear little significance to the later-developing verbal, social, and other abstract functions that constitute intelligence in later years.

In reality, the I.Q. scores do fluctuate to some degree. Large shifts in I.Q. are usually associated with the child's motivation, emotional independence, cultural milieu, and home emotional climate. The I.Q. scores of children in socioeconomically disadvantaged environments tend to decrease with age; those in superior environments tend to increase.

Aptitude Tests. Because most intelligence tests concentrate on the more abstract verbal and numerical abilities, there is also a need for tests measuring the more concrete and practical intellectual skills. Mechanical aptitudes were among the first for which special tests were developed. Tests of clerical aptitude, measuring chiefly perceptual speed and accuracy, and tests of musical and artistic aptitudes followed.

Multiple-aptitude batteries provide a profile of scores on separate tests. An example is the Differential Aptitude Tests (DAT), which yields scores in eight abilities: verbal reasoning, numerical ability, abstract reasoning, clerical speed and accuracy, mechanical reasoning, space relations, spelling, and grammar. Multiple-aptitude batteries are most useful in testing older children and adolescents.

Educational Tests

Readiness Tests. Readiness tests are designed to assess a child's qualifications for schoolwork. The importance of prior learning is paramount, as the acquisition of simple concepts equips the child for learning more complex concepts at any age.

Special emphasis is placed on those abilities found to be most important to learning to read; some attention is also given to the prerequisites of numerical thinking and to the sensorimotor control required in learning to write. Among the functions covered are visual and auditory discrimination, motor control, verbal comprehension, vocabulary, quantitative concepts, and general information. A well-known example is the Metropolitan Readiness Tests.

Tests of Special Education Disabilities. Reading tests are customarily classified as survey and diagnostic tests. Survey tests indicate the general level of the child's achievement in reading. These tests mainly screen children in need of remedial instruction. Diagnostic tests are designed to analyze the child's performance and identify specific sources of difficulty. These tests yield more than one score, and some include detailed checklists of specific types of errors. Information about possible emotional difficulties and a complete case history are essential.

Educational Achievement Batteries. Achievement tests measure the effects of a course of study. Many achievement tests gauge the attainment of relatively broad educational goals, cutting across subject matter specialties. An outstanding example is the Sequential Tests of Educational Progress (STEP). These tests are available at several levels, extending from the fourth grade of elementary school to the sophomore year of college and beyond. At each level there are seven tests: multiple-choice tests in reading, writing, mathematics, science, social studies, and listening and an essay-writing test. The main emphasis is on the application of learned skills to the solution of new problems.

Creativity Tests. The growing recognition that creative talent is not synonymous with intelligence, as measured by traditional intelligence tests, has been accompanied by vigorous efforts to develop specialized tests of creativity. The tests involve various aspects of fluency, flexibility, and originality. An example of a test that is effective with young children is the improvements test, in which the child is given toys, such as a nurse kit, a fire truck, and a stuffed dog, and is asked to think of ways of changing each toy so that it will be more fun to play with.

Personality Tests

In comparison with tests of ability, personality tests are much less satisfactory with regard to norms, reliability, and validity. Any information obtained from personality tests should be verified and supplemented by other sources, such as interviews with the child and his or her associates, direct observation of behavior, and case history.

Self-report Inventories. Self-report inventories are a series of questions concerning emotional problems, worries, interests, motives, values, and interpersonal traits. Several inventories designed for children and adolescents are basically checklists of personal problems. The questions pertain directly to the information that the examiner wishes to elicit about the child's feelings and actions, and the responses are accepted at face value. A clear example of this approach is the Mooney Problem Check List. The problem areas covered in the junior high school form include health and physical development, school, home and family, money, work and the future, boy–girl relations, relations with people in general, and self-centered concerns. Personality inventories find their major usefulness to be screening and identifying children in need of further evaluation.

Projective Techniques. In projective techniques, the subject is assigned an unstructured task that permits an almost unlimited variety of possible responses. The test stimuli are typically vague and equivocal, and the instructions are brief and general. These techniques are based on the hypothesis that the way in which the person perceives and interprets the test materials reflects basic characteristics of his or her personality. The test stimuli thus serve as a screen on which the subject projects his or her own ideas.

One of the most widely used projective techniques is the Rorschach test, in which the subject is shown a set of bilaterally symmetrical inkblots and asked to tell what he or she sees or what the blot represents. Rorschach norms have been developed for children between the ages of 2 and 10 years and for adolescents between the ages of 10 and 17.

A somewhat more structured test is the Children's Apperception Test (CAT), an adaptation of the Thematic Apperception Test (TAT). In the CAT, pictures of animals are substituted for pictures of people, on the assumption that children respond more readily to animal characters. The pictures are designed to evoke fantasies relating to problems of feeding and other oral activities, sibling rivalry, parent–child relations, aggression, toilet training, and other childhood experiences. Another example is the Blacky Pictures, a set of cartoons showing a small dog, his parents, and a sibling. Based on a psychoanalytic theory of psychosexual development, the cartoons depict situations suggesting various types of sexual conflicts. Still another type of picture test is illustrated by the Rosenzweig Picture–Frustration Study. This test presents a series of cartoons in which one person frustrates another. In a blank space provided, the child writes what the frustrated person might reply.

Drawings, toy tests, and other play techniques represent other applications or projective methods. Play and dramatic objects, such as puppets, dolls, toys, and miniatures, have also been used. The objects are usually selected because of their associative value and often include dolls representing adults and children, bathroom and kitchen fixtures, and other household furnishings. Play with such articles is expected to reveal the child's attitudes toward his or her family, sibling rivalries, fears, aggressions, and conflicts. They are particularly useful in eliciting sexual abuse problems in children.

When evaluated as standardized tests, most projective techniques have fared quite poorly and thus should be regarded not as tests but as aids to the clinical interviewer.

References

Andersen J C, Williams S, McGee R, Silva P A: DSM-III Disorders in Preadolescent Children. *Arch Gen Psych 44*:69, 1987.

Benton A L, Hamsher K de S, Varney N R, Spreen O: *Contributions to Neuropsychological Assessment: A Clinical Manual.* Oxford University Press, New York, 1983.

Call J D: Toward a nosology of psychiatric disorders in infancy. In *Frontiers of Infant Psychiatry*, J D Call, E Galenson, R L Tyson, editors, p 117, Basic Books, New York, 1983.

Chess S: *An Introduction to Child Psychiatry*, ed 2. Grune & Stratton, New York, 1969.

Gittelman R: The role of psychological tests for differential diagnosis in child psychiatry. J Am Acad Child Psychiatry *19*:413, 1980.

Hillard J R, Slomowitz M, Levi L S: A retrospective study of adolescents, visits to a general hospital psychiatric emergency service. Am J Psych *144*:432, 1987.

Kashani J H, Beck N C, Hoeper E W, Fallahi C, Corcoran C M, McAllister J A, Rosenberg T K, Reid J C: Psychiatric disorders in a community sample of adolescents. Am J Psych *144*:584, 1987.

Kashani J H, Carlson G: Seriously depressed preschoolers. Am J Psych *144*:348, 1987.

Kaufman A S, Kaufman N L: *Kaufman Assessment Battery for Children: Interpretive Manual*. American Guidance Service, Circle Pines, MN 1983.

Kazdin, A E: Assessment Techniques for childhood depression: A critical appraisal. J Am Acad Child Psychiatry *20*:358, 1981.

Ollendick, T H, Heresen M, editors: *Handbook of Child Psychopathology*. Plenum, New York, 1983.

Puig-Antich J, Chambers W J, Tabrizi M A: The clinical assessment of current depressive episodes in children and adolescents: Interviews with parents and children. In *Affective Disorders in Childhood and Adolescence—An Update*, D P Cantwell, G A Carlson, editors, p 157. S P Medical & Scientific Books, New York, 1983.

Puig-Antich J, Perel J M, Lupatkin W, Chambers W J, Talerizi M A, King J, Goetz R, Davies M, Stiller R L: Imipramine in prepubertal major depressive disorders. Arch Gen Psych *44*:81, 1987.

Sattler J M: *Assessment of Children's Intelligence*, ed 2. Saunders, Philadelphia, 1982.

Simmons J E: *Psychiatric Examination of Children*, ed 2. Lea & Febiger, Philadelphia, 1974.

33

Mental Retardation

DEFINITION

Mental retardation is a behavioral syndrome that does not have a single etiology, mechanism, course, or prognosis. The definition of mental retardation has evolved through the years and is still in the process of refinement. It has reflected the views and attitudes of society toward mental retardation, as well as the diagnostic techniques and the state of medical knowledge.

There are two major conceptual approaches in defining mental retardation: the biomedical and sociocultural and adaptational models. The adherents of the biomedical model, particularly in the United States, maintain that the presence of basic changes in the brain is essential to the diagnosis of mental retardation. Alternatively, the proponents of the sociocultural adaptational model emphasize the social functioning and general ability to adapt to accepted norms.

Table 1 focuses on the developmental impairment in infancy and preschool years, learning difficulties in school age, and poor social-vocational adjustment in adulthood. This table includes the criteria of both DSM-III-R and the American Association of Mental Deficiency (AAMD). According to the 1983 AAMD definition, mental retardation refers to significantly subaverage general intellectual functioning resulting in or associated with concurrent impairments in adaptive behavior and manifested during the developmental period. The AAMD definition is virtually identical with the DSM-III-R definition, which describes the essential features of mental retardation as: (1) significantly subaverage general intellectual functioning accompanied by (2) significant deficits or impairments in adaptive functioning, (3) with onset before the age of 18. See Table 2 for the DSM-III-R criteria for mental retardation. The diagnosis is made regardless of whether there is a coexisting physical or other mental disorder.

"General intellectual functioning" is determined by results of a standardized test of intelligence, and the term "significantly subaverage" is defined as an I.Q. of approximately 70 or below, or two standard deviations below the mean for the particular test.

NOMENCLATURE

The term "mental retardation" is often used interchangeably with "mental deficiency." The World Health Organization (WHO) has recommended the term "mental subnormality," which includes two separate and distinct categories: mental retardation and mental deficiency. Mental retardation, according to WHO nosology, is reserved for subnormal functioning secondary to identifiable underlying pathological causes, whereas mental deficiency is often used as a legal term, applied to individuals with an I.Q. of less than 70.

The term "feeble-mindedness" was often used in the past, especially in American literature, and is still in use in Great Britain, where it generally denotes the mild forms of mental retardation. "Oligophrenia" is commonly used in the USSR, Scandinavia, and other Western European countries. "Amentia" is no longer used in modern psychiatry, except occasionally to refer to a terminal stage of a degenerative illness.

CLASSIFICATION

The degrees or levels of mental retardation are expressed in various terms. DSM-III-R presents four subtypes of mental retardation, reflecting the degree of intellectual impairment: mild mental retardation, moderate mental retardation, severe mental retardation, and profound mental retardation. The degrees of mental retardation by I.Q. range are indicated in Table 3.

In addition, DSM-III-R lists "unspecified mental retardation" as a subtype reserved for those persons who are strongly suspected of having mental retardation but cannot be tested by standard intelligence tests or are too impaired or uncooperative to be tested. This subtype may be applicable to infants whose significantly subaverage intellectual functioning is clinically judged, but for whom the available tests (e.g., Bayley, Cattell) do not yield numerical I.Q. values. This subtype should not be used when the intellectual level is presumed to be above 70.

EPIDEMIOLOGY

The prevalence of mental retardation at any one time is estimated to be about 1 percent of the population. The incidence of mental retardation is difficult to calculate accurately because of the impossibility of stating when an individual is diagnosed as having mental retardation. In many cases, retardation may be "latent" for a long time before the person's limitations are recognized, or because of good adaptation, the formal diagnosis is not warranted at a particular point in the person's life. The highest incidence is in school-aged children, with the peak at ages 10 to 14.

Table 1
Developmental Characteristics of the Mentally Retarded*
This table integrates chronological age, degree of retardation, and level of intellectual, vocational, and social functioning.

Degree of Mental Retardation	Preschool Age 0–5 Maturation and Development	School Age 6–20 Training and Education	Adult 21 and over Social and Vocational Adequacy
Profound	Gross retardation; minimal capacity for functioning in sensorimotor areas; needs nursing care; constant aid and supervision required	Some motor development present; may respond to minimal or limited training in self-help	Some motor and speech development; may achieve very limited self-care; needs nursing care
Severe	Poor motor development; speech minimal; generally unable to profit from training in self-help; little or no communication skills	Can talk or learn to communicate; can be trained in elemental health habits; profits from systematic habit training; unable to profit from vocational training	May contribute partially to self-maintenance under complete supervision; can develop self-protection skills to a minimal useful level in controlled environment
Moderate	Can talk or learn to communicate; poor social awareness; fair motor development; profits from training in self-help; can be managed with moderate supervision	Can profit from training in social and occupational skills; unlikely to progress beyond 2nd grade level in academic subjects; may learn to travel alone in familiar places	May achieve self-maintenance in unskilled or semi-skilled work under sheltered conditions; needs supervision and guidance when under mild social or economic stress
Mild	Can develop social and communication skills; minimal retardation in sensorimotor areas; often not distinguished from normal until later age	Can learn academic skills up to approximately 6th grade level by late teens; can be guided toward social conformity	Can usually achieve social and vocational skills adequate to minimum self-support, but may need guidance and assistance when under unusual social or economic stress

*Adapted from *Mental Retardation Activities of the U.S. Department of Health, Education and Welfare*, p 2. United States Government Printing Office, Washington, D.C., 1963. DSM-III-R criteria are adapted essentially from this chart.

Mental retardation is approximately 1½ times more common among males than females.

ETIOLOGICAL FACTORS AND SYNDROMES

Based on current knowledge, approximately 25 percent of the cases of mental retardation are known to be caused by biological abnormalities. Chromosomal and metabolic disorders, such as Down's syndrome and phenylketonuria, are the most common disorders manifesting mental retardation. Mental retardation associated with these disorders is usually diagnosed at birth or relatively early in childhood, and the severity is generally moderate to profound.

No specific biological causes can be identified in the remaining 75 percent of the cases. The level of intellectual impairment of individuals with no known causes is usually mild, with I.Q.s between 50 and 70. The diagnosis of mild retardation is not usually made before grade school. In mild mental retardation, a familial pattern is often seen in parents and siblings.

The lower socioeconomic classes are overrepresented in the cases of mild retardation, and the significance of this is not clear. However, psychosocial deprivation, such as deprivation in social, linguistic, and intellectual stimulation, has been suspected as contributing to mental retardation without known biological etiology. Current knowledge suggests that three sets of etiologic factors are involved, either singly or in combination: genetic factors, environmental biological factors (e.g., malnutrition), and early child-rearing experiences.

PRENATAL FACTORS

Important prerequisites for the overall development of the fetus include the mother's physical and psychological health during pregnancy and her nutritional state. Maternal chronic illnesses and conditions affecting the normal development of the fetus's central nervous system include uncontrolled diabetes, anemia, emphysema, hypertension, and chronic usage of alcohol and narcotic substances. Maternal infection during pregnancy, especially viral infections, has been known to cause fetal damage and mental retardation. The degree of fetal damage depends on variables such as the type of viral infection, the gestational age of the fetus, and the severity of the illness. Although numerous infectious diseases have been reported to affect the fetus's central nervous system, the following three infectious disorders have been definitely identified as high-risk conditions for mental retardation: rubella (German measles), cytomegalic inclusion disease, and syphilis.

Rubella (German Measles)

Rubella has replaced syphilis as the major cause of congenital malformations and mental retardation due to maternal infection. The children of affected mothers may present a number of abnormalities, including congenital heart disease, mental retardation, cataracts, deafness, microcephaly, and microphthalmia. Tim-

Table 2
Diagnostic Criteria for Mental Retardation

A. Significantly subaverage general intellectual functioning: an IQ of 70 or below on an individually administered IQ test (for infants, a clinical judgment of significantly subaverage intellectual functioning, since available intelligence tests do not yield numerical IQ values).

B. Concurrent deficits or impairments in adaptive functioning, i.e., the person's effectiveness in meeting the standards expected for his or her age by his or her cultural group in areas such as social skills and responsibility, communication, daily living skills, personal independence, and self-sufficiency.

C. Onset before the age of 18.

Table from DSM-III-R, *Diagnostic and Statistical Manual of Mental Disorders,* ed 3, revised. (Current Classification of Mental Disorders, 1987.) Copyright American Psychiatric Association, Washington, D.C., 1987. Used with permission.

Table 3
Severity of Mental Retardation by I.Q. Range*

Severity of Mental Retardation	I.Q. Range	Percentage of Retarded Population
Mild	50–55 to approx. 70	85
Moderate	35–40 to 50–55	10
Severe	20–25 to 35–40	3–4
Profound	Below 20 or 25	1–2

*Adapted from DSM-III-R, *Diagnostic and Statistical Manual of Mental Disorders,* ed 3, revised. (Current Classification of Mental Disorders, 1987.) Copyright American Psychiatric Association, Washington, D.C., 1987. Used with permission.

ing is crucial, as the extent and the frequency of the complications are inversely related to the duration of pregnancy at the time of maternal infection. When mothers are infected in the first trimester of pregnancy, 10 to 15 percent of the children will be affected, but the incidence rises to almost 50 percent when the infection occurs in the first month of pregnancy. The situation is often complicated by subclinical forms of maternal infection, which often go undetected. Maternal rubella can be prevented by immunization.

Cytomegalic Inclusion Disease

In many cases, cytomegalic inclusion disease remains dormant in the mother. Some children are stillborn, and others develop jaundice, microcephaly, and hepatosplenomegaly and have radiographic findings of intracerebral calcification. Children with mental retardation from this disease frequently have cerebral calcification, microcephaly, or hydrocephalus. The diagnosis is confirmed by positive throat and urine cultures of the virus and the recovery of inclusion-bearing cells in the urine.

Syphilis

Syphilis in pregnant women used to be the main cause of various neuropathological changes in their offspring, including mental retardation. Today, the incidence of syphilitic com-

plications of pregnancy fluctuates with the incidence of syphilis in the general population. Some recent alarming statistics from several major cities in the United States indicate that there is still no room for complacency.

Other Diseases

Brain damage due to toxoplasmosis transmitted from the pregnant mother to the fetus is another universally recognized, but relatively rare, complication of pregnancy that often results in mental retardation and a variety of brain malformations. Damage to the fetus from maternal hepatitis has also been reported.

Currently, AIDS has become an important public health issue, and extensive research is being conducted to study its effects on fetuses and newborn infants. The pregnancy of a woman who has a confirmed case of AIDS results in fetal death, still birth, spontaneous abortion, or death of the baby within a few years. Because the virus is known to affect the brain tissue directly, it is presumed that children born to such mothers may show signs of brain damage with varying degrees of mental retardation.

The role of other maternal infections during pregnancy—such as influenza, common-cold viruses, pneumonia, and urinary tract infections—in causing mental retardation is being investigated, and the results are not yet conclusive.

Complications of Pregnancy

Toxemia of pregnancy and uncontrolled maternal diabetes present hazards to the fetus and may sometimes result in mental retardation. Maternal malnutrition during pregnancy often results in prematurity and other obstetrical complications. Vaginal hemorrhage, placenta previa, premature separation of the placenta, and prolapse of the cord may damage the fetal brain by causing anoxia.

The potential teratogenic effect of pharmacological agents administered during pregnancy was widely publicized after the thalidomide tragedy (a drug which produced a high percentage of deformed babies when given to pregnant women). So far, with the exception of metabolites used in cancer chemotherapy, no usual doses are known to damage the fetus's central nervous system, but caution and restraint in prescribing drugs to pregnant women are certainly indicated. The use of lithium and excessive alcohol consumption during pregnancy were recently implicated in some congenital malformations, especially of the cardiovascular system (e.g. Ebstein's syndrome).

CHROMOSOMAL ABNORMALITIES

Abnormalities in autosomal chromosomes are associated with mental retardation, although aberrations in sex chromosomes are not always associated with mental retardation (e.g., Turner's syndrome with XO and Kleinfelter's syndrome with XXY, XXXY, or XXYY variations). Some children with Turner's syndrome have normal to superior intelligence.

Down's Syndrome

Down's syndrome was first described by the English physician Langdon Down in 1866 and was based on the physical characteristics associated with subnormal mental functioning. Since then,

Down's syndrome has remained the most investigated and the most discussed syndrome in mental retardation. The children with this syndrome were originally called *mongoloid* based on their physical characteristics of slanted eyes, epicanthal folds, and flat nose.

Despite a plethora of theories and hypotheses advanced in the past 100 years, the cause of Down's syndrome is still unknown. There is agreement on very few predisposing factors in chromosomal disorders—among them, the increased age of the mother, possibly the increased age of the father, and x-ray radiation. The problem of cause is complicated even further by the recent recognition of three types of chromosomal aberrations in Down's syndrome:

1. Patients with trisomy 21 (3 of chromosome 21, instead of the usual 2) represent the overwhelming majority; they have 47 chromosomes, with an extra chromosome 21. The mothers' karyotypes are normal. A nondisjunction during miosis, occurring for yet unknown reasons, is held responsible for this disorder.
2. Nondisjunction occurring after fertilization in any cell division results in mosaicism, a condition in which both normal and trisomic cells are found in various tissues.
3. In translocation, there is a fusion of 2 chromosomes, mostly 21 and 15, resulting in a total of 46 chromosomes, despite the presence of an extra chromosome 21. The disorder, unlike trisomy 21, is usually inherited, and the translocation chromosome may be found in unaffected parents and siblings. These asymptomatic carriers have only 45 chromosomes.

The incidence of Down's syndrome in the United States is about 1 in every 700 births. In his original description, Down mentioned the frequency of 10 percent among all mentally retarded patients. Interestingly, today, around 10 percent of patients with Down's syndrome are in institutions for the mentally retarded. For a middle-aged mother (more than 32 years old), the risk of having a Down's syndrome child with trisomy 21 is about 1 in 100 births, but when translocation is present, the risk is about one in three. These facts assume special importance in genetic counseling.

Amniocentesis, in which a small amount of amniotic fluid is removed from the amniotic cavity transabdominally between the 14th and 16th week of gestation, has been useful in diagnosing various infant abnormalities, especially Down's syndrome. Amniotic fluid cells, mostly fetal in origin, are cultured for cytogenetic and biochemical studies. Many serious hereditary disorders can be predicted with this method, and therapeutic abortion is the only method of prevention. Amniocentesis is recommended for all pregnant women over the age of 35. Fortunately, most chromosomal anomalies occur only once in a family.

Mental retardation is the overriding feature of Down's syndrome. The majority of patients belong to the moderately and severely retarded groups, with only a minority having an I.Q. above 50. Mental development seems to progress normally from birth to 6 months of age. I.Q. scores gradually decrease from near normal at 1 year of age to about 30 at older ages. This decline in intelligence may be real or apparent. It could be that infantile tests do not reveal the full extent of the defect, which may become manifest when more sophisticated tests are used in early childhood. According to many sources, patients with Down's syndrome are placid, cheerful, and cooperative, which facilitates their adjustment at home. The picture, however, seems to change in adolescents, especially those in institutions, who may develop various emotional difficulties, behavior disorders, and (rarely) psychotic illnesses.

The diagnosis of Down's syndrome is made with relative ease in an older child but is often difficult in newborn infants. The most important signs in a newborn include general hypotonia, oblique palpebral fissures, abundant neck skin, a small flattened skull, high cheek bones, and a protruding tongue. The hands are broad and thick, with a single palmar transversal crease, and the little fingers are short and curved inward. Moro's reflex is weak or absent. More than 100 signs or stigmata are described in Down's syndrome, but rarely are all found in one person.

Life expectancy used to be about 12 years. With the advent of antibiotics, however, few young patients succumb to infections, but most of them do not live beyond the age of 40, when they already have many signs of senescence, which are similar to those of Alzheimer's disease. Despite numerous therapeutic recommendations, no treatment has proved effective.

Cat-cry (Cri-du-Chat) Syndrome

Children with cat-cry syndrome are missing part of the fifth chromosome. They are severely retarded and show many stigmata often associated with chromosomal aberrations, such as microcephaly, low-set ears, oblique palpebral fissures, hypertelorism, and micrognathia. The characteristic cat-like cry—due to laryngeal abnormalities—that gave the syndrome its name gradually changes and disappears with increasing age.

Other syndromes of autosomal aberrations associated with mental retardation are much less prevalent than is Down's syndrome. Various types of autosomal and sex chromosome aberration syndromes are included in Table 4.

GENETIC DEFECTS

Phenylketonuria (PKU)

Phenylketonuria (PKU) was first described by Folling in 1934 as the paradigmatic inborn error of metabolism. PKU is transmitted as a simple recessive autosomal Mendelian trait and occurs in approximately 1 in every 10,000 to 15,000 live births. To the parents who already have had a child with PKU, the chance of having another child with PKU is one in every four to five successive pregnancies. Although the disease is reported predominantly in people of North European origin, a few cases have been described in blacks, Yemenite Jews, and Asians. The frequency among institutionalized defectives is about 1 percent.

The basic metabolic defect in PKU is an inability to convert phenylalanine, an essential amino acid, to paratyrosine, because of the absence or inactivity of the liver enzyme phenylalanine hydroxylase, which catalyzes the conversion. Two other types of hyperphenylalaninemia have recently been described. One is due to a deficiency of an enzyme, dihydropteridine reductase, and the other to a deficiency of a cofactor, biopterin. The first defect can be detected in fibroblasts, and biopterin can be measured in body fluids. Both of these rare disorders carry a high risk of fatality.

The majority of patients with PKU are severely retarded, but some are reported to have borderline or normal intelligence. Eczema, vomiting, and convulsions are present in about a third of all cases. Although the clinical picture varies, typical PKU children are hyperactive and exhibit erratic, unpredictable behavior, which makes them difficult to manage. They frequently have temper tantrums and often display bizarre movements of their bodies and upper extremities and twisting hand mannerisms, and their behavior sometimes resembles that of autistic or schizophrenic children. Verbal and nonverbal communication is usually severely

Table 4
Thirty-Five Important Syndromes with Multiple Handicaps*

Syndrome	Diagnostic Manifestations			Mental Retardation	Short Stature	Genetic Transmission
	Craniofacial	Skeletal	Other			
Aarskog syndrome	Hypertelorism; broad nasal bridge, anteverted nostrils, long philtrum	Small hands and feet; mild interdigital webbing; short stature	Scrotal "shawl" above penis		+	X-linked semidominant
Apert syndrome (acrocephalosyndactyly)	Craniosynostosis; irregular midfacial hypoplasia; hypertelorism	Syndactyly; broad distal thumb and toe		±		Autosomal dominant
Cerebral gigantism (Sotos syndrome)	Large head; prominent forehead; narrow anterior mandible	Large hands and feet	Large size in early life; poor coordination	±		?
Cockayne syndrome	Pinched facies; sunken eyes; thin nose; prognathism; retinal degeneration	Long limbs, with large hands and feet; flexion deformities	Hypotrichosis; photosensitivity; thin skin; diminished subcutaneous fat; impaired hearing	+	+	Autosomal recessive
Cohen syndrome	Maxillary hypoplasia with prominent central incisors	Narrow hands and feet	Hypotonia; obesity	+	±	? Autosomal recessive
Cornelia de Lange syndrome	Synophrys (continuous eyebrows); thin down-turning upper lip; long philtrum; anteverted nostrils; microcephaly	Small or malformed hands and feet; proximal thumb	Hirsutism	+	+	?
Cri-du-chat syndrome	Epicanthic folds and/or slanting palpebral fissures; round facial contour; hypertelorism; microcephaly	Short metacarpals or metatarsals; four-finger line in palm	Catlike cry in infancy	+	+	?
Crouzon syndrome (craniofacial dysostosis)	Proptosis with shallow orbits; maxillary hypoplasia; craniosynostosis					Autosomal dominant
Down's syndrome	Upward slant to palpebral fissures; mid-face depression; epicanthic folds; Brushfield spots; brachycephaly	Short hands; clinodactyly of 5th finger; four-finger line in palm	Hypotonia; loose skin on back of neck	+	+	21 Trisomy
Dubowitz syndrome	Small facies; lateral displacement of inner canthi; ptosis; broad nasal bridge; sparse hair; microcephaly		Infantile eczema; high-pitched hoarse voice	±	++	? Autosomal recessive

Syndrome			Craniofacial/primary features	Skeletal/other features	Associated features	Inheritance
Fetal alcohol syndrome	+	+	Short palpebral fissures; midfacial hypoplasia; microcephaly		± Cardiac defect, fine motor dysfunction	
Fetal hydantoin syndrome (Dilantin)	±	±	Hypertelorism; short nose; occasional cleft lip	Hypoplastic nails, especially 5th	Cardiac defect	
Goldenhar syndrome			Malar hypoplasia; macrostomia; micrognathia; epibulbar dermoid and/or lipodermoid; malformed ear with preauricular tags	± Vertebral anomalies		?
Incontinentia pigmenti		±	± Dental defect; deformities of ears; ± Patchy alopecia		Irregular skin pigmentation in fleck, whorl, or spidery form	? Dom. X-linked ? Lethal in males
Laurence-Moon-Biedl syndrome		+	Retinal pigmentation	Polydactyly; syndactyly	Obesity; seizures; hypogenitalism	Autosomal recessive
Linear nevus sebaceus syndrome		+	Nevus sebaceus, face or neck		+— Seizures	?
Lowe syndrome (oculocerebrorenal syndrome)		+	Cataract		Renal tubular dysfunction	X-linked recessive
Möbius syndrome (congenital facial diplegia)		±	Expressionless facies; ocular palsy	± Clubfoot; syndactyly	Hypotonia	?
Neurofibromatosis		±	± Optic gliomas; acoustic neuromas	± Bone lesions; pseudarthroses	Neurofibromas; café-au-lait spots; seizures	Autosomal dominant
Noonan syndrome		±	Webbing of posterior neck; malformed ears; hypertelorism	Pectus excavatum; cubitus valgus	Cryptorchidism; pulmonic stenosis	?
Prader-Willi syndrome		+	± Upward slant to palpebral fissures	Small hands and feet	Hypotonia, especially in early infancy; then polyphagia and obesity; hypogenitalism	?
Robin complex			Micrognathia; glossoptosis; cleft palate, U-shaped		± Cardiac anomalies	?
Rubella syndrome		±	Cataract; retinal pigmentation; ocular malformations		Sensorineural deafness; patent ductus arteriosus	
Rubinstein-Taybi syndrome		+	Slanting palpebral fissures; maxillary hypoplasia; microcephaly	Broad thumbs and toes	Abnormal gait	?
Seckel syndrome		+	Facial hypoplasia; prominent nose; microcephaly	Multiple minor joint and skeletal abnormalities		Autosomal recessive
Sjögren-Larsson syndrome		+	Spasticity, especially of legs		Ichthyosis	Autosomal recessive

Table 4 *continued*

Syndrome	Diagnostic Manifestations			Mental Retardation	Short Stature	Genetic Transmission
	Craniofacial	Skeletal	Other			
Smith-Lemli-Opitz syndrome	Anteverted nostrils and/or ptosis of eyelid	Syndactyly of 2nd and 3rd toes	Hypospadias; cryptorchidism	+	+	Autosomal recessive
Sturge-Weber syndrome	Flat hemangioma of face, most commonly trigeminal in distribution		Hemangiomas of meninges with seizures	±		?
Treacher Collins syndrome (mandibulofacial dysostosis)	Malar and mandibular hypoplasia; downslanting palpebral fissures; defect or lower eyelid; malformed ears					Autosomal dominant
Trisomy 18	Microstomia; short palpebral fissures; malformed ears; elongated skull	Clenched hand, 2nd finger over 3rd; low arches on fingertips; short sternum	Cryptorchidism; congenital heart disease	+	+	Trisomy 18
Trisomy 13	Defects of eye, nose, lip, ears, and forebrain of holoprosencephaly type	Polydactyly; narrow hyperconvex fingernails	Skin defects, posterior scalp	+	+	Trisomy 13
Tuberous sclerosis	Hamartomatous pink to brownish facial skin nodules	± Bone lesions	Seizures; intracranial calcification	±		Autosomal dominant
Waardenburg syndrome	Lateral displacement of inner canthi and puncta		Partial albinism; white forelock; heterochromia of iris; vitiligo; +/- deafness			Autosomal dominant
Williams syndrome	Full lips; small nose with anteverted nostrils; iris dysplasia	Mild hypoplasia of nails	± Hypercalcemia in infancy; supravalvular aortic stenosis	+	+	?
Zellweger cerebrohepatorenal syndrome	High forehead; flat facies		Hypotonia; hepatomegaly; death in early infancy	+	+	Autosomal recessive

*Table by Syzmanski L, Crocker A, and adapted from Smith D W: Patterns of malformation. In *Nelson Textbook of Pediatrics*, ed 11. V C Vaughan III, R J McKay Jr, R E Behrman, editors, p. 2035. Saunders, Philadelphia, 1979.

impaired or nonexistent. Their coordination is poor, and they have many perceptual difficulties.

This disease was previously diagnosed on the basis of a urine test: phenylpyruvic acid in the urine reacts with ferric chloride solution to yield a vivid green color. However, this test has its limitations, as it may not detect the presence of phenylpyruvic acid in urine before the baby is 5 or 6 weeks old, and it may give positive responses with other aminoacidurias. Currently, a more reliable screening test that is widely used is the Guthrie inhibition assay, which uses a bacteriological procedure to detect blood phenylalanine.

Early diagnosis is important, as a low phenylalanine diet, in use since 1955, significantly improves both behavior and developmental progress. The best results seem to be obtained with early diagnosis and the start of dietary treatment before the child is 6 months of age.

Dietary treatment is not without risk, however. Phenylalanine is an essential amino acid, and its omission from the diet may lead to such severe complications as anemia, hypoglycemia, edema, and even death. Dietary treatment of PKU can often be discontinued at the age of 5 or 6 years, although no alternative metabolic pathway capable of keeping the blood phenylalanine levels in the normal range has yet been discovered. Children who are diagnosed before the age of 3 months and are placed on an optimal dietary regimen may have normal intelligence. For untreated older children and adolescents with PKU, a low phenylalanine diet will not influence the level of mental retardation. However, the diet will decrease their irritability and abnormal EEG changes and will increase their social responsiveness and attention span.

The parents of PKU children and some of these children's normal siblings are heterozygous carriers. The disease can be detected by a phenylalanine tolerance test, which may be important to the genetic counseling of these people.

Maple Syrup Urine Disease (Menkes' Disease)

The clinical symptoms of Menkes' disease appear during the first week of life. The infant deteriorates rapidly and develops decerebrate rigidity, seizures, respiratory irregularity, and hypoglycemia. If untreated, most patients die in the first months of life, and the survivors are severely retarded. Some variants have been reported, with transient ataxia and only mild retardation.

Treatment follows the general principles established for PKU and consists of a diet very low in the three involved amino acids—leucine, isoleucine, and valine.

Other Enzyme Deficiency Disorders

Several enzyme deficiency disorders associated with mental retardation have been identified, and still more diseases are being added as new discoveries are made. Some of these include Hartnup disease, galactosemia, and glycogen storage diseases. Thirty important syndromes with inborn errors of metabolism, hereditary transmission patterns, defective enzymes, clinical signs, and relationship to mental retardation, are listed in Table 5.

ACQUIRED CHILDHOOD DISEASES

Occasionally a child's developmental status changes dramatically as a result of a specific disease or physical trauma. In retrospect, it is sometimes difficult to ascertain the full normalcy of the child's developmental progress before the insult, but the adverse effects on the child's development or loss of skills undoubtedly have a new origin.

Infection

The most serious infections affecting cerebral integrity are encephalitis and meningitis. Measles encephalitis has been virtually eliminated by the universal use of measles vaccine, and the incidences of other bacterial infections of the central nervous system have been markedly reduced with antibacterial agents. Most episodes of encephalitis are caused by viral organisms. It is sometimes necessary to assess retrospectively a probable encephalitic component in a past obscure illness that had high fever and lasting encephalopathy. Meningitis that was diagnosed late and followed by antibiotic treatment or obstructive complications can seriously affect a child's cognitive development. Thrombotic and purulent intracranial phenomena secondary to septicemia are rarely seen today, except in small infants.

Head Trauma

The most well-known causes of head injury in children that produce developmental handicaps, including seizures, are motor vehicle accidents. More head injuries, however, are caused by household accidents, such as falls from tables, from open windows, or on stairways. Child abuse is also a cause of head injury.

Other Issues

Brain damage from cardiac arrest during anesthesia is rare. One cause of complete or partial decortication is asphyxia associated with near-drowning. Chronic exposure to lead is a well-established cause of compromised intelligence and learning skills. Intracranial tumors of various types and origins, in themselves or from the effects of surgery and chemotherapy, can also adversely affect brain function.

ENVIRONMENTAL AND SOCIOCULTURAL INFLUENCES

It is well known that mild retardation is significantly more prevalent among persons of culturally deprived, lower socioeconomic classes and that many of the family members or relatives are affected with similar degrees of mental retardation. No biological causes have been identified in these cases.

In any case, it is clear that children in poor, socioculturally deprived families are subjected to potentially pathogenic and developmentally adverse conditions. The prenatal environment is compromised by poor medical care and poor maternal nutrition. Teenage pregnancies are frequent and are associated with obstetrical complications, prematurity, and low birth weight. Poor postnatal medical care, malnutrition, exposure to such toxic substances as lead, and physical traumata are frequent. Family instability, frequent moves, and multiple but inadequate caretakers are common. Furthermore, the mothers in such families are often poorly educated and ill equipped to give the child appropriate stimulation.

Another unresolved issue is the influence of severe parental mental illness. It has been hypothesized that such illness adversely affects the child's care and stimulation and other aspects of the environment, thus putting the child at a developmental risk. Chil-

Table 5
Thirty Important Syndromes with Inborn Errors of Metabolism*

Name of Disorder		Hereditary Transmission†	Enzyme Defect	Prenatal Diagnosis	Mental Retardation	Clinical Signs
I. LIPID METABOLISM						
Niemann-Pick disease						
Group A/infantile		A.R.	Sphingomyelinase	+	±	Hepatosplenomegaly
Group B/adult			Unknown	–	+	Pulmonary infiltration
Groups C and D/ intermediate						
Infantile Gaucher disease		A.R.	β-Glucosidase	+	±	Hepatosplenomegaly, pseudobulbar palsy
Tay-Sachs disease		A.R.	Hexosaminidase A	+	+	Macular changes, seizures, spasticity
Generalized gangliosidosis		A.R.	β-Galactosidase	+	+	Hepatosplenomegaly, bone changes
Krabbe disease		A.R.	Galactocerebroside β-Galactosidase	+	+	Stiffness, seizures
Metachromatic leukodystrophy		A.R.	Cerebroside sulfatase	+	+	Stiffness, developmental failure
Wolman disease		A.R.	Acid lipase	+	–	Hepatosplenomegaly, adrenal calcification, vomiting, diarrhea
Farber lipogranulomatosis		A.R.	Acid ceramidase	+	+	Hoarseness, arthropathy, subcutaneous nodules
Fabry disease		X.R.	α-Galactosidase	+	+	Angiokeratomas, renal failure
II. MUCOPOLYSACCHARIDE METABOLISM						
Hurler's syndrome	MPS I	A.R.	Iduronidase	+	+	Varying degrees of bone changes, hepatosplenomegaly, joint restriction, etc.
Hunter's disease	II	X.R.	Iduronate sulfatase	+	+	
Sanfilippo disease	III	A.R.	Various sulfatases (types A-D)	+	+	
Morquio disease	IV	A.R.	N-Acetylgalactosamine-6-sulfate sulfatase	+	–	
Maroteaux-Lamy disease	VI	A.R.	Arylsulfatase B	+	±	
III. OLIGOSACCHARIDE AND GLYCOPROTEIN METABOLISM						
I-cell disease		A.R.	Glycoprotein N-acetylglucosaminylphosphotransferase	+	+	Hepatomegaly, bone changes, swollen gingivae
Mannosidosis		A.R.	Mannosidase	+	+	Hepatomegaly, bone changes, facial coarsening
Fucosidosis		A.R.	Fucosidase	+	+	Same as above

IV. AMINO ACID METABOLISM

Disorder	Transmission	Enzyme/defect			Clinical features
Phenylketonuria	A.R.	Phenylalanine hydroxylase	−	−	Eczema, blonde hair, musty odor
Homocystinuria	A.R.	Cystathionine β-synthetase	+	+	Ectopia lentis, Marfan-like phenotype, cardiovascular anomalies
Tyrosinosis	A.R.	Tyrosine amine transaminase	−	+	Hyperkeratotic skin lesions, conjunctivitis
Maple syrup urine disease	A.R.	Branched chain ketoacid decarboxylase	+	+	Recurrent ketoacidosis
Methylmalonic acidemia	A.R.	Methyl malonyl-CoA mutase	+	+	Recurrent ketoacidosis, hepatomegaly, growth retardation
Propionic acidemia	A.R.	Propionyl-CoA carboxylase	+	+	Same as above
Nonketotic hyperglycinemia	A.R.	Glycine cleavage enzyme	+	+	Seizures
Urea cycle disorders	A.R. mostly	Urea cycle enzymes	+	+	Recurrent acute encephalopathy, vomiting
Hartnup disorder	A.R.	Renal transport disorder	−	−	None consistent

V. OTHERS

Disorder	Transmission	Enzyme/defect			Clinical features
Galactosemia	A.R.	Galactose-1-phosphate uridyltransferase	−	+	Hepatomegaly, cataracts, ovarian failure
Wilson hepatolenticular degeneration	A.R.	Unknown factor in copper metabolism	−	±	Liver disease, Kayser-Fleischer ring, neurologic problems
Menkes kinky-hair disease	X.R.	Same as above	+	−	Abnormal hair, cerebral degeneration
Lesch-Nyhan disease	A.R.	Hypoxanthine guanine phosphoribosyltransferase	+	+	Behavioral abnormalities

*Table by Syzmanski L, Crocker A, and adapted from Leroy J 3: Heredity, development, and behavior. In *Developmental-Behavioral Pediatrics*, Levine et al., editors, p. 315. Saunders, Philadelphia, 1983.
†A.R. = autosomal recessive transmission. X.R. = x-linked recessive transmission.

dren of parents with affective disorder and schizophrenia are known to be at risk for developing these or related disorders. Recent studies also suggest a higher prevalence among these children of motor and other developmental delays, but not necessarily frank retardation.

MENTAL DISORDERS AND MENTAL RETARDATION

Personality and Behavioral Patterns

The most common misconception among professionals and the general public has been the belief that mentally retarded persons are a behaviorally homogeneous group. In fact, retarded persons display more personality styles and behaviors than do the nonretarded. For example, a mildly retarded individual who is living independently with some supervision and who is partially self-supporting has more in common with a nonretarded co-worker than with a profoundly retarded person who is totally dependent on others' care. Another misconception is the belief that the maladaptive behaviors of retarded persons are the result of mental retardation and organicity rather than their life experiences.

All behaviors and personality patterns exhibited by retarded persons are seen also in nonretarded persons. However, certain behavioral patterns may be expected to be more frequently associated with mental retardation because of retarded persons' cognitive and other deficits and life experiences. Egocentricity and concreteness of thinking are often seen in retarded persons and are related to cognitive deficits, particularly difficulties in concept formation and abstract thinking.

Organicity, that is, definite neurological abnormalities, usually cannot be readily linked to behavioral patterns, especially in mildly or moderately impaired persons. Such neurological abnormalities are more common in profoundly retarded individuals. They might be associated with motor hyperactivity and short attention span. Contrary to another misconception, aggressive behavior is not organically based and is not an especially common behavioral feature of retarded individuals.

Environmental and experiential influences are probably the main factors responsible for the retarded individuals' behavior. Impersonal, dehumanizing, and understaffed custodial institutions have been the most pathogenic in this respect. The institution staff often rewards passivity, compliance, and lack of initiative. Some individuals, however, thrive on the staff's negative attention, which they can elicit through inappropriate behaviors, including aggression. Overprotection by care-givers, especially parents, is often responsible for the retarded individual's dependency, low frustration tolerance, sense of inadequacy, and low self-esteem.

Vulnerability to Mental Disorders

Negative self-image and low self-esteem are probably almost universal personality features of retarded persons, particularly the mildly or moderately retarded. They are well aware of being different from others, of not meeting their parents' and society's expectations, and of progressively falling behind their peers and even their younger siblings.

Defenses against an intolerable sense of inadequacy, low self-

image, and anxiety may often be maladaptive and pathological and may lead to inappropriate behavior. Some retarded adolescents or young adults may thus resort to delinquency and aggressive behaviors.

The conflict between the expected self-image and the real self-image may be a source of lifelong stress and anxiety among mildly retarded individuals who are aware of their handicap. Prolonged dependence on care and support from others prevents most retarded individuals from developing a self-image as a separate person and, in a sense, prevents true separation-individuation. Communication difficulties further increase such persons' vulnerability to feeling inadequate and frustrated. Inappropriate behaviors such as aggression or withdrawal are common. The low self-esteem of mildly or moderately retarded individuals may predispose them to depression.

No reliable data are available on the incidence of psychiatric disorders in mentally retarded persons, mainly because of methodological difficulties. However, several reports indicate a very high risk of psychiatric illness in such persons, with the incidence ranging from 40 percent to 75 percent.

Among mildly and moderately retarded adults, the most frequent diagnoses are adjustment disorders, mood disorders, and psychoses; and among children, these are mood disorders, anxiety disorders, and pervasive developmental disorders.

DIAGNOSIS

History

In most cases, the history from the parents and primary caretaker is the only source of information about the retarded person, and so every effort and caution should be taken to ensure its accuracy. The history of the pregnancy, labor, and delivery, the consanguinity of the parents, and the presence of hereditary disorders in their families deserve particular attention. The parents may also provide information about the child's developmental milestones. This area is especially subject to distortions because of parental bias and anxiety. A history is particularly helpful in assessing the emotional climate of the family and their sociocultural background, which are important to the evaluation of clinical findings.

Psychiatric Interview

Two factors are of paramount importance when interviewing the patient: the interviewer's attitude and the manner of communication with the patient. The interviewer should not be guided by the patient's mental age, as it cannot fully characterize the person. A mildly retarded adult with a mental age of 10 is not a 10-year-old child. When addressed as if they were children, some retarded individuals become justifiably insulted, angry, and uncooperative. More passive and dependent individuals, on the other hand, may assume the child's role that they think is expected of them. In both cases, no valid diagnostic data can be obtained.

The patient's verbal abilities, including receptive and expressive language, should be assessed as soon as possible from observing verbal and nonverbal communication between the care-givers and the patient and also from the history. In this regard, it is often helpful first to see the patient and the care-givers together. If the patient uses sign language, the care-giver may have to stay during the interview as an interpreter.

Retarded individuals have the lifelong experience of failing in many areas, and they may be quite anxious before seeing an interviewer. The interviewer and the care-giver should attempt to give such patients a clear, supportive, and concrete explanation of the diagnostic process, particularly those patients with sufficient receptive language. Giving patients the impression that their bad behavior is the cause for the referral should be avoided. Support and praise should be offered in language appropriate to the patient's age and understanding. Leading questions should be avoided, as retarded individuals may be suggestible and wish to please others. Subtle directiveness, structure, and reinforcements may be necessary to keep them on the task or topic.

The child's control over motility patterns should be ascertained, and clinical evidence of distractibility and distortions in perception and memory may be evaluated. The use of speech, reality testing, and the ability to generalize from experiences are important to note.

The nature and the maturity of the child's defenses—particularly exaggerated or self-defeating uses of avoidance, repression, denial, introjection, and isolation—should be observed. Sublimation potential, frustration tolerance, and impulse control—especially over motor, aggressive, and sexual drives—should be assessed. Also important are self-image and its role in the development of self-confidence, as well as the assessment of tenacity, persistence, curiosity, and the willingness to explore the unknown.

In general, the psychiatric examination of the retarded child should reveal how the child has coped with the stages of personality development. In regard to failure or regression, it is possible to develop a personality profile that allows the logical planning of management and remedial approaches.

Physical Examination

Various parts of the body may have certain characteristics that are commonly found in the mentally retarded and have prenatal causes. For example, the configuration and the size of the head offer clues to a variety of conditions, such as microcephaly, hydrocephalus, and Down's syndrome. The patient's face may have some of the stigmata of mental retardation, which greatly facilitate the diagnosis. Such facial signs are hypertelorism, a flat nasal bridge, prominent eyebrows, epicanthal folds, corneal opacities, retinal changes, low-set and small or misshapen ears, a protruding tongue, and a disturbance in dentition. Facial expression, such as dull appearance, may be misleading and should not be relied on without other supporting evidence. The color and the texture of the skin and hair, a high-arched palate, the size of the thyroid gland, and the size of the child and his or her trunk and extremities are further areas to be explored. The circumference of the head should be measured as part of the clinical investigation.

Dermatoglyphics or the handprinting patterns may offer another diagnostic tool, as uncommon ridge patterns and flexion creases are often found in retarded children. Abnormal dermatoglyphics may be found in chromosomal disorders and in children who were infected prenatally with rubella. Table 5 lists the multiple handicaps associated with the syndromes discussed.

Neurological Examination

When neurological abnormalities are present, their incidence and severity generally rise in inverse proportion to the degree of retardation. That is, many severely retarded children have no neurological abnormalities, but conversely, about 25 percent of all children with cerebral palsy have normal intelligence.

Disturbances in motor areas are manifested in abnormalities of muscle tone (spasticity or hypotonia), reflexes (hyperreflexia), and involuntary movements (choreoathetosis). A smaller degree of disability in this area is revealed in clumsiness and poor coordination.

Sensory disturbances may include hearing difficulties, ranging from cortical deafness to mild hearing deficits. Visual disturbances may range from blindness to disturbances of spatial concepts, design recognition, and concept of body image.

The infants with the poorest prognosis are those who manifest a combination of inactivity, general hypotonia, and exaggerated response to stimuli. In older children, hyperactivity, short attention span, distractibility, and a low frustration tolerance are often hallmarks of brain damage.

In general, the younger the child is at the time of investigation, the more caution is indicated in predicting future ability, as the recovery potential of the infantile brain is very good. Following the child's development at regular intervals is probably the most reliable approach.

A pneumoencephalogram is somewhat hazardous and rarely used in the evaluation for mental retardation and has been replaced by CT scans. The occasional findings of internal hydrocephalus, cortical atrophy, or porencephaly in a severely retarded, brain-damaged child are not considered important to the general picture.

Skull x-rays are usually taken routinely but are illuminating only in a relatively few conditions, such as craniosynostosis, hydrocephalus, and others that result in intracranial calcifications (e.g., toxoplasmosis, tuberous sclerosis, cerebral angiomatosis, and hypoparathyroidism).

An electroencephalogram (EEG) is best interpreted with caution in cases of mental retardation. The exceptions are patients with hypsarrhythmia or grand mal seizures, in whom the EEG may help establish the diagnosis and suggest treatment. In most other conditions, a diffuse cerebral disorder produces nonspecific EEG changes, characterized by slow frequencies with bursts of spikes and sharp or blunt wave complexes. The confusion over the significance of the EEG in the diagnosis of mental retardation is best illustrated by the reports of frequent EEG abnormalities in Down's syndrome, which range from 25 percent to the majority of patients examined.

Laboratory Tests

Laboratory tests include examination of the urine and the blood for metabolic disorders. Enzymatic abnormalities in chromosomal disorders, particularly Down's syndrome, promise to become useful diagnostic tools. The determination of the karyotype in a suitable genetic laboratory is indicated whenever a chromosomal disorder is suspected.

Hearing and Speech Evaluations

Hearing and speech evaluations should be done routinely. The development of speech may be the most reliable criterion in investigating mental retardation. Various hearing impairments are often present in the mentally retarded; however, in some instances, the impairments may simulate mental retardation. Unfortunately, the commonly used methods of hearing and speech evaluation require the patient's cooperation and thus are often unreliable in the severely retarded.

Psychological Assessment

Examining physicians may use several screening instruments for infants and toddlers. As in many areas of mental retardation, there is a heated controversy over the predictive value of infant psychological tests. The correlation of abnormalities during infancy with later abnormal functioning is reported by some as very low and by others as very high. It is generally agreed that the correlation rises in direct proportion to the age of the child at the time of the developmental examination.

Copying geometric figures, the Goodenough Draw-a-Person Test, the Kohs Block Test, and geometric puzzles all may be used as a quick screening test of visual-motor coordination.

Psychological testing, performed by an experienced psychologist, is a standard part of an evaluation for mental retardation. The Gesell, Bayley, and Cattell tests are most commonly used with infants. For children, the Stanford–Binet and the Wechsler Intelligence Scale for Children are the most widely used in this country. Both tests have been criticized for penalizing the culturally deprived child, for testing mainly potential for academic achievement rather than for adequate social functioning, and for their unreliability in children with I.Q.s of less than 50. Some people have tried to overcome the language barrier of the mentally retarded by devising picture vocabulary tests, of which the Peabody Vocabulary Test is the most widely used.

The tests often found useful in detecting brain damage are the Bender–Gestalt and the Benton Visual Retention tests. These tests are also useful for mildly retarded children. In addition, a psychological evaluation should assess perceptual, motor, linguistic, and cognitive abilities. Information about motivational, emotional, and interpersonal factors is also important.

DIFFERENTIAL DIAGNOSIS

Children who come from deprived homes that provide inadequate stimulation may manifest motor and mental retardation that can be reversed if an enriched, stimulating environment is provided in early childhood. A number of sensory handicaps, especially deafness and blindness, may be mistaken for mental retardation if, during testing, no compensation for the handicap is allowed. Speech deficits and cerebral palsy often make a child seem retarded, even in the presence of borderline or normal intelligence.

Chronic, debilitating diseases of any kind may depress the child's functioning in all areas. Convulsive disorders may give an impression of mental retardation, especially in the presence of uncontrolled seizures.

Chronic brain syndromes may result in isolated handicaps, failure to read (alexia), failure to write (agraphia), failure to communicate (aphasia), and several others that may exist in a person of normal and even superior intelligence.

In children with specific developmental disorders, there is a delay or failure of development in a specific area, such as reading or language, but the children develop normally in other areas. In contrast, children with mental retardation show general delays in many areas of develoment.

A pervasive developmental disorder is manifested as distortions in the timing, rate, and sequence of many basic psychological functions necessary to the development of social skills and language. Also present are severe qualitative abnormalities that are not normal for any stage of development. In mental retardation, however, generalized delays in development are present, and such children behave as if they were passing through an earlier normal developmental stage. Mental retardation may coexist with specific developmental disorders and frequently with pervasive developmental disorders.

The most controversial differential diagnostic problem concerns children with severe retardation, brain damage, early infantile autism, childhood schizophrenia, and, according to some, Heller's disease. The confusion stems from the fact that details of the child's early history are often unavailable or unreliable, and when they are evaluated, many children with these conditions display similar bizarre and stereotyped behavior, mutism, or echolalia, and they function on a retarded level. By the time these children are usually seen, it does not matter from a practical point of view whether the child's retardation is secondary to a primary early infantile autism or schizophrenia, or whether the personality and behavioral distortions are secondary to brain damage or retardation. When ego functions are delayed in development or are atrophic on any other basis, the physician must first concentrate on overcoming the child's unrelatedness. The child must be reached before remedial educational measures can be successful.

TREATMENT

Mental retardation is associated with several heterogeneous groups of disorders and a multitude of psychosocial factors. The best treatment of mental retardation is the preventive medicine model of primary, secondary, and tertiary prevention.

Primary Prevention

Primary prevention refers to efforts and actions taken to eliminate or reduce the factors and conditions that lead to the development of the disorders associated with mental retardation. Such measures include (1) education to increase the general public's knowledge and awareness of mental retardation, (2) continuing efforts of health professionals to ensure and upgrade public health policies, (3) legislation to provide optimal maternal and child health care, and (4) the eradication of the known disorders associated with central nervous system damage. Family and genetic counseling will help reduce the incidence of mental retardation in a family with a history of a genetic disorder with mental retardation. For the children and mothers of low socioeconomic status, proper prenatal and postnatal medical care and various supplementary enrichment programs and social service assistance may help minimize medical and psychosocial complications.

Secondary and Tertiary Prevention

Once a disorder or condition associated with mental retardation has been identified, the disorder should be treated so as to shorten the course of the illness (secondary prevention) and to minimize the sequelae or consequent handicaps (tertiary prevention).

Hereditary metabolic or endocrine disorders, such as PKU and hypothyroidism, can be effectively treated in an early stage by dietary control or hormone replacement therapy.

Mentally retarded children frequently develop emotional and behavioral difficulties requiring psychiatric treatment. These children's limited cognitive and social capabilities require modified psychiatric treatment modalities based on the children's level of intelligence. Play therapy and opportunities for social group interaction often may help them express their inner conflicts.

Behavior therapy, especially positive reinforcement, has proved effective in modifying certain maladaptive behaviors. Occasionally, psychotropic medication can help remove or modify certain target behavioral symptoms, such as hyperactive and impulsive behavior, anxiety, or depression.

The parents need continuous counseling or, if indicated, family therapy. The parents should be allowed opportunities to express their feelings of guilt, despair, anguish, recurring denial, and anger regarding the child's disorder and future. The psychiatrist should be prepared to give the parents all the basic and current medical information regarding the etiology, treatment, and other pertinent areas (e.g., special training and correction of sensory defects).

References

Chess S, Hassibi M: *Principles and Practice of Child Psychiatry.* ed 2. p 296. Plenum, New York, 1986.

Crocker A C: Current strategies in prevention of mental retardation. Pediat Ann *11*:450, 1982.

Crocker A C, Cushna B: Ethical considerations and attitudes in the field of developmental disorders. In *Developmental Disorders: Evaluation, Treatment and Education,* Johnston R B, Magrab P R, editors, p. 495. University Park Press, Baltimore, 1976.

Crocker A C, Nelson, R P: Mental retardation. In *Developmental-Behavioral Pediatrics,* M D Levine, W B Carey, A C Crocker, R T Gross, editors, p 756. Saunders, Philadelphia, 1983.

Edgerton B R, Bollinger M, Herr B: The cloak of competence: After two decades. Am J Ment Defic *88*:345, 1984.

Frankenburg W F: Infant and preschool developmental screening. In *Developmental-Behavioral Pediatrics,* M D Levine, W B Carey, A C Crocker, R T Gross: editors, p 927. Saunders, Philadelphia, 1983.

Menolascino F J, editor: *Psychiatric Approaches to Mental Retardation.* Basic Books, New York, 1970.

Pueschel S M, Rynders J E, editors: *Down Syndrome: Advances in Biomedicine and Behavioral Sciences.* Ware Press, Cambridge, MA, 1982.

Ruedrich S C, Wadle C V, Sallach H S, Hahn R K, Menolascino F J: Adrenocortical function and depressive illness in mentally retarded patients. Am J Psych *144*:597, 1987.

Stack L S, Haldipur D V, Thompson M: Stressful life events and psychiatric hospitalization of mentally retarded patients. Am J Psych *144*:661, 1987.

Syzmanski L S, Tanguay P E, editors: *Emotional Disorders of Mentally Retarded Persons.* University Park Press, Baltimore, 1980.

Wolfensberger W: *The Principle of Normalization in Human Services.* National Institute on Mental Retardation, Toronto, 1972.

34

Pervasive Developmental Disorders

DEFINITION

Pervasive developmental disorder was first officially recognized in DSM-III as a distinct childhood psychiatric disorder group in 1980. The later DSM-III-R classification recognizes only one subgroup of the general category pervasive developmental disorders, namely, autistic disorder, also known as infantile autism and Kanner's syndrome.

These disorders present clinical features of distortions, deviations, or delays in attention, perception, reality testing, and the development of social, language, and motor behaviors. Autistic disorder is characterized by behavioral abnormalities and includes three major clusters of developmental and behavioral diagnostic criteria: (1) impairments in reciprocal social interaction, (2) impairments in communication and imaginative activity, and (3) a markedly restricted repertoire of activities and interests. In diagnosing autistic disorder, DSM-III-R requires specifying the age at onset of autistic disorder: infantile (before 36 months) childhood (after 36 months), or age unknown or not otherwise specified.

The category of pervasive developmental disorder not otherwise specified is reserved for the diagnosis of cases that meet the general description of a pervasive developmental disorder but not the specific criteria for autistic disorder. The DSM-III-R criteria for the diagnoses of autistic disorder and pervasive developmental disorder not otherwise specified (NOS) are presented in Tables 1 and 2, respectively.

AUTISTIC DISORDER

Historical Overview

Henry Maudsley (1867) was the first psychiatrist who paid serious attention to very young children with severe mental disorders involving a marked deviation, delay, and distortion in the developmental processes. Initially, all such disorders were considered "psychoses." In 1943, Leo Kanner, in his classic paper *Autistic Disturbances of Affective Contact* coined the term "infantile autism" and provided a clear and comprehensive account of the early childhood syndrome. He described children who exhibited "extreme autistic aloneness," failure to assume an anticipatory posture, delayed or deviant language development with echolalia

and pronominal reversal (using "you" for "I"), monotonous repetitions of noises or verbal utterances, excellent rote memory, limited range in the variety of spontaneous activities, stereotypies and mannerisms, "anxiously obsessive desire for the maintenance of sameness" and a "dread of change and incompleteness," and abnormal relationships with people and a preference for pictures or inanimate objects. Kanner suspected the syndrome to be more frequent than it seemed and suggested that some of these children had been confused with mentally retarded or schizophrenic children.

There has been confusion about whether infantile autism was the earliest possible manifestation of schizophrenia or a discrete clinical entity, but the evidence points toward establishing infantile autism and schizophrenia as separate entities.

Epidemiology

Prevalence.   Autistic disorder occurs at a rate of 4 to 5 cases per 10,000 children (or 0.04 to 0.05 percent) under age 12 or 15, with a much higher rate among children with a maternal history of rubella infection during pregnancy, thereby producing mental retardation. If severe mental retardation with some autistic features is included, the rate can rise as high as 20 per 10,000. In most cases, autism begins before 36 months but may not be evident to parents, depending on their awareness and the severity of the disease.

Sex Distribution.   Infantile autism is found more frequently in boys. Three to five times more boys than girls have autism. But autistic girls tend to be more seriously affected and more likely to have a family history of cognitive impairment.

Social Class.   Early studies suggested that a higher socioeconomic status was common in families with autistic children; however, those findings were probably based on referral biases. Over the past 20 years, an increasing proportion of cases have been found in the lower socioeconomic classes. This may well be due to an increased awareness of the syndrome and the increased availability of child mental health workers for such individuals.

Etiology and Pathogenesis

Autistic disorder is a developmental behavioral syndrome that is currently considered to have multiple causes.

Table 1
Diagnostic Criteria for Autistic Disorder

At least eight of the following sixteen items are present, these to include at least two items from A, one from B, and one from C.

Note: Consider a criterion to be met *only* if the behavior is abnormal for the person's developmental level.

A. Qualitative impairment in reciprocal social interaction as manifested by the following:

(The examples within parentheses are arranged so that those first mentioned are more likely to apply to younger or more handicapped, and the later ones, to older or less handicapped, persons with this disorder.)

(1) marked lack of awareness of the existence or feelings of others (e.g., treats a person as if he or she were a piece of furniture; does not notice another person's distress; apparently has no concept of the need of others for privacy)

(2) no or abnormal seeking of comfort at times of distress (e.g., does not come for comfort even when ill, hurt, or tired; seeks comfort in a stereotyped way, e.g., says "cheese, cheese, cheese" whenever hurt)

(3) no or impaired imitation (e.g., does not wave bye-bye; does not copy mother's domestic activities; mechanical imitation of others' actions out of context)

(4) no or abnormal social play (e.g., does not actively participate in simple games; prefers solitary play activities; involves other children in play only as "mechanical aids")

(5) gross impairment in ability to make peer friendships (e.g., no interest in making peer friendships; despite interest in making friends, demonstrates lack of understanding of conventions of social interaction, for example, reads phone book to uninterested peer)

B. Qualitative impairment in verbal and nonverbal communication, and in imaginative activity, as manifested by the following:

(The numbered items are arranged so that those first listed are more likely to apply to younger or more handicapped, and the later ones, to older or less handicapped, persons with this disorder.)

(1) no mode of communication, such as communicative babbling, facial expression, gesture, mime, or spoken language

(2) markedly abnormal nonverbal communication, as in the use of eye-to-eye gaze, facial expression, body posture, or gestures to initiate or modulate social interaction (e.g., does not anticipate being held, stiffens when held, does not look at the person or smile when making a social approach, does not greet parents or visitors, has a fixed stare in social situations)

(3) absence of imaginative activity, such as playacting of adult roles, fantasy characters, or animals; lack of interest in stories about imaginary events

(4) marked abnormalities in the production of speech, including volume, pitch, stress, rate, rhythm, and intonation (e.g., monotonous tone, questionlike melody, or high pitch)

(5) marked abnormalities in the form or content of speech, including stereotyped and repetitive use of speech (e.g., immediate echolalia or mechanical repetition of television commercial); use of "you" when "I" is meant (e.g., using "You want cookie?" to mean "I want a cookie"); idiosyncratic use of words or phrases (e.g., "Go on green riding" to mean "I want to go on the swing"); or frequent irrelevant remarks (e.g., starts talking about train schedules during a conversation about sports)

(6) marked impairment in the ability to initiate or sustain a conversation with others, despite adequate speech (e.g., indulging in lengthy monologues on one subject regardless of interjections from others)

C. Markedly restricted repertoire of activities and interests, as manifested by the following:

(1) stereotyped body movements, e.g., hand-flicking or twisting, spinning, head-banging, complex whole-body movements

(2) persistent preoccupation with parts of objects (e.g., sniffing or smelling objects, repetitive feeling of texture of materials, spinning wheels of toy cars) or attachment to unusual objects (e.g., insists on carrying around a piece of string)

(3) marked distress over changes in trivial aspects of environment, e.g., when a vase is moved from usual position

(4) unreasonable insistence on following routines in precise detail, e.g., insisting that exactly the same route always be followed when shopping

(5) markedly restricted range of interests and a preoccupation with one narrow interest, e.g., interested only in lining up objects, in amassing facts about meteorology, or in pretending to be a fantasy character

D. Onset during infancy or childhood.

Specify if childhood onset (after 36 months of age).

Table from DSM-III-R, *Diagnostic and Statistical Manual of Mental Disorders,* ed 3, revised. (Current Classification of Mental Disorders, 1987.) Copyright American Psychiatric Association, Washington, D.C., 1987. Used with permission.

Both psychodynamic theories and organic theories of causation have been postulated. The current evidence indicates that there are usually significant biological abnormalities underlying the disorder.

Psychodynamic and Family Causation. In his initial report, Kanner noted that few parents of autistic children were "really warmhearted" and that for the most part, the parents and other family members were preoccupied with intellectual abstractions and tended to express little genuine interest in their children. This finding, however, has not been replicated over the past 40 years. Other theories, such as parental rage and rejection and parental reinforcement of autistic symptoms, have also not been substantiated. Recent studies comparing parents of autistic children with parents of normal children have not shown significant differences in infant- and child-rearing skills. There has been no satis-

Table 2
Diagnostic Criteria for Pervasive Developmental Disorder Not Otherwise Specified

This category should be used when there is a qualitative impairment in the development of reciprocal social interaction and of verbal and nonverbal communication skills, but the criteria are not met for Autistic Disorder, Schizophrenia, or Schizotypal or Schizoid Personality Disorder. Some people with this diagnosis will exhibit a markedly restricted repertoire of activities and interests, but others will not.

Table from DSM-III-R, *Diagnostic and Statistical Manual of Mental Disorders*, ed 3, revised. (Current Classification to Mental Disorders, 1987.) Copyright American Psychiatric Association, Washington, D.C., 1987. Used with permission.

factory evidence that any particular kind of deviant family functioning or psychodynamic constellation of factors leads to the development of autistic disorder.

Organic-Neurological-Biological Abnormalities. Autistic children show more evidence of perinatal complications than do comparison groups of normal children or those with other disorders. Perinatal stress seems to increase the risk of developing infantile autism. The finding that autistic children have significantly more minor congenital physical anomalies than do their siblings or normal controls suggests that complications of pregnancy in the first trimester are significant. Four to 32 percent of autistics will develop grand mal seizures at some point in life, and about 20 to 25 percent of autistics show ventricular enlargement on computed tomography scans. Various EEG abnormalities are found in 10 percent to 83 percent of autistic children, and although there is no EEG finding specific to infantile autism, there is some indication of failed cerebral lateralization.

Biochemical Abnormalities. Elevated serum serotonin levels are found in about one third of autistic children; however, these levels are also raised in about one third of nonautistic children with severe mental retardation. In a small sample of patients, a significant correlation was found between high serotonin blood levels and a decrease in cerebrospinal fluid 5-hydroxyindoleacetic acid (5-HIAA). Also, the main serotonin metabolite 5-hydroxy-N, N-dimethyltryptamine (bufotenine) was found in the urine of autistics and their families, but not in controls.

Genetic Studies. Approximately 2 percent of siblings of autistics are afflicted by infantile autism, a rate 50 times greater than in the general population. The concordance rate for autism in monozygotic pairs is 35 percent, whereas the concordance rate in dizygotic pairs is zero. Clinical reports and studies suggest that the nonautistic members of these families share various language or other cognitive problems with the autistic person, but they are less severe.

Clinical Description

Physical Characteristics

Appearance. Kanner was struck by autistic children's intelligent and attractive appearance. They also tend to be shorter between the ages of 2 and 7 than is the normal population.

Handedness. There is a failure of lateralization in most autistic children because of a developmental lag. That is, they remain ambidextrous at an age when cerebral dominance is established in normal children. There is also a greater incidence of abnormal dermatoglyphics (e.g., fingerprints) than in the general population which may suggest a disturbance in neuroectodermal development.

Intercurrent physical illness. There is a higher incidence of upper respiratory infections, excessive burping, febrile seizures, constipation, and loose bowel movements in younger autistic children than in controls. Many autistic children react differently to illness than do normal children, which may reflect an immature or abnormal autonomic nervous system. In addition, autistic children may not develop an elevated temperature with infectious illness, may not complain of pain either verbally or by gesture, and may not show the malaise of an ill child. Interestingly, their behavior and relatedness may improve to a noticeable degree when they are ill, and in some cases this may be a clue to physical illness.

Behavioral Characteristics

Failure to develop relatedness (autism). All autistic children fail to develop the usual relatedness to their parents and other people. As infants, many lack a social smile and anticipatory posture for being picked up as an adult approaches. Abnormal eye contact is a common finding. The social development of autistic children is characterized by a lack of attachment behavior and a relatively early failure of person-specific bonding. These children often do not seem to recognize or differentiate the most important people in their lives—parents, siblings, or teachers. And they may show virtually no separation anxiety upon being left in an unfamiliar environment with strangers.

When they have reached school age, autistic children's withdrawal may have diminished or not be as obvious, particularly in the better-functioning children. Instead, their failure to play with peers and to make friends, social awkwardness and inappropriateness, and, particularly, failure to develop empathy are observed.

In late adolescence, those autistics who make the most progress often have a desire for friendships. However, their ineptness of approach and inability to respond to other's interests, emotions, and feelings are major obstacles in developing friendships. Autistic adolescents and adults generally have ordinary sexual feelings, but their lack of social competence and skills prevent most of them from developing a sexual relationship. It is extremely rare for autistics to get married.

Disturbances of communication and language. Gross deficits and deviances in language development are among the principal criteria for diagnosing infantile autism. Autistic children are not simply reluctant to speak, and their speech abnormalities are not due to lack of motivation. Language deviance as much as language delay is characteristic of autistic disorder. In contrast with normal or mentally retarded children, autistic children make little use of "meaning" in their memory and thought processes. When autistic individuals do learn to converse fluently, they lack social competence, and their conversations are not characterized by reciprocal responsive interchanges.

In the first year of life, the autistic child's amount and pattern of babbling may be reduced or abnormal. Some children emit noises (e.g., clicks, sounds, screeches, or nonsense syllables) in a stereotyped fashion with no seeming intent at communication.

Unlike normal young children, who always have better receptive language skills and understand much before they can speak, verbal autistic children usually say more than they understand.

Words or even entire sentences may drop in and out of a child's vocabulary. Such children may use a word once and then not use it again for a week, month, or years. Their speech is usually in the form of echolalia, both immediate or delayed, or stereotyped phrases out of context. These abnormalities are often associated with pronominal reversal; that is, the child asks "Do you want the toy?" when he means he wants it. Difficulties in articulation are also noted. Use of peculiar voice quality and rhythm are observed clinically in many cases. About 50 percent of autistic children never develop useful speech. Some of the brighter children show a particular fascination with letters and numbers. A few literally teach themselves to read at preschool age, often astonishingly well. In virtually all cases, however, these children read without any comprehension whatsoever.

Abnormalities in play. In the first years of an autistic child's life, much of the normal child's exploratory play is absent or minimal. Toys and objects are often manipulated differently from their intended use. Play tends to be stereotyped, nonfunctional, and nonsocial. Play patterns are rigid and limited, with little variety, creativity, and imagination and few symbolic features. Autistic children cannot imitate or use abstract pantomime.

Stereotypies and ritualistic behaviors, insistence on sameness, and resistance to change. The activities and play, if any, of the autistic child are rigid, repetitive, and monotonous. Ritualistic and compulsive phenomena are common and, in early and middle childhood, usually take the form of rigid and ritualized routines. They often spin, bang, and line up objects and become attached to inanimate objects. In addition, many autistic children, particularly those who are more intellectually impaired, exhibit various abnormalities of movements. Stereotypies, mannerisms, and grimacing are more frequent when the child is left alone and may decrease when placed in a structured situation. Autistic children are resistant to transition and change. Moving to a new house, moving furniture in a room, and serving breakfast before bath, when the reverse was the routine, may result in panic or temper tantrums.

Responses to sensory stimuli. Autistic children may be overresponsive or underresponsive to sensory stimuli (e.g., to sound or pain). They may selectively ignore spoken language directed at them, and so they are often thought to be deaf. However, they may show unusual interest in the sound of a wristwatch. Many have a diminished pain threshold or an altered response to pain. Indeed, these children may injure themselves rather severely and not cry.

Many autistic children seem to enjoy music. They frequently will hum a tune or sing a song or commercial before saying words or using speech. Some particularly enjoy vestibular stimulation—spinning, swinging, or up and down movements.

Other behavioral symptoms. Hyperkinesis is a common behavior problem in young autistic children. Hypokinesis is less frequent, and when present, it often alternates with hyperactivity. Aggressiveness and temper tantrums are observed, often for no apparent reason, or are prompted by change or demands. Self-injurious behavior includes head banging, biting, scratching, and hair pulling. Short attention span, or a complete inability to focus on a task, insomnia, feeding and eating problems, enuresis, and encopresis are also frequent.

Intellectual Functioning. About 40 percent of the children with infantile autism have I.Q. scores below 50 to 55 (moderate, severe, or profound retardation); 30 percent have scores of 50 to approximately 70 (mild retardation); and 30 percent have scores 70 or more. Epidemiological and clinical studies show that the risk of autism increases as the I.Q. decreases. About one fifth of autistic children have a normal nonverbal intelligence. The I.Q. scores of autistic children tend to show problems with verbal sequencing and abstraction skills rather than with visuospatial or rote memory skills, suggesting the importance of defects in language-related functions.

Unusual or precocious cognitive or visuomotor abilities are present in some autistic children. These may exist even within the overall retarded functioning and are referred to as "splinter functions" or "islets of precocity." Perhaps the most striking examples are the idiot-savants who have prodigious rote memories or calculating abilities. Here, the specific abilities usually remain beyond the capabilities of normal peers. Other precocious abilities in young autistic children include an early ability to read well (although they are not able to understand what they read), memorizing and reciting, or musical abilities (singing tunes or recognizing different musical pieces).

Differential Diagnosis

The major differential diagnoses are childhood onset of schizophrenic disorder; mental retardation with behavioral symptoms; developmental language disorder, receptive type; congenital deafness or severe hearing disorder; psychosocial deprivation; and disintegrative (regressive) psychoses.

Because children with a pervasive developmental disorder usually have many concurrent problems, Michael Rutter suggested a stepwise approach to use in the differential diagnosis (Table 3).

Childhood Onset of Schizophrenic Disorder. Whereas there is a wealth of literature on infantile autism, there are only few data on children under age 12 who meet the DSM-III-R criteria for schizophrenic disorder. Childhood schizophrenia is rare under the age of 5. It is accompanied by hallucinations or delusions, with a lower incidence of seizures and mental retardation and a more even I.Q. than that of autistics.

Mental Retardation with Behavioral Symptoms. About 40 percent of autistic children are moderately, severely, or profoundly retarded, and retarded children may have behavioral symptoms that include autistic features. DSM-III-R states that when both disorders are present, both should be diagnosed. The main differentiating features between autistic disorder and mental retardation are that (1) mentally retarded children usually relate to adults and other children in accordance with their mental age; (2) they use the language they do have to communicate with others; and (3) they have a relatively even profile of retardedness without splinter functions.

Developmental Language Disorder: Receptive Type. There is a subgroup of children who have autistic-like features and may present a diagnostic problem. Table 4 summarizes the major differences.

Acquired Aphasia with Convulsion. Acquired aphasia with convulsion is a rare condition and is sometimes difficult to differentiate from autistic disorder or disintegrative psychosis.

Table 3
Procedure for Differential Diagnosis on a Multiaxial System

1. Determine intellectual level
2. Determine level of language development
3. Consider whether child's behavior is appropriate for
   (i) chronological age
   (ii) mental age
   (iii) language age
4. If not appropriate, consider differential diagnosis of psychiatric disorder according to
   (i) pattern of social interaction
   (ii) pattern of language
   (iii) pattern of play
   (iv) other behaviors
5. Identify any relevant medical conditions
6. Consider whether there are any relevant psychosocial factors

From Rutter M, Hersov L: *Child and Adolescent Psychiatry: Modern Approaches.* ed 2. Blackwell Scientific Publications, Oxford, London, Edinburgh, 1985. Used with permission.

Table 4
Infantile Autism vs. Developmental Language Disorder: Receptive Type

Criteria	Infantile Autism	Developmental Language Disorder
Incidence	2–4 in 10,000	5 in 10,000
Sex ratio (M:F)	3–4:1	Equal or almost equal sex ratio
Family history of speech delay or language problems	Present in about 25% of cases	
Associated deafness	Very infrequent	Not infrequent
Nonverbal communication (gestures, etc.)	Absent or rudimentary	Present
Language abnormalities (e.g., echolalia, stereotyped phrases out of context)	More common	Less common
Articulatory problems	Less frequent	More frequent
Level of intelligence	Often severely impaired	Though may be impaired, less frequently severe
Patterns of I.Q. tests	Uneven, lower on verbal scores than dysphasics; lower on comprehension subtest than dysphasics	More even, though verbal I.Q. lower than performance I.Q.
Autistic behaviors, impaired social life, stereotypies and ritualistic activities	More common and more severe	Absent or, if present, less severe
Imaginative play	Absent or rudimentary	Usually present

From Campbell M, Green W H: Pervasive developmental disorders of childhood. In *Comprehensive Textbook of Psychiatry*, ed 4, p 1681. H I Kaplan and B J Sadock, editors. Williams & Wilkins, Baltimore, 1985.

Children with this condition develop normally for several years before losing both their receptive and expressive language over a period of weeks or months. Most of them develop a few seizures and generalized EEG abnormalities at the onset, which usually do not persist. A profound disorder of language comprehension then follows, characterized by a deviant speech pattern and speech impairment. Some children recover, but with considerable residual language impairment.

Congenital Deafness or Severe Hearing Impairment. Because autistic children often are mute or show a selective disinterest in spoken language in infancy, they are often thought to be deaf. The following may be differentiating features: Autistic children may babble only infrequently, whereas deaf infants have a history of relatively normal babbling which then gradually tapers off and may stop from 6 months to 1 year of age.

Deaf children respond only to loud sounds, whereas autistic children may ignore loud or normal sounds and respond to soft or low sounds. Most importantly, audiogram or auditory evoked potentials indicate significant hearing loss in deaf children. Unlike autistic children, deaf children usually relate to their parents, seek their affection, and, as infants, enjoy being held.

Psychosocial Deprivation. Severe disturbances in the physical and emotional environment (e.g., maternal deprivation, psychosocial dwarfism, hospitalism, or failure to thrive) can cause children to appear apathetic, withdrawn, and alienated. Language and motor skills can be delayed. These children almost always rapidly improve when placed in a favorable and enriched psychosocial environment, which is not the case with an autistic child.

Disintegrative (Regressive) Psychoses. The disintegrative psychoses usually begin between ages 3 and 5 years.

These conditions are even rarer than is infantile autism. The child's development in these disorders is usually within normal limits until the onset of illness, when there is severe regression and decline in intelligence and all areas of behavior, accompanied by stereotypies and mannerisms. The illness progresses over a period of a few months. It may follow a mild illness or a known viral infection. In others, a lipoidosis, leukodystrophy, or Heller's disease (dementia infantilis) is found at autopsy.

Prognosis and Outcome

Autistic disorder has a chronic course and a guarded prognosis. As a general rule, the autistic children with higher I.Q.s (above 70) and those who use communicative language by ages 5 to 7 have the best prognosis. Adult outcome studies indicate that approximately two thirds of autistic individuals remain severely handicapped and live in complete or semidependence, either with their relatives or in long-term institutions. Only 1 or 2 percent acquire a normal and independent status with gainful employment, and 5 to 20 percent achieve a borderline normal status. The prognosis is improved if the environment or home is supportive and capable of meeting the excessive needs of such a child.

Although a decrease of symptoms is noted in many cases, severe self-mutilation or aggressiveness and regression may develop in others. Approximately 4 to 32 percent develop grand mal seizures in late childhood or adolescence, and these adversely affect the prognosis.

Treatment of Autistic Disorder

The goals of treatment are to decrease behavioral symptoms and to aid in the development of delayed, rudimentary, or nonexistent functions, such as language and self-care skills. In addition, the parents, often distraught, need support and counseling.

Insight-oriented individual psychotherapy has proved ineffective. Educational and behavioral methods are currently considered to be the treatments of choice.

Structured classroom training in combination with intrusive behavioral methods is the most effective treatment method for many autistic children and is superior to other types of behavioral approaches. Well-controlled studies indicate that gains in the areas of language and cognition, as well as decreases in maladaptive behaviors, are achieved using this method. Careful training and individual tutoring of parents in the concepts and skills of behavior modification, and the resolution of parents' problems and concerns, within a problem-solving format, may yield considerable gains in the child's language, cognitive, and social areas of behavior. However, the training programs are rigorous and require a great deal of the parents' time. The autistic child requires as much structure as possible, and a daily program for as many hours as feasible is desirable.

Although no drug has been proven specific to autistic disorder, psychopharmacotherapy is a valuable adjunct to comprehensive treatment programs. Administration of haloperidol (Haldol) both reduces behavioral symptoms and accelerates learning. The drug decreases hyperactivity, stereotypies, withdrawal, fidgetiness, abnormal object rela-

tions, irritability, and labile affect. There is supportive evidence that when used judiciously, haloperidol remains an effective long-term drug. Under careful clinical monitoring, tardive and withdrawal dyskinesias are not frequent, and in the studies to date, they always have been reversible.

Fenfluramine, a drug with antiserotonergic properties, has been reported to decrease behavioral symptoms and reduce autistism, pending clinical validation of the reported efficacy in a large number of autistic children.

PERVASIVE DEVELOPMENTAL DISORDER NOT OTHERWISE SPECIFIED

Pervasive developmental disorder not otherwise specified should be diagnosed when a child manifests a qualitative impairment in the development of reciprocal social interaction and verbal and nonverbal communication skills but does not meet the criteria for autistic disorder, schizophrenia, or schizotypal or schizoid personality disorder. Some children with this diagnosis may often exhibit a markedly restricted repertoire of activities and interests. This condition usually shows a better outcome than does autistic disorder.

Treatment of Pervasive Developmental Disorder NOS

These children require a broad ego-educative approach that helps the development of particular adaptive skills. Behavior therapy is effective in altering specific behaviors, including social interactions and responses, self-mutilative behavior, imitative behavior, and communication.

The major tranquilizers have been used to influence specific behaviors of such children—for example, chlorpromazine for reducing hyperactivity, and trifluoperazine for overcoming marked apathy and hypoactivity. However, drugs have not generally been shown to be effective in reversing the global state of a child with a pervasive developmental disorder or with childhood schizophrenia or in improving the outcome of the life course. Allopurinol combined with a low purine diet in patients manifesting hyperuricosuria has been useful in some cases.

The therapeutic program should delineate the child's specific failures in the development and organization of thought, feeling, and social response and try to improve his or her skills in each area of adaptive failure. The psychotherapy itself must try to improve the child's language, thought, and social response before it can proceed to issues of inner emotional and motivational conflict.

Educating these children requires clear-cut objectives and a structured therapeutic design throughout the day, every day, and for long periods of time. Casual, irregular, or infrequent adult contacts with such children are ineffective. Help for the children and their families should be provided as early as possible.

Changes in therapeutic setting may also be profitable. Thus, residential or inpatient care and separation from the family may be used for varying periods of time. Day treatment and specialized schooling may be helpful at other times.

Table 5
Infantile Autism vs. Schizophrenic Disorder

Criteria	Infantile Autism	Schizophrenic Disorder (with onset before puberty)
Age of onset	Before 36 months	Not under 5 years of age
Incidence	2–4 in 10,000	Unknown, possibly same or even rarer
Sex ratio (M:F)	3–4:1	1.67:1 (nearly equal, or slight preponderance of males)
Family history of schizophrenia	Not raised or probably not raised	Raised
Social class	Overrepresentation of upper classes (artifact)	More common in lower classes
Pre- and perinatal complications and cerebral dysfunction	More common in autism	
Behavioral characteristics	Failure to develop relatedness; absence of speech or echolalia; stereotyped phrases; language comprehension absent or poor; insistence on sameness and stereotypies	Hallucinations and delusions; thought disorder
Adaptive functioning	Usually always impaired	Deterioration in functioning
Level of intelligence	In majority of cases subnormal, frequently severely impaired (70% ≤ 70)	Usually within normal range, mostly dull normal (15% ≤ 70)
Pattern of I.Q.	Marked unevenness	More even
Grand mal seizures	4–32%	Absent or lower incidence

From Campbell M, Green W H: Pervasive developmental disorders of childhood. In *Comprehensive Textbook of Psychiatry*, ed 4, p 1680. H I Kaplan and B J Sadock, editors. Williams & Wilkins, Baltimore, 1985.

SCHIZOPHRENIA WITH ONSET IN CHILDHOOD

There is much evidence to establish schizophrenia as a separate entity. Profound disturbances in very young children are expressed in a limited number of ways. A small subgroup of autistic children may be early-onset schizophrenics who have not yet reached the developmental stages at which the symptoms necessary to diagnose schizophrenic disorder can be expressed. A few cases have been reported of children who, at a young age, fulfilled the criteria for infantile autism and, when older, fit the diagnostic criteria for schizophrenia, with the possible exception of lack of deterioration from a previous level of functioning.

According to DSM-III-R, schizophrenia occurring in childhood is manifested by oddities of behavior, typically hallucinations, delusions, and loosening of associations or incoherence. Hallucinations and delusions exclude the diagnosis of autistic disorder. Moreover, during some phase of the illness, schizophrenia always involves deterioration from a previous level of functioning in such areas as work, social relations, and self-care.

Schizophrenia must be differentiated from infantile autism (Table 5). The majority of autistic children are impaired in all areas of adaptive functioning, from early life onward. The onset is always before the age of 3 years, whereas the onset of schizophrenic disorder is usually in adolescence or young adulthood. There are practically no reports of an onset of schizophrenia before the age of 5 years, but children under the age of 12 can be diagnosed as having schizophrenia.

References

Anderson L T, Campbell M, Grega D M, Perry R, Small A M, Green W H: Haloperidol and infantile autism: Effects on learning and behavior symptoms. Am J Psychiatry *141*:123, 1984.

DeMyer M K, Hintgen J N, Jackson R K: Infantile autism reviewed: A decade of research. Schizo Bull 7:388, 1981.

Fish B, Ritvo E R: Psychoses of childhood. In *Basic Handbook of Child Psychiatry*, vol 2, J D Noshpitz, editor, p 249. Basic Books, New York, 1979.

Folstein S, Rutter M: Infantile autism: A genetic study of 21 twin pairs. J Child Psychiatry *18*:297, 1977.

Green W H, Campbell M, Hardesty A S, Grega D M, Padron-Gayol M, Shell J, Erlenmeyer-Kimling L: A comparison of schizophrenic and autistic children. J Am Acad Child Psychiatry *23*:399, 1984.

Hermelin B: Coding and the sense modalities. In *Early Childhood Autism: Clinical, Education and Social Aspects*, ed 2. L Wing, editor, p 35, Pergamon, Oxford, England, 1976.

Ritvo E R, Freeman B J, Geller E, Yuwiler A: Effects of fenfluramine on 14 outpatients with the syndrome of autism. J Am Acad Child Psychiatry *22*:549–558, 1983.

Rutter M: Cognitive defects in the pathogenesis of autism. J Child Psychol Psychiatry *24*:513, 1983.

Rutter M: Infantile autism and other pervasive developmental disorders. In *Childhood Adolescent Psychiatry: Modern Approaches*, ed 2. M Rutter, L Hersov, editors, p 545. Blackwell Scientific Publications, Oxford, England, 1985.

Rutter M: The treatment of autistic children. J Child Psychol Psychiatry *26*:193, 1985.

35

Specific Developmental Disorders

35.1

Developmental Arithmetic Disorder

INTRODUCTION

Developmental arithmetic disorder is one of the academic skills disorders contained in the DSM-III-R category of specific developmental disorders. In the past, this disorder had been known by various terms: acalculia, Gerstmann's syndrome, congenital arithmetic disability, dyscalculia, and arithmetic disorder.

DEFINITION

Developmental arithmetic disorder has the following clinical characteristics and criteria: The individual's performance in daily activities requiring arithmetic skills is markedly below his or her intellectual capacity and these impaired arithmetic skills and performance are confirmed by an individually administered standardized test (Table 1).

According to DSM-III-R, there are a number of different types of skills that may be impaired in developmental arithmetic disorder, including linguistic skills (such as understanding or naming mathematical terms, understanding or naming mathematical operations or concepts, and translating written problems into mathematical symbols), perceptual skills (such as recognizing or reading numerical symbols or arithmetic signs and clustering objects into groups), attention skills (such as copying figures correctly, remembering to add in "carried" numbers, and observing operational signs), and mathematical skills (such as following sequences of mathematical steps, counting objects, and learning multiplication tables).

EPIDEMIOLOGY

The prevalence of developmental arithmetic disorder is not known, but the disorder is less common than is developmental reading disorder. The ratio of the disorder between boys and girls is unknown as well. It is commonly accepted that some children are born with exceptionally gifted mathematical talents and display advanced mathematical competence from early childhood. This view suggests that persons may be born with an inability to learn arithmetic skills.

ETIOLOGY

The cause of developmental arithmetic disorder is not known. An early theory proposed a neurological deficit in the right cerebral hemisphere, particularly in the occipital lobe areas. These regions are responsible for processing visual-spatial stimuli which, in turn, are responsible for mathematical skills. However, the validity of this theory has not been supported in subsequent neuropsychiatric studies.

The current view on etiology is multifactorial. Maturational, cognitive, emotional, educational and socioeconomic factors account in varying degrees and combinations for developmental arithmetic disorder.

CLINICAL FEATURES

Most children with developmental arithmetic disorder can be diagnosed during the second and third grade in elementary school. The affected child's performance in handling basic number concepts, such as counting or adding even one-digit numbers, is significantly below the age-expected norms, whereas the child shows normal intellectual skills in other areas.

During the first two or three years of elementary school, a child with developmental arithmetic disorder may appear to make some progress in mathematics by relying on rote memory. But soon, as arithmetic progresses into more complex and higher levels requiring discrimination and manipulation of spatial and numerical relationships, the presence of the disorder becomes conspicuous.

Some investigators have classified arithmetic disorder into several subcategories: (1) difficulty in learning to count meaningfully, (2) difficulty in mastering cardinal and ordinal systems, (3) difficulty in performing arithmetic operations, and (4) difficulty in envisioning clusters of objects as groups. In addition, there may be difficulties in associating auditory and visual symbols, understanding the conservation of quantity, remembering sequences of arithmetic steps, and choosing principles for problem-solving activities. Children with these problems are, however, presumed to have good auditory and verbal abilities.

Table 1
Diagnostic Criteria for Developmental Arithmetic Disorder

A. Arithmetic skills, as measured by a standardized, individually administered test, are markedly below the expected level, given the person's schooling and intellectual capacity (as determined by an individually administered IQ test).

B. The disturbance in A significantly interferes with academic achievement or activities of daily living requiring arithmetic skills.

C. Not due to a defect in visual or hearing acuity or a neurologic disorder.

Table from DSM-III-R, *Diagnostic and Statistical Manual of Mental Disorders,* ed 3, revised. (Current Classification of Mental Disorders, 1987.) Copyright American Psychiatric Association, Washington, D.C., 1987. Used with permission.

The relationship between developmental arithmetic disorder and other language and academic skills disorders is not yet clear. Although children with developmental language disorder, receptive or expressive, are not necessarily affected by developmental arithmetic disorder, the two conditions may often coexist, as they are associated in terms of sharing impairments in both coding and encoding processes.

Some children with developmental arithmetic disorder may also have reading and spelling difficulties. Children with cerebral palsy may have developmental arithmetic disorder with normal overall intelligence.

Associated features include delayed developmental milestones, academic difficulties in nonarithmetic areas, and secondary behavioral or emotional problems. Other features include developmental receptive language disorder, developmental reading disorder, developmental expressive writing disorder, developmental coordination disorder, and memory and attention deficits. Often, younger grade-school children with arithmetic disorder present these associated features as their chief complaints. Such children should be evaluated to determine whether developmental arithmetic disorder is indeed the primary difficulty or the associated feature of another developmental disorder.

COURSE AND PROGNOSIS

Developmental arithmetic disorder is usually apparent by the time the child is 8-years-old (third grade). In some children the disorder is apparent as early as 6 years (first grade), and in others it may not occur until age 10 (fifth grade) or later. Thus far, not much systematic study data have been available to present clear patterns of developmental and academic progress of children who were diagnosed with this disorder in early school grades. However, untreated children with a moderate developmental arithmetic disorder or those children whose arithmetic difficulties cannot be resolved by intensive remedial interventions may develop complications, which include continuing academic difficulties, poor self-concept, depression, and frustration. These may then lead to a reluctance to attend school, outright truancy, or a conduct disorder.

DIAGNOSIS

In a typical case of developmental arithmetic disorder, a careful inquiry into school performance history will reveal the child's earlier difficulties with arithmetic subjects. The definite diagnosis can be made only after the child takes an individually administered standardized arithmetic test and scores markedly below the expected level, considering the child's schooling and intellectual capacity as measured by a standardized intelligence test. A pervasive developmental disorder or mental retardation should also be ruled out before confirming the primary diagnosis of developmental arithmetic disorder. Attention deficit disorder and conduct disorder may be associated with arithmetic problems, and in these cases, both diagnoses should be made.

DIFFERENTIAL DIAGNOSIS

Arithmetic difficulties seen in mental retardation will be accompanied by a generalized impairment in overall intellectual functioning. In unusual cases of mild mental retardation, arithmetic skills may be significantly below the expected level, given the person's schooling and level of mental retardation. In such cases, the additional diagnosis of developmental arithmetic disorder should be made, as treatment of the arithmetic difficulties can be particularly helpful to the child's chances for employment in adulthood. Inadequate schooling, however, can often cause the child's poor arithmetic performance on a standardized arithmetic test. If so, it is likely that most of the other children in the same class will have similarly poor arithmetic performances. Conduct disorder and attention-deficit hyperactivity disorder may be present with developmental arithmetic disorder and should be ruled out as the primary condition.

TREATMENT

The current most effective treatment for developmental arithmetic disorder is remedial educational intervention. Controversy continues as to the comparative effectiveness of various remedial educational treatments. However, the current consensus is that the treatment methods and materials are useful only when they fit the particular child, the subtype of the disorder, and the severity and feasibility of the particular teaching plans. Project MATH, a multimedia self-instructional or group-instructional in-service training program, has been found to be successful for certain children with developmental arithmetic disorder. Poor coordination may accompany the disorder, so physical therapy and sensory integration activities may be helpful.

References

Badian N A: Dyscalculia and nonverbal disorders of learning. In *Progress in Learning Disabilities,* vol 5, H R Myklebust, editor, p 235. Grune & Stratton, New York, 1983.

Johnson D, Myklebust H: *Learning Disabilities: Educational Principles and Practices.* Grune & Stratton, New York, 1967.

Kosc L: Neuropsychological implications of diagnoses and treatment of mathematical learning disabilities. Top Lang Learn Disord *1*:19, 1981.

McCleod T M, Crump W D: The relationship of visuospatial skills and verbal ability to learning disabilities in mathematics. J Learn Dis *11*:237, 1978.

McEntire E: Learning disabilities and mathematics. Top Learn Learn Disabil *1*:1, 1981.

Rourke B P, Strang J D: Subtypes of reading and arithmetic disabilities: A neuropsychological analysis. In *Developmental Neuropsychiatry*, M Rutter, editor, p 473. Guilford Press, New York, 1983.

Yule W, Lansdown R, Urbanowicz M: Predicting educational attainment for WISC-R in a primary school sample. Brit J Psychol *21*:43, 1982.

35.2 _____
Developmental Expressive Writing Disorder

INTRODUCTION

The ability to transfer one's thoughts into written words and sentences requires multimodal sensory-motor coordination and information processing. Developmental expressive writing disorder—as do other academic skills disorders—affects a child's academic competence from fairly early in grade school, through high school, and eventually to adulthood, when the disorder irreversibly jeopardizes the affected individual's access to most of the more gainful and intellectually productive occupations.

Developmental expressive writing disorder is a new diagnostic entity in DSM-III-R. Clinically, it is viewed as a distinct and specific developmental disorder.

DEFINITION

DSM-III-R defines developmental expressive writing disorder as an academic skills disorder first occurring during childhood, characterized by poor performance in writing and composition (spelling words and expressing thoughts), considering the level of the person's schooling and intellectual capacity. That level is measured by a standardized test on which the person scores below the expected level.

This disorder is not due to a defect in visual or hearing acuity or a neurological disorder (Table 1). Rather, this diagnosis is made only if the impairment significantly interferes with academic achievement or with activities of daily living that require expressive writing skills.

EPIDEMIOLOGY

No precise figures about the prevalence of developmental expressive writing disorder are available. However, the clinical features of this disorder are frequently manifested by individuals who also have an expressive or receptive language disorder or a reading disorder. There appears to be no difference in the incidence rate between males and females. There are some indications that affected persons are more frequently from families with a history of this disorder among its members.

ETIOLOGY

Developmental expressive writing disorder is a new disorder that has received research attention only recently. Its etiology is not known. Psychiatrists are becoming more aware of and interested in this disorder because of the adverse consequences that affected individuals suffer as a result of expressive writing incompetence.

One etiological hypothesis holds that developmental expressive writing disorder results from the combined effects of one or more of the following disorders: developmental expressive language disorder, developmental receptive language disorder, and developmental reading disorder. This view suggests the possible existence of neurological and cognitive defects or malfunction somewhere in the central information-processing areas.

Hereditary predisposition of the disorder has been suggested based on empirical findings that most children with developmental expressive writing disorder have relatives with the disorder.

Temperamental characteristics may play some role in developmental expressive writing disorder, especially such characteristics as short attention span and easy distractibility.

CLINICAL FEATURES

Children with developmental expressive writing disorder present difficulties very early in grade school, in spelling words and expressing their thoughts according to age-appropriate grammatic norms. Their spoken and written sentences contain an unusually large number of grammatical errors or poor paragraph organization. During and after the second grade, these children commonly make simple grammatical errors in writing a short sentence. For example, they frequently fail, despite constant reminders, to start the first letter of the first word in a sentence with a capital letter and to end a sentence with a period.

As they grow older and progress toward higher grades in school, such children's spoken and written sentences be-

Table 1

Diagnostic Criteria for Developmental Expressive Writing Disorder

A. Writing skills, as measured by a standardized, individually administered test, are markedly below the expected level, given the person's schooling and intellectual capacity (as determined by an individually administered IQ test).

B. The disturbance in A significantly interferes with academic achievement or activities of daily living requiring the composition of written texts (spelling words and expressing thoughts in grammatically correct sentences and organized paragraphs).

C. Not due to a defect in visual or hearing acuity or a neurologic disorder.

Table from DSM-III-R, *Diagnostic and Statistical Manual of Mental Disorders*, ed 3, revised. (Current Classification of Mental Disorders, 1987.) Copyright American Psychiatric Association, Washington, D.C., 1987. Used with permission.

come more conspicuously primitive, odd, and inferior to those of their expected grade level: Their word choices are erroneous and inappropriate; their paragraphs are disorganized and not in proper sequence; and their ability to spell correctly becomes increasingly more difficult as their vocabulary becomes more abstract and larger in number and characters.

Associated features of developmental expressive writing disorder include refusal or reluctance to go to school and to do assigned written homework, poor academic performance in other areas (e.g., mathematics), general disinterest in school work, truancy, and conduct disorder.

Most children with this disorder become frustrated and angry over their feelings of inadequacy and failure in their academic performance. They may thus develop a chronic depression as a result of their growing sense of isolation, estrangement, and despair.

Adults with developmental expressive writing disorder who do not receive remedial intervention continue to have difficulties in social adaptation involving writing skills, as well as a continuing sense of incompetence, inferiority, isolation, and estrangement. Some of them even try to avoid or procrastinate writing a response letter or a simple greeting card for fear that their writing incompetence may be exposed. When their coping mechanism fails, the severity of psychopathology is likely to be increased. Most of them choose occupations that require minimal writing skills, such as in trade, custodianship, or other menial work; seldom do they achieve or hold a socially desirable occupational position requiring a high level of expressive writing. Common associated disorders are developmental reading disorder, developmental expressive and receptive language disorder, developmental arithmetic disorder, developmental coordination disorder, and disruptive behavior disorders.

COURSE AND PROGNOSIS

In severe cases, the disorder is apparent by age 7 (second grade); in less severe cases, the disorder may not be apparent until age 10 (fifth grade) or later. Most individuals with mild and moderate developmental expressive writing disorder fare rather well if they receive timely remedial educational intervention early in grade school. Severe developmental expressive writing disorder requires continuing extensive remedial treatment through the late part of high school and even into college.

The prognosis depends on the severity of the disorder, the age or grade when the remedial intervention was started, the length and continuity of treatment, and the presence or absence of associated or secondary emotional or behavioral problems.

Those individuals who later become well compensated or who completely recover from developmental expressive writing disorder are usually from families of favorable socioeconomic backgrounds.

DIAGNOSIS

The diagnosis is made on the basis of the individual's consistently poor performance on the composition of written text. Performance is markedly below the individual's intellectual capacity, as confirmed by an individually administered standardized expressive writing test. The presence of a major disorder, such as pervasive developmental disorder or mental retardation, obviates the diagnosis of developmental expressive writing disorder. Other disorders to be differentiated from developmental writing disorder are developmental expressive and receptive language disorders, reading disorder, and impaired vision and hearing.

Dyslexia is characterized by an inability to read, and dysgraphia by an inability to write. From a diagnostic procedural viewpoint, it is important that any person suspected of having developmental expressive writing disorder first be given a standardized intelligence test, such as the Revised Wechsler Intelligence Scale for Children (WISC-R) or the Revised Wechsler Adult Intelligence Scale (WAIS-R), in order to determine his or her intellectual capacity before administering a standardized expressive writing test.

TREATMENT

The best treatment to date is remedial educational intervention. Although controversy continues as to the effectiveness of various remedial expressive writing modalities, an intensive and continuous administration of individually tailored one-to-one expressive and creative writing therapy appears to show the most favorable treatment outcomes.

The treatment of this disorder requires an optimal patient–therapist relationship, as in psychotherapy. The success or failure in sustaining the patient's motivation greatly affects the treatment's long-term efficacy.

Associated and secondary emotional and behavioral problems should be given prompt attention, with appropriate psychiatric treatment and parental counseling.

References

Johnson D, Myklebust H: *Learning Disabilities: Educational Principles and Practices.* Grune & Stratton, New York, 1967.
Orton S: *Reading, Writing, and Speech Problems in Children.* Norton, New York, 1937.
Persell C H: *Education and Inequality: A Theoretical and Empirical Synthesis.* Free Press, New York, 1977.
Weiss C E, Lillywhite H S: *Communicative Disorders: Prevention and Early Intervention.* Mosby, St. Louis, 1981.

35.3 ——————
Developmental Reading Disorder

INTRODUCTION

Developmental reading disorder, which involves delay and impairment in reading competence, has been referred to by various and, at times, confusing terms: alexia, dyslexia, developmental reading disorder, reading backwardness, learning disability, specific reading disability, and developmental word blindness. Despite decades of research effort, there still is controversy about the disorder's pathogenesis, nature, and effective treatment.

DEFINITION

Developmental reading disorder is characterized by a marked impairment in the development of word recognition skills and reading comprehension that cannot be explained by mental retardation or inadequate schooling and that is not due to a visual or hearing defect or a neurological disorder. According to DSM-III-R, the diagnosis should be made only if this impairment significantly interferes with academic achievement or with activities of daily living that require reading skills. This disorder is also referred to as dyslexia.

EPIDEMIOLOGY

It is estimated that 2 to 8 percent of school-age children in the United States are affected by this disorder. Developmental reading disorder is two to four times more common in boys than in girls. In the adult form (reading backwardness or reading retardation), there is no difference in incidence between males and females.

ETIOLOGY

Developmental reading disorder tends to be more prevalent among family members than in the general population, leading to the speculation that the disorder may have a genetic origin. However, family and twin studies have not supplied definitive evidence to support this theory.

Studies in the 1930s attempted to explain developmental reading disorder with the cerebral hemispheric function model, which suggested positive correlations of reading disorder with left-handedness, left-eyedness, or mixed laterality. But subsequent epidemiological studies did not find any consistent association between reading disorder and laterality of handedness or eyedness. However, right-left confusion has been shown to be associated with reading difficulties. The reversal of cerebral asymmetry may result in the transference of language lateralization to a cerebral hemisphere that is less differentiated to accommodate language function, thereby leading to a developmental reading disorder.

There tends to be a high incidence of developmental reading disorder among children with cerebral palsy who are of normal intelligence. A slightly increased incidence of developmental reading disorder is also seen among epileptic children. Complications during pregnancy, prenatal and perinatal difficulties including prematurity, and low birth weight are more common in the histories of children with reading disorders.

Secondary reading disorders may be seen in children with postnatal brain lesions in the left occipital lobe resulting in right visual field blindness. They may also be seen in children with lesions in the splenum of the corpus callosum that block the transmission of visual information from the intact right hemisphere to the language areas of the left hemisphere.

Developmental reading disorder may be one manifestation of developmental delay or maturational lag. Temperamental attributes have been reported to be closely associated with developmental reading disorder. Compared with nonreading-disordered children, children with developmental reading disorder often have more difficulty concentrating and a shorter attention span.

Some studies suggest an association between malnutrition and cognitive function. Children who were malnourished for a long time during early childhood show subaverage performances in various cognitive tests. Their cognitive performances are lower than those of their siblings who grew up in the same family environment but who were not subjected to the same degree of malnutrition.

Severe developmental reading disorder is often associated with psychiatric problems. Developmental reading disorder may be the result of a preexisting psychiatric disorder or the cause of emotional and behavior disorders; however, it is not always easy to ascertain the causal relationship between a developmental reading disorder and a coexisting psychiatric disorder.

CLINICAL FEATURES

Developmental reading disorder is usually apparent by age 7 (second grade). In severe cases, evidence of reading difficulty may be apparent as early as age 6 (first grade). Sometimes, developmental reading disorder may be compensated for in the early elementary grades, particularly when it is associated with high scores on intelligence tests. In this case, the disorder may not be apparent until age 9 (fourth grade) or later.

The acquisition of reading skill is a complex intermodal operation involving cognitive and perceptual processes and requiring intact and balanced functioning of the central nervous system. These components include a neurological base that is mature and intact enough to integrate information arriving through various processing systems and to relegate disturbing stimuli to the background; the emotional maturity necessary for the postponement of immediate gratification for long-term gain; sufficient freedom from conflict to permit the investment of energy in the task, rather than maintaining defenses against anxiety; and a sociocultural value system that views reading as basic to survival.

Reading-disordered children make many errors in their oral reading. The faulty reading is characterized by omission, additions, and distortions of words. Such children have difficulty distinguishing between printed letter characters and sizes, especially those that differ only in spatial orientation and length of line. The problems in managing printed or written language may pertain to individual letters, sentences, and even a whole page. Their reading speed is slow, often with minimal comprehension. Most children with developmental reading disorder have an age-appropriate ability to copy from written or printed text, but nearly all of them are poor spellers.

Associated problems include language difficulties, shown often as impaired sound discrimination and difficulties in properly sequencing words. The reading-disordered child may start a word in the middle or at the end of a printed or written sentence. At times such children transpose letters that are to be read because of poorly established left-to-right tracking sequence. Failures in both memory recall and sustained elicitation result in poor recall of letter names and sounds.

Most children with developmental disorder dislike reading and writing and avoid them. Their anxiety is heightened when they are confronted with demands that involve printed language.

ASSOCIATED FEATURES

Deficits in expressive language and speech discrimination are usually present in developmental reading disorder and may be severe enought to warrant the additional diagnosis of developmental expressive or receptive language disorder. Developmental expressive writing disorder is often present. In some cases there is a discrepancy between verbal and performance intelligence scores. Visual perceptual deficits are seen in only about 10 percent of cases. Disruptive behavior disorders may also be present, particularly in older children and adolescents.

Most reading-disordered children who do not receive remedial education develop a sense of shame and humiliation from their continuing failure and subsequent frustration. These feelings become more intense as time progresses. Older children tend to be angry and depressed, and their aggression may be directed against society, perhaps leading to the development of a conduct disorder.

COURSE AND PROGNOSIS

Even without any remedial assistance, many reading-disordered children may acquire a little information about printed language during their first two years in grade school. By the end of the first grade, some may have learned how to read a few words. If no remedial educational intervention is given by the third grade, however, these children will remain reading impaired. Under the best circumstances, a child is identified as being at risk for a reading disorder during the kindergarten year or early in the first grade.

When remediation is instituted early, it can sometimes be discontinued by the end of the first or second grade. In more severe cases and depending on the pattern of deficits and strengths, remediation may be continued into the middle and high school years. Most children who have either compensated satisfactorily or completely recovered from earlier developmental reading disorder are from families of socioeconomically advantaged backgrounds.

DIAGNOSIS

The main diagnostic feature of a developmental reading disorder is a markedly decreased performance in reading skills that are below the individual's intellectual capacity. Other characteristic features include difficulties with the recall, evocation, and sequencing of printed letters and words; with the processing of sophisticated grammatical constructions; and with the making of inferences (Table 1). Clinically, the observer is impressed by the interaction between emotional and specific features. The experience of school failure seems to confirm preexisting doubts that some children have about themselves. The energy of some

Table 1
Diagnostic Criteria for Developmental Reading Disorder

A. Reading achievement, as measured by a standardized, individually administered test, is markedly below the expected level, given the person's schooling and intellectual capacity (as determined by an individually administered IQ test).

B. The disturbance in A significantly interferes with academic achievement or activities of daily living requiring reading skills.

C. Not due to a defect in visual or hearing acuity or a neurologic disorder.

Table from DSM-III-R, *Diagnostic and Statistical Manual of Mental Disorders,* ed 3, revised. (Current Classification of Mental Disorders, 1987.) Copyright American Psychiatric Association, Washington, D.C., 1987. Used with permission.

children is so bound to their conflicts that they are unable to exploit their assets. The psychiatric evaluation should assess the need for psychiatric intervention and decide on an appropriate treatment.

The diagnosis of developmental reading disorder cannot be established without confirmation by a standardized reading achievement test, and pervasive developmental disorders and mental retardation must be ruled out.

DIFFERENTIAL DIAGNOSIS

Reading difficulties may be primarily caused by the generalized impairment in intellectual functioning seen in mental retardation, which can be checked by administering a standardized intelligence test.

Inadequate schooling resulting in poor reading skills can be determined by finding out whether other children in the same school have similarly poor reading performance on standardized reading tests.

Hearing and visual impairments should be ruled out with screening tests.

Reading disorder often accompanies other emotional and behavioral disorders, especially attention-deficit hyperactivity disorder, conduct disorder, and depression.

PSYCHOEDUCATIONAL TESTS

In addition to standardized intelligence tests, psychoeducational diagnostic tests should be administered. The diagnostic battery may include a standardized spelling test, the writing of a composition, assessment of the processing and use of oral language, design copying, a judgment of the adequacy of pencil use. A screening projective battery may include human-figure drawings, picture-story tests, and sentence completion. The evaluation should also include a systematic observation of behavior variables.

TREATMENT

There is a general consensus that the treatment of choice for developmental reading disorder is a remedial educational approach; however, there is considerable controversy as to the relative efficacy of various remedial teaching strategies.

One frequently used methodology, developed by Samuel Orton, urges therapeutic attention to the mastery of simple phonetic units, followed by the blending of those units into words and sentences. An approach that systematically engages the several senses is recommended. The rationale for this and similar methods is that children's difficulties in managing letters and syllables are basic to their failures to learn to read; therefore, if they are taught to cope with graphemes, they will learn to read.

As in psychotherapy, the therapist–patient relationship is important to a successful treatment outcome in remedial educational therapy.

Reading-disordered children should be placed in a grade as close as possible to their social functional level and given special remedial work in reading. Coexisting emotional and behavioral problems should be treated by appropriate psychotherapeutic means. Parental counseling may also be helpful.

References

Bender L: Specific reading disability as a maturational lag. Bull Orton Soc 7:9, 1957.
Benton A: Dyslexia: Evolution of a concept. Bull Orton Soc 30:10, 1980.
Benton A, Pearl D: Dyslexia: An Appraisal of Current Knowledge. Oxford University Press, New York, 1978.
Doehring D, Trites R, Patel P, Fiedorowicz C: Reading Disabilities. Academic Press, New York, 1981.
Downing J, Leong C: Psychology of Reading. Macmillan, New York, 1982.
Duffy F H, Geschwind N: Dyslexia: A Neuroscientific Approach to Clinical Evaluation. Little, Brown, Boston, 1985.
Gaddes W H: Learning Disability and Brain Function: A Neuropsychological Approach. Springer-Verlag, New York, 1980.
Geschwind N: Asymmetries of the brain: New development. Bull Orton Soc 29:67, 1979.
Knights R M, Bakker D J: Treatment of Hyperactive and Learning Disordered Children. University Park Press, Baltimore, 1980.
Silver A A, Hagin R A: A Scanning Instrument for the Identification of Learning Disability. Walker Educational Book, New York, 1980.
Yule W, Rutter M: Reading and other learning difficulties. In M Rutter, L Hersov, editors, p 444. Child and Adolescent Psychiatry: Modern Approaches, ed 2. Blackwell Scientific Publications, Oxford, England, 1985.

35.4 _____
Developmental Articulation Disorder

INTRODUCTION

Developmental articulation disorder is characterized by frequent and recurrent misarticulations of speech sounds, resulting in abnormal speech. Language development is within normal limits. A variety of terms have been used to indicate this condition: baby talk, lalling, dyslalia, functional speech disorder, infantile perseveration, infantile articulation, delayed speech, lisping, oral inaccuracy, lazy speech, specific developmental speech disorder, and oral inaccuracy. In most mild cases, intelligibility may not be seriously affected, and spontaneous recovery is common. Severe cases may result in completely unintelligible speech and require lengthy and intensive treatment.

DEFINITION

DSM-III-R defines developmental articulation disorder as a consistent failure to make correct articulations of speech sounds at the developmentally appropriate age. The condition cannot be accounted for by pervasive developmental disorder, mental retardation, impairment of the oral speech mechanism, or neurological, intellectual, or hearing impairments. The disorder is manifested by frequent misarticulations, substitutions, or omissions of speech sounds, giving the impression of "baby talk" (Table 1). It is not due to any anatomical structural, physiological, auditory, or neurological abnormalities. The disorder refers to a number of different articulation difficulties ranging in severity from mild to severe. Speech may be completely intelligible, partially intelligible, or unintelligible. Only one speech sound or phoneme (the smallest sound unit) or many speech sounds may be affected.

EPIDEMIOLOGY

The prevalence of developmental articulation disorder is conservatively estimated to be approximately 10 percent of children below 8 years of age and approximately 5 percent of children 8 years of age and above. The disorder is two to three times more common in boys than in girls.

ETIOLOGY

The cause of developmental articulation disorder is unknown. It is generally believed that a simple developmental lag or maturational delay in the neurological process underlying speech, rather than an organic dysfunction, is at fault.

A disproportionately high frequency of developmental articulation disorder has been found among children from large families and from lower socioeconomic status families, suggesting the possible causal effects of inadequate speech stimulation and reinforcement in these families.

Constitutional factors, rather than environmental factors, seem to be of major importance in determining whether a child has developmental articulation disorder. The high proportion of children with the disorder who have relatives with a similar disorder suggests that the disorder may have a genetic component.

Table 1
Diagnostic Criteria for Developmental Articulation Disorder

A. Consistent failure to use developmentally expected speech sounds. For example, in a three-year-old, failure to articulate p, b, and t, and in a six-year-old, failure to articulate r, sh, th, f, z, and l.

B. Not due to a Pervasive Developmental Disorder, Mental Retardation, defect in hearing acuity, disorders of the oral speech mechanism, or a neurologic disorder.

Table from DSM-III-R, *Diagnostic and Statistical Manual of Mental Disorders*, ed 3, revised. (Current Classification of Mental Disorders, 1987.) Copyright American Psychiatric Association, Washington, D.C., 1987. Used with permission.

Poor motor coordination, laterality, and handedness have been proved not to contribute to developmental articulation disorder.

CLINICAL FEATURES

In severe cases, this disorder is first recognized at about age 3 years. In less severe cases, the disorder may not be apparent until age 6 years. The essential features of developmental articulation disorder include articulation that is judged to be defective when compared with the dialect of children at the same age level and that cannot be attributed to abnormalities in intelligence, hearing, or physiology of speech mechanism. In very mild cases, only one phoneme may be affected. Single phonemes are usually affected, most commonly those acquired late in the normal language acquisition process.

According to DSM-III-R, the speech sounds that are most frequently misarticulated are those acquired later in the developmental sequence (r, sh, th, f, z, l, and ch). But in more severe cases or in younger children, sounds such as b, m, t, d, n, and h may be mispronounced. One or many speech sounds may be affected, but vowel sounds are not among them.

The child with developmental articulation disorder is not able to articulate certain phonemes correctly and may distort, substitute, or even omit the affected phonemes. With omissions, the phonemes are absent entirely—for example, "bu" for "blue," "ca" for "car," or "whaa?" for "what's that?" With substitutions, difficult phonemes are replaced with incorrect ones—for example, "wabbit" for "rabbit," "fum" for "thumb," or "whath dat?" for "what's that?" With distortions, the correct phoneme is approximated but is articulated incorrectly. Rarely do additions—usually of the vowel "schwa" or "uh"—occur—for example, "puhretty," for "pretty," "what's uh that uh?" for "what's that?"

Omissions are thought to be the most serious types of misarticulation, with substitutions the next most serious type, and distortion the least serious type. Omissions are most frequently found in the speech of younger children and usually occur at the end of words or in clusters of consonants ("ka" for "car," "scisso" for "scissors"). Distortions, which are found mainly in older children, result in a sound that is not part of the speaker's dialect. Distortions may be the last type of misarticulation remaining in the speech of children whose articulation problems have mostly remitted. The most common types of distortions are the *lateral slip* in which the child pronounces s sounds with the air stream going across the tongue, producing a whistling effect, and the *palatal lisp* in which the s sound is formed with the tongue too close to the palate, producing a shh sound effect. The misarticulations of children with developmental articulation disorder are often inconsistent and random. A phoneme may be pronounced correctly in one situation and incorrectly another time. Misarticulations are most common at the ends of words, in long and syntactically complex sentences, and during rapid speech.

Omissions, distortions, and substitutions also occur normally in the speech of young children learning to talk. However, whereas young normal children soon replace these misarticulations, children with developmental articulation disorder do not. Even as children with developmental articulation disorder grow and finally acquire the correct phoneme, they may use it only in newly acquired words and may not correct earlier learned words that they have been mispronouncing for some time.

By the third grade, most children eventually outgrow developmental articulation disorder. After the fourth grade, however, spontaneous recovery is unlikely, and so it is important to try to remediate the disorder before the development of complications.

In most mild cases, recovery from developmental articulation disorder is spontaneous, and often the child's beginning kindergarten or school precipitates the improvement. Speech therapy is clearly indicated for those children who have not shown a spontaneous improvement by the third or fourth grade. For those children whose articulation is significantly unintelligible and are clearly troubled by their inability to speak clearly, speech therapy should be initiated at an early age.

According to DSM-III-R, other specific developmental disorders are commonly present, including developmental expressive language disorder, developmental receptive language disorder, developmental reading disorder, and developmental coordination disorder. Functional enuresis may also be present.

A delay in reaching speech milestones (such as "first word" and "first sentence") has been reported in some children with developmental articulation disorder, but most children with this disorder begin speaking at the appropriate age.

Children with developmental articulation disorder may have various concomitant social, emotional, and behavioral problems. About one third of children with this condition have a psychiatric disorder, such as attention-deficit hyperactivity disorder, separation anxiety disorder, avoidant disorder, adjustment disorders, and depression. Those children with a severe degree of articulation impairment or whose disorder is chronic and nonremitting are the ones most likely to suffer from psychiatric problems.

DIAGNOSIS

The essential feature of developmental articulation disorder is an articulation defect characterized by the consistent failure to use developmentally expected speech sounds of certain consonants, including omissions, substitutions, and distortions of phonemes, which are generally late-learned phonemes. The disorder cannot be attributed to structural or neurological abnormalities and is accompanied by normal language development.

DIFFERENTIAL DIAGNOSIS

The differential diagnostic process for developmental articulation disorder involves three steps: First, determine that the misarticulations are severe enough to be considered abnormal, and rule out the normal misarticulations of young children. Second, determine that there are no physical abnormalities to account for the articulation errors, and rule out dysarthria, hearing impairment, or mental retardation. And third, establish that expressive language is within normal limits, and rule out developmental language disorder and pervasive developmental disorders.

A rough guideline for a clinical assessment of children's articulation is that normal 3-year-olds correctly articulate m, n, ng, b, p, h, t, k, q, and d; normal 4-year-olds correctly articulate f, y, ch, sh, and z; and normal 5-year-olds correctly articulate th, s, and r.

Neurological, oral structural, and audiometric examinations may be necessary to rule out physical factors that may cause certain types of articulation disorders.

Table 2
Differential Diagnosis of Articulation Disorders

Criteria	Articulation Disorder Due to Structural or Neurological Abnormalities (Dysarthria)	Articulation Disorder Due to Hearing Impairment	Developmental Articulation Disorder	Articulation Disorder Associated with Mental Retardation, Infantile Autism, Developmental Dysphasia, Acquired Aphasia, or Deafness
Language development	Within normal limits	Within normal limits unless hearing impairment is serious	Within normal limits	Not within normal limits
Examination	Possible abnormalities of lips, tongue, or palate; muscular weakness, incoordination, or disturbance of vegetative functions, such as sucking or chewing	Hearing impairment shown on audiometric testing	Normal	
Rate of speech	Slow; marked deterioration of articulation with increased rate	Normal	Normal; possible deterioration of articulation with increased rate	
Phonemes affected	Any phonemes, even vowels	F, th, sh, and s	R, ch, th, ch, dg, j, f, v, s, and z are most commonly affected	

Table by Lorian Baker, Ph.D., and Dennis Cantwell, M.D.

Children with dysarthria, an articulation disorder caused by structural or neurological abnormalities, differ from children with developmental articulation disorder, in that dysarthria is very difficult and sometimes impossible to remedy. Drooling, slow or uncoordinated motor behavior, abnormal chewing or swallowing, and awkward or slow protrusion and retraction of the tongue are indications of dysarthria. A slow rate of speech is another indication of dysarthria (Table 2).

PROGNOSIS

Recovery is frequently spontaneous, particularly in children whose misarticulations involve only a few phonemes. Spontaneous recovery is rare after the age of 8 years.

TREATMENT

Speech therapy is considered the most successful treatment for most articulation errors. Speech therapy is indicated when the child's articulation intelligibility is poor, when the affected child is over 8 years of age, when the speech problem is apparently causing problems with peers, learning, and self-image, when the articulation impairment is so severe that many consonants are misarticulated, and when errors involve omissions and substitutions of phonemes, rather than distortions.

Monitoring of the child's peer relationships, school behavior, and parental counseling may be necessary for the timely implementation of psychiatric treatment when the need arises.

References

Bloodstein O: *Speech Pathology: An Introduction*. Houghton Mifflin, Boston, 1979.

Fey M, Leonard L, Wilcox, K: Speech style modification in language-impaired children. J Speech Hearing Disorder 46:91, 1981.

Hixon T, Shriberg L: *Introduction to Communication Disorders*. Wiley, New York, 1980.

Metter J E: *Speech Disorders: Clinical Evaluation and Diagnosis*. SP Medical and Scientific Books, New York, 1985.

Paul R, Shriberg L: Associations between phonology and syntax in speech delayed children. J Speech Hearing Res. 25:536, 1982.

Powers M H: Clinical and educational procedures in functional disorders of articulation. In *Handbook of Speech Pathology*, L E Travis, editor, p 877. Prentice-Hall, Englewood Cliffs, NJ, 1969.

Sander, E R: When are speech sounds learned? J Speech Hear Disord 37:55, 1972.

Weiss C E, Lillywhite H S: *Communicative Disorders: Prevention and Early Intervention*. Mosby, St. Louis, 1981.

Wiig E, Semel E: *Clinical Evaluation of Language Functions*. Chas. Merrill, Columbus, OH, 1980.

Wintz H: *Articulatory Acquisition and Behavior*. Prentice-Hall, Englewood Cliffs, NJ, 1969.

35.5 _____

Developmental Language Disorders: Developmental Expressive Language Disorder and Developmental Receptive Language Disorder

INTRODUCTION

Language disorders are categorized into three major types: (1) failure to acquire any language, (2) an acquired language disability secondary to trauma or neurological disorder, and (3) delayed language acquisition, also called developmental language disorder. The most common language disorder, developmental language disorder, is divided into two types: developmental expressive language disorder and developmental receptive language disorder.

DEVELOPMENTAL EXPRESSIVE LANGUAGE DISORDER

Definition

According to DSM-III-R, the essential feature of developmental language disorder is marked impairment in the development of expressive language that cannot be explained by mental retardation or inadequate schooling and that is not due to a pervasive developmental disorder, hearing impairment, or a neurologic disorder. The diagnosis should be made only if this impairment significantly interferes with academic achievement or with activities of daily living that require the expression of verbal (or sign) language (Table 1).

Epidemiology

The prevalence of developmental expressive language disorder ranges from 3 percent to 10 percent of school-age children. The disorder is two to three times more common in boys than in girls. The disorder is also more prevalent among children whose relatives have a family history of developmental articulation disorder or other developmental disorders.

Etiology

The cause of developmental expressive language disorder is not known. Subtle cerebral damage or maturational lags in cerebral development have been postulated as being the underlying causes, but there is no evidence supporting these theories.

The roles of unknown genetic factors have been suspected because the relatives of children with developmental learning disorders have a relatively high incidence of developmental expressive language disorder.

Table 1
Diagnostic Criteria for Developmental Expressive Language Disorder

A. The score obtained from a standardized measure of expressive language is substantially below that obtained from a standardized measure of nonverbal intellectual capacity (as determined by an individually administered IQ test).

B. The disturbance in A significantly interferes with academic achievement or activities of daily living requiring the expression of verbal (or sign) language. This may be evidenced in severe cases by use of a markedly limited vocabulary, by speaking only in simple sentences, or by speaking only in the present tense. In less severe cases, there may be hesitations or errors in recalling certain words, or errors in the production of long or complex sentences.

C. Not due to a Pervasive Developmental Disorder, defect in hearing acuity, or a neurologic disorder (aphasia).

Table from DSM-III-R, *Diagnostic and Statistical Manual of Mental Disorders*, ed 3, revised. (Current Classification of Mental Disorders, 1987.) Copyright American Psychiatric Association, Washington, D.C., 1987. Used with permission.

Clinical Features

Severe forms of the disorder usually occur before age 3 years. Less severe forms may not occur until early adolescence, when language ordinarily becomes more complex. The essential feature of the child with developmental expressive language disorder is a marked impairment in the development of age-appropriate expressive language, which results in the use of verbal or sign language that is markedly below the expected level, considering the child's nonverbal intellectual capacity. The child's language understanding (decoding) skills remain relatively intact.

The disorder becomes conspicuous by about age 18 months when the child fails to utter spontaneously or even to echo single words or sounds. Even simple words, such as "mama" and "dada," are absent from the child's active vocabulary, and the child points or uses gestures to indicate his or her desires. The child seems to want to communicate, maintains eye contact, relates well to his or her mother, and enjoys games such as pat-a-cake and peek-a-boo.

The child's repertoire of vocabulary is severely limited. At 18 months, the child can, at most, comprehend simple commands and can point to common objects when they are named. When the child finally begins to speak, the language deficit becomes more apparent. Articulation is usually immature. Numerous articulation errors are present but are inconsistent, particularly with such sounds as th, r, s, z, y, and l, which are either omitted or are substituted for other sounds.

By the age of 4, most children with this disorder can speak in short phrases, but they appear to forget old words as they learn new ones. After beginning to speak, they acquire language more slowly than do normal children. Their use of various grammatical structures is also markedly lower than the age-expected level. Their developmental milestones may also be slightly delayed. Developmental articulation disorder is often present. Developmental coordination disorder and functional enuresis are not uncommon associated features.

Complications

Emotional problems involving poor self-image, frustration, and depression may develop in school-age children. Children with the disorder may also have a learning impairment, manifested by reading retardation, that may result in serious difficulties in various academic subjects. The major learning difficulties are in perceptual skills or skills of recognizing and processing symbols in the proper sequences.

Other behavioral symptoms and problems that may appear in children with developmental expressive language disorder include hyperactivity, short attention span, withdrawing behavior, thumb sucking, temper tantrums, bed-wetting, disobedience, accident proneness, and conduct disorder. Neurological abnormalities have been reported in a number of children. These associated features include soft neurological signs, depressed vestibular responses, and EEG abnormalities.

Course and Prognosis

In general, the prognosis for developmental expressive language disorder is favorable. The rapidity and degree of recovery depend on the severity of the disorder, the child's motivation to participate in therapies, and the timely institution of speech and other therapeutic interventions. As many as 50 percent of children with a mild developmental expressive language disorder recover spontaneously without any sign of language impairment, but children with a severe developmental expressive language disorder may later display the features of mild to moderate impairment.

Diagnosis

The presence of markedly below age-level verbal or sign language, accompanied by a low score on standardized expressive verbal and nonverbal intellectual tests, is diagnostic. The disorder is not caused by a pervasive developmental disorder, as the child shows a desire to communicate. If there is any language, it is severely retarded; vocabulary is limited; grammar is simple; and articulation is variable. Inner language or the appropriate use of toys and household objects is present.

In order to confirm the diagnosis, the child should be tested with standardized expressive language and nonverbal intellectual tests. Observations of the disordered child's verbal and sign language patterns in various settings (e.g., in the school yard, classroom, home, and playrooms) and during interactions with other children will help ascertain the severity and specific areas of the child's impairment, as well as aid in the early detection of behavioral and emotional complications.

A careful family history should include the presence or absence of developmental expressive language disorder among relatives.

An audiogram is indicated for very young children and for those children whose hearing acuity appears to be impaired.

Differential Diagnosis

In mental retardation, there is an overall impairment in intellectual functioning, as shown in below-normal intelligence tests scores in all subtest areas. The nonverbal intellectual capacity and functioning of children with developmental expressive language disorder are within normal limits.

In developmental receptive language disorder, comprehension of language (decoding) is markedly below the expected age-appropriate level, whereas in developmental expressive language disorder, language comprehension remains within normal limits.

In pervasive developmental disorders, in addition to the cardinal cognitive characteristics, the affected children have no inner language, symbolic or imagery play, appropriate use of gesture, or capacity to form warm and meaningful social relationships. In contrast, all of these characteristics are present in children with developmental expressive language disorder.

Children with acquired aphasia or dysphasia have a history of an earlier normal language development, and the disordered language has its onset following head trauma or other neurological disorders (e.g., seizure disorders).

Children with elective mutism have a history of normal language development, and their speech is limited only to certain family members (e.g., mother, father, and siblings). More girls than boys are affected by elective mutism, and the affected children are mostly shy and withdrawn outside the family.

Treatment

Language therapy should be started immediately upon diagnosis of the disorder. Such therapy consists of behaviorally reinforced exercises and practice with phonemes (sound units), vocabulary, and sentence construction. The goal is to increase the number of phrases by using block-building methods and conventional speech therapies.

Psychotherapy is not usually indicated unless the language-disordered child shows signs of concurrent or secondary behavioral or emotional difficulties.

Interpretive and supportive parental counseling may be indicated in some cases. The parents may need help to reduce intrafamilial tension arising from difficulties in rearing the language-disordered child and to increase their awareness and understanding of the child's disorder.

DEVELOPMENTAL RECEPTIVE LANGUAGE DISORDER

Definition

According to DSM-III-R, the essential feature of developmental receptive language disorder is marked impairment in the development of language comprehension that cannot be explained by mental retardation or inadequate schooling and that is not due to a pervasive developmental disorder, hearing impairment, or neurologic disorder. The diagnosis should be made only if this impairment significantly interferes with academic achievement or with activities of daily living that require comprehension of verbal (or sign) language (Table 2).

Table 2
Diagnostic Criteria for Developmental Receptive Language Disorder

A. The score obtained from a standardized measure of receptive language is substantially below that obtained from a standardized measure of nonverbal intellectual capacity (as determined by an individually administered IQ test).

B. The disturbance in A significantly interferes with academic achievement or activities of daily living requiring the comprehension of verbal (or sign) language. This may be manifested in more severe cases by an inability to understand simple words or sentences. In less severe cases, there may be difficulty in understanding only certain types of words, such as spatial terms, or an inability to comprehend longer or more complex statements.

C. Not due to a Pervasive Developmental Disorder, defect in hearing acuity, or a neurologic disorder (aphasia).

Table from DSM-III-R, *Diagnostic and Statistical Manual of Mental Disorders,* ed 3, revised. (Current Classification of Mental Disorders, 1987.) Copyright American Psychiatric Association, Washington, D.C., 1987. Used with permission.

Epidemiology

The prevalence of developmental receptive language disorder ranges from 3 percent to 10 percent of school-age children. No familial pattern is known. The disorder is about two to three times more common in boys than in girls.

Etiology

The cause of this disorder is not known. Earlier theories listed perceptual dysfunction, subtle cerebral damage, maturational lag, and genetic factors as probable etiological factors, but there is no definitive supporting evidence for these theories. Several studies suggest the possible presence of underlying impairment of auditory discrimination, as most children with developmental receptive language disorder are more responsive to environmental sounds than to speech sounds.

Clinical Features

The disorder typically appears before the age of 4 years. Severe forms are apparent by age 2; mild forms may not become evident until age 7 (second grade) or older, when language becomes more complex. Children with developmental receptive language disorder show markedly delayed and below-normal ability to comprehend (decode) verbal or sign language, although they do have age-appropriate nonverbal intellectual capacity. In most cases of the disorder, verbal or sign expression (encoding) of language is also impaired. The clinical features of developmental receptive language disorder in children between the ages of 18 and 24 months are almost indistinguishable from those of developmental expressive language disorder: the child fails to make spontaneous utterances of a single phoneme (sound unit) or to mimic another person's words.

Many children with developmental receptive language disorder have auditory sensory difficulties or are unable to process visual symbols, such as the meaning of a picture. There are deficits in integrating both auditory or visual symbols—for example, recognizing the basic common attributes of a toy truck and a toy passenger car. Whereas a child with developmental expressive language disorder at 18 months can comprehend simple commands and can point to familiar household objects when told to do so, the child of the same age with developmental receptive language disorder is not able either to point to common objects or to obey simple commands. A child with developmental receptive language disorder usually appears to be deaf; however, the child does hear and responds normally to nonlanguage sounds from the environment, but not to spoken language. If the child starts to speak at a later time, his or her speech will contain numerous articulation errors, such as omissions, distortions, and substitution of a phoneme or phonemes. Their language acquisition is much slower than in normal children.

Developmental receptive language–disordered children also have difficulty recalling earlier visual and auditory memory and recognizing and reproducing symbols in proper sequence. In some cases, bilateral EEG abnormalities are seen. Most children with developmental receptive language disorder have a partial hearing defect for true tones, increased threshold of auditory arousal, and inability to localize sound sources. Seizure disorder and reading disorder are more common among relatives of children with developmental receptive language disorder than they are in the general population.

Associated features include developmental articulation disorder, developmental expressive language disorder, and academic skills disorder. Less commonly present are functional enuresis, developmental coordination disorder, attention-deficit hyperactivity disorder, and other social and behavioral problems.

Course and Prognosis

The overall prognosis for developmental receptive language disorder is less favorable than that for developmental expressive language disorder. The prognosis is fair in mild cases. In severe cases with auditory perceptual problems and difficulties in sensory integration, memory recall, and sequencing, the prognosis is guarded.

Diagnosis

The presence of markedly below age-appropriate level of comprehension of verbal or sign language with fairly intact age-appropriate nonverbal intellectual capacity, the confirmation of the language difficulties by standardized receptive language tests, and the absence of pervasive developmental disorders confirms the diagnosis of developmental receptive language disorder. In most cases, developmental receptive language disorder coexists with developmental expressive language disorder. Therefore, both standardized receptive and expressive language tests should be given to any child suspected of having developmental receptive language disorder.

An audiogram is indicated in all suspected developmental receptive language–disordered children in order to rule out or confirm the presence of deafness and to determine the types of auditory deficits.

Table 3
Differential Diagnosis*

	Hearing Impairment	Mental Retardation	Infantile Autism	Expressive Lang Disorder	Receptive Lang Disorder	Elective Mutism	Developmental Articulation Disorder
Language comprehension	−	−	−	−	−	+	+
Expressive language	−	−	−	−	−	Variable	+
Audiogram	−	+	+	+	Variable	+	+
Articulation	−	−	Variable	Variable	−	+	−
Inner language	+	+ (Limited)	−	+	+ (Slightly limited)	+	+
Uses gestures	+	+ (Limited)	−	+	+	Variable	+
Echoes	−	+	+ (inappropriate)	+	+	+	+
Attends to sounds	Loud or low frequency only	+	−	+	Variable	+	+
Watches faces	+	+	−	+	+	+	+
Performance I.Q.	+	−	+	+	+	+	+

Table by Lorian Baker, Ph.D., and Dennis Cantwell, M.D.
*+ = **Normal**; − = **abnormal**.

A careful history of the child and family and observation of the child in various settings will help clarify the diagnosis.

Differential Diagnosis

In developmental expressive language disorder, comprehension of spoken language (decoding) remains within age norms. Children with developmental articulation disorders (e.g., stuttering and cluttering) have normal expressive and receptive language competence, despite their having articulation impairments. Hearing impairment should be ruled out. Most children with developmental receptive language disorder have a history of variable and inconsistent responses to sounds; that is, they respond more often to environmental sounds than to speech sounds (Table 3).

Mental retardation, acquired aphasia, and pervasive developmental disorders should also be ruled out.

Treatment

Speech and language therapy is indicated for children with developmental receptive language disorder. The form of such treatment is still being debated. Some therapists believe that such children should be isolated in a nondistracting setting and should be taught single specific linguistic structures. Others believe that such children should learn in a natural setting with a group of children and should be taught several language structures simultaneously.

Psychotherapy is often necessary because these children frequently have emotional and behavioral problems. Particular attention should be paid to improving the child's self-image and social skills. Family counseling in which parents are taught appropriate patterns of interaction with the child can also be helpful.

References

Aram D M, Nation J E: *Child Language Disorders*. Mosby, St. Louis, 1982.
Cantwell D P, Baker L: Psychiatric and learning disorders in children with communication disorders. Adv in Learn Behav Disabil 4:511, 1984.
Cantwell D P, Baker L: Speech and language disorder: Developmental and disorders. In *Child and Adolescent Psychiatry: Modern Approaches*, M Rutter, L Hersov, editors, p 526. Blackwell Scientific Publications, Oxford, England, 1985.
Fundudis I, Kolvin I, Garside R F: A follow-up of speech retarded children. In *Language and Language Disorders in Childhood* (book supplement), J Child Psychol Psychiatry 2:97, 1980.
Holland A, editor: *Language Disorders in Children: Recent Advances*. College Hill Press, San Diego, 1984.
Laney M: *Reading in Childhood Language Disorders*. Wiley, New York, 1978.
Morehead D, Morehead A, editors: *Normal and Deficient Child Language*. University Park Press, Baltimore, 1976.
Myklebust H R: Childhood aphasia: Identification, diagnosis, and remediation. In *Handbook of Speech Pathology and Audiology*, L E Travis, editor. Appleton-Century-Crofts, New York, 1971.
Rutter M, Martin J A, editors: *The Child with Delayed Speech*. Heinemann, London, 1972.
Siegel L S: Reproductive, perinatal and environmental factors as predictors of the cognitive and language development of preterm and fullterm infants. Child Dev 53:963, 1982.

35.6 _____
Developmental Coordination Disorder

INTRODUCTION

DSM-III-R includes developmental coordination disorder for the first time as a specific developmental disorder. It was also included in the ninth revision of the International Classification of Diseases (ICD-9).

There are relatively few studies of children with developmental coordination disorder, fewer than those on other developmental disorders, such as developmental language and academic skills disorders. It is not a well-documented condition.

DEFINITION

According to DSM-III-R, the essential feature of developmental coordination disorder is a marked impairment in the development of motor coordination that cannot be explained by mental retardation and that is not due to a known physical disorder. This diagnosis should be made only if this impairment significantly interferes with academic achievement or with activities of daily living (Table 1).

EPIDEMIOLOGY

In some studies, the prevalence rate has been estimated as high as 6 percent of children between the ages of 5 and 11 years. The ratio between boys and girls is not known; however, as in most developmental disorders, more boys than girls are affected. No data available suggest an increased incidence of this disorder among the relatives of children with developmental coordination disorder.

ETIOLOGY

Two groups of possible etiological factors have been suggested: developmental and organic.

The developmental hypothesis views developmental coordination disorder as resulting from the delayed development of perceptual-motor skills. It suggests that the affected children will recover eventually from coordination disorder as they catch up from their maturational lags.

According to the organic hypothesis, certain minimal cerebral insults predispose children to developmental coordination disorder. Such insults include perinatal complications, such as maternal toxemia of pregnancy, hypoxia, malnutrition, low birth weight, and other intrauterine events that may cause brain or physical trauma of the fetus or neonate.

Table 1
Diagnostic Criteria for Developmental Coordination Disorder

A. The person's performance in daily activities requiring motor coordination is markedly below the expected level, given the person's chronological age and intellectual capacity. This may be manifested by marked delays in achieving motor milestones (walking, crawling, sitting), dropping things, "clumsiness," poor performance in sports, or poor handwriting.

B. The disturbance in A significantly interferes with academic achievement or activities of daily living.

C. Not due to a known physical disorder, such as cerebral palsy, hemiplegia, or muscular dystrophy.

Table from DSM-III-R, *Diagnostic and Statistical Manual of Mental Disorders*, ed 3, revised. (Current Classification of Mental Disorders, 1987.) Copyright American Psychiatric Association, Washington, D.C., 1987. Used with permission.

CLINICAL FEATURES

The clinical signs suggesting the existence of developmental coordination disorder are evident as early as infancy, when the affected child begins to attempt tasks requiring motor coordination. The essential clinical feature is the child's markedly impaired performance in motor coordination. The difficulties in motor coordination may vary with the child's age and developmental stage.

In infancy and early childhood, the disorder may be manifested as delays in normal developmental milestones, such as turning over, crawling, sitting, standing, walking, buttoning shirts, and zipping up pants. Between the ages of 2 and 4 years, clumsiness appears in almost all activities requiring motor coordination. Such children cannot hold objects and drop them easily; their gait is unsteady; they often trip over their own feet; and they may bump into other children while attempting to go around them.

In older children, the impaired motor coordination may be shown in table games, such as putting together puzzles or building blocks, and in any type of ball game. Although there are no specific features that are pathognomonic of developmental coordination disorder, developmental milestones are frequently delayed. Many children with this disorder may also have a speech disorder. Older children may also have secondary problems of school difficulties, including behavioral and emotional problems, that require appropriate therapeutic interventions.

COURSE AND PROGNOSIS

There are no reliable data available on the prospective longitudinal outcomes of both treated and untreated children with developmental coordination disorder. Some studies suggest a favorable outcome among those children who have an average or above-average intellectual capacity because they are able to learn to compensate for their coordination deficits. In general, the clumsiness persists into adolescence and adult life.

In very severe cases that remain untreated, there may be a number of secondary complications, such as repeated failures in both nonacademic and academic school tasks, repeated problems in attempting to integrate with a peer group, and inability to play games and sports. These problems may lead to low self-esteem, unhappiness, withdrawal, and, in some cases, increasingly severe behavioral problems as a reaction to the frustration engendered by the disability. All levels of adaptive functioning can be expected in these children. Commonly associated features include delays in other nonmotor milestones, developmental articulation disorder, and developmental receptive and expressive language disorders.

DIAGNOSIS

The diagnosis of developmental coordination disorder requires a careful history of the child's early motor behavior, including the direct observation of motor activities. The diagnosis is confirmed by below-normal scores on the performance subtests of standardized intelligence tests and by normal or above-normal scores on the verbal subtests. The individual's chronological age and intellectual capacity must be taken into account, and there should be no known neurological or neuromuscular disorder. However, slight reflex abnormalities and other soft neurological signs may occasionally be found on examination.

DIFFERENTIAL DIAGNOSIS

In mental retardation, there is an overall decrease in performance involving both verbal and nonverbal motor areas. Pervasive developmental disorders should be ruled out, as motor coordination difficulties, such as an abnormal gait and delays in motor milestones, sometimes are present in these disorders. Neurological and neuromuscular disorders, such as cerebral palsy, muscular dystrophy, and hemplegia, may be associated with problems in coordination, and a conventional neurological examination will reveal definite neural damage and abnormal findings.

TREATMENT

The various treatments include perceptual motor training, neurophysiological techniques of exercise for motor dysfunction, and modified physical education methods. The Montessori technique (developed by Maria Montessori) may be useful with many preschool children, as it emphasizes the development of motor skills. No single exercise or training method seems to be more advantageous or effective than another. Secondary behavioral or emotional problems and coexisting language and speech disorders must be managed by appropriate treatment methods.

Parental counseling helps reduce the parents' anxiety and guilt over the child's impairment and increases their awareness and confidence to cope with the child.

SPECIFIC DEVELOPMENTAL DISORDER NOT OTHERWISE SPECIFIED

This DSM-III-R residual category covers disorders in the development of language, speech, academic, and motor skills that cannot be classified as any of the specific developmental disorders discussed previously in this chapter.

See Table 2 for the diagnostic criteria and examples of specific developmental disorder not otherwise specified.

Table 2
Diagnostic Criteria for Specific Developmental Disorder Not Otherwise Specified

Disorders in the development of language, speech, academic, and motor skills that do not meet the criteria for a Specific Developmental Disorder. Examples include aphasia with epilepsy acquired in childhood ("Landau syndrome") and specific developmental difficulties in spelling.

Table from DSM-III-R, *Diagnostic and Statistical Manual of Mental Disorders,* ed 3, revised. (Current Classification of Mental Disorders, 1987.) Copyright American Psychiatric Association, Washington, D.C., 1987. Used with permission.

References

Arnheim D D, Sinclair W A: *The Clumsy Child.* Mosby, St. Louis, 1975.

Breaner M W, Gillman S, Zangwill O L, Farrell M: Visuo-motor disability in school children. Br Med J *4*:259, 1967.

Drillien C M: Etiology and outcome in low-birth-weight infants. Dev Med Child Neurol *14*:563, 1972.

Gordon N: *Pediatric Neurology for the Clinician.* Heinemann, Philadelphia, 1976.

Prechtl H F, Stemmer C J: The choreiform syndrome in children. Dev Med Child Neurol *4*:119, 1962.

Stott D H: A general test of motor impairment for children. Dev Med Child Neurol *8*:523, 1966.

36

Disruptive Behavior Disorders

INTRODUCTION TO DISRUPTIVE BEHAVIOR DISORDERS

Disruptive behavior disorders are a new classification in DSM-III-R characterized by behavior that is socially disruptive and more distressing to others than to the persons with the disorders. There are three subclasses: conduct disorder, attention-deficit hyperactivity disorder (ADHD), and oppositional defiant disorder, which are discussed in Sections 36.1, 36.2, and 36.3.

36.1

Conduct Disorder

DEFINITION AND DIAGNOSTIC CRITERIA

The essential feature of conduct disorder is a repetitive and persistent pattern of conduct in which either the basic rights of others or major age-appropriate societal norms or rules are violated. The conduct is more serious than the ordinary mischief and pranks of children and adolescents. DSM-III-R lists three subtypes of conduct disorder: solitary aggressive type, group type, and undifferentiated type. The DSM-III-R diagnostic criteria for conduct disorder is listed in Table 1. This diagnosis is only given to individuals below the age of 18 years.

EPIDEMIOLOGY

Conduct disorder is a fairly common disorder during childhood and adolescence. It is estimated that approximately 9 percent of males and 2 percent of females under the age of 18 years have the disorder. The disorder is more common among boys than among girls, and the ratio ranges from 4 to 1 to 12 to 1. Conduct disorder is more common in children of parents with antisocial personality and alcohol dependence than it is in the general population. The prevalence of conduct disorder and antisocial behavior is significantly related to socioeconomic factors.

Table 1
Diagnostic Criteria for Conduct Disorder

A. A disturbance of conduct lasting at least six months, during which at least three of the following have been present:

(1) has stolen without confrontation of a victim on more than one occasion (including forgery)

(2) has run away from home overnight at least twice while living in parental or parental surrogate home (or once without returning)

(3) often lies (other than to avoid physical or sexual abuse)

(4) has deliberately engaged in fire-setting

(5) is often truant from school (for older person, absent from work)

(6) has broken into someone else's house, building, or car

(7) has deliberately destroyed others' property (other than by fire-setting)

(8) has been physically cruel to animals

(9) has forced someone into sexual activity with him or her

(10) has used a weapon in more than one fight

(11) often initiates physical fights

(12) has stolen with confrontation of a victim (e.g., mugging, purse-snatching, extortion, armed robbery)

(13) has been physically cruel to people

Note: The above items are listed in descending order of discriminating power based on data from a national field trial of the DSM-III-R criteria for Disruptive Behavior Disorders.

B. If 18 or older, does not meet criteria for Antisocial Personality Disorder.

Table from DSM-III-R, *Diagnostic and Statistical Manual of Mental Disorders*, ed 3, revised. (Current Classification of Mental Disorders, 1987.) Copyright American Psychiatric Association, Washington, D.C., 1987. Used with permission.

ETIOLOGY

No single factor can account for children's antisocial behavior and conduct disorder. Rather, a variety of biopsychosocial factors contribute to its development.

Parental Factors

It has long been recognized that certain parental attitudes and faulty child-rearing practices influence the development of children's maladaptive behaviors. Chaotic home conditions are associated with conduct disorder and delinquency. However, broken homes per se are not etiologically significant; it is the strife between the parents that contributes to conduct disorder. Parental psychiatric impairments, particularly sociopathy and alcoholism, are viewed as important causal factors. Recent studies suggest that many of the parents suffer from more serious psychopathology, including psychoses that are often overlooked, and their obvious antisocial and addictive behaviors often mask other underlying psychopathology. Psychodynamic hypotheses suggest that children unconsciously act out their parents' antisocial wishes.

Sociocultural Theory

The current theories suggest that socioeconomically deprived children, unable to achieve status and obtain material goods through legitimate routes, are forced to resort to socially unacceptable means to achieve these goals and that such behavior is normal and acceptable under circumstances of socioeconomic deprivation, as the children are adhering to the values of their own subculture.

Other Factors

Attention-deficit hyperactivity disorder, CNS dysfunction or damage, parental rejection, early institutional living, inconsistent management with harsh discipline, frequent shifting of parental figures (foster parents, relatives, or stepparents), and illegitimacy can predispose a child to the development of conduct disorder. Early extremes of temperament also appear to play an important role in the development of conduct disorder. Longitudinal temperament studies suggest that many behavioral deviations are initially a straightforward response to a poor fit between, on the one hand, a child's temperament and emotional needs and, on the other hand, parental attitudes and child-rearing practices.

DIFFERENTIAL DIAGNOSIS

Isolated acts of antisocial behavior do not justify a diagnosis of conduct disorder. Rather, antisocial behavior should be repetitive and persistent for a period of 6 months or more to justify a diagnosis of conduct disorder. Children with conduct disorder usually have impaired social and school functioning that may not be apparent in an isolated act of antisocial behavior.

Oppositional disorder includes some of the features of conduct disorder, such as disobedience and defiant and oppositional behavior to authority figures. However, unlike conduct disorder, oppositional disorder does not violate the basic rights of others and major age-appropriate societal norms or rules. Bipolar disorder must also be ruled out. The irritability and antisocial behavior associated with manic episodes are usually brief, whereas the symptoms of conduct disorder tend to persist over time. Attention deficit–hyperactive disorder and specific developmental disorder are common associated diagnoses of conduct disorder, and these should be noted when present.

TYPES OF CONDUCT DISORDER

Conduct Disorder, Solitary Aggressive Type

Description. In addition to fulfilling the behavioral symptoms of the diagnostic criteria (Table 1), affected children manifest the predominant features of aggressive physical or verbal behavior, usually toward adults and peers. Their aggressive behavior is solitary and not a group activity. These children usually make little attempt to conceal their antisocial behavior. Sexual behavior and the regular use of tobacco, liquor, or nonprescribed drugs begin unusually early for such children.

The aggressive antisocial behavior may take the form of bullying, physical aggression, and cruel behavior toward peers. Such children may be hostile, verbally abusive, impudent, defiant, and negativistic toward adults. Persistent lying, frequent truancy, and vandalism are common. In severe cases, there is often destructiveness, stealing, and physical violence.

Many of these children fail to develop social attachment, as manifested by their difficulty in or lack of sustained normal peer relationships. Such children are often socially withdrawn or isolated. Some of them may befriend a much older or younger person or have superficial relationships with other antisocial youngsters. Most of them have low self-esteem, although they may project an image of "toughness." Characteristically, they will not put themselves out for others even if it has an obvious immediate advantage. Their egocentrism is shown by their readily manipulating others for favors without any effort to reciprocate. They lack concern for the feelings, wishes, and welfare of others. They seldom have feelings of guilt or remorse for their callous behavior and try to blame others.

Not only have these children frequently encountered unusual frustrations, particularly of their dependency needs, but they also have escaped any consistent pattern of discipline. Their deficient socialization is revealed not only in their excessive aggressiveness but also in their lack of sexual inhibition, which is frequently expressed aggressively and openly. Their general behavior is unacceptable in almost any social setting. They are generally viewed as bad kids and are frequently punished. Unfortunately, such punishment almost invariably increases their maladaptive expression of rage and frustration, rather than ameliorating the problem.

In evaluation interviews, solitary aggressive conduct–disordered children are typically uncooperative, hostile, and provocative. They volunteer hardly any information regarding their personal difficulties. If confronted, they may deny any behavioral problems. Finally, when they are cornered in the interview, they may attempt to justify their misbehavior, are suspicious and angry about the source of the examiner's information, or even bolt from the room. Most often, they become angry at the examiner and express their resentment of the examination with open belligerence or sullen withdrawal. Their hostility is not limited to adult authority figures but is expressed with equal venom toward their age-mates and younger children. In fact, they often bully those who are smaller and weaker than they. By boasting, lying, and expressing little interest in the listener's response, such children reveal their profoundly narcissistic orientation.

Evaluation of the family situation often reveals severe marital disharmony, which initially may center on disagreements over management of the child. Because of a tendency toward family instability, there is often a stepparent or stepparents in the picture. Many children with this type of conduct disorder are only children of unplanned or unwanted pregnancies. The parents, especially the father, are often diagnosed as having antisocial personality disorder or alcoholism.

The solitary aggressive child and his or her family demonstrate a stereotyped pattern of impulsive and unpredictable verbal and physical hostility. The child's aggressive behavior rarely seems directed toward any definable goal and offers little pleasure, success, or even sustained advantages with peers or authority figures. The child strikes out wildly at the world, grabbing and slashing, with very little idea of what he or she would like to gain through such behavior.

Treatment. Many clinical studies report difficulties in successfully treating children with conduct disorder of the solitary aggressive type. The age at which treatment begins is important to its success, not only because of the tendency of this behavioral pattern to become increasingly internalized and fixed in the face of the counterhostility that these youngsters engender in others, but also because of the greater ease with which overt aggressiveness can be managed in a younger child. Most therapists find it difficult to be patient with and sympathetic to these hostile youngsters.

Whenever feasible, family involvement is essential. Unless the parents can come to feel some acceptance of and warmth toward the youngster and provide consistent guidelines for acceptable behavior, even the most intensive work with the child will probably not be helpful. Conjoint marital therapy and family therapy with these families is demanding. The therapist often feels overwhelmed by the intensity of the hostile interactions among the family group members and frustrated by the parents' inability to reach and follow through on their decisions regarding their child. The therapist is often faced with a confusing barrage of accusations, verbal attacks, and manipulations aimed at forcing him or her into an alliance with one family member against another. Countertransference reactions of irritation, confusion, and helplessness are understandable. Firmness and impartiality are essential but difficult to maintain in the atmosphere of mutual recrimination and contradictory accounts of family interactions. Occasionally, the entire family achieves a temporary united front, but all too often it is based on a shared desire to attack the therapist.

In order to treat the child effectively, it is often necessary to remove him or her from the home. Even in a placement in a foster home or institution, the youngster can be expected to continue his or her extraordinary aggressiveness, testing of limits, and provocation. Those who are entrusted with caring for the solitary aggressive child must be prepared to offer acceptance and affection for long periods of time with very little positive feedback. Expectations for more socialized behavior from the youngster are initially minimal and are only gradually increased.

Behavior modification in a hospital setting has had some success, with varying degrees of lasting effects.

Medications are of limited value and only for the temporary and symptomatic amelioration of severe behaviors, such as phenothiazines for agitation and violent temper outbursts and methylphenidate for concurrent attention-deficit hyperactivity disorder. However, medication cannot substitute for the consistent and affectionate therapeutic atmosphere that the child needs for the development of internal controls, restoration of positive self-image, and new adaptive skills.

Conduct Disorder, Group Type

Description. The DSM-III-R criteria for conduct disorder, group type, list the predominant feature as conduct problems occurring mainly as a group activity in the company of friends who have similar problems and to whom the individual is loyal. Physical aggression may be included in this condition.

The group antisocial behavior invariably occurs outside the home. It includes repeated truancy, vandalism, and serious physical aggression or assault against others, such as mugging, gang fighting, and beating.

Children with this disorder usually have age-appropriate friendships. They are likely to show concern for the welfare of their friends or own gang members and are unlikely to blame them or inform on them.

Clinical Features. In most cases, there is a history of adequate or even excessive conformity during early childhood that ended when the youngster became a member of the delinquent peer group, usually in preadolescence or during adolescence. Also present in the history is some evidence of earlier problems, such as marginal or poor school performance, mild behavior problems, or neurotic symptoms.

Some degree of family social or psychological pathology is usually evident. Patterns of paternal discipline are rarely ideal and may vary from harshness and excessive strictness to inconsistency or relative absence of supervision and control. The mother has often protected the child from the consequences of early mild misbehavior but does not seem actively to encourage delinquency. Delinquency, also called juvenile delinquency, is most often associated with conduct disorder but may also be the result of other psychological or neurological disorders. There is usually evidence of a relatively warm relationship between the mother and the child, especially in infancy and early childhood. Some degree of marital disharmony may be present, and there is typically an absence of genuine family cohesion and comfortable interdependence. The group delinquent is likely to be from a large family living under poor economic circumstances.

Such children's misdeeds usually occur in the company of a peer group. The parents often recognize the role of the peer group in the youngsters' difficulties and complain of their wish to spend all their time with their friends. Frequently, the parents use this accurate observation to discount the predisposing factors within the family and the community that underlie such children's selection of unsuitable companions.

The specific delinquent acts and the circumstances under which they occur may provide important clues to the diagnosis. Truancy, stealing, and relatively minor criminal or antisocial acts are usually the rule, but there may be occasional violent crimes against persons and even destructive acts of vandalism. Some of the youngsters' misdeeds seem bold and almost playful—cops and robbers in reality.

The important and constant dynamic features in this condition are the significant influence of the peer group on such youngsters' behavior, and their extreme dependency needs to maintain their membership in the gang.

Course and Prognosis. Very few youngsters in this category of conduct disorder remain delinquent beyond adolescence, they even may give it up during adolescence. They may relinquish their delinquent behavior in response to fortuitous positive happenings, such as academic or athletic success, romantic attachments, or role modeling of an interested adult. Other youngsters may be dissuaded from the repetitive pattern through the unpleasantness of arrest and appearance in a juvenile court. Such occurrences may also awaken the family to their responsibilities for the child.

Treatment. Traditional individual psychotherapy alone has proved to be relatively ineffective, partly because of adolescents' common resistance to this type of therapy. Some delinquent youngsters respond better to the accepting, permissive, and dynamically-oriented counseling approach. Cognitive approach in a group setting has shown favorable results. These groups use a core of reformed delinquents who understand the rationalizations, denials, and self-justifications of the gang member seeking help and who vigorously confront the youngster with the realities of his or her behavioral predicament and the inevitability of negative consequences. The relatively high success rate in treating delinquent youngsters with the group-oriented approach is explained by the group conduct–disordered youngsters' natural tendency to turn to peers for advice and emotional support. Occasionally, such youngsters need to be separated from their previous peer group and to be transplanted to an entirely new environment, as in training schools, Outward Bound, and therapeutic camping programs.

Many youngsters with group conduct disorder do not receive psychiatric treatment at all but are, instead, remanded to training schools or reformatories. A high percentage of these youngsters improve spontaneously as they become interested in heterosexual relationships, assume family responsibilities, and secure employment. Because their basic capacity for human relatedness is intact, they often discover their own passage out of delinquency.

Therapeutic optimism is very much warranted in this group of youngsters. Any approach that alters the attitudes of the entire group or that separates the youngsters from their delinquent peer group and offers them contact with strong adult leaders and less delinquent peers is quite likely to improve the group's antisocial or criminal behavior.

Conduct Disorder, Undifferentiated Type

Conduct disorder, undifferentiated type, is a category reserved for children or adolescents with a conduct disorder with clinical features that cannot be classified as either a solitary aggressive or a group type.

References

Berger M: Personality development and temperament. In *Temperamental Differences in Infants and Young Children*. R Porter, G M Collins, editors, p 176. Pitmann, London, 1982.
Farrington, D P: The family backgrounds of aggressive youths. In *Aggression and Antisocial Behavior in Childhood and Adolescence*, L Herzov, M Berger, D Shaffer, editors. Pergamon, Oxford, England, 1978.
Hutchings B, Mednick S A: Registered, criminality on the adoptive and biological parents of registered male criminal adoptees. In *Genetics, Environment and Psychopathology*, S A Mednick, F Schlesinger, J Higgins, B Bell, editors. North Holland/Elsevier, Amsterdam, 1974.
Johnson R E: *Juvenile Delinquency and Its Origin: An Integrated Theoretical Approach*. Cambridge University Press, Cambridge, England, 1979.
Lamb M E: Parental influences on early socioemotional development. J Child Psychol Psychiat, *23*:185, 1982.
Lewis D O, editor: *Vulnerabilities to Delinquency*. Spectrum, New York, 1981.
Lewis D O, Shanok S S, Grant M, Ritvo E: Homicidally aggressive young children: Neuropsychiatric and experiental correlates. Am J Psychiatry *140*:148, 1983.
Lewis D O, Shanok S S, Lewis M L, Unger L, Goldman C: Conduct disorder and its synonyms: Diagnosis of dubious validity and usefulness. Am J Psychiatry *141*:514, 1984.
McAuley R: Annotation: Training parents to modify conduct problems in their children. J Child Psychol Psychiat 23:335, 1982.
Robins L: *Deviant Children Grown Up*. Williams & Wilkins, Baltimore, 1966.

36.2 ————
Attention-Deficit Hyperactivity Disorder

DEFINITION

Attention-deficit hyperactivity disorder (ADHD) is a cluster of symptoms characterized by a short attention span resulting in poor concentration, impulsivity, and hyperactivity. In order to make the diagnosis, the behavioral disturbances must be present for at least 6 months and must first have appeared before the age of 7. DSM-III-R classifies the disorder under the new category heading of disruptive behavior disorders. The diagnostic criteria for attention-deficit hyperactivity disorder are presented in Table 1.

Various terms have been used to describe children affected by this disorder: hyperkinetic reaction of childhood, hyperkinetic syndrome, hyperactive child syndrome, minimal brain dysfunction, minimal cerebral dysfunction, minimal brain damage, minor cerebral dysfunction, and, more recently by DSM-III, attention deficit disorder with or without hyperactivity.

EPIDEMIOLOGY

Reports on the incidence of ADHD in the United States have varied from 2 to 20 percent of grade school children. However, a more conservative figure is about 3 to 5 percent of prepubertal elementary school children. In Great Britain, the incidence is lower, less than 1 percent. There is a greater incidence in boys than in girls, with the ratio being from three to one to five to one. It is more common in firstborn boys. The parents of children with ADHD show an increased incidence of hyperkinesis, sociopathy, alcoholism, and hysteria. Although the onset is usually by the age of 3, the diagnosis generally is not made until the child is in elementary school and the formal learning situation requires structured behavior patterns, including developmentally appropriate attention span and concentration.

ETIOLOGY

Neurobiological Factors

The majority of children with ADHD do not show evidence of gross structural damage or disease in the central nervous system (CNS) when examined by conventional neurological methods. On the other hand, most children with neurological disorders or brain injuries do not display any specific features of hyperactivity. Research efforts to find a neurophysiological or neurochemical basis have not yielded any definite findings. Nevertheless, some children with the disorder may have minimal and subtle brain damage from adverse circulatory, toxic, metabolic, or mechanical insults to the CNS during fetal and perinatal periods. That may account for the association of learning disorders in children with attention-deficit hyperactivity disorder.

Table 1
Diagnostic Criteria for Attention-deficit Hyperactivity Disorder

Note: Consider a criterion met only if the behavior is considerably more frequent than that of most people of the same mental age.

A. A disturbance of at least 6 months during which at least eight of the following are present:

   (1) often fidgets with hands or feet or squirms in seat (in adolescents, may be limited to subjective feelings of restlessness)
   (2) has difficulty remaining seated when required to do so
   (3) is easily distracted by extraneous stimuli
   (4) has difficulty awaiting turn in games or group situations
   (5) often blurts out answers to questions before they have been completed
   (6) has difficulty following through on instructions from others (not due to oppositional behavior or failure of comprehension), e.g., fails to finish chores
   (7) has difficulty sustaining attention in tasks or play activities
   (8) often shifts from one uncompleted activity to another
   (9) has difficulty playing quietly
   (10) often talks excessively
   (11) often interrupts or intrudes on others, e.g., butts into other children's games
   (12) often does not seem to listen to what is being said to him or her
   (13) often loses things necessary for tasks or activities at school or at home (e.g., toys, pencils, books, assignments)
   (14) often engages in physically dangerous activities without considering possible consequences (not for the purpose of thrill-seeking), e.g., runs into street without looking

Note: The above items are listed in descending order of discriminating power based on data from a national field trial of the DSM-III-R criteria for Disruptive Behavior Disorders.

B. Onset before the age of 7.

C. Does not meet the criteria for a Pervasive Developmental Disorder.

Table from DSM-III-R, *Diagnostic and Statistical Manual of Mental Disorders*, ed 3, revised. (Current Classification of Mental Disorders, 1987.) Copyright American Psychiatric Association, Washington, D.C., 1987. Used with permission.

Hypersensitivity and idiosyncratic responses to food additives (e.g., colorings and perservatives) have been suggested as causes of the disorder, but these claims have not been scientifically validated.

Genetic Inheritance

A genetic basis of ADHD has been suggested by data that show a concordance in some twins. Siblings of hyperactive children are also at greater risk for hyperactivity than are half siblings.

Brain Damage

It has long been speculated that some of the children affected by ADHD may have received minimal and subtle brain damage to the CNS during fetal and perinatal periods The brain damage may have been caused by adverse circulatory, toxic, metabolic, mechanical assault, and other effects; as well as by stress and physical insult to the brain during early infancy, caused by infection, inflammation, and trauma. This minimal, subtle, and subclinical severity of brain damage may be responsible for the genesis of learning disorders and ADHD.

Maturational Lag

The human brain normally undergoes major growth spurts at several ages: 3 to 10 months, 2 to 4 years, 6 to 8 years, 10 to 12 years, and 14 to 16 years. Some children have a maturational delay in this developmental sequence and may show a clinical picture of ADHD that is temporary and disappears as maturational lags catch up to normal milestones at around puberty.

Psychosocial Factors

Children in institutions frequently are overactive with poor attention spans. These symptoms result from prolonged emotional deprivation and disappear when deprivational factors are removed, such as placement in a foster home or adoption. Stressful psychic events, a disruption of family equilibrium, or other anxiety-inducing factors contribute to the initiation or perpetuation of the disorder. Predisposing factors may include the child's temperament, genetic-familial factors, and the demands of society to adhere to a routinized way of behaving and performing. Socioeconomic status does not seem to be a predisposing factor.

CLINICAL FEATURES

The disorder may have its onset in infancy. Such infants are unduly sensitive to stimuli and are easily upset by noise, light, temperature, or other environmental changes. At times, the reverse occurs, and the children are placid and limp, sleep much of the time, and appear to develop slowly in the first months. It is more common, though, for such infants to be active in the crib, sleep little, and show increased crying. Hyperkinetic children are far less likely than are normal children to reduce their locomotor activity when their environment is structured by social limits. In school, ADHD children may rapidly attack a test but answer only the first two questions. They may be unable to wait to be called on in school and may respond for everyone else, and at home they cannot be put off for even a minute.

These children are often explosively irritable. This irritability may be set off by relatively minor stimuli, which may puzzle and dismay them. They frequently are emotionally labile, easily set off to laughter or to tears, and their mood and performance are apt to be variable and unpredictable. Impulsiveness and an inability to delay gratification are characteristic. They are often accident prone.

Concomitant emotional difficulties are frequent. The fact that other children grow out of this kind of behavior and hyperkinetic children do not grow out of it at the same time and rate, the variability of their performance, the temporary response to pressures, the fact that most such children are not retarded and have no excuse for their behavior, the general nuisance and inexplicability of their behavior—all may lead to adults' dissatisfaction and pressure. The resulting negative self-concept and reactive hostility are worsened by the children's frequent recognition that they are not right inside.

The characteristics most often cited are, in order of frequency: (1) hyperactivity, (2) perceptual motor impairment, (3) emotional lability, (4) general coordination deficit, (5) disorders of attention (short attention span, distractibility, perseveration, failure to finish things, inattention, poor concentration), (6) impulsivity (action before thought, abrupt shifts in activity, lack of organization, jumping up in class), (7) disorders of memory and thinking, (8) specific learning disabilities, (9) disorders of speech and hearing, and (10) equivocal neurological signs and electroencephalographic irregularities.

Approximately 75 percent of children diagnosed as having this condition fairly consistently show behavioral symptoms of aggression and defiance. But whereas defiance and aggression generally are associated with adverse intrafamily relationships, hyperactivity is more closely related to developmental lags in sensorimotor coordination, language, and impaired performance on cognitive tests requiring concentration. Some studies claim that several relatives of hyperactive children show features of antisocial personality.

School difficulties, both learning and behavioral, are common, sometimes coming from concomitant developmental language or specific learning disorders or from the children's distractibility and fluctuating attention, which hamper their acquisition, retention, and display of knowledge. These difficulties resemble specific learning disorders, especially when evaluated on group tests. The adverse reactions of school personnel to the behavior characteristic of the syndrome, and the lowering of self-regard because of felt inadequacies, may combine with the adverse comments of peers to make school a place of unhappy defeat. This, in turn, may lead to acting-out antisocial behavior and self-defeating, self-punitive behaviors.

DIAGNOSIS

The principal sign of hyperactivity should alert clinicians to the possibility of ADHD. A detailed prenatal history of the child's early developmental patterns and direct observation will usually reveal excessive motor activity. Hyperactivity may be seen in some situations (e.g., school), but not in others (e.g., while watching a favorite television program), and it may be less obvious in structured situations than in unstructured situations. However, it should not be an isolated, brief, and transient behavioral manifestation under stress but should have been present over a long time. Other distinguishing features of this condition are short attention span and easy distractibility. In school, these children cannot follow instructions and often demand extra attention from their teachers. At home, they often do not follow through on their parents' requests. They are prone to act impulsively, show emotional lability, and are explosive and irritable.

Specific developmental disorders—such as those involving reading, arithmetic, language, and coordination—may be found in association with the attention deficit disorders. The history is important, as it may give clues to prenatal (including genetic), natal, and postnatal factors that may have affected the central nervous system structure or function. Rates of development and deviations in development and parental reactions to significant or stressful behavioral transitions should be ascertained, as they may help determine the degree to which parents have contributed to or reacted to the child's inefficiencies and dysfunctions.

School history and teachers' reports are important in evaluating whether such children's difficulties in learning and school behavior are primarily due to their attitudinal or maturational problems or to their poor self-image because of felt inadequacies. This information may also reveal how the children have handled these problems. How they have related to siblings, peers, and adults, and to free and structured activities gives valuable diagnostic clues to the presence of attention-deficit hyperactivity disorder and helps identify the complications of the disorder.

The mental status examination may show a secondarily depressed mood but no thought disturbance, impaired reality testing, or inappropriate affect. There may be great distractibility, perseverations, and a concrete and literal mode of thinking. There may be indications of visual-perceptual, auditory-perceptual, language, or cognition problems. Occasionally there may be evidence of a basic, pervasive, organically based anxiety, often referred to as body anxiety.

A neurological examination may reveal visual-motor-perceptual or auditory-discriminatory immaturity or impairments without overt signs of disorders of visual or auditory acuity. These children may show problems with motor coordination and difficulties with copying age-appropriate figures, rapid alternating movements, right-left discrimination, ambidexterity, reflex asymmetries, and a variety of subtle nonfocal neurological signs (soft signs). An EEG should be obtained to recognize the child with frequent bilaterally synchronous discharges resulting in short absence spells. Such a child may react in school with hyperactivity out of sheer frustration. The child with an unrecognized temporal lobe seizure focus can present a secondary behavior disorder. In these instances, several features of the attention-deficit hyperactivity disorder are often present. Identification of the focus requires an EEG obtained in drowsiness and in sleep.

COURSE AND PROGNOSIS

The course of the condition is highly variable: Symptoms may persist into adolescence or adult life; they may remit at puberty; or the hyperactivity may disappear, but the decreased attention span and impulse control problems may persist.

The overactivity is usually the first symptom to remit, and distractibility the last. Remission is not likely before the age of 12. If it does occur, it is usually between the ages of 12 and 20. Remission may be accompanied by a productive adolescence and adult life, satisfying interpersonal relationships, and few significant sequelae. The majority of patients with ADHD, however, undergo partial remission and are vulnerable to antisocial, other personality disorders, and mood disorders. Learning problems often continue.

In about 15 to 20 percent of cases, the symptoms of

attention-deficit hyperactivity disorder persist into adulthood. Such persons may show diminished hyperactivity but remain somewhat impulsive and accident prone. Although their educational attainment is lower than that of persons without ADHD, their early employment history is not different from those with a similar education.

DIFFERENTIAL DIAGNOSIS

A temperamental constellation consisting of high activity level and short attention span should be first considered. It is often difficult to differentiate these temperamental characteristics from the cardinal symptoms of attention-deficit hyperactivity disorder before age 3, mainly because of the overlapping features of a normally immature nervous system and the emerging signs of visual-motor-perceptual impairments frequently seen in ADHD.

Anxiety states in the overanxious child or a nonspecific anxiety disorder needs to be evaluated. Anxiety may accompany ADHD as a secondary feature, and anxiety by itself may be manifested by overactivity and easy distractibility.

Many children with attention-deficit hyperactivity disorder develop secondary depression in reaction to their continuing frustration over their failure to learn and their consequent low self-esteem. This must be distinguished from a primary depressive disorder, which is more likely to show hypoactivity and withdrawal.

The various forms of conduct disorder with overactivity and aggression may be confused with attention-deficit hyperactivity disorder, which is often associated with and secondary to these disorders. Frequently, conduct disorder and ADHD coexist, and so both must be diagnosed.

TREATMENT

Medication

The pharmacological agents for this condition are the central nervous system stimulants, primarily dextroamphetamine sulfate (Dexedrine), methylphenidate (Ritalin), and pemoline (Cylert). A child may respond favorably to one of these drugs and unfavorably to the other, better to one drug than to the other, or even better to another medication. The appropriate dosage also varies.

The mechanism of action of the stimulants is unknown but they have an idiosyncratic action in that they decrease motor activity and increase attention span. These drugs are controversial because of the central nervous system stimulants' possible suppression of height and weight. Some investigators have reported a height and weight rebound after the medication is stopped. These possible adverse effects must be weighed against the favorable effects, case by case. There is also a debate about the habit formation and abuse potential of these drugs; however, if used judiciously and within the recommended dose range, their benefits outweigh their risks for abuse.

Another recommended medication was originally introduced as an antidepressant—imipramine hydrochloride (Tofranil). But the manufacturer does not advise it for ADHD or, for any reason, for children younger than age 6, as children react more strongly to its cardiotoxic effects than do adults. An advantage of imipramine is that it has no abuse potential. These drugs work by blocking the reuptake of catecholamines. They should be used with great care in children because of their potential toxic effects.

Psychotherapy

The use of medication only rarely satisfies the comprehensive therapeutic needs of ADHD children and their families and so should be accompanied by psychological support. At the very least, this support should give the children the opportunity to explore the meaning of the medication to them, helping dispel misconceptions (such as "I'm crazy") because medication is used and making it clear that the medication is only an adjuvant. These children need to understand that perfection is not the goal and that they have an equal right with all other human beings to be occasionally unpredictable, disagreeable, and difficult.

When such children are not only allowed but also helped to structure their environment, their anxiety diminishes. Thus, their parents and teachers should set up a predictable structure of reward and punishment using a behavior therapy model and applying it to the physical, temporal, and interpersonal environment. An almost universal requirement is to help the parents recognize that permissiveness is not helpful to their child. They also should be helped to recognize that despite their children's deficiencies in some areas, they face the normal tasks of maturation, including the need to introject standards and to form a normal, flexible superego. Therefore, children with ADHD do not benefit from being exempted from the requirements, expectations, and planning applicable to other children.

Evaluation of Therapeutic Progress

Monitoring starts with the initiation of medication. Because school performance is most markedly affected, special attention and efforts should be given to establishing and maintaining a close collaborative working relationship with the children's school.

In most patients, stimulants reduce overactivity, distractibility, impulsiveness, explosiveness, and irritability. There is no evidence that the medications directly improve any existing impairments in learning, although the attention deficits diminish so that the children can learn more effectively. That is, medication provides the preconditions for improved academic performance, but whether academic performance will actually improve depends on what the school has to offer in the way of individual remedial instruction.

UNDIFFERENTIATED ATTENTION-DEFICIT DISORDER

This disorder results from ADHD that has not remitted by the time the patient is 18 years of age. The history indicates that the patient had an illness during childhood

Table 2
Diagnostic Criteria for Undifferentiated Attention-deficit Disorder

This is a residual category for disturbances in which the predominant feature is the persistence of developmentally inappropriate and marked inattention that is not a symptom of another disorder, such as Mental Retardation or Attention-deficit Hyperactivity Disorder, or of a disorganized and chaotic environment. Some of the disturbances that in DSM-III would have been categorized as Attention Deficit Disorder without Hyperactivity would be included in this category. Research is necessary to determine if this is a valid diagnostic category and, if so, how it should be defined.

Table from DSM-III-R, *Diagnostic and Statistical Manual of Mental Disorders*, ed 3, revised. (Current Classification of Mental Disorders, 1987.) Copyright American Psychiatric Association, Washington, D.C., 1987. Used with permission.

that met the criteria for ADHD. In adults, residual signs of the illness include impulsivity and attention deficit (e.g., difficulty in organizing and completing work, inability to concentrate, increased distractibility, and sudden decision making without thought of consequences). Many of those patients suffer from a secondary depression which is associated with low self-esteem related to their impaired performance and affects both occupational and social functioning. The treatment of this disorder is the use of amphetamines (5 to 40 mg per day) or methylphenidate (5 to 60 mg per day). A positive response is an increased attention span, decreased impulsiveness, and improved mood. Psychopharmacologic therapy may need to be continued indefinitely. Because of the abuse potential of these drugs, clinicians should carefully monitor drug response and patient compliance. DSM-III-R recognizes the need for more research on this category (Table 2).

References

Biederman J, Munir K, Knee D, Armentano M, Auter S, Waternaux C, Tsuang M: High rate of affective disorders in probands with attention deficit disorder and in their relatives: A controlled family study. Am J Psych *144*:330, 1987

Loney J, Kramer J, Milich R: The hyperkinetic child grows up: Predictors of symptoms, delinquency, and achievement at follow-up. In K D Gadow, J Loney, editors: *Psychosocial Aspects of Drug Treatment for Hyperactivity*, p 381. Westview Press, Boulder, CO, 1981.

Rutter M, Graham P, Yule W: A neuropsychiatric study in childhood. Am J Psychiatry *139*:1, 1982.

Silver L B: A proposed view on the etiology of the neurological learning disability syndrome. J Learn Disabil *4*:123, 1971.

Taylor E: Syndromes of overactivity and attention deficit. In *Child and Adolescent Psychiatry: Modern Approaches*, ed 2. M Rutter, L Hersov, editors, p 424. Blackwell Scientific Publications, Oxford, England, 1985.

Trites R L, Lapraed K: Evidence for an independent syndrome of hyperactivity. Child Psychol Psychiatry *24*:573, 1983.

Weiss G, Minde K, Werry J, Douglas V, Nemeth E: Studies on the hyperactive child, vol 7: Five year follow-up. Arch Gen Psychiat *24*:409, 1971.

36.3 ————
Oppositional Defiant Disorder

DEFINITION AND DIAGNOSTIC CRITERIA

The essential feature of oppositional defiant disorder is a pattern of negativistic, hostile, and defiant behavior, often directed toward parents or teachers. These actions, however, do not include the more serious violations of the basic rights of others seen in the various conduct disorders. The DSM-III-R diagnostic criteria for oppositional defiant disorder are given in Table 1. Oppositional defiant disorder was previously called oppositional disorder in DSM-III.

EPIDEMIOLOGY

Oppositional, negativistic behavior may be developmentally normal in early childhood. Epidemiological studies of negativistic traits in nonclinical populations found them in between 16 and 22 percent of school-age children. Although the disorder can begin as early as 3 years of age, it typically begins by 8 years of age and usually not later than adolescence.

DSM-III-R states that the disorder is more prevalent in males before puberty and that the sex ratio probably equalizes after puberty. Another authority suggests that girls may be diagnosed as having oppositional disorder more frequently than boys (using the DSM-III criteria), as boys are more often given the diagnosis of conduct disorder.

There are no distinct family patterns, but almost all parents of oppositional children are themselves overconcerned with issues of power, control, and autonomy. Some families contain several obstinate characters, controlling and depressed mothers, and passive-aggressive fathers. In many cases, the patients were unwanted children.

ETIOLOGY

Asserting one's own will and opposing that of others is crucial to normal development. It is related to establishing one's autonomy, forming an identity, and setting inner standards and controls. The most dramatic example of normal oppositional behavior peaks between 18 and 24 months, "the terrible twos," when the toddler behaves negativistically as an expression of growing autonomy. Pathology begins when this developmental phase persists abnormally; authority figures overreact; or oppositional behavior recurs considerably more frequently than in most children of the same mental age.

Children may have constitutional or temperamental predispositions to strong will, strong preferences, or greater assertiveness. If power and control are issues for the parents or if they exercise authority for their own needs, a struggle can ensue that sets the stage for the development of an oppositional defiant disorder. What begins for the infant as

Table 1
Diagnostic Criteria for Oppositional Defiant Disorder

Note: Consider a criterion met only if the behavior is considerably more frequent than that of most people of the same mental age.

A. A disturbance of at least 6 months during which at least five of the following are present:
  (1) often loses temper
  (2) often argues with adults
  (3) often actively defies or refuses adult requests or rules, e.g., refuses to do chores at home
  (4) often deliberately does things that annoy other people, e.g., grabs other children's hats
  (5) often blames others for his or her own mistakes
  (6) is often touchy or easily annoyed by others
  (7) is often angry and resentful
  (8) is often spiteful or vindictive
  (9) often swears or uses obscene language
  Note: The above items are listed in descending order of discriminating power based on data from a national field trial of the DSM-III-R criteria for Disruptive Behavior Disorders.

B. Does not meet the criteria for Conduct Disorder, and does not occur exclusively during the course of a psychotic disorder, Dysthymia, or a Major Depressive, Hypomanic, or Manic Episode.

Table from DSM-III-R, *Diagnostic and Statistical Manual of Mental Disorders,* ed 3, revised. (Current Classification of Mental Disorders, 1987.) Copyright American Psychiatric Association, Washington, D.C., 1987. Used with permission.

an effort to establish self-determination becomes transformed into a defense against overdependency on the mother and a protective device against intrusion into the ego's autonomy. In later childhood, environmental traumata, illness, or chronic incapacity, such as mental retardation, may trigger oppositionalism as a defense against helplessness, anxiety, and loss of self-esteem. Another normative oppositional stage occurs in adolescence as an expression of the need to separate from the parents and to establish an autonomous identity.

Classical psychoanalytic theory implicates in the etiology of this disorder unresolved conflicts that developed during the anal period. Behavioral theorists have suggested that oppositionalism is a reinforced, learned behavior through which the child exerts control over authority figures—for example, by having a temper tantrum when some undesired act is requested, the child coerces the parents to withdraw their request. In addition, increased parental attention—for example, long discussions about the behavior—may also reinforce the behavior.

CLINICAL DESCRIPTION

DSM-III-R notes that children with this disorder commonly argue with adults, frequently lose their temper, swear, and are often angry, resentful, and easily annoyed by others. They frequently actively defy adults' requests or rules and deliberately annoy other people. They tend to blame others for their own mistakes and difficulties. Manifestations of the disorder are almost invariably present in the home but may not be present at school or with other adults or peers. In some cases, from the beginning of the disturbance, features of the disorder are displayed outside the home; in other cases, they start in the home but later are displayed outside the home. Typically, symptoms of the disorder are more evident in interactions with adults or peers whom the child knows well. Thus, children with the disorder are likely to show little or no signs of the disorder when examined clinically. Usually they do not regard themselves as oppositional or defiant but justify their behavior as a response to unreasonable circumstances. The disorder appears to cause more distress to those around the children than to the children themselves.

Chronic oppositional defiant disorder almost always interferes with interpersonal relationships and school performance. These children are often friendless and perceive human relationships as unsatisfactory. Despite adequate intelligence, they do poorly or fail in school, as they withhold participation, resist external demands, and insist on solving problems without others' help.

Secondary to these difficulties are low self-esteem, poor frustration tolerance, depressed mood, and temper outbursts. Adolescents may abuse alcohol and illegal psychoactive agents. Often this disturbance evolves into a conduct disorder or a mood disorder.

DIFFERENTIAL DIAGNOSIS

Because oppositional behavior is both normal and adaptive at specific developmental stages, these periods of negativism must be distinguished from the disorder itself. Developmental-stage oppositional behavior is of shorter duration than is oppositional defiant disorder and is not considerably more frequent or more intense than that of other children of the same mental age.

Oppositional defiant behavior that occurs temporarily in reaction to a severe stress should be diagnosed as an adjustment disorder.

When features of oppositional defiant disorder appear during the course of a conduct disorder, schizophrenic disorder, or mood disorder, the diagnosis of oppositional defiant disorder should not be made.

Oppositional and negativistic behaviors also may be present in pervasive developmental disorder, attention-deficit hyperactivity disorder, chronic brain syndromes, and mental retardation. Whether a concomitant diagnosis of oppositional defiant disorder should be given depends on the severity, pervasiveness, and duration of such behavior.

TREATMENT

The primary treatments for this disorder are individual psychotherapy for the child with counseling and direct training of the parents in child management skills.

Behavior therapists emphasize teaching parents how to alter their behavior in order to discourage their child's oppositional behavior and encourage his or her appropriate behavior. Behavior therapy focuses on selectively reinforcing and praising appropriate behavior and ignoring or not reinforcing undesired behavior.

Clinicians who treat these patients with individual psychotherapy note that family patterns are rigid and difficult to alter unless the children themselves have a new type of object relationship with the therapist. Within the therapeutic relationship, children can relive the autonomy-threatening experiences that produced their defenses. In the safety of a noncontrolling relationship, they can understand the self-destructive nature of their behavior and risk expressing themselves directly. Their self-esteem must be restored before their automatic defenses against external control can be relinquished. In this way, independence may replace habitual defenses against intrusion and control. Once a therapeutic relationship has been formed on the basis of respect for the patient's separateness, the patient is ready to understand the source of his or her defenses and to try new coping behaviors.

References

Doke L A, Flippo J R: Aggressive and oppositional behavior. In *Handbook of Child Psychopathology*, T Ollendick, editor, p 222. Plenum, New York, 1982.

Farrington D P: The family backgrounds of aggressive youths. In *Aggression and Antisocial Behavior in Childhood and Adolescence*, L Herzov, M Berger, D Shaffer, editors. Pergamon, Oxford, England, 1978.

Glueck S, Glueck E: *Unraveling Juvenile Delinquency*. Commonwealth Fund, New York, 1950.

Group for the Advancement of Psychiatry: *Psychopathological Disorders in Childhood. Theoretical Considerations and a Proposed Classification*. Group for the Advancement of Psychiatry, New York, 1966.

Levy D M: Oppositional syndromes and oppositional behavior. In *Psychopathology of Childhood*, P Hoch, J Zubin, editors, p 204. Grune & Stratton, New York, 1955.

Lewis D O, Shanok S S, Grant M, Ritvo E: Homicidally aggressive young children: Neuropsychiatric and experiential correlates. Am J Psychiatry *140*:148, 1983.

Lewis D O, Shanok S S, Lewis M L, Unger L, Goldman C: Conduct disorder and its synonyms: Diagnosis of dubious validity and usefulness. Am J Psychiatry *141*:514, 1984.

Robins L: *Deviant Children Grown Up*. Williams & Wilkins, Baltimore, 1966.

37

Anxiety Disorders of Childhood or Adolescence

Anxiety disorders include three disorders of childhood or adolescence in which anxiety is the predominant clinical feature. In separation anxiety disorder and avoidant disorder of childhood or adolescence, the anxiety is focused on specific situations. In overanxious disorder, the anxiety is generalized to a variety of situations. See Table 1 for a description of the anxiety disorders described in this chapter.

SEPARATION ANXIETY DISORDER

Definition

Separation anxiety disorder is a clinical syndrome whose predominant feature is excessive anxiety on separation from the major attachment figures or from home or other familiar surroundings. When so separated, such children may experience anxiety to the point of panic, beyond that expected at their developmental level.

According to DSM-III-R, a diagnosis of separation anxiety order should not be made if the anxiety occurs exclusively during the course of another illness, such as pervasive developmental disorder or any other psychotic disorder.

Epidemiology

This disorder is ubiquitous in early childhood and occurs equally in both sexes. The onset may be as early as preschool years, but most cases begin around 11 or 12 years, especially the most extreme form of the disorder, refusing to go to school.

Etiology

Psychosocial. Young children, immature and dependent on a mothering figure, are particularly prone to anxiety related to separation. Because children undergo a series of developmental fears—fear of being annihilated, fear of losing their mother, fear of their impulses, fear of losing their body parts and body integrity, and fear of the punishing anxiety of the superego and of guilt—most have transient experiences of separation anxiety based on one or another of these fears. However, well-defined separation anxiety disorders are most frequently seen in early infancy, when they are defined as anaclitic depression or depression due to loss of the mothering figure. At the point of necessary separation from the

parent to enter school, the syndrome of school phobia or school refusal occurs.

Thus, the syndrome is common in childhood, especially in mild forms that do not reach the physician's office. It is only when the symptoms have become established and disturb the child's general adaptation to family life, peers, and school that they come to the attention of professionals.

Learning. Phobic anxiety may be communicated from parents to children by direct modeling. If a parent is fearful, there is a greater likelihood of the child's developing a phobic adaptation to new situations, especially to the school environment. Some parents appear to teach their children to be anxious by overprotecting them from expected dangers or by exaggerating the dangers. For example, the parent who cringes in a room during a lightning storm teaches a child to do the same. The parent who is frightened of mice or insects conveys the affect of fright to the child. Conversely, the parent who becomes angry at a child during an incipient phobic concern about animals may inculcate a phobic concern in the child by the very intensity of the anger expressed.

Genetics. There is probably a genetic basis for the intensity with which separation anxiety is experienced by individual children. Family studies have shown that the biological offspring of adults with anxiety disorder are more prone to suffer in their childhood from separation anxiety. There is also an overlap between separation anxiety disorder and depression in children, and some clinicians view this disorder as a variant of depression.

Clinical Features

According to DSM-III-R, the essential feature of this disorder is extreme anxiety precipitated by separation from parents, home, or other familiar surroundings. The child's anxiety may approach terror or panic. The distress is greater than normally expected for the child's developmental level and cannot be explained by any other disorder. In many cases, the disorder is a kind of phobia, although the phobic concern is a general one and not directed to a particular symbolic object. Because the disorder is associated with childhood, it is not included among the phobic disorders of adulthood, which imply a much greater structuralization of the personality.

Morbid fears, preoccupations, and ruminations are characteristic of this disorder. Such children become fearful that someone close to them will be hurt or that something terrible will happen to them when they are away from important caring figures. Many children worry that they or

Table 1
Common Characteristics of Anxiety Disorders of Childhood or Adolescence*

Criteria	Separation Anxiety Disorder	Avoidant Disorder	Overanxious Disorder
Minimum duration to establish diagnosis	More than 2 weeks	At least 6 months	not specified
Age of onset	Preschool to 18 yrs	2½ years 18 years	3 years or older
Precipitating stresses	Separation from significant parental figures, other losses, travel	Pressure for social participation	Unusual pressure for performance, damage to self-esteem, feelings of lack of competence
Peer relations	Good when no separation involved	Tentative, overly inhibited	Overly eager to please, peers sought out and dependent relationship established
Sleep	Difficulty in falling asleep, fear of dark, nightmares	Difficulty in falling asleep at times	Difficulty in falling asleep
Psychophysiological symptoms	Stomachaches, nausea, vomiting, flu-like symptoms, headaches, palpitations, dizziness, faintness	Blushing, body tension	Stomachaches, nausea, vomiting, lump in the throat, shortness of breath, dizziness, palpitations
Differential diagnosis	Overanxious disorder, schizophrenic disorder, depressive disorder, conduct disorders, pervasive developmental disorder, major depression, panic disorder with agoraphobia	Adjustment disorder with withdrawal, overanxious disorder, separation anxiety disorder, major depression, dysthymia, avoident personality disorder, borderline personality disorder	Separation anxiety disorder, attention-deficit hyperactivity disorder, avoidant disorder, adjustment disorder with anxious mood, obsessive-compulsive disorder, psychotic disorder, mood disorder

*****Adapted from Table by Sidney Werkman, M.D.**

their parents will have an accident or become ill. Fears about getting lost and about being kidnapped and never again finding their parents are common.

Adolescents may not directly express any anxious concern about separation from a mothering figure. Yet their behavior patterns often reflect a separation anxiety in that they may express discomfort about leaving home, engage in solitary activities, and continue to use the mothering figure as a helper in buying clothes and entering social and recreational activities.

The separation anxiety disorder in children often is manifested at the thought of travel or in the course of travel away from home. Such children may refuse to go to camp, a new school, or even a friend's house. Frequently, there is a continuum between mild anticipatory anxiety before separation from an important figure and pervasive anxiety after the separation has occurred. Premonitory signs include irritability, difficulty in eating, whining, clinging behavior, staying in a room alone, clinging to parents, and following the parent everywhere. Often, when a family moves, the child displays separation anxiety by intense clinging to the mother figure. Sometimes geographic relocation anxiety is expressed in feelings of acute homesickness or psychophysiological symptoms that break out when the child is away from home or is going to a new country. The child yearns to return home and becomes preoccupied with fantasies of how much better his or her old home was. Integration into the new life situation may become extremely difficult.

Sleep difficulties are frequent and may require that someone remain with the children until they fall asleep. Children often go to their parent's bed or even sleep at the parents' door when the bedroom is barred to them. Nightmares and morbid fears are other expressions of this anxiety.

Associated features include fear of the dark and imaginary, bizarre worries. Children may see eyes staring at them and become preoccupied with mythical figures or monsters reaching out for them in their bedrooms.

Many children are demanding and intrusive in adult affairs and require constant attention to allay their anxieties. Symptoms emerge when separation from an important parent figure becomes necessary. If separation is not threatened, many children with this disorder do not experience interpersonal difficulties. They may, however, look sad and cry easily. They sometimes complain that they are not loved, express a wish to die, or complain that siblings are favored over them. They frequently develop gastrointestinal symptoms of nausea, vomiting, or stomachaches and have pains in various parts of the body, sore throats, and flu-like symptoms. In older children, typical cardiovascular and respiratory symptoms of palpitations, dizziness, faintness, and strangulation are reported.

Course and Prognosis

Typically, periods of exacerbation and remission alternate over a period of several years. The course of this disorder depends on the presence or absence of a reliable mothering figure. When the mothering figure is absent in infancy for a short period of time, separation anxiety disorder may develop, only to be reversed on the return of the mothering figure. In later childhood, symptoms of separation anxiety disorder are not so easily reversed, even with the return of the mothering figure. However, the availability of an adequate substitute caring figure may minimize or reverse the expression of symptoms.

When a reliable mothering figure is not available for a period of months, or when the internalized representation of a rejecting or unavailable mothering figure has become crystallized, the separation anxiety disorder may persist over a long period of time or may be exacerbated by specific stresses. Once established, both the separation anxiety and the symptoms developed to avoid this anxiety may be sustained for many years. In severe cases, such children may be unable to attend school or function independently in various areas. In a very few cases, inpatient care may be necessary to offer children an opportunity to escape noxious influences in the home and to profit from a supportive, reliable environment. Cases left untreated become chronic, with fear and physical symptoms evolving into somatoform disorders or depression.

Predisposing Factors

The character structure pattern in many children who develop this disorder includes conscientiousness, eagerness to please, and a tendency toward conformity. Families tend to be close-knit and caring, and such children often seem to be spoiled or the objects of parental overconcern.

External life stresses often coincide with the development of the disorder. The death of a relative, illness in the child, a change in the child's environment, or a move to a new neighborhood or new school are frequently noted in the histories of children with this disorder.

Diagnosis

The diagnosis is made when any of the primary symptoms listed in Table 2 are present for at least 2 weeks. The disorder is considered to be mild when the child shows more than occasional concerns about separating from parents or home but can function in a new situation despite evidence of anxiety. The disorder is considered to be moderate when the child has panic reactions to separation but can perform adequately for a while, although acute symptoms develop intermittently; for example, the child may have to be picked up from school or camp or be accompanied on errands. In severe separation anxiety disorder, the child has panic reactions to threatened or actual separation and refuses to go to school or to stay home alone.

The history frequently reveals important episodes of separation in the child's life, particularly because of illness and hospitalization, illness of the parent, loss of a parent, or geographic relocation. The period of infancy should be scrutinized for evidence of separation-individuation disorders or lack of an adequate mothering figure. The use of fantasies, dreams, play material, and observation of the child are of great help in making the diagnosis. Not only the content of thought but also the way in which thoughts are expressed should be examined. For example, children may express fears that their parents will die, even when their behavior does not show evidence of motor anxiety. Similarly, their difficulty in describing events or their bland denial of obviously anxiety-provoking events may indicate the presence of a separation anxiety disorder. Difficulty with memory in expressing separation themes, or patent distortions in the recital of such themes, may give clues to the disorder's presence.

Table 2
Diagnostic Criteria for Separation Anxiety Disorder

A. Excessive anxiety concerning separation from those to whom the child is attached, as evidenced by at least three of the following:

(1) unrealistic and persistent worry about possible harm befalling major attachment figures or fear that they will leave and not return

(2) unrealistic and persistent worry that an untoward calamitous event will separate the child from a major attachment figure, e.g., the child will be lost, kidnapped, killed, or be the victim of an accident

(3) persistent reluctance or refusal to go to school in order to stay with major attachment figures or at home

(4) persistent reluctance or refusal to go to sleep without being near a major attachment figure or to go to sleep away from home

(5) persistent avoidance of being alone, including "clinging" to and "shadowing" major attachment figures

(6) repeated nightmares involving the theme of separation

(7) complaints of physical symptoms, e.g., headaches, stomachaches, nausea, or vomiting, on many school days or on other occasions when anticipating separation from major attachment figures

(8) recurrent signs or complaints of excessive distress in anticipation of separation from home or major attachment figures, e.g., temper tantrums or crying, pleading with parents not to leave

(9) recurrent signs of complaints of excessive distress when separated from home or major attachment figures, e.g., wants to return home, needs to call parents when they are absent or when child is away from home

B. Duration of disturbance of at least 2 weeks.

C. Onset before the age of 18.

D. Occurrence not exclusively during the course of a Pervasive Developmental Disorder, Schizophrenia, or any other psychotic disorder.

Table from DSM-III-R, *Diagnostic and Statistical Manual of Mental Disorders*, ed 3, revised. (Current Classification of Mental Disorders, 1987.) Copyright American Psychiatric Association, Washington, D.C., 1987. Used with permission.

Differential Diagnosis

According to DSM-III-R, some degree of separation anxiety is a normal phenomenon, and clinical judgment must be used in distinguishing this from separation anxiety disorder. In overanxious disorder, anxiety is not focused on separation. In pervasive developmental disorders or schizophrenia, anxiety about separation may occur but is viewed as caused by these conditions rather than as a separate disorder. In major depression occurring in children, the diagnosis of separation anxiety should also be made when the criteria for both disorders are met. Panic disorder with agoraphobia is uncommon before age 18, and the fear is of being incapacitated by a panic attack rather than of separation from parental figures. In some adult cases, however, many of the symptoms of separation anxiety disorder may be present. In conduct disorder, truancy is common, but the child stays away from home and does not have anxiety about separation.

Treatment

For the treatment of school phobia, which may present as a psychiatric emergency, a comprehensive treatment plan involves the child, the parents, and the child's peers and school. The child should be encouraged to attend school, if only to be in a nonthreatening setting or to be with peers in nonacademic situations. There should be graded contact with the object of anxiety under the tutelage of a benevolent adult. This form of behavior modification can be applied to any type of separation anxiety.

Anxiety disorders in general respond to psychotherapy directed toward increasing the child's autonomy by exploring the unconscious meaning of symptoms. Family therapy helps the parents understand the need for consistent, supportive love as well as the importance of preparing for any important change in life, such as illness, surgery, or geographic relocation.

Pharmacotherapy is useful for panic and separation anxiety. The heterocyclic antidepressants such as imipramine (Tofranil), are usually begun in doses of 25 mg daily, increased by additional 25 mg doses up to a total of 150 to 200 mg daily, until a therapeutic effect is noted. With 200 mg daily, if no effect is noted, the plasma levels of imipramine and its active metabolite, desmethylimipramine, should be studied to determine whether a therapeutic blood level has been attained. Aside from its antidepressant effect, imipramine has been postulated to yield results that reduce panic and fear related to separation. Diphenhydramine (Benadryl) can be useful to break a dangerous cycle of sleep disturbances.

AVOIDANT DISORDER

Definition

According to DSM-III-R, avoidant disorder is characterized by a persistent and excessive shrinking from contact with unfamiliar people that is of sufficient severity to interfere with social functioning in peer relationships, is of least 6 months' duration, and is coupled with a clear desire for social involvement with familiar people, such as family members and peers the person knows well. Relationships with family members and other familiar figures are warm and satisfying. This diagnosis should not be made if the person is 18 or older.

Epidemiology

Avoidant disorder is not common and is clinically observed more frequently in boys than in girls, possibly because of the socially sanctioned role models of passivity and withdrawal in girls. The syndrome may develop as early as 2½ years of age, after stranger anxiety or a normal developmental phenomenon should have disappeared. Modeling of a shy, retiring parent is frequently noted in such situations, and girls may go through many years of

avoiding social situations without overt anxiety if parents support their shyness. Boys, on the other hand, are frequently expected to be more independent and aggressive. Therefore, if shyness is a predominant characteristic in their personality makeup, boys will begin to suffer symptoms earlier than girls will. Anxiety disorders are more common in the mothers of children with avoidant disorder than in the general population.

Etiology

Temperamental differences may account for some of the predisposition to this disorder, particularly if the parent supports the child's shyness and withdrawal. Devastating losses early in childhood, sexual traumas, or other kinds of physical abuse or neglect may also contribute to avoidant disorder. Children who have chronic medical problems in childhood, such as rheumatic fever or orthopedic handicaps, may not learn the age-related social skills shared by their peers because they have not been involved in typical social interactions with their age-mates. Likewise, children who have grown up in foreign countries or have moved a great deal may not learn the necessary social skills that allow them to integrate effectively into the social world of their peers.

Clinical Features

Children with avoidant disorder excessively hold back from establishing interpersonal contacts or satisfactory relationships with strangers, to an extent that noticeably interferes with their peer functioning. The avoidance of involvement with strangers persists even after prolonged exposure to new relationships. These children are slow to warm up, although many of them participate actively in social groups that offer considerable support and structure. Typically, these children relate warmly and naturally in their home situation. However, they may be clinging, whining, and overly demanding with caretakers, making great demands on those who are with them.

Embarrassment and timidity are conveyed in their voices, and they may tend to whisper and stand behind people or hide behind furniture in an attempt not to be noticed. Blushing, difficulties in speech, and easy embarrassment are characteristic. Underneath these behaviors—and often expressed in close relationships—are anger, sullen resentment, rage, or grandiosity. There is no evidence of a pattern of intellectual impairment or fundamental difficulty in communication, even when such children seem inarticulate.

When pressured into social participation, children with avoidant disorder may become tearful and anxious. They may cling to their caretakers and refuse to become involved in new activities. In adolescence, the long delay in the development of psychosexual maturity may be evidenced by difficulty in peer relationships and in the establishment of appropriate social, sexual, and aggressive adolescent activities. Extreme inhibition in recreational activities is common, and a great deal of support is necessary to encourage participation. At times, shyness and inhibition complicate the learning process. In such cases, a child's true abilities become apparent only under extremely favorable educational conditions.

Diagnosis

The diagnosis should not be made before the age of 2½ years, when the normal stranger anxiety phase has passed. It is diagnosed on the basis of excessive shrinking from contact with unfamiliar people for a period of 6 months or longer. Children with avoidant disorder may have great difficulty in separating from a parent figure especially to meet unfamiliar persons. Often the parent must come into the examination room at the beginning of the session because the child demands to know exactly where the parent is during the session. See Table 3 for the DSM-III-R criteria for avoidant disorder.

Differential Diagnosis

Avoidant disorder often shades into the realm of avoidant personality disorder, adjustment disorder with withdrawal, and borderline personality. Adjustment disorder with withdrawal is clearly related to a recent psychosocial stressor, in contrast with avoidant disorder, which tends to be a long-term situation with no acute, overt stress precipitating it. In the overanxious disorder of childhood, the anxiety is not limited to contact with strangers, as in avoidant disorder. In the separation anxiety disorder, the anxiety is due to separation from the primary caretaker rather than to forced contact with strangers. The avoidant personality disorder is diagnosed only after the behavior pattern has persisted for many years. Borderline syndromes show more serious character pathology and a greater and more diffuse variety of symptoms, which are not characterized primarily by the avoidance of contact with strangers and new situations. In major depression and dysthymia, the patient is withdrawn, but generally to all persons, including familiar ones.

Treatment

Psychotherapy with the explicit approval of the parent figure is the treatment of choice at the start. A great deal of work is directed toward helping the child separate from the

Table 3
Diagnostic Criteria for Avoidant Disorder of Childhood or Adolescence

A. Excessive shrinking from contact with unfamiliar people, for a period of 6 months or longer, sufficiently severe to interfere with social functioning in peer relationships.

B. Desire for social involvement with familiar people (family members and peers the person knows well), and generally warm and satisfying relations with family members and other familiar figures.

C. Age at least 2½ years.

D. The disturbance is not sufficiently pervasive and persistent to warrant the diagnosis of Avoidant Personality Disorder.

Table from DSM-III-R, *Diagnostic and Statistical Manual of Mental Disorders*, ed 3, revised. (Current Classification of Mental Disorders, 1987.) Copyright American Psychiatric Association, Washington, D.C., 1987. Used with permission.

parent and recognize that independent activity can be safe and fulfilling. In working with the parents, the therapist should show empathically and sensitively how the child is controlling the parent by means of shyness. The parent can then give the child opportunities to experience manageable anxiety and thus be able to give up some of the secondary gains of shyness. The development of skills in dancing, music performance, singing, or writing may be valuable ego supports for such children.

On occasion, antianxiety medication on a short-term basis may decrease anxiety in order to overcome the avoidant behavior. What is most needed, however, is a restructuring of relationships in a supportive therapeutic environment that directs the child toward facing new situations and mastering anxiety in order to achieve a higher level of independent functioning.

Parents often require therapy because they may be unwilling to support the newly assertive child, especially if shyness fulfilled unconscious needs in the parents to keep the child infantalized.

OVERANXIOUS DISORDER

Definition

According to DSM-III-R, the essential feature of overanxious disorder is excessive and unrealistic anxiety or worry for a period of 6 months or longer. Children with this disorder tend to be extremely self-conscious, to worry about future events (e.g., examinations, the possibility of injury, or inclusion in peer group activities) or about meeting expectations (e.g., deadlines, keeping appointments, or performing chores), and to be concerned about the discomforts or dangers of a variety of situations. For example, routine visits to the doctor may be anticipated with excessive worry about minor procedures. Such children may also be overly anxious about competence in a number of areas and especially about what others think of them. In general, the disorder presents a picture of excessive worrying and fearful behavior.

Epidemiology

Some evidence suggests that overanxious disorder is most common in small families of upper socioeconomic status and in firstborn children. Although both boys and girls develop this disorder, some workers believe that it is more common in boys than in girls; however, DSM-III-R describes the disorder as equally common in males and females. It may also be more common in urban than in rural areas.

Etiology

There is some evidence of a familial pattern, in that children with the disorder are more likely to have mothers who also suffer from anxiety disorders. Unconscious conflicts related to fixations at the oedipal psychosexual phase of development have been postulated. The disorder is often associated with situations in which there is great concern about performance, even when the child is functioning at an adequate level. In such families, children come to believe that they must meet their parents' high expectations.

Clinical Description

According to DSM-III-R, the principal characteristics of the disorder are that such children are always worried, especially about future events that require meeting expectations (e.g., examinations, parties, and sports). They are greatly concerned about their competence and about being judged negatively. At times, these worries may have an obsessive or ruminative pattern. Physical signs and symptoms (e.g., insomnia, nail biting, palpitations, respiratory and gastrointestinal distress) are common. The children may always appear nervous or tense.

Associated features include social and simple phobias. Children with this disorder may refuse to attend school because of their anxiety there. They often seem hypermature because of their "precocious" concerns. Perfectionist tendencies, with obsessional self-doubt, may be evident; the children may be excessively conformist and overzealous in seeking approval. They may be reluctant to engage in age-appropriate activities in which there are demands for performance, such as sports. Many of these children are accident prone and seem to exaggerate the extent of pain, deformity, or

Table 4
Diagnostic Criteria for Overanxious Disorder

A. Excessive or unrealistic anxiety or worry, for a period of 6 months or longer, as indicated by the frequent occurrence of at least four of the following:

(1) excessive or unrealistic worry about future events
(2) excessive or unrealistic concern about the appropriateness of past behavior
(3) excessive or unrealistic concern about competence in one or more areas, e.g., athletic, academic, social
(4) somatic complaints, such as headaches or stomachaches, for which no physical basis can be established
(5) marked self-consciousness
(6) excessive need for reassurance about a variety of concerns
(7) marked feelings of tension or inability to relax

B. If another Axis I disorder is present (e.g., Separation Anxiety Disorder, Phobic Disorder, Obsessive Compulsive Disorder), the focus of the symptoms in A are not limited to it. For example, if Separation Anxiety Disorder is present, the symptoms in A are not exclusively related to anxiety about separation. In addition, the disturbance does not occur only during the course of a psychotic disorder or a Mood Disorder.

C. If 18 or older, does not meet the criteria for Generalized Anxiety Disorder.

D. Occurrence not exclusively during the course of a Pervasive Developmental Disorder, Schizophrenia, or any other psychotic disorder.

Table from DSM-III-R, *Diagnostic and Statistical Manual of Mental Disorders,* ed 3, revised. (Current Classification of Mental Disorders, 1987.) Copyright American Psychiatric Association, Washington, D.C., 1987. Used with permission.

potential handicap that may result from illness or accidents, and they may have unnecessary medical examinations as a result.

Course and Prognosis

Because of the high level of verbal and intellectual abilities of many children with overanxious disorder, the relatively effective mothering experiences in their lives, and their strong desires to relate, the course of the disorder is often benign. However, unusually stressful life experiences may contradict such a prognosis. Rarely does the disorder result in an inability to meet at least the minimal demands of school, home, and social life, but youngsters with overanxious disorder may have a great deal of inner stress that persists into adult life as an anxiety disorder, such as generalized anxiety disorder or social phobia.

Diagnosis

The symptoms include the presence of persistent anxiety and worrying about future events, together with a concern about competence in a variety of areas. Difficulty in falling asleep, combined with frightening dreams, and somatic complaints—such as headaches, gastrointestinal symptoms, and respiratory symptoms for which no medical basis can be established—are typically noted. The disorder must be present for at least 6 months and must not be a symptom of another disorder, such as separation anxiety disorder, avoidant disorder, phobic disorder, obsessive-compulsive disorder, depressive disorder, schizophrenia, or a pervasive developmental disorder. Table 4 lists the DSM-III-R diagnostic criteria for overanxious disorder.

Differential Diagnosis

Overanxious disorder is distinct from separation anxiety disorder, which emphasizes separation from a familiar person. Panic disorder is characterized by recurrent panic attacks and a fear of future attacks. Obsessive-compulsive disorder has more highly structured obsessions and compulsions than does overanxious disorder, and pervasive developmental disorder has an earlier age of onset and the classic diagnostic criteria of that illness. Depression has predominant mood symptoms and signs. Coterminous and overlapping diagnoses may include dream anxiety disorder, functional enuresis, learning disability, and almost any of the personality disorders coded on Axis II. Overanxious disorder should not be diagnosed when the anxiety is a symptom of a psychotic disorder or a mood disorder.

Treatment

Antianxiety medications, such as diazepam (Valium), may be useful in acute situations when accompanied by a discussion of their use and the concomitant psychotherapeutic involvement of the parents. Acute anxiety accompanied by insomnia can be effectively treated by the short-term use of such sedatives as diphenhydramine (Benadryl). Buspirone has been found to be effective.

When such children complain of psychophysiological symptoms, they should be given the benefit of a thorough medical or pediatric examination. If the findings of such an examination are normal, their symptoms should be discussed and treated as somatic equivalents of anxiety. The patient should be assured that such symptoms will disappear when the basis for anxiety is resolved.

These children are excellent candidates for insight therapy, either individually or with their families. Many believe this to be the treatment of choice. Themes of sibling rivalry, wishes to excel, and oedipal struggles tend to emerge. The prognosis in such children with treatment is usually excellent.

References

Adams P L, Fras I: *Beginning Child Psychiatry*. Brunner/Mazel, New York, 1987.

Anthony E J: Communicating therapeutically with the child. J Am Child Psychiatry 3:106, 1964.

Bowlby J: *Attachment and Loss,* 3 vols. Basic Books, New York, 1969, 1973, 1980.

Compton A: A study of the psychoanalytic theory of anxiety. J Am Psychoanal Assoc 20:3, 1972.

Freud S: Introductory lectures on psychoanalysis. In *Complete Psychological Works of Sigmund Freud,* vol 16, p 393. Hogarth Press, London, 1963.

Last C G, Francis G, Hersen M, Kazdin A E, Strauss C C: Separation anxiety and school phobia: A comparison using DSM-III criteria. Am J Psych 144:653, 1987.

O'Brien J: School problems: School phobia and learning disabilities. Psychiatr Clin North Am 5:297, 1982.

Simeon J G, Ferguson H B: Recent developments in the use of antidepressants and anxiolytic medications. Psychiatric Clin North Amer 8:893, 1985.

Thomas A, Chess S, Birch H S: *Temperament and Behavior Disorders in Children*. New York University Press, New York, 1968.

38

————— Eating Disorders

INTRODUCTION TO EATING DISORDERS

According to DSM-III-R, these disorders are characterized by gross disturbances in eating behavior; it includes anorexia nervosa, bulimia nervosa, pica, and rumination disorder of infancy. Anorexia nervosa and bulimia nervosa are apparently related disorders, typically beginning in adolescence or early adult life. Pica and rumination disorder of infancy are primarily disorders of young children and are probably unrelated to anorexia nervosa and bulimia nervosa.

38.1 —————
Pica

DEFINITION AND DIAGNOSTIC CRITERIA

Pica is the repeated ingestion of nonnutritive substances, such as dirt, clay, plaster, and paper. The DSM-III-R diagnostic criteria are given in Table 1.

EPIDEMIOLOGY

Pica rarely occurs in adults. DSM-III-R states that it is occasionally seen in young children, in persons with mental retardation, and in pregnant females. However, pica may be more common that this statement implies. Several studies report between 10 percent and 32.3 percent of children between 1 and 6 years of age have pica. The incidence diminishes with age, and the disorder is apparently seen equally frequently in both sexes.

Clay eating (geophasia) and starch (e.g., Argo starch) eating appear to have an increased incidence among pregnant women in certain subcultures. In one study, 55 percent of pregnant females in Georgia had geophasia, and in another, 41 percent of pregnant black females ate starch, and 27 percent ate clay.

ETIOLOGY

There are three commonly suggested causes of pica: (1) the result of an inadequate mother–child relationship that results in unsatisfied oral needs expressed in the persistent search for inedible substances; (2) a specific nutritional deficiency causing the indiscriminant ingestion of nonfood items; and (3) cultural factors suspected to be important to geophasia (earth or clay eating) and starch eating by some pregnant women.

CLINICAL DESCRIPTION

Eating nonedible substances after 18 months of age is usually considered abnormal. The onset of pica is usually between age 12 and 24 months, and the incidence declines with age. The specific substances ingested vary somewhat with their accessibility, and they increase with the child's mastery of locomotion and the resultant increased independence and decreased parental supervision. Typically, young children ingest paint, plaster, string, hair, and cloth; older children have access to dirt, animal feces, stones, and paper.

Clinical implications may be benign or life threatening, according to the objects ingested. Among the most serious complications are lead poisoning, usually from lead-based paint, intestinal parasites following ingestion of soil or feces, anemia and zinc deficiency following the ingestion of clay, severe iron deficiency following the ingestion of large quantities of starch, and intestinal obstruction from the ingestion of hair balls, stones, or gravel.

With the exception of mentally retarded individuals, pica usually remits by adolescence. Pica associated with pregnancy is usually limited to the pregnancy itself.

DIFFERENTIAL DIAGNOSIS

DSM-III-R notes that nonnutritive substances may be eaten by patients with autistic disorder, schizophrenia, and certain physical disorders, such as Kleine–Levin syndrome, and that in such cases pica should not be noted as an

Table 1
Diagnostic Criteria for Pica

A. Repeated eating of a nonnutritive substance for at least 1 month.

B. Does not meet the criteria for either Autistic Disorder, Schizophrenia, or Kleine-Levin syndrome.

Table from DSM-III-R, *Diagnostic and Statistical Manual of Mental Disorders,* ed 3, revised. (Current Classification of Mental Disorders, 1987.) Copyright American Psychiatric Association, Washington, D.C., 1987. Used with permission.

additional diagnosis. Some clinicians believe that to be unfortunate because only a small minority of autistic and schizophrenic persons ingest nonedible items.

The eating of bizarre and sometimes potentially dangerous substances (e.g. animal food, toilet water, and garbage) is a frequent behavioral abnormality among children with psychosocial dwarfism.

TREATMENT

There is no definitive treatment for pica. Treatments basically emphasize psychosocial, environmental, behavioral, and/or family guidance approaches.

An effort should be made to ameliorate any significant psychosocial stressors that are present. When lead is present in the surroundings, it must be eliminated or rendered inaccessible, or the child must be moved to new surroundings.

Several behavioral techniques have been used with some effect. The most rapidly successful seems to be mild aversion therapy or negative reinforcement (e.g., mild electric shock, unpleasant noise, or an emetic drug). Positive reinforcement, modeling, behavioral shaping, and overcorrection treatment have also been used.

Increasing parental attention, stimulation, and emotional nurturance may have positive results. One study found that pica was negatively correlated with involvement with play materials and occurred more frequently in impoverished environments.

In some patients, correction of an iron or zinc deficiency has resulted in the elimination of pica.

Medical complications (e.g., lead poisoning) that develop secondarily to the pica must also be treated.

References

Blinder B J, Chaitin B, Goldstein R, editors: *The Eating Disorders.* Pergamon Press, New York, 1987.

Cooper M: *Pica.* Thomas, Springfield, IL, 1957.

Danford D E, Smith C J, Huber A M: Pica and mineral status in the mentally retarded. Am J Clin Nut *35*:958, 1982.

Lourie R S, Millican F K. Pica. In *Modern Perspectives in International Child Psychiatry,* J G Howells, editor, p 445. Brunner/Mazel, New York, 1971.

Millican F K, Dublin C C, Lourie R S: Pica. In *Basic Handbook of Child Psychiatry,* Noshpitz J D, editor, vol 2, p 660. Basic Books, New York, 1979.

Millican F K, Lourie R S, Laymen E M: Emotional factors in the etiology and treatment of lead poisoning. Am J of Diseases of Children *91*:144, 1956.

Provence S, Lipton R C: *Infants and Institutions.* International Universities Press, New York, 1962.

38.2 _____
Rumination Disorder of Infancy

DEFINITION AND DIAGNOSTIC CRITERIA

Rumination is an extremely rare but fascinating illness that has been recognized for hundreds of years. This regurgitation disorder, which can be fatal, occurs predominantly in infancy and seldom in adults. An awareness of the disorder is important so that it may be correctly diagnosed and so that unnecessary surgical procedures or inappropriate treatment can be avoided.

Rumination is derived from the Latin word *ruminare,* which means to chew the cud. The Greek equivalent is *merycism,* which describes the act of regurgitation of food from the stomach into the mouth, rechewing the food, and reswallowing it.

The DSM-III-R criteria for rumination disorder of infancy are given in Table 1. DSM-III-R notes that the essential feature of this disorder is repeated regurgitation of food, with weight loss or failure to gain expected weight, developing after a period of normal functioning. Partially digested food is brought up into the mouth without nausea, retching, disgust, or associated gastrointestinal disorder. The food is then ejected from the mouth or reswallowed. A characteristic position of straining and arching the back, with the head held back, is observed. The infant makes sucking movements with his or her tongue and gives the impression of gaining considerable satisfaction from the activity. An associated feature that is usually present is that the infant is generally irritable and hungry between episodes of rumination.

EPIDEMIOLOGY AND PREVALENCE

Rumination is a rare disorder. It seems most common among infants between 3 months and 1 year of age and mentally retarded children and adults. Adults with rumination usually maintain a normal weight. It is apparently equally common in males and females. There are no reliable figures on predisposing factors or familial patterns.

ETIOLOGY

Several etiologies have been proposed. The psychodynamic theories hypothesize various disturbances in the mother-child relationship. The mothers of these infants are usually immature, involved in a marital conflict, and unable to give much attention to the baby. This results in insufficient emotional gratification and stimulation for the infant, who thus seeks gratification from within. The rumination is interpreted as an attempt by the infant to recreate the feeding process and provide gratification that the mother does not provide. Overstimulation and tension have also been suggested as causing rumination.

Table 1
Diagnostic Criteria for Rumination Disorder of Infancy

A. Repeated regurgitation, without nausea or associated gastrointestinal illness, for at least 1 month following a period of normal functioning.

B. Weight loss or failure to make expected weight gain.

Table from DSM-III-R, *Diagnostic and Statistical Manual of Mental Disorders*, ed 3, revised. (Current Classification of Mental Disorders, 1987.) Copyright American Psychiatric Association, Washington, D.C., 1987. Used with permission.

A dysfunctional autonomic nervous system has also been implicated. As more sophisticated and accurate investigative techniques are refined, a substantial number of children diagnosed as ruminators are shown to have gastroesophageal reflux or a hiatal hernia.

Behaviorists attribute rumination to the positive reinforcement of the pleasurable self-stimulation, as well as the attention the baby receives from others as a consequence of the disorder.

CLINICAL DESCRIPTION

Initially, rumination may be difficult to distinguish from the regurgitation, which frequently occurs in normal infants. In the fully developed case, however, the diagnosis is obvious. Food or milk is regurgitated without nausea, retching, or disgust and is subjected to what appears to be innumerable pleasurable sucking and chewing movements. The food is then reswallowed or ejected from the mouth.

Although spontaneous remissions are common, severe secondary complications may develop, such as progressive malnutrition, dehydration, and lowered resistance to disease. Failure to thrive, with growth failure and developmental delays in all areas, may occur. Mortality as high as 25 percent has been reported in severe cases.

An additional complication is that the mother or caretaker is often discouraged by the failure to feed the infant successfully and may become alienated, if not already so. Further alienation often occurs as the noxious odor of the regurgitated material leads to avoidance of the infant.

DIFFERENTIAL DIAGNOSIS

Rumination must be differentiated from congenital anomalies or infections of the gastrointestinal tract that may cause regurgitation of food. Pyloric stenosis is usually associated with projectile vomiting and is evident before 3 months of age.

TREATMENT

It is difficult to evaluate the effectiveness of treatments, as most are single case reports and are not randomly assigned to controlled studies. Any concomitant medical complications must also be treated.

Treatments include improvement of the child's psychosocial environment, more "tender loving care" from the mother or caretakers, and psychotherapy for the mother or both parents.

When anatomical abnormalities such as hiatal hernia are present, surgical repair may be necessary.

Behavioral techniques have also been used effectively. Aversive conditioning involves administering a mild electric shock or squirting an unpleasant substance (e.g., lemon juice) in the mouth whenever rumination occurs, and this appears to be the most rapidly effective treatment. Rumination is eliminated within 3 to 5 days. In the aversive-conditioning reports on rumination, the infants were doing well at 9- or 12-month follow-ups, with no recurrence of the rumination and with weight gains, increased activity levels, and greater general responsiveness to people.

One study showed that if subjects were allowed to eat as much as they wanted, the rate of rumination decreased.

References

Blinder B J, Chaitin B, Goldstein R, editors: *The Eating Disorders*. Pergamon Press, New York, 1987.

Davis P K, Cuvo A J: Chronic vomiting and rumination in intellectually normal and retarded individuals: Review and evaluation of behavioral research. Behav Res Severe Dev Disabil *1*:31, 1980.

Flanagan C H: Rumination in infancy—Past and present. With a case report. J Am Acad Child Psychiatry *16*:40, 1977.

Linscheid T R, Cunningham C E: A controlled demonstration of the effectiveness of electric shock in the elimination of chronic infant rumination. J Applied Behav Anal *10*:500, 1977.

Rast J, Johnston J M, Drum C, Conrin J: The relation of food quantity to rumination behavior. J Applied Behav Anal *14*:221, 1981.

38.3 _____
Anorexia Nervosa and Bulimia Nervosa

ANOREXIA NERVOSA

Definition

Anorexia nervosa is an eating disorder characterized by self-imposed dietary limitations, peculiar patterns of handling food, significant weight loss, and an intense fear of obesity and gaining weight. There is a significant disturbance in body image (anorexics claim to feel fat even when emaciated). There must be a weight loss of at least 15 percent of the original body weight. Anorexics refuse to maintain body weight over a minimal normal weight for their age and height. In order to make the diagnosis of anorexia, there must be no known physical illness to account for the weight loss. Usually there is a single episode of anorexia, with eventual full recovery. Anorexic patients diet incessantly and often abuse diuretics and laxatives. In women, there is amenorrhea. It is one of the few psychiatric illnesses that may have a course that leads to death.

Epidemiology and Prevalence

The only incidence study of anorexia nervosa conducted in this country reported an average incidence of 0.37 per 100,000 population per year.

Recent prevalence studies have shown anorexia nervosa to be a common disorder in the age group most at risk—10 years (prepuberty) to 30 years—and especially in the higher socioeconomic classes. It most commonly occurs during early to late adolescence.

Various studies report that about 4 to 6 percent of anorexics are males. The morbidity risk for a sister of an anorexic patient is about 7 percent, which greatly exceeds normal expectations. Often mothers or fathers had an explicit history of significantly low adolescent weight or a weight phobia. The available evidence does not permit any conclusions about the role of heredity in the development of anorexia. As many as 1 in 100 and as few as 1 in 800 females between the ages of 12 and 18 years may develop the disorder.

Etiology

The psychological theories concerning the causes of anorexia nervosa have centered mostly on phobias and psychodynamic formulations. One investigator postulated that anorexia nervosa constitutes a phobic-avoidance response to food, resulting from the sexual and social tensions generated by the physical changes associated with puberty. The resulting malnutrition leads to a reduction in sexual interest, which in turn leads to greater self-starvation.

An early psychodynamic theory was that anorexic patients reject, through starvation, a wish to be pregnant and have fantasies of oral impregnation. Other dynamic formulations have included a dependent seductive relationship with a warm but passive father and guilt over aggression toward an ambivalently regarded mother. Others have described disturbances of body image (denial of their emaciation), disturbances in self-perception (lack of recognition or denial of fatigue, weakness, and hunger), and a sense of ineffectiveness caused by false learning experiences.

No adequate studies have been conducted to establish definite predisposing factors in anorexia nervosa. In the descriptive literature of this illness, several different stressful life situations have been noted to occur shortly before the onset of anorexia nervosa. Above-average scholastic achievement, model perfectionism, and an unrealistic fear of failure are often characteristics of these patients. About one third of anorexics are mildly overweight before the onset of the illness.

Clinical Features

The onset of anorexia nervosa occurs between the ages of 10 and 30. The onset is uncommon before age 10 and after age 30, and often those cases outside this age range are not typical, and so their diagnoses should be questioned. After the age of 13 years, the frequency of onset increases rapidly, with the maximum frequency at 17 to 18 years of age. About 85 percent of all anorexic patients develop the illness between the ages of 13 and 20 years.

Most of the aberrant behavior directed toward losing weight occurs in secret. The anorexic patients usually refuse to eat with their families or in public places. They lose weight by a drastic reduction in their total food intake, with a disproportionate decrease in high-carbohydrate and fatty foods.

Unfortunately, the term anorexia is a misnomer because the loss of appetite is usually rare until late in the illness. Evidence that the patients are constantly thinking about food is their passion for collecting recipes and preparing elaborate meals for others. Some patients cannot continuously control their voluntary restriction of food intake, and so they have eating binges. These binges usually occur secretly and often at night. Self-induced vomiting frequently follows the eating binge. Patients abuse laxatives and even diuretics in order to lose weight. Ritualistic exercising, extensive cycling, and walking, jogging, or running are common activities.

Patients with this disorder exhibit peculiar behavior regarding food. They hide food all over the house and frequently carry large quantities of candies in their pockets and purses. While eating meals, they try to dispose of food in their napkins or hide it in their pockets. They cut their meat into very small pieces and spend a great deal of time rearranging the food items on their plate. If the patients are confronted about their peculiar behavior, they often deny that their behavior is unusual or flatly refuse to discuss it.

An intense fear of gaining weight and becoming obese is present in all patients with this illness and undoubtedly contributes to their lack of interest in and even resistance to therapy.

Obsessive-compulsive behavior, depression, and anxiety are the other psychiatric symptoms in anorexia nervosa most frequently noted in the literature. Somatic complaints, especially epigastric discomfort, are usual. Compulsive stealing, usually of candies and laxatives but occasionally of clothes and other items, is common.

Poor sexual adjustment is frequently described in patients with this disorder. Many adolescent anorexics have delayed psychosocial sexual development, and adults often have a markedly decreased interest in sex accompanying the onset of the illness. An unusual minority subgroup of anorexics have a premorbid history of promiscuity or drug abuse or both, and during the illness, they do not show a decreased interest in sex.

Patients usually come to medical attention when their weight loss becomes apparent. As the weight loss becomes profound, physical signs such as hypothermia (as low as 35°C), dependent edema, bradycardia, hypotension, and lanugo (the appearance of neonatal-like hair) appear, and there are a variety of metabolic changes (Figure 1).

Many female anorexics come to medical attention because of amenorrhea, which often appears before their weight loss is noticeable. Most studies have shown an impaired luteinizing hormone (LH) response to gonadotropin-releasing hormone during the acute stage of emaciation. The LH returns to normal with weight gain in most anorexics. Abnormal LH secretory pattern patients often continue to have eating problems.

Abnormal thyroid function is found in other malnourished states and thus cannot be considered a defect specific to anorexia nervosa.

A reduced metabolic clearance rate of cortisol and the incomplete supression of adrenocorticotrophic hormone (ACTH) and cortisol levels by dexamethasone have been reported in patients with protein calorie malnutrition, as well in anorexia nervosa patients.

There is a remarkable variability of fasting growth hormone levels in patients with anorexia nervosa. About one third have elevated basal growth hormone levels.

The noradrenergic neurotransmitter system is involved both in the control of feeding behavior and in primary depression. There also is a relationship between the urinary secretion of 3-methoxy-4-hydroxy phenylglycol (MHPG), a major metabolite of brain norepinephrine, and the symptom of depression in anorexia nervosa patients. An increase in urinary MHPG correlates with a decrease in depression ratings after weight gain.

Some anorexic patients induce vomiting or abuse purgatives and diuretics, causing concern about hypokalemic alkalosis. Impaired water diuresis may be noted.

Electrocardiographic changes, such as flattening or inversion of the T waves, ST segment depression, and lengthening of the QT interval, have been noted in the emaciated stage of anorexia nervosa. EKG changes may also occur as a result of potassium loss, which may lead to death. Gastric dilation is a rare complication of anorexia. In some of these patients, aortography has shown a superior mesenteric artery syndrome.

Course and Prognosis

The course of anorexia nervosa varies greatly—from spontaneous recovery without treatment, recovery after a variety of treatments, a fluctuating course of weight gains followed by relapses, to a gradually deteriorating course resulting in death due to complications of starvation. The short-term response of patients to almost all hospital treatment programs is good. Studies have shown a range of mortality rates from 5 percent to 18 percent.

The most consistent indicator of a good outcome is an early age onset of the illness and few previous hospitalizations. Such factors as childhood neuroticism, parental conflict, bulimia, vomiting, laxative abuse, and various behavioral manifestations (e.g., obsessive-compulsive, hysterical, depressive, psychosomatic, neurotic, and denial symptoms) have been related to poor outcome in some studies but have not been significant in affecting outcome in other studies. The expected outcome can vary from complete recovery, with normal weight maintenance and unusually effective functioning, to an inability to maintain weight, with a gradual starvation course and, eventually, an inability to function because of extreme weakness and severe preoccupation with losing weight and thoughts of food.

Diagnosis

The diagnosis of anorexia nervosa should be made only after finding the features listed in Table 1. Patients with this disorder are often secretive, deny their symptoms, and resist treatment. In almost all cases, it is necessary to have relatives or intimate acquaintances confirm their history. The mental status examination usually shows a patient who is alert and very knowledgeable on the subject of nutrition and who is also preoccupied with food and weight.

It is necessary that the patient have a thorough general physical and neurological examination. If the patient is vomiting, a hypokalemic alkalosis may be present. Because most patients are dehydrated, it is necessary initially to obtain serum electrolytes and then again periodically during hospitalization.

Differential Diagnosis

It is extremely important to ascertain that the patient does not have a medical illness that can account for the weight loss (e.g., brain tumor, cancer). Weight loss, peculiar eating behavior, and

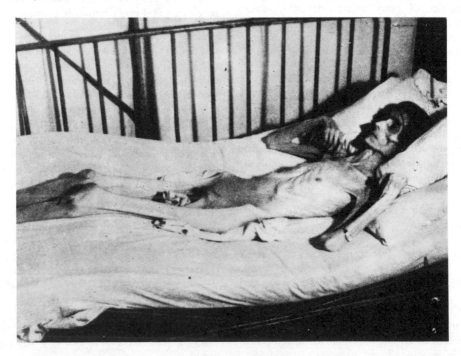

Figure 1. Patient with anorexia nervosa. (Courtesy Katherine Halmi, M.D.)

Table 1
Diagnostic Criteria for Anorexia Nervosa

A. Refusal to maintain body weight over a minimal normal weight for age and height, e.g., weight loss leading to maintenance of body weight 15% below that expected; or failure to make expected weight gain during period of growth, leading to body weight 15% below that expected.

B. Intense fear of gaining weight or becoming fat, even though underweight.

C. Disturbance in the way in which one's body weight, size, or shape is experienced, e.g., the person claims to "feel fat" even when emaciated, believes that one area of the body is "too fat" even when obviously underweight.

D. In females, absence of at least three consecutive menstrual cycles when otherwise expected to occur (primary or secondary amenorrhea). (A woman is considered to have amenorrhea if her periods occur only following hormone, e.g., estrogen, administration.)

Table from DSM-III-R, *Diagnostic and Statistical Manual of Mental Disorders,* ed 3, revised. (Current Classification of Mental Disorders, 1987.) Copyright American Psychiatric Association, Washington, D.C., 1987. Used with permission.

vomiting can occur in several psychiatric illnesses. Depressive disorders and anorexia nervosa have several features in common, such as depressed feeling, crying spells, sleep disturbance, obsessive ruminations, and occasional suicidal thoughts. These disorders, however, have several distinguishing features. Generally, a patient with a depressive disorder has a decreased appetite, whereas an anorexic claims to have a normal appetite and to feel hungry. It should be emphasized that only in the severe stages of anorexia nervosa does the patient actually have a decreased appetite. In contrast with depressive agitation, the hyperactivity seen in anorexia nervosa is planned and ritualistic. The preoccupation with the caloric content of food, recipes, and the preparation of gourmet feasts is typical of the anorexic patient and is not present in the patient with a depressive disorder. And in depressive disorder, there is no intense fear of obesity or disturbance of body image, as there is in anorexia nervosa.

Weight fluctuations, vomiting, and peculiar food handling may occur in somatization disorder. On rare occasions, a patient fulfills the criteria for both a somatization disorder and anorexia nervosa; in such a case, both diagnoses should be made. Generally, the weight loss in a somatization disorder is not as severe as that in anorexia nervosa, nor does the patient with a somatization disorder express a morbid fear of becoming overweight, as is common in the anorexic patient. Amenorrhea for 3 months or longer is unusual in a somatization disorder.

Delusions about food in schizophrenia are seldom concerned with the caloric content of food. A patient with schizophrenia is rarely preoccupied with a fear of becoming obese and does not have the hyperactivity that is seen in the anorexic patient. Schizophrenics have bizarre eating habits, and not the entire syndrome of anorexia nervosa.

Anorexia nervosa must be differentiated from bulimia, a disorder in which episodic binge eating, followed by depressive moods, self-deprecating thoughts, and often self-induced vomiting, occurs while the patient maintains his or her weight within a normal range. Furthermore, in bulimia there is seldom a 15 percent weight loss. Both conditions occasionally occur together.

Treatment

The immediate aim of treatment in anorexia nervosa is to restore the patient's nutritional state to normal, because the complications of emaciation, dehydration, and electrolyte imbalance may cause death. Usually, a hospitalized treatment program that provides considerable environmental structure is necessary for the weight restoration stage of treatment.

The general management of anorexia nervosa patients during a hospitalized treatment program should take into account the following: Each patient should be weighed daily early in the morning after emptying the bladder. The daily fluid intake and urine output should be recorded. If vomiting is occurring, it is especially important to obtain serum electrolytes regularly and to watch for the development of hypokalemia. Because food is regurgitated after meals, it is possible to control the vomiting by making the bathroom inaccessible for at least 2 hours after meals or by having an attendant in the bathroom to prevent such activities. Anorexics' constipation is relieved when they begin to eat normally. Occasionally, it may be necessary to give stool softeners, but never laxatives. If diarrhea occurs, it usually means that the patient is surreptitiously taking laxatives. Because of the rare complication of stomach dilation and the possibility of circulatory overload if the patient immediately starts eating an enormous amount of calories, it is advisable to start patients on about 500 calories over the amount required to maintain their present weight (usually 1,500 to 2,000 calories a day). It is wise to give these calories in six equal feedings throughout the day, so that the patients do not have to eat a large amount of food in one sitting. There may be an advantage in starting patients on a liquid food supplement, such as Sustagen, because they may be less apprehensive about gaining weight slowly with the formula than by eating food.

After discharge from the hospital, it is usually necessary to continue some type of outpatient supervision of whatever problems are identified in the patients and their families.

Most patients are uninterested in and even resistant to psychiatric treatment and are brought to a doctor's office unwillingly by agonizing relatives or friends. The patients rarely accept the advice for hospitalization without arguing and criticizing the program being offered. At this time, emphasizing the benefits, such as relief of insomnia or depressive signs and symptoms, may help persuade the patients to admit themselves willingly to the hospital. The relatives' support and confidence in the doctor and the treatment team are essential when firm recommendations must be carried out. The patients' families should be warned that they will resist admission and, for the first several weeks of treatment, will make many dramatic pleas for the family's support for release from the program. Only when the risk of death from complications of malnutrition is likely should a compulsory admission or commitment be obtained. On rare occasions, patients may prove wrong the doctor's statements about the probable failure of outpatient treatment. Such patients may gain a specified amount of weight by the time of each outpatient visit; however, this behavior is uncommon, and usually a period of inpatient care is necessary.

There is now a nursing treatment program that contains many of the positive reinforcements and privileges used in behavior therapy programs. In this program, total bed rest is instituted and then progressively relaxed through a series of rewards as the patients cooperate and gain weight.

Behavioral conditioning has been used along with family therapy. The usefulness of behavioral contingencies in conjunction with other therapies in treating anorexia nervosa has become widely recognized.

Pharmacologic agents have also been successful, such as chlorpromazine (Thorazine). More recently, heterocyclic antidepressants (e.g., amitriptyline) have been effective in treating anorexia nervosa. Another drug that has been used to treat anorexia nervosa is cyproheptadine (Periactin).

In some cases, electroconvulsive therapy (ECT) has been reported to be successful, especially when there is a strong depressive component.

The classical psychodynamically oriented therapy approach has not been effective in anorexia nervosa, particularly in inducing weight gain or in changing the abnormal eating behavior.

Family therapy has been used in treating this disorder to examine the interactions among family members and the possible secondary gain for the patient as a result of the disorder.

BULIMIA NERVOSA

Definition

Bulimia is an episodic, uncontrolled, compulsive, and rapid ingestion of large quantities of food over a short period of time (binge eating). Physical discomfort, such as abdominal pain or feelings of nausea, terminates the bulimic episode, which is followed by feelings of guilt, depression, or self-disgust. The person regularly uses laxatives or diuretics or induces vomiting or other artificial or extreme means of purging.

Epidemiology

Bulimia usually begins in adolescence or early adult life and is more common in females than in males. Some studies suggest a prevalence rate of 4 percent in women, compared with less than 0.5 percent in men. No familial incidence has been noted, but obesity may be found in other family members. Obesity in adolescence may predispose to the disorder in adulthood.

Etiology

There is no specific etiologic cause of bulimia. Disorders of the hypothalamic pituitary axis have been postulated, but no abnormal hormonal levels have been found. There may be a relationship between bulimia and depression because some bulimics respond to antidepressant medication. Although definite precipitating factors are vague, there is an association with adolescent life events (e.g., going away to school or getting a job).

Clinical Features

According to DSM-III-R, the essential features of bulimia nervosa are recurrent episodes of binge eating; a feeling of lack of control over eating behavior during the eating binges; self-induced vomiting; the use of laxatives or diuretics, strict dieting, fasting, or vigorous exercise in order to prevent weight gain; and persistent overconcern with body shape and weight.

Vomiting is common and is usually induced by sticking a finger down the throat, although some patients are able to vomit at will. Vomiting decreases the abdominal pain and feeling of being bloated and allows the patients to continue eating without fear of gaining weight. Depression often follows the episode and has been called "postbinge anguish." During their binges, the patients eat food that is sweet, high in calories, and generally of smooth texture or soft, such as cakes or pastry. The food is eaten secretly and rapidly and is sometimes not even chewed.

Most bulimics are within their normal weight range, but some may be either underweight or overweight. Bulimics are concerned about their body image and their appearance, worry about how others see them, and are concerned about their sexual attractiveness. Most bulimics are sexually active compared with anorexics, who are not interested in sex.

Course and Prognosis

The usual course of bulimia is chronic over a period of many years, with occasional remissions. Bulimia is rarely incapacitating except in a few persons who spend their entire day in binge eating and self-induced vomiting, which can lead to dehydration and electrolyte imbalance and which may require hospitalization. Dental caries may result from the action of the vomitus on tooth enamel.

Diagnosis

The diagnostic criteria for bulimia nervosa are listed in Table 2.

Table 2
Diagnostic Criteria for Bulimia Nervosa

A. Recurrent episodes of binge eating (rapid consumption of a large amount of food in a discrete period of time).

B. A feeling of lack of control over eating behavior during the eating binges.

C. The person regularly engages in either self-induced vomiting, use of laxatives or diuretics, strict dieting or fasting, or vigorous exercise in order to prevent weight gain.

D. A minimum average of two binge eating episodes a week for at least 3 months.

E. Persistent overconcern with body shape and weight.

Table from DSM-III-R, *Diagnostic and Statistical Manual of Mental Disorders*, ed 3, revised. (Current Classification of Mental Disorders, 1987.) Copyright American Psychiatric Association, Washington, D.C., 1987. Used with permission.

Differential Diagnosis

A diagnosis of bulimia nervosa cannot be made if anorexia nervosa is present, but episodic bulimic symptoms can occur in anorexia nervosa. If a patient meets all the criteria for the diagnosis of anorexia nervosa, then a diagnosis of anorexia nervosa should be given. Bulimia does not lead to a severe weight loss, and amenorrhea is rare, two symptoms that are necessary for a diagnosis of anorexia nervosa.

Bulimia nervosa should not be diagnosed if the patient meets positive criteria for schizophrenia. It is necessary to ascertain that the patient has no neurological disease state, such as epileptic-equivalent seizures, central nervous system tumors, Klüver-Bucy-like syndromes, and Kleine-Levin syndrome. The pathological features manifested by the Klüver-Bucy syndrome are visual agnosia, compulsive licking and biting, examination of objects by the mouth, inability to ignore any stimulus, placidity, altered sexual behavior (hypersexuality), and altered dietary habits, especially hyperphagia. This syndrome is exceedingly rare and is unlikely to cause a problem in differential diagnosis. Kleine-Levin syndrome consists of periodic hypersomnia, lasting for 2 to 3 weeks, and hyperphagia. As in bulimia, the onset is usually during adolescence, but this syndrome is more common in males. Borderline personalities sometimes binge eat, but it is associated with the other signs of the borderline syndrome.

Treatment

The treatment of bulimia nervosa in obese patients by means of psychotherapy is frequently stormy and always prolonged, although some obese bulimics who have had prolonged psychotherapy do surprisingly well. Effective positive reinforcement, informational feedback, and contingency contracting with bulimic women with anorexia nervosa are useful. A program of desensitization to the thoughts and feelings that bulimic patients have just before binge eating, in conjunction with a behavioral contract, may be a promising approach to the treatment of bulimia.

Several investigators have reported good results with imipramine. Pharmacotherapy requires further study.

EATING DISORDER NOT OTHERWISE SPECIFIED

The DSM-III-R diagnostic classification of eating disorder not otherwise specified is a residual category used

Table 3
Diagnostic Criteria for Eating Disorder Not Otherwise Specified

Disorders of eating that do not meet the criteria for a specific Eating Disorder.

Examples:

(1) a person of average weight who does not have binge eating episodes, but frequently engages in self-induced vomiting for fear of gaining weight
(2) all of the features of Anorexia Nervosa in a female except absence of menses
(3) all of the features of Bulimia Nervosa except the frequency of binge eating episodes

Table from DSM-III-R, *Diagnostic and Statistical Manual of Mental Disorders,* ed 3, revised. (Current Classification of Mental Disorders, 1987.) Copyright American Psychiatric Association, Washington, D.C., 1987. Used with permission.

for eating disorders that do not meet the criteria for a specific eating disorder. The DSM-III-R diagnostic criteria and examples are given in Table 3.

References

Blinder B J, Chaitin B, Goldstein R, editors: *The Eating Disorders*. Pergamon Press, New York, 1987.
Crisp A H, Hsu L K G, Harding B, Hartshorn J: Clinical features of anorexia nervosa: A study of 102 cases. J Psychosom Research 24:179, 1980.
Darby P L, Garfinkel P E, Garner D M, Coscina D V, editors: *Anorexia Nervosa: Recent Developments*. Alan R. Liss, New York, 1983.
Emmett S W, editor: *Theory and Treatment of Anorexia Nervosa and Bulimia: Biomedical, Sociocultural, and Psychological Perspectives*. Brunner/Mazel, New York, 1985.
Garfinkel P E, Garner D M, Rose J, Darby P L, Brandes O S, O'Hanlon J, Walsh N: A comparison of characteristics in the families of patients with anorexia nervosa and normal controls. Psychol Med 13:821, 1983.
Halmi K A: The state of research on anorexia nervosa and bulimia. Psychiat Dev 1:247, 1983.
Hudson J E, Pope H G Jr, editors: *The Psychobiology of Bulimia*. American Psychiatric Press, Washington, DC, 1987.
Johnson C, Strober M, Garner D M: Bulimia: A bio-psycho-social disorder. Int J Eating Disorders, 1987.
Kaye W H, Gwirtsman H E, editors: *A Comprehensive Approach to the Treatment of Normal-Weight Bulimia*. American Psychiatric Press, Washington, DC, 1985.
Pope H G Jr., Hudson J E: *New Hope for Binge Eaters: Advances in the Understanding and Treatment of Bulimia*. Harper & Row, New York, 1984.
Toner B B, Garfinkel P E, Garner D M: Cognitive style of patients with bulimic and diet-restricting anorexia nervosa. Am J Psych 144:510, 1987.
Wamholdt F S, Kaslow N J, Swift W J, Ritholz M: Short-term course of depressive Symptoms in patients with eating disorders. Am J Psych 144:362, 1987.

39

Gender Identity Disorders

INTRODUCTION

Gender identity refers to the sense of oneself as being male or female. The person with a healthy gender identity is able to say with certainty, "I am male" or "I am female." Gender role is the public expression of gender identity. According to DSM-III-R, gender role is everything that one says or does to indicate to others or to oneself the degree to which one is male or female. A distinction should be made to the term sex, which is strictly limited to the anatomical and physiological characteristics that indicate whether one is a man or a woman (e.g., penis, vagina).

Gender identity disorders are rare and should be differentiated from feelings of inadequacy in fulfilling the expectations of one's gender role. Normally, there is concordance between one's physically assigned sex and one's gender role.

According to DSM-III-R, gender identity disorders are classified under the heading of disorders first appearing during childhood or adolescence. Even though persons who present clinically with gender identity problems may be of any age, most cases begin in childhood.

CLASSIFICATION

DSM-III-R provides three diagnoses for males and females with gender identity disorders: (1) gender identity

Table 1
Diagnostic Criteria for Gender Identity Disorder Not Otherwise Specified

Disorders in gender identity that are not classifiable as a specific Gender Identity Disorder.

Examples:

(1) children with persistent cross-dressing without the other criteria for Gender Identity Disorder of Childhood
(2) adults with transient, stress-related cross-dressing behavior
(3) adults with the clinical features of Transsexualism of less than 2 years' duration
(4) people who have a persistent preoccupation with castration or peotomy without a desire to acquire the sex characteristics of the other sex

Table from DSM-III-R, *Diagnostic and Statistical Manual of Mental Disorders,* ed 3, revised. (Current Classification of Mental Disorders, 1987.) Copyright American Psychiatric Association, Washington, D.C., 1987. Used with permission.

disorder of childhood, (2) transsexualism, and (3) gender identity disorder of adolescence or adulthood, nontranssexual type (GIDAANT). Persons with gender identity disorder feel persistent discomfort and that their assigned gender is inappropriate. Those persons with a persistent preoccupation with and a desire to have sex reassignment surgery (SRS)—or to use hormones to achieve that end—are labeled transsexuals; those without that persistent preoccupation are labeled nontranssexuals (GIDAANT). Gender identity disorder not otherwise specified (NOS) is the classification for those who do not fit into the other diagnostic categories (Table 1).

DSM-III-R places gender identity disorders on a continuum: Persons with mild cases are aware that they are male or female but are uncomfortable about it. Persons with severe cases not only are uncomfortable with their assigned sex but actually feel that they belong to the opposite sex (e.g., transsexualism).

EPIDEMIOLOGY

There is almost no information about the prevalence of gender identity disorders among children, teenagers, and adults. Most estimates of prevalence are based on the number of people seeking sex reassignment surgery, and those indicate a male preponderance. The ratio of boys to girls reported in three child gender identity clinics were 30 to 1, 17 to 1, and 6 to 1, indicating little experience with girls. This disparity might indicate a greater male vulnerability to gender identity disorders, or a greater sensitivity to and worry about cross-gender identified boys than cross-gender identified girls. According to DSM-III-R, the estimated prevalence of transsexualism is 1 per 30,000 for males and 1 per 100,000 for females.

ETIOLOGY

Biologic

For mammals, the resting state of tissue is initially female, and as the fetus develops, a male will be produced only if androgen (set off by the Y chromosome) is added. That implies that maleness and masculinity depend on fetal and perinatal androgens. Lower animals' sexual behavior is governed by sex steroids, and as one ascends the evolutionary scale, this effect diminishes. Sex steroids influence the expression of sexual behavior in the mature man or woman.

That is, testosterone can increase libido and aggressiveness in females, and estrogen can decrease libido and aggressiveness in males. But masculinity and femininity and gender identity are more a product of postnatal life events than of prenatal hormonal organization.

Psychosocial

Children develop a gender identity consonant with their sex of rearing (also known as assigned sex), which is based on the temperament of the child, the qualities of the parents, and the interaction between them. There are culturally acceptable gender roles: Boys are not expected to be effeminate, and girls are not expected to be tomboys. There are boys' games (e.g., cops and robbers) and girls' games (e.g., dolls and doll houses). These roles are learned, although some investigators believe that some boys are temperamentally more delicate and sensitive and that some girls are more aggressive and energized—traits that stereotypically are known in our culture as feminine or masculine, respectively. Freud believed that fixation at the phallic psychosexual stage of development, when the oedipal conflict is primary, could lead to gender identity problems. The greater the identification is with the opposite-sex parent, compared with that of the same-sex parent, the greater will be the risk of gender confusion. According to Freud, a boy who is too closely attached to his mother and who has too little paternal involvement will be feminine. And a girl who is too closely attached to her father and who has too little maternal input will be masculine. Steven Levine suggested that children who have been abused physically or sexually, or those who have never had a consistent relationship with a nurturant parent, may adapt by trying to live out their fantasy that they would have been better treated if they were a member of the opposite sex.

GENDER IDENTITY DISORDER OF CHILDHOOD

According to DSM-III-R, the essential feature of gender identity disorder is a persistent and intense distress in a child about his or her assigned sex and the desire to be, or insistence that he or she is, of the other sex. Girls and boys show an aversion to normative stereotypic feminine or masculine clothing and repudiate their respective anatomic characteristics. Table 2 lists the DSM-III-R criteria for this disorder.

At the extreme of gender disorder in children are those boys who, by the standards of their cultures, are as feminine as are the most feminine of girls and those girls who are as masculine as are the most masculine of boys. No sharp line can be drawn on the continuum of gender disorder between children who deserve a formal diagnosis and those who do not. Its prevalence is therefore unknown. DSM-III-R comments that girls with this disorder regularly have male companions and an avid interest in sports and rough-and-tumble play; they show no interest in dolls or playing "house" (unless they play the father or another male role). More rarely, a girl with this disorder refuses to urinate in a sitting position, claims that she has, or will grow, a penis, does not want to grow breasts or menstruate, and asserts that she will grow up to become a man (not merely in role).

According to DSM-III-R, boys with this disorder usually are preoccupied with female stereotypic activities. They may have a preference for dressing in girls' or women's clothes or may improvise such items from available material when the genuine articles are not available. (The cross-dressing typically does not cause sexual excitement, as in transvestic fetishism.) They often have a compelling desire to participate in the games and pastimes of girls. Female dolls are often their favorite toys, and girls are regularly their preferred playmates. When playing "house," such boys take the role of a female. Their gestures and actions are often judged against a standard of cultural stereotype to be feminine, and such boys are usually subjected to male peer group teasing and rejection, whereas the same rarely occurs among girls until adolescence. Boys with this dis-

Table 2
Diagnostic Criteria for Gender Identity Disorder of Childhood

For Females:

A. Persistent and intense distress about being a girl, and a stated desire to be a boy (not merely a desire for any perceived cultural advantages from being a boy), or insistence that she is a boy

B. Either (1) or (2):

  (1) persistent marked aversion to normative feminine clothing and insistence on wearing stereotypical masculine clothing, e.g., boys' underwear and other accessories

  (2) persistent repudiation of female anatomic structures, as evidenced by at least one of the following:

    (*a*) an assertion that she has, or will grow, a penis

    (*b*) rejection of urinating in a sitting position

    (*c*) assertion that she does not want to grow breasts or menstruate

C. The girl has not yet reached puberty.

For Males:

A. Persistent and intense distress about being a boy and an intense desire to be a girl or, more rarely, insistence that he is a girl.

B. Either (1) or (2):

  (1) preoccupation with female stereotypical activities, as shown by a preference for either cross-dressing or simulating female attire, or by an intense desire to participate in the games and pastimes of girls and rejection of male stereotypical toys, games, and activities

  (2) persistent repudiation of male anatomic structures, as indicated by at least one of the following repeated assertions:

    (*a*) that he will grow up to become a woman (not merely in role)

    (*b*) that his penis or testes are disgusting or will disappear

    (*c*) that it would be better not to have a penis or testes

C. The boy has not yet reached puberty.

Table from DSM-III-R, *Diagnostic and Statistical Manual of Mental Disorders,* ed 3, revised. (Current Classification of Mental Disorders, 1987.) Copyright American Psychiatric Association, Washington, D.C., 1987. Used with permission.

order may assert that they will grow up to become women (not merely in role). In rare cases, a boy with this disorder claims that his penis or testes are disgusting or will disappear or that it would be better not to have a penis or testes at all.

Some children refuse to attend school because of teasing or pressure to dress in attire stereotypical of their assigned sex. Most children with this disorder deny being disturbed by it, except that it brings them into conflict with expectations of their family or peers.

Course and Outcome

The prognosis for gender disorder depends on the age of onset and the intensity of the symptoms. Boys begin to develop the disorder before age 4, and peer conflict develops during the early school years, at about the age of 7 or 8. Grossly feminine mannerisms may lessen as the child grows older, especially if attempts are made to discourage such behavior. Cross-dressing may be part of the disorder, and 75 percent of boys who cross-dress begin to do so before age 4. The age of onset is also early for females, but most give up masculine behavior by adolescence.

In both sexes, homosexuality is likely to develop in one-third to two-thirds of cases, although fewer girls than boys develop a homosexual orientation, for reasons that are not clear. Levine reported that follow-up studies of gender-disturbed boys consistently indicate that homosexual orientation, not transsexualism, is the usual adolescent outcome. Transsexualism occurs in less than 10 percent of cases. Retrospective data on homosexual men indicate a high frequency of cross-gender identifications and feminine gender role behavior during childhood.

Treatment

Gender disorders and other mental illness, particularly borderline personality, often coexist, and in those cases, attention needs to be directed to both conditions. Attempts to inculcate culturally acceptable behavioral patterns in boys, by role modeling adults or peers, have been successful in some cases.

For treatment, Green employs a one-to-one play relationship with the child and parental counseling in conjunction with group meetings of children with the same problem and their parents. Parents' encouragement of the child's atypical behavior (e.g., dressing a boy in girl's clothing or not giving him haircuts) needs to be examined in therapy. It is important to note ethical considerations in regard to the attempt to modify such behavior.

TRANSSEXUALISM

According to DSM-III-R, the essential features of transsexualism are a persistent discomfort and sense of inappropriateness regarding one's assigned sex in a person who has reached puberty. In addition, there is a persistent preoccupation, for at least 2 years, with getting rid of one's primary and secondary sex characteristics and acquiring the sex characteristics of the other sex. Therefore, the diagnosis

of transsexualism should not be made if the disturbance is limited to brief periods of stress. The wish to live as a member of the other sex is always present (Table 3).

Most retrospective studies of transsexuals report gender identity problems during childhood; however, prospective studies of children with gender identity disorder indicate that very few develop into transsexuals. Transsexualism is much more common in males (1 per 30,000 men) than in females (1 per 100,000 women).

The diagnosis is easily made clinically. As DSM-III-R notes, people with this disorder usually complain that they are uncomfortable wearing the clothes of their assigned sex and therefore dress in clothes of the other sex. They engage in activities associated with the other sex. These people find their genitals repugnant, which may lead to persistent requests for sex reassignment surgery (SRS). That desire may override all other wishes, and in time, they attempt the following: Males take estrogen to create breasts and other feminine contours; have electrolysis to remove their male hair; and have SRS, which includes removal of the testes and penis and the creation of an artificial vagina. Females bind their breasts or have a mastectomy, hysterectomy, and oophorectomy; take testosterone to build up their muscle mass and deepen their voice; and have SRS, in which an artificial phallus is created. These procedures may make the transsexual indistinguishable from members of the other sex. Some investigators describe behavior in sex-reassigned persons that is almost a caricature of male and female roles.

Course and Prognosis

Transsexualism, which usually begins in childhood, is chronic. Impaired social and occupational functioning as a result of the person's wanting to participate in the desired (and opposite) gender role is common. Depression is also a common problem, especially if the person feels hopeless about obtaining a sex change with surgery or hormones. Male transsexuals have been known to castrate themselves, not as a suicide attempt, but as a way of forcing a surgeon to deal with their problem.

Subtypes

DSM-III-R defines three transsexual subtypes according to sexual orientation: (1) asexual, referring to persons who give no

Table 3
Diagnostic Criteria for Transsexualism

A. Persistent discomfort and sense of inappropriateness about one's assigned sex.

B. Persistent preoccupation for at least 2 years with getting rid of one's primary and secondary sex characteristics and acquiring the sex characteristics of the other sex.

C. The person has reached puberty.

Specify history of sexual orientation: **asexual, homosexual, heterosexual,** or **unspecified.**

Table from DSM-III-R, *Diagnostic and Statistical Manual of Mental Disorders,* ed 3, revised. (Current Classification of Mental Disorders, 1987.) Copyright American Psychiatric Association, Washington, D.C., 1987. Used with permission.

history of sexual activity or pleasure derived from the genitals; (2) homosexual, in which there is sexual arousal from same-sex partners; and (3) heterosexual. Persons in the homosexual group often deny they are homosexual because they believe themselves to be members of the opposite sex. Thus, a man will claim he is not a homosexual because he feels like a woman and thus is heterosexual if defined by his identity. But if defined by his anatomy and that of his male partner, he is homosexual.

Like transsexual men, transsexual women do not deny their anatomic sex but are preoccupied with the sense of really being men who are attracted to women; they too are classified as asexual, homosexual, or heterosexual.

Despite the detailed subdivision of DSM-III-R, clinicians should be aware that the overwhelming majority of transsexuals believe themselves to be heterosexual. The common statement among this group is, "I am a woman trapped in a man's body," or vice versa.

Treatment

A psychiatric evaluation to determine the presence of another mental disorder is essential. Some clinicians believe that the transsexual's belief of being of the opposite sex should be classified as a delusion. According to DSM-III-R, however, the insistence by a person that he or she is of the other sex is not a delusion, because what is invariably meant is that the person feels *like* a member of the other sex rather than truly believing that he or she *is* a member of the other sex.

Other illnesses may accompany transsexualism. Personality disorders, especially borderline personality, have been found to be highly represented in this group. Depression is also common. Psychotherapy is useful for those conditions; however, so far, there has been no psychological treatment reported that will make transsexuals satisfied with their anatomic sex. The psychiatrist can either do nothing or can comply with the patient's wish for a sex change. Sex reassignment surgery is more successful male to female than female to male, mainly because of the surgical techniques. Surgical treatment is definitive, and because there is no turning back, careful standards preceding the surgery have been developed, which include the following: (1) There must be a trial of cross-gender living for at least 3 months and sometimes up to 1 year. For some transsexuals, the real-life test may make them change their minds because they find it uncomfortable to relate to friends, workers, and lovers in that role. (2) They must receive hormone treatments, with estradiol and progesterone in male-to-female change and testosterone in female-to-male change. Many transsexuals like the changes in their bodies that occur as a result of this treatment, and some will stop at this point. About 50 percent of transsexuals who meet the above criteria go on to SRS. Outcome studies are highly variable in terms of how success is defined and measured (e.g., successful intercourse, body image satisfaction).

About 70 percent of male-to-female and 80 percent of female-to-male SRS patients report satisfactory results. Unsatisfactory results correlate with preexisting mental disorder. Suicide in postoperative SRS patients has been reported in up to 2 percent of cases. SRS is a highly controversial measure that is undergoing much scrutiny.

GENDER IDENTITY DISORDER OF ADOLESCENCE OR ADULTHOOD, NONTRANSSEXUAL TYPE (GIDAANT)

DSM-III-R has a new diagnosis to describe persons with gender disorders who are not interested in changing their anatomic sex or in acquiring the characteristics of the other sex but who are uncomfortable with their assigned sex. An essential feature of this disorder is cross-dressing in the role of the other sex, either in fantasy or reality (Table 4).

According to DSM-III-R, cross-dressing phenomena range from occasional solitary wearing of female clothes to extensive feminine identification in males and masculine identification in females and involvement in a transvestic subculture. More than one article of clothing of the other sex is involved, and the person may dress entirely as a member of the opposite sex. The degree to which the cross-dressed person appears as a member of the other sex varies, depending on mannerisms, body habitus, and cross-dressing skill. When not cross-dressed, the person usually appears as an unremarkable member of his or her assigned sex.

This disorder differs from transvestic fetishism in that the cross-dressing is not for the purpose of sexual excitement. It differs from transsexualism in that there is no persistent preoccupation (for at least 2 years) with getting rid of one's primary and secondary sex characteristics and acquiring the sex characteristics of the other sex.

Some people with this disorder once had transvestic fetishism but no longer become sexually aroused by cross-dressing. Other people with this disorder are homosexuals who cross-dress. This disorder is common among female impersonators.

INTERSEXUAL DISORDERS

Intersexual disorders include a variety of syndromes that produce persons with gross anatomic or physiologic aspects of the opposite sex. Although not an official DSM-III-R term, intersexual disorders is used by clinicians, and such persons should be classified on Axis III (physical disorders and conditions).

Turner's Syndrome

In Turner's syndrome, one sex chromosome is missing (XO). The result is an absence (agenesis) or minimal development (dysgenesis) of the gonads; no significant sex hormones, male or female, are produced in fetal life or postnatally. The sexual tissues thus remain in a female resting state. Because the second X chromosome, which seems responsible for full femaleness, is missing, these girls have an incomplete sexual anatomy and, lacking adequate estrogens, develop no secondary sex characteristics without treatment. They often suffer other stigmata, such as web neck, low posterior hairline margin, short stature, and cubitus valgus. The infant is born with normal-appearing female external genitals and so is unequivocally assigned to the female sex and is thusly reared. All these children develop as unremarkably feminine, heterosexually oriented girls; however, later medical management is necessary to assist them with their infertility and absence of secondary sex characteristics.

Table 4
Diagnostic Criteria for Gender Identity Disorder of Adolescence or Adulthood Nontranssexual Type (GIDAANT)

A. Persistent or recurrent discomfort and sense of inappropriateness about one's assigned sex.

B. Persistent or recurrent cross-dressing in the role of the other sex, either in fantasy or actuality, but not for the purpose of sexual excitement (as in Transvestic Fetishism).

C. No persistent preoccupation (for at least 2 years) with getting rid of one's primary and secondary sex characteristics and acquiring the sex characteristics of the other sex (as in Transsexualism).

D. The person has reached puberty.

Specify history of sexual orientation: **asexual, homosexual, heterosexual,** or **unspecified.**

Table from DSM-III-R, *Diagnostic and Statistical Manual of Mental Disorders,* ed 3, revised. (Current Classification of Mental Disorders, 1987.) Copyright American Psychiatric Association, Washington, D.C., 1987. Used with permission.

Klinefelter's Syndrome

A person (usually XXY) with Klinefelter's syndrome has a male habitus, under the influence of the Y chromosome, but this effect is weakened by the presence of the second X chromosome. Although born with a penis and testes, the testes are small and infertile, and the penis may also be small. In adolescence, some of these patients develop gynecomastia and other feminine-appearing contours. Their sexual desire is usually weak. Sex assignment and rearing should lead to a clear sense of maleness, but these patients often have gender disturbances, ranging from a complete reversal, as in transsexualism, to homosexuality or an intermittent desire to put on women's clothes. As a result of lessened androgen production, the fetal hypogonadal state in some patients seems not to have completed the central nervous system organization that should underlie masculine behavior. In fact, in many of these patients, there is a wide spread of psychopathology, ranging from emotional instability to mental retardation.

Congenital Virilizing Adrenal Hyperplasia (Adrenogenital Syndrome)

Congenital virilizing adrenal hyperplasia results from an excess of androgen acting on the prenatal fetus. When the condition occurs in females, excessive adrenal fetal androgens from the adrenal gland cause androgenization of the external genitals, ranging from mild clitoral enlargement to external genitals that look like a normal scrotal sac, testes, and a penis; but hidden behind these external genitals are a vagina and a uterus. These patients are otherwise normally female. At birth, if the genitals look male, the child is assigned to the male sex and is so reared. The result is a clear sense of maleness and unremarkable masculinity; but, if the child is diagnosed as a female and is so reared, a sense of femaleness and femininity will result. If the parents are uncertain to which sex their child belongs, a hermaphroditic identity will result. The resultant gender identity reflects the rearing practices, but androgens may help determine behavior, based on the finding that those children raised unequivocally as girls have a tomboy quality more intense than that found in a control series. The girls nonetheless do have a heterosexual orientation.

Pseudohermaphroditism

Infants may be born with ambiguous genitals, which is an obstetrical emergency because the sex assignment will determine gender identity. Male pseudohermaphroditism is incomplete differentiation of the external genitals, even though a Y chromosome is present. Testes are present but rudimentary. Female pseudohermaphroditism is virilized genitals in an individual who is XX, the most common cause being the adrenogenital syndrome described above.

The genitals' appearance at birth determines the sex assignment, and the core gender identity is male, female, or hermaphroditic, depending on the family's conviction as to the child's sex. Usually a panel of experts determine the sex of rearing, basing their decision on buccal smears, chromosome studies, and parental wishes. Assignment should usually be made within 24 hours so that the parents can adapt accordingly. If surgery is necessary to correct the genital deformity, it is generally done before the age of 3.

True hermaphroditism is characterized by the presence of both testes and ovaries in the same person, a rare condition.

Androgen Insensitivity Syndrome

Androgen insensitivity syndrome, a congenital X-linked recessive trait disorder—also known as testicular feminization syndrome—results from an inability of target tissues to respond to androgens. Unable to respond, the fetal tissues remain in their female resting state, and the central nervous system is not organized to masculinity. The infant at birth appears to be an unremarkable female, although she is later found to have cryptorchid testes, which produce the testosterone to which the tissues do not respond, and minimal or absent internal sexual organs and vagina. Secondary sex characteristics at puberty are female because of the small but sufficient amounts of estrogens typically produced by the testes. These patients invariably sense themselves as females and are feminine.

References

Green R: Gender identity in childhood and later sexual orientation: Followup of 78 males. Am J Psychiatry *142*:399, 1985.

Lothstein L M: *Female to Male Transsexualism: Historical, Clinical, and Theoretical Issues.* Routledge Kegan Paul, Boston, 1983.

Lothstein L M, Levine S B: Expressive psychotherapy with gender dysphoric patients. Arch Gen Psychiatry *38*:924, 1981.

McEwan L, Ceber S, Davis J: Male-to-female surgical genital reassignment. In *Transsexualism and Sex Reassignment,* W A W Walters, M J Ross, editors, p 103. Oxford University Press, Melbourne, 1986.

Money J, Ehrhardt A A: *Man and Woman. Boy and Girl: Differentiation and Dimorphism of Gender Identity from Conception to Maturity.* Johns Hopkins University Press, Baltimore, 1972.

Pauley I B, Edgerton M T: The gender identity movement: A growing surgical-psychiatric liaison. Arch Sex Behavior *15*:315, 1986.

Steiner B W, editor: *Gender Dysphoria: Development, Research and Management.* Plenum, New York, 1984.

Stoller R J: *Presentations of Gender.* Yale University Press, New Haven, CT, 1986.

Walker P, Berger J, Green R, Laub D, Reynolds C, Wollman L: Standards of care. The hormonal and surgical reassignment of gender dysphoric persons. Arch Sex Behavior *14*:79, 1985.

Zucker K J, Green R: Treatment of the gender identity disorder of childhood. In *APA Task Force on the Treatment of Psychiatric Disorders,* T B Karasu, editor. American Psychiatric Press, Washington, DC, 1987.

40

Tic Disorders

INTRODUCTION

As delineated by DSM-III-R, the tic disorders include Tourette's disorder, chronic motor or vocal tic disorder, transient tic disorder, and tic disorder not otherwise specified (NOS). The DSM-III-R diagnostic criteria for these disorders are given in Tables 1 through 4.

Tics are involuntary, sudden, rapid, recurrent, nonrhythmic, stereotyped motor movements or vocal productions. They are experienced as irresistible but can be voluntarily suppressed for varying lengths of time, from minutes to hours. DSM-III-R notes: Both motor and vocal tics may be classified as either simple or complex, although the boundaries are not well defined. Common simple motor tics are eye-blinking, neck-jerking, shoulder-shrugging, and facial grimacing. Common simple vocal tics are coughing, throat-clearing, grunting, sniffing, snorting, and barking. Common complex motor tics are facial gestures, grooming behaviors, hitting or biting self, jumping, touching, stamping, and smelling an object. Common complex vocal tics are repeating words or phrases out of context, coprolalia (use of socially unacceptable words, frequently obscene), palilalia (repeating one's own sounds or words), and echolalia (repeating the last-heard sound, word, or phrase of another person or a last-heard sound). Other complex tics include echokinesis (imitation of the movements of someone who is being observed).

Stresses, such as intense self-consciousness and anxious anticipation, may exacerbate tics. On the other hand, absorption in an activity may attenuate tics. Although most authorities state that tics disappear during sleep, one recent study suggests that at least some individuals with Tourette's disorder continue to have tics during sleep.

Tics appear to be more common in the families of individuals with tic disorders than in the general population. They are about three times more frequent in males than in females.

DIFFERENTIAL DIAGNOSIS

Tics must be reliably differentiated from other disordered movements (e.g., dystonic, choreiform, athetoid, myoclonic, and hemiballismic movements) and the neurological diseases of which they are characteristic (e.g., Huntington's chorea, Parkinsonism, Sydenhams's chorea, and Wilson's disease), as described in Table 5. Tremors, mannerisms, and a stereotypy or habit disorder (e.g., head banging or body rocking) must also be distinguished from tic disorders. The voluntary nature of stereotypy or habit disorder and the fact that such movements do not cause subjective distress differentiate it from tic disorders. Compulsions also are intentional behaviors.

Both autistic and mentally retarded children may exhibit symptoms similar to those seen in the tic disorders, including Tourette's disorder. Tardive dyskinesia must also be considered in those patients who are receiving or have received medications that may cause this untoward effect.

Stimulant medications (e.g., methylphenidate, amphetamine, and pemoline) have been reported to exacerbate preexisting tics and to precipitate the development of new tics and Tourette's disorder. This has been reported primarily in some children and adolescents being treated for attention-deficit hyperactivity disorder. In most but not all cases, after discontinuing the drug, the tics remitted or returned to premedication levels. Some authorities believe that stimulants should not be used to treat children with attention-deficit hyperactivity disorder if a child has or has had tics or Tourette's disorder, that they should be used very cautiously if there is a family history of tics or Tourette's disorder, and that they should be discontinued immediately if a child develops tics. Other experts suggest that children and adolescents who develop tics while on stimulants probably are predisposed genetically and would have developed tics regardless of their treatment with stimulants. Until the situation is clarified, there should be great caution and frequent clinical monitoring of children at risk for tics who are given stimulants.

ETIOLOGY

Dysregulation of the neurochemical systems of the central nervous system is probably the most important etiological factor in the majority of tics. Head trauma also may sometimes precipitate the onset of a tic disorder. Other etiologies have been proposed, including psychoanalytic explanations, which postulate various psychodynamic mechanisms, and learning theory explanations, which invoke drive-reducing conditioned avoidance responses and classical operant conditioning models.

Stimulants may exacerbate existing tics or cause new tics probably as a result of the release of dopamine from nigrostriatal dopaminergic nerve terminals. In addition, the dopamine blocker, haloperidol, is effective in treating tics. The combination of these two factors suggests a dysregulation of dopamine, resulting in a relative hyperdopaminergia in the etiology of tics.

Table 1
Diagnostic Criteria for Transient Tic Disorder

A. Single or multiple motor and/or vocal tics.

B. The tics occur many times a day, nearly every day for at least 2 weeks, but for no longer than 12 consecutive months.

C. No history of Tourette's or Chronic Motor or Vocal Tic Disorder.

D. Onset before age 21.

E. Occurrence not exclusively during Psychoactive Substance Intoxication or known central nervous system disease, such as Huntington's chorea and postviral encephalitis.

Specify: single episode or **recurrent.**

Table from DSM-III-R, *Diagnostic and Statistical Manual of Mental Disorders,* ed 3, revised. (Current Classification of Mental Disorders, 1987.) Copyright American Psychiatric Association, Washington, D.C., 1987. Used with permission.

Table 2
Diagnostic Criteria for Chronic Motor or Vocal Tic Disorder

A. Either motor or vocal tics, but not both, have been present at some time during the illness.

B. The tics occur many times a day, nearly every day, or intermittently throughout a period of more than 1 year.

C. Onset before age 21.

D. Occurrence not exclusively during Psychoactive Substance Intoxication or known central nervous system disease, such as Huntington's chorea and postviral encephalitis.

Table from DSM-III-R, *Diagnostic and Statistical Manual of Mental Disorders,* ed 3, revised. (Current Classification of Mental Disorders, 1987.) Copyright American Psychiatric Association, Washington, D.C., 1987. Used with permission.

Abnormalities in noradrenergic regulation have also been implicated by the favorable response of some cases of Tourette's disorder to clonidine, a noradrenergic blocker, and the worsening of tics caused by anxiety and stress.

Although there is increasing evidence of genetic and disturbed neurochemical functioning, biological heterogeneity (which results in a similar final pathway of symptom expression) must still be considered. No one explanation satisfactorily accounts for the variations in clinical course, response to pharmacological treatment, and family history.

CLASSIFICATION

DSM-III-R emphasizes precise and specific symptom patterns, time frameworks, and age of onset in classifying the tic disorders. Although similar to the DSM-III criteria used for these disorders, the DSM-III-R criteria are different enough to be confusing and to make it difficult or impossible to compare studies utilizing the different diagnostic criteria.

Table 3
Diagnostic Criteria for Tourette's Disorder

A. Both multiple motor and one or more vocal tics have been present at some time during the illness, although not necessarily concurrently.

B. The tics occur many times a day (usually in bouts), nearly every day or intermittently throughout a period of more than 1 year.

C. The anatomic location, number, frequency, complexity, and severity of the tics change over time.

D. Onset before age 21.

E. Occurrence not exclusively during Psychoactive Substance Intoxication or known central nervous system disease, such as Huntington's chorea and postviral encephalitis.

Table from DSM-III-R, *Diagnostic and Statistical Manual of Mental Disorders,* ed 3, revised. (Current Classification of Mental Disorders, 1987.) Copyright American Psychiatric Association, Washington, D.C., 1987. Used with permission.

Table 4
Diagnostic Criteria for Tic Disorder Not Otherwise Specified

Tics that do not meet the criteria for a specific Tic Disorder. An example is a Tic Disorder with onset in adulthood.

Table from DSM-III-R, *Diagnostic and Statistical Manual of Mental Disorders,* ed 3, revised. (Current Classification of Mental Disorders, 1987.) Copyright American Psychiatric Association, Washington, D.C., 1987. Used with permission.

The exact relationships among the tic disorders are unknown. DSM-III-R and many therapists postulate a continuum of severity, beginning with transient tics and progressing to Tourette's disorder. Although this is clearly true for many cases, it is uncertain whether all transient tics, which develop and usually disappear during childhood, are related to Tourette's disorder or whether some of them are primarily determined by psychological conflicts or are learned responses.

TRANSIENT TIC DISORDER

Definition and Diagnosis

The DSM-III-R criteria for establishing the diagnosis of transient tic disorder are as follows: (1) The tics are single or multiple motor and/or vocal tics; (2) the tics occur many times a day nearly every day for at least 2 weeks but for no longer than 12 consecutive months; (3) there is no history of Tourette's or chronic motor or vocal tic disorder; (4) the onset is before age 21; and (5) the tic does not occur exclusively during psychoactive substance intoxication or known CNS disease. The diagnosis should also specify whether there has been single or recurrent episodes (Table 1).

Transient tic disorder can be distinguished from chronic motor or vocal tic disorder and Tourette's disorder only by following the symptom's progression over time.

Table 5
Clinical Characteristics of Some Movement Disorders to Be Differentiated from Tics

Disease or syndrome	Age of onset	Associated symptoms and findings	Course without treatment	Types of movements
Athetoid type of cerebral palsy (including status marmoratus)	Birth-3	Often other neurological deficits, including mental retardation	Static after age 3	Athetoid, Choreoathetoid
Dystonia musculorum deformans	5–15	Occasionally familial, common in Russian Jews	Progressive and death in 10–15 years, rare remissions occur	Torsion dystonia
Encephalitis lethargica (von Economos encephalitis)	Any age	Other evidence or history of encephalitis, Parkinsonian symptoms, rare cases of klazomania associated with coprolalia, no recent occurrence of this encephalitis	Improving static or relapsing (chronic)	Any
Hallervorden-Spatz disease	About 10	Familial, may be associated with optic atrophy, club feet, retinitis pigmentosa, dysarthria, dementia, emotional lability	Progressive to death in 5–20 years	Choreic, athetoid, myoclonic
Huntington's chorea (including senile chorea)	30–50, but 1% in early childhood	Familial dementia; EEG abnormalities	Progressive to death 10–50 years	Choreiform
Pelizaeus-Merzbacher disease	Infancy	Familial, predominantly males, often neurological abnormalities	Progressive to ages 5–6, then may remit or be static	Choreoathetoid
Status dysmyelinatus	1st year	Abnormal movements, which are gradually replaced by rigidity	Progressive to death in second decade	Athetoid
Sydenham's chorea (including chorea gravidarum and in senlens)	Childhood, usually 5–15 (in pregnancy any age)	Females more frequent than males, 75% associated with rheumatic fever, eosinophilia, EEG abnormalities	Self-limited, though habit spasms may be sequelae	Choreiform
Wilson's disease (hepatolenticular degeneration)	Usually 10–25	Kayser-Fleischer rings, liver cirrhosis, other organ involvement, serum and urine abnormalities, mild dementia	Progressive to death in several years	Any
Lesch-Nyhan	Usually 2nd year	Hypoxanthine phosphoribosyl transferase enzyme defect, recessive sex-linked in males, mental retardation	Progressive to death in several years	Spasticity, selfmutilation, biting, screaming, coprolalia

Table from Shapiro A K, Shapiro E S: *Tics, Tourette Syndrome and Other Movement Disorders: A Pediatrician's Guide.* Tourette Syndrome Association, Inc., Bayside, NY, 1980. Used with permission.

Epidemiology

Transient, tic-like habit movements or nervous muscular twitches are common in children. From 5 to 24 percent of school-age children have a history of tics. The prevalence of tics as defined here is unknown.

Etiology

Transient tics have probably either organic or psychogenic origins, with some tics combining elements of both. Organic tics are probably most likely to progress to Tourette's disorder and have an increased family history of tics, whereas psychogenic tics are most likely to remit spontaneously. Those that progress to chronic motor or vocal tic disorder are most likely to have components of both.

Clinical Description

The average age of onset of tics is 7 years but may occur as early as 2 years. The most common tic is an eye blink or another facial tic. The most common tics involve the face and then the neck, with a descending gradient of frequency to the feet.

The most commonly described tics are as follows: (1) face and head: grimacing; puckering of forehead; raising eyebrows; blinking eyelids; winking; wrinkling nose; trembling nostrils; twitching mouth; displaying teeth; biting lips and other parts; extruding tongue; protracting lower jaw; nodding, jerking, or shaking the head; twisting neck; looking sideways; and head rolling. (2) arms and hands: jerking hands, jerking arms, plucking fingers, writhing fingers, and clenching fists. (3) body and lower extremities: shrugging shoulders; shaking foot, knee, or toe; peculiarities of gait; body writhing; and jumping. (4) respiratory and alimentary: hiccuping, sighing, yawning, snuffing, blowing through nostrils, whistling inspiration, exaggerated breathing, belching, sucking or smacking sounds, and clearing throat.

Clinical Course and Prognosis

Most individuals with transient tic disorder do not progress to a more serious tic disorder. Their tics either disappear permanently or, in some cases, may recur during periods of special stress. Only a small percentage go on to develop chronic motor or vocal tic disorder or Tourette's disorder.

Treatment

It is initially unclear whether the tics will disappear spontaneously, progress or become chronic. As focusing attention on tics often may exacerbate them, it is often recommended to the family that at first they disregard them as much as possible. But if the tics are so severe as to impair the patient or if they are accompanied by significant emotional disturbance, complete psychiatric and pediatric neurological examinations are recommended. Treatment will depend on the results of the evaluation. Psychopharmacology is not recommended unless the symptoms are unusually severe and disabling. Several studies have found that behavioral techniques, particularly habit reversal treatments, have been effective in treating transient tics.

CHRONIC MOTOR OR VOCAL TIC DISORDER

Definition and Diagnostic Criteria

The DSM-III-R criteria for establishing the diagnosis of chronic motor or vocal tic disorder are (1) the presence of either motor or vocal tics, but not both as in Tourette's disorder; (2) the tics' occurrence many times daily nearly every day or intermittently for more than 1 year; (3) onset before age 21; and (4) occurrence not exclusively during psychoactive substance intoxication or known CNS disease (Table 2).

This diagnosis is, in fact, composed of two mutually exclusive diagnoses, chronic motor tic disorder and chronic vocal tic disorder.

Epidemiology

The combined incidence of both chronic motor tic disorder and Tourette's disorder has been estimated at 1.6 percent of the population.

Chronic tic disorders are less well studied and may be rarer than is Tourette's disorder.

Clinical Course and Prognosis

Onset appears to be in early childhood. The types of tics and their locations are similar to those in transient tic disorder. Chronic vocal tic disorder is considerably rarer than is chronic motor tic disorder. Chronic vocal tics also are usually much less conspicuous than are those in Tourette's disorder. They often are not loud or intense and consist of grunts or other noises caused by thoracic, abdominal, or diaphragmatic contractions; the tics are not primarily from the vocal cords.

Children whose tics start between the ages of 6 and 8 years seem to have the best outcomes. Symptoms usually last for 4 to 6 years and stop in early adolescence. Those children whose tics involve the limbs or the trunk tend to do less well than do those with only facial tics.

Treatment

The treatment depends on the severity and frequency of the tics; the subjective distress; the impact on school or work, job performance, socialization; and the presence of any other concomitant psychiatric disorders.

Psychotherapy may be indicated in order to focus on what may be the primary emotional conflict or to minimize the secondary emotional problems caused by the tics. Several studies have found that behavioral techniques, particularly habit reversal treatments, have been effective in treating chronic tic disorder. Minor tranquilizers have not been successful. Haloperidol (Haldol) has been helpful in some cases, but the risks must be weighed against the possible clinical benefits because of the adverse effects of this drug, including the development of tardive dyskinesia.

TOURETTE'S DISORDER

History

Gilles de la Tourette first described Tourette's disorder in 1885 while studying under Charcot at the Salpétrière Clinic in Paris.

Definition and Diagnosis

The DSM-III-R criteria for diagnosing Tourette's disorder are as follows: (1) the presence of both multiple motor and one or more vocal tics at some time during the illness, not necessarily concurrently; (2) the tics' occurrence many times daily (usually in bouts) nearly every day or intermittently for more than 1 year; (3) a change in the tics' anatomic location, number, frequency, complexity, and severity over time; (4) age of onset prior to 21 years; and (5) occurrence not exclusively during psychoactive substance intoxication or known CNS disease (see Table 3).

Epidemiology

The prevalence of full-blown Tourette's disorder has been estimated to be minimally 1 per 2,000 (0.05 percent). If Tourette's disorder and multiple tics are considered to be part of a genetically determined spectrum, one review estimates the prevalence of this diathesis would approach 1 per 200 to 300 persons.

Sons of mothers with Tourette's disorder appear to have the highest risk of developing the disorder. There may also be a genetic association between Tourette's disorder and attention-deficit hyperactivity disorder and obsessive-compulsive disorder. The ratio of males to females with this disorder is approximately three to one.

Etiology

There is a higher prevalence of tics in families with Tourette's disorder than in the general population. Evidence for a genetic component includes a higher incidence of Tourette's disorder among monozygotic than dizygotic twins, and an increased incidence of Tourette's disorder and tics in families of patients with this disorder.

The primary etiology appears to be a dysregulation of neurochemical systems in the brain.

Clinical Course and Prognosis

Typically, prodromal behavioral symptoms—such as irritability, attentional difficulties, and poor frustration tolerance—are evident before or coincide with the onset of tics. Over 25 percent of the subjects in some studies received stimulants for a diagnosis of attention-deficit hyperactivity disorder before their having been diagnosed as suffering from Tourette's disorder.

The first tics usually begin between the ages of 2 and 10 years and almost always before the age of 14 years. The mean age of onset is between 7 and 8 years. The most frequent initial symptom is an eye-blink tic, followed by a head tic or facial grimace. Most of the complex motor and vocal symptoms emerge only several years after the initial symptoms. Coprolalia (obscene words) usually begins in early adolescence and occurs in about one-third of cases. Mental coprolalia, in which there is a sudden, intrusive socially unacceptable thought or obscene word, may also occur. In some severe cases, physical injury—including retinal detachment and orthopedic problems—has resulted from severe tics.

Obsessions, compulsions, attentional difficulties, impulsivity, and personality problems have been associated with Tourette's disorder. It is still being debated whether these problems usually develop secondarily to the patient's tics or are caused primarily by the same underlying pathobiological condition.

Many tics have an aggressive or sexual component, which may result in serious social consequences for the ticquer. Phenomenologically, the tics resemble a failure of censorship, both conscious and unconscious, with increased impulsivity and a too-ready transformation of thought into action.

Untreated, Tourette's disorder is usually a chronic, life-long disease with relative remissions and exacerbations. Initial symptoms may decrease, persist, or increase, and old symptoms may be replaced by new ones. Severely afflicted individuals may have serious emotional problems, including serious depression. Some of these difficulties appear to be associated with the disorder, whereas others result from severe social, academic, and vocational consequences, which are frequent sequelae of the disorder. In some cases, despair over the disruption of social and occupational functioning is so severe that individuals may contemplate and attempt suicide. On a more positive note, some children with Tourette's disorder have satisfactory peer relations, function well in school, and have adequate self-esteem; they may need no treatment and can be monitored by their pediatrician.

Treatment

Pharmacological treatments are most effective for Tourette's disorder. Psychotherapy is usually ineffective as a primary treatment modality, although it may help the patient cope with the symptoms of this disorder and any concommitant personality and behavioral difficulties that may arise.

Several behavioral techniques, including massed (negative) practice, self-monitoring, incompatible response training, presentation and removal of positive reinforcement, and habit reversal treatment were reviewed by S. A. Hobbs. He reported that tic frequencies were reduced in many cases, particularly with habit reversal treatment, but relatively few studies have reported clinically significant change. In general, behavioral treatments were much more effective in treating transient and chronic tic disorders, whereas relatively few cases of Tourette's disorder responded favorably. Behavioral therapy currently seems most useful in reducing stresses which may aggravate Tourette's disorder. Whether there is a synergistic effect when behavioral therapy is combined with pharmacotherapy has not been sufficiently investigated.

Pharmacotherapy. Haloperidol (Haldol) is the most frequently prescribed drug for Tourette's disorder. Up to 80 percent of patients have a favorable response, with their symptoms decreasing by as much as 70 to 90 percent of baseline frequencies. Follow-up studies, however, suggest that only 20 to 30 percent of patients continue on long-term maintenance. Discontinuation is often based on adverse effects of the drug.

Haloperidol appears to be most effective at relatively low doses. The initial daily average dosage for adolescents and adults is usually between 0.25 mg and 0.5 mg of haloperidol. Haloperidol is not approved for use in children under 3 years of age. For children between 3 and 12, it is recommended that a total daily dosage of between 0.05 mg per kg and 0.075 mg per kg be administered in divided doses either two or three times a day. Thus, this dosage would impose a daily limit of 3 mg of haloperidol for a 40 kg child. The dosage for all patients should be increased slowly so as to minimize the likelihood of an acute dystonic reaction. The maximum effective dosage in adolescents and adults is often in the range of 3 to 4 mg a day, but some patients require higher doses of up to 10 to 15 mg a day.

Patients, and their parents when appropriate, must be made aware of the drug's possible immediate and long-term adverse effects. It is particularly important to forewarn them of the possibilities of acute dystonic reactions and Parkinsonian symptoms. While prophylactic use of an anticholinergic agent is not recommended, it is appropriate to prescribe diphenhydramine (Benadryl) or benztropine mesylate (Cogentin) to the patient so that it is available should an acute dystonic reaction or Parkinsonian effects occur at home or on vacation. Other effects of special concern are cognitive dulling, which can impair school performance and learning, and the risk of developing tardive dyskinesia. School phobias in children and disabling social phobias in adults have been reported during the early phase of treatment, but they usually remit within a few weeks after discontinuing haloperidol.

Pimozide (Orap), an inhibitor of postsynaptic dopamine receptors, was approved recently to treat Tourette's disorder. Reportedly it is about as effective as haloperidol. Its use is only for those patients with severe symptoms that have not responded to haloperidol. It should not be used to treat simple tics or tics other than those associated with Tourette's disorder. Pimozide is a neuroleptic and has adverse effects similar to those of other neuroleptics. Furthermore, adverse cardiac effects are unusually frequent, and deaths have occurred at high doses. Electrocardiograms must be performed at baseline and periodically during treatment. There is very little experience in administering this drug to children under age 12.

The initial dose of pimozide is usually 1 mg to 2 mg daily in divided doses and may be increased every other day. Most patients are maintained at less than 0.2 mg per kg a day or 10 mg a day, whichever is less. It is recommended that a dose of 0.3 mg per kg a day or 20 mg a day never be exceeded.

Although not presently approved for use in Tourette's disorder, clonidine, a noradrenergic antagonist, has been reported in several studies to be efficacious, with 40 to 70 percent of patients benefiting from this medication. It has been used by some clinicians after carefully considering its risks and benefits and fully informing the patient, and

when appropriate the parents, of the situation. Clonidine has a slower onset of action than does haloperidol, and improvement may continue for over a year in some cases. In addition to the improvement in tic symptoms, patients may experience less tension, a greater sense of well-being, and longer attention span.

The benzodiazepines may be useful in diminishing anxiety in some patients, but they do not appear to reduce significantly the frequency of tics.

TIC DISORDER NOT OTHERWISE SPECIFIED (NOS)

Tic disorder not otherwise specified (NOS) is a residual category for tics that do not meet the criteria for a specific tic disorder (Table 4). All tic disorders with onset after age 21 must be diagnosed as tic disorder NOS.

References

Cohen D J, Leckman J F, editors: Tourette's syndrome: Advances in treatment and research. J Am Acad Child Psych *23*:123, 1984.

Cohen D J, Leckman J F, Shaywitz B A: The tourette syndrome and other tics. In *The Clinical Guide to Child Psychiatry*, D Shaffer, A A Ehrandt, L L Greenhill, editors, p 3. Free Press, New York, 1985.

Friedhoff A J, Chase T N, editors: *Gilles de la Tourette Syndrome*. Raven Press, New York, 1982.

Fulop G, Phillips R A, Shapiro A K, Gomes J A, Shapiro E, Nordhic J W: ECG changes during haloperidol and pimozide treatment of Tourette's disorder. Am J Psych *144*:673, 1987.

Glaze D G, Jankovic J, Frost J D: Sleep in Gilles de la Tourette syndrome: Disorder of arousal. Neurology *32*:153, 1982.

Hobbs S A, Dorsett P G, Dahlquist L M: Tic disorders. In *Behavior Therapy with Children and Adolescents: A Clinical Approach*, M Hersen, V B Van Hasselt, editors, p 241. Wiley, New York, 1987.

Kidd K K, Prasoff B A, Cohen D J: The familial pattern of Gilles de la Tourette Syndrome. Arch Gen Psychiatry *37*:1336, 1980.

Shapiro A K, Shapiro E S: *Tic, Tourette Syndrome and Other Movement Disorders: A Pediatrician's Guide*. Tourette Syndrome Association, Inc., Bayside, NY, 1980.

Shapiro A K, Shapiro E S: The treatment and etiology of tics and Tourette syndrome. Compr Psychiatry *22*:193, 1981.

Shapiro A K, Shapiro E S, Bruun R D, Sweet R D: *Gilles de la Tourette Syndrome*. Raven Press, New York, 1978.

Shapiro A K, Shapiro E S, Young J G, Feinberg T E: *Tourette and Tic Disorders*. Raven Press, New York, 1987.

Weiden P, Bruun R: Worsening of Tourette's disorder due to neuroleptic-induced akathisia. Am J Psych *144*:504, 1987.

41

Elimination Disorders

INTRODUCTION

Bowel and bladder control usually develop gradually and sequentially. The normal sequence of attaining these milestones is (1) development of nocturnal fecal continence, (2) development of diurnal fecal continence, (3) development of diurnal bladder control, and (4) development of nocturnal bladder control.

Acquisition of these milestones is influenced by physiological maturation; intellectual capacity; cultural attitudes toward toilet training, including age at which it is initiated and the specific techniques employed; and the psychological makeup of each parent–child dyad.

FUNCTIONAL ENCOPRESIS

Definition and Diagnostic Criteria

Functional encopresis is fecal soiling past the time that bowel control is physiologically possible and after toilet training should have been accomplished. The DSM-III-R criteria for functional encopresis are given in Table 1. The feces may be of normal, near normal, or liquid consistency. This permits the inclusion of some, but not all, cases of overflow incontinence, the cause of the majority of encopresis seen by pediatricians, under the rubric of functional encopresis. DSM-III-R states that the child's chronological and mental age must be at least 4 years and that fecal mishaps must have occurred at least once monthly for at least 6 months.

DSM-III-R also provides for specifying whether the encopresis is primary or secondary type. Encopretics are classified as primary type if the encopresis continues after both chronological and mental ages have reached at least 4 years and there has not been a prior period of fecal continence lasting at least 1 year. Encopresis that develops anytime after a yearlong period of continence is termed secondary type encopresis.

Epidemiology

About 1 percent of 5-year-olds may be diagnosed as having functional encopresis. It appears to be more common in lower socioeconomic classes and is three to four times more frequent in males. About one quarter of encopretic children are also enuretic. Most encopresis occurs during waking hours; cases associated with nocturnal encopresis have a poorer prognosis.

Although most cases of encopresis are not associated with voluminous fecal impaction, about one fourth of encopretics have an associated constipation that results in encopresis of the overflow type.

Etiology

Inadequate or lack of appropriate toilet training may delay the child's attainment of continence. There is also evidence that some encopretic children suffer from lifelong inefficient and ineffective gastrointestinal motility. Either of these alone, but especially in combination, offer an opportunity for a power struggle between child and parent over issues of autonomy and control; such battles often aggravate the disorder and frequently cause secondary behavioral difficulties. Occasionally there may be a special fear of using the toilet, which must be resolved.

Encopretics who are clearly able to control their bowel function adequately and who deposit feces of relatively normal consistency in abnormal places usually also have a psychiatric difficulty.

Encopresis may be associated with other neurodevelopmental problems, including easy distractibility, short attention span, low frustration tolerance, hyperactivity, and poor coordination.

Psychogenic Megacolon. Many encopretic children also retain feces and become constipated either voluntarily or secondary to painful defecation. The resulting chronic rectal distention from large, hard fecal masses may cause loss of tone in the rectal wall and desensitization to pressure. Thus, many of these children become unaware of the need to defecate, and so overflow encopresis occurs with usually relatively small amounts of liquid or soft stool leaking out. Olfactory accommodation may diminish or eliminate sensory cues.

Secondary encopresis sometimes appears to be a regression following such stresses as the birth of a sibling, parental separation, change in domicile, or the start of school.

Clinical Description

The natural course is usually self-limited, and encopresis rarely continues beyond early to middle adolescence.

Encopresis is a particularly repugnant symptom to most people and may lead to severe intrafamilial tensions and social ostracism. The encopretic child is often scapegoated

Table 1
Diagnostic Criteria for Functional Encopresis

A. Repeated passage of feces into places not appropriate for that purpose (e.g., clothing, floor), whether involuntary or intentional. (The disorder may be overflow incontinence secondary to functional fecal retention.)

B. At least one such event a month for at least 6 months.

C. Chronologic and mental age, at least 4 years.

D. Not due to a physical disorder, such as aganglionic megacolon.

Specify primary or secondary type.

> **Primary type:** the disturbance was not preceded by a period of fecal continence lasting at least 1 year.

> **Secondary type:** the disturbance was preceded by a period of fecal continence lasting at least 1 year.

Table from DSM-III-R, *Diagnostic and Statistical Manual of Mental Disorders,* ed 3, revised. (Current Classification of Mental Disorders, 1987.) Copyright American Psychiatric Association, Washington, D.C., 1987. Used with permission.

and ridiculed by peers and shunned by adults. Psychologically, the patient may appear blunted to the effect of the disorder on other people, but most encopretics have abysmally low self-esteem and realize that they are unwanted.

Other than these psychosocial complications, the major difficulties are problems with the lower gastrointestinal tract secondary to fecal retention, including impaction and anal fissures.

Differential Diagnosis

Based on DSM-III-R criteria, overflow incontinence secondary to functional fecal retention would be considered to be "functional encopresis." The characteristic features of this are frequent liquid stools and hard fecal masses in the colon and rectum on abdominal palpation and rectal examination. Some children have a coexisting anal fissure or history of anal fissure and bleeding with associated pain on defecation. Although these children may need both pediatric and psychiatric treatment, technically, the associated structural organic cause excludes them from the diagnosis of functional encopresis.

Organic causes of encopresis also must be eliminated. The chief differential problem is that of aganglionic megacolon or Hirschsprung's disease, in which the patient may have an empty rectum and no desire to defecate but may still have an overflow of feces.

Treatment

By the time a child is brought in for treatment, there is considerable family discord and distress. Family tensions regarding the symptom must be reduced, and a nonpunitive atmosphere must be created. Similar efforts should be made to reduce the child's embarrassment at school. Multiple changes of underwear with a minimum of fuss should be arranged.

Psychotherapy is useful for easing family tensions, to treat the encopretics' reactions to their symptoms (e.g., low

self-esteem and social isolation), to address the psychodynamic causes present in those children who have bowel control but continue to deposit their feces in inappropriate locations, and to treat those cases of secondary encopresis that are reactions to psychological stressors.

Behavioral techniques have been used with great success, including "star charts," with the child inserting a star on a chart whenever he or she is dry, and other behavioral reinforcers.

In cases of overflow incontinence secondary to fecal retention, proper bowel hygiene should be taught, and pain on defecation caused by fissures or hard stool should be eliminated or reduced; this may be done in consultation with a pediatrician.

FUNCTIONAL ENURESIS

Definition and Diagnostic Criteria

Enuresis is manifested as a repetitive and inappropriate passage of urine. The voiding may be involuntary or voluntary. For instance, persons with daytime enuresis may intentionally fail to inhibit the reflex to pass urine, and some persons admit to being awake and choosing to urinate in bed rather than get up and go to the toilet. Second, a minimum chronological age of 5 years and a minimum mental age of 4 years are required. The DSM-III-R criteria for the diagnosis of functional enuresis are given in Table 2.

Enuretics are characterized as "primary" if they have never been continent for a minimum of 1 year and "secondary" if their enuresis began after 1 year of dryness. The clinician should further note whether the enuresis is "diurnal," that is, occurring during the daytime, or nocturnal, the most common form, or both. These subclassifications have practical diagnostic and therapeutic applications.

Table 2
Diagnostic Criteria for Functional Enuresis

A. Repeated voiding of urine during the day or night into bed or clothes, whether involuntary or intentional.

B. At least two such events per month for children between the ages of 5 and 6, and at least one event per month for older children.

C. Chronologic age at least five, and mental age at least 4.

D. Not due to a physical disorder, such as diabetes, urinary tract infection, or a seizure disorder.

Specify primary or secondary type.

> **Primary type:** the disturbance was not preceded by a period of urinary continence lasting at least one year.

> **Secondary type:** the disturbance was preceded by a period of urinary continence lasting at least one year.

Specify nocturnal only, diurnal only, or **nocturnal and diurnal.**

Table from DSM-III-R, *Diagnostic and Statistical Manual of Mental Disorders,* ed 3, revised. (Current Classification of Mental Disorders, 1987.) Copyright American Psychiatric Association, Washington, D.C., 1987. Used with permission.

Epidemiology

More males than females of all ages are enuretic. Prevalence is estimated to be 7 percent of boys and 3 percent of girls at age 5, 3 percent of boys and 2 percent of girls at age 10, and 1 percent of boys and almost no girls at age 18.

Diurnal enuresis is much less common than nocturnal enuresis. Only about 2 percent of 5-year-olds have diurnal enuresis at least weekly. Unlike nocturnal enuresis, diurnal enuresis is more common in girls than in boys.

Psychiatric problems are present in only about 20 percent of enuretic children, and they are most common in enuretic girls and in children who wet both day and night.

Etiology

Normal bladder control is acquired gradually and is influenced by neuromuscular and cognitive development, socioemotional factors, toilet training, and, possibly, genetic factors. Difficulties in one or more of these areas may delay urinary continence. Although an organic etiology precludes a diagnosis of functional enuresis, the correction of an anatomical defect or the cure of an infection does not always cure the enuresis, which suggests that the etiology may still be functional in some of these cases.

In a longitudinal study of child development, those children who were enuretic were about twice as likely to have concomitant developmental delays.

About 75 percent of enuretic children have a first-degree relative who is or was enuretic. The concordance rate is higher in monozygotic than in dizygotic twins. Although there may be a genetic component, much could be accounted for by greater tolerance of enuresis in these families, as well as other psychosocial factors.

Most enuretics have a bladder with a normal anatomical capacity when anesthetized but a "functionally small bladder." Thus, enuretic children feel an urge to void with less urine in the bladder than do normal children and hence urinate more frequently and in smaller quantities than do normal children.

Psychosocial stressors appear to precipitate some cases of secondary enuresis. In young children, this disorder has been particularly associated with the birth of a sibling, hospitalization between the ages of 2 to 4, the start of school, the breakup of a family because of divorce or death, and a move to a new domicile.

Clinical Description

Functional enuresis is usually self-limited. The child eventually can remain dry without psychiatric sequelae. Most enuretics find their symptom ego dystonic and have enhanced self-esteem and improved social confidence when they become continent.

About 80 percent of enuretics are primary, never having achieved a yearlong period of dryness. Secondary enuresis usually begins between ages 5 and 8 years; if it occurs much later, especially during adulthood, organic causes must be investigated. There is some evidence that secondary enuresis in children is more frequently associated with a concomitant psychiatric difficulty than is primary enuresis.

Enuresis does not appear to be related to a specific stage of sleep or time of night, rather, bedwetting appears randomly. In most cases, quality of sleep is normal. There is little evidence that enuretics sleep more soundly than do other children.

Relapses occur in enuretics who are becoming dry spontaneously as well as in those who are being treated.

The significant emotional and social difficulties of enuretics usually result from the primary symptom and include poor self-image, decreased self-esteem, social embarrassment and restriction, and intrafamilial conflict.

Differential Diagnosis

Although the large majority of enuretics are functional, possible organic causes must be ruled out. Organic factors are found most often in children with both nocturnal and diurnal enuresis combined with urinary frequency and urgency. They include (1) genitourinary pathology—structural, neurological, and infectious—for example, obstructive uropathy, spina bifida occulta, and cystitis; (2) other organic disorders that may cause polyuria and enuresis, for example, diabetes mellitus or diabetes insipidus; (3) disturbances of consciousness and sleep, for example, seizures, intoxication, and somnambulism during which the person urinates; and (4) side effects from treatment with antipsychotics, for example, thioridazine (Mellaril).

Treatment

Because there is usually no identifiable cause in functional enuresis and because it tends to remit spontaneously even if not treated, some success has been achieved by a number of methods.

Appropriate Toilet Training. First, appropriate toilet training with parental reinforcement should have been attempted, especially in primary enuresis. If toilet training was not given, parents and patient should be guided in this undertaking. Record keeping is helpful in determining a baseline and following the child's progress and may itself be a reinforcer. A "star chart" may be particularly helpful. Other useful techniques include restricting fluids before bed and night lifting to toilet-train the child.

Behavioral Therapy. Classical conditioning with the bell (or buzzer) and pad apparatus is the most effective and generally safe treatment for enuresis. Dryness results in over 50 percent of cases. This treatment is equally effective in children with and without concomitant psychiatric disorders, and there is no evidence of "symptom substitution." Difficulties may include child and family compliance, improper use of the apparatus, and relapse.

Bladder training—the encouragement or reward for delaying micturition for increasing lengths of time during waking hours—has also been used. Although sometimes effective, this method is decidedly inferior to the bell and pad.

Pharmacotherapy. Drugs should rarely be used in treating enuresis and then only as a last resort in intractable cases causing serious socioemotional difficulty for the sufferer. Imipramine (Tofranil) is both efficacious and has been approved for use in treating childhood enuresis, primarily on a short-term basis. Initially, up to 30 percent of enuretics may stay dry, and up to 85 percent may wet less frequently. This, however, does not often last. Tolerance often develops after 6 weeks of therapy, and once the drug is discontinued, relapse and enuresis at former frequencies usually occur within a few months. A more serious problem is the adverse effects of the drug, which include cardiotoxiocity.

Psychotherapy. Although there have been many psychological and psychoanalytic theories regarding enuresis, controlled studies have found that psychotherapy alone is not an effective treatment of the enuresis. Psychotherapy, however, may be useful in dealing with emotional and family difficulties that arise secondary to the symptom or with coexisting psychiatric problems.

References

Anders T F, Freeman E D: Enuresis. In *Basic Handbook of Child Psychiatry,* J Nospitz editor, vol 2, p 546. Basic Books, New York, 1979.

Fleisher D R: Diagnosis and treatment of disorders of defecation in children. Pediatr Ann 5:72, 1976.

Foxman B, Valdez R B, Brook R H: Childhood enuresis: Prevalence, perceived impact, and prescribed treatments. Pediatr 77:482, 1986.

Hersov L: Faecal soiling. In *Child and Adolescent Psychiatry: Modern Approaches,* ed 2. M Rutter, L Hersov, editors, p 482. Blackwell Scientific Publications, Oxford, England, 1985.

Kisch E H, Pfeffer C R: Functional encopresis: Psychiatric in patient treatment. Am J Psychother 38:264, 1984.

Kolvin I, MacKeith R C, Meadow S R, editors: Bladder control and enuresis. Clinics in Developmental Medicine nos. 48/49. Spastics International Medical Publications, London, 1973.

Landman G B: Locus of control and self-esteem in children with encopresis. J Dev Behav Pediatr 7:11, 1986.

Levine M D, Mazonson P, Bakow H: Behavioral symptom substitution in children cured of encopresis. Am J Dis Child 134:663, 1980.

Schmitt B D: Daytime wetting (diurnal enuresis). Pediatr Clin North Am 29:9, 1982.

Shaffer D: Enuresis. In *Child and Adolescent Psychiatry: Modern Approaches,* ed 2. M Rutter, L Hersov, editors, p 465. Blackwell Scientific Publications, Oxford, England, 1985.

42

Speech Disorders Not Elsewhere Classified

42.1
Cluttering

DEFINITION

DSM-III-R defines cluttering as a disorder of speech fluency involving both the rate and rhythm of speech, which results in impaired speech and intelligibility. In this disorder, speech is erratic and dysrhythmic, consisting of rapid and jerky spurts that usually involve faulty phrasing patterns (e.g., alternating pauses and bursts of speech that produce groups of words unrelated to the sentence's grammatic structure). Cluttering is a new disorder classification in the DSM-III-R category of developmental language and speech disorders.

EPIDEMIOLOGY

Research on this disorder has been sparse, and no precise prevalence figure is currently available. However, it is estimated that the disorder is less common than is stuttering. Cluttering is slightly more common in males than in females.

ETIOLOGY

The cause of cluttering is not known. There appears to be higher rate of clutterers among the family members of the affected individual than among the general population. Some clinical reports indicate that this condition may be present among elementary school children learning English as a second language.

CLINICAL FEATURES

The onset of the disorder is between ages 2 and 8 years. It develops over a period of weeks or months and worsens under emotional stress or pressured situations. Speech is fast, and at times the rapid and jerky spurts make speech sounds unintelligible. Between the rapid bursts of strings of words are pauses that are unrelated to the completion of the sentence, thereby making the presentation of sentences fragmented and incomplete.

About two thirds of children may recover spontaneously as they approach early adolescence. Cluttering has fewer associated features, such as social isolation, tics, and depression, than does stuttering. In a small number of severe cases, secondary emotional disorders may ensue as a result of poor peer interaction or negative familial response to the child's problem.

DIAGNOSIS AND DIFFERENTIAL DIAGNOSIS

Except in children younger than 2 to 2½ years, the fully developed disorder is manifested as described in Table 1.

Cluttering should be differentiated from stuttering, another developmental speech disorder which is characterized by frequent repetitions or prolongations of sounds or syllables, thereby markedly impairing the fluency of speech. A major differential diagnostic feature is that in cluttering, the affected individual is usually unaware of the disturbance, whereas after the initial phase of stuttering, the individual is painfully aware of the speech disorder.

TREATMENT

In most moderate to severe cases, speech therapy is indicated. Psychotherapy is indicated when the affected child shows frustration, anxiety, depression, and difficulties in social adjustment with peers and in school. Family ther-

Table 1
Diagnostic Criteria for Cluttering

A disorder of speech fluency involving both the rate and the rhythm of speech and resulting in impaired speech intelligibility. Speech is erratic and dysrhythmic, consisting of rapid and jerky spurts that usually involve faulty phrasing patterns (e.g., alternating pauses and bursts of speech that produce groups of words unrelated to the grammatical structure of the sentence).

Table from DSM-III-R, *Diagnostic and Statistical Manual of Mental Disorders,* ed 3, revised. (Current Classification of Mental Disorders, 1987.) Copyright American Psychiatric Association, Washington, D.C., 1987. Used with permission.

apy may be helpful in enabling the parents to understand their reactions to the disorder and to be supportive of the child.

The long-term effects of speech therapy and various psychotherapeutic approaches are not yet documented; however, such therapies should ameliorate the condition.

References

Bloom L, Lahey M: *Language Development and Language Disorders.* Wiley, New York, 1978.

Chess S, Rosenberg M: Clinical differentiation among children with initial language complaints. J Autism Child Schizoph *4*:99, 1974.

Templin M, Darley F: *The Templin Darley Tests of Articulation.* Bureau of Education Research and Service, University of Iowa, Iowa City, 1969.

Wylie H L, Franchack P, McWilliams B J: Characteristics of children with speech disorders seen in a child guidance center. Percept Motor Skills *20*:1101, 1955.

42.2 _____
Stuttering

DEFINITION

According to DSM-III-R, stuttering is a developmental speech disorder characterized by frequent repetitions or prolongation of sounds or syllables, markedly impairing the fluency of speech. Unusual hesitations and pauses disrupt the rhythmic flow of speech. The cause of the condition is not known. The term "stammering" is used synonymously with stuttering.

EPIDEMIOLOGY

Approximately 5 percent of all children have a persistent problem with stuttering that continues into adolescence. The disorder is about three times more common in boys than in girls, and it persists longer in boys as well. The prevalence appears to vary in different cultures and is slightly higher in cultures characterized by competitive pressure.

ETIOLOGY

Although precise etiological factors are not known, many theories have been proposed: (1) theories that explain the stuttering block, (2) theories related to conditions under which the disorder has its onset, (3) learning theories, (4) cybernetic model theory, and (5) brain function theories.

Stuttering Block Theories

Stuttering block theories can be grouped into three areas: genogenic, psychogenic, and semantogenic.

The basic premise of the genogenic model is that the stutterer is biologically different from the nonstutterer. An example is the theory of cerebral dominance, which states that children are predisposed to stutter by a conflict between the two halves of the cerebrum for control of the speech organs' activity. The current consensus is that there may be some sort of constitutional predisposition toward stuttering but that environmental stresses work together with this somatic variant to produce stuttering.

Most psychogenic theories emphasize obsessive-compulsive mechanisms and a variety of psychosocial factors, such as a dysfunctional family. Stuttering is seen as a neurosis caused by the persistence into later life of early pregenital oral-sadistic and anal-sadistic components.

According to the semantogenic theories, stuttering is a learned pathological response to the mislabeling of normal early syllable and word repetitions.

Onset Theories

Onset theories fall into three subgroups: the breakdown, the repressed-need, and the anticipatory-struggle theories.

The breakdown theories view stuttering as a momentary failure of the complicated coordinations involved in speech. Most such theories regard constitutional or organic factors—that is, the genogenic factors discussed above—as the causes of the breakdown.

The repressed-need theory is based on psychoanalytic concepts and defines stuttering as a neurotic symptom rooted deeply in unconscious needs. Early theories suggested that stuttering satisfies oral gratifications or reflects oral-aggressive or anal-aggressive concerns.

The theme of the anticipatory-struggle theory is that stutterers interfere in some manner with the way they talk because of their belief in the difficulty of speech; that is, stutterers anticipate difficulty with speech.

Learning Theories

Learning theories use feedback models. The stimulus–response theories of learning use the relatively precise language of behavioral science to define the process by which stuttering is learned and maintained, by identifying the motivational factors, stimulus variables, and reinforcing conditions. One of the central problems in applying learning principles to stuttering is to explain the nature of the reinforcement that causes it to persist despite repeated punishment.

Cybernetic Model

In the cybernetic model, speech is seen as an automatic process that depends on feedback for regulation. Stuttering may be caused by a breakdown in feedback or in the sensor receptors of this feedback. The observations that stuttering is reduced by white noise and that delayed auditory feedback produces artificial stuttering in normal speakers support this view.

Brain Function Theories

Research on cerebral hemispheric lateralization and specialization suggests that incomplete lateralization of language may result in stuttering. Several studies using electroencephalography report that stuttering males demonstrated right hemisphere alpha suppression across stimulus words and tasks, as contrasted with left hemisphere alpha suppression for nonstuttering males and females. The earlier concern that forcing left-handed children to use their right hand caused stuttering has not been validated.

Recent family and twin studies strongly suggest that stuttering is a genetically inherited neurological disorder. However, the available data are not conclusive at this time.

CLINICIAL FEATURES AND COURSE

Stuttering usually appears before the age of 12 years, in most cases between 18 months and 9 years, with two sharp peaks of onset between the ages of 2 to 3½ and 5 to 7 years. Stuttering does not suddenly begin; it typically occurs over a period of weeks or months with a repetition of initial consonants, whole words that are usually the first words of a phrase, or long words. As the disorder progresses, the repetitions become more frequent with consistent stuttering on the most important words or phrases. Even after it develops, stuttering may be absent during oral readings, singing, or talking to pets or inanimate objects.

Four gradually evolving phases in the development of stuttering have been identified.

Phase 1 occurs during the preschool period. Initially, the difficulty tends to be episodic, appearing for periods of weeks or months between long interludes of normal speech. There is a high percentage of recovery from these periods of stuttering. During this phase, children stutter most often when excited or upset, when they seem to have a great deal to say, or under other conditions of communicative pressure.

Phase 2 usually occurs in the elementary school years. The disorder is chronic, with few if any intervals of normal speech. Such children become aware of their speech difficulty and regard themselves as stutterers. In this phase, the stuttering occurs mainly on the major parts of speech—nouns, verbs, adjectives, and adverbs.

Phase 3 is usually seen after age 8 and up to adulthood. It occurs most often in late childhood and early adolescence. During this phase, the stuttering comes and goes largely in response to specific situations, such as reciting in class, speaking to strangers, making purchases in stores, and using the telephone. Certain words and sounds are regarded as more difficult than others.

Phase 4 is typically seen in late adolescence and adulthood. Stutterers show a vivid, fearful anticipation of stuttering. They fear words, sounds, and situations. Word substitutions and circumlocutions are common. Stutterers avoid situations requiring speech and show other evidence of fear and embarrassment.

The course of stuttering is usually chronic, with some periods of partial remission lasting for weeks or months and exacerbations occurring most frequently when under pressure to communicate. Fifty to 80 percent of children with stuttering, mostly mild cases, recover spontaneously.

In chronic cases of school-age children, impairment in peer relationships may develop as a result of teasing and social ostracism. These children may face academic difficulties if they avoid speaking in class. Later major complications include the affected individual's limitation in occupational choice or advancement.

The disorder is more common among family members of the affected child than in the general population.

Stutterers may develop associated clinical features: vivid, fearful anticipation of stuttering with avoidance of particular words, sounds, or situations in which stuttering is anticipated; eye blinks; tics; and tremors of the lips or jaw. Frustration, anxiety, and depression are common among chronic stutterers.

DIAGNOSIS

The diagnosis of stuttering is not difficult when the clinical features are apparent and well developed and each of the four phases can be readily recognized. Diagnostic difficulties may arise, however, when trying to determine the existence of stuttering in young children, as some children pass through a period during the preschool years when speech is not fluent. It may not be clear whether this nonfluent pattern is part of normal speech and language development for some children, or whether it represents the initial stage in the development of stuttering. Because 50 to 80 percent of stutterers remit spontaneously, it is best to be reassuring and to minimize focusing on the impairment during this early developmental period. Table 1 outlines the DSM-III-R diagnostic criteria for stuttering.

DIFFERENTIAL DIAGNOSIS

Spastic dysphonia is a stuttering-like speech disorder and is distinguished from stuttering by the presence of an abnormal pattern of breathing.

Cluttering is another developmental speech disorder characterized by erratic and dysrhythmic speech patterns of rapid and jerky spurts of words and phrases. In cluttering, affected individuals are usually unaware of the disturbance, whereas after the initial phase of the disorder, stutterers are acutely aware of their speech difficulties.

TREATMENT

Until the end of the 19th century, the most common treatments for stuttering were distraction, suggestion, and relaxation. More recent approaches using distraction include teaching stutterers to talk in time to rhythmic movements of the arm, hand, or fingers. Stutterers are also advised to speak slowly in a sing-song or monotone. These approaches, however, remove the stuttering only temporarily. Suggestion techniques, such as hypnosis, also stop stuttering but, again, only temporarily. Relaxation techniques are based on the premise that it is almost impossible to be relaxed and at the same time to stutter in the usual manner. Because of their lack of long-term benefits, distraction, suggestion, and relaxation approaches as such are not currently used.

Table 1
Diagnostic Criteria for Stuttering

Frequent repetitions or prolongations of sounds or syllables that markedly impair the fluency of speech.

Table from DSM-III-R, *Diagnostic and Statistical Manual of Mental Disorders*, ed 3, revised. (Current Classification of Mental Disorders, 1987.) Copyright American Psychiatric Association, Washington, D.C., 1987. Used with permission.

Classical psychoanalysis, insight-oriented psychotherapy, group therapy, and other psychotherapeutic modalities have not been successful in treating stuttering. However, if stutterers have a poor self-image, anxiety, depression, or show evidence of an established neurotic process or another emotional disability, individual psychotherapy is indicated and effective for the associated condition.

Family therapy should also be considered if there is evidence of family dysfunction, family contribution to the stutterer's symptoms, or family stress caused by trying to cope with or to help the stutterer.

Most of the modern treatments of stuttering are based on the view that stuttering is essentially a learned form of behavior that is not necessarily associated with a basic neurotic personality or neurological abnormalities. These approaches work directly with the speech difficulty to minimize the issues that maintain and strengthen the stuttering, to modify or decrease the severity of the stuttering by eliminating the secondary symptoms, and to encourage the stutterer to speak, even if stuttering, in a relatively easy and effortless fashion, thereby avoiding fears and blocks.

One example of this approach is the self-therapy proposed by the Speech Foundation of America. Self-therapy is based on the premise that stuttering is not a symptom but a behavior that can be modified. Stutterers are told that they can learn to control their difficulty partly by modifying their feelings about and attitudes toward stuttering and partly by modifying the deviant behaviors associated with their stuttering blocks. This approach includes desensitization, reducing the emotional reaction to and fears of stuttering, and substituting positive action to control the moment of stuttering. The basic principle is that stuttering is something one is doing and that stutterers can learn to change what they are doing.

Whichever therapeutic approach is used, individual and family assessments and supportive interventions may be helpful. A team assessment of the child or adolescent and his or her family should be made before any approaches to treatment are begun.

References

Andrew G, Guitar B, Howie P: Meta-analysis of the effects of stuttering treatment. J Speech Hear Disord *45*:287, 1980.

Kavanaugh J, Strange W: *Speech and Language in the Laboratory, School, and Clinic*. MIT Press, Cambridge, MA, 1978.

Koller W C: Dysfluency (stuttering) in extrapyramidal disease. Arch Neurol *40*:175, 1983.

Metter J E: *Speech Disorders: Clinical Evaluation and Diagnosis*. S P Medical and Scientific Books, New York, 1985.

Ryan B P: *Programmed Therapy for Stuttering in Children and Adults*. Thomas, Springfield, IL, 1974.

Schwartz M F: *Stuttering Solved*. Lippincott, Philadelphia, 1976.

Shames G: Dysfluency and stuttering. Pediatr Clinics North Am *15*:691, 1968.

Sheehan J: *Stuttering: Research and Therapy*. Harper & Row, New York, 1970.

Travis L, editor: *Handbook of Speech Pathology and Audiology*. Appleton-Century-Crofts, New York, 1971.

Van Riper C: *The Nature of Stuttering*. Prentice-Hall, Englewood Cliffs, NJ, 1971.

43

Other Disorders of Infancy, Childhood, or Adolescence

43.1

Elective Mutism

DEFINITION AND DIAGNOSTIC CRITERIA

Elective mutism is characterized by a persistent refusal to talk in one or more major social situations, including at school, despite the ability to comprehend spoken language and to speak. The DSM-III-R criteria for elective mutism are given in Table 1.

EPIDEMIOLOGY

Elective mutism is an uncommon disorder. It is present in less than 1 percent of patients referred to child mental health-related services. The sex ratio is unusual. Although most childhood psychiatric disorders are more prevalent in boys, elective mutism is as common or slightly more common in girls.

Many of these children have a history of delayed onset of speech. A history of enuresis or encopresis is also more common in children with elective mutism than in the general population or in children with other speech disorders. Compulsive traits, negativism, temper tantrums, and oppositional and aggressive behavior, particularly in the home, have been reported frequently in these children. Out of the home, they are often excessively shy and reticent.

Etiology

Elective mutism is a psychologically determined inhibition or refusal to speak. Maternal overprotection may pre-dispose to its development. Children with elective mutism usually speak freely at home; they have no significant biological disability. Some children seem predisposed to develop elective mutism after early emotional or physical traumata, and so some clinicians refer to this phenomenon as traumatic mutism rather than elective mutism.

CLINICAL DESCRIPTION

The most common pattern is that such children speak almost exclusively with the nuclear family at home but not elsewhere, especially not at school. Consequently, they may have significant academic difficulties and even failure. They may not form social relationships, and teasing and scapegoating by peers may cause them to refuse to go to school.

Some children with elective mutism will communicate with gestures, such as nodding or shaking the head or saying "umm-hum" or "no." Most cases last only a few weeks or months, but some may persist for years. In one follow-up study, about half the subjects improved within 5 to 10 years. Children who do not improve by age 10 appear to have a more chronic course and a worse prognosis.

Some mute children appear to develop negativistic and sadistic relationships with adults and use their defiant muteness to punish them. This behavior seems to improve concomitantly with increasing speech in the environments where the child previously had been mute.

DIFFERENTIAL DIAGNOSIS

Very shy children may exhibit a transient muteness in new, anxiety-provoking situations. These children often have a history of not speaking in the presence of strangers and clinging to their mothers. Most of these children who are mute upon entering school improve spontaneously and may be described as having transient adaptational shyness.

Elective mutism must also be distinguished from organic and developmental disabilities, childhood psychoses, and other emotional disorders. In these disorders, however, the symptoms are more widespread, and there is not one situation in which the child communicates essentially normally; there may be an inability to speak rather than a refusal to

Table 1
Diagnostic Criteria for Elective Mutism

A. Persistent refusal to talk in one or more major social situations (including at school).

B. Ability to comprehend spoken language and to speak.

Table from DSM-III-R, *Diagnostic and Statistical Manual of Mental Disorders,* ed 3, revised. (Current Classification of Mental Disorders, 1987.) Copyright American Psychiatric Association, Washington, D.C., 1987. Used with permission.

speak. In mutism secondary to hysteria, the mutism is also pervasive.

Children introduced into an environment where a different language is spoken may be reticent to begin using the new language. Elective mutism should be diagnosed only when children also refuse to converse in their native language and when they have gained communicative competence in the new language.

TREATMENT

Psychotherapy, counseling, behavioral therapies, hypnosis, speech therapy, and family therapy have been used with varying success. A multimodal approach using individual, behavioral, and family interventions is most likely to be successful.

References

Brown J B, Lloyd H: A controlled study of children not speaking in school. J Assoc Workers Maladjusted Children, p 49, 1975.

Cantwell P D, Baker L: Speech and language: Development and Disorders. In *Child and Adolescent Psychiatry. Modern Approaches*, M Rutter, L Hersov, editors, p 531. Blackwell Scientific Publications, Oxford, England, 1985.

Fundudis, T, Kolvin I, Garside R: *Speech Retarded and Deaf Children: Their Psychological Development*. Academic Press, London, 1979.

Hasselman S: Elective mutism in children 1877–1981. A literary summary. Acta Paedopsychiatry *49*:297, 1983.

Hayden T L: Classification of elective mutism. J Am Acad Child Psychiat *19*:18, 1980.

Kolvin I, Fundudis T: Elective mute children: Psychological development and background factors. J Child Psychol Psychiatry *22*:219, 1981.

Laybourne P C: Elective mutism. In *Basic Handbook of Child Psychiatry*, vol 2, J D Noshpitz, editor. p 464. Basic Books, New York, 1979.

Wilkins R: A comparison of elective mutism and emotional disorders in children. Brit J Psychiatry *146*:198, 1985.

Wright H L: A clinical study of children who refuse to talk in school. J Am Acad Child Psychol *7*:603, 1968.

43.2 _____
Identity Disorder

DEFINITION AND DIAGNOSTIC CRITERIA

DSM-III-R defines identity disorder as severe subjective distress over an inability to reconcile aspects of the self into a relatively coherent and acceptable sense of self. The disturbance is manifested by uncertainty about a variety of issues relating to identity, including long-term goals, career choice, friendship patterns, values, and loyalties. These symptoms last for at least 3 months. The diagnosis is not valid if the reaction is symptomatic of a mood disorder or a psychotic disorder. The DSM-III-R criteria for the diagnosis of identity disorder are given in Table 1.

EPIDEMIOLOGY

There is no reliable information on predisposing factors, familial pattern, sex ratio, or prevalence. It appears, however, that identity disorder is more common in modern society than in earlier times. This may be because of the current greater exposure through the media and education to more moral, behavioral, and life-style possibilities and because of the increased conflicts between adolescent peer values and those of parents or society.

ETIOLOGY

The cause of identity disorder is hypothesized to be psychological. Adolescents are unable to use effectively the intrapsychic and social moratoriums provided by society and do not achieve ego identity, in the Eriksonian sense. The normal intrapsychic transformations necessary for ego mastery result in persistent regressive phenomena leading to crisis formation and, if not relieved by adequate growth responses, identity diffusion.

CLINICAL DESCRIPTION: COURSE AND PROGNOSIS

The onset of identity disorder is most frequently in late adolescence, as the individual separates from the nuclear family and attempts to establish an independent identity and value system. The onset is usually manifested by a gradual increase in anxiety, depression, regressive phenomena—such as loss of interest in friends, school, or activities—irritability, sleep difficulties, and changes in eating habits.

The essential features seem to revolve around the question "Who am I?" According to DSM-III-R, there is severe subjective distress regarding the inability to integrate aspects of the self into a relatively coherent and acceptable

Table 1
Diagnostic Criteria for Identity Disorder

A. Severe subjective distress regarding uncertainty about a variety of issues relating to identity, including three or more of the following:

    (1) long-term goals
    (2) career choice
    (3) friendship patterns
    (4) sexual orientation and behavior
    (5) religious identification
    (6) moral value systems
    (7) group loyalties

B. Impairment in social or occupational (including academic) functioning as a result of the symptoms in A.

C. Duration of the disturbance of at least 3 months.

D. Occurrence not exclusively during the course of a Mood Disorder or of a psychotic disorder, such as Schizophrenia.

E. The disturbance is not sufficiently pervasive and persistent to warrant the diagnosis of Borderline Personality Disorder.

Table from DSM-III-R, *Diagnostic and Statistical Manual of Mental Disorders,* ed 3, revised. (Current Classification of Mental Disorders, 1987.) Copyright American Psychiatric Association, Washington, D.C., 1987. Used with permission.

sense of self. In particular, there is confusion and ambivalence about long-term goals, sexuality, career choice, religious matters, morality, friendship patterns, and group loyalties. These conflicts are experienced as irreconcilable aspects of the self that the adolescent is unable to integrate into a coherent identity. If the symptoms are not recognized and resolved, a full-blown identity crisis may develop. As described by Erikson, the youth manifests severe doubting and an inability to make decisions (abulia), a sense of isolation and inner emptiness, a growing inability to relate to others, disturbed sexual function, a distorted time perspective with a sense of urgency, and the assumption of a negative identity.

The associated features frequently include marked discrepancy between the adolescent's self-perception and the views that others have of the adolescent; moderate anxiety and depression, usually related to inner preoccupation rather than external realities; and self-doubt and uncertainty about the future, with either difficulty in making choices or impulsive experimentations in an attempt to establish an independent identity.

The course is usually relatively brief, as developmental lags are responsive to support, acceptance, and the provision of a psychosocial moratorium. An extensive prolongation of adolescence with continued identity disorder may lead to the chronic state of identity diffusion that usually indicates disturbance of early developmental stages and the presence of borderline personality organization, mood disorder, or schizophrenia. The disorder usually resolves by the mid-20s. If it persists, the individual may be unable to make career commitments or lasting attachments.

DIFFERENTIAL DIAGNOSIS

Identity disorder should not be diagnosed if the identity problems are secondary to another mental disorder (e.g., borderline personality disorder, schizophreniform disorder, schizophrenic disorder, or mood disorder). At times, what initially appears to be an identity disorder may be the prodromal manifestations of one of these disorders.

It has been suggested that intense but normal conflicts associated with maturing, such as adolescent turmoil or mid-life crisis, may be confusing, but they are usually not associated with such marked deterioration in school, vocational, or social functioning or with such severe subjective distress. There is considerable evidence, however, that adolescent turmoil often is not a phase that is outgrown but is indicative of true psychopathology.

TREATMENT

Individual psychotherapy directed toward encouraging growth and development is usually considered the therapy of choice. Adolescents, particularly in the regressed state of an identity disorder, react similarly to borderline personalities and respond well to the technique in which the transference is permitted to develop in the context of a controlled regression without gratifying or infantilizing the patient. The patients' feelings and wishes are recognized, and the patients are encouraged to examine their longings and feelings of deprivations and to try to understand, with the empathic help of the therapist, what is happening to them.

References

Blos P: *On Adolescence*. Free Press, Glen Cove, NY, 1962.
Egan J: Etiology and treatment of borderline personality disorder in adolescents. Hosp and Comm Psychiatry 37:6, 613, 1986.
Erikson E H: The problems of ego identity. J Am Psychoanal Assoc 4:428, 1956.
Goldberg A: On the prognosis and treatment of narcissism. J Am Psychoanal Assoc 22:243, 1974.
Grinker R R, Holzman P S: Schizophrenic pathology in young adults. Arch Gen Psychiatry 28:168, 1973.
Masterson J F: *The Psychiatric Dilemma of Adolesence*. Little, Brown, Boston, 1967.
Puig-Antich J: Major depression and conduct disorder in prepuberty. J Am Acad of Child Psych 21:118, 1982.
Robson K S: *The Borderline Child. Approaches to Etiology, Diagnosis, and Treatment*. McGraw-Hill, New York, 1983.
Soloff P H, George A, Nathan R S, Schulz P M: Progress in pharmacotherapy of borderline disorders. Arch Gen Psychiatry 43:7, 691, 1986.
Stone M H: *The Borderline Syndromes*. McGraw-Hill, New York, 1980.

43.3 ————

Reactive Attachment Disorder of Infancy and Early Childhood

DEFINITION AND DIAGNOSTIC CRITERIA

The DSM-III-R criteria for reactive attachment disorder of infancy and early childhood are given in Table 1. The reader is referred to this table for a summary of the characteristics of this disorder.

EPIDEMIOLOGY

Reactive attachment disorder of infancy and early childhood is essentially a new diagnosis that covers a broad range of conditions and etiologies. There are no specific data on prevalence, sex ratio, or familial pattern available at this time. Although cases so diagnosed come from all socioeconomic classes, studies of certain subgroups (e.g., infants that do not thrive) suggest an increased vulnerability among the lower classes. This would be congruent with the greater likelihood of psychosocial deprivation, single-parent households, family disorganization, and economic difficulties in these families.

It is also important to realize that a caretaker may be fully satisfactory for one child but that another child under his or her care may develop a reactive attachment disorder.

ETIOLOGY

The etiology is included in the disorder's definition. It is presumed that grossly pathogenic care of the infant or young child by the caretaker causes the markedly disturbed

Table 1
Diagnostic Criteria for Reactive Attachment Disorder of Infancy or Early Childhood

A. Markedly disturbed social relatedness in most contexts, beginning before the age of 5, as evidenced by either (1) or (2):

(1) persistent failure to initiate or respond to most social interactions (e.g., in infants, absence of visual tracking and reciprocal play, lack of vocal imitation or playfulness, apathy, little or no spontaneity; at later ages, lack of or little curiosity and social interest)

(2) indiscriminate sociability, e.g., excessive familiarity with relative strangers by making requests and displaying affection

B. The disturbance in A is not a symptom of either Mental Retardation or a Pervasive Developmental Disorder, such as Autistic Disorder.

C. Grossly pathogenic care, as evidenced by at least one of the following:

(1) persistent disregard of the child's basic emotional needs for comfort, stimulation, and affection. *Examples:* overly harsh punishment by caregiver; consistent neglect by caregiver.

(2) persistent disregard of the child's basic physical needs, including nutrition, adequate housing, and protection from physical danger and assault (including sexual abuse)

(3) repeated change of primary caregiver so that stable attachments are not possible, e.g., frequent changes in foster parents

D. There is a presumption that the care described in C is responsible for the disturbed behavior in A; this presumption is warranted if the disturbance in A began following the pathogenic care in C.

Note: If failure to thrive is present, code it on Axis III.

Table from DSM-III-R, *Diagnostic and Statistical Manual of Mental Disorders,* ed 3, revised. (Current Classification of Mental Disorders, 1987.) Copyright American Psychiatric Association, Washington, D.C., 1987. Used with permission.

social relatedness usually evident. The emphasis is on an unidirectional etiology; that is, the caretaker does something inimical or neglects to do something essential for the infant or child. It is suggested, however, that in evaluating a patient for whom such a diagnosis is appropriate, the contributions of each member of the caretaker-child dyad, as well as their interactions, be considered. Thus, such things as infant and child temperament, deficient or defective bonding, a developmentally disabled or sensorially impaired child, and a particular caretaker–child mismatch should be weighed. Parental mental retardation; lack of parenting skills because of personal upbringing, social isolation, or deprivation, and lack of opportunities to learn about caretaking behavior; and premature parenthood (during early and middle adolescence), with an inability to recognize obligations to respond to and care for the infant's needs and in which the parents' own needs take precedence over their infant's or child's needs may increase the likelihood of the child's developing a reactive attachment disorder.

Frequent changes of the primary caretaker, as might occur in institutionalization, repeated lengthy hospitalizations, or multiple foster home placements, may also cause a reactive attachment disorder.

CLINICAL DESCRIPTION

DSM-III-R defines the distinguishing symptom of this disorder as a markedly disturbed social relatedness in most contexts. It is evidenced by a persistent failure to initiate or respond appropriately to most social interactions or by indiscriminate sociability, such as excessive familiarity with relative strangers (e.g., making requests and displaying affection). The clinical picture varies greatly according to the child's chronological and mental ages.

Perhaps the most typical clinical picture of the infant with this disorder is the nonorganic failure to thrive. In these infants, hypokinesis, dullness, listlessness, or apathy with a poverty of spontaneous activity are usually seen. They look sad, unhappy, joyless, or miserable. Some infants also appear frightened and watchful with a radar-like gaze. Despite this, these infants may exhibit delayed responsiveness to a stimulus that would elicit fright or withdrawal in a normal infant.

Most of these infants appear significantly malnourished, and many have protruding abdomens. Occasionally, foul-smelling, celiac-like stools are reported. In unusually severe cases, a clinical picture of marasmus may appear (Figure 1). The infant's weight is often below the third percentile and markedly below their appropriate weight for height. If serial weights are available, it may be noted that weight percentiles have progressively decreased because of an actual weight loss or a failure to gain weight as height increases. Head circumference is usually normal for the age. Muscle tone may be poor. The skin may be colder and paler or more mottled than the normal child's. Laboratory values are usually within normal limits, except those abnormal findings coincident with any malnutrition, dehydration, or concurrent illness. Bone age is usually retarded. Growth hormone levels are usually normal or elevated, suggesting that growth failure in these children is secondary to caloric deprivation and malnutrition. These children both improve physically and gain weight rapidly after hospitalization.

Socially, these infants usually show little spontaneous activity and a marked diminution of both initiative toward others and/or a lack of reciprocity in response to the caretaking adult or examiner. Both the mother and infant may be indifferent to their separation upon hospitalization or termination of subsequent hospital visits. These infants frequently show none of the normal upset, fretting, or protest about hospitalization. Older infants usually show little interest in their environment. They may have little interest in playing or in toys, even if encouraged. However, they rapidly or gradually take an interest in and relate to their caretakers in the hospital.

Classical psychosocial dwarfism or psychosocially determined short stature is a syndrome that is usually first manifested in children 2 to 3 years of age. These children typically are unusually short and have frequent growth hor-

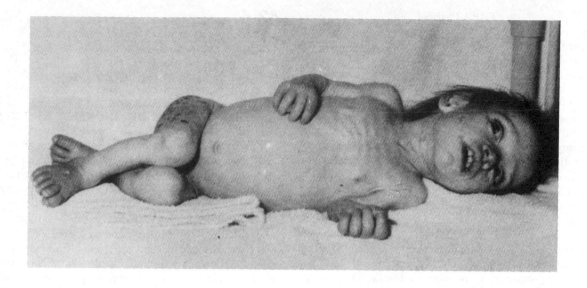

Figure 1. Marasmus precipitated by a mild chest infection in an infant with failure to thrive secondary to maternal deprivation. (Reproduced with permission from Davis J A, Dobbing J, editors: *Scientific Foundation of Paediatrics,* 1st ed. William Heinemann Medical Books, Philadelphia 1974.)

mone abnormalities and severe behavioral disturbances. All of these symptoms are the result of an inimical caretaker–child relationship and resolve without any medical or psychiatric treatment upon being removed from the home and placed in a more favorable domicile.

There is evidence that the "affectionless character" may occur when there is a failure or lack of opportunity to form attachments before age 2 to 3 years. The affectionless character is unable to form lasting relationships, and this is sometimes accompanied by a lack of guilt, an inability to obey rules, and a need for attention and affection. Some such children are indiscriminately friendly. This disorder is usually not reversible.

DIFFERENTIAL DIAGNOSIS

DSM-III-R notes that the pervasive developmental disorders, mental retardation, various severe neurological abnormalities, and psychosocial dwarfism are the primary considerations in the differential diagnosis. Autistic disorder in children with onset under 5 years of age is manifested by severe impairment in reciprocal social interaction, significant impairment in communication (both verbal and through gestures), and a markedly restricted repertoire of activities and interests. These difficulties are typically present from birth or become evident at the mental age at which specific behaviors should develop. Moderate, severe, and profound mental retardation are present in about 50 percent of these children, whereas most children with reactive attachment disorder are mildly retarded or have normal intelligence. There is no evidence that autism is caused by parental pathology, and most parents of autistic children do not differ significantly from parents of normal children. Unlike children with reactive attachment disorder, autistic children do not frequently improve rapidly when removed from their homes and placed in a hospital or other more favorable environment.

Mentally retarded children may evidence delay in all social skills. These children may be differentiated from children with reactive attachment disorder, as their social relatedness should be appropriate to their mental age and they should show a sequence of development similar to that seen in normal children.

Sensory deficits should be ruled out. If such deficits are responsible for the children's impaired relatedness, caretakers may need to be shown how to give appropriate stimulation and how to facilitate communication. This will usually ameliorate difficulties secondary to the sensory deficit.

PROGNOSIS

The prognosis depends on the severity of the pathological caretaking of the infant or child and the length of time spent in the inimical environment. If the patient remains in or returns to the home after evaluation, the adequacy of corrective measures in changing caretaking behavior must also be considered. Outcomes range from the extremes of death to the normal development of the child. In general, the longer the child stays in the inimical environment without adequate intervention, the worse the prognosis will be. For those children who have multiple problems stemming from the abnormal caretaking, physical recovery is usually more complete than is emotional or educational recovery.

TREATMENT

There are some general principles of treatment. Often, the first decision is whether to hospitalize an infant or child or to attempt treatment while the child remains in the home. Usually the severity of the child's physical and emotional state or the severity of the pathological caretaking will determine the strategy. The overriding choice must be for the child's safety. The patient must be given appropriate psychological and, if necessary, pediatric treatment. Concomitantly, the treatment team must begin to alter the unsatisfactory relationship between the caretaker and the child. This usually requires extensive and intensive long-term psychological therapy with the mother or, in intact households, both parents, whenever possible.

Possible interventions include but are not limited to the following: (1) psychosocial support services, including hiring homemaker, improving the physical condition of the apartment or obtaining more adequate housing, improving the family's financial status, and decreasing the family's isolation; (2) psychotherapeutic interventions, including individual psychotherapy, psychotropic medications, and family or marital therapy; (3) educational-counseling services, including mother-infant or mother-toddler groups, and counseling to increase awareness and understanding of the child's needs and to increase parenting skills; and (4) provisions for close monitoring of the progression of the patient's emotional and physical well-being. Should these interventions be unfeasible, be inadequate, or fail, placement with relatives, in foster care, adoption, or a group home or residential treatment facility must be considered.

References

Ainsworth M D S: The development of infant–mother attachment. In *Review of Child Development Research*, vol 3, B M Caldwen, H N Ricciuhi, editors, p 1. University of Chicago Press, Chicago, 1973.

Bowlby J: *Attachment and Loss,* 3 vols. Basic Books, New York, 1969, 1973, 1980.

Campbell M, Green W H, Caplon R, David R: Psychiatry and endocrinology in children: Early infantile autism and psychosocial dwarfism. In *Handbook of Psychiatry and Endocrinology,* P J V Beumont, G D Burrows, editors, p 15. Elsevier, Amsterdam, 1982.

Ferholt J B: A psychodynamic study of psychosomatic dwarfism. J Am Acad Child Psychiat *14*:49, 1985.

Green W H, Campbell M, David R: Psychosocial dwarfism: A critical review of the evidence. J Am Acad Child Psychiat *23*:39, 1984.

Greenspan S I: *Psychopathology and Adaptation in Infancy and Early Childhood: Principles of Clinical Diagnosis and Preventive Intervention.* International Universities Press, New York, 1981.

Klaus M H, Kennell J M: *Parent–Infant Bonding,* ed 2. Mosby, St. Louis, 1982.

Rutter M: *Maternal Deprivation Reassessed,* ed 2. Penguin Books, Middlesex, England, 1981.

Taylor P M, editor: *Parent–Infant Relationships.* Grune & Stratton, New York, 1980.

43.4 ————

Stereotypy and Habit Disorder

DEFINITION AND DIAGNOSTIC CRITERIA

Stereotypy and habit disorder is a new diagnosis first appearing in DSM-III-R; its diagnostic criteria are given in Table 1. Habit disorders include thumb or finger sucking, nail biting, or nose or skin picking. There is a criterion of severity, namely, that the disorder must cause physical injury or markedly interfere with normal activities; thus, mild nailbiting is precluded from this diagnosis. Stereotypy and habit disorder cannot be part of a pervasive developmental disorder or a tic disorder, but it is permissible for the individual to be mentally retarded. Because stereotypies are especially prevalent in individuals with mental retardation and pervasive developmental disorder, and these two diagnoses frequently coexist (about 75 percent of pervasive developmental-disordered individuals are mentally retarded), this may be an unfortunate exclusion. Indeed, it would seem as important and useful in planning treatment to know that a child with a pervasive developmental disorder had a coexisting severe stereotypy or habit disorder as it would to know that a mentally retarded individual had such a coexisting disorder.

EPIDEMIOLOGY

The diagnosis is a compilation of many different symptoms and various subgroups (e.g., head bangers, body rockers, repetitive hand movers, and nail biters), which will have to be studied separately to obtain data concerning prevalence, sex ratio, and familial patterns. It is clear, however, that most of these stereotypies and habit patterns are more prevalent in the mentally retarded, in males, and in individuals with severe sensory impairments, such as blindness or deafness.

The provisions that the disorder must cause physical injury or markedly interfere with normal activities may cause some confusion. In one pediatric clinic, up to 20 percent of children had a history of rocking, head banging, or swaying in one form or another. Deciding which cases are severe enough to confirm a diagnosis may be difficult. Injury in some cases will depend more on the parental care, supervision, and quality of environment (e.g., a padded crib) than on the intensity of the stereotypy.

ETIOLOGY

The etiologies of these disorders are essentially unknown, but there are several theories. Many of the behaviors may be associated with normal development. For example, up to 80 percent of normal children show rhythmic activities that phase out by the age of 4 years. These rhythmic patterns seem to be purposeful, to provide sensorimotor stimulation and tension release, and to be satisfying

Table 1
Diagnostic Criteria for Stereotypy and Habit Disorder

A. Intentional, repetitive, nonfunctional behaviors, such as hand-shaking or -waving, body-rocking, head-banging, mouthing of objects, nail-biting, picking at nose or skin.

B. The disturbance either causes physical injury to the child or markedly interferes with normal activities, e.g., injury to head from head-banging; inability to fall asleep because of constant rocking.

C. Does not meet the criteria for either a Pervasive Developmental Disorder or a Tic Disorder.

Table from DSM-III-R, *Diagnostic and Statistical Manual of Mental Disorders, ed 3, revised.* (Current Classification of Mental Disorders, 1987.) Copyright American Psychiatric Association, Washington, D.C., 1987. Used with permission.

and pleasurable to the children. These movements may increase at times of frustration, boredom, or tension.

The progression from what are perhaps viscissitudes of normal development to stereotypies and habit disorders is thought to reflect disordered development, as in mental retardation (or pervasive developmental disorder) or psychological conflict. It has also been suggested that such behaviors as head banging may result from maternal neglect or abuse and lack of psychosocial and physical stimulation.

CLINICAL DESCRIPTION

Individuals may suffer from one or more symptoms of stereotypy and habit disorder; thus, the clinical picture varies considerably. Most commonly, one symptom predominates. However, when several severe symptoms are present, it tends to be among the more severely afflicted persons with mental retardation or pervasive developmental disorder. These individuals frequently have other significant psychiatric disorders, especially behavioral disorders.

DSM-III-R notes that in extreme cases, severe mutilation and life-threatening injuries may result, or secondary infection and septicemia may follow self-inflicted trauma.

Head Banging

Head banging is an example of a stereotypy disorder. Typically, head banging begins during infancy, between 6 and 12 months of age. The head is struck with a definite rhythmic and monotonous continuity against the crib or other hard surface. Infants appear to be absorbed in the activity which may persist until they become exhausted and fall asleep. The head banging is transitory in many children, but in some cases, it may persist into middle childhood.

Head banging that is a component of temper tantrums is different and ceases once the tantrums and their secondary gains are controlled.

Nail Biting

Nail biting, an example of a habit disorder, may begin as early as 1 year of age and increase in incidence until age 12.

Usually all the nails are bitten. Most cases are not sufficiently severe to meet the DSM-III-R diagnostic criteria. The ones that are, are those that cause physical damage to the finger itself, usually by associated biting of the cuticle and/or by secondary infections of the finger and nail bed. Nail biting seems to occur or increase in intensity when the individual is either anxious or bored. Some of the most severe nail biting occurs in the severely and profoundly mentally retarded and in some paranoid schizophrenic patients. Some nail biters, however, have no obvious emotional disturbance.

DIFFERENTIAL DIAGNOSIS

DSM-III-R notes that these symptoms cannot be caused by a more pervasive disorder, such as autistic disorder. This is likely to be the most difficult differential diagnosis among moderately, severely, and profoundly mentally retarded individuals who have associated autistic symptomatology. DSM-III-R also directs that this diagnosis not be used if these symptoms arise during the course of a tic disorder. Stereotypy and habit disorder are distinguishable from tics in that they consist of voluntary movements and are not spasmodic. Moreover, unlike children with a tic disorder, those with stereotypy and habit disorder are not distressed by the symptoms.

Stereotypy and habit disorder may be diagnosed concurrently with psychoactive substance- (e.g., amphetamine)-induced organic mental disorder, severe sensory impairments, CNS and degenerative disorders (e.g., Lesch-Nyhan syndrome), severe schizophrenic disorder, or obsessive-compulsive disorder.

TREATMENT

Treatment obviously should be related to the specific symptom or symptoms being treated, their causes, and the individual's mental age. Here only general principles will be reviewed.

The psychosocial environment should be changed for those infants, young children, and mentally retarded persons for whom lack of adequate caretaking, little opportunity for physical expression, boring inactivity, and self-stimulation seem to be important causes. In these cases, increased nurturance and stimulation may be helpful. Such measures as padding hard surfaces may be important for severe head bangers.

Behavioral techniques, including reinforcement and behavioral shaping, are successful in some cases. There is a large, specialized literature addressing these problems in the seriously retarded.

Psychotherapy has been used primarily in older, mentally normal individuals in whom intrapsychic conflict or interpersonal difficulties seem prominent.

Finally, for those cases in which severe physical damage occurs, especially in the severely retarded, psychopharmacology must be considered. Phenothiazines have been the most frequently used drugs; however, the psychiatrist must be particularly aware of adverse effects, including tardive dyskinesia and impairment of cognition.

UNDIFFERENTIATED ATTENTION-DEFICIT DISORDER

DSM-III-R includes undifferentiated attention-deficit disorder as a residual category for disturbances in which the predominant feature is the persistence of developmentally inappropriate and marked inattention that is not a symptom of another disorder such as mental retardation or attention-deficit hyperactivity disorder, or of a disorganized and chaotic environment. It notes that some cases that would have been given the DSM-III diagnosis of attention deficit disorder without hyperactivity would be classified here. Diagnostic criteria have not been advanced by DSM-III-R, pending additional study to determine the validity of this diagnosis. For additional information, see Section 36.2 on Attention-deficit Hyperactivity Disorder.

References

Cerny R: Thumb and finger sucking. Aust Dent J 26:167, 1981.
DeLissovoy V: Head banging in early childhood. Child Dev 33:43, 1962.
Evans J: Rocking at night. J Child Psychol Psychiat Allied Discipl 2:71, 1961.
Malone A J, Massler M: Index of nailbiting in children. J Abnormal and Social Psychol 47:193, 1952.
Matthews L H, Leibowtiz J M, Matthews J R: Tics, Habits and mannerisms. In *Handbook of Clinical Child Psychology*, C E Walker, M C Roberts, editors, p 406. Wiley, New York, 1983.
Schroeder S R, Schroeder C S, Rojahn J, Mulick J A: Self-injurious behavior: An analysis of behavior management techniques. In *Handbook of Behavior Modification with the Mentally Retarded*. p 61. Plenum, New York, 1981.
Silberstein R M, Blackman S, Mandell W: Autoerotic head banging: A reflection on the opportunism of infants. J Am Acad Child Psychiat 5:235, 1966.
Werry J, Corlielle J, Fitzpatrick J: Rhythmic motor activities in children under five: Etiology and prevalence. J Am Acad Child Psychiatry 22:329, 1983.

44

Child Psychiatry: Special Areas of Interest

44.1

Mood Disorders

INTRODUCTION

The essential feature of mood disorders, which were previously called affective disorders, is a disturbance of mood, generally either depression or elation, which colors the whole psychic life and is not caused by any other physical or mental disorder.

It is generally agreed that these disorders may occur during childhood and adolescence, and there is substantial evidence for major depressive disorder and dysthymia in both age groups. Mania and hypomania appear to occur much more frequently in adolescents than in children.

The adult mood disorders were reviewed in detail in Chapter 17. Hence, only those issues that pertain specifically to children and adolescents will be considered here.

DEFINITION AND DIAGNOSTIC CRITERIA

Major Depressive Episode

The DSM-III-R diagnostic criteria for children and adolescents differ from those for adults in two of the nine symptoms that are given as indicative of depression (Table 1). Symptom 1, the depressed mood that must be present most of the day, nearly every day for at least 2 weeks in adults, may be an irritable mood in children and adolescents rather than a depressed mood. Symptom 3, significant weight gain or loss, and decrease or increase in appetite nearly every day may be reflected in children as a failure to make expected weight gains. The amount of weight that most children would be expected to gain over a 2-week period is too insignificant to measure accurately in most situations. Thus, in clinical practice, this would become a useful diagnostic criterion primarily in depressions of longer duration.

Dysthymia (Depressive Neurosis)

DSM-III-R notes that the boundaries of dysthymia with major depression are unclear, particularly in children and adolescents. The onset is usually during childhood, adolescence, or early adulthood and was referred to in the past as depressive personality. There are two significant differences in the diagnostic criteria for dysthymia for children and adolescents and those for adults. Children and adolescents may exhibit an irritable mood instead of, or in addition to, the depressed mood required for adults. And the mood disturbance in children and adolescents needs be present for only 1 rather than 2 years. DSM-III-R also directs that early onset be specified for children and adolescents. It should be noted that if a major depressive disorder develops while dysthymia is still present, both diagnoses should be given.

Occasionally, youngsters fulfill the criteria for dysthymia except that their episodes last only 2 weeks to several months, with symptom-free intervals lasting for over 2 to 3

Table 1
Symptoms of Depression

1. depressed mood (or can be irritable mood in children and adolescents) most of the day, nearly every day, as indicated either by subjective account or observation by others

2. markedly diminished interest or pleasure in all, or almost all, activities most of the day, nearly every day (as indicated either by subjective account or observation by others of apathy most of the time)

3. significant weight loss or weight gain when not dieting (e.g., more than 5% of body weight in a month), or decrease or increase in appetite nearly every day (in children, consider failure to make expected weight gains)

4. insomnia or hypersomnia nearly every day

5. psychomotor agitation or retardation nearly every day (observable by others, not merely subjective feelings of restlessness or being slowed down)

6. fatigue or loss of energy nearly every day

7. feelings of worthlessness or excessive or inappropriate guilt (which may be delusional) nearly every day (not merely self-reproach or guilt about being sick)

8. diminished ability to think or concentrate, or indecisiveness, nearly every day (either by subjective account or as observed by others)

9. recurrent thoughts of death (not just fear of dying), recurrent suicidal ideation without a specific plan, or a suicide attempt or a specific plan for committing suicide

Table adapted from DSM-III-R, *Diagnostic and Statistical Manual of Mental Disorders,* ed 3, revised. (Current Classification of Mental Disorders, 1987.) Copyright American Psychiatric Association, Washington, D.C., 1987. Used with permission.

months. These minor affective presentations in children are likely to indicate more severe mood disorder episodes in the future. Current knowledge suggests that the longer, the more recurrent, the more frequent, and perhaps the less related to environmental stress these episodes are, the greater likelihood there is of severe mood disorder in the future.

An important exception to this is that when minor depressive episodes follow a significant stressful life event by less than 3 months, they do not indicate future affective episodes, and so they should be diagnosed as an adjustment disorder with depressive mood or uncomplicated bereavement.

Manic Episode

The DSM-III-R diagnostic criteria for a manic episode and manic and hypomanic syndromes in children and adolescents are identical to those in adults. Mania and hypomania are quite rare in prepubertal children.

Cyclothymia

The only DSM-III-R diagnostic criterion for cyclothymia that is different for children and adolescents from that for adults is the duration of the illness. Rather than a period of 2 years of numerous alternating hypomanic and depressed mood episodes, only 1 year is required. Some investigators believe that cyclothymia is a mild form of bipolar disorder, and it is likely that most cyclothymic adolescents go on to develop a full-fledged bipolar illness.

Schizoaffective Disorder

The DSM-III-R criteria for schizoaffective disorder in children, adolescents, and adults are identical. Although some adolescents and probably children do fit the criteria for schizoaffective disorder, little is now known about the natural course of their illness, family history, psychobiology, and treatment.

EPIDEMIOLOGY

The prevalence rate among 10-year-olds for the combined DSM-III criteria for major depression and dysthymic disorder, which are slightly different from the DSM-III-R criteria, was reported to be 1.7 percent.

It has been conservatively estimated that on general child and adolescent services in general hospitals, about 5 percent of prepubertal children and 15 percent of adolescents would be diagnosed as having mood disorders of all types.

ETIOLOGY

There is considerable evidence that the mood disorders are the same fundamental disease or disease group, regardless of age of onset. Both genetic and environmental factors appear to be important.

Genetic Factors

Mood disorders in children, adolescents, and adult patients tend to cluster in the same families. The more first- and second-degree relatives that have mood disorder, the more of their offspring are likely to be affected, and the younger their age of onset is likely to be. Having one depressed parent probably doubles the risk to the offspring, and having both parents depressed quadruples the risk of a child's developing a mood disorder before age 18, when compared with the risk in children with two unaffected parents.

Some evidence indicates that the number of recurrences of parental depression does increase the likelihood that their children will be affected, but this may be related, at least in part, to the effective loading of that parent's own family tree. Similarly, children with the most severe episodes of major depressive disorder—the endogenous subtype—have shown more evidence of denser and deeper familial aggregation for major depression than has the non-endogenous major depressive proband group.

Environmental Factors

The finding that identical twins do not have a 100 percent concordance rate suggests a role for nongenetic factors. So far, there is little evidence that parental marital status, size of sibship, socioeconomic status, parental separation, divorce or marital functioning, or familial constellation or structure play much of a role in causing depressive disorders in children. There is, however, some evidence that male children whose fathers died before they were 13 years old are more likely than are controls to develop depression.

The psychosocial deficits that are found in depressed children improve following sustained recovery from the depression. These deficits appear to have been secondary to the depression itself and to have been compounded by the long duration in this age group of most dysthymic or depressive episodes, during which poorly or unaccomplished developmental tasks accumulated. It is likely that among preschoolers, in whom depressive-like clinical presentations are described, the role of environmental influence will receive more experimental support.

PSYCHOBIOLOGY

Studies of prepubertal major depression and adolescent mood disorders have revealed biological abnormalities.

Prepubertal children in an episode of major depression have been shown to secrete significantly more growth hormone during sleep than do normal children and those with nondepressed emotional disorders. They also secrete significantly less growth hormone in response to insulin-induced hypoglycemia than does the latter group. Both abnormalities have been found to remain abnormal and basically unchanged after at least 4 months of full, sustained clinical response, the last month in a drug-free state.

In contrast, although occasional cases of cortisol hypersecretion are found among prepubertal children in a major depressive episode, the majority have normal cortisol secretion during and after the depressive episode.

Investigators have reported an inherited biochemical trait that may be present in some children whose parents suffer from bipolar or unipolar depression. There may be a receptor supersensitivity to the neurotransmitter acetylcholine in those children who are at risk for later developing a major mood disorder. The test for this abnormality demonstrates that skin cells, especially fibroblasts grown *in vitro,* show an increased density of muscarinic cholinergic receptors which are then shown to be sensitive to acetylcholine. This test, which must be validated by further studies, is important because 25 percent of children with a manic depressive parent develop either a bipolar or a unipolar disorder later in life. Early detection could identify this subgroup and enable clinicians more easily to distinguish depression from substance abuse and antisocial behavior, which often mask or are confused with depression. In addition, clinicians are reluctant to use antidepressants in children and adolescents without a clear indication for their use, and this test would help provide this.

Despite frequent subjective sleep complaints, prepubertal children do not show polysomnographic abnormalities during a major depressive episode. In adolescents, as well as in adults, rapid eye movement (REM) latency is shortened during major depressive episodes.

CLINICAL DESCRIPTION AND CLINICAL COURSE

The onset of a major depressive episode in children tends to be insidious and retrospectively difficult to pinpoint. When the first episode occurs during adolescence, it is more likely to have a more clearly delineated or acute onset. Typically, mania, hypomania, and cyclothymia begin during or after puberty, although the onset of depressive or dysthymic illness is likely to have occurred prepubescently in many of these youngsters.

Adolescent onset of mood disorder may be difficult to diagnose when first seen if there have been attempts at self-medication with illicit drugs or alcohol. In a recent study, 17 percent of the youngsters with mood disorder first presented to medical attention as substance abusers. Only after detoxification could the psychiatric symptoms be properly assessed and the correct affective diagnosis be made.

DSM-III-R notes that in prepubertal children with a major depressive episode, somatic complaints, psychomotor agitation, and mood-congruent hallucinations (usually only a single voice talking to the child) are particularly frequent. It also notes that separation anxiety and overanxious and avoidant disorders commonly coexist with a major depressive episode.

In adolescents, DSM-III-R notes that negativistic or frankly antisocial behavior and use of alcohol or illicit drugs may be present and justify the additional diagnoses of oppositional defiant disorder, conduct disorder, or psychoactive substance abuse or dependence. Feelings of wanting to leave home or of not being understood and approved of, restlessness, grouchiness, and aggression are common. Sulkiness, a reluctance to cooperate in family ventures, and withdrawal from social activities, with retreat to one's room, are frequent. School difficulties are likely. There may be inattention to personal appearance and increased emotionality, with particular sensitivity to rejection in love relationships.

Children can be reliable reporters about their own behavior, emotions, relationships, and difficulties in psychosocial functions. They may, however, refer to dysphoria by many names. Thus, it is necessary to ask about feeling sad, empty, low, down, blue, very unhappy, like crying, or having a bad feeling inside that is there most of the time. Depressed children will usually identify one or more of these terms as the persistent dysphoric feeling they have had. The duration and periodicity of depressive mood should be carefully assessed in order to differentiate relatively universal, short-lived, and sometimes frequent periods of sadness, usually after a frustrating event, from true, persistent depressive mood. The younger the child, the more imprecise his or her time estimates are likely to be.

Mood disorders tend to be more chronic if they have begun early. Childhood onset may represent the most severe forms of affective illness and tends to appear in families with a high incidence of mood disorder and alcoholism. Such children are more likely to develop secondary complications such as conduct disorder, alcoholism, substance abuse, and antisocial behavior.

Functional impairment associated with depressive syndrome in childhood extends to practically all areas of the child's psychosocial world; school performance and behavior, peer relationships, and family relations all suffer. Only highly intelligent and academically oriented children with no more than a moderate depression can compensate for their difficulty in learning by substantially increasing their time and effort. Otherwise, school performance is invariably affected by a combination of difficulty in concentrating, slowed down thinking, lack of interest and motivation, fatigue, sleepiness, depressive ruminations, and preoccupations. Depression in a child may be misdiagnosed as a learning disability. Learning problems secondary to depression, even when long standing, correct themselves rapidly after recovery from the depressive episode.

Children and adolescents with major depressive syndrome may have hallucinations and delusions. In most cases, these psychotic symptoms are thematically consistent with the depressed mood, occur within the depressive episode (usually at its worst), and do not include such types of hallucinations as conversing voices or a commenting voice, which are more specific to schizophrenia. These cases are referred to as psychotic depressions, whereas depressive hallucinations usually consist of a single voice speaking to the subject from outside his or her head, with derogatory or suicidal content. Depressive delusions center on themes of guilt, physical disease, death, nihilism, deserved punishment, personal inadequacy, or sometimes persecution. These delusions are rare in prepuberty, probably because of cognitive immaturity, but are present in about half of psychotically depressed adolescents.

A parallel situation exists for psychotic mania. Delusions and hallucinations may involve grandiose evaluations of the patient's own power, worth, knowledge, family, or relationships, persecutory delusions, or flight of ideas with gross impairment of reality testing.

Suicide

Suicide and, more commonly, suicidal ideation and gestures occur frequently in depressed children and adolescents. Suicide is the third leading cause of death in adolescence. The suicide rate is higher among male children and in children whose families have recently moved or have been dislocated.

PROGNOSIS

Mood disorders with childhood or adolescent onset are likely to recur and, if not sucessfully treated, will produce considerable short- and long-term difficulties and complications: poor academic achievement, arrest or delay in psychosocial development patterns, complicating negative reinforcement, suicide, drug and alcohol abuse as a means of self-medication, and development of conduct disorders. Follow-up studies to date indicate a continued risk for mood disorder.

DIFFERENTIAL DIAGNOSIS

Psychotic forms of depression, mania, and schizoaffective disorders must be differentiated from schizophrenic disorders. Organic mood syndromes can sometimes be differentiated from the mood disorders only after detoxification. Anxiety symptoms and conduct-disordered behaviors can coexist with depression and frequently can pose problems in differentiating these cases from nondepressed emotional and conduct disorders.

Of particular importance is the distinction between agitated depression or mania and attention-deficit hyperactivity disorder, in which the persistent excessive activity and restlessness may be confused. Prepubertal children do not present with classical forms of agitated depression, such as hand wringing and pacing. Instead, their inability to sit still and their frequent temper tantrums are the most common symptoms. Sometimes the correct answer becomes evident only after successful tricyclic antidepressant treatment is discontinued. If the child has no difficulty concentrating and is not hyperactive while recovered from the depressive episode in a drug-free state, it is highly unlikely that an attention-deficit hyperactivity disorder was present.

TREATMENTS

Hospitalization

The important immediate consideration is often whether hospitalization is indicated. When the patient is suicidal, hospitalization is indicated to provide maximum protection against the patient's own self-destructive impulses and behavior. This consideration may also be important when there is a coexisting drug abuse, dependency, or addiction.

Psychotherapy

Child psychotherapy as generally practiced does not appear to be very effective in treating the depressive symptomatology or any other aspect of the child's psychopathology, as long as the youngster is severely depressed.

It is usually prudent to defer a decision for psychotherapeutic intervention until after the youngster has recovered from the major depressive disorder. The best indication for individual or group treatment is the lack of spontaneous gradual improvement in relationships after the mood disorder has remitted. Other times, familial crises are precipitated by the child's recovery, indicating that the patient's illness had fulfilled certain family needs and that the family's psychodynamic equilibrium has been upset by the recovery. The indication for family therapy in such cases is clear.

Psychopharmacology

Evidence from recent studies suggests that the initial treatment of choice for prepubertal major depression may be an antidepressant, such as imipramine. The use of this drug requires careful baseline studies, gradual titration of the drug, and monitoring of EKG changes, blood pressure, side effects, and, whenever possible, serum levels. Because imipramine toxicity produces serious cardiac arrhythmias, seizures, coma, and death and the therapeutic-toxicity ratio is low, extremely careful monitoring is essential. The clinical response appears to be correlated with plasma level. Because imipramine has not yet been approved for use in depressed children and because of its potentially serious side effects and toxicity, it is recommended that clinicians use this drug in children only after careful study or consultation with a clinician experienced in its use.

In all cases, it is important to educate the youngster and his or her caretakers to be alert for the beginning of future episodes so they may be reported without delay to the treating physician. Then, treatment can be instituted without delay.

References

Adams P L, Fras I: *Beginning Child Psychiatry*. Brunner/Mazel, New York, 1987.
Cantwell D P, Carlson G A, editors: *Affective Disorders in Childhood and Adolescence: An Update*. Spectrum Publications, New York, 1983.
French A, Berlin I, editors: *Depression in Children and Adolescents*. Human Sciences Press, New York, 1979.
Golombek H, Garfinkel B D, editors: *The Adolescent and Mood Disturbance*. International Universities Press, New York, 1983.
Pfeffer C R: *The Suicidal Child*. Guilford Press, New York, 1986.
Rutter M, Izard C E, Read P B, editors: *Depression in Young People*. Guilford Press, New York, 1986.
Schulterbrand J G, Raskin A, editors: *Depression in Childhood: Diagnosis, Treatment, and Conceptual Models*. Raven Press, New York, 1977.
Thomas A, Chess S: Genesis and evolution of behavioral disorders: From infancy to early adult life. Am J Psychiat *141*:1, 1984.
Weissman M M, Leckman J F, Merikangas K R: Depression and anxiety disorders in parents and children. Arch Gen Psychiatry *41*:845, 1984.

44.2 _____
Child Abuse

INTRODUCTION

The abuse of children ranges from the deprivation of food, clothing, shelter, and parental love to incidences in which children are physically abused and mistreated by an adult, resulting in obvious trauma to the child and often leading to death. Child abuse is a medical-social disease that is assuming epidemic proportions and is becoming more entrenched in the population. It is considered by some to be one aspect of the social violence that is insidiously creeping into society and is reflected in all statistics on crime.

EPIDEMIOLOGY

The National Center on Child Abuse and Neglect in Washington, D.C., has estimated that 1 million children are maltreated each year. There are 2,000 to 4,000 deaths annually in the United States due to child abuse and neglect. About 125,000 children are victims of sexual abuse each year. The actual occurrence rates are likely to be higher than these estimates because many maltreated children go unrecognized and undiagnosed. Of those children physically abused, 32 percent are under 5 years of age; 27 percent are between 5 and 9 years; 27 percent are between 10 and 14 years; and 14 percent are between 15 and 18 years. More than 50 percent of abused or neglected children were born prematurely or had low birth weight.

ETIOLOGY

Many abused children are perceived by their parents as being different, slow in development or mentally retarded, bad, selfish, or hard to discipline. Children who are hyperactive are particularly vulnerable to abuse, especially if born to parents with limited capacities for nurturant behavior.

The perpetrator of the battered child syndrome is more often the woman than the man. One parent is usually the active batterer, and the other parent passively accepts the battering. Of the perpetrators studied, 80 percent were regularly living in the homes of the children they abused. More than 80 percent of the children studied were living with married parents, and approximately 20 percent were living with a single parent. The average age of the mother who abused her children is reported to be around 26 years; the average age of the father is 30 years. Most abused children come from poor homes, and the families tend to be socially isolated.

The abusive parents have inappropriate expectations of their children, with a reversal of dependency needs. That is, the parent deals with the child as if the child were older than the parent. The parent often turns to the child for reassurance, nurturing, comfort, and protection and expects a loving response. Ninety percent of these parents were severely physically abused by their own mothers or fathers. Sexual abuse is usually by men, although women acting in concert with men or alone have also been involved, especially in child pornography.

DIAGNOSIS

A maltreated child often presents no obvious signs of being battered but has multiple minor physical evidences of emotional and, at times, nutritional deprivation, neglect, and abuse. The maltreated child is often taken to a hospital or private physician and has a history of failure to thrive, malnutrition, poor skin hygiene, irritability, withdrawal, and other signs of psychological and physical neglect. The more severely abused children are seen in hospital emergency rooms with external evidences of body trauma, bruises, abrasions, cuts, lacerations, burns, soft tissue swellings, and hematomas. Hypernatremic dehydration, after periodic water deprivation by psychotic mothers, has been reported as a form of child abuse. Inability to move certain extremities, because of dislocations and fractures associated with neurological signs of intracranial damage, can also indicate inflicted trauma. Other clinical signs and symptoms attributed to inflicted abuse may include injury to the viscera. Abdominal trauma may result in unexplained ruptures of the stomach, bowel, liver, or pancreas, with manifestations of an acutely injured abdomen. Those with the most severe maltreatment injuries arrive at the hospital or physician's office in coma or convulsions, and some arrive dead.

SEXUAL ABUSE OF CHILDREN

The sexual abuse and exploitation of children has become an increasingly widespread type of child abuse, with psychosocial, legal, and medical implications. More than 5,000 cases of incest are reported annually. However, most cases of sexual abuse involving children are never revealed because of the victim's guilt feelings, shame, ignorance, and tolerance, compounded by some physicians' reluctance to recognize and report sexual abuse, the court's insistence on strict rules of evidence, and the families' fears of dissolution if discovered.

Sexual abuse has been reported in schools, day-care centers, and group homes, where the adult caretakers have been found to be the major offenders. The incidence of sexual abuse and child pornography is much higher than previously assumed.

Children may be sexually abused as early as infancy and through adolescence. Approximately 50 percent of abuse is by family members, with incest the principal form of sexual abuse. The most common abuse is by fathers, stepfathers, uncles, and older siblings. Mother-son incest is associated with more overtly severe maternal psychopathology than is father-daughter incest. Features that have been described as common in many homes include a passive, sick, absent, or in some other way incapacitated mother; a daughter who takes on the maternal role in the family; alcohol abuse in the father; and overcrowding (Table 1).

The psychological and physical effects of sexual or physical abuse can be devastating and long lasting. Children who are stimulated sexually by an adult feel anxiety and

Table 1
Sexual Abuse

Reported cases in U.S., 1985	123,000
Prevalence of male abuse	3–31 percent
Prevalence of female abuse	6–62 percent
Perpetrators	
Father/stepfather	7–8 percent
Uncles/older siblings	16–42 percent
Friends	32–60 percent
Strangers	1 percent
Sexual Activity	
Coitus	16–29 percent
Oral sex and intercourse	3–11 percent
Touching genitals	13–33 percent
Age	Peak between ages 9 and 12
	25 percent below age 8
High-risk factors	Child living in single-parent home
	Marital conflict
	History of physical abuse
	Increase in sexual abuse
Reported motivation of abuser	Pedophilic impulses
	No other sexual object
	Inability to delay gratification

Data from Finklehor D: The sexual abuse of children: Current research reviewed. Psych Ann *17*:4, 1987. Figures may total more than 100 percent because of overlapping studies.

overexcitement, lose confidence in themselves, and become mistrustful of adults. Seduction, incest, and rape are important predisposing factors to later symptom formation, such as phobias, anxiety, and depression. Such children tend to be hyperalert to external aggression, as shown by an inability to deal with their own aggressive impulses toward others or with others' hostility directed toward them.

PHYSICIAN'S RESPONSIBILITY

In cases of suspected child abuse and neglect, the physician should (1) diagnose the suspected maltreatment; (2) intervene and admit the child into the hospital; (3) make an assessment—history, physical examination, skeletal survey, and photographs; (4) report the case to the appropriate department of social service and child protection unit or central registry; (5) request a social worker's report and appropriate surgical and medical consultations; (6) confer within 72 hours with members of the child abuse committee; (7) arrange a program of care for the child and the parents; and (8) arrange for social service follow-up.

TREATMENT

Child

Ideally, each abused child should be given an intervention plan based on the assessment of (1) the factors re-

sponsible for the parent's psychopathology; (2) the overall prognosis for the parents' achieving adequate parenting skills; (3) the time estimated to achieve meaningful change in the parent's ability to parent; (4) an estimate of whether the parent's dysfunction is confined to this child or involves other children; (5) the extent to which the parent's overall malfunctioning, if this is the case, is acute or chronic (reflects a lifelong pattern); (6) the extent to which the mother's malfunctioning is confined to infants, as opposed to older children (that is, the incidence of abuse is inversely related to the child's age); (7) the parent's willingness to participate in the intervention plan; (8) the availability of personnel and physical resources to implement the various intervention strategies; and (9) the risk of the child's sustaining additional physical abuse by remaining in the home.

Parents

On the basis of the information obtained, several options can be selected to improve the parents' functioning: (1) eliminate or diminish the social or environmental stresses; (2) lessen the adverse psychological impact of the social factors on the parents; (3) reduce the demands on the mother to a level that is within her capacity, through day-care placement of the child or provision of a housekeeper or baby sitter; (4) provide emotional support, encouragement, sympathy, stimulation, instruction in maternal care, and aid in learning to plan for, assess, and meet the needs of the infant (supportive case work); and (5) resolve or diminish the parents' inner psychic conflicts (psychotherapy).

PREVENTION

In general, child abuse prevention and treatment programs should try to (1) prevent the separation of parents and child if possible, (2) prevent the placement of children in institutions, (3) encourage the parents' attainment of self-care status, and (4) encourage the family's attainment of self-sufficiency. As a last resort and to prevent further abuse and neglect, it may be necessary to remove children from families who are unwilling or unable to profit from the treatment program. In regard to sexual abuse, the licensing of day-care centers and the psychological screening of those persons who work in them should be mandatory so as to prevent further abuses. Education of the medical profession and members of allied health fields as well as all who come in contact with children will aid in early detection. And pro-

viding support services to stressed families will aid in preventing the problem in the first place.

References

Finkelhor D: *A Sourcebook on Child Sexual Abuse*. Sage Publications, Beverly Hills, CA, 1986.

Fontana V J: *The Maltreated Child: The Maltreatment Syndrome in Children*, ed 4. Thomas, Springfield, IL, 1979.

Fontana V J: The "maltreatment syndrome" in children. N Engl J Med *269*:1389, 1963.

Fontana V J: A multidisciplinary approach to the treatment of child abuse. Pediatr *57*:760, 1976.

Fontana V J: *Somewhere a Child is Crying*. Macmillan, New York, 1973.

Green A H: *Child Maltreatment*. Jason Aronson, New York, 1980.

Green A H: Dimensions of psychological trauma in abused children. J Amer Acad Child Psychiatr 22:231, 1983.

Kaplan S J, Zitrin A: Psychiatrists and child abuse. J Am Acad Child Psychiatry 22:253, 1983.

Kempe C H, Silverman F N, Steele B N, Droegemueller W, Silver H K: The battered child syndrome. JAMA *181*:17, 1962.

45

_____ # Psychiatric Treatment of Children and Adolescents

45.1 _____

Individual Psychotherapy

THEORETICAL ASSUMPTIONS

The choice of intervention with an individual youngster should be based on the clinician's understanding of the child's problem and should stem from an individualized assessment of the child and his family. But, regardless of how individualized such an evaluation is, any rational assessment requires that the data of observation be organized within a coherent framework. Typically, such systematizing schemata are derived from the therapist's preferred theory of personality development and organization, rendering it vital that the clinician be vigilant that these theories not distort the clinical observations or inappropriately influence the therapeutic interventions. Currently, four major theoretical systems underlie the bulk of child psychotherapy: (1) psychoanalytic theories of the evolution and resolution of emotional disturbance, (2) social-learning-behavioral theories, (3) family systems-oriented transactional theories of psychopathology and treatment, and (4) developmental theories.

Classical Psychoanalytic Theory

Classical psychoanalytic theory conceives of exploratory psychotherapy's working, with patients of all ages, by reversing the evolution of psychopathological processes. A principal difference noted with advancing age is a sharpening distinction between psychogenetic and psychodynamic factors. The younger the child, the more the genetic and the dynamic forces are intertwined.

The development of these pathological processes is generally thought to begin with experiences that have proved to be particularly significant to the patient, and have affected him adversely. Although in one sense the experiences were real, in another sense they may have been misinterpreted or imagined. In any event, for the patient they were traumatic experiences that caused unconscious complexes. Being inaccessible to conscious awareness, these unconscious elements readily escape rational adaptive maneuvers, and are subject to a pathological misuse of adaptive and defensive mechanisms. The end result is the development of distressing symptoms, character attitudes, or patterns of behavior that constitute the emotional disturbance.

Increasingly, the psychoanalytic view of emotional disturbances in children has assumed a developmental orientation. Thus, the maladaptive defensive functioning is directed against conflicts between impulses that are characteristic of a specific developmental phase and environmental influence, or the child's internalized representations of the environment. In this framework, the disorders are the result of environmental interferences with maturational time tables or conflicts with the environment engendered by developmental progress. The result is difficulty in achieving or resolving developmental tasks and achieving the capacities specific to later phases of development, which can be expressed in various ways, such as Anna Freud's lines of development and Erikson's concept of sequential psychosocial capacities.

Psychoanalytic psychotherapy is a modified form of psychotherapy which is expressive and exploratory and endeavors to reverse this evolution of emotional disturbance, through a reenactment and desensitization of the traumatic events by free expression of thoughts and feelings, in an interview-play situation. Ultimately, the therapist helps the patient understand the warded-off feelings, fears, and wishes that have beset him.

Whereas the psychoanalytic psychotherapeutic approach seeks improvement by exposure and resolution of buried conflicts, suppressive-supportive-educative psychotherapy works in an opposite fashion. It aims to facilitate repression. The therapist, capitalizing on the patient's desire to please, encourages the patient to substitute new adaptive and defensive mechanisms. In this type of therapy, the therapist uses interpretations minimally; instead, the therapist emphasizes suggestion, persuasion, exhortation, operant or classical reinforcement, counseling, education, direction, advice, abreaction, environmental manipulation, intellectual review, gratification of the patient's current dependent needs, and similar techniques.

Learning-Behavioral Theories

All behavior, regardless of whether it is adaptive or maladaptive, is a consequence of the same basic principles of behavior acquisition and maintenance. It is either learned or unlearned, and what renders behavior abnormal or disturbed is its social significance.

Although the theories and their derivative therapeutic intervention techniques have become increasingly complex over the years, it is still possible to subsume all learning within two global basic mechanisms. One is classical respondent conditioning, akin to Pavlov's famous experiments, and the second is operant instrumental learning, which is to be associated with Skinner, even though it is basic to both Thorndike's law of effect regarding the influence of reinforcing consequences of behavior, and to Freud's pain-pleasure principle. Both of these basic mechanisms assign the highest priority to the immediate precipitants of behavior, deemphasizing those remote underlying causal determinants that are important in the psychoanalytic tradition. The theory asserts quite simply that there are but two types of abnormal behavior. On the one hand, there are the behavioral deficits that result from a failure to learn, and, on the other hand, there is deviant maladaptive behavior that is a consequence of learning inappropriate things.

Such concepts have always been an implicit part of the rationale underlying all child psychotherapy. Intervention strategies derive much of their success, particularly with children, from rewarding previously unnoticed good behavior, thereby highlighting it and making it more frequent.

Family Systems Theory

Although families have long been an interest of children's psychotherapists, their understanding of transactional family processes has been greatly enhanced by conceptual contributions from cybernetics, systems theory, communications theory, object relations theory, social role theory, ethology, and ecology.

The bedrock premise entails the family's functioning as a self-regulating open system that possesses its own unique history and structure. Its structure is constantly evolving as a consequence of the dynamic interaction between the family's mutually interdependent subsystems and individuals who share a complementarity of needs. From this conceptual foundation, a wealth of ideas has emerged under rubrics such as the family's development, life cycle, homeostasis, functions, identity, values, goals, congruence, symmetry, myths, rules, roles (spokesperson, symptom bearer, scapegoat, affect barometer, pet, persecutor, victim, arbitrator, distractor, saboteur, rescuer, breadwinner, disciplinarian, nurturer), structure (boundaries, splits, pairings, alliances, coalitions, enmeshed, disengaged), double bind, scapegoating, pseudomutuality, and mystification. Increasingly, it is being noted that appreciation of the family system sometimes explains why a minute therapeutic input at a critical junction may result in far-reaching changes, whereas in other situations huge quantities of therapeutic effort appear to be absorbed with minimal evidence of change.

Developmental Theories

Underlying child psychotherapy is the assumption that in the absence of unusual interferences, children mature in basically orderly, predictable ways that are codifiable in a variety of interrelated psychosociobiological sequential systematizations. The central and overriding role of a de-velopmental frame of reference in child psychotherapy distinguishes it from adult psychotherapy. The therapist's orientation should entail something more than knowledge of age-appropriate behavior derived from such studies as Gesell's descriptions of the morphology of behavior. It should encompass more than psychosexual development with ego-psychological and sociocultural amendments, exemplified by Erikson's epigenetic schema. It extends beyond familiarity with Piaget's sequence of intellectual evolution as a basis for acquaintance with the level of abstraction at which children of various ages may be expected to function or for assessing their capacity for a moral orientation.

TYPES OF PSYCHOTHERAPY

Among the common bases for classification of child therapy is identification of the element presumed to be helpful for the young patient.

Isolating a single therapeutic element as the basis for classification tends to be somewhat artificial, because most, if not all, of the factors are present in varying degrees in every child psychotherapeutic undertaking. For example, there is no psychotherapy in which the relationship between therapist and patient is not a vital factor; nevertheless, child psychotherapists commonly talk of relationship therapy to describe a form of treatment in which a positive, friendly, helpful relationship is viewed as the primary, if not the sole, therapeutic ingredient. Probably one of the best examples of pure relationship therapy is to be found outside of a clinical setting in the work of the Big Brother Organization.

Remedial, educational, and patterning psychotherapy endeavors to teach new attitudes and patterns of behavior to children who persist in using immature and inefficient patterns, which are often presumed to be due to a maturational lag.

Supportive psychotherapy is particularly helpful in enabling a well-adjusted youngster to cope with the emotional turmoil engendered by a crisis. It is also used with those quite disturbed youngsters whose less than adequate ego functioning may be seriously disrupted by an expressive-exploratory mode or by other forms of therapeutic intervention. At the beginning of most psychotherapy, regardless of the patient's age and the nature of the therapeutic interventions, the principal therapeutic elements perceived by the patient tend to be the supportive ones, a consequence of therapists' universal efforts to be reliably and sensitively responsive. In fact, some therapy may never proceed beyond this supportive level, whereas others develop an expressive-exploratory or behavioral modification flavor on top of the supportive foundation.

Release therapy, described initially by David Levy, facilitates the abreaction of pent-up emotions. Although abreaction is an aspect of many therapeutic undertakings, in release therapy the treatment situation is structured to encourage only this factor. It is indicated primarily for preschool-age children who are suffering from a distorted emotional reaction to an isolated trauma.

Preschool-age children are sometimes treated through the parents, a process called filial therapy. The therapist using this strategy should be alert to the possibility that apparently successful filial treatment can obscure a significant diagnosis. The first case of filial therapy was that of Little Hans reported on by Freud in 1905. Hans was a 5-year-old phobic child who was treated by Hans's father under Freud's supervision.

Psychotherapy with children is often psychoanalytically oriented, which means that it endeavors through the vehicle of self-understanding to enable the child to develop his potential further. This development is accomplished by liberating for more constructive use the psychic energy that is presumed to be expended in defending against fantasied dangers. The child is generally unaware of these unreal dangers, his fear of them, and the psychological defenses he uses to avoid both the danger and the fear. With the awareness that is facilitated, the patient can evaluate the usefulness of his defensive maneuvers and relinquish the unnecessary ones that constitute the symptoms of his emotional disturbance.

This form of psychoanalytic psychotherapy is to be distinguished from child psychoanalysis, a more intensive and less common treatment, in which the unconscious elements are interpreted systematically from outside in, resulting in the orderly sequence of affect-defense-impulse. Under these circumstances, the therapist anticipates unconscious resistances and allows transference manifestations to mature to a full transference neurosis, through which neurotic conflicts are resolved.

Although interpretations of dynamically relevant conflicts are emphasized in psychoanalytic descriptions, this does not imply the absence of elements that are predominant in other types of psychotherapies. Indeed, in all psychotherapy, the child should derive support from the consistently understanding and accepting relationship with the therapist, while varying degrees of remedial educational guidance and emotional release are inevitably present.

Interrelationship of Behavioral and Psychodynamic Therapies

Probably the most vivid examples of the integration of psychodynamic and behavioral approaches, even though they are not always explicitly conceptualized as such, are to be found in the milieu therapy of child psychiatric residential and day treatment facilities. Behavioral change is initiated in the residential setting, and its repercussions are explored concurrently in individual psychotherapeutic sessions, so that the action in one arena and the information stemming from it augment and illuminate what transpires in the other arena.

Other Types of Psychotherapy. Cognitive therapy has been used with children, adolescents, and adults. This approach attempts to correct cognitive distortions, particularly negative conceptions of oneself, and is used mainly in depression.

DIFFERENCES BETWEEN CHILDREN AND ADULTS

Logic suggests that psychotherapy with children, who generally are more flexible than adults and have simpler defenses and other mental mechanisms, should consume less time than comparable treatment of adults. Experience does not usually confirm this expectation, because of the relative absence in children of some elements that contribute to successful treatment.

A child, for example, typically does not seek help. As a consequence, one of the first tasks for the therapist is to stimulate the child's motivation for treatment. Children commonly begin therapy involuntarily, often without the benefit of true parental support. Although the parents may want their child helped or changed, this desire is often generated by frustrated anger with the child. Typically, this anger is accompanied by relative insensitivity to what the therapist perceives as the child's need and the basis for a therapeutic alliance. Thus, whereas adult patients frequently perceive advantages in getting well, children may envision therapeutic change as nothing more than conforming to a disagreeable reality, which heightens the likelihood of perceiving the therapist as the parent's punitive agent. This is hardly the most fertile soil in which to nurture a therapeutic alliance.

Children tend to externalize internal conflicts in search of alloplastic adaptations and to find it difficult to conceive of problem resolution except by altering an obstructing environment. The passive, masochistic boy who is the constant butt of his schoolmates' teasing finds it inconceivable that this situation could be rectified by altering his mode of handling his aggressive impulses, rather than by someone's controlling his tormentors, a view that may be reinforced by significant adults in his environment.

The tendency of children to reenact their feelings in new situations facilitates the early appearance of spontaneous and global transference reactions that may be troublesome. Concurrently, the eagerness that children have for new experiences, coupled with their natural developmental fluidity, tend to limit the intensity and therapeutic usefulness of subsequent transference developments.

Children have a limited capacity for self-observation, with the notable exception of some obsessive children who resemble adults in this ability. These obsessive children, however, usually isolate the vital emotional components. In the exploratory-interpretative psychotherapies, development of a capacity for ego splitting—that is, simultaneous emotional involvement and self-observation—is most helpful. Only by means of identification with a trusted adult, and in alliance with that adult, are children able to approach such an ideal. The therapist's sex, or the relatively superficial aspects of the therapist's demeanor, may be important elements in the development of a trusting relationship with a child.

Regressive behavioral and communicative modes can be wearing on child therapists. Typically motor-minded, even when they do not require external controls, children may demand a degree of physical stamina that is not of consequence in therapy with adults. The age appropriateness of such primitive mechanisms as denial, projection, and isolation hinders the process of working through, which relies on a patient's synthesizing and integrating capacities, both of which are immature in children. Also, environmental pressures on the therapist are generally greater in psychotherapeutic work with children than in work with adults.

Although children compare unfavorably with adults in many of the qualities that are generally considered desirable in therapy, children have the advantage of active maturational and developmental forces. The history of psychotherapy for children is punctuated by efforts to harness these assets and to overcome the liabilities. Recognition of the importance of play constituted a major forward stride in these efforts.

THE PLAYROOM

The structure, design, and furnishing of the playroom suitable for child psychotherapy is most important. The number of toys should be few, simple, and carefully selected to facilitate the communication of fantasy. Others suggest that a wide variety of playthings be available, to increase the range of feelings that the child may express. These contrasting recommendations have been attributed to differences in therapeutic methods. Some therapists tend to avoid interpretation even of conscious ideas, whereas others recommend the interpretation of unconscious content directly and quickly. Therapists tend to change their preferences in equipment as they accumulate experience and develop confidence in their abilities.

Although special equipment—such as genital dolls, amputation dolls, and see-through anatomically complete (except for genitalia) models—has been used in therapy, many therapists have observed that the unusual nature of such items risks making children wary and suspicious of the therapist's motives. Until the dolls available to the children in their own homes include genitalia, the psychic content that these special dolls are designed to elicit may be more available at the appropriate time with conventional dolls.

Although individual considerations should be decisive, the following equipment can constitute a well-balanced playroom or play area: multigenerational families of flexible but sturdy dolls of various races; additional dolls representing special roles and feelings, such as policeman, doctor, and soldier; dollhouse furnishings with or without a dollhouse; toy animals; puppets; paper, crayons, paint, and blunt-ended scissors; clay or something comparable; tools like rubber hammers, rubber knives, and guns; building blocks, cars, trucks, and airplanes; and eating utensils. These toys should enable children to communicate through play. It is wise to avoid mechanical toys because they break readily and thereby contribute to children's guilt feelings and to clutter.

A special drawer or box should be available to each individual child in which to store items the child brings to the therapy session or to store projects, such as drawings and stories, for future retrieval. Of course, limits have to be set, so that this private storage capacity is not used to hoard communal play equipment, depriving the therapist's other patients. Some therapists assert that an absence of such arrangements evokes material about sibling rivalry; however, others feel that this is a rationalization for not respecting the child's privacy, inasmuch as there are other ways of facilitating the expressions of such feelings.

INITIAL APPROACH

A variety of approaches can be derived from the therapist's individual style and perception of the child's needs. The range extends from those in which the therapist endeavors to direct the child's thought content and activity—as in release therapy, some behavior therapy, and certain educational patterning techniques—to those exploratory methods in which the therapist endeavors to follow the child's lead. Even though the child determines the focus, it remains the therapist's responsibility to structure the situation. Encouraging a child to say whatever he wishes and to play freely, as in exploratory psychotherapy, establishes a definite structure. The therapist has created an atmosphere in which he hopes to get to know all about the child—the good side, as well as the bad side, as children would put it. The therapist may communicate to the child that he does not intend to get angry or to be pleased in response to what the child says or does, but that the therapist will try to understand him. Such an assertion does not imply that therapists do not have emotions, but it assures the young patient that the therapist's personal feelings and standards are subordinate to understanding the youngster.

THERAPEUTIC INTERVENTIONS

Therapeutic interventions with children encompass a range comparable to those used with adults in psychotherapy. If the amount of therapist activity is used as the basis for a classificatory continuum, at the least active end are the questions posed by the therapist requesting elaboration of the patient's statements or behavior. Closely aligned is the process of clarification of the patient's manifest productions by means of questions, recapitulation, and reorganization that can arrange the child's productions in a logical, temporal sequence, so frequently neglected by children. Also, clarification can serve as a preliminary step toward the specific goal of the therapy by recapitulating the child's productions so as to highlight motivational possibilities, target behaviors, or whatever may be appropriate for the particular type of therapy. Next on the continuum of therapeutic activity are the exclamations and confrontations in which the therapist more pointedly directs attention to some data of which the patient is cognizant. Then there are interpretations, designed to expand the patient's conscious awareness of himself by making explicit those elements that have previously been implicitly expressed in his thoughts, feelings, and behavior. Beyond interpretation, the therapist may educatively offer the patient information that is new because the patient has not been exposed to it previously. At the most active end of the continuum there is advising, counseling, and directing, designed to help the patient adopt a course of action or a conscious attitude.

Nurturing and maintaining a therapeutic alliance may require some education of the child regarding the process of therapy. Another educational intervention may entail assigning labels to affects that have not been part of the youngster's past experience. Rarely does therapy have to compensate for a real absence of education regarding acceptable decorum and playing games. Usually, children are in therapy not because of the absence of educational efforts, but because repeated educational efforts have failed. Therefore, therapy generally does not need to include additional teaching efforts, despite the frequent temptation to offer them.

Adults' natural educational fervor with children is often accompanied by a paradoxical tendency to protect them from learning about some of life's realities. In the past, this tendency contributed to the stork's role in childbirth, the dead having taken a long trip, and similar fairy-tale explanations for natural phenomena about which adults were uncomfortable in communicating with children. Although adults are more honest with children today, therapists can find themselves in a situation in which their overwhelming urge to protect the hurt child may be as disadvantageous to the child as was the stork myth.

The temptation to offer oneself as a model for identification may stem also from helpful educational attitudes toward children. Although there are instances in which this may be an appropriate therapeutic strategy, therapists should not lose sight of the pitfalls in this apparently innocuous strategy.

PARENTS

Psychotherapy with children is characterized by the need for parental involvement. This involvement does not necessarily reflect parental culpability for the youngster's emotional difficulties, but is a reality of the child's dependent state. This fact cannot be stressed too much because of what could be considered an occupational hazard shared by many who work with children. This hazard is the motivation to rescue children from the negative influence of their parents, sometimes related to an unconscious competitive desire to be a better parent than the child's or one's own parents.

There are varying degrees of parental involvement in child psychotherapy. With preschool-age children, the entire therapeutic effort may be directed toward the parents, without any direct treatment of the child. At the other extreme, children can be seen in psychotherapy without any parental involvement beyond the payment of fees and perhaps transporting the child to the therapy sessions. Most therapists agree that only relatively rare neurotic children who have reached the oedipal phase of development can sustain therapy by themselves. Even in such instances, however, the majority of practitioners prefer to maintain an informative alliance with the parents for the purpose of obtaining additional information about the child.

Probably the most frequent arrangements are those that were developed in child guidance clinics—that is, parent guidance focused on the child or on the parent-child interaction, or therapy for the parents' own individual needs concurrent with the child's therapy. The parents may be seen by the child's therapist or by someone else. In recent years, there have been increasing efforts to shift the focus from the child as the primary patient, to the concept of the child as the family's emissary to the clinic. In such family therapy, all or selected members of the family are treated simultaneously as a family group. Although the preferences of specific clinics or practitioners for either an individual or family therapeutic approach may be unavoidable, the final decision as to which therapeutic strategy of combination to use should be derived from the clinical assessment.

CONFIDENTIALITY

Consideration of parental involvement highlights the question of confidentiality in psychotherapy with children. There are advantages to creating an atmosphere in which the child can feel that his

words and actions will be viewed by the therapist as simultaneously both serious and tentative. In other words, the child's communications do not bind him to a commitment; nevertheless, they are too important to be communicated to a third party without the patient's permission. Although such an attitude may be conveyed implicitly, there are occasions in which it is wise to explicitly discuss confidentiality with the child. It can be risky to promise a child that the therapist will not tell parents what transpires in therapeutic sessions. Although the therapist has no intention of disclosing such data to the parents, the bulk of what children do and say in psychotherapy is common knowledge to the parents. Therefore, should the child be so motivated, it is easy for him to manipulate the situation so as to produce circumstantial evidence that the therapist has betrayed his confidence. Accordingly, if confidentiality requires specific discussion during treatment, the therapist may not want to go beyond indicating that he is not in the business of telling parents what goes on in therapy, as his role is to understand children and to help them.

It is also important to try to enlist the parents' cooperation in respecting the privacy of the child's therapeutic sessions. This respect is not always readily honored, as parents quite naturally are not only curious about what transpires, but may also be threatened by the therapist's apparently privileged position.

Routinely reporting to children the essence of all communications with the third parties regarding the child underscores the therapist's reliability and his respect for the child's autonomy. In certain types of treatment, this report may be combined with soliciting the child's guesses about these transactions. Also, it may be fruitful to invite children, particularly older ones, to participate in discussions about them with third parties.

INDICATIONS AND CONTRAINDICATIONS FOR PSYCHOTHERAPY

The present level of knowledge does not permit the compilation of a meaningful list of the multifaceted indications for child psychotherapy. Existing diagnostic classifications cannot serve as the basis for such a list because of invariable deficiencies in nosological specificity and comprehensiveness. In general, psychotherapy is indicated for children with emotional disorders that appear to be permanent enough to impede maturational and developmental forces. Psychotherapy may also be indicated when the child's development is not impeded, but is inducing reactions in the environment that are considered pathogenic. Ordinarily, such disharmonies are dealt with by the child with his parents' assistance, but, when these efforts are persistently inadequate, psychotherapeutic interventions may be indicated.

Psychotherapy should be limited to those instances in which there are positive indicators pointing to its potential usefulness. If psychotherapy, despite contraindications, is invariably recommended after every child psychiatric evaluation by a particular therapist or clinic, this fact suggests not only unsatisfactory professional practice and a disservice to patients, but also an indiscriminate use of psychotherapy.

Psychotherapy is contraindicated if the emotional disturbance is judged to be an intractable one that will not respond to treatment. This is an exceedingly difficult judgment, but one that is essential, considering the excess of the demand for psychotherapy over its supply. Because the potential for error in such prognostic assessments is so great, therapists should bring to them both professional humility and a readiness to offer a trial of therapy. There are times when the essential factor in intractability is the therapist. Certain patients may elicit a reaction from one therapist that is a contraindication for psychotherapy with this therapist, but not necessarily with another.

Another contraindication is evidence that the therapeutic process will interfere with reparative forces. A difficult question is posed by suggestions that the forces mobilized as a consequence of psychotherapy may have dire social or somatic effects. An example is the circumstance in which psychotherapy may upset a precarious family equilibrium, thereby causing more difficulty than the original problem posed.

References

Adams P L: *A Primer of Child Psychotherapy*. Little, Brown, Boston, 1982.
Berline I N: Some transference and countertransference issues in the playroom. Am Acad Child Adol Psychiatry 26:101, 1987.
Carek D M: *Principles of Child Psychotherapy*. Thomas, Springfield, IL, 1972.
Dulcan M K: Brief psychotherapy with children and their families: The state of the art. J Am Acad Child Adol Psychiatry 25:544, 1984.
Glenn J, editor: *Child Analysis and Therapy*. Jason Aronson, New York, 1978.
Looney J G: Treatment planning in child psychiatry. J Am Acad Child Psychiatry 23:529, 1984.
McDermott J F, Harrison S I, editors: *Psychiatric Treatment of the Child*. Jason Aronson, New York, 1977.
Ornstein A: Making contact with the inner world of the child. Compreh Psychiatry 17:3, 1976.
Rutter M: Psychological therapies in child psychiatry: Issues and prospects. Psychol Med 12:723, 1982.
Shapiro T, Esman A H: Psychotherapy with children and adolescents. Psychiat Clin No Am 8:909, 1985.

45.2 ▬▬▬▬
Group Therapy with Children

INTRODUCTION

The characteristics of developmental stages have influenced the growth of group psychotherapy techniques perhaps more than any other factor.

PRESCHOOL AND EARLY SCHOOL-AGE GROUPS

Work with the preschool group is usually structured by the therapist through the use of a particular technique, such as puppets or artwork, or it is couched in terms of a permissive play atmosphere. In therapy with puppets, the children project onto the puppets their fantasies in a way not unlike ordinary play. The main value lies in the cathexis afforded the child, especially if he shows difficulty in expressing his feelings. Here the group aids the child less by interaction with other members than by action with the puppets.

In play group therapy, the emphasis rests on the interactional qualities of the children with each other and with the therapist in the permissive playroom setting. The therapist should be a person who can allow the children to produce fantasies verbally and in play, but who also can use active restraint when the children undergo excessive tension. The toys are the traditional ones used in individual play therapy. The children use the toys to act out aggressive impulses and to relive with the group members and with the therapist their home difficulties. The children catalyze each other, and obtain libido-activating stimulation from this catalysis and from their play materials. The therapist interprets a child to the group in the context of the transference to the therapist and to other group members.

The children selected for group treatment show in common a social hunger, the need to be like their peers and to be accepted by them. Usually, the therapist excludes the child who has never realized a primary relationship, as with his mother, inasmuch as individual psychotherapy can better help this child. Usually, the children selected include those with phobic reactions, effeminate boys, shy and withdrawn children, and children with primary behavior disorders.

Modifications of these criteria have been used in group therapy for autistic children, along with parent group therapy and art therapy.

A modification of group therapy was used for physically handicapped toddlers who showed speech and language delays. This experience of twice-a-week group activities involved the mothers and their children in a mutual teaching-learning setting. The experience proved effective to the mothers, who received supportive psychotherapy in this group experience; their formerly hidden fantasies about the children emerged, to be dealt with therapeutically.

LATENCY-AGE GROUPS

Activity group therapy assumes that poor and divergent experiences have led to deficits in appropriate personality development in the behavior of children; therefore, corrective experiences in a therapeutically conditioned environment will modify them. Because some latency-age children present deep disturbances, involving neurotic traits (fears, high anxiety levels, and guilt), an activity-interview group psychotherapy modification evolved. This format uses interview techniques, verbal explanations of fantasies, group play, work, and other communications.

In this type of group therapy, as with pubertal and adolescent groups, the children verbalize in a problem-oriented manner, with the awareness that problems brought them together, and that the group aims to change them. They report dreams, fantasies, and day dreams, as well as traumatic and unpleasant experiences. Both these experiences and the group behavior undergo open discussion. Therapists vary in their use of time, of co-therapists, and of food and materials. Most groups are after school and last at least 1 hour, although some leaders prefer 90 minutes. Some therapists serve food in the last 10 minutes, and others prefer serving times when the children are more together for talking. Food, however, does not become a major feature, never becoming central to the group's activities.

PUBERTAL AND ADOLESCENT GROUPS

Similar group therapy methods can be used with pubertal children, who are often grouped monosexually, rather than mixed. Their problems resemble those of late latency-age children, but they are also beginning, especially the girls, to feel the impact and pressures of early adolescence. In a way, these groups offer help during a transitional period. The group appears to satisfy the social appetite of pre-adolescents, who compensate for feelings of inferiority and self-doubt by the formation of groups. This form of therapy puts to advantage the influence of the process of socialization during these years. Because children of this age experience difficulties in conceptualizing, pubertal therapy groups tend to use play, drawing, psychodrama, and other nonverbal modes of expression. The therapist's role is active and directive, as opposed to the older, more passive role assigned him.

Activity group psychotherapy has been the recommended type of group therapy for latency-age and pubertal children who do not have significantly neurotic personality patterns. The children, usually of the same sex and in groups of not more than eight, freely act out in a setting especially designed and planned for its physical and milieu characteristics. Samuel Slavson, one of the pioneers in group psychotherapy, pictured the group as a substitute family in which the passive, neutral therapist becomes the surrogate for parents. The therapist assumes different roles, mostly in a nonverbal manner, as each child interacts with him and with other group members. Recent therapists, however, tend to see the group as a form of peer group, with its attendant socializing processes, rather than as a reenactment of the family. Late adolescents, from 16 years of age and up, may be included in groups of adults when indicated. Group therapy has been very useful in the treatment of substance abuse problems. Combined therapy (the use of group and individual therapy) has also been used successfully with adolescents.

PARENT GROUPS

In the group treatment, as with most treatment procedures for children, parental difficulties present obstacles. Sometimes uncooperative parents refuse to bring a child or to participate in their own therapy. The extreme of this situation reveals itself when severely disturbed parents use the child as their channel of communication in working out their own needs. In such circumstances, the child finds himself in the intolerable position of receiving positive group experiences that seem to create havoc at home.

Parents groups, therefore, can be a valuable aid to the group therapy of their children. The parent of a child in therapy often has difficulty in understanding the nature of his child's ailment, of discerning the line of demarcation between normal and pathological behavior, in relating to the medical establishment, and in coping with feelings of guilt. A parents' group assists them in these areas, and helps the members formulate guidelines for action.

OTHER GROUP THERAPY SITUATIONS

Some residential and day treatment units frequently use group therapy techniques in their work. Group therapy in school for underachievers and for the underprivileged has relied on reinforcement and on modeling theory, in addition to traditional techniques, and has been supplemented by parent groups.

With the opportunity for more controlled conditions, residential treatment units have been used for specific studies in group therapy, such as behavioral contracting. Behavioral contracting with reward-punishment reinforcement provides positive reinforcements among preadolescent boys with severe concerns in basic trust, with low self-esteem, and with dependency conflicts. Somewhat akin to formal residental treatment units are social group work homes. The children undergo many psychological assaults before placement, so that supportive group therapy offers ventilation and catharsis, but more often it succeeds in letting these children become aware of the enjoyment of sharing activities and developing skills.

Public schools—also a structured environment, although usually considered not the best site for group therapy—have been used by a number of workers. Group therapy as group counseling readily lends itself to school settings. One such group used gender- and problem-homogeneous selection for groups of six to eight students, who met once a week during school hours over a time span of 2 to 3 years.

From the foregoing, one can gather that there are many indications for the use of group psychotherapy as a treatment modality. Some indications can be described as situational; the therapist may work in a reformatory setting, where group psychotherapy has seemed to reach the adolescents better than does individual treatment. Another indication is time economics; more patients can be reached within a given time span by the use of groups than by individual therapy. Using groups best helps the child at a given age and developmental stage, and with a given type of problem. In the young age group, the child's social hunger and his potential need for peer acceptance help to determine his suitability for group therapy. Criteria for unsuitability are controversial, and have been progressively loosened.

References

Abramowitz C V: The effectiveness of group psychotherapy with children. Arch Gen Psychiatry *33*:320, 1976.

Blotcky M, Sheinbein M, Wiggins K, Forgotson J: A verbal group technique for ego-disturbed children: Action to words international. J Psychoanal Psychother *8*:203, 1980.

Kraft I A: Group therapy. In *Basic Handbook of Child Psychiatry,* J D Noshpitz, editor, vol 3, p 159. Basic Books, New York, 1979.

Kraft I A: Some special considerations in adolescent group psychotherapy. Int J Group Psychother *2*:196, 1961.

Rose S D: *Treating Children in Groups.* Jossey/Bass, San Francisco, 1972.

Scheidlinger S: Group treatment of adolescents. Am J Orthopsychiatry *55*:102, 1985.

Scheidlinger S: Short-term group psychotherapy for children: An overview. Int J Group Psychother *34*:573, 1984.

Slavson S R, Schiffer M: *Group Psychotherapies for Children.* International Universities Press, New York, 1985.

Sugar M, editor: *The Adolescent in Group and Family Therapy.* Brunner/Mazel, New York, 1975.

Yalom I D: *Inpatient Group Psychotherapy.* Basic Books, New York, 1983.

45.3 _____
Residential and Day Treatment

RESIDENTIAL TREATMENT

Introduction

There are over 20,000 emotionally disturbed children in residential treatment centers in the United States, and the number is increasing. Such centers serve a very real need in that they provide a structured living environment in which children may form strong attachments to and receive commitments from the staff. Special education for the children and treatment of their families are expressions of this commitment.

Staff and Setting

Staffing patterns include various combinations of child care workers, teachers, social workers, psychiatrists, pediatricians, nurses, and psychologists, making the cost of residential treatment very high.

The Joint Commission on Mental Health of Children made the following structural and setting recommendations:

In addition to space for therapy programs, there should be facilities for a first-rate school and a rich evening activity program, and there should be ample space for play, both indoors and out. Facilities should be small, seldom exceeding 60 in capacity, with 100 a maximum limit, and should make provision for children to live in small groups. The centers should be located near the families they serve and be readily accessible by public transportation. They should be located for ready access to special medical and educational services and to various community resources, including consultants. They should be open institutions whenever possible; locked buildings, wards, or rooms should only rarely be required. In designing residential programs, the guiding principle should be this: Children should be removed the least possible distance—in space, in time, and in the psychological texture of the experience—from their normal life setting.

Indications

Most children who are referred for residential treatment have already been seen by one or more professional persons, such as a school psychologist or pediatrician or members of a child guidance clinic, juvenile court, or state welfare agency. Unsuccessful previous attempts at outpatient treatment and foster home or other custodial placement often precede residential treatment. The age range of the children varies from institution to institution, but most children are between 5 and 15 years of age. Boys are referred more frequently than are girls.

An initial review of the data enables the intake staff to determine whether a particular child is likely to benefit from their treatment program. Often for every one child accepted for admission, three are rejected. The next step usually is interviews with the child and his or her parents by various staff members, such as a therapist, a group living worker, and a teacher. Psychological testing and neurological examinations are given when indicated, if they have not already been done. The child and parents should be prepared for these interviews.

Group Living

Most of the children's time in a residential treatment setting is spent in group living. The group living staff consists of child care workers who offer a structured environment that constitutes a therapeutic milieu. The environment places boundaries and limitations on the children. Tasks are defined within the limits of the children's abilities; incentives, such as additional privileges, encourage them to progress rather than regress. In milieu therapy, the environment is structured; limits are set; and a therapeutic atmosphere is maintained.

The children often select one or more staff members with whom to form a relationship through which the children express, consciously and unconsciously, many of their feelings about their parents. The child care staff should be trained to recognize such transference reactions and to respond to them in a way that is different from the children's expectations, based on their previous or even current relationship with their parents.

To maintain consistency and balance, the group living staff must communicate freely and regularly with one another and with the other professional and administrative staff members of the residential setting, particularly the children's teachers and therapists. The child care staff members must recognize any tendency toward becoming the good (or bad) parent in response to a child's splitting behavior. This tendency may be manifested as a pattern of blaming other staff members for a child's disruptive behavior. Similarly, the child care staff must recognize and avoid such individual and group countertransference reactions as sadomasochistic and punitive behavior toward a child.

The structured setting should offer a corrective emotional experience and opportunities for facilitating and improving the children's adaptive behavior, particularly when such deficiencies as speech and language deficits, intellectual retardation, inadequate peer relationships, bed wetting, poor feeding habits, and attention deficits are present. Some of these deficits are the basis of the children's poor school academic performance and unsocialized behavior, including temper tantrums, fighting, and withdrawal.

Behavior modification principles have also been used, particularly in group work with children. Behavior therapy is part of the residential center's total therapeutic effort.

Education

Children in residential treatment frequently have severe learning disabilities as well as disruptive behavior. Usually they cannot function in a regular community school and consequently need a special on-grounds school setting. The educational process in residential treatment is complex, and Table 1 shows some of its components.

A major goal of the on-grounds school is to motivate the children to learn.

Therapy

Traditional modes of psychotherapy have a place in residential treatment, including intensive, individual psychotherapy with the child; group therapy with selected children; individual or group therapy or both for parents; and, in some cases, family therapy. However, several modifications need to be kept in mind.

The child relates to the total staff of the setting and, therefore, needs to know that what transpires in the therapist's office is shared with all professional staff members. The therapist informs the child that what they discuss and do in individual therapy will not be revealed to other family members or to other children in the residential center but will be shared with the professional staff members within the setting itself.

The Parents

Concomitant work with the parents is essential. The child usually has a strong tie to the parent, no matter how disturbed this parent is. Sometimes the child idealizes the parent, who repeatedly fails the child. Sometimes the parent has an ambivalent or unrealistic expectation that the child will return home. In some instances, the parent must be helped to enable the child to live in another setting when this is in the child's best interests. Most residential treatment centers offer individual or group therapy with the parents, couples or marital therapy, and, in some cases, conjoint family therapy.

DAY TREATMENT

Introduction

The concept of daily comprehensive therapeutic experiences without removing the children from their homes or families derived in part from experiences with a therapeutic nursery school. The development of day hospital programs for children followed, and the number of programs continues to grow.

The main advantage of day treatment is that the children remain with their families, and so the families can be more involved in the treatment. Day treatment is also much less expensive than is residential treatment. At the same time, the risks of day treatment are the child's social isolation and confinement to a narrow band of social contacts within the program's disturbed peer population.

Indications

The primary indication for day treatment is the need for a more structured, intensive, and specialized treatment program than can be provided on an outpatient basis. At the same time, the home in which the child is living should be able to provide an environment that is at least not de-

structive to the child's development. Children who are likely to benefit from day treatment may have a wide range of diagnoses, including infantile autism, borderline conditions, conduct disorder, attention-deficit hyperactivity disorder, and mental retardation. Exclusion symptoms include behavior that is likely to be destructive to the children themselves or to others under the treatment conditions. Thus, some children who threaten to run away, set fires, attempt suicide, hurt others, or disrupt to a significant degree the life of their family while they are at home may not be suitable for day treatment.

The same ingredients that lead to a successful residential treatment program apply to day treatment. These ingredients include clear administrative leadership, team collaboration, open communication, and an understanding of the children's behavior. Indeed, there are advantages in having a single agency offer both residential and day treatment.

A major function of the child care staff in day treatment for psychiatrically disturbed children is to provide positive experiences and a structure that will enable the children and their families to internalize controls and to function better in regard to themselves and to the outside world. Again, the methods used are essentially similar to those found in the full residential treatment program.

Because the age, needs, and range of diagnoses of children who may benefit from some form of day treatment vary, a broad spectrum of day treatment programs has developed. Some programs specialize in the special educational and structured environmental needs of mentally retarded children. Others offer the special therapeutic efforts required to treat autistic or schizophrenic children. Still other programs provide the total spectrum of treatment usually found in full residential treatment, of which they may be a part. The children may then move from one part of the program to another and may be in residential treatment or day treatment according to their needs. The school program is always a major component of day treatment, and the psychiatric treatment varies according to the child's needs and diagnosis.

Results

The results of day treatment have not yet been adequately evaluated. The assessment of the long-term effectiveness of day treatment is fraught with difficulties, whether one is making the assessment from the point of view of the child's maintenance of gains, the therapist's view of what has been accomplished, or society's concerns for such matters as cost–benefit ratios.

At the same time, the advantage of day treatment has encouraged further development of these programs. Moreover, the lessons learned from day treatment programs have moved the mental health disciplines toward having the services follow the children, rather than perpetuating discontinuities of care. The experiences of day treatment for the psychiatric conditions of children and adolescents have also encouraged pediatric hospitals and departments to adapt this model for the medical nursing care of children with physical disorders, particularly those with chronic physical illnesses.

Table 1
The Educational Process in Residential Treatment

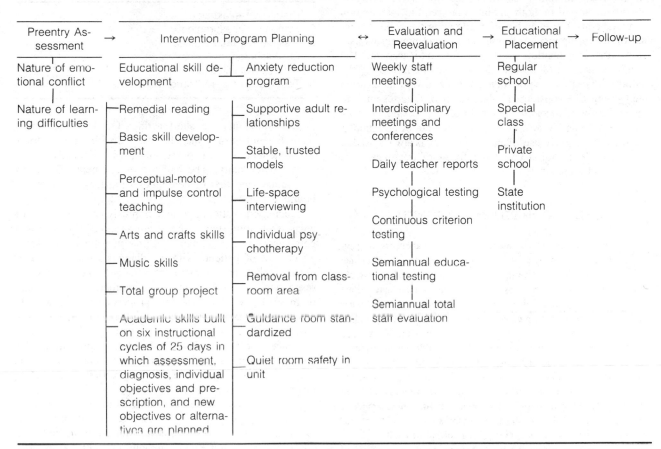

Preentry Assessment	→	Intervention Program Planning		↔	Evaluation and Reevaluation	→	Educational Placement	→	Follow-up
Nature of emotional conflict		Educational skill development	Anxiety reduction program		Weekly staff meetings		Regular school		
Nature of learning difficulties		Remedial reading	Supportive adult relationships		Interdisciplinary meetings and conferences		Special class		
		Basic skill development	Stable, trusted models		Daily teacher reports		Private school		
		Perceptual-motor and impulse control teaching	Life-space interviewing		Psychological testing		State institution		
		Arts and crafts skills	Individual psychotherapy		Continuous criterion testing				
		Music skills	Removal from classroom area		Semiannual educational testing				
		Total group project	Guidance room standardized		Semiannual total staff evaluation				
		Academic skills built on six instructional cycles of 25 days in which assessment, diagnosis, individual objectives and prescription, and new objectives or alternatives are planned	Quiet room safety in unit						

Table by Lewis M: Residential Treatment. In *Comprehensive Textbook of Psychiatry*, ed 4, H I Kaplan and B J Sadock, editors, p 1800. Williams & Wilkins, Baltimore, 1985.

References

Dingman P R: Day programs for children: A note on terminology. Ment Hyg 53:646, 1969.

Evangelakis M G: *A Manual for Residential and Day Treatment of Children.* Thomas, Springfield, IL, 1974.

Hunger D S, Webster C D, Konstantareas M M, Sloman L: Ten years later: What becomes of the psychiatrically disturbed child in day treatment. J Child Care 1:45, 1982.

LaVietes R, Cohen R, Reems R, Ronall R. Day treatment center and school: Seven years' experience. Am J Orthopsychiatry 35:160, 1965.

Lewis M, Brown T E: Child care in the residential treatment of the borderline child. Child Care Q 9:41, 1980.

Lewis M, Lewis D O, Shanok S S, Klatskin E, Osborn J R: The undoing of residential treatment. J Am Acad Child Psychiatry 19:160, 1980.

Prentice-Dunn S, Wilson D R, Lyman R D: Client factors related to outcome in a residential and day treatment program for children. J Clin Child Psychol 10:188, 1981.

Vaughan W J, Davis F E: Day hospital programming in a psychiatric hospital for children. Am J Orthopsychiatry 33:542, 1963.

Zang L D: The antisocial aggressive school-age child: Day hospitals. In *Handbook of Treatment of Mental Disorders and Adolescence*, B Wolman, J Egan, A Ross, editors, p 317. Prentice-Hall, Englewood Cliffs, NJ, 1978.

45.4 ————
Organic Therapies

INTRODUCTION

Organic therapy in children and adolescents has emerged from the shadow of adult psychiatry. More attention to cognitive variables and more extensive psychostimulant research with children have begun to influence and contribute to the parent field. The recognition and treatment of disorders like major depression, once considered to be limited to older age groups, have extended conceptions from general psychiatry to the pediatric area.

THERAPEUTIC CONSIDERATIONS

A thorough diagnostic assessment first must be conducted (Table 1). Does the child have a disorder of a type and severity that warrants organic therapy? Other medical or social conditions causing such symptoms should be considered. Equally important are an evaluation and understanding of the patient's social and family context, which may influence the choice of therapy. Psychiatric disorders in one or both parents may require intervention simultaneously or even before medicating the child. Parental or school opposition to medication can prevent its use, and careful evaluation must take this into account. The family's and child's own ideas about what caused the child's illness may color their attitudes toward medication and so must be considered. The history of drug response in other family members may be helpful in assessing the risk–benefit ratio and in selecting which member of a particular class of drugs to choose. Pharmacotherapy is always used in treatment as an adjunct to other forms of treatment; it is never used alone.

CHILDHOOD PHARMACOKINETICS

Children appear to be more efficient metabolizers of psychoactive drugs than are adults, and so they may require or tolerate slightly higher doses on a milligram per kilogram of body weight basis. This is clearly the case with lithium, which may reflect children's greater renal clearance. One explanation for the other differential effects is the greater liver–body weight ratio in children (e.g., 30 percent greater for a 6-year-old than an adult). Stimulants seem to have a somewhat shorter half-life in children than in adults. Children convert imipramine to desmethylimipramine more actively than do adults. In children, it is expected that the desmethylated metabolite is the predominant active moiety. Although children clear imipramine more rapidly via demethylation, their clearance of the sum of imipramine and desmethylimipramine following imipramine administration is at a rate similar to that of adults.

Studies of the serum levels of both these different classes of drugs demonstrate wide variability of serum levels among subjects receiving the same milligram-per-kilogram dose. Similarly, this same variation has been seen in adults with these drugs as well as with most other psychotherapeutic agents. With imipramine, depressed children also require the same plasma levels associated with a favorable response in adults.

INDICATIONS

Attention-Deficit Hyperactivity Disorder (ADHD)

The best-documented indication for pharmacologic treatment in child psychiatry is attention-deficit hyperactivity disorder (ADHD). The symptoms usually prompting therapy are developmentally inappropriate inattention and impulsivity that do not respond to social control.

The first choice among organic therapies is a stimulant, of which there are three: methylphenidate (Ritalin), dextroamphetamine (Dexedrine), or pemoline (Cylert). The dosage of the stimulant can be titrated about every 3 to 5 days (every week in the case of pemoline) until either a therapeutic benefit is achieved or side effects prohibit a further increase. The physician should use the lowest effective dose. Doses are usually limited to the day, with their frequency based on the drug's half-life. Compared with the long half-lives of the antidepressants and antipsychotics, all

Table 1
Stepwise Process of Organic Therapy

1. Diagnostic evaluation
2. Symptom measurement
3. Risk/benefit ratio analysis
4. Establishment of a contract of therapy
5. Periodic reevaluation
6. Termination/tapered drug withdrawal

of the stimulants are short acting. Of the three drugs, methylphenidate has the shortest half-life (2½ hours is about the mean). As a consequence, it is frequently administered twice daily. The half-life of amphetamines is intermediate, and that of pemoline is the longest (about 12 hours).

Decreased restlessness and impulsivity as well as increased attention span, concentration, and compliance with commands are the hallmarks of treatment response. About 75 percent of patients with the diagnosis will respond to either amphetamine or methylphenidate. Some children will respond to one stimulant but not to another. Although many of these drugs' pharmacologic properties are known, the mechanism of action has not been elucidated. It should be emphasized that the actions of stimulants are not specific to hyperactive children. Normal children show similar behavioral responses, and so stimulant responsiveness does not confirm a diagnosis of attention-deficit hyperactivity disorder.

Stimulants are contraindicated in children with thought disorder or psychosis, as they may exacerbate those conditions. Stimulants are also contraindicated for mental retardates, ticquers, and highly anxious children. They have been associated with precipitation or aggravation of Tourette's disorder. The common side effects of stimulants are listed in Table 2.

If stimulants are not effective or if the side effects are severe, a second line of drugs is the tricyclic antidepressants. Those who respond do so rapidly (e.g., within 1 to 2 days); however, the response may be short-lived and not as striking as that with stimulants. The dosage used has been lower than that for antidepressant activity. Antipsychotics such as haloperidol have also been tried but the risk of tardive dyskinesia must be considered.

The dietary management of hyperactivity has received a great amount of public attention, but controlled studies have not substantiated its benefit. Similarly, in most controlled studies, caffeine was not found superior to a placebo for attention-deficit hyperactivity disorder.

Tourette's Disorder

Tourette's disorder, characterized by both multiple skeletal muscle tics and multiple vocal tics, is one of the clearest indications for pharmacotherapy. Although patients have some ability to suppress these movements voluntarily, most obtain significant additional relief from haloperidol (Haldol). The suggested dose range for 3- to 12-year-old children is 0.02 to 0.2 mg per kg a day. Haloperidol is now the standard treatment against which other proposed treat-

Table 2
Common Dose-Related Side Effects of Stimulants

1. Insomnia
2. Decreased appetite
3. Irritability or nervousness
4. Weight loss

---

ments should be judged. Recently, improvements have been demonstrated with pimozide, a calcium-channel-binding antipsychotic, and clonidine, a presynaptic alpha-adrenergic blocking agent.

Infantile Autism

Autistic children's hyperactivity, agitation, crying, screaming, and lability of mood make caring for them very difficult, and drugs can manage only their symptomatic behavior. Antipsychotics cannot relieve the main symptoms of gross deficits in communication and social unresponsiveness. Low doses of relatively less sedating antipsychotics (e.g., haloperidol 0.5 to 16 mg a day) seem to ameliorate the secondary symptoms.

Fenfluramine, a sympathomimetic amine, has been claimed to be useful but has not been demonstrated in controlled studies to be better than a placebo. It may be helpful in some cases, however. Naltrexone, an opioid antagonist, has shown some promise.

Schizophrenic Disorders

Children with signs and symptoms comparable with those found in adult schizophrenia probably benefit from antipsychotics, but there have been no controlled studies in this area. There is evidence that antipsychotics cause the same toxic side effects in children as in adults, including tardive dyskinesia. Consequently, the risk-benefit ratio is high, and great care must be taken to determine the need for continued antipsychotic use. Schizophrenia with onset in late adolescence is treated like the adult disorder.

Mood Disorders

Major depression has recently been recognized to occur in childhood and adolescence, not just in adulthood. The role of pharmacologic therapy in this disorder has not been ruled out. Depressed children with endogenous features may respond, with improvement in mood, to imipramine in dosages ranging from 1.0 to 2 mg per kg a day. The side effects are similar to those experienced by adults. The margin of benefit over a placebo is not as clear as it is in adults. Whether MAO inhibitors are any better has not yet been determined. There is no current indication for ECT in children.

Bipolar patients' retrospective accounts indicate that a sizable minority (30 percent) first become ill in adolescence or earlier. Although lithium has had very limited study, a trial is warranted in those who meet the DSM III R criteria for the disorder and have not responded to more con-

servative management. Dosages of lithium to achieve blood levels of 0.6 to 1.2 meq per liter, similar to that for adult patients, are suggested, and doses may approximate adult doses to achieve this. Side effects and complications are similar to those seen in adults.

Conduct Disorder

Little is known about the organic treatment of conduct disorder. There is considerable overlap between conduct disorder and attention-deficit hyperactivity disorder, making it unclear in many studies which was responding to the drug treatment. The role of organic therapy in pure conduct disorders, therefore, has yet to be defined. Recent trials with lithium and haloperidol in hospitalized conduct-disordered children report beneficial effects.

The older anticonvulsants do not appear beneficial, even to those who also have seizure disorders. There have been some claims for the efficacy of carbamazepine (Tegretol) and propranolol (Inderal), but they need further study. Stimulants may be effective for aggressiveness in those with attention-deficit hyperactivity disorder but may not be helpful in severe conduct disorder, and compliance or abuse is a problem in this group.

Antipsychotics decrease the severity of aggression, but their utility is limited by sedation and possible cognitive impairment.

Enuresis

Tricyclic antidepressants, particularly imipramine, control enuretic symptoms but do not provide a cure. They are indicated in some situations as adjunctive therapy in children 6 years or older. Initially, an oral dose of 25 mg a day given 1 hour before bedtime should be tried. The dosage may be increased to 50 mg in those children under 12, and 75 mg in those over 12, but should not exceed 2.0 mg per kg a day. The action that relieves the symptoms is not known. What is known is that the anticholinergic effect is irrelevant to enuresis control, as other peripherally acting anticholinergics are not efficacious. By the end of a week of an adequate amount of the drug, 60 percent or more of the children will have experienced relief, but this may wear off, or tolerance may occur in half of these responders. However, the use of bell-and-pad conditioning is preferable, as the risk is minimal, and it produces long-lasting results.

Mental Retardation

Recent surveys have found that roughly half of institutionalized mentally retarded persons receive antipsychotic drugs, which most likely reflects their overutilization. Mental retardation by itself is not an indication for psychotropic drug use, although some behaviors, such as hyperactivity or stereotypy, may be alleviated by stimulants or antipsychotics. Low doses of haloperidol appear to offer the greatest benefit with the least cognitive impairment.

Thioridazine and haloperidol may be useful in reducing unwanted behavior, such as self-stimulation, aggression, and motor activity. However, besides the risk of tardive dyskinesia, there are other risks: antipsychotics may impair the effectiveness of behavioral training and other rehabilitative efforts, such as workshop performance, if the patient has side effects that produce somnolence.

Anxiety Disorders of Childhood or Adolescence

Imipramine has been shown to be useful as an adjunct in the treatment of school-phobic children, and it may be useful in separation anxiety in general. There are not enough anecdotal reports of school-phobic children's benefiting from chlordiazepoxide and from amphetamine to justify their use in clinical practice. Antianxiety agents are overprescribed in these disorders.

Sleep Terror

Sleep terror disorder consists of repeated episodes of abrupt awakening with intense anxiety marked by autonomic arousal. It occurs during stage IV sleep. The child, who appears confused and disoriented, will not usually respond to comfort measures during the episode. Diazepam, in 2- to 5-mg doses, reduces the proportion of stage IV sleep and has been shown to be helpful.

Obsessive-Compulsive Disorder

Obsessive-compulsive disorder is a rare condition in children. It is marked by obsessive thoughts and compulsive actions, which can be very disabling. Clomipramine, not currently available in the United States, appears to relieve obsessive-compulsive symptoms, whether or not there is coexisting depression.

Specific Developmental Disorders

No pharmacologic agent has been shown to make a clinically significant improvement in any specific developmental disorder. However, many children with psychiatric disorders also have learning disabilities, and many who have learning disabilities also have behavioral problems. This, as well as the importance of school and learning in children's lives, raises questions about the cognitive effects of psychotropics. Table 3 summarizes the effects of drugs on cognitive tests of learning functions.

In children with learning disabilities but no other psychiatric diagnosis, methylphenidate has been shown to facilitate performance on several standard cognitive, psycholinguistic, memory, and vigilance tests but has shown no improvement in academic achievement ratings or teacher ratings. Cognitive impairment from psychotropic drugs, especially antipsychotics, may be an even greater problem in mentally retarded persons.

Eating Disorders

Eating disorders are characterized by compulsive binge-eating episodes or by anorexia. There now are reports indicating that antidepressant drugs are beneficial.

MEDICATION EFFECTS AND COMPLICATIONS

Antidepressants

The side effects of antidepressants in children are usually similar to those in adults and result from imipramine's anticholinergic properties. They include dry mouth, constipation, palpitations, tachycardia, loss of accommodation, and sweating. The most serious side effects are cardiovascular, although in children, diastolic hypertension is more common, and postural hypotension occurs more rarely than in adults. EKG changes are more apt to be seen in children on high doses. Slowed cardiac conduction (PR interval >0.20 seconds or QRS interval >0.12) may necessitate lowering the dose. FDA guidelines limit doses to a maximum of 5 mg per kg a day. The drug can be very toxic in an overdose, and in small children, ingestions of 200 to 400 mg can be fatal. When the dose is lowered too rapidly, withdrawal effects are manifested mainly by gastrointestinal symptoms: cramping, nausea, vomiting, and sometimes also apathy and weakness. The treatment is a slower tapering off of the dosage.

Antipsychotics

The best studied of the antipsychotics given to pediatric age groups are chlorpromazine (Thorazine), thioridazine

Table 3
Effects of Psychotropic Drugs on Cognitive Tests of Learning Functions*†

Drug Class	Continuous Performance Test (Attention)	Matching Familiar Figures (Impulsivity)	Test Function Paired Associates (Verbal Learning)	Porteus Maze (Planning Capacity)	Short Term Memory‡	WISC (Intelligence)
Stimulant	↑	↑	↑	↑	↑	↑
Antidepressants	↑	0		0	0	0
Neuroleptics	↕		↓	↓	↓	0

*Adapted from M G Aman: Drugs, learning and the psychotherapies. In *Pediatric Psychopharmacology. The Use of Behavior Modifying Drugs in Children*, J S Werry, editor, Bruner/Mazel, New York, 1978.
† ↑ Improved, ↕ inconsistent, ↓ worse, and 0 no effect.
‡Various Tests: digit span, word recall, etc.

(Mellaril), and haloperidol (Haldol). It is widely held in adult psychiatry that high- and low-potency antipsychotics differ in their side effect profiles. The phenothiazine derivatives (chlorpromazine and thioridazine) have the most pronounced sedative and atropinic actions, whereas the high-potency antipsychotics are more commonly thought to be associated with extrapyramidal reactions, such as parkinsonian symptoms, akathisia, and acute dystonias. Caution is warranted in assuming that this is also true in children. In particular, when comparisons are made at low dosage levels of equivalent potency, differences may not be detected.

Even if the frequency of these side effects differs among the medications, they always are caused by antipsychotics. Demonstrations in children of impaired cognitive function and, most importantly, of tardive dyskinesia, call for great caution in their use. Tardive dyskinesia, characterized by persistent abnormal involuntary movements of the tongue, face, mouth, or jaw, and which may also involve the extremities—is a known hazard of giving antipsychotics to patients of all age groups. There is no known effective treatment. Tardive dyskinesia has not been reported in patients taking less than 375 or 400 g of chlorpromazine equivalents. Nonpersistant choreiform movements of the extremities and trunk, on the other hand, are very common after an abrupt discontinuation of antipsychotics in children and so need to be watched so as to distinguish them from the persistent dyskinesias.

It is recommended that whenever clinically feasible, children on antipsychotics be periodically withdrawn in order to assess current clinical need and the possible development of tardive dyskinesia.

Stimulants

Problems with retarded growth associated with taking stimulants have been reported, although there is no evidence for them. The current thinking is that any growth suppression is temporary and that children taking stimulants will eventually reach their normal height.

USE OF OTHER ORGANIC THERAPIES

There is little convincing evidence that dietary manipulation, is a successful treatment for childhood psychiatric disorders, but it would be premature to dismiss it without good research. Studies of starvation and/or protein caloric malnutrition emphasize the importance of adequate nutrition to growth and development and suggest that infant malnutrition does have behavioral sequelae. Concepts such as dietary self-selection as a reflection of metabolic differences, and oligoantigenic diets, are now being studied.

Electroconvulsive therapy has been used in the past with children and adolescents, but little, if any, benefit has been reported. Most reports have been confined to children with psychotic disorders rather than children with mood disorders. Whether there is any indication for ECT in this age group has not been documented with controlled trials. No side effects or complications unique to childhood have been reported.

There is no accepted indication in child psychiatry for psychosurgery.

Table 4 lists a comprehensive overview of representative psychoactive drugs with their indication and dosages.

Table 4
Representative Psychoactive Drugs. Indications and Dosages

Psychoactive Agents	Indications	Dosage/day	
		mg	mg/kg
STIMULANTS	Attention-deficit hyperactivity disorder		
dextroamphetamine* (Dexedrine)		2.5–40	
methylphenidate** (Ritalin)		10–60	0.3–1.0
magnesium pemoline* (Cylert)		37.5–112.5	
NEUROLEPTICS			
Phenothiazines			
chlorpromazine (Thorazine)	Schizophrenic disorders; conduct disorder, aggressive type; attention-deficit hyperactivity disorder (not responding to stimulant drug)	10–200 (800[†])	2.0 maximum
thioridazine (Mellaril)	(as above)	10–200 (800[†])	
trifluoperazine (Stelazine)	Schizophrenic disorders; autistic disorder	1–20 (40[†])	
Butyrophenones			
haloperidol (Haldol)	Schizophrenic disorders; autistic disorder; Tourette's disorder; chronic motor or vocal tic disorder; conduct disorder, aggressive type; attention-deficit hyperactivity disorder (not responding to stimulant drug); mental retardation with severe aggressiveness against self or others	0.5–16	0.02–0.20

Table 4 *continued*
Representative Psychoactive Drugs. Indications and Dosages

Psychoactive Agents	Indications	Dosage/day	
		mg	mg/kg
Thioxanthenes			
thiothixene (Navane)	Schizophrenic disorders	5–42	0.3
Dihydroindolones			
molindone (Moban)	Schizophrenic disorders; autistic disorder; conduct disorder, aggressive type	1–40 (200[†])	
Dibenzoxazepines			
loxapine	Schizophrenic disorders	20–100	
Diphenylbutyl-piperidines			
pimozide	Tourette's disorder	1–4	
ANTIDEPRESSANTS			
Tricyclics			
imipramine	Functional enuresis; attention-deficit hyperactivity disorder; depressive disorders; school phobia	25–50 (75[†])	1.0–2.0 5.0 maximum
amitriptyline	Depressive disorders	45–110	1.5
nortriptyline	Depressive disorders	20–50	
OTHERS			
Lithium	Bipolar disorders	500–2,000 (and/or blood level 0.4–1.2mEq/L)	
	Conduct disorder, aggressive type; mental retardation with severe aggressiveness against self or others		
Benzodiazepines			
chlordiazepoxide			
diazepam		2–10 (20[†])	

Table prepared by Magda Campbell, M.D., Director of Child and Adolescent Services, NYU Medical Center.
  * **3 years of age or older**
** **6 years of age or older**
† **Maximum dose for older adolescents**

References

Campbell M: Drug treatment of infantile autism: The past decade. In *The Third Generation of Progress*, H Y Meltzer, editor, p 1225. Raven Press, New York, 1987.

Campbell M, Green W H, Deutsch S I: *Child and Adolescent Psychopharmacology*. Sage Publications, Beverly Hills, CA, 1985.

Campbell M, Perry R, Green W H: The use of lithium in children and adolescents. Psychosomatics *25*:95, 1984.

Campbell M, Small A M, Green W H, Jennings S J, Perry R, Bennett W G, Anderson L: Behavioral efficacy of haloperidol and lithium carbonate: A comparison in hospitalized aggressive children with conduct disorder. Arch Gen Psychiatry *41*:650, 1984.

Gittelman-Klein R: Pharmacotherapy of childhood hyperactivity: An update. In *The Third Generation of Progress*, H Y Meltzer, editor. Raven Press, New York, 1987.

Gittelman R, Koplewicz H: Pharmacotherapy of childhood anxiety. In *Anxiety Disorders of Childhood*, R Gittleman, editor, p 188. Guilford Press, New York, 1986.

Gualtieri C T, Quade D, Hicks R E, Mavo J P Schroeder S R: Tardive dyskinesia and other clinical consequences of neuroleptic treatment in children and adolescents. Am J Psychiatry *141*:20, 1984.

Klein D F, Gittelman R, Quitkin F, Rifkin A: *Diagnosis and Drug Treatment of Psychiatric Disorders: Adults and Children*, ed 2. Williams & Wilkins, Baltimore, 1980.

Psychopharmacology Bulletin. Special Feature: Rating scales and assessment instruments for use in pediatric psychopharmacology research *21*:765, 1985.

Ryan N D, Puig-Antich J, Cooper T, Rabinovich H, Ambrosini P, Davies M, King J, Torres D, Fried J: Imipramine in adolescent major depression: Plasma level and clinical response. Acta Psychiatr Scand *73*:275, 1986.

Werry J S, editor: *Pediatric Psychopharmacology: The Use of Behavior Modifying Drugs in Children*, Brunner/Mazel, New York, 1978.

45.5 _____

Psychiatric Treatment of Adolescents

INTRODUCTION

Puberty and the stress of adolescence affect psychopathology in that both precipitate psychiatric illness in vulnerable adolescents and color their clinical presentations. It is a unique time of life that requires special treatment approaches.

DIAGNOSIS

Adolescents can be assessed in both their specific stage-appropriate function and their general progress in accomplishing the tasks of adolescence. For almost all adolescents in our culture, at least until their late teens, school performance is the prime barometer of healthy function. Intellectually normal adolescents who are not functioning satisfactorily in some form of schooling are demonstrating significant psychological problems whose nature and causes should be identified.

Questions to be asked in regard to adolescents' stage-specific tasks are: What degree of separation from their parents have the adolescents achieved? What sort of identities are evolving? How do they perceive their past? Do they perceive themselves as being responsible for their own development or as being only the passive recipients of their parents' influences? How do they perceive themselves with regard to the future, and how do they anticipate their future responsibilities for themselves and others? Can they think about the differing consequences of different ways of living? How do they express their sexual and affectionate interests? These tasks occupy all of adolescence and normally are performed at different points during the early or late phase.

Adolescents' object relations must be evaluated. Do they perceive and accept both the good and bad qualities in their parents? Do they see their peers and boyfriends or girlfriends as separate individuals with needs and identities of their own, or do they exist only for their own needs?

A respect for and, if possible, some actual understanding of the adolescent's subcultural and ethnic background are essential. For example, in some groups, depression is acceptable, but in others, overt depression is a sign of weakness and is masked by antisocial acts, drug misuse, and self-destructive risks. It is not true, however, that a psychiatrist must be of the same race or group identity as the adolescent in order to be effective. Respect and knowledgeable concern are human qualities, not group-restricted ones.

PARENT INTERVIEWS

Whenever circumstances permit, both the adolescent and the parents should be interviewed. Other family members may also have to be included, depending on their degree of involvement in the youngster's life and difficulties. It is advisable, however, to see the adolescent first; this preferential treatment helps avoid the appearance of being the parents' agent.

Interview Techniques

All patients test and mistrust, but in adolescents these manifestations are likely to be crude, intense, provocative, and prolonged. Clinicians must establish themselves credibly as essentially the adolescent's agent, a task that they will have to repeat frequently. They should have the adolescents tell their own stories, without interrupting to check out discrepancies, as that will sound like correcting and disbelief. They should obtain explanations and theories from the patients about what happened, why these behaviors or feelings occur, when things changed, and what caused the identified problems to begin when they did.

Language is crucial. Even when a teenager and a doctor come from the same socioeconomic class, their language is seldom the same. Psychiatrists should use their own language, explain any specialized terms or concepts, and ask for an explanation of unfamiliar in-group jargon or slang.

Drug use and suicidal thoughts or attempts must be discussed specifically and in a matter-of-fact manner. Adolescents are usually honest about the existence and seriousness of their suicidal ideation. Many of them will deny or minimize their drug use, but others who may honestly answer straight questions will not volunteer such information unless asked specifically about each drug and the amount and frequency of its use.

Adolescents' sexual history and current sexual activities are increasingly important information for adequate evaluation. The nature of adolescents' sexual behavior is often a vignette of their whole personality structure and ego development.

TREATMENT MODALITIES

Usually no specific therapy is the only one for a particular disorder. The best choice, then, is often what best fits the characteristics of the individual adolescent and the family or social milieu. Adolescents' real dependency needs may press clinicians to strive harder to maintain even the sickest youngsters in a satisfactory home. But for the same reason, clinicians may be forced to remove adolescents from pathogenic homes even when the severity of their illness alone would not dictate it, because the youngsters are not developmentally capable of handling the double burden of working to overcome their illness while also being traumatized at home. Also, adolescents' striving for autonomy may so complicate problems of compliance with therapy that they force involuntary inpatient treatment of difficulties for which such treatment may not be necessary at a different stage of life. Thus, the following discussion is less a set of guidelines than a brief summary of what each modality can or should offer.

Individual Psychotherapy

Few, if any, adolescent patients will be trusting or open without considerable time and testing, and so it is helpful to anticipate this by letting the patients know that this is to be expected and is natural and healthy. Pointing out the likelihood of therapeutic problems—for instance, impatience and disappointment with the psychiatrist, with therapy, with the time required, and with the often-intangible results—may help keep them under control. Therapeutic goals should be stated in terms that adolescents understand and value. Although they may not see the point in exercising self-control, enduring dysphoric emotions, or forgoing impulsive gratification, they may value feeling more confident and gaining more real control over their lives and the events that affect them.

Typical adolescent patients need a real relationship with a therapist whom they can perceive as a real person. The therapist becomes another parent because adolescents still need appropriate parenting or reparenting. Thus, the professional who is impersonal and anonymous is a less useful model than is the one who can accept and respond rationally to an angry challenge or confrontation without fear or false conciliation, can impose limits and controls when the adolescents cannot, can admit mistakes and ignorance, and can openly express the gamut of human emotions. The failure to take a stand regarding self-damaging and self-destructive behavior or a passive response to manipulative and dishonest behavior is perceived as indifference or collusion.

Individual outpatient therapy is appropriate for adolescents whose problems are manifested in conflicted emotions and nondangerous behavior, who are not too disorganized to be maintained outside a structured setting, and whose family or other living environment is not so disturbed as to negate the influence of therapy. Such therapy characteristically focuses on intrapsychic conflicts and inhibitions; on the meanings of emotions, attitudes, and behavior; and on the influence of the past and the present.

Antianxiety agents can be used in adolescents whose anxiety may be high at certain times during psychotherapy.

Group Therapy

In many ways, group therapy is a natural setting for adolescents. Most are more comfortable with peers than with adults. A group diminishes the sense of unequal power between the adult therapist and the adolescent patient. Participation varies, depending on the adolescent's readiness. Not all interpretations and confrontations need come from the parent-figure therapist; group members are often adept at picking up symptomatic behavior in one another, and adolescents may find it easier to hear and consider critical or challenging comments from their peers.

Group therapy usually addresses interpersonal and present life issues. But some adolescents may be too fragile or have symptoms or social traits too likely to elicit peer group ridicule, and so they may need individual therapy to attain enough ego strength to struggle with peer relationships. Conversely, others may need to resolve interpersonal issues in a group before they can tackle intrapsychic ones in the intensity of one-to-one therapy.

Family Therapy

Family therapy is the primary modality when the adolescent's difficulties are mainly a reflection of a dysfunctional family (e.g., simple school phobics, runaways). The same may be true when developmental issues, such as adolescent sexuality or striving for greater autonomy, trigger family conflict. Or the family pathology may be more severe, as in cases of incest and child abuse. In these instances, the adolescent usually needs individual therapy as well, but family therapy is mandatory if the adolescent is to remain in or return to the home. Serious character pathology, such as that underlying antisocial or borderline personality disorders, develops out of highly pathogenic early parenting. Family therapy is strongly indicated whenever possible in such disorders, but most authorities would consider it adjunctive to intensive individual psychotherapy when individual psychopathology has become sufficiently internalized that it would persist regardless of current family status.

Treatment in Institutional Settings

Residential treatment schools are often preferable for long-term therapy, but hospitals are more suitable for acute emergencies, although some adolescent inpatient hospital units also provide educational, recreational, and occupational facilities for longer-term patients. Adolescents whose families are too disturbed or incompetent, who are dangerous to themselves or others, who are out of control in ways that preclude further healthy development, or who are seriously disorganized require, at least temporarily, the external controls of a structured environment.

Long-term inpatient therapy is the treatment of choice for those severe disorders that are considered wholly or largely psychogenic in origin, such as major ego deficits that are caused by early massive deprivation and that respond poorly or not at all to medication. Severe borderline personality disorganization, for example, regardless of the behavioral symptomatology, requires a full-time corrective environment in which regression is possible and safe, and failed ego development can take place. Psychosis in adolescence often requires hospitalization, but psychotic adolescents also often respond to appropriate medication, so that therapy is usually feasible in an outpatient setting except during acute exacerbations. Schizophrenic adolescents who show a chronic, deteriorating course may require hospitalization periodically.

Day Hospitals

In day hospitals, which are increasingly popular, the adolescent spends the day in the center participating in therapy, usually both individual and group, and in the educational and other programs but goes home in the evenings. Compared with full hospitalization, day hospitals are less expensive and are usually preferred by the patient.

SPECIFIC CLINICAL PROBLEMS

Atypical Puberty

Pubertal changes that occur within 2 or 2½ years earlier or later than the average age are within the normal range. But body image is so important to adolescents that extremes of the norm may be terribly distressing to some, either because markedly early maturation may subject them to social and sexual pressures for which they are unready or because late maturation may make them feel inferior and may exclude them from some peer activities. Medical reassurance, even if based on examination and testing to rule out pathophysiology, may be insufficient. Their distress may show as sexual or delinquent acting out, withdrawal, or problems at school of such a degree as to warrant therapeutic intervention. Therapy may also be prompted by similar disturbances in some adolescents who fail to achieve the peer-valued stereotypes of physical development despite normal pubertal physiology.

Drug Use

Some experimentation with drugs is almost ubiquitous among adolescents, certainly if one includes alcohol. But the majority do not become abusers, particularly of prescription or illegal drugs.

Regular drug use of any degree represents disturbance. Drug abuse is sometimes a defense against depression or schizophrenic deterioration and sometimes a sign of characterological disorder in teenagers whose ego deficits render them unequal to the stresses of puberty and the tasks of adolescence. However, many drugs, especially cocaine, have a physiologically reinforcing action that acts independently of preexisting psychopathology. Regardless of why the abuse developed, it becomes a problem in itself. Ego development depends on confronting and learning to cope adaptively with reality. Drugs become both a substitute for and an avoidance of reality, thus impairing ego development and perpetuating their use to conceal even poorer coping skills.

When drug use covers an underlying illness or is a maladaptive response to current stresses or disturbed family dynamics, treatment of the underlying cause may take care of the drug use. Outpatient psychotherapy, however, is generally useless with chronic abusers, who require a structured setting where drugs are not available.

Suicide

Suicide is now the third leading cause of death among adolescents. It is the final common pathway for a number of different disorders, and its high incidence reflects grave psychopathology. Some authorities consider that in adolescence, in contrast with adulthood, schizophrenia more often underlies suicide than major mood disorder. Among adolescents who are not psychotic, a higher suicidal risk occurs in those adolescents who have a history of parental suicide, who are unable to form stable attachments, who display impulsive behavior or episodic dyscontrol, and who abuse drugs. Many adolescent suicides show a common pattern of long-standing family and social problems throughout childhood and of escalation of subjective distress under the pressures and stresses of puberty and adolescence, followed by a suicide attempt precipitated by the sudden perceived loss of some person or social support felt to be the one source of meaning or closeness.

Normal developmental losses—of childhood dependency, of the parents of childhood—can also cause psychogenic depression in adolescents. The more rapid and extreme mood swings in adolescence, coupled with the adolescent's difficulty seeing beyond the intensity of the moment, contribute to catastrophic despair and impulsive suicide attempts over losses that adults could weather. Normally persistent magical thinking may impair the sense of permanency of one's own death, allowing adolescents to contemplate suicide more lightly.

Both during evaluation and treatment, suicidal thoughts, plans, and past attempts must be discussed directly when the concern arises and information is not volunteered. Chronic or recurring thoughts should be taken seriously, and a contract should be negotiated with the adolescent not to attempt suicide without first calling and talking about it with the psychiatrist. Adolescents are usually honest about making and keeping, or refusing, such contracts; if they refuse, closed hospitalization is indicated. This sign of serious, protective concern may be as therapeutic as is the opportunity to conduct or plan further treatment in a safe environment.

Major Mood Disorders

Major depressions are not uncommon in adolescents, but a typical adult-like clinical presentation is. Adolescents tend toward action-oriented defenses; they externalize onto the environment and act out to avoid the pain of loss or of feeling helpless and hopeless. Adolescents may mask their symptoms of depression with delinquent behavior, promiscuity, poor school performance, anger and irritability and power struggles at home, running away, and drug abuse. The vegetative signs of depression may not be evident even when there is a biogenic component.

A family history of major depression or alcoholism coupled with no childhood history of psychiatric or behavioral problems suggest that the underlying depression may respond to antidepressant medication.

Bipolar disorder can be manifested first in adolescence, but here, too, the developmental state usually colors the clinical picture. Bursts of severe rebellion, overconfidence, grandiosity, and sudden sexual acting out are some of the adolescent behavioral equivalents of the adult syndrome. The masking symptoms can be difficult to distinguish, except with time, from the ones covering the depression alone. The depressive equivalents may be more chronic, whereas the manifestations of bipolar illness are periodic, and the cycles are often rapid compared with those of adults. Antidepressants and lithium are indicated.

Violence may also indicate a mood disorder. Outbursts of violence may be manifestations of sudden episodic dyscontrol which may be responsive to antidepressants or lithium. Regarding the use of any psychotropic medications, whatever the illness, adolescents are less predictable than are adults in their response and in effective dosage levels. Electroconvulsive therapy is not used for adolescent depressive disorders.

Schizophrenia

The original term, "dementia precox," arose out of the recognition that what is now called schizophrenia frequently appeared first in adolescence. The illness is not fundamentally different when it occurs in adolescents, compared with other age groups. Some suggest that the earlier the onset, the greater the genetic or constitutional vulnerability and the lesser the ego strength for coping with life demands that normally intensify with age will be.

Adolescence does sometimes blur the clinical picture. As with depression, adolescents with schizophrenia tend toward action-oriented defenses (e.g., drug abuse), but paradoxically, they may initially also appear depressed. In James Masterson's research, schizophrenia was the most difficult condition to diagnose correctly on the initial evaluation. The differential diagnosis between that and serious character disorders or depression was often not clarified until the illness could be followed further. Adolescents with schizophrenia are responsive, sometimes idiosyncratically, to the dosage of the major antipsychotics. Compliance may be especially problematic because of adolescents' resistance to adult orders. Some cases may benefit from prolonged, intensive psychoanalytic psychotherapy.

References

Aichhorn A: *Wayward Youth*. Viking Press, New York, 1965.

Blos P: *On Adolescence*. Free Press, New York, 1962.

Erikson E H: The problem of ego identity. J Am Psychoanal Assoc *4*:56, 1966.

Feinstein S C, Miller D: Psychoses of adolescence. In *Basic Handbook of Child Psychiatry*, J D Noshpitz, editor. Basic Books, New York, 1979.

Freud A: Adolescence. Psychoanal Study Child 16:225, 1958.

Freud A: *The Ego and the Mechanism of Defense*. International Universities Press, New York, 1946.

Group for the Advancement of Psychiatry: *Normal Adolescence*, vol 6, Report 68, February 1968.

Masterson J F: *The Psychiatric Dilemma of Adolescence*. Little Brown, Boston, 1967.

Peterson A C, Taylor B. The biological approach to adolescence. In *Handbook of Adolescent Development*, J Adelson, editor. Wiley, New York, 1980.

Schowalter J E, Anyan W R: *The Family Handbook of Adolescence*. Knopf, New York, 1979.

46

Geriatric Psychiatry

INTRODUCTION

Psychological changes accompany the passing of years, including such well-known features as slowness of thinking, mild nonprogressive impairment of recent memory, reduction of surgency of enthusiasm, an increase in cautiousness, changes in sleep patterns with a tendency to take daytime naps, and a relative libidinal shift from genitality to the alimentary tract and interior of the body.

DEFINITION

Agedness—if one may use this term to denote the psychopathology of and attending to the later period of life—is a crisis in slow motion. Most changes are gradual and progressive. From ages 30 to 40, the change in nerve conduction velocity and cardiac output, for example, are quantitatively the same as those from ages 60 to 70. According to the theory of aging, the body dies a little every day.

Old age may be considered as yet another of the developmental phases in a person's life span—developmental in the sense that it is not static—and the defensive responses to the resulting physical and psychosocial deficits may be both old and new. Every phase in the human life cycle has specific traumatic elements that are germane and unique to that particular age group. The aged, however, have accumulated many scars from their exposure to all the sources of human suffering.

The elderly tend to be defined according to their separateness from the mainstream of humanity rather than according to their continuity. By its very nature, old age is visible and thus is easily labeled as a diagnostic entity for which remedies may be denied and neglect begun.

DIAGNOSIS

Precise psychiatric diagnosis in the elderly may not be simple. Psychiatric illnesses may be manifested by physical symptoms and signs, such as loss of weight, constipation, dry mouth, changes in heart rate and blood pressure, and tremors. Disorders of awareness, mood, perception, thinking, and thought content are usually present and prominent.

Medical Assessment

A number of common and important physical conditions should be kept in mind when examining an elderly psychiatric patient, because these conditions are known to cause mental symptoms. Toxins of bacterial and metabolic origin are common in old age. Bacterial toxins usually originate in occult or inconspicuous foci of infection, such as suspected pneumonic conditions and urinary infections. The most common metabolic intoxication causing mental symptoms in the aged is uremia. Mild diabetes, hepatic failure, and gout also may easily be missed as causative agents. Alcohol and drug misuse cause many mental disturbances in late life, but these abuses, with their characteristic effects, are easily determined by taking a history.

Cerebral anoxia, resulting from cardiac insufficiency or emphysema or both, often precipitates mental symptoms in old people. Anoxic confusion may follow surgery, a cardiac infarct, gastrointestinal bleeding, or occlusion or stenosis of the carotid arteries. Nutritional deficiencies may not only be symptomatic of emotional illness but also cause mental symptoms. Vitamin deficiencies are not common. All in all, various deficiencies should be considered in the physical assessment of the aged.

Mental Assessment

In obtaining a psychiatric history from an elderly patient, the psychiatrist should stress a number of components particularly germane to this age group.

Overt behavior may be manifested in the patient's motor activity, walk, expressive movements, and the form of speaking. Or it can be observed by the examining physician, and the history can be obtained from meaningful others.

Mood disorder may be inferred from the patient's movements. But the psychiatrist must be aware of the presence of euphoria, sadness, despair, anxiety, tension, loss of feelings, and a paucity of ideation. The patient often complains of somatic sensations that may, in a sense, substitute for the expression of an emotion.

The evaluation of the patient's mental content should be extensive and detailed and include the patient's own description of his or her feelings and account of the onset.

Abnormalities of cognitive functioning may be the result

of many depressive or schizophrenic disturbances, but they are most often due to some cerebral dysfunctioning or deterioration. In many instances, intellectual difficulties are not obvious, and so a searching evaluation may be necessary.

PSYCHIATRIC CONDITIONS

Mental disorders in old age are quite common. The causes are multiple, complex, and complicated by the frequent presence of organic brain involvement.

Organic Mental Disorders

Organic mental disorders are mental states associated with the impaired function or death of brain tissues. The disorders have distinct features: disorientation to time, place, and person; impairment of intellectual functioning; disturbances and impairment of memory; impairment of judgment; defects in comprehension or grasp; evidence of impaired immediate recall; and emotional lability.

Alzheimer's disease patients constitute 50 percent of the 1.3 million people in nursing homes. It is a common type of senile brain disorder, affecting millions of people throughout the world, and is associated with more than 100,000 deaths in the United States each year. The confusion and memory disturbances of patients with Alzheimer's disease lead to total incapacity. The most serious symptom of Alzheimer's disease closely correlates with the accumulation in neuronal cells of abnormal protein structures, known as neurofibrillary tangles, that are destroyed and replaced by neuritic plaques. (Alzheimer's disease and organic mental disorders are discussed in Chapter 11.)

Various drugs used in medicine can cause psychiatric symptoms in all classes of patients, but especially among the elderly. These symptoms may result if the drug is prescribed in too large a dose, if the patient is particularly sensitive to the medication, or if the patient does not follow the instructions for its use. Common symptoms include confusion, delirium, disorientation, and depression. Schizophrenic-like symptoms may appear if the patient begins to hallucinate or becomes paranoid.

Recent reports by several investigators have implicated certain drugs as producing psychiatric symptoms in the elderly. These symptoms are generally depression, agitation, and delirium. Some of the medications are the following: transdermal scopolamine, eye drops containing atropine, cimetidine (Tagamet), ibuprofen (Motrin, Advil), indomethacin (Indocin), levodopa (Dopar), timolol (Timoptic), trazodone (Desyrel), and rantidine (Zantac).

Psychiatric symptoms usually cease after the drug is withdrawn, but the clinician must also be alert to withdrawal reactions to a drug, especially if the drug is stopped abruptly.

Schizophrenic Disorders

There is much confusion over late-onset schizophrenias in the elderly. This confusion is based on the dispute over the connection among paraphrenic, paranoid, and schizophrenic disorders. At present, no one view is generally accepted. Late paraphrenia is the Europeans' diagnosis for those patients with a paranoid symptom complex in which there are no signs of organic dementia or sustained confusion. Delusional and hallucinatory symptoms do not seem to be caused by major mood disorders.

On the whole, paranoid symptoms seem to be a defense against the patients' gradual loss of mastery. Thus, elderly men, especially those with prostatism or postoperative conditions, express delusions about their wives' infidelity. Women often complain about being spied on, being subjected to stimulation by concealed electrical appliances, or being poisoned by fumes. These symptoms represent face-saving defenses against their gradual loss of control and the resulting fear. Implicit in all of them is a cry for help.

Aged schizophrenic persons respond quite well to the phenothiazines; however, as with all medication for the elderly, it should be judiciously administered. One should begin with small doses and gradually work up to the individual patient's tolerance, remembering all the time that elderly persons' metabolism and detoxifying mechanisms are not as efficient as those of younger schizophrenia patients.

Schizophrenic and paranoid symptoms in the elderly almost always respond to antipsychotic medications. For example, chlorpromazine or thioridazine, beginning with 10 mg three times a day and working up to 50 mg four times a day, may be sufficient to reduce excitation, restlessness, and agitation.

Mood Disorders

Depressions are unusually common in later life. Late-onset depressives, in comparison with early-onset depressives, have better-adjusted personalities emotionally, socially, and psychosexually. The majority of first depressive attacks, especially severe attacks, appear in the second half of life. The highest first incidence occurs between 55 and 65 in men and between 50 and 60 in women. Regardless of the presence of predominantly neurotic or psychotic symptoms, the onset follows closely the occurrence of some traumatic event. All these precipitating events can be classified as various kinds of loss, such as bereavement, the moving away of children, loss of status, retirement from a job, threatened loss through physical illness, and the illness of the spouse. The precipitants occur more frequently in late-onset depression than in early-onset depression.

Antidepressant drugs, particularly the tricyclics, are useful in treating depressive disorders. Those cases resistant to drugs may benefit from a course of electroconvulsive therapy.

Manic and Hypomanic Disorders. Manic and hypomanic disorders are less frequent than are depressions. Nevertheless, they may appear in late life. The patient and his or her family may fail to recognize the hypomanic phase of a bipolar disorder, as it may be ascribed to the aggressiveness, overactivity, and poor judgment of a senile brain. It usually follows a depressive disorder, which may have been so brief as to have escaped the attention of those near the patient. Hostile or paranoid behavior is usually present. Lithium has been used successfully in these conditions in the elderly.

Neuroses. There is a widespread belief that most neuroses and personality disorders improve with age. Certainly, old people are less often referred by their physicians and their families to psychiatrists or clinics. And community mental health centers report that the elderly make up only a small percentage of their patient load.

Nevertheless, the neuroses occupy a conspicuous place in the disorders of later life. Indeed, the incidence of neuroses is far greater than that of the psychoses, yet little attention is paid to them because, in the neuroses, there is no total break with reality.

Hypochondriasis. Hypochondriasis is the inordinate preoccupation with one's bodily functions, and it is understandably an especially common disorder in the aged. Hypochondriacal overconcern is often mitigated by reeducation in the activities permitted by a person's physical limitations and by conventions in certain socioeconomic groups that accept an excessive concern with bodily functions as normal behavior. However, with fewer worthwhile things than in the past to hold the attention and to divert one from self-concern, it becomes easier to notice and to talk about minor ailments and accidents. In general, the older that people are, the more experience they have had with illness, operations, and accidents, whether their own or those of other people, and the easier it is for them to feel ill or in danger themselves. Then, too, bodily concern helps save face when one is beset by failures. "I am ill and, therefore, cannot . . ." is a rationalization more universally acceptable than is the truthful but prestige-shattering "I cannot."

Anxiety Disorders. Anxiety disorders are not entirely new experiences for old people. In all probability, they had similar reactions, perhaps rather frequently, whenever their security was threatened or whenever they faced emotional deprivation. Because insecurity and realistic anxiety-producing situations are common in later life, anxiety states can easily arise. Recent evidence suggests that cells in the locus ceruleus that produce norepinephrine and serotonin (which account for biological symptoms of anxiety) decrease in number. That may account for a decrease in anxiety symptoms in some persons as they age and also may explain the symptoms of depression that are caused by the smaller number of neurotransmitters.

Obsessive-Compulsive Disorders. Obsessive-compulsive disorders and patterns in later life are similar to those occurring in earlier life. Compulsive persons can be recognized by their overconscientiousness, perfectionism, orderliness, overattention to details, and doubts about themselves and their adequacies. Some of these character traits may be considered praiseworthy, but they can also become symptoms that undermine people's efficiency and immobilize them. Such symptoms may take the form of excessive cleanliness and orderliness, and inflexible rituals to guard against mistakes, danger, or evil thoughts. There may be endless counting; a compulsion to do certain things over and over again—such as checking and rechecking gas jets, locks, or faucets; rituals in food, dress, excretion, and evacuation; and excessive washing of hands.

Any attempt to stop these compulsive acts may arouse acute and intolerable anxiety, as these symptoms are an effort by the patient to ward off complete disintegration. Therapy, therefore, should be directed at both the environment and the symptoms themselves.

Hysterical Neuroses. Hysterical neuroses are not common in later years. The classical hysterical picture of giving up the function of a bodily part—as in hysterical paralysis, blindness, or deafness—so that the rest of the organism can continue to function unimpaired is relatively rare in the elderly. What one does see is an exaggeration of minor physical symptoms.

Sleep Disturbances. Contrary to the popular myth, elderly persons need as much, if not more, sleep than they did in their earlier mature years. However, complaints about sleeplessness are common. To some extent, these complaints can be traced to sleep disturbances rather than to sleeplessness. These sleep disturbances may be due to the need for more frequent visits to the bathroom, with resulting problems in again falling asleep. Furthermore, many elderly persons—retired, unemployed, inactive, and non-involved—succumb to the practice of taking catnaps during their waking hours, a habit that may interfere with what they describe as a good night's sleep.

When the insomnia is not accompanied by delirium or a psychotic reaction, the problem usually will respond to standard hypnotics. When the insomnia is accompanied by a psychotic or depressive reaction, phenothiazine or tricyclic medication often will induce sleep.

THERAPY

Psychotherapy

The remedial measures for most difficulties can be gratifying. One must make allowance for the reduced vigor, agility, and learning capacity of the elderly patient, but beyond that, therapy can be conducted along the lines of therapy at any age level.

The type of therapy to be used in treating the older patient depends on a number of factors. First, one should assess the patient's physical state in order to determine how much treatment he or she will be able to take. Second, one must evaluate the patient's suitability for therapy from the viewpoint of his or her earlier adaptation and maladjustments, capacity for establishing a workable relation with the therapist, and the degree to which these characteristics can be modified. Third, one must determine whether the presenting symptoms are something new in the life of the patient or a continuation of a long-existing neurotic personality structure. All of these determinations require the judgment of a trained psychiatrist, whose responsibility is to decide what type of treatment is to be instituted and who is to do the therapy.

The overall treatment goals for geriatric patients are to maximize their mental, physical, and social capacities. Remotivation techniques challenge the patients' desire to withdraw from life or to die. They are encouraged to establish new social relations and reestablish old ones and to develop and redevelop former interest in church, recreation, games, and household activities in close proximity to other people. They are encouraged to engage in mutual helping relations and to take an active interest in the lives of others.

Pharmacotherapy

The following principles are useful guidelines regarding the use of psychotropic drugs for the elderly.

Before prescribing a psychotropic drug, the physician should make a comprehensive evaluation that includes a review of the patient's medical and psychiatric history, current stress factors, use of prescribed and over-the-counter medications, mental status and physical examination results, and other test results as indicated. It is especially useful to have the elderly patient or his or her family bring to the physician all currently used medications, because multiple drug usage may be contributing to the symptoms. If the patient is taking psychotropic drugs at the time of the comprehensive evaluation, it is helpful, whenever possible, to discontinue those medications and to reevaluate the patient during a drug-free baseline period. This is because the psychotropic drugs, alone or in combination with other drugs, may be contributing to the patient's symptoms.

The comprehensive evaluation may reveal a recent stress, such as a death in the family, that may account for a change in the patient's behavior. The patients's symptoms may, therefore, respond better to environmental support or psychotherapy than to a major tranquilizer.

Most psychotropic drugs should be given in equally divided doses three or four times over a 24-hour period, because elderly patients may not be able to tolerate a sudden rise in drug blood level resulting from one large daily dose. Any changes in blood pressure, pulse rate, and other side effects should be watched. For patients with insomnia, however, giving the major portion of an antipsychotic or antidepressant at bedtime takes advantage of its sedating and soporific effects. Liquid preparations are useful for elderly patients who cannot or who refuse to swallow tablets.

Patients should be frequently reassessed to determine the need for maintenance medication, changes in dosage, and the development of side effects. An antiparkinsonian drug to counteract the extrapyramidal side effects of a major tranquilizer should be used only as needed and not prophylactically, as it may aggravate the anticholinergic side effects of the major tranquilizer and other medications. If an antiparkinsonian drug is used, it should be discontinued on a trial basis after 4 to 6 weeks, as only 18 to 20 percent of patients whose antiparkinsonian drug is discontinued have a recurrence of the extrapyramidal side effects. If the extrapyramidal side effects are mild, decreasing the dosage of the antipsychotic may circumvent the need for an antiparkinsonian drug.

If an antipsychotic is indicated for such symptoms as agitation, delusions, and hallucinations, it is best to choose the drug that is least likely to aggravate concurrent medical problems. For example, an elderly psychotic patient whose cardiovascular system is impaired may be particularly sensitive to the hypotensive side effect of a phenothiazine drug, such as chlorpromazine. Haloperidol, because it produces less hypotension and sedation than does a phenothiazine

drug, may be preferable for such a patient. Likewise, a phenothiazine, rather than haloperidol, is better for the elderly patient who has difficulty in motor coordination because haloperidol produces more extrapyramidal side effects than does a phenothiazine.

Elderly persons, particularly if they have an organic brain disease, are especially susceptible to the side effects of antipsychotics. Two side effects merit discussion here. The first, tardive dyskinesia, is characterized by disfiguring and involuntary buccal and lingual masticatory movements. Akathisia, choreiform body movements, and rhythmic extension and flexion movements of the fingers may also be noticeable. Examination of the patient's protruded tongue for fine tremors and vermicular movements is a useful diagnostic procedure.

The second side effect is a toxic confusional state, resulting from the anticholinergic properties of a single drug or in combination, such as an antipsychotic, an antiparkinsonian drug, and a tricyclic antidepressant. Also referred to as the central anticholinergic syndrome, it is characterized by a marked disturbance in short-term memory, impaired attention, disorientation, anxiety, visual and auditory hallucinations, increased psychotic thinking, and peripheral anticholinergic side effects. The syndrome is sometimes difficult to recognize, particularly in patients who were psychotic, confused, and agitated before they developed the side effect. The onset may be signaled by a worsening of the preexisting psychotic symptoms, and so the syndrome may be incorrectly attributed to a worsening of the psychosis, which leads the physician to increase the medication, resulting in the symptoms' increase again. The anticholinergic properties of the antiparkinsonian agent may be a causative factor. Because many elderly patients take both an antipsychotic and an antiparkinsonian drug, the most efficacious treatment may be to discontinue the antiparkinsonian drug or to reduce or discontinue the antipsychotic or both. The confusional state usually clears within 1 or 2 days after the drug or drugs are discontinued.

The elderly patient with mild to moderate anxiety may be a candidate for an antianxiety agent. The effective dosage is usually less than in other adult patients. Chlordiazepoxide or diazepam in doses of 5 or 10 mg, two or three times a day, is often effective. Such drugs can also be used at bedtime for their hypnotic effect. Compared with the barbiturates, the benzodiazepines have a higher ratio of therapeutic effectiveness to side effects and so are considered safer. However, they can also be addictive and can produce paradoxical reactions characterized by confusion, disorientation, excitement, and aggravated psychiatric symptoms.

Depression is the most common psychiatric disorder of the elderly; indeed, elderly white men have the highest suicide rate of any group. Depressions are fairly common among the elderly and generally respond to psychotherapy. The tricyclic antidepressants, such as amitriptyline and imipramine, can be used in initial doses of 50 to 75 mg a day and be gradually increased according to the patient's response and development of side effects. Careful cardiac monitoring is nevertheless mandatory. The tricyclic antidepressants, like other psychotropic drugs, have more side effects in older patients than in younger patients. These include anticholinergic side effects: exacerbation of psychotic symptoms, extrapyramidal symptoms, and tremors; the central anticholinergic syndrome; and cardiotoxicity. Elderly patients vary in regard to the optimal dosage and the development of side effects. Patients who do not respond to one tricyclic antidepressant may respond to another. If a patient is still significantly depressed despite intensive psychotherapy and a trial on one or more antidepressants, hospitalization should be considered. In the hospital, a monoamine oxidase inhibitor, such as phenelzine, or electroconvulsive therapy may be considered.

The reader is referred to Chapter 31 on Biological Therapies for a comprehensive survey of organic therapy.

References

Butler R N, Lewis M I: *Aging and Mental Health, Positive Psychosocial Approaches*. Mosby, St. Louis, 1973.

Committee on Leadership for Academic Geriatric Medicine: *Academic Geriatrics for the Year 2000*. Division of Health Promotion and Disease Prevention, Institute of Medicine, National Academy Press, Washington, DC, 1986.

Eslinger P, Damasio A, Benton A, Van Allen M: Neuropsychologic detection of abnormal mental decline in older persons. JAMA *253*:670, 1985.

Greenblatt D J, Abernethy D R, Shader R I: Pharmacokinetic aspects of drug therapy in the elderly. Therapeutic Drug Monitoring 8:249, 1986.

Jarvik L F, editor: *APA Task Force on Treatment of Organic Mental Disorders*. American Psychiatric Association, Washington, DC, 1987.

Lazarus L W, Groves L: Brief psychotherapy with the elderly: A study of process and outcome. In *Treating the Elderly with Psychotherapy: The Scope for Change in Later Life*, J Sadavoy, M Leszcz, editors. International Universities Press, New York, 1987.

Lazarus L W, Newton N, Cohler B: Frequency and presentation of depressive symptoms in patients with primary degenerative dementia. Am J Psych *144*:41, 1987.

Osgood N J: *Suicide in the Elderly*. Aspen Systems Corp, Rockville, MD, 1985.

Plotkin D A, Gershon S C, Jarvik L F, Meltzer H Y: *Antidepressant Drug Treatment in the Elderly in Psychopharmacology: The Third Generation of Progress*. Raven Press, New York, 1987.

Roth M: Multidimensional diagnosis in gerontopsychiatry. In *Geropsychiatric Diagnostics and Treatment*, M Bergener, editor, p 125. Springer, New York, 1983.

47

Forensic Psychiatry

INTRODUCTION

The intermix of law and psychiatry, called forensic psychiatry, includes problems of credibility of witnesses; culpability of accused persons; competency to make a will, contract, to take care of oneself or one's property, or to stand trial; compensation of injured persons; and custody of children.

Other noteworthy areas are assisting in jury selection and preparing presentencing evaluations for probationary status. In addition, the issue of professional negligence, or malpractice, has become an important concern for psychiatrists and other physicians.

THE JUDICIAL PROCESS

Before considering the specific issues that arise with respect to psychiatry and the law, it is helpful to review the rules of procedure and evidence that apply to all judicial matters.

First, the legal process is adversarial, not cooperative, in contrast with that of medicine. Under the adversary system, each side is expected to put its best foot forward, with the judge or jury deciding between them on the basis of the evidence offered. The issues are polarized. In effect, an attorney is a salesperson selling in a case. Likewise, once experts decide to join the undertaking, they, too, become proponents of a cause, although they may use neutral language. Attorneys put experts or other witnesses on the stand only if they will represent the interests of their clients.

The rules of evidence generally are rules of exclusion. An objection can be made either to the form in which the question is asked or to the substance of the evidence being elicited. A witness is considered to belong to one side or the other. Hence, attorneys may ordinarily not ask leading questions—questions that suggest the answer desired—of persons they call as witnesses, but opposing attorneys on cross-examination may ask leading questions, as the witnesses are assumed to be unfriendly. Thus, in a cross-examination of a psychiatrist, the cross-examiner usually tries to impugn the psychiatric method of gathering information and forming conclusions.

THE PSYCHIATRIST IN COURT

The most common role of psychiatrists in court proceedings is as an expert, a medical specialist on mental disorders. Psychiatrists thus may be asked to testify on issues of competency, testamentary capacity, diagnosis, treatment, or criminal responsibility.

The Psychiatrist as Expert Witness

When psychiatric experts testify, they should present their information in three clearly distinguishable portions. First, they should present and discuss their psychological theories as they relate to the legal question at hand. Second, they should describe their data base in detail, including such things as exact quotations of what the patient has said, information about the patient that has been revealed in documents, and data obtained from the patient's family and significant persons who know him or her. Third, the diagnostic and legal inferences drawn in regard to the issue at trial should be identified so that their logic may be tested thoroughly and without confusion by the fact finders.

During the pretrial conferences with counsel, the psychiatrist should help him or her prepare to deal with the opposing side's expert. In addition, the confusion of seemingly disparate expert views can be diminished by having the various psychiatrists make their examinations and write their reports together.

The trial court may appoint its own expert witnesses and can reveal to the jury such appointments. Unlike the situation when they are serving one side or the other, the court-appointed experts' reports go to both parties.

Hearsay. The law of evidence bars hearsay—that is, an out-of-court statement offered to prove the truth of the matter asserted.

But there are exceptions to the hearsay rule. One such exception allows a treating physician to repeat a patient's statement to him or her about the patient's medical history or symptoms. But conventional doctrine has excluded from the exception, as not within its guarantee of truthfulness, statements made to a physician who is consulted solely for the purpose of testifying as an expert witness.

In criminal cases, the character of the accused often comes to the attention of the attorney for consideration in plea bargaining, and may be considered by the judge in a presentencing or probation report. Ironically, testimony that may have been inadmissible at the trial may find its way into a presentencing report.

Court-mandated Evaluations. In several legal situations, clinicians are asked to be consultants to the court, which raises the issue of for whom they work. Because clinical information may have to be revealed to the court, clinicians may not enjoy the same confidential relationship with their patients that they have in private practice. Clinicians who make such court-ordered evaluations are under an ethical and, in some states, a legal obligation to so inform the patients at the outset of the examination and to make sure that the patients understand this condition.

Evaluation of Witnesses' Credibility. It is up to the trial judge to grant a psychiatric examination requested by one of the parties to the action. Before ordering such an examination, the trial judge will ask for evidence showing that such an examination is necessary to determine the merits of the case and that the imposition on or inconvenience to the witness does not outweigh the examination's value. Many courts limit psychiatric examinations to complaining witnesses in rape and other sex offense cases, in which corroborative proof is nearly always circumstantial. In incest cases, for example, the father and the daughter may jointly deny the incest that the mother persistently alleges; the father may steadfastly deny the act, and in some cases, the mother may support his denial; or after accusing her father, the daughter may retract her accusation. Psychiatrists say that only a thorough psychiatric examination of the family can eliminate such confusion. Recognizing that false sex charges may stem from the psychic complexes of a victim who appears normal to a layperson, the courts permit psychiatrists to expose mental defects, hysteria, and pathological lying in complaining witnesses. The liberal attitude in this area is probably due to the gravity of the charge, to the general lack of corroborating evidence, and perhaps to a popular feeling that sex is peculiarly within the ken of psychiatrists.

Testimonial Privilege. Testimonial privilege is the right to maintain secrecy or confidentiality in the face of a subpoena. This privilege belongs to the patient, not to the physician, and so it can be waived by the patient. Currently, 38 of the 50 states have statutes providing some kind of physician–patient privilege. Psychiatrists, also licensed to practice medicine, may claim medical privilege, but they have found that it is so riddled with qualifications that it is practically meaningless. Purely federal cases have no psychotherapist–patient privilege. Moreover, the privilege does not exist at all in military courts, regardless of whether the physician is military or civilian, or whether the privilege is recognized in the state where the court-martial takes place. There are numerous exceptions to the privilege, which are often viewed as implied waivers. In the most common exception, the patient is said to waive the privilege by injecting his or her condition into the litigation, thereby making the condition an element of his or her claim or defense. Another exception involves proceedings for hospitalization, in which the interests of both the patient and the public are said to call for a departure from confidentiality. Yet another exception is made in child custody and child protection proceedings, in regard to the best interest of the child. Furthermore, the privilege does not apply to actions between a therapist and a patient. Thus, in a fee dispute or a malpractice claim, the complainant's lawyer can obtain the necessary therapist's records to resolve the dispute.

In summary, the confidentiality of a physician–patient or psychotherapist–patient communication is protected from disclosure in a courtroom only by showing that the communication is not relevant or material to the issues in the case.

CONFIDENTIALITY

A long-held premise of medical ethics binds the physician to hold secret all information given to him or her by a patient. This obligation is what is meant by confidentiality. Understanding confidentiality requires an awareness that it applies to certain populations and not to others. That is, one can identify a group that is "within" the circle of confidentiality, meaning that sharing information with the members of this group does not require specific permission from the patient. Within this circle are other staff treating the patient, clinical supervisors, and consultants. Parties outside the circle include the patient's family, attorney, and previous therapist. Sharing information with such people does require the patient's permission. Nevertheless, there are innumerable instances in which the psychiatrist may be asked to divulge information imparted by the patient. Although it is a court demand for information that worries psychiatrists most, the most frequent demand is by one such as an insurer, who cannot compel disclosure but who can withhold a benefit without it. But apart from statutory disclosure requirements and judicial compulsion, there is no legal obligation to furnish information, even to law enforcement officials.

Generally the patient himself or herself makes disclosures or authorizes the psychiatrist to make them so as to receive a benefit, such as employment, welfare benefits, or insurance.

THIRD-PARTY PAYERS, SUPERVISION, AND RESEARCH

Increased insurance coverage for health care is precipitating the concern with confidentiality and the conceptual model of psychiatric practice. Today, insurance covers about 70 percent of all health care bills, and to provide coverage, an insurance carrier must be able to obtain information with which it can assess the administration and cost of various programs.

In regard to supervision, confidentiality considered as an absolute would impede the quality control of care. Quality control necessitates a review of individual patients and therapists, as well as discriminate disclosure. The therapist in training also must breach the confidence of his or her patient to discuss the case with a supervisor. And a judicially ordained right to treatment envisions individualized treatment for institutionalized patients based on a program submitted for review to a mental health board.

WRITING ABOUT PATIENTS

In general, professionals have multiple loyalties: to clients, to society, and to the profession. Through their writings, they can share their acquired knowledge and experience, providing information that may be valuable to other professionals and to the public. But it is not easy to write about a psychiatric patient without breaching the confidentiality of this relationship. Unlike physical ailments, which can be discussed without anyone's recognizing the patient, a psychiatric history usually entails a discussion of distinguishing characteristics.

DISCLOSURE TO SAFEGUARD THE PATIENT OR OTHERS

In some situations, the psychiatrist becomes an informer in order to protect the patient or others.

There are times, albeit few in number, when a report by a psychotherapist may be crucial, but there may be a conflict between the therapist's responsibility to an individual patient and to others.

In some situations, the physician must report to the authorities, as it is specifically required by law. The classic example of mandatory reporting is that of a patient with epilepsy who operates a motor vehicle. Another example of mandatory reporting—one in which penalties are imposed for failing to report—involves child abuse. By law, therapists are obliged to report suspected cases of child abuse to public authorities. Expanded definitions of what constitutes child abuse under the law have been amended in some jurisdictions to include emotional as well as physical child abuse. Under this legislation, practitioners who learn that their patient is engaged in sexual activity with a child are obliged to report it, although nothing may be gained by notifying the authorities. Other examples of mandatory reporting include many dangerous or contagious diseases, firearm and knife wounds, and patients in drug abuse treatment programs. In the absence of a specific statute that mandates reporting, a report is optional. As a general principle, a person has no duty to come to the aid of another unless there is a special relationship that mandates this duty.

Does the establishment of a therapist–patient relationship obligate the therapist to care for the safety of not only the patient but also others? This issue was raised in the case of _Tarasoff v. Regents of University of California_ in 1966. In this case, Prosenjit Poddar, a student and a voluntary outpatient at the mental health clinic of the University of California, told his therapist his intention to kill a girl readily identified as Tatiana Tarasoff. Realizing the seriousness of the intention, the therapist, with the concurrence of a colleague, concluded that Poddar should be committed for observation under a 72-hour emergency psychiatric detention provision of the California commitment law. The therapist notified the campus police both orally and in writing that Poddar was dangerous and should be committed.

Concerned about the breach of confidentiality, the therapist's supervisor vetoed the recommendation and ordered all records relating to Poddar's treatment destroyed. At the same time, the campus police temporarily detained Poddar but released him on his assurance that he would "stay away from that girl." Poddar stopped going to the clinic when he learned from the police of his therapist's recommendation to commit him. Two months later, he carried out his previously announced threat to kill Tatiana. The girl's parents thereupon sued the university for negligence.

As a consequence, the California Supreme Court, which deliberated the case for the unprecedented time of some 14 months, ruled that a physician or a psychotherapist who has reason to believe that a patient may injure or kill someone must notify the potential victim, his or her relatives or friends, or the authorities.

The discharge of the duty imposed on the therapist to protect the intended victim against such danger may take one or more various steps, depending on the case. Thus, said the court, it may call for the therapist to warn the intended victim or others likely to notify the victim of the danger, to notify the police, or to take whatever other steps are reasonably necessary under the circumstances.

The Tarasoff decision has not drastically affected psychiatrists, as it has long been their practice to warn the appropriate persons or law enforcement authorities when a patient presents a distinct and immediate threat to someone. According to the American Psychiatric Association, confidentiality may, with careful judgment, be broken in the following ways: (1) A patient will probably commit murder, and the act can be stopped only by the psychiatrist's notification of the police. (2) A patient will probably commit suicide, and the act can be stopped only by the psychiatrist's notification of the police. (3) A patient, such as a bus driver or airline pilot, who has potentially life-threatening responsibilities, shows marked impairment of judgment.

The Tarasoff ruling does not require therapists to report fantasies; rather, it simply means that when they are convinced that a homicide is in the making, it is their duty to exercise good judgment.

LAWS GOVERNING HOSPITALIZATION

Civil Commitment

It is preferable to have a patient voluntarily enter a mental hospital or the psychiatric inpatient service of a general hospital, for the same reason that the patient's prognosis is better if he or she voluntarily enters psychotherapy as an outpatient: because he or she needs help.

All of the states provide for some form of involuntary hospitalization. Such action is usually taken when psychiatric patients present a danger to themselves and to others in their environment to the degree that their urgent need for treatment in a closed institution is evident.

The statutes governing hospitalization of the mentally ill have generally been designated as commitment laws. However, psychiatrists have long considered the term an undesirable one because commitment legally means a warrant for imprisonment. The American Bar Association and the American Psychiatric Association have thus recommended that the term be replaced by the less offensive and more accurate "hospitalization," which has been adopted by most of the states. Although this change in terminology will not correct the attitudes of the past, the emphasis on hospitalization and treatment is more in keeping with psychiatrists' views.

Procedures of Admission

There are four procedures of admission to psychiatric facilities that have been endorsed by the American Bar Association as safeguarding civil liberties and insuring that no individual can be railroaded into a mental hospital. Although each of the 50 states has the power to enact its own laws regarding psychiatric hospitalization, the procedures outlined are gaining much acceptance.

Informal Admission. Informal admission operates on the general hospital model in which the patient is admitted to a psychiatric unit of a general hospital on the same basis as a medical or surgical patient might be admitted. Under such circumstances, the ordinary doctor–patient relationship applies, with the patient free to enter and to leave, even against medical advice.

Voluntary Admission (Operates in Psychiatric Hospitals). In voluntary admission, patients apply in writing for admission to a psychiatric hospital. They may come to the hospital on the advice of their personal physician, or they may seek help on the basis of their own decision. In either case, the patients are examined by a psychiatrist on the staff of the hospital and are admitted if that examination reveals the need for hospital treatment.

Temporary Admission (Emergency Admission or Certificate of One Physician). Temporary admission is used for patients who are so senile or confused that they require hospitalization and are not able to make decisions of their own, or for patients who are so acutely disturbed that they must be immediately admitted to a psychiatric hospital on an emergency basis.

Under this procedure, a person is admitted to the hospital on the written recommendation of one physician. Once having been brought to the psychiatric hospital, the need for hospitalization must be confirmed by a psychiatrist on the hospital staff.

This procedure is temporary because patients cannot be hospitalized against their will for more than 15 days.

Involuntary Admission (Certificate of Two Physicians). Involuntary admission involves the question of whether such patients are a danger to themselves, such as suicidal patients, or a danger to others, such as homicidal patients. Because these individuals do not recognize their need for hospital care, the application for admission to a hospital may be made by a relative or friend.

Once the application is made, such patients must be examined by two physicians, and if they confirm the need for hospitalization, the patients can then be admitted.

There is an established procedure for written notification to the next of kin whenever involuntary hospitalization is involved. Furthermore, the patients have access at any time to legal counsel, who can bring the case before a judge. If the judge does not feel that hospitalization is indicated, he or she can order the patient's release.

Involuntary admission allows the patient to be hospitalized for 60 days. After this time, if the patient is to remain hospitalized, the case must be reviewed periodically by a board consisting of psychiatrists, nonpsychiatric physicians, lawyers, and other citizens not connected with the institution. In New York State, this board is called the Mental Health Information Service. The power of the state to commit mentally ill persons in need of care is known as *parens patriae,* also known as police power, in that it prevents mentally ill persons from doing harm to themselves or to others.

Despite the clear-cut procedures and safeguards for hospitalization available to patients, to their families, and to the medical and legal professions, involuntary admissions are viewed by some as an infringement of civil rights.

Persons who have been hospitalized involuntarily and who believe that they should be released have the right to file a petition for a writ of *habeas corpus.* Under law, a writ of *habeas corpus* may be proclaimed on behalf of anyone who claims that he or she is being deprived illegally of liberty. This legal procedure asks a court to decide whether hospitalization has been accomplished without due process of the law, and the case must be heard by a court at once, regardless of the manner or form in which it is filed. Hospitals are obligated to submit these petitions to the court immediately.

Involuntary Discharge, Involuntary Termination, and Abandonment

Under a variety of circumstances, patients may have to be discharged from a hospital against their will—if they have intentionally broken a major hospital rule (e.g., smuggled drugs, assaulted another patient), refused treatment, or been restored to health but still wish to remain hospitalized. Some people may wonder why many patients wish to remain in a psychiatric hospital. But for some patients, such a protective environment is preferable to the streets, jail, or their family's home. Although the focus here is on discharge from an inpatient unit, similar issues are involved in unilateral termination with an outpatient.

Abandonment as a Cause of Action. A serious potential pitfall of involuntary termination of hospitalization is the charge of abandonment. This claim can be a particularly fertile ground for malpractice litigation when the inevitable bad feelings are combined with a poor outcome. Such a situation therefore requires the clinician to exercise special care.

The Ended Relationship: Alliance Threat. An involuntary discharge entails all the pain of the termination process with far less opportunity for perspective, healing, and growth. Most importantly, in this situation the clinician directly opposes the patient's proclaimed wishes, thereby severely straining the therapeutic alliance.

Documentation and Consultation. Consultation and documentation of the rationale for the action are the two safeguards against liability.

Going the Extra Mile. "Going the extra mile" refers to smoothing the way for the patient to obtain care in the future. Termination does not mean abandonment when a good-faith transfer of services is made through an appropriate referral to another hospital or therapist. Furthermore, when possible, the patient should be told that the door is open for a negotiated return at some future time after restitution has been made or the problem has otherwise been redressed.

The Emergency Exception. The one circumstance in which the clinician cannot terminate a patient is a state of emergency. A typical example is a patient who attacks a therapist. The therapist cannot terminate the patient, no matter how severe the assault, until the emergency situation has been resolved (e.g., by hospitalizing the patient or arranging for seclusion or restraint). Only then can the therapist terminate the relationship and transfer the patient.

RIGHT TO TREATMENT

Among the rights of patients, that of the standard of quality of care is fundamental. It has been litigated in much-publicized cases in recent years under the slogan of "right to treatment."

In 1966, Judge David Bazelon, speaking for the District of Columbia Court of Appeals in *Rouse v. Cameron,* noted that the purpose of involuntary hospitalization is treatment and concluded that the absence of treatment draws into question the constitutionality of the confinement. Treatment in exchange for liberty is the logic of the ruling. In that case, the patient was discharged on a writ of *habeas corpus,* the basic legal remedy to ensure liberty.

Alabama Federal District Court Judge Frank Johnson was more venturesome in the decree he rendered in 1971 in *Wyatt v. Stickney.* The Wyatt case was a class-action proceeding, brought under newly developed rules that sought not release but treatment. Judge Johnson ruled that persons civilly committed to a mental institution have a constitutional right to receive such individual treatment as will give each of them a reasonable opportunity to be cured or to improve his or her mental condition. Johnson set out minimum requirements for staffing, specified physical facilities and nutritional standards, and required individualized treatment plans. Shortly thereafter, Texas Federal District Judge William Justice set out standards for state training schools.

The new codes, more detailed than the old ones, include the right to be free from excessive or unnecessary medication; the right to privacy and dignity; the right to the least restrictive environment; the unrestricted right to be visited by attorneys and private physicians; and the right not to be subjected to lobotomy, electroconvulsive treatments, or other procedures without fully informed consent. Patients can be required to perform therapeutic tasks but not hospital chores unless they volunteer for them and are paid the federal minimum wage. This requirement is an attempt to eliminate the practice of *peonage,* in which psychiatric patients were forced to work at menial tasks, without payment, for the benefit of the state.

In a number of states today, medication or electroschock therapy cannot be forcibly administered to a patient without first obtaining court approval, which may take as much as 10 days. The right to refuse treatment is a legal doctrine that holds that a person cannot be forced to have treatment against his or her will unless it is a life-and-death emergency.

In the 1976 case of *O'Connor v. Donaldson,* the U.S. Supreme Court ruled that harmless mental patients cannot be confined against their will without treatment if they can survive outside. According to the Court, a finding of mental illness alone cannot justify a state's confining persons in a hospital against their will. Instead, patients must be considered dangerous to themselves or others. A question has been raised about psychiatrists' ability to accurately predict dangerousness, as well as the risk to the psychiatrists, who may be sued for monetary damages if a person is thereby deprived of his or her civil rights.

The ethical controversy over applications of the law to psychiatric patients came to the fore through Thomas Szasz, a professor of psychiatry at the State University of New York. In his book *The Myth of Mental Illness,* Szasz argued that the various psychiatric diagnoses are totally devoid of significance and contended that psychiatrists have no place in the courts of law and that all forced confinement of people because of mental illness is unjust. Szasz's opposition to suicide prevention and the imposition of treatment, with or without confinement, is interesting but is viewed by the psychiatric community with strong misgivings.

SECLUSION AND RESTRAINT

Seclusion refers to the placement and retention of an inpatient in a bare room for the purpose of containing a clinical situation that may result in a state of emergency. Restraint refers to measures designed to confine a patient's bodily movements, such as the use of leather cuffs and anklets or straitjackets. The use of seclusion and restraint raises important issues of safety. The American Psychiatric Association's *Task Force Report on Seclusion and Restraint* provides standards for the use of these interventions. Clinicians practicing in institutions that employ such measures should be familiar with this report as well as with local statutes. Finally, clinicians facing a genuine emergency should act conservatively. A patient can always be released from restraints or seclusion, whereas the harm caused by uncontained violence may be irreversible.

INFORMED CONSENT

Lawyers representing an injured claimant now invariably add to a claim of negligent performance or procedures (malpractice) an informed consent claim as another possible area of liability. Ironically, it is one claim under which the requirement of expert testimony may be avoided. The usual claim of malpractice requires the litigant to produce an expert to establish that there was a departure from accepted medical practice. But in a case in which there was no informed consent, the fact that the treatment was technically well performed and effected a complete cure is immaterial. However, as a practical matter, unless there are adverse consequences, a complainant will not get very far with a jury in an action based only on an allegation that the treatment was performed without consent.

In classical tort (a tort is a wrongful act) theory, an intentional touching to which one has not given consent is a battery. Thus, the administration of electroconvulsive therapy or chemotherapy, though it may be therapeutic, is a battery when done without consent. Indeed, any unauthorized touching outside conventional social intercourse constitutes a battery. It is an offense to the dignity of the person, an invasion of his or her right of self-determination for which punitive and actual damages may be imposed. Justice Benjamin Cardozo wrote: "Every human being of adult years and sound mind has a right to determine what shall be done with his own body; and a surgeon who performs an operation without his patient's consent commits [a battery] for which he is liable in damages."

According to Cardozo, it is not the effectiveness or the timeliness of the treatment that allows taking care of another but the consent to it. Thus, a mentally competent adult may refuse treatment, even though it is effective and of little risk. But for example, when gangrene sets in and the patient is psychotic, treatment—even of such momentous proportions as amputation—may be ordered to save the patient's life. The state is also said to have a compelling interest in preventing its citizens from committing suicide.

In the case of minors, the parent or guardian is the person legally empowered to consent to medical treatment.

However, most states by statute list specific diseases or conditions that a minor can consent to have treated— venereal disease, pregnancy, contraception, drug dependency, alcoholism, and contagious diseases. And in an emergency, a physician can treat a minor without parental consent. The trend is to adopt what is referred to as the "mature minor rule," allowing minors to consent to treatment under ordinary circumstances. As a result of the Gault decision, all juveniles must now be represented by counsel, must be able to confront witnesses, and must be given proper notice of any charges. Emancipated minors have the rights of an adult when it can be demonstrated that they are living as an adult with control over their own lives.

In the past, to obviate a claim of battery, physicians needed only to relate what they proposed to do and obtain the patient's consent thereto. However, simultaneously with the growth of product liability and consumer law, the courts began to require that physicians also relate sufficient information to allow the patient to decide whether such a procedure is acceptable in light of the risks and benefits and the available alternatives, including no treatment at all. This duty of full disclosure gave rise to the phrase "informed consent is no consent." In general, informed consent requires that there be (1) an understanding of the nature and the foreseeable risks and benefits of a procedure, (2) a knowledge of alternative procedures, (3) awareness of the consequences of withholding consent, and (4) the recognition that the consent is voluntary.

Consent Forms

The basic function of a consent form is as a written document that informed consent has been obtained. However, there are several problems inherent in its design and use. Consent forms are usually designed by attorneys whose aim is to protect the institution from liability. Therefore, such forms are often exhaustive and require a level of reading comprehension that is beyond that of many patients. Paradoxically, if such a form truly covered all possible eventualities, it would probably be too long to be comprehensible, and if it were short enough to be comprehensible, it might be incomplete. Some theorists have recommended that the form be replaced by a standardized discussion and a progress note.

CHILD CUSTODY

The action of a court in a child custody dispute is now predicated on the best interests of the child. The maxim reflects the idea that a natural parent does not have an inherent right to be named as the custodial parent, but the presumption, although a bit eroded, remains in favor of the mother in the case of young children. By a rule of thumb, the courts presume that the welfare of a child of tender years is generally best served by maternal custody when the mother is a good and fit parent. The best interest of the mother may be served by naming her as the custodial parent, as a mother may never resolve the impact of the loss or death of a child, but her best interest is not to be equated *ipso facto* with the best interest of the child. Care and

protection proceedings refer to the court's intervention in the welfare of a child when the parents are unable to do so.

As has been widely reported, more and more fathers are asserting custodial claims. In about 5 percent of the cases, they are named custodians. The movement supporting women's rights is also enhancing the chances of paternal custody. With more and more women going outside the home to work, the traditional rationale for maternal custody has less force than it did in the past.

Every state today has a statute allowing a court, usually a juvenile court, to assume jurisdiction over a neglected or abused child and to remove the child from parental custody. Most states provide several grounds for assuming jurisdiction, such as parental abuse, an environment injurious to the child's welfare, and the danger of the child's being brought up to lead an idle, dissolute, or immoral life. If the court removes the child from parental custody, it usually orders that the care and custody of the child be supervised by the welfare or probation department.

TASK-SPECIFIC COMPETENCE

Technically, there is no such thing as competence or general competence. The concept has meaning only in terms of the task, decision, or procedure that the individual is facing. Moreover, although psychiatrists often give opinions on competence, only a judge's ruling converts the opinion into a "finding"; that is, a patient is not competent or incompetent until the court says so.

TESTAMENTARY AND CONTRACTUAL CAPACITY

Psychiatrists may be asked to evaluate patients' testamentary capacity, that is, their competency to make a will. Three psychological abilities are necessary to demonstrate this competency. Patients must know (1) the nature and extent of their bounty (property); (2) that they are making a will; and (3) who their natural beneficiaries are— that is, their spouse, children, and other relatives.

Quite often, when a will is being probated, one of the heirs or some other person challenges its validity. A judgment in such cases must be based on a reconstruction of what the testator's mental state was at the time the will was written. The expert gathers evidence for this reconstruction from persons who knew the testator at the time he or she wrote the will, from data from documents, and from expert psychiatric testimony.

An incompetency proceeding and the appointment of a guardian may be considered necessary when a member of the family is spending the family's assets. The guardianship process may be used when property is in danger of dissipation, as in the case of the aged, the retarded, alcoholics, and psychotics. The issue is whether such persons are capable of managing their own affairs. However, a guardian appointed to take control of the property of one deemed incompetent cannot make a will for the ward. When one is unable or does not exercise one's right to make a will, the law in all states provides for the distribution of one's property to the heirs; if there are no heirs, the estate will go to the public treasury. Witnesses at the signing of the will, which may include a psychiatrist, may attest that the testator was rational at the time the will was executed. In unusual cases the lawyer may videotape the signing to safeguard the will from attack.

Competency is determined on the basis of a person's ability to make a sound judgment. The diagnosis of a mental disorder is not, in itself, sufficient to warrant a finding of incompetency. Rather, the mental disorder must cause an impairment in judgment regarding the specific issues involved. Once declared incompetent, individuals are deprived of certain rights: they cannot make contracts, marry, start a divorce action, drive a vehicle, handle their own property, or practice their profession. Incompetency is decided at a formal courtroom proceeding, and the court usually appoints a guardian who will best serve the patient's interests. Another hearing is necessary to declare the patient competent. It should be noted that admission to a mental hospital does not automatically mean the individual is incompetent; a separate hearing for that is usually required.

In reference to contracts, competency is essential, as a contract is an agreement between parties to do some specific act. The contract will be declared invalid if, when it was signed, one of the parties was unable to comprehend the nature of his or her act. The marriage contract is subject to the same standard and thus can be voided if either party did not understand the nature, duties, obligations, and other characteristics entailed at the time they were married. In general, however, the courts are unwilling to declare a marriage void on the basis of incompetency.

Whether the competence is related to wills, contracts, or the making or breaking of marriages, the fundamental concern is the person's state of awareness and his or her capacity to comprehend the significance of the particular commitment he or she was making—at the time it was made.

Competence to Inform

Competence to inform is a relatively new concept involving the patient's interaction with the clinician and is useful in ambiguous situations that may have a poor outcome. The clinician first explains to the patient the value of being honest with him or her and then attempts to determine whether the patient is competent to weigh the risks and benefits of withholding information about suicidal or homicidal intent. This process must be documented.

A conservator handles the fiscal or contractual affairs of the person under his or her control, but not with respect to medical or surgical treatment.

CRIMINAL LAW AND PSYCHIATRY

Criminal Responsibility

According to criminal law, a socially harmful act is not the sole criterion of a crime. Rather, the objectionable act must have two components: voluntary conduct (*actus reus*) and evil intent (*mens rea*). There cannot be a *mens rea* if the offender's mental status is so deficient, so abnormal, or so diseased as to have deprived him or her of the capacity for rational intent. The law can be invoked only when an illegal intent is implemented. Neither behavior, however harmful, nor the intent to do harm is, in itself, grounds for criminal action.

Until quite recently, in most American jurisdictions a person could be found not guilty by reason of insanity if he or she suffered from a mental illness, did not know the difference between right and wrong, and did not know the nature and consequences of his or her acts.

M'Naghten Rule. The precedent for determining legal responsibility was established in the British courts in 1843. The so-called M'Naghten rule, which has, until recently, determined responsibility in most of the United States, holds that people are not guilty by reason of insanity if they labored under a mental disease such that they were unaware of the nature, quality, and consequences of their act or if they were incapable of realizing that their act was wrong. Moreover, to absolve people from punishment, a delusion has to be one that if true, would be an adequate defense. If the deluded idea does not justify the crime, then presumably such persons are to be held responsible, guilty, and punishable. The M'Naghten rule is known commonly as the right-wrong test.

The M'Naghten rule derives from the famous M'Naghten case dating back to 1843. At that time, Edward Drummond, the private secretary of Sir Robert Peel, was murdered by Daniel M'Naghten. M'Naghten had been suffering from delusions of persecution for several years. He had complained to many people about his delusional persecutors, and finally he decided to correct the situation by murdering Sir Robert Peel. When Drummond came out of Peel's home, M'Naghten shot Drummond, mistaking him for Peel. He was later adjudged insane and committed to a hospital. The case aroused great interest, causing the House of Lords to debate the problems of criminality and insanity. In response to questions about what guidelines could be used to determine whether a person should plead insanity as a defense against criminal responsibility, the English judiciary wrote:

1. To establish a defense on the ground of insanity it must be clearly proved that, at the time of committing the act, the party accused was laboring under such a defect of reason, from disease of the mind, as not to know the nature and quality of the act he was doing, or if he did know it, he did not know he was doing what was wrong.
2. Where a person labors under partial delusions only and is not in other respects insane and as a result commits an offense he must be considered in the same situation as to responsibility as if the facts with respect to which the delusion exists were real.

The jury, as instructed under the prevailing law, found the defendant not guilty by reason of insanity.

The M'Naghten rule does not ask whether the accused knows the difference in general between right and wrong; it asks whether the defendant understood the nature and quality of his act and if he knew the difference between right and wrong with respect to his act. It asks specifically whether he knew what he was doing was wrong or, perhaps, thought he was right, that is, whether he was under a delusion causing him to act in legitimate self-defense.

Irresistible Impulse.   In 1922, a committee of jurists in England reexamined the M'Naghten rule and suggested broadening the concept of insanity in criminal cases to include the concept of the irresistible impulse. This means that a person charged with a criminal offense is not responsible for his act if the act was committed under an impulse that the person was unable to resist because of mental disease. The courts have chosen to interpret this law in such a way that it has been called the "policeman-at-the-elbow" law. In other words, the court will grant the impulse to be irresistible only if it determines that the accused would have gone ahead with the act even if he had had a policeman at his elbow. To most psychiatrists this law is unsatisfactory because it covers only a small and very special group of those who are mentally ill.

Durham Rule.   In 1954, in the case of *Durham v. United States,* a decision was handed down by Judge David Bazelon, a pioneering jurist in forensic psychiatry in the District of Columbia Court of Appeals, that resulted in the product rule of criminal responsibility: An accused is not criminally responsible if his unlawful act was the product of mental disease or defect.

In the Durham case, Judge Bazelon expressly stated that the purpose of the rule was to get good and complete psychiatric testimony. He sought to release the criminal law from the theoretical straitjacket of the M'Naghten test. However, judges and juries in cases using the Durham rule became mired in confusion over the terms "product," "disease," and "defect." In 1972, some 19 years after its adoption, the Court of Appeals for the District of Columbia, in *United States v. Brawner,* discarded it. The court—all nine members, including Judge Bazelon—decided in a 143-page opinion to throw out its Durham rule and to adopt in its place the test recommended in 1962 by the American Law Institute in its Model Penal Code, which is the law in the federal courts today.

Model Penal Code.   In its Model Penal Code, the American Law Institute recommended the following test of criminal responsibility: (1) A person is not responsible for criminal conduct if at the time of such conduct, as a result of mental disease or defect, he lacked substantial capacity either to appreciate the criminality [wrongfulness] of his conduct or to conform his conduct to the requirement of the law; (2) As used in this article, the terms "mental disease or defect" do not include an abnormality manifested only by repeated criminal or otherwise antisocial conduct.

There are five operative concepts in subsection 1 of the American Law Institute rule: (1) mental disease or defect, (2) lack of substantial capacity, (3) appreciation, (4) wrongfulness, and (5) conformity of conduct to the requirements of law. The second subsection of the rule, stating that repeated criminal or antisocial conduct is not of itself to be taken as mental disease or defect, aims to keep the sociopath or psychopath within the scope of criminal responsibility.

The test of criminal responsibility and other tests grading criminal liability refer to the time of the offense's commission, whereas the test of competency to stand trial refers to the time of the trial.

Although much has been written on the insanity plea, it is actually asserted as a defense in only a small percentage of cases, and it is upheld in only a fraction of those.

The verdict of a District of Columbia jury in 1982 finding the would-be assassin of President Ronald Reagan, John W. Hinckley, Jr., not guilty by reason of insanity ignited moves to limit or abolish this special plea. Hinckley's trial by jury also turned out to be a trial of law and psychiatry. The psychiatrists and the law allowing their testimony were made the culprits for the unpopular verdict. "The psychiatrists spun sticky webs of pseudo-scientific jargon," wrote a prominent columnist, "and in these webs the concept of justice, like a moth, fluttered feebly and was trapped." The American Bar Association (ABA) and the American Psychiatric Association (APA) quickly issued statements calling for a change in the law. Over 40 bills were introduced in the Congress to amend the law, but none was passed. But they helped defuse the public criticism. At present, Hinckley is hospitalized indefinitely at the federal St. Elizabeth's Hospital in Washington, D.C.

Attempts at reform have included the plea of guilty but mentally ill, which is already used in some jurisdictions. This standard has the advantage of identifying guilt while allowing some adaptation to psychiatric conditions. For example, it allows for treatment in restricted settings while permitting the courts to maintain an active role.

The American Medical Association proposed yet another reform: limiting the insanity exculpation to cases in which the individual is so ill as to lack the necessary criminal intent (*mens rea*). This approach would all but eliminate the insanity defense and place a large burden on the prisons to accept large numbers of mentally ill persons.

The ABA and the APA in their statements of 1982 recommended a defense of nonresponsibility, which focuses solely on whether the defendant, as a result of mental disease or defect, is unable to appreciate the wrongfulness of his or her conduct. These proposals would limit evidence of mental illness to cognition and exclude it on control (but there would apparently still be a defense available under a not-guilty plea—such as extreme emotional disturbance, automatism, provocation, or self-defense—that could be established without psychiatric testimony on mental illness). The APA also urged that "mental illness" be limited to "severely" abnormal mental conditions. These proposals remain controversial, and it is likely that this issue will rise again with each sensational case in which the insanity defense is employed.

Competence to Stand Trial

The U.S. Supreme Court stated that the prohibition against trying someone who is mentally incompetent is fundamental to our system of justice. Accordingly, the Court has approved a test of competence that seeks to ascertain whether a criminal defendant "has sufficient present ability to consult with his lawyer with a reasonable degree of rational understanding—and whether he has a rational as well as factual understanding of the proceedings against him."

MALPRACTICE

Malpractice is the term commonly used to refer to professional negligence. It has also been loosely used to cover intentional or willful invasion of another's legally protected interest, such as battery or treatment without consent. An action based on negligence, whatever the specific situation, involves basic problems of the relation among the parties, risk, and reason.

Four Elements of Malpractice

In order to claim malpractice, the patient, or plantiff, must be able to demonstrate that four elements of malpractice are present. These elements can be mnemonically summarized as the four D's of malpractice: Dereliction (negligence) of a Duty Directly causing Damages.

In negligence, (1) a standard of care requisite under the particular circumstances must exist; (2) a duty must have been owed by the defendant or by someone for whose conduct the defendant is answerable; (3) the duty must have been owed to the plantiff; and (4) a breach of the duty must be the legal cause of the plantiff's asserted damage or injury.

The requisite standard of care under the circumstances may be established in the federal or state constitution, statutes, administrative regulations, court decisions, or the custom of the community. However, the law, with few exceptions, does not specifically define the particular duties. And it is not possible to define the way in which a person ought to act under various circumstances and conditions. As a general rule, professionals have the duty to exercise the degree of skill ordinarily used under similar circumstances by other similar professionals.

Complainants in a malpractice action must prove their allegations by a preponderance of evidence. To sustain the burden of proof, the plaintiff must show (1) an act or omission on the part of the defendant or of someone for whose conduct he or she is answerable, (2) a causal relation between the conduct and the damage or injury allegedly suffered by the plaintiff, and (3) the negligent quality of the conduct. Because most professional conduct is not within the common knowledge of the layperson, expert testimony usually must provide such information.

In relative frequency of malpractice suits, psychiatry ranks eighth among the medical specialties, and in almost every suit for psychiatric malpractice in which liability was imposed, tangible physical injury was demonstrated. The number of suits against psychiatrists is said to be small because of the patient's reluctance to expose a psychiatric history, the skill of the psychiatrist in dealing with the patient's negative feelings, and the difficulty in linking injury with treatment. Psychiatrists have been sued for malpractice for faulty diagnosis or screening, improper certification in commitment, suicide, harmful effects of electroconvulsive treatments and psychotropic drugs, improper divulgence of information, and sexual intimacy with patients (Figure 1).

Sexual intimacy with patients is a significant problem, and it is both illegal and unethical. Serious legal and ethical questions extend to a psychotherapist's even dating or marrying a patient after discharging him or her from therapy.

Preventing Liability

Although it is impossible to eliminate malpractice, some preventive approaches have proved valuable in clinical practice. (1) Clinicians should provide only those kinds of care that they are qualified to offer. They should not overload their practices or overstretch their abilities; they should take reasonable care of themselves; and they should treat their patients with respect. (2) The documentation of good care is a strong deterrent to liability. Such documentation should include the decision-making process, the clinician's rationale for treatment, and an evaluation of costs and benefits. (3) A consultation affords protection against liability because it allows the clinician to obtain information about his or her peer group's standard of practice. It also provides a second opinion, enabling the clinician to submit his or her judgment to the scrutiny of a peer. A clinician who takes the trouble to obtain a consultation in a difficult and complex case is unlikely to be viewed by a jury as careless or negligent. (4) The informed consent process refers to a discussion of the inherent uncertainty of psy-

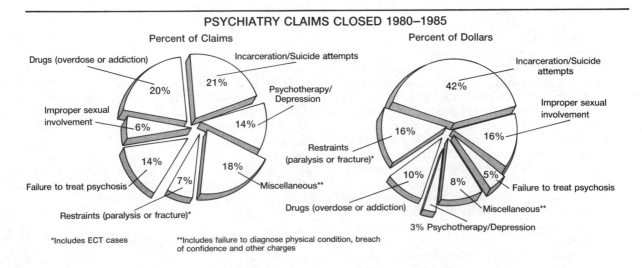

Figure 1   Figure from American Psychiatric Association: Psychiatric News 22:12, 1987. Used with permission.

chiatric practice. Such a dialogue helps prevent a liability suit.

CONSULTATION

Because of the many legal problems with which psychiatrists must deal, the APA in 1982 established the Prepaid Legal Consultation Program. For an annual fee, members of the program can take advantage of an unlimited number of telephone consultations and legal memoranda provided by a Washington, D.C., law firm. Various state psychiatric societies have also initiated such programs. In their operation to date, the most frequently raised issues are (1) malpractice (risks of particular drugs or forms of therapy, commitment and voluntary hospitalization, liability for acts of others, consent forms, insurance coverage, suicide, and duty to warn), (2) business-related matters (billing and bill collection, employment contracts with hospitals or clinics, staff privileges, and advertising), and (3) confidentiality and privilege. Other areas in which members sought advice pertained to patients' access to records, professional incorporation, tax matters, relationships with nonphysician health care providers, office sharing and leases, record keeping, testimony as a witness or expert witness, the meaning of various legal standards, third party issues (most involving private insurance), and referrals to attorneys.

References

Barton W E, Sanborn C F, editors: *Law and the Mental Health Professions: Friction at the Interface*. International Universities Press, New York, 1978.

Bloch S, Chodoff P, editors: *Psychiatric Ethics*. Oxford University Press, New York, 1981.

Bloom J S, Faulkner L R: Competency determinations in civil commitment. Am J Psychiatry *144*:193, 1987.

Ciccone R J, Clemens C: Forensic psychiatry and applied clinical ethics: Theory and practice. Am J Psychiatry *141*:395, 1984.

Gutheil T G, Appelbaum P S: *Clinical Handbook of Psychiatry and the Law*. McGraw-Hill, New York, 1982.

Halleck S L: *Law in the Practice of Psychiatry*. Plenum, New York, 1980.

Hargreaver W A, Shumway M, Knutsen E J, Weinstein A, Senter N: Effects of the *Jamison–Farabee* consent decree: Due process protection for involuntary psychiatric patients treated with psychoactive medication. Am J Psychiatry *144*:188, 1987.

Keliz J, James W S: Medicine court: Rogers in practice. Am J Psychiatry *144*:62, 1987.

Mills M J, Sullivan G, Eth S: Protecting third parties: A recode after Tarasoff. Am J Psychiatry *144*:68, 1987.

Sadoff R L: *Forensic Psychiatry: A Practical Guide for Lawyers and Psychiatrists*. Thomas, Springfield, IL, 1975.

Simon R I: *Psychiatric Interventions and Malpractice*. Thomas, Springfield, IL, 1982.

Simon R I: *Clinical Psychiatry and the Law*. American Psychiatric Press, Washington, DC, 1987.

Slovenko R: *Psychiatry and Law*. Little, Brown, Boston, 1973.

Winslade W J, Ross J W: *The Insanity Plea*. Scribner's, New York, 1983.

Yates A. Should young children testify in cases of sexual abuse? Am J Psychiatry *144*:476, 1987.

Appendix: Thirty Clinical Case Vignettes

The following clinical case vignettes are brief illustrations of various diagnostic categories. They have been drawn from the *DSM-III Case Book,* published by the American Psychiatric Association (1981), edited by R. L. Spitzer, M.D., A. E. Skodol, M.D., M. Gibbon, M.S.W., and J.B.W. Williams, D.S.W., and used with permission. Each vignette is followed by a short discussion which highlights the signs and symptoms presented by the patient. The diagnoses and discussions have been modified to conform to the criteria as listed in DSM-III-R.

Case 1: Schizophreniform Disorder

The patient is a 19-year-old white male who, until admission, was working in a mailroom while waiting to apply to college. The onset of his illness is not clear. According to him, he has not been "the same" since his mother died of a cerebral hemorrhage 9 months before his admission. According to his father, however, he exhibited a normal mourning response to his mother's death and changed only 3 months ago. At that time, shortly after his girl friend had rejected him for another man, he began to think that male co-workers were making homosexual advances to him. He began to fear that he was homosexual and that his friends believed he was homosexual. He finally developed the conviction that there was a disorder of his reproductive system: he had one normal testicle that produced sperm and his other testicle was actually an ovary that produced eggs. He thought this was evidence that a "woman's body resides inside my man's body." He began to gamble and was convinced that he had won $400,000 and was not paid by his bookie, and that he was sought after by talk-show hosts to be a guest on their shows and tell his unusual story (all not true). He claimed that he had a heightened awareness, an "extra sense," and that sounds were unusually loud. He had difficulty sleeping at night, but no appetite disturbance.

On admission his speech was somewhat rapid, and he jumped from topic to topic. His affect was neither irritable, euphoric, nor expansive. He said he was now seeking treatment because "there is a war between my testicles, and I prefer to be a male."

When he was 10, his pediatrician became concerned that he had an undersized penis. This led to a complete endrocrine workup and examinations of his genitals every 4 months for the next 4 years. At that time it was concluded that there were no significant abnormalities.

During high school he was a poor student with poor attendance. He claims always to have had many friends. He has never received psychiatric treatment. He admits to occasional marijuana and phencyclidine use in the past, but denies any use of hallucinogens.

The patient is the oldest child in a family of six children. His parents met when they were both patients in a psychiatric hospital.

Discussion

The significant features of this man's illness include bizarre somatic delusions, grandiose delusions, and disorganization in his speech (jumped from topic to topic). Although the grandiose delusions and pressured speech suggest the possibility of a manic episode, this is ruled out by the absence of either an elevated, expansive, or irritable mood.

When did his illness begin? Although he says he has not been the same since his mother died 9 months ago, he does not describe any change in himself that is out of keeping with normal bereavement. Furthermore, his father claims that his abnormal behavior began only 3 months ago. Giving the patient the benefit of the doubt, we date the onset of the illness at 3 months before admission. The presence of the characteristic symptoms of schizophrenia in an illness of less than 6 months' duration indicates schizophreniform disorder.

DSM-III-R Diagnosis:
Axis I: Schizophreniform Disorder

Case 2: Organic Personality Syndrome

A 34-year-old white male former schoolteacher lives in a halfway house. For the last 2 years he has been unemployed and separated from his wife and children, who avoid him. Two years ago he was in a serious auto accident which resulted in a coma, from which he made a gradual recovery with only supportive medical treatment. Now he has no significant neurological signs except for very minor loss in one visual field. Verbal and performance I.Q. is about 120.

According to the family he has changed since the accident. He is frequently impulsive and argumentative, often misses buses and trains to familiar places, and gets lost. He displays poor social judgment and financial irresponsibility, e.g., he makes long-distance phone calls (including one to the Pope at the Vatican) and then sends the bills to his family.

When seen, the patient was disheveled and joked frequently, but with an undercurrent of bitterness and hostility. A computerized tomography (CT) scan demonstrated large areas of brain tissue destruction, principally in the frontal lobes.

Discussion

The apparently abrupt change in this man's functioning following his recovery from coma secondary to head trauma obviously indicates an organic brain syndrome. Although there is some evidence of memory impairment (often misses buses and trains and gets lost), his high I.Q. is inconsistent with the generalized loss in intellectual functioning of a dementia. Instead, the most prominent features are impulsivity, argumentativeness, poor judgment, and deterioration in self-care, all of which have led to severe occupational and social impairment. These changes in personality, associated with a specific organic factor known to be etiologic to the disturbance (history of trauma and CT scan indicating frontal lobe brain damage), indicate an organic personality syndrome.

DSM-III-R Diagnosis:
Axis I: Organic Personality Syndrome
Axis III: Frontal-lobe brain damage secondary to trauma

Case 3: Alcoholic Hallucinosis

A 44-year-old unemployed male who lived alone in a single-room occupancy hotel was brought to the emergency room by police, to whom he had gone for help, complaining that he was frightened by hearing voices of men in the street below his window talking about him and threatening him with harm. When he looked out the window, the men had always "disappeared."

The patient had a 20-year history of almost daily alcohol use, was commonly "drunk" each day, and often experienced the "shakes" on awakening. On the previous day he had reduced his intake to one pint of vodka, because of gastrointestinal distress. He was fully alert and oriented on mental status examination.

Discussion

Vivid auditory hallucinations that occur in a clear state of consciousness following reduction or cessation of alcohol use indicate alcohol hallucinosis. This is distinguished from alcohol withdrawal delirium by the absence of clouded sensorium and disturbance in attention.

The additional diagnosis of alcohol dependence is made because of the chronic pathological pattern of alcohol use (daily intoxication) and withdrawal (experiencing morning "shakes"). Alcohol hallucinosis apparently develops only in people with a long history of alcohol dependence.

DSM-III-R Diagnosis:
Axis I: Alcohol Hallucinosis
         Alcohol Dependence

Case 4: Psychotic Depression

Sandy, a bright 9-year-old boy, was taken to the pediatric emergency room after his mother found him in the bathroom pressing a knife to his stomach. Examination revealed no more than a minor scratch. Upon questioning, the child told the psychiatric resident that he wanted to die because he didn't want to continue to live the way he did. When specifically questioned, he reported that he was feeling sad, bad, and angry most of the time, that he wasn't having any fun anymore, and that he felt very tired all the time. He had no difficulty falling asleep, but regularly woke up at about 3:00 A.M. and then again at 5:30 A.M. and couldn't fall asleep again. He also reported that he had heard a single voice talking to him, telling him to kill himself with a knife to his belly. He identified the voice as that of his grandfather, who had died 4 years previously from a stroke. He had been hearing such a voice for the last month.

Sandy's mother corroborated his report from her observations and added that the onset was about 6 months ago and that he had gotten progressively worse. Four months ago he began to steal from her and became quite disobedient and had temper tantrums. During the last 2 weeks he had resisted going to school and cried all the way there. She also reported that he had been very preoccupied with the separation of his parents 2 years earlier, and felt it was all his fault. His teacher had reported to her that his attention span was rapidly decreasing and that he had withdrawn from friends and appeared quite sluggish.

Discussion

This case illustrates that a major depressive episode, identical with that seen in adults, can occur in a prepubertal child. There is the persistent depressed mood (feeling sad and bad), loss of pleasure, and such associated depressive symptoms as suicidal ideation and impulses, loss of energy, hypoactivity (appeared quite sluggish), sleep disturbance, inappropriate guilt, and diminished concentration. The fifth-digit subclassification of "with psychotic features" is made because of the presence of auditory hallucinations, although it is not clear whether the child recognizes that the voice is a product of his imagination, which would indicate intact reality testing and, therefore, strictly speaking, no psychotic features.

Although in this case there is also a disturbance of conduct (stealing and disobedience) and school refusal, these are considered age-specific associated features of the depressive episode and do not indicate the need for an additional diagnosis, such as a conduct disorder.

DSM-III-R Diagnosis:
Axis I: Major Depression, Single Episode, with
         Psychotic Features

Case 5: Induced Psychotic Disorder

Ms. B. is a 43-year-old married housewife who entered the hospital in 1968 with a chief complaint of being concerned about her "sex problem"; she stated that she needed hypnotism to find out what was wrong with her sexual drive. Her husband supplied the history; he complained that she had had many extramarital affairs, with many different men, all through their married life. He insisted that in one 2-week period she had had as many as a hundred different sexual experiences with men outside the marriage. The patient herself agreed with this assessment of her behavior, but would not speak of the experiences, saying that she "blocks" the memories out. She denied any particular interest in sexuality, but said that apparently she felt a compulsive drive to go out and seek sexual activity despite her lack of interest.

The patient had been married to her husband for over 20 years. He was clearly the dominant partner in the marriage. The patient was fearful of his frequent jealous rages, and apparently it was he who suggested that she enter the hospital in order to receive hypnosis. The patient maintained that she could not explain why she sought out other men, that she really did not want to do this. Her husband stated that on occasion he had tracked her down, and when he had found her, she acted as if she did not know him. She confirmed this and believed it was due to the fact that the episodes of her sexual promiscuity were blotted out by "amnesia."

When the physician indicated that he questioned the reality of the wife's sexual adventures, the husband became furious and accused the doctor and a ward attendant of having sexual relations with her.

Neither an amytal interview nor considerable psychotherapy with the wife was able to clear the "blocked out" memory of periods of sexual activities. The patient did admit to a memory of having had two extramarital relationships in the past, one 20 years before the time of admission and the other just a year before admission. She stated that the last one had actually been planned by her husband, and that he was in the same house at the time. She continued to believe that she had actually had countless extramarital sexual experiences, though she remembered only two of them.

Discussion

One's first impression is that an amnestic syndrome, either psychogenic or organic, should be considered. However, the plot thickens as evidence accumulates that the husband, the chief informant, has persecutory delusions that his wife is repeatedly unfaithful to him. Apparently, under his influence, his wife has accepted this delusional belief, explaining her lack of memory of the events by believing that she has "amnesia." It would seem that she has adopted his persecutory delusion and does not really have any kind of "amnesia." Since there are none of the essential features of schizophrenia (e.g., bizarre delusions, hallucinations, or incoherence), and because the delusional system developed as a result of a close relationship with another person who had an established disorder with persecutory delusions, the diagnosis is induced psychotic disorder, formerly called shared paranoid disorder in DSM-III and *folie à deux*.

An interesting twist to this case is that it is the patient who, by virtue of her alleged extramarital activity, is the source of the persecution of the husband. It is more common in an induced psychotic disorder for the person who has adopted the other's delusional system to believe that he or she is also being persecuted.

DSM-III-R Diagnosis:
Axis I: Induced Psychotic Disorder

Case 6: Somatization Disorder

A perplexed internist asked for a psychiatric consultation on a 50-year-old divorced and unemployed secretary. When first encountered the patient was lying in bed in a contorted position, with occasional jerking movements of her arms, one every few seconds. Within 10 minutes she was sitting up and explaining that she had been having "a seizure" that was "still there, in my spine. At any minute it can break out and overwhelm me again." Her present difficulties began 2½ months previously with nausea, abdominal cramps, and pain in the extremities that kept her bedridden for several days.

The patient reported having abdominal pain since age 17, necessitating exploratory surgery that yielded no specific diagnosis. She had several pregnancies, each with severe nausea, vomiting, and abdominal pain; she ultimately had a hysterectomy for a "tipped uterus." Since age 40 she had experienced dizziness and "blackouts," which she eventually was told might be multiple sclerosis or a brain tumor. She continued to be bedridden for extended periods of time, with weakness, blurred vision, and difficulty urinating. At age 43 she was worked up for a hiatal hernia because of complaints of bloating and intolerance of a variety of foods. She also had additional hospitalizations for neurological, hypertensive, and renal workups, all of which failed to reveal a definitive diagnosis.

She has been divorced since age 32 and has worked very sporadically. She lives with her only child, an adult son. They lead a rather vagabond life, settling for a few months at a time in a residential hotel, then moving on to another city. They have no significant relationships other than with each other. She avoids heterosexual encounters, explaining that "sex has never turned me on."

Discussion

This is a chronic, polysymptomatic disorder of physically unexplainable symptoms involving multiple organ systems. There are gastrointestinal symptoms (nausea, abdominal cramps, vomiting, bloating, food intolerance), conversion or pseudoneurological symptoms (seizure, blurred vision, and blackouts), female reproductive symptoms (nausea and vomiting during pregnancy), psychosexual symptoms (sexual indifference), pain (extremity, abdominal), and cardiopulmonary symptoms (dizziness). These symptoms have led to numerous medical workups and hospitalizations. This clinical picture, far more common in women than in men, in the past referred to as hysteria or Briquet's syndrome, is now called somatization disorder.

Although conversion symptoms are present (e.g., seizure), the diagnosis of conversion disorder is not made since the full clinical picture of somatization disorder is present. In this case there is no evidence of voluntary production of the symptoms, which would suggest factitious disorder with physical symptoms. Frequently, although not invariably, somatization disorder is associated with histrionic personality disorder. In this case there is no evidence to justify that additional diagnosis.

DSM-III-R Diagnosis:
Axis I: Somatization Disorder

Case 7: Atypical Psychosis

This 42-year-old socialite has never had any psychiatric problems before. A new performance hall is to be formally opened with the world premiere of a new ballet; and the patient, because of her position on the cultural council, has taken on the responsibility for coordinating that event. However, construction problems, including strikes, have made it uncertain that the finishing details will meet the deadline. The set designer has been volatile, threatening to walk out on the project unless the materials meet his meticulous specifications. The patient has had to attempt to calm this volatile man while attempting to coax disputing groups to negotiate. She has also had increased responsibilities at home since her housekeeper has had to leave to visit a sick relative.

In the midst of these difficulties, the patient's best friend is decapitated in a tragic auto crash. The patient herself is an only child, and her best friend had been very close to her since grade school. People have often commented that the two women were like sisters. Immediately following the funeral, the patient becomes increasingly tense and jittery, and able to sleep only 2 to 3 hours a night. Two days later she happens to see a woman driving a car just like the one that her friend had driven. She immediately becomes puzzled, and after a few hours she becomes convinced that her friend is alive, that the accident had been staged, along with the funeral, as part of a plot. Somehow the plot is directed toward deceiving the patient, and she senses that somehow she is in great danger and must solve the mystery to escape alive. She begins to distrust everyone except her husband, and begins to believe that the phone is tapped and the rooms "bugged." She pleads with her husband to help save her life. She begins to hear a high-pitched, undulating sound, which she fears is an ultrasound beam aimed at her. She is in a state of sheer panic, gripping her husband's arm in terror, as he brings her to the emergency room the next morning.

Discussion

Our initial impression was that this was a rather straightforward example of brief reactive psychosis. A severe psychosocial stressor (the death and funeral of her friend) preceded the development of psychotic symptoms (persecutory delusions and, later, auditory hallucinations) in a thus far short-lived illness. On further reflection, however, we realized that the psychotic symptoms did not begin *immediately* after the stressor, as is the case in brief reactive psychosis, but two days later. Moreover, although the patient was tense and jittery, she displayed no evidence of emotional turmoil—that is, rapid shifts from one dysphoric affect to another without the persistence of any one affect.

Since the predominant symptoms are persecutory de-

lusions, acute delusional disorder needs to be considered; but that diagnosis requires a duration of illness of at least 1 week. Furthermore, some clinicians would regard the patient's delusion of an ultrasound "beam aimed at her" as bizarre, which would rule out a delusional disorder and suggest schizophreniform disorder. We are therefore left with the residual category of atypical psychosis. If the illness persists for more than a week or two (but less than 6 months), the diagnosis can be changed to acute delusional disorder or schizophreniform disorder.

DSM-III-R Diagnosis:
Axis I: Atypical Psychosis (Provisional)
              R/O Acute Delusional Disorder, Schizophreni-
              form Disorder

Case 8: Schizophrenia

Susan, a 15-year-old, was seen at the request of her school district authorities for advice on placement. She had recently moved into the area with her family and, after a brief period in a regular class, was placed in a class for the emotionally disturbed. She proved very difficult, with a very poor understanding of schoolwork at about the fifth-grade level, despite an apparently good vocabulary; and she disturbed the class by making animal noises and telling fantastic stories, which made the other children laugh at her.

At home Susan is aggressive, biting or hitting her parents or brother if frustrated. She is often bored, has no friends, and finds it difficult to occupy herself. She spends a lot of time drawing pictures of robots, spaceships, and fantastic or futuristic inventions. Sometimes she has said she would like to die, but she has never made any attempt at suicide, and apparently has not thought of killing herself. Her mother says that from birth she has been different, and that the onset of her current behavior has been so gradual that no definite date can be assigned to it.

Susan's prenatal and parental history are unremarkable. Her milestones were delayed, and she did not use single words until 4 or 5 years of age. Ever since she entered school there has been concern about her ability. Repeated evaluations have suggested an I.Q. in the lower 70s, with achievement somewhat behind even that expected at this level of ability. Because her father was in the military, there have been many moves; and results of her earlier evaluations are not available.

The parents report that Susan has always been difficult and restless, and that several doctors have said she is not just mentally retarded but suffers from a serious mental disorder. The results of an evaluation done at the age of 12, because of difficulties in school, showed "evidence of bizarre thought processes and fragmented ego structure." At this time she was sleeping well at night and was not getting up with nightmares or bizarre requests, though this apparently had been a feature of her earlier behavior. Currently she is reported to sleep very poorly and tends to disturb the household by getting up and wandering around at night. Her mother emphasizes Susan's unpredictability, the funny stories that she tells, and the way in which she will talk to herself in "funny voices." Her mother regards the stories Susan tells as childish make-believe and pre-occupation and pays little attention to them. She says that since Susan went to see the movie *Star Wars* she has been obsessed with ideas about space, spaceships, and the future.

Her parents are in their early 40s. Her father, having retired from military service, now works as an engineer. Susan's mother has many unusual beliefs about herself. She claims to have grown up in India and to have had a very bizarre early childhood full of dramatic and violent episodes. Many of these episodes sound highly improbable. Her husband refuses to let her talk about her past in his presence and tries to play down this material and Susan's problems. The parents appear to have a rather restricted relationship in which the father plays the role of a taciturn, masterful head of household and the mother bears the brunt of everyday family duties. The mother, in contrast, is loquacious and very circumstantial in her history-giving. She dwells a great deal on her strange childhood experiences. Susan's brother is now 12 and apparently is a normal child with an average school career. He does not spend much time in the house or with the family, but prefers to play with his friends. He is ashamed of Susan's behavior and tries to avoid going out with her.

In the interview Susan presented as a tall, overweight, pasty-looking child, dressed untidily and with a somewhat disheveled appearance. She complained vociferously of her insomnia, though it was very difficult to elicit details of the sleep disturbance. She talked at length about her interests and occupations. She says she made a robot in the basement that ran amok and was about to cause a great deal of damage, but she was able to stop it by remote control. She claims to have built the robot from spare computer parts, which she acquired from the local museum. When pressed on details of how this worked, she became increasingly vague, and when asked to draw a picture of one of her inventions, drew a picture of an overhead railway and went into what appeared to be complex mathematical calculations to substantiate the structural details, but which in fact consisted of meaningless repetitions of symbols (e.g., plus, minus, divide, multiply). When the interviewer expressed some gentle incredulity, she blandly replied that many people did not believe that she was a supergenius. She also talked about her unusual ability to hear things other people cannot hear, and said she was in communication with some sort of creature. She thought she might be haunted, or perhaps the creature was a being from another planet. She could hear his voice talking to her and asking her questions; he did not attempt to tell her what to do. The voice was outside her own head, but was inaudible to others. She did not regard the questions being asked her as upsetting. They did not make her angry or frightened.

Her teacher comments that although Susan's reading is apparently at the fifth-grade level, her comprehension is much lower. She tends to read what is not there and sometimes changes the meaning of the paragraph. Her spelling is at about the third-grade level, and her mathematics a little bit below that. She works hard at school, though very slowly. If pressure is placed on her, she becomes upset, and her work deteriorates.

Discussion

At the present time Susan exhibits several psychotic symptoms. She apparently is delusional in that she believes that she has made a complicated invention and that she is in communication with "some sort of creature." She has auditory hallucinations of voices talking to her and asking her questions. The presence of delusions and hallucinations, in the absence of a specific organic etiology or of a full affective syndrome, raises the question of schizophrenia.

The DSM-III-R criteria for schizophrenia require deterioration from a previous level of functioning in such areas as work, social relations, and self-care. The major intent of this particular criterion was to exclude cases in which the illness did not seem to be associated with any impairment in functioning. For example, there are rare instances in which an individual may harbor a bizarre delusion for many years without any noticeable impairment in functioning, and it seemed advisable to differentiate such a condition from schizophrenia. (Such an unusual case would probably end up with a diagnosis of atypical psychosis.) The problem in this case is not the absence of functional impairment, but whether or not there has been deterioration. Susan's mother says that she was "different" from birth, her developmental milestones were delayed, and she did not use single words until 4 or 5 years of age. Is her current psychotic behavior a deterioration from this level of functioning? Perhaps it is difficult or impossible to make such a judgment when serious psychopathology is present at a very early age. Should such cases not be diagnosed as schizophrenia, even if the characteristic schizophrenic symptoms are present at a later age? Some would argue that schizophrenia should be diagnosed only when a psychotic illness develops in an individual with a relatively intact personality. According to this view, Susan should not be diagnosed as having schizophrenia. Others would argue that frequently, as in Susan's case, the prodromal phase of severe forms of schizophrenia may be evident in early childhood. We take the latter view, partly because we think that a history of severe disturbance at an early age may not be that unusual in cases that later seem to develop a typical schizophrenic illness. Therefore, our diagnosis of Susan is schizophrenia, chronic. Although her delusions have a grandiose quality, they seem too diffuse to justify paranoid type. In the absence of prominent catatonic features or frequent incoherence, we are left with undifferentiated type.

DSM-III-R Diagnosis:
Axis I: Schizophrenia, Chronic, Undifferentiated Type

Case 9: Alcohol Dementia

A medical student on rotation at a chronic-disease hospital was assigned to present at rounds a 56-year-old retired chief petty officer. The patient was a long-time heavy consumer of alcoholic beverages. Following his divorce many years previously, his drinking had become exceptionally heavy, and he underwent a change in personality. He was often belligerent, even when sober, and on several occasions had assaulted members of his family. This disturbing behavior had necessitated two brief admissions to mental hospitals. The patient persisted in his heavy drinking, and on several other occasions had been admitted to hospitals for tremulousness and hallucinations associated with alcohol withdrawal. As far as was known, he had never had major trauma or a stroke. Finally, because of his inability to care for himself properly, he had been sent to live in a nursing home; but because of his belligerent and disruptive behavior, admission to this hospital had been found necessary 7 years earlier.

When examined by the student, the patient was somewhat peevish and inattentive. His consciousness was not clouded, however, and he was not hallucinating. He knew the name of the hospital, but not the correct date. He could not retain the names of five objects after a brief interval of distraction. He remembered events of his youth and young manhood, but not those of more recent years. He remembered the dispute between President Truman and General MacArthur, but had no recollection of the Watergate affair. His language was normal, but he could not copy the drawing of a two- or three-dimensional figure. He could not do even the simplest of calculations, and he interpreted proverbs very concretely. Neurological examinations revealed somewhat diminished ankle jerks, and there was mild unsteadiness of gait. Laboratory tests failed to reveal any positive evidence for the etiology of the disturbance.

Discussion

The short-term and recent memory disturbances suggest an amnestic syndrome; but the marked loss of intellectual abilities, the personality change, the poor judgment, and other disturbances of higher cortical functioning (e.g., inability to copy drawings and do calculations, and concrete responses to proverbs) all indicate the presence of the more global disturbance, a dementia.

The differential diagnosis of dementia involves a search for specific causes, such as trauma (particularly important with a history of alcohol dependence) and brain tumor. In this case, the absence of a history of trauma and the failure of the laboratory tests to reveal the etiology of the dementia make prolonged heavy drinking the most likely etiologic agent; thus, the diagnosis is dementia associated with alcoholism.

DSM-III-R Diagnosis:
Axis I: Dementia Associated with Alcoholism

Case 10: Alcohol Withdrawal

A 43-year-old divorced carpenter is examined in the hospital emergency observation ward. The patient's sister is available to provide some information. The sister reports that the patient has consumed large quantities of cheap wine daily for over 5 years. Evidently the patient had a reasonably stable home life and job record until his wife left him for another man 5 years previously. The sister indicates that the patient drinks more than a fifth of wine a day, and that this has been an unvarying pattern since the divorce. He often has had blackouts from drinking and has missed work; consequently, he has been fired from several jobs. Fortu-

nately for him, carpenters are in great demand, and he has been able to provide marginally for himself during these years. However, 3 days ago he ran out of money and wine and had to beg on the street to buy a meal. The patient has been poorly nourished, eating perhaps one meal a day and evidently relying on the wine as his prime source of nourishment.

The morning after his last day of drinking (3 days ago), he felt increasingly tremulous, his hands shaking so grossly that it was difficult for him to light a cigarette. Accompanying this was an increasing sense of inner panic, which had made him virtually unable to sleep. A neighbor became concerned about the patient when he seemed not to be making sense and clearly was unable to take care of himself. The neighbor contacted the sister, who brought him to the hospital.

On examination, the patient alternates between apprehension and chatty, superficial warmth. He is quite keyed up and talks almost constantly. At times he recognizes the doctor, but at other times he thinks the doctor is his older brother. Twice during the examination he calls the doctor by his older brother's name and asks when he arrived, evidently having lost track entirely of the interview up to that point. He has a gross hand tremor at rest, and there are periods when he picks at "bugs" he sees on the bed sheets. He is disoriented for time and thinks that he is in a supermarket parking lot rather than in a hospital. He indicates that he feels he is fighting against a terrifying sense that the world is ending in a holocaust. He is startled every few minutes by sounds and scenes of fiery car crashes (evidently provoked by the sound of rolling carts in the hall). Efforts at testing memory and calculation fail because his attention shifts too rapidly. An electroencephalogram indicates a pattern of diffuse encephalopathy.

Discussion

This carpenter, with a long history of heavy alcohol use, develops severe withdrawal symptoms after he stops drinking. He has a gross hand tremor, anxiety, disorientation to time and place, misinterpretations (thinking the doctor is his brother), visual hallucinations (picking at "bugs" on the bed sheets), difficulty sustaining attention, and synesthesias (he sees scenes of car crashes provoked by the sound of rolling carts in the hall).

Although the treatment will initially be directed at the alcohol withdrawal delirium, the additional diagnosis of alcohol dependence is warranted by the pathological pattern of use (need for daily use, consumption of more than a fifth of alcohol each day, blackouts) and the patient's social and occupational impairment (fired from several jobs).

DSM-III Diagnosis:
Axis I: Alcohol Withdrawal Delirium
          Alcohol Dependence

Case 11: Codeine Dependence

A 42-year-old executive in a public relations firm was referred for psychiatric consultation by his surgeon, who discovered him sneaking large quantities of a codeine-containing cough medicine into the hospital. The patient had been a heavy cigarette smoker for 20 years and had a chronic, hacking cough. He had come into the hospital for a hernia repair, and found the pain from the incision unbearable when he coughed.

An operation on his back 5 years previously had led his doctor to prescribe codeine to help relieve the incisional pain at that time. Over the intervening 5 years, however, he had continued to use codeine-containing tablets and had increased his intake to 60 to 90 5-mg tablets daily. He stated that he often "just took them by the handful—not to feel good, you understand, just to get by." He had tried several times to stop using codeine, but had failed. During this period he lost two jobs because of lax work habits and was divorced by his wife of 11 years.

Discussion

The presence of tolerance to codeine, that is, markedly increased amounts are needed to achieve the desired effect (his taking 60 to 90 tablets a day), indicates psychiatric substance dependence. The diagnosis is coded as opioid dependence, because codeine is classified as an opioid. However, the name of the specific substance, codeine, rather than the class of substance, opioid, is recorded. The course is classified as continuous since there has been more or less regular maladaptive use for over 6 months.

DSM-III-R Diagnosis:
Axis I: Codeine Dependence, Continuous

Case 12: Psychogenic Amnesia

Psychiatric consultation was requested by an emergency-room physician on an 18-year-old male who had been brought into the hospital by the police. The youth appeared exhausted and showed evidence of prolonged exposure to the sun. He identified the current date incorrectly, giving it as September 27 instead of October 1. It was difficult to get him to focus on specific questions, but with encouragement he supplied a number of facts. He recalled sailing with friends, apparently about September 25, on a weekend cruise off the Florida coast, when bad weather was encountered. He was unable to recall any subsequent events and did not know what had become of his companions or how he had gotten to the hospital. He had to be reminded several times that he was in a hospital, since he expressed uncertainty as to his whereabouts. Each time he was told, he seemed surprised.

There was no evidence of head injury or dehydration. Electrolytes and cranial nerve examination were unremarkable. Because of the patient's apparent exhaustion, he was permitted to sleep for 6 hours. Upon awakening, he was much more attentive, but was still unable to recall events after September 27, including how he had come to the hospital. There was no longer any doubt in his mind that he was in the hospital, however; and he was able to recall the contents of the previous interview and the fact that he had fallen asleep. He was able to remember that he was a student at a southern college, maintained a B average, had a small group of close friends, and reported a good relationship with his family. He denied any previous psychiatric history and did not abuse drugs or alcohol.

Because of the patient's apparently sound physical condition, a sodium amytal interview was performed. During this interview he related that neither he nor his companions were particularly experienced sailors capable of coping with the ferocity of the storm they had encountered. Although he had taken the precaution of securing himself to the boat with a life jacket and tie line, his companions had failed to do this and had been washed overboard in the heavy seas. He had completely lost control of the boat and felt he was saved only by virtue of good luck and his lifeline. Over a 3 day period, he had been able to consume a small supply of food that was stowed away in the cabin. He never saw either of his sailing companions again. He had been picked up on October 1 by a Coast Guard cutter and brought to shore, and subsequently the police had brought him to the hospital.

Discussion

The differential diagnosis of acute memory loss begins with a consideration of an organic mental disorder, such as delirium, dementia, or amnestic syndrome, which may be due to head trauma, cerebrovascular accidents, or drug use. The normal physical and neurological examination and the absence of a history of drug use rule out these possibilities in this patient. With the amytal interview it becomes clear that the amnestic period developed following a particularly traumatic and life-threatening experience. Amnesia (memory loss that is too extensive to be considered "forgetfulness") that is not due to an organic mental disorder justifies the diagnosis psychogenic amnesia. In this case, the circumscribed nature of the amnesia and the perplexity and disorientation during the amnestic period, all following a traumatic event, are quite characteristic of the diagnosed disorder.

DSM-III-R Diagnosis:
Axis I: Psychogenic Amnesia

Case 13: Conversion Disorder

A 46-year-old married housewife was referred by her husband's psychiatrist for consultation. In the course of discussing certain marital conflicts that he was having with his wife, the husband had described "attacks" of dizziness that his wife experienced that left her quite incapacitated.

In consultation, the wife described being overcome with feelings of extreme dizziness, accompanied by slight nausea, four or five nights a week. During these attacks, the room around her would take on a "shimmering" appearance, and she would have the feeling that she was "floating" and unable to keep her balance. Inexplicably, the attacks almost always occurred at about 4:00 P.M. She usually had to lie down on the couch and often did not feel better until 7:00 or 8:00 P.M. After recovering, she generally spent the rest of the evening watching TV; and more often than not, she would fall asleep in the living room, not going to bed in the bedroom until 2:00 or 3:00 in the morning.

The patient had been pronounced physically fit by her

internist, a neurologist, and an ENT specialist on more than one occasion. Hypoglycemia had been ruled out by glucose tolerance tests.

When asked about her marriage, the patient described her husband as a tyrant, frequently demanding and verbally abusive of her and their four children. She admitted that she dreaded his arrival home from work each day, knowing that he would comment that the house was a mess and the dinner, if prepared, not to his liking. Recently, since the onset of her attacks, when she was unable to make dinner he and the four kids would go to McDonald's or the local pizza parlor. After that, he would settle in to watch a ball game in the bedroom, and their conversation was minimal. In spite of their troubles, the patient claimed that she loved her husband and needed him very much.

Discussion

This woman complains of a variety of physical symptoms (dizziness, nausea, visual disturbances, loss of balance) that all suggest a physical disorder; but thorough examinations by a number of medical specialists have failed to detect a physical disorder that could account for the symptoms. With a specific physical disorder ruled out, the differential diagnosis is between undiagnosed physical symptoms and a mental disorder.

The context in which these symptoms occur suggests the role of psychological factors in their development: they recur at virtually the same time each day, closely associated with the husband's arrival home from work; the symptoms enable the patient to avoid both her husband's angry tirades and her responsibility for preparing evening meals. Since there is no evidence that the patient is voluntarily producing the symptoms (e.g., taking a drug that would induce such symptoms or claiming to have the symptoms when they are not present), diagnoses of a factitious disorder or malingering are ruled out. The disorder is a somatoform disorder—a mental disorder with physical symptoms that suggest a physical disorder.

Since the patient's complaints are not part of a long-standing polysymptomatic disturbance involving many organ systems, somatization disorder is excluded. The symptoms are all limited to an alteration in physical functioning; hence, the diagnosis is conversion disorder.

DSM-III-R Diagnosis:
Axis I: Conversion Disorder

Case 14: Somatoform Pain Disorder

A 29-year-old married woman was presented as the neurology patient of a Psychiatric Specialty Board examination. Three months previously she had been riding in a car driven by her husband that was involved in a minor traffic accident. She was thrown forward, but was kept from hitting the window or dashboard by her seat belt. Three days later she began to complain of a stiff neck and sharp, radiating pains down both arms, her spine to the small of her back, and both legs. Because an orthopedic consultation failed to uncover the cause of the pain, she was referred to the neurology clinic.

The patient was an attractive, statuesque woman in obvious distress who described her injury and her symptoms in vivid detail, tracing the course of her pains down her arms and legs with her hands. She smiled frequently at the young psychiatrist and at the two examiners who were observing him. She performed each test of neurologic function with precision and appeared to relish the attention. The neurologic examination findings were totally normal.

The psychiatrist inquired into the patient's past history and present life. There was no previous history of emotional disturbance. The patient currently worked as a computer programmer. She had been married for 4 years and had no children. Until recently her marriage had been smooth, except that her husband sometimes complained that they were "mismatched" sexually, in that he seemed considerably more interested in frequent and "imaginative" sex, while she seemed satisfied with weekly intercourse without variation or much foreplay.

Two weeks before the accident the patient had discovered a woman's phone number in her husband's wallet. When she confronted him with it, he admitted that he had seen several women over the preceding year, mainly for "sexual release." The patient was bitterly hurt and disappointed for several days, then began to get angry and attacked him for his "hang-ups." At the time of the accident, they had been arguing in the car on the way to a friend's house for dinner. After the accident they decided to try harder to please each other in their marriage, including sexually; but because of the pains that the patient was experiencing, they had not been able to have any sexual contact.

The young psychiatrist passed the exam.

Discussion

The absence of physical findings and the apparent genuineness of the symptoms rule out physical disorder, malingering, and a factitious disorder. This leaves us with the pain as an undiagnosed physical symptom or somatoform pain disorder. The issue then revolves around positive evidence for the role of psychological factors in initiating the disorder.

It is difficult to escape the conclusion that this woman's pain serves the function of enabling her to avoid an activity that is noxious to her, having to deal with both her husband's increasing sexual demands and their apparent sexual incompatibility. Further positive evidence of the role of psychological factors is the temporal relationship between the onset of the symptoms and the discovery of and argument about the husband's extramarital sexual activity.

DSM-III-R Diagnosis:
Axis I: Somatoform Pain Disorder

Case 15: Hypochondriasis

A 38-year-old radiologist is evaluated after returning from a 10-day stay at a famous out-of-state diagnostic center to which he had been referred by a local gastroenterologist after "he reached the end of the line with me." He reports that he underwent extensive physical and laboratory examinations there, including x-ray examinations of the entire gastrointestinal tract, esophagoscopy, gastroscopy, and colonoscopy. Although he was told that the results of the examinations were negative for significant physical disease, he appears resentful and disappointed rather than relieved at the findings. He was seen briefly for a "routine" evaluation by a psychiatrist at the diagnostic center, but had difficulty relating to the psychiatrist on more than a superficial level.

On further inquiry concerning the patient's physical symptoms, he describes occasional twinges of mild abdominal pain, sensations of "fullness," "bowel rumblings," and a "firm abdominal mass" that he can sometimes feel in his left lower quadrant. Over the last few months he has gradually become more aware of these sensations and convinced that they may be due to a carcinoma of the colon. He tests his stool for occult blood weekly and spends 15 to 20 minutes every 2 to 3 days carefully palpating his abdomen as he lies in bed at home. He has secretly performed several x-ray studies on himself in his own office after hours.

Although he is successful in his work, has an excellent attendance record, and is active in community life, the patient spends much of his limited leisure time at home alone in bed. His wife, an instructor at a local school of nursing, is angry and bitter about this behavior, which she describes as "robbing us of what we've worked so hard and postponed so much fun for." Although she and the patient share many values and genuinely love each other, his behavior causes a real strain on their marriage.

When the patient was 13 years old, a heart murmur was detected on a school physical exam. Since a younger brother had died in early childhood of congenital heart disease, the patient was removed from gym class until the murmur could be evaluated. The evaluation proved the murmur to be benign, but the patient began to worry that the evaluation might have "missed something" and considered his occasional sensations of "skipping a beat" as evidence that this was so. He kept his fears to himself, and they subsided over the next 2 years, but never entirely left him.

As a second year medical student he was relieved to share some of his health concerns with his classmates, who also worried about having the diseases they were learning about in pathology. He realized, however, that he was much more preoccupied with and worried about his health than they were. Since graduating from medical school, he has repeatedly experienced a series of concerns, each following the same pattern: noticing a symptom, becoming increasingly preoccupied with what it might mean, and having a negative physical evaluation. At times he returns to an "old" concern, but is too embarrassed to pursue it with physicians he knows, as when he discovered a "suspicious" nevus only one week after he had persuaded a dermatologist to biopsy one that proved to be entirely benign.

The patient tells his story with a sincere, discouraged tone, brightened only by a note of genuine pleasure and enthusiasm as he provides a detailed account of the discovery of a genuine but clinically insignificant ureteral anomaly as the result of an intravenous pyelogram he had ordered himself. Near the end of the interview he explains that his coming in for evaluation now is largely at his own insistence, precipitated by an encounter with his 9-year-old son. The boy had accidentally walked in while he was palpating his own abdomen for "masses" and asked, "What do you think it is this time, Dad?" As he describes his shame and anger (mostly at himself) about this incident, his eyes fill with tears.

Discussion

It is apparent that this doctor's symptoms are not due to any physical disorder. Preoccupation with physical symptoms without an organic basis can be seen in psychotic disorders, such as schizophrenia or major depression with psychotic features, but there is no evidence of any psychotic features in this case. This suggests, therefore, a somatoform disorder—a mental disorder with physical symptoms suggesting physical disorder, but for which there is positive evidence, or a strong presumption, that the symptoms are linked to psychological factors.

A variety of physical symptoms without organic basis is seen in somatization disorder. In this case the symptoms are few, whereas in somatization disorder there is a large number of different symptoms that appear in many different organ systems. Furthermore, in somatization disorder the preoccupation is generally with the symptoms themselves. In this case the disturbance is preoccupation with the fear of having a serious disease resulting from the unrealistic interpretation of physical signs or sensations. The persistence of this irrational fear, despite medical reassurance, to the point that it interferes with social and/or occupational functioning indicates hypochondriasis.

DSM-III-R Diagnosis:
Axis I: Hypochondriasis

Case 16: Exhibitionism

A 27-year-old engineer requested consultation because of irresistible urges to exhibit his naked penis to female strangers.

The patient, an only child, had been reared in an orthodox Jewish environment. Sexuality was strongly condemned by both parents as being "dirty." His father, a schoolteacher, was authoritarian and punitive, but relatively uninvolved in the home. His mother, a housewife, was domineering, controlling, and intrusive. She was preoccupied with cleanliness and bathed the patient until he was 10 years old. The patient remembers that he feared he might have an erection in his mother's presence during one of his baths; however, this did not occur. His mother was opposed to his meeting and dating girls during his adolescence. He was not allowed to bring girls home; according to her, the proper time to bring a woman home was when she was "your wife, and not before." Despite his mother's antisexual values, she frequently walked about the house partially disrobed in his presence. To his shame, he found himself sexually aroused by this stimulation, which occurred frequently throughout his development.

As an adolescent the patient was quiet, withdrawn, and studious; teachers described him as a "model child." He was friendly but not intimate with a few male classmates. Puberty occurred at 13, and his first ejaculation occurred at that age during sleep. Because of feelings of guilt, he resisted the temptation to masturbate, and between the ages of 13 and 18 orgasms occurred only with nocturnal emissions.

He did not begin to date women until he moved out of his parents' home, at age 25. During the next 2 years he dated from time to time, but was too inhibited to initiate sexual activity.

At age 18, for reasons unknown to himself, during the week before final exams, he first experienced an overwhelming desire to engage in the sexual activity for which he now sought consultation. He sought situations in which he was alone with a woman he did not know. As he would approach her, he became sexually excited. He would then walk up to her and display his erect penis. He found that her shock and fear further stimulated him, and usually he would then ejaculate. At other times he fantasized past encounters while masturbating.

He felt guilty and ashamed after exhibiting himself and vowed never to repeat it. Nevertheless, the desire often overwhelmed him, and the behavior recurred frequently, usually at periods of tension. He felt desperate, but was too ashamed to seek professional help. Once, when he was 24, he had almost been apprehended by a policeman, but managed to run away.

For the last 3 years the patient has managed to resist his exhibitionistic urges. Recently, however, he met a young woman, who has fallen in love with him and is willing to have sexual intercourse with him. Never having had intercourse before, he felt panic lest he fail in the attempt. He likes and respects his potential sexual partner, but also condemns her for being willing to engage in premarital relations. He has once again started to exhibit himself and fears that, unless he stops, he will eventually be arrested.

Discussion

One could discuss at great length the childhood experiences that may have contributed to the development of this disorder in this patient. Regarding the diagnosis, however, there can be little discussion. The repetitive exposing of his genitals to strangers for the purpose of achieving sexual excitement with no attempt at further sexual activity establishes the diagnosis of exhibitionism.

Many clinicians would assume that there is also a coexisting personality disorder, but without more information about the patient's personality functioning, such a diagnosis cannot be made.

DSM-III-R Diagnosis:
Axis I: Exhibitionism

Case 17: Inhibited Female Orgasm

The patient, a 25-year-old female laboratory technician, has been married to a 32-year-old cabdriver for 5 years. The couple has a two-year-old son, and the marriage appears harmonious.

The presenting complaint is the wife's lifelong inability to experience orgasm. She has never achieved orgasm, although during sexual activity she has received what should have been sufficient stimulation. She has tried to masturbate, and on many occasions her husband has manually stimulated her patiently for lengthy periods of time. Although she does not reach climax, she is strongly attracted to her husband, feels erotic pleasure during lovemaking, and lubricates copiously. According to both of them, the husband has no sexual difficulty.

Exploration of her thoughts as she nears orgasm reveals a vague sense of dread of some undefined disaster. More generally, she is anxious about losing control over her emotions, which she normally keeps closely in check. She is particularly uncomfortable about expressing any anger or hostility.

Physical examination reveals no abnormality.

Discussion

This woman's sexual difficulties are limited to the orgasm phase of the sexual response cycle (she has no difficulty in desiring sex or in becoming excited). During lovemaking there is what would ordinarily be an adequate amount of stimulation. The report of a "vague sense of dread of some undefined disaster" as she approaches orgasm is evidence that her inability to have orgasms represents a pathological inhibition. There is no suggestion of any other Axis I disorder or any physical disorder that could account for the disturbance. Thus, the diagnosis is inhibited female orgasm.

If with treatment it became apparent that the fear of loss of control was a symptom of a personality disorder, such as obsessive-compulsive personality disorder, the diagnosis of a psychosexual dysfunction would nonetheless prevail. It is only when a sexual disturbance is judged to be symptomatic of another Axis I disorder, such as major depression, that the diagnosis of a psychosexual dysfunction is not made.

DSM-III-R Diagnosis:
Axis I: Inhibited Female Orgasm

Case 18: Intermittent Explosive Disorder

A 31-year-old housewife sought help because of a 2-to-3-year history of temper outbursts associated with increasing marital discord. During the past few years she had had increasing difficulty with her husband, whom she suspected of having an affair with his secretary. She ruminated angrily about his possible deception whenever he claimed to be working late. During such ruminative episodes, she felt her tension "building up," and would often attempt to "discharge it" by calisthenics; but she still found herself "exploding" when her husband eventually came home. On one occasion she threw a glass at him; on another, she banged on the walls of her house with her high-heeled shoes, causing the plaster to crumble; and on yet another occasion she put her hand through a window when her husband left abruptly after one of her outbursts. Before each outburst she tried to remain calm, but often experienced a headache and a feeling of "strangeness" when she saw her husband coming home. At this point she would usually lose control and become violent. Following the outburst she felt depressed and remorseful, recognizing that her outbursts were "crazy"—even if her suspicions were justified. She also admitted that when the children cried or were impatient when she was in one of her ruminative periods, she was overzealous in her discipline and often found herself slapping them or punishing them more harshly than she ordinarily would. On one occasion she had lost her temper when one of her children would not go to sleep and had slapped him hard enough to cause a bruise on his face.

The episodes of loss of control occurred one to two times a month, but had seemed to be increasing over the past year. Between these episodes the patient was generally calm and displayed no signs of aggressiveness.

Past history revealed that at the age of 8 the patient had been knocked unconscious for a short period of time in a roller-skating accident, but had no medical intervention for this injury. Apparently she had sustained repeated head injuries, to the point where the family urged her to "wear a football helmet" because she was so clumsy.

An electroencephalogram (EEG) was done after the patient entered therapy and revealed a nonspecific abnormality, a 6 to 14-second dysrhythmia. During the course of her treatment she confronted her husband, who finally acknowledged that he was having an affair with his secretary.

Discussion

This woman entered therapy because she realized that, even if her suspicions about her husband were warranted, her angry outbursts were inappropriate and markedly at variance with her normally unaggressive behavior. Each outburst was preceded by a mounting sense of tension and followed by feelings of remorse. These features suggest an impulse disorder, specifically, intermittent explosive disorder.

The diagnosis in this case hinges on two issues. Do the outbursts result in "serious assaultive acts or destruction of property," and is the behavior "grossly out of proportion to any precipitating psychosocial stressors?" The patient had on one occasion broken a window with her fist and on another bruised her child's face. These acts just make it past our threshold for serious assault and destruction of property, although some more worldly clinicians might be unimpressed. (One could argue that no degree of rage is "out of proportion" to the provocation of a lying, unfaithful husband.) But what about her losing control with her child when he refused to go to sleep? We are inclined to think that this behavior is grossly out of proportion to the provocation. Therefore, we propose the provisional diagnosis intermittent explosive disorder, because of our own uncertainty about the boundary between this disorder and the "normal" temper outbursts to which relations between spouses and between parents and children may give rise. In this case, particularly because of the potential for child abuse, we think it better to err on the side of making a diagnosis that justifies treatment directed at the patient's loss of impulse control.

The EEG abnormality suggests an underlying disorder of the central nervous system, as is often the case in patients with this disorder. This is the basis for noting on Axis III the history of head injury and the EEG abnormality.

DSM-III-R Diagnosis:

Axis I: Intermittent Explosive Disorder (Provisional)
Axis III: History of head injury and nonspecific EEG abnormality

Case 19: Factitious Disorder with Psychological Symptoms

J. P. is a muscular 24-year-old man who presented himself to the admitting office of a state hospital. He told the admitting physician that he had taken 30 200-mg tablets of Thorazine in the bus on the way over to the hospital. After receiving medical treatment for the "suicide attempt," he was transferred to the inpatient ward.

On mental status examination the patient told a fantastic story about his father's being a famous surgeon who had a patient die in surgery and whose husband then killed his father. J. P. then stalked his father's murderer several thousand miles across the United States and he found him, but was prevented from killing him at the last moment by the timely arrival of his 94-year-old grandmother. He also related several other intriguing stories involving his $14,000 sports car, which had a 12-cylinder diesel engine, and about his children, two sets of identical triplets. All these stories had a grandiose tinge, and none of them could be confirmed. The patient claimed that he was hearing voices, as on the TV or in a dream. He answered affirmatively to questions about thought control, thought broadcasting, and other Schneiderian first-rank symptoms; he also claimed depression. He was oriented and alert and had a good range of information except that he kept insisting that it was the Germans (not the Russians) who had invaded Afghanistan. There was no evidence of any associated features of mania or depression, and the patient did not seem either elated, depressed, or irritable when he related these stories.

It was observed on the ward that the patient bullied the other patients and took food and cigarettes from them. He was very reluctant to be discharged, and whenever the subject of his discharge was brought up, he renewed his complaints about "suicidal thoughts" and "hearing voices." It was the opinion of the ward staff that the patient was not truly psychotic, but merely feigned his symptoms whenever the subject of disposition was brought up. They thought that he wanted to remain in the hospital primarily so that he could bully the other patients and be a "big man" on the ward.

Discussion

Although this patient would have us believe that he is psychotic, his story, almost from the start, seems to conform to no recognizable psychotic syndrome. That his symptoms are not genuine is confirmed by the observation of the ward staff that he seemed to feign his symptoms whenever the subject of disposition was brought up.

Why does this fellow try so hard to act crazy? His motivation is not to achieve some understandable goal, such as, for instance, avoiding the draft, as would be the case in malingering; this goal becomes understandable only with knowledge of his individual psychology (the suggestion that he derives satisfaction from being the "big man" on the ward). The diagnosis is, therefore, factitious disorder with psychological symptoms.

DSM-III-R Diagnosis:
Axis I: Factitious Disorder with Psychological Symptoms

Case 20: Separation Anxiety Disorder

Tina is a small, sweet-faced, freckled, 10-year-old who has been referred by a pediatrician who was unsuccessful in treating her for refusing to go to school. Her difficulties began on the first day of school one year ago when she cried and hid in the basement. She agreed to go to school only when her mother promised to go with her and stay to have lunch with her at school. For the next three months, on school days Tina had a variety of somatic complaints, such as headaches and "tummyaches," and each day would go to school only reluctantly, after much cajoling by her parents. Soon thereafter she could be gotten to school only if her parents lifted her out of bed, dressed and fed her, and drove her to school. Often she would leave school during the day and return home. Finally, in the spring the school social-worker consulted Tina's pediatrician, who instituted a be-havior-shaping program with the help of her parents. Because this program was of only limited help, the pediatrician had referred Tina now, at the beginning of the school year.

According to her mother, despite Tina's many absences from school last year, she performed well. During this time she also happily participated in all other activities, including Girl Scout meetings, sleepovers with several friends (usual-ly also with her sister), and family outings. Her mother wonders if her taking a part-time bookkeeping job 2 years ago, and the sudden death of a maternal grandfather to whom Tina was particularly close, might have been responsible for the child's difficulties.

When Tina was interviewed, she at first minimized any problems about school, insisting that "everything is okay," and that she got good grades and liked all the teachers. When this subject was pursued, she became angry and gave a lot of "I don't know" responses as to why, then, she often refused to go to school. Eventually she said that kids teased her about her size, calling her "Shrimp" and "Shorty"; but she gave the impression, as well as actually stated, that she liked school and her teachers. She finally admitted that what bothered her was leaving home. She could not specify why, but hinted that she was afraid something would happen, though to whom or to what she did not say; but she con-fessed that she felt uncomfortable when all of her family was out of sight.

On the Rorschach there was evidence of obsessive rumination about catastrophic events involving injury to members of her family and themes concerning family dis-ruption.

Discussion

All of Tina's problems involve a fear of going to school. The question is: Is it school that she is really afraid of, or is it separating herself from her parents? The evidence that she is really afraid of school is her claim that the other children tease her and her willing participation in other activities away from home, such as sleepovers and Girl Scout meet-ings. But Tina herself concludes that it is really her fear that something bad will happen when her family is out of her sight that is behind her refusal to go to school. We are inclined to accept this explanation. An enforced 6 hours away from her family every day is apparently more trou-bling to her than an occasional hour at a Girl Scout meeting or a sleepover, usually with her sister.

In the absence of a more pervasive disorder, the ex-cessive anxiety concerning separation from the family and unrealistic worry about harm befalling them, reluctance to go to school, and complaints of physical symptoms on school days, over a period of more than two weeks, all indicate separation anxiety disorder. We would not quarrel with a clinician who wished to make this diagnosis pro-visional pending further clarification of Tina's distress about being teased. If she is excessively fearful of the possibility of being humiliated or embarrassed in public, then the diagnosis of social phobia should be considered as an alternative or as an additional diagnosis.

DSM-III-R Diagnosis:
Axis I.   Separation Anxiety Disorder

Case 21: Bulimia Nervosa

Alice is a single 17-year-old who lives with her parents, who insisted that she be seen because of binge eating and vomiting. She achieved her greatest weight of 180 pounds at 16 years of age. Her lowest weight since she reached her present height of 5'9" has been 150 pounds, and her present weight is about 160 pounds.

Alice states she has been dieting since age ten and says she has always been very tall and slightly chubby. At age 12 she started binge eating and vomiting. She was a serious competitive swimmer at that time, and it was necessary for her to keep her weight down. She would deprive herself of all food for a few days and then get an urge to eat. She could not control this urge, and would raid the refrigerator and cupboards for ice cream, pastries, and other desserts. She would often do this at night, when nobody was looking, and would eat, for example, a quart of ice cream, an entire pie, and any other desserts she could find. She would eat until she felt physical discomfort and then would become de-pressed and fearful of gaining weight, following which she would self-induce vomiting. When she was 15 she was having eating binges and vomiting 4 days a week. Since age 13 she has gone through only one period of 6 weeks without gaining weight or eating binges or vomiting. She quit school this year (at age 17) for a period of 5 months, during which she just stayed home, overeating and vomiting. She then went back to school and tried to do better in her schoolwork. She has obtained average or below-average grades in junior high and high school.

For the past 2 years Alice has been drinking wine and beer on weekends. She drinks mostly with girl friends; she dates infrequently. Alice states that she wants to date, but is ashamed of the way she looks. At times in the past she has taken Dexedrine to lose weight. Several months ago she was hospitalized for 2 weeks to control her binge eating. During this time she was very depressed and cut her wrists several times while hospitalized.

Alice is neatly dressed, well oriented, and answers inquiries rationally. During the interview she indicates that she realizes she has a serious problem with binge eating and vomiting, but feels rather hopeless about getting the behavior under control.

Discussion

Clearly Alice has a gross disturbance in eating behavior, an eating disorder. She consumes large quantities of food over a short period of time (binge eating). The food she eats during the binges is typically high in calories (ice cream, pastries, and other desserts), she eats it in secret (at night when nobody is looking), and the binge ends in self-induced vomiting and feelings of self-reproach. Alice has had frequent fluctuations in weight due to the binges, and dieting and control of her weight have been a chronic preoccupation. Furthermore, she is aware that the eating pattern is abnormal and that she is unable to control it. These are the characteristic features of bulimia nervosa.

Although binge eating can be an associated feature of anorexia nervosa, there is no suggestion here of the severe weight loss characteristic of that disorder. Since depressive symptoms are typically associated with bulimia nervosa, we see no advantage in adding the diagnosis of adjustment disorder with depressed mood to characterize the more recent depressive episode, triggered, perhaps, by Alice's hospitalization; but we would not quarrel with a clinician who added this diagnosis.

Mention is made of Alice's drinking wine and beer and using Dexedrine. There is, however, no clear pattern of maladaptive use or resulting impairment in social or occupational functioning to justify a diagnosis of substance abuse.

DSM-III-R Diagnosis:
Axis I: Bulimia Nervosa

Case 22: Tourette's Disorder

Alan, a 10-year-old boy, is brought for a consultation by his mother because of "severe compulsions." The mother reports that the child at various times has to run and clear his throat, touch the doorknob twice before entering any door, tilt his head from side to side, rapidly blink his eyes, and touch the ground with his hands all of a sudden by flexing his whole body. These "compulsions" began 2 years ago. The first was the eye-blinking, and then the others followed, with a waxing and waning course. The movements occur more frequently when the patient is anxious or under stress. The last symptom to appear was the repetitive touching of the doorknobs. The consultation was scheduled after the child began to make the middle finger sign while saying "fuck."

When examined, Alan reported that he did not know most of the time when the movements were going to occur except for the touching of the doorknob. Upon questioning

he said that before he felt he had to touch the doorknob, he got the thought of doing it and tried to push it out of his head, but he couldn't because it kept coming back until he touched the doorknob several times. Then he felt better. When asked what would happen if someone did not let him touch the doorknob, he said he would just get mad, and that his father had tried to stop him and he had had a temper tantrum. During the interview the child grunted, cleared his throat, turned his head, and rapidly blinked his eyes several times. At other times he tried to make it appear as if he had voluntarily been trying to perform these movements.

Past history and physical and neurological examinations were totally unremarkable except for the abnormal movements and sounds. The mother reported that her youngest uncle had had similar symptoms when he was an adolescent, but she could not elaborate any further. She stated that she and her husband had always been "very compulsive," by which she meant only that they were quite well organized and stuck to routines.

Discussion

The mother describes Alan's difficulties as "compulsions," because she realizes that he is compelled to perform senseless acts. In true compulsions, however, there are also mounting anxiety and the sense that the compulsion will ward off an undesirable future event or situation. For example, in a hand-washing or counting compulsion the patient may have the feeling that something terrible will happen unless the compulsion is acted upon. In this case there is only mounting frustration until the act is performed, and then a sense of relief. Hence, these are not compulsions, but a variety of motor and verbal tics that often look purposeful but in fact serve no purpose. In an effort to avoid embarrassment, the patient sometimes tries to disguise them as voluntary, purposeful movements.

The combination of motor and verbal tics with a duration of over 1 year establishes the diagnosis of Tourette's disorder.

DSM-III-R Diagnosis:
Axis I: Tourette's Disorder

Case 23: Attention-deficit Hyperactivity Disorder

Eight-year-old Fred was referred to a school counselor because his teacher "could not handle" his behavior. The boy was reported to be inattentive, often not listening or being easily distracted. He was inappropriately active in the classroom, often fidgeting in his seat and needing to get up to sharpen his pencil or go to the bathroom. His teachers complained that he frequently yelled out answers to questions in class without waiting to hear them to their conclusion. He had difficulty concentrating and organizing his schoolwork and needed constant supervision to get his homework done.

Discussion

This child shows signs of developmentally inappropriate inattention (often not listening, easily distracted, difficulty concentrating on schoolwork), impulsivity (calling out in class, difficulty organizing schoolwork, needing constant supervision), and hyperactivity (constant fidgeting and difficulty staying seated). When the disturbances are not due to a more serious disorder, such as schizophrenia or severe or profound mental retardation, these are the hallmarks of attention-deficit hyperactivity disorder.

DSM-III-R Diagnosis:
Axis I: Attention-Deficit Hyperactivity Disorder

Case 24: Narcissistic Personality Disorder

A 25-year-old, single, graduate student complains to his psychoanalyst of difficulty completing his Ph.D. in English Literature and expresses concerns about his relationships with women. He believes that his thesis topic may profoundly increase the level of understanding in his discipline and make him famous, but so far he has not been able to get past the third chapter. His mentor does not seem sufficiently impressed with his ideas, and the patient is furious at him, but also self-doubting and ashamed. He blames his mentor for his lack of progress, thinks that he deserves more help with his grand idea, and that his mentor should help with some of the research. The patient brags about his creativity and complains that other people are "jealous" of his insight. He is very envious of students who are moving along faster than he and regards them as "dull drones and ass kissers." He prides himself on the brilliance of his class participation and imagines someday becoming a great professor.

He becomes rapidly infatuated with women and has powerful and persistent fantasies about each new woman he meets, but after several experiences of sexual intercourse feels disappointed and finds them dumb, clinging, and physically repugnant. He has many "friends," but they turn over quickly, and no one relationship lasts very long. People get tired of his continual self-promotion and lack of consideration of them. For example, he was lonely at Christmas and insisted that his best friend stay in town rather than visit his family. The friend refused, criticizing the patient's self-centeredness; and the patient, enraged, decided never to see this friend again.

Discussion

This patient's narcissistic personality traits are clear: grandiosity about the importance of his thesis, entitlement in expecting his mentor to do some of his work, and over-idealization and devaluation of women. Because these traits significantly interfere both with his academic achievement and with friendships and heterosexual relations, a diagnosis of narcissistic personality disorder is appropriate.

Although it is not specifically stated that these traits are of long duration, this is a reasonable assumption. (There is no description in the literature of episodic narcissism!)

DSM-III-R Diagnosis:
Axis II: Narcissistic Personality Disorder

Case 25: Dependent Personality Disorder

The patient is a 34-year-old single man who lives with his mother and works as a draftsman. He presents with feelings of unhappiness after breaking up with his girlfriend. His mother had disapproved of their marriage plans, ostensibly because the woman was of a different religion. The patient felt trapped and forced to choose between his mother and girl friend; and since "blood is thicker than water," he had decided not to go against his mother's wishes. Nonetheless, he is angry at himself and at her and believes that she will never let him marry and is possessively hanging on to him. His mother "wears the pants" in the family and is a strongly domineering woman who is used to getting her way. The patient is afraid of her and criticizes himself for being weak, but also admires his mother and respects her judgment—"Maybe Carol wasn't right for me after all." The patient alternates between resentment and a "Mother knows best" attitude. He feels that his own judgment is poor.

The patient works at a job several grades below his education and talent. On several occasions he has turned down promotions because he didn't want the responsibility of having to supervise other people or make independent decisions. He has worked for the same boss for 10 years, gets on well with him, and is, in turn, highly regarded as a dependable and unobtrusive worker. The patient has two very close friends who go back to early childhood. He has lunch with one of them every single workday and feels lost if his friend is sick and misses a day.

The patient is the youngest of four children and the only boy. He was "babied and spoiled" by his mother and elder sisters. He had considerable separation anxiety as a child—difficulty falling asleep unless his mother stayed in the room, mild school refusal, and unbearable homesickness when he occasionally tried "sleepovers." As a child he was teased by other boys because of his lack of assertiveness and was often called a baby. He has lived at home his whole life except for one year of college (he returned because of homesickness). His heterosexual adjustment has been normal except for his inability to leave his mother in favor of another woman.

Discussion

This patient has allowed his mother to make the important decision as to whether he should marry his girl friend, and this seems to be merely one instance of a pattern of subordinating his own needs and wishes to those of his domineering mother. At work he demonstrates lack of confidence and reluctance to rely on his own judgment and abilities by avoiding promotions and working below his potential. These personality traits are severe enough to interfere significantly with his social and occupational functioning and therefore justify the diagnosis dependent personality disorder.

DSM-III-R Diagnosis:
Axis II: Dependent Personality Disorder

Case 26: Passive-Aggressive Personality Disorder

A 34-year-old psychiatrist is 15 minutes late for his first appointment. He had recently been asked to resign from his job in a mental health center because, according to his boss, he had frequently been late for work and meetings, missed appointments, forgot about assignments, was late with his statistics, refused to follow instructions, and seemed unmotivated. The patient was surprised and resentful—he thought he had been doing a particularly good job under trying circumstances and experienced his boss as excessively obsessive and demanding. Nonetheless, he reported a long-standing pattern of difficulties with authority.

The patient had a childhood history of severe and prolonged temper tantrums that were a legend in his family. He had been a bossy child who demanded that other kids "play his way" or else he wouldn't play at all. With adults, particularly his mother and female teachers, he was sullen, insubordinate, oppositional, and often unmanageable. He had been sent to an all-boys' prep school that had primarily male teachers, and he gradually became more subdued and disciplined. He continued, however, to stubbornly want things his own way and to resent instruction or direction from teachers. He was a brilliant but erratic student, working only as hard as he himself wanted to, and he "punished" teachers he didn't like by not doing their assignments. He was argumentative and self-righteous when criticized, and complained that he was not being treated fairly.

The patient is unhappily married. He complains that his wife does not understand him and is a "nitpicker." She complains that he is unreliable and stubborn. He refuses to do anything around the house and often forgets to complete the few errands he has accepted as within his responsibility. Tax forms are submitted several months late; bills are not paid. The patient is sociable and has considerable charm, but friends generally become annoyed at his unwillingness to go along with the wishes of the group: for example, if a restaurant is not his choice, he may sulk all night or forget to bring his wallet.

Discussion

Whenever this patient feels that demands are being made on him, either socially or occupationally, he passively resists through such characteristic maneuvers as procrastination (e.g., tax returns are late, bills are not paid), stubbornness (e.g., unwillingness to go along with the wishes of his friends), and forgetfulness (e.g., forgets errands for wife and assignments at work). His behavior has resulted in impaired work performance and marital difficulties. Such a long-standing pattern of resistance to demands for adequate performance in role functioning is a prototype of passive-aggressive personality disorder.

Although passive-aggressive behavior is quite common in situations in which assertive behavior is not encouraged or is actually punished (e.g., in the military service), the diagnosis is made only if the behavior occurs in situations in which more assertive behavior is possible. Passive-aggressive traits may be seen as an associated feature of other personality disorders; but the diagnosis passive-aggressive personality disorder is not made when another personality disorder is present.

This case demonstrates that neither a high IQ nor membership in a mental health profession conveys immunity to this disorder.

DSM-III-R Diagnosis:
Axis II: Passive-Aggressive Personality Disorder

Case 27: Obsessive-Compulsive Personality Disorder

The patient is a 45-year-old lawyer who seeks treatment at his wife's insistence. She is fed up with their marriage: she can no longer tolerate his emotional coldness, rigid demands, bullying behavior, sexual disinterest, long work hours, and frequent business trips. The patient feels no particular distress in his marriage, and has agreed to the consultation only to humor his wife.

It soon develops, however, that the patient is troubled by problems at work. He is known as the hardest-driving member of a hard-driving law firm. He was the youngest full partner in the firm's history, and is famous for being able to handle many cases at the same time. Lately, he finds himself increasingly unable to keep up. He is too proud to turn down a new case, and too much of a perfectionist to be satisfied with the quality of work performed by his assistants. He finds himself constantly correcting their briefs, displeased with their writing style and sentence structure, and therefore unable to stay abreast of his schedule. People at work complain that his attention to detail and inability to delegate responsibility are reducing his efficiency. He has been through two or three secretaries a year for 15 years. No one can tolerate working for him for very long because he is so critical of any mistakes made by others. When assignments get backed up, he cannot decide which to address first, starts making schedules for himself and his staff, but then is unable to meet them and works 15 hours a day. He finds it difficult to be decisive now that his work has expanded beyond his own direct control.

The patient discusses his children as if they were mechanical dolls, but also with a clear underlying affection. He describes his wife as a "suitable mate" and has trouble understanding why she is dissatisfied. He is punctilious in his manners and dress and slow and ponderous in his speech, dry and humorless, with a stubborn determination to get his point across.

The patient is the product of two upwardly mobile, extremely hard-working parents. He grew up feeling that he was never working hard enough, that he had much to achieve and very little time. He was a superior student, a bookworm, and awkward and unpopular in adolescent social pursuits. He has always been competitive and a high achiever. He has trouble relaxing on vacations, develops elaborate activities schedules for every family member, and becomes impatient and furious if they refuse to follow his plans. He likes sports but has little time for them and refuses to play if he can't be at the top of his form. He is a ferocious competitor on the tennis courts and a poor loser.

Discussion

Although the marital problem is the entry ticket, it is clear that this fellow has many personality traits that are quite maladaptive. He is cold and rigid and excessively perfectionistic. He is indecisive, but insists that others do things his way; his interpersonal relationships suffer because of his excessive devotion to work. It is hard to imagine a more prototypical case of obsessive-compulsive personality disorder!

The additional notation of marital problem is not made in this case since the patient's marital problems are clearly symptomatic of his mental disorder.

DSM-III-R Diagnosis:
Axis II: Obsessive-Compulsive Personality Disorder

Case 28: Avoidant Personality Disorder

The patient is a 26-year-old teacher's aide who seeks counseling. For several years she has been feeling increasingly lonely and "lost," particularly since her 2-year-older sister married and moved out of town three months ago. This sister and one close friend from high school have been the patient's only real social contacts; otherwise she has no other girl friends, and she is extremely afraid of men. As far back as she can remember, she has felt she has very little to offer others. She has always anticipated that men, even if attracted to her, would quickly find fault with her and "drop" her. Although she would like to be married, she characteristically cuts off potential relationships with men after two or three dates because of her fear of eventual rejection. Her relationships with others are superficial and usually structured through work with civic groups or her church club. She is rarely critical of others or able to get angry at them, except concerning social or political issues. She champions the causes of minorities, ecology, and liberalism against the rich and the powerful, but she is more likely to volunteer to spend a Saturday stuffing leaflets in envelopes than canvassing door-to-door to collect money.

At work the patient is regarded as competent and responsible and apparently does not demand the kind of unconditional acceptance from her 4-year-old students that she demands from adults. She has for several years considered seeing a counselor, but this is her first attempt to get professional help.

Discussion

Although the exacerbation of the patient's long-standing problems since her sister moved away has caused her to seek treatment at this time, this does not represent a new illness (such as adjustment disorder).

Throughout most of her life this patient has had significant difficulty establishing relationships with other people. Social isolation is commonly seen in schizotypal personality disorder, but the absence of oddities of behavior and thinking rules out that diagnosis. In schizoid personality disorder the isolation is apparently the result of a basic emotional coldness and indifference to others. In this case, however, there is obviously a strong desire for affection and acceptance, which is inhibited by anticipation of rejection—the characteristic features of avoidant personality disorder. The patient also displays low self-esteem (she feels she has little

to offer others), another characteristic feature of this disorder.

For most people, the departure of a married sister to another city would not be a major psychosocial stressor. It is only because of the patient's personality disorder that she was particularly vulnerable to this stressor. This patient clearly functions more effectively at work than socially.

DSM-III-R Diagnosis:
Axis II: Avoidant Personality Disorder

Case 29: Autistic Disorder

Richard, aged three and a half, a firstborn child, was referred at the request of his parents because of his uneven development and abnormal behavior. Delivery had been difficult, and he had needed oxygen at birth. His physical appearance, motor development, and self-help skills were all age-appropriate; but his parents had been uneasy about him from the first few months of life because of his lack of response to social contact and the usual baby games. Comparison with their second child, who, unlike Richard, enjoyed social communication from early infancy, confirmed their fears.

Richard appeared to be self-sufficient and aloof from others. He did not greet his mother in the mornings, or his father when he returned from work, though, if left with a baby-sitter, he tended to scream much of the time. He had no interest in other children and ignored his younger brother. His babbling had no conversational intonation. At 3 years he could understand simple practical instructions. His speech consisted of echoing some words and phrases he had heard in the past, with the original speaker's accent and intonation; but he could use one or two such phrases to indicate his simple needs. For example, if he said "Do you want a drink?" he meant he was thirsty. He did not communicate by facial expression or use gesture or mime, except for pulling someone along and placing his or her hand on an object he wanted.

He was fascinated by bright lights and spinning objects, and would stare at them while laughing, flapping his hands, and dancing on tiptoe. He also displayed the same movements while listening to music, which he had liked from infancy. He was intensely attached to a miniature car, which he held in his hand, day and night; but he had no imaginative, pretend play with this or any other toy. He could assemble jigsaw puzzles rapidly (with one hand because of the car held in the other), whether the picture side was exposed or hidden. From age 2 he had collected kitchen utensils and arranged them in repetitive patterns all over the floors of the house. These pursuits, together with occasional periods of aimless running around, made up his whole repertoire of spontaneous activities.

The major management problem was Richard's intense resistance to any attempt to change or extend his interests. Removing his toy car, disturbing his puzzles or patterns (including retrieving, for example, an egg whisk or a spoon for its legitimate use in cooking) or even trying to make him look at a picture book precipitated temper tantrums that could last an hour or more with screaming, kicking, and biting himself or others. These tantrums could be cut short by restoring the *status quo*. Otherwise, playing his favorite music or a long car ride were sometimes effective.

His parents had wondered if Richard could be deaf, but his love of music, his accurate echoing, and his sensitivity to some very soft sounds, such as that made by unwrapping a chocolate in the next room, convinced them that this was not the cause of his abnormal behavior. Psychological testing gave him a mental age of 3 years in non-language-dependent skills (fitting and assembly tasks), but only 18 months in language comprehension.

Discussion

Richard demonstrates a lack of responsiveness and gross impairment that began in the first few months of life. His speech has continued to be peculiar in that it consists entirely of echoing the words and phrases of others. His responses to the environment are often bizarre (flapping his hands and dancing on tiptoe in response to bright lights, or spinning objects, and temper tantrums when his routines are interfered with). These behaviors are the characteristic signs of autistic disorder.

DSM-III-R Diagnosis:
Axis I: Autistic Disorder

Case 30: Mania

The patient was first admitted to the hospital at the age of 22. For 3 or 4 months before admission she felt depressed and had anorexia, with a weight loss of about ten pounds, and both initial and terminal insomnia. About 2 months before admission she began to feel increasingly energetic, requiring only 2 to 5 hours of sleep at night, and to experience her thoughts as racing. She began to see symbolic meanings in things, especially sexual meanings, and experienced marked ideas of reference, involving, particularly, innocent comments on television shows. During the month preceding admission she became increasingly euphoric and irritable and began experiencing both visual and auditory hallucinations. She believed that there was a hole in her head through which radar messages were being sent to her. These messages could control her thoughts or produce emotions of anger, sadness, or the like, that were beyond her control. She also believed that her thoughts could be read by people around her and that alien thoughts from other people were intruding themselves via the radar into her own head. She described hearing voices, which sometimes spoke about her in the third person and at other times ordered her to perform various functions, particularly sexual activity.

Before her recent illness the patient had been asymptomatic and had been a successful student at a prestigious university. There she had done well academically and had had a large circle of friends of both sexes. She could not recall any particular precipitants of her symptoms, saying that they seemed to arise almost at random in the midst of an uneventful period in her second year of college.

Upon admission to the hospital the patient was started on chlorpromazine and lithium carbonate. Over the course of about 3 weeks she experienced a fairly rapid reduction in hyperactivity, euphoria, pressured speech, delusions, and hallucinations. After 4 weeks the chlorpromazine dosage was gradually reduced and then discontinued. She was maintained thereafter on lithium carbonate alone. At the time of her discharge, her manic symptoms had disappeared, but she displayed hypersomnia of about 10 hours per night; mild anorexia; definite diurnal variation, worse in the mornings; and mild psychomotor retardation. These symptoms, however, were not severe enough to require hospitalization, and the patient was discharged to live with friends.

Approximately 8 months after her discharge, the patient was taken off lithium carbonate by her psychiatrist at college. She continued asymptomatic for approximately 3 or 4 weeks, but then began to experience a gradual reappearance of symptoms similar to those that had precipitated her previous hospitalization. About 2 weeks after this she was readmitted to the hospital with a syndrome almost identical with that which had characterized her on her first admission. She again responded uneventfully to a regimen of chlorpromazine and lithium initially, with her medication gradually being reduced to lithium alone. At the time of her discharge she again displayed mild depressive symptoms.

The patient's father had had a severe episode of depression, characterized by hypersomnia, anorexia, profound psychomotor retardation, and suicidal ideation, when in his 40s. The patient's paternal grandmother had committed suicide during what also appeared to be a depressive episode.

Discussion

This woman was functioning at a high level before the development of a depressive period, followed shortly by an episode with characteristic manic symptoms: increased energy, less need for sleep, racing thoughts, euphoria, and irritability. At the height of the illness she developed bizarre delusions (her emotions were controlled by radar messages sent through a hole in her head) and hallucinations (voices commanding her to perform sexual acts). In the absence of any evidence of a specific organic factor that could account for the disturbance, such as the use of a stimulant, this disturbance is a manic episode. The occurrence of a manic episode (even in the absence of a full depressive episode) is sufficient for a diagnosis of bipolar disorder, manic. Because the content of the delusions and hallucinations has no apparent relationship to such typical manic themes as inflated worth or identity, the subclassification is "with psychotic features (mood-incongruent)."

DSM-III-R Diagnosis:
Axis I: Bipolar Disorder, Manic, with Psychotic Features
              (Mood-Incongruent)

Index

Page numbers in **boldface** type indicate major discussions; those followed by *t* or *f* denote tables or figures, respectively.

Symbiotic phase, Mahler's theory of, 28*t*
Symbolization, 82
  definition, 312*t*
Sympathomimetic(s), 274
  delirium, diagnostic criteria, 239*t*
  delusional disorder, diagnostic criteria, 239*t*
  for depression, 517
  intoxication, diagnostic criteria, 238*t*
  organic mental disorder with, 218, 250*t*
  withdrawal, diagnostic criteria, 239*t*
Synapses, **68-69**
  axoaxonic, 68-69
  axodendritic, 68-69
  axosomatic, 68-69
  chemical, 68
  cholinergic, 74
  conjoint, 68
  dendroaxonic, 69
  dendrodendritic, 69
  dopaminergic, 71-72
  electrical, 68
  humoral, 68
  noradrenergic (adrenergic), 73
  serotonergic, 74
Synaptic transmission, 68*f*, 68
Syncope, 414
Syndrome(s), DSM-III-R definition, 188
Synesthesia, definition, 173
Syphilis
  and mental retardation, 544
  tertiary, 206
  tests for, 164
Systematic desensitization, 87-88, **486-487**
Systemic lupus erythematosus, 78, **207**, 336, 421, 424*t*
Szasz, Thomas, 24
  The Myth of Mental Illness, 666

Tactual Performance Test, 131
Taijin kyofusho, 101*t*
Tangentiality, 260
  definition, 171
Tarasoff case, 122, 664
Tardive dyskinesia, 72, 73, 75, 77, 268, 609, 651, 660
  with antipsychotics, **507**
  differential diagnosis, 509*t*
Taurine, 75
Tay-Sachs disease, 550*t*
TCA. *See* Tricyclic antidepressant(s)
Technetium scan, 166
Telephone scatalogia, 362
Temazepam. *See also* Benzodiazepine(s)
Temporal lobe epilepsy, 59
Temporomandibular joint pain, biofeedback therapy, 485
Tension, definition, 170
Tension headache, **417**
  biofeedback therapy, 485
Tension reduction theory, 88
Teratogen(s), and mental retardation, 544
Terminally ill. *See* Dying patient
Termination
  emergency exception, 665
  going the extra mile, 665
Test(s). *See also* Intelligence testing; Laboratory tests; Neuropsychiatric test(s);

Personality testing; *specific test*
  battery, 123, 131
  classification of, 123
  of children, 539-540
  comprehensive, 131
  for developmental reading disorder, 568
  in factitious disorder(s), 399
  findings, integration of, 128
  group, 123
  individual, 123
  and normality, 23
  objective, 123
  projective, 89, 123
    for children, 540
    in schizophrenia, 261
  in psychiatric report, 162
  in schizophrenia, 261
  standardization, 123
Testamentary capacity, **667-668**
Testicular feminization syndrome, 608
Testimonial privilege, 663
Testosterone
  and aggression, 400
  for sexual disorders, 375-376
Test-retest reliability, 103
Tetrahydroaminoacridine, 204
Δ-9-Tetrahydrocannabinol, 246
Thalamus, 64*f*, **66**
Thanatology, 51
Thanatos, 90, 135, 454
Thematic Apperception Test, 123, **125**, 149, 540
Therapeutic alliance, 153, **467**
  with child, 641-642
  and involuntary discharge, 665
Therapeutic community, 100
Therapeutic interventions, with children, 641-642
Thinking. *See also* Magical thinking
  abstract, 82, 158
    definition, 171
  adolescent's, 43
  animistic, 82
  definition, 170
  disturbances in form of, 170-171
  hypotheticodeductive, 82
  illogical, definition, 171
  parataxic mode, 150
  primary process, 135
  prototaxic mode, 150
  secondary process, 139
  syntaxic mode, 150
Thinking process, assessment, in children, 538
Thioridazine (Mellaril), 500, 501
  affinity for neurotransmitter receptors, 501*t*
  for children, indications and dosage, 651*t*
  effects and complications in children, 650-651
  in mental retardation, 649-650
  molecular structure, 499*f*
  potency, 502*t*
Thiothixene (Navane), 499
  affinity for neurotransmitter receptors, 501*t*
  for children, indications and dosage, 652*t*
  molecular structure, 499*f*
  potency, 502*t*

Thioxanthene(s), 502*t*
  for children, indications and dosage, 652*t*
  definition, 499
Third-party payers, and confidentiality, 663
Thomas, Alexander, 32, 105, 432
Thorndike, Edward L., 86
Thorndike's law of effect, 639
Thought
  concrete, 43
  content of, 158
    disturbances of, 171-172
  disorders of content, in schizophrenia, 260
  disorders of form, in schizophrenia, 260
  disorders of process, in schizophrenia, 260-261
  formal operational, 43
  form of, specific disturbances in, 171
  operational, 82
  preoccupation of, definition, 172
  preoperational, 39, 82
  stream of, 158
  trend of, definition, 172
Thought blocking, 261
Thought broadcasting, definition, 172
Thought deprivation, definition, 171
Thought insertion, definition, 172
Thought process
  in delusional disorder(s), 272
  in depressive episode, 294
  in manic episode, 295
  in mental status examination, 158
  in psychiatric report, 161
Thought withdrawal, definition, 172
Thyroid disorder(s), 208
Thyroid function test, 163
Thyroid stimulating hormone, in mood disorder(s), 290
Thyrotoxicosis. *See* Hyperthyroidism
Thyrotropin-releasing hormone, in schizophrenia, 257
Thyrotropin-releasing hormone stimulation test, 163
TIA. *See* Transient ischemic attacks
Tic(s)
  definition, 170, 609
  motor, 609
  organic, 611
  psychogenic, 611
  and stimulants, 609
  vocal, 609
Tic disorder(s), 328, **609-614**, 629. *See also specific disorder(s)*
  chronic motor, diagnostic criteria, 610*t*
  chronic motor or vocal, **612**
  chronic vocal, diagnostic criteria, 610*t*
  classification, 610
  differential diagnosis, 609
  DSM-III-R categories and codes, 180*t*
  etiology, 609-610
  not otherwise specified, 614
    diagnostic criteria, 610*t*
  transient, **610-612**
    clinical features, 611-612
    course, 612
    definition, 610
    diagnosis, 610
    diagnostic criteria, 610*t*
    epidemiology, 611